Pearson's Massage Therapy

Blending Art with Science

PATRICIA J. BENJAMIN, PHD, NCTMB

PEARSON

Boston Columbus Indianapolis New York San Francisco Upper Saddle River
Amsterdam Cape Town Dubai London Madrid Milan Munich Paris Montreal Toronto
Delhi Mexico City Sao Paulo Sydney Hong Kong Seoul Singapore Taipei Tokyo

Library of Congress Cataloging-in-Publication Data

Benjamin, Patricia J.
  Pearson's massage therapy : blending art with science / Patricia J.
Benjamin.
     p. ; cm.
  Includes bibliographical references and index.
  ISBN-13: 978-0-13-229668-7
  ISBN-10: 0-13-229668-3
  1. Massage therapy--Textbooks. I. Title. II. Title: Massage therapy.
  [DNLM: 1. Massage--ethics. 2. Massage--methods. 3. Practice Management.
WB 537 B468pa 2011]
  RM721.B475 2011
  615.8'2--dc22

                                              2009051990

Notice: The author and the publisher of this volume have taken care that the information and technical recommendations contained herein are based on research and expert consultation, and are accurate and compatible with the standards generally accepted at the time of publication. Nevertheless, as new information becomes available, changes in clinical and technical practices become necessary. The reader is advised to carefully consult manufacturers' instructions and information material for all supplies and equipment before use, and to consult with a health care professional as necessary. This advice is especially important when using new supplies or equipment for clinical purposes. The author and publisher disclaim all responsibility for any liability, loss, injury, or damage incurred as a consequence, directly or indirectly, of the use and application of any of the contents of this volume.

Publisher: Julie Levin Alexander
Assistant to Publisher: Regina Bruno
Editor-in-Chief: Mark Cohen
Associate Editor: Melissa Kerian
Assistant Editor: Nicole Ragonese
Development Editor: Lynda Hatch
Senior Media Editor: Amy Peltier
Media Project Manager: Lorena Cerisano
Managing Production Editor: Patrick Walsh
Production Liaison: Yagnesh Jani
Production Editor: Kate Boilard, Laserwords Maine
Manufacturing Manager: Ilene Sanford
Manufacturing Buyer: Pat Brown
Senior Art Director: Maria Guglielmo

Cover/Interior Designer: Wanda España/Wee Design
Medical Illustrator: Marcelo Oliver, BodyScientific International
Front Cover Image: Corbis/Inspirestock
Director of Marketing: David Gesell
Executive Marketing Manager: Katrin Beacom
Marketing Specialist: Michael Sirinides
Marketing Assistant: Judy Noh
Manager, Rights and Permissions: Zina Arabia
Manager, Visual Research: Beth Brenzel
Manager, Cover Visual Research and Permissions: Karen Sanatar
Image Permission Coordinator: Jan Marc Quisimbing
Composition: Laserwords, Maine
Printer/Binder: Webcrafters, Inc.
Cover Printer: Lehigh Phoenix Color/Hagerstown

10 9 8 7 6 5 4 3 2 1

www.pearsonhigered.com

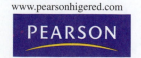

ISBN-13: 978-0-13-229668-7
ISBN-10: 0-13-229668-3

Brief Contents

Welcome!

Welcome to *Pearson's Massage Therapy*. This is a learning tool for a new generation, but it results from years of experience, wisdom, and research on the part of the author and countless therapists who have molded this book with their suggestions, feedback, and original writings. Truly this represents the culmination of great ideas from the world's massage community. In crafting this text, we aimed to reflect the needs of students and educators alike. Here are our basic premises.

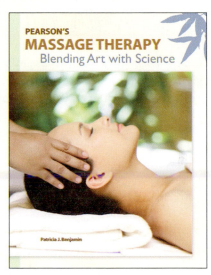

- **Students are visual and kinesthetic learners.** We have designed this book with a wealth of beautiful anatomical illustrations and clear, step-by-step sequences that zero in on techniques. Our goal is to provide an engaging visual link between the book and hands-on practice.

- **Video is a dynamic way of demonstrating techniques.** We produced a complete video library in connection with this book. The DVD is included in the back of the text and will bring the study of the techniques and professional aspects of massage into three dimensions.

- **Instructors can shine when provided with world-class resources.** We have invested in a full battery of instructional support materials to facilitate dynamic presentations, well-organized lectures, and successful testing experiences.

- **Online learning is a viable option.** With this book and the component resource materials, we have built a program that can support online instruction. This book is available as an e-text, and all support materials are available for instructor download via the web.

This is a comprehensive text for entry-level massage therapy programs. It covers the wide variety of competencies and prepares you for employment in a range of settings when you graduate. The book's title conveys that successful massage therapists excel at blending the art and science of the profession. Massage therapists must be knowledgeable about the human body in health and disease, skillful in interpersonal relationships, ethical in their behavior, and shrewd in building their careers. This is in addition to mastering theory, physical skills, and finally putting it all together in applications that accomplish client goals. Our text reflects the highest curricular standards, the expectations of employers, and the demands of a growing profession. It provides the foundations, guidance, and the know-how that you will need in order to master the essential task of *blending art with science* and becoming an outstanding massage therapist.

Pearson's Massage Therapy takes a holistic approach by addressing many different learning styles to maximize your potential. You will use your mind, hands, and heart in acquiring the fundamental skills needed to start your new career. Professional knowledge and skills cannot be downloaded like a computer software program. It will take effort to transform yourself from the inside out. This book is your guide for that transformation.

Now please turn the page to get a glimpse of what makes this book an ideal guide to the fundamentals, techniques, and profession of massage therapy.

A "NEXT-GENERATION" LEARNING TOOL

Pearson's Massage Therapy prepares therapists for careers in today's world. This debut edition features several important elements that will foster a successful, engaging, and interactive teaching and learning experience. Here are some exciting features:

Practice Sequences with Corresponding Videos

Practice Sequences are step-by-step suggested applications. These sections can be used as starting points for mastering the techniques and coming up with routines that work best for each student. Each *Practice Sequence* is demonstrated in full, vibrant detail on the student DVD. The video segments can be viewed in class or at home. So that students can track their progress, the DVD, as well as Appendix F, provides *Performance Evaluation Forms* for every *Practice Sequence*.

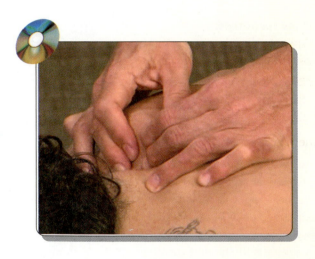

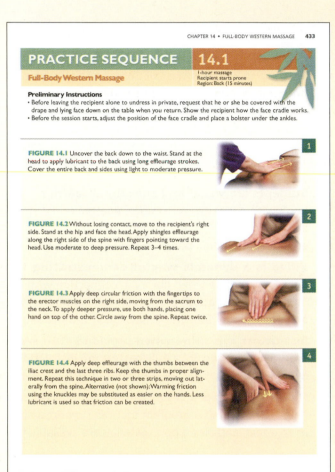

PRACTICE SEQUENCE 14.1

Full-Body Western Massage

1-hour massage
Recipient starts prone
Region: Back (15 minutes)

Preliminary Instructions
• Before leaving the recipient alone to undress in private, request that he or she be covered with the drape and lying face down on the table when you return. Show the recipient how the face cradle works.
• Before the session starts, adjust the position of the face cradle and place a bolster under the ankles.

FIGURE 14.1 Uncover the back down to the waist. Stand at the head to apply lubricant to the back using long effleurage strokes. Cover the entire back and sides using light to moderate pressure.

FIGURE 14.2 Without losing contact, move to the recipient's right side. Stand at the hip and face the head. Apply shingles effleurage along the right side of the spine with fingers pointing toward the head. Use moderate to deep pressure. Repeat 3–4 times.

FIGURE 14.3 Apply deep circular friction with the fingertips to the erector muscles on the right side, moving from the sacrum to the neck. To apply deeper pressure, use both hands, placing one hand on top of the other. Circle away from the spine. Repeat twice.

FIGURE 14.4 Apply deep effleurage with the thumbs between the iliac crest and the last three ribs. Keep the thumbs in proper alignment. Repeat this technique in two or three strips, moving out laterally from the spine. Alternative (not shown): Warming friction using the knuckles may be substituted as easier on the hands. Less lubricant is used so that friction can be created.

A LOGICAL FORMAT FROM START...

Each chapter begins with a consistent set of features that help readers set their goals.

- **Chapter Outline** provides an organized overview of the material to be covered.

- **Learning Outcomes** points readers toward intended goals.

- **Key Terms** identifies essential words and concepts.

- **Massage in Action** points readers to the appropriate video content on the DVD.

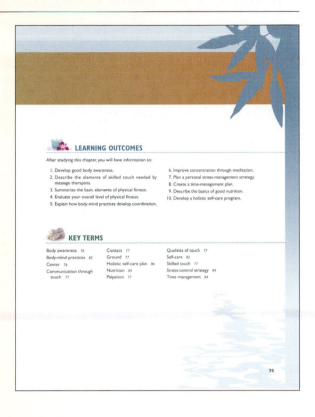

...TO FINISH

Each chapter concludes with a built-in study guide that helps prepare students to succeed in their training and beyond.

Chapter Highlights summarizes each chapter's information in a user-friendly, bulleted outline.

Exam Review presents several different tools to help readers confirm their mastery of the content. Features include:

- **Key Terms** – a matching exercise for studying and applying essential vocabulary

- **Memory Workout** – a fill-in-the-blank review of main concepts

- **Test Prep** – a multiple-choice mock exam

- **Video Challenge** – a quiz based on selected segments on the video DVD.

- **Comprehension Exercises** – a series of short-answer questions that key in on important ideas.

- **For Greater Understanding** – suggested field-based activities that employ various learning styles to help readers apply chapter concepts

A WEALTH OF LEARNING TOOLS ON EVERY PAGE

Photoreal Illustrations

Over 650 full-color illustrations provide first-class reinforcement for visual learners. The photoreal style is clear, focused, and detailed, without background distractions.

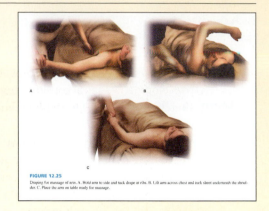

FIGURE 12.25

Draping for massage of arm. A. Hold arm to side and tuck drape at ribs. B. Lift arm across chest and tuck sheet underneath the shoulder. C. Place the arm on table ready for massage.

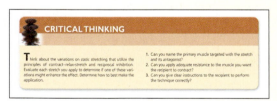

Case for Study

Real-world, critical-thinking scenarios that challenge readers to analyze a situation and solve the problem.

Practical Application

Activities that involve observation, role play, creativity, and planning.

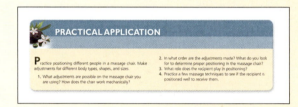

Critical Thinking

Situations that students can analyze and evaluate on a deeper level, by contemplating thoughtful questions, asking intelligent questions, broadening their knowledge base, and making informed decisions.

Reality Check

A report-from-the-real-world feature, in which a new massage therapist asks for advice from a more experienced colleague who provides an insightful view into the profession by responding to questions, feelings, and doubts often left unmentioned.

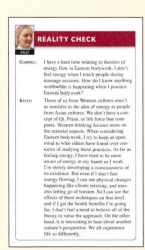

Massage Connection

Found throughout Chapter 6, *Anatomy & Physiology, Pathology, and Kinesiology*, this feature targets the fundamental link between human science and its application to therapeutic massage.

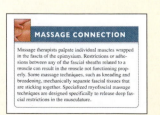

viii

ORGANIZED FOR STUDENT SUCCESS

Pearson's Massage Therapy is divided into five parts covering the essential competencies.

PART I: FOUNDATIONS

An overview of the massage therapy profession, important elements of personal and professional development, ethical considerations, and a review of basic sciences relevant to massage therapy. It addresses foundation knowledge apart from hands-on skills.

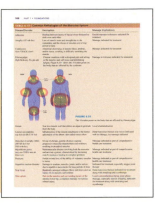

> ***Chapter 6: Anatomy & Physiology, Pathology, and Kinesiology*** provides an at-a-glance reference for the essential sciences related to massage therapy. It allows students to find basic information in tables and illustrations. Note that this chapter is not intended to take the place of science textbooks in specific classes, but to act as a handy reference for students.

PART II: KNOWLEDGE FOR PLANNING MASSAGE SESSIONS

Background specific to planning effective and safe massage therapy sessions. It takes the view that no matter where massage therapists work, they owe it to clients to provide a safe environment and to tailor sessions to meet client expectations and goals.

PART III: MASSAGE GUIDELINES AND APPLICATIONS

Coverage of the physical setup for massage and an introduction to basic Western techniques. It presents essential hands-on skills and their application for table and seated sessions.

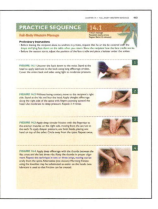

> ***Chapter 14: Full-Body Western Massage*** explains how individual techniques are organized logically into massage routines that address the entire body. It presents a suggested full-body Practice Sequence that can be used to demonstrate basic principles, or as a starting point for learning full-body massage.

PART IV: ADJUNCT THERAPIES AND SPECIAL APPLICATIONS

A look at therapies that complement Western massage, massage technique specializations, and popular forms of bodywork from Asia. It offers approaches for enhancement of basic Western massage and adaptations to address needs of special populations.

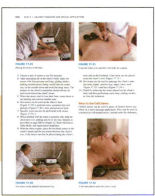

> ***Chapter 17 Spa Applications*** presents common spa treatments. Detailed instructions are provided for applying herbal wraps, skin treatments, temperature therapy, and massage sessions common in spa settings.

PART V: CAREER AND PRACTICE DEVELOPMENT

This section describes what it takes to get started in a successful massage therapy career—from envisioning a future practice to making that dream come true. It covers career planning, finding employment, developing a private practice, and the ethics of the business side of massage.

A COMPLETE VIDEO LIBRARY IN YOUR HANDS

The DVD videos provide a dynamic learning tool. They can be viewed at home as a study tool and review of chapter material; in class to illustrate concepts and spark discussion; or prior to practicing hands-on skills in technique classes.

Here is a list of segments that are included:

- Advertising
- AMI for the Back
- Biomechanical Analysis
- Body Mechanics
- Bookkeeping
- Business Plan
- Claims for Massage Therapy
- Cold Application for Knee
- Developing a Business Plan
- Documentation and SOAP Notes
- Effleurage
- Emotional Intelligence
- Employment Interview
- Ethical Decision-Making Model
- Ethical Judgment
- Ethics
- First Impressions
- First-Year Budget
- Friction
- Full-Body Western Massage
- Gait Analysis
- General Reflexology Session
- General Session of Polarity Therapy
- Gentle Hand and Arm Massage
- Getting Started in Your Career

- Goal-Oriented 6-Step Planning
- Greeting Clients
- Health Care
- Health History Forms
- Holistic Self-Care Plan
- Hot Application on Upper Back
- Hygienic Hand Washing
- Ice Massage for Elbow
- Image Detractors
- Infant Massage
- Informed Voluntary Consent
- Intervention Model
- Joint Movements
- Licensing and Credentials
- Lymphatic Facilitation for the Head and Neck
- Lymphatic Facilitation for the Lower Extremity
- Massage for the Elderly in a Semi-Reclining Position
- Massage Therapy 1970–80s
- Myofascial Massage of the Back
- Natural Healing
- Observation: Posture, Biomechanics, and Gait
- Organizations
- Performance Evaluation Forms

- Personal Care
- Petrissage
- Positioning and Draping
- Post-Event Sports Massage for Run/Walk Event
- Posture Analysis
- Pregnancy Massage
- Professional Boundaries
- Professional Dress, Posture, and Speech
- Qi Gong Twenty Form Routine
- Research
- Roles and Responsibilities
- Seated Massage
- Selling Products
- Sports and Fitness
- Tapotement
- Tips and Gifts
- Today's Eclectic Profession
- Touch without Movement
- Trigger Point Therapy for Tension Headaches
- Variety of Workplaces for Massage Therapists
- Vibration
- Wellness Massage Pyramid
- Writing SOAP Notes

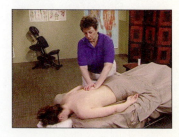
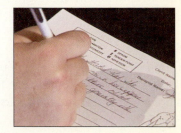
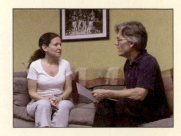

ONLINE RESOURCES AT YOUR FINGERTIPS

No massage therapy textbook has as extensive a selection of web-based resources as *Pearson's Massage Therapy*.

Instructor Resource Center

All instructional ancillary resources are available online for instant download by educators by clicking on ***www.myhealthprofessionskit.com*** and then selecting this book from the massage therapy discipline. Here instructors will find an instructor's manual, PowerPoint lecture slides, an electronic test bank, and an image library.

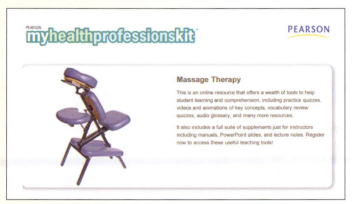

CourseSmart e-text

We realize that massage therapy students are conscious about avoiding placing undue strain on their bodies. We also know that students are often on tight budgets. Introducing CourseSmart, a value-priced e-text option that relieves the stress of carrying an extra book. Students can download this textbook for a reduced price at ***www.coursesmart.com*** and they can begin taking advantage of these benefits:

- Instant access
- Full-text searching
- Highlighting and printing capabilities

CourseSmart is a "green" solution that literally saves tons of paper every year. Pearson is proud of this initiative as a measure of our commitment to the environment.

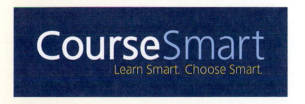

TOOLS TO HELP INSTRUCTORS SHINE

Pearson's Massage Therapy offers a rich array of ancillary materials to benefit instructors and help infuse a spark in the classroom. The full complement of supplemental teaching materials is available to all qualified instructors from your Pearson representative.

Instructor's Resource Manual

This manual contains a wealth of material to help faculty plan and manage their courses. It includes:

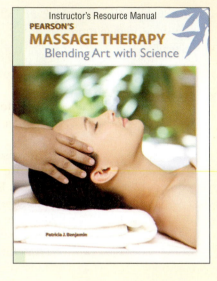

- Comprehensive lecture notes that contain abstracts, factoids, and teaching strategies.
- A wealth of worksheets and handouts.
- A complete test bank of nearly 600 questions.

Test Bank

A complete test bank of nearly 600 questions that allows instructors to generate customized exams and quizzes.

PowerPoints

A comprehensive, turn-key lecture package in PowerPoint format containing discussion points, with embedded color images.

Image Library

Every photograph and illustration contained in the textbook.

A WORD ABOUT NATIONAL CERTIFICATION

Through our Vue division, Pearson is pleased to provide a variety of national certification exams. While this book is not directly correlated to these exams, it can serve as a useful study reference. Visit **http://www.vue.com/fsmtb/** or **http://www.vue.com/ncbtmb/** for information.

 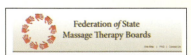

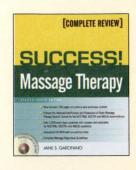

To help prepare you for any of these important certification exams, you may wish to purchase our bestselling test prep book, *SUCCESS! in Massage Therapy* by Jane Garofano. The book is organized based on the national exam format and contains review content and a variety of mock exams. Order online or at your local bookstore (ISBN: 0135072220)

Acknowledgments

How can one even begin to acknowledge all those who have contributed to *Pearson's Massage Therapy: Blending Art with Science*? Producing a comprehensive textbook like this involves many people both known and unknown to the primary author. Everyone who touched this project in any way has my gratitude for their efforts. A few who stand out will be acknowledged here.

First is Frances M. Tappan (1917–1999), who many years ago invited me to join her on the adventure of writing massage therapy textbooks. She provided the spark that started me on the journey that has led to this point.

Thanks to all those who contributed to *Tappan's Handbook of Healing Massage Techniques* and *Professional Foundations for Massage Therapists*. These two textbooks laid the groundwork for *Pearson's Massage Therapy*.

Various people have lent their expertise and knowledge, and provided a depth of understanding and accuracy that would otherwise be missing from this text. They include Beverly Schoenberger, Polarity Therapy; Barbara Esher and John f. Johnson, Asian Bodywork Therapy Theory; Will Parks, Acupressure Massage Integration; Xie Ling Welch, Qi Gong; Christopher Alvarado, Myofascial Massage; Dale Perry, Lymphatic Facilitation; Paula Stone, Reflexology; and Ann L. Mihina and Sandra K. Anderson, Spa Applications.

Massage therapists who appear in the DVD video massage segments include Christopher Alvarado, Bobbe Bermann, Danielle Bianchi, Annette Chamness, Larry Clemmons, Maria Durbin-Cooper, Wayne Hussey, Connie Love, John Magruder, Will Parks, Dale Perry, Xie Ling Welch, and Patricia Vater, who coordinated the demonstrations. Other massage therapists appearing in the videos include Joli Behr-Cook, Jennifer van Dam, Caleb Edmond, Julie Favaro, and Jeff Mann.

Reviewers who made thoughtful criticisms and suggestions on draft pages have added greatly to the quality and relevance of the book. This includes official reviewers as well as colleagues who offered their opinions on different aspects of this text. It is a better book because of your comments.

Thanks to the production staff at Pearson—especially Mark Cohen, Editor-in-Chief of Health Professions, and to Development Editor, Lynda Hatch, who has kept me more or less on schedule and who improved the text in so many ways.

Last, but not least, I want to acknowledge the support and encouragement of family and friends, who pitched in as needed many times. This includes my mother, Mary Benjamin, and my sister, Debra Benjamin, who appear in a few figures as clients. Special appreciation is reserved for Martha Fourt who stepped up whenever I needed a model, photographer, editor, go-fer, or any other task—usually on short notice.

Thanks to all.

Patricia J. Benjamin

About the Author

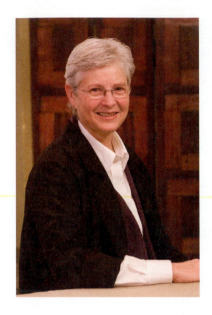

Patricia J. Benjamin, PhD, NCTMB, is a licensed massage therapist, educator, author, and appreciative massage and bodywork client. She has a deep respect for massage therapy as an art, science, and wellness practice. She has studied its traditions and watches for trends in the massage therapy profession today.

Building on her earlier background in sports and fitness, Dr. Benjamin graduated from the Chicago School of Massage Therapy in the mid-1980s. She was drawn to massage as an active, hands-on therapy whose foundations dovetail with her former career in health, physical education, and recreation. After having a full-time massage therapy practice, she gravitated back to education, first as an association education director, and then as a teacher and massage school administrator. Over the years, she has served on various committees involved in the development of ethical standards and national certification for massage therapists, and the accreditation of massage programs.

Dr. Benjamin has taught at the high school and college levels, and enjoys developing curriculum materials for the career-oriented courses offered in vocational programs. She holds master's and advanced study degrees in education with a specialty in curriculum development from Northern Illinois University. A doctorate in recreation and leisure studies from Purdue University has deepened her appreciation of the many facets of wellness and grounded her in a variety of research methods.

Frances M. Tappan approached Patricia Benjamin to join her as coauthor of *Healing Massage Techniques* for its 3rd edition (1998). Since Dr. Tappan's passing in 1999, Dr. Benjamin has continued to update and improve *Tappan's Handbook of Healing Massage Techniques*, and it remains a standard in the field today. Dr. Benjamin authored *Professional Foundations for Massage Therapists* (2009) as a resource for students to learn about the profession, its history, varied competencies, ethics, and business practices.

In her leisure time, Dr. Benjamin enjoys reading historical fiction and nonfiction, gardening, tai chi and qi gong, Zen archery, and swimming. Her outdoor pursuits include hiking, canoeing, and a new interest in birding. She currently resides in Chicago, Illinois.

Our Development Team

The fresh and unique vision, format, and content contained within the pages of *Pearson's Massage Therapy: Blending Art with Science* comes as a result of an incredible collaboration of expert educators from all around. This book represents the collective insights, experience, and thousands of hours of work performed by members of this development team. Their influence will continue to have an impact for decades to come. Let us introduce the members of our team.

CONTRIBUTORS

Text

Ann L. Mihina—Spa Applications
Sandra K. Anderson—Spa Applications
    Chapter 17 Spa Applications is adapted from their
      book, *Natural Spa and Hydrotherapy* (2009).
Christopher Alvarado—Myofascial Massage
    Licensed Massage Therapist
    Evanston, Illinois
Barbara Esher—Asian Bodywork Therapy Theory
    Senior Instructor and Curriculum Coordinator for the
      Shiatsu Program and Asian Bodywork
    Baltimore School of Massage
    Baltimore, Maryland
John F. Johnson—Asian Bodywork Therapy Theory
    Shiatsu Instructor
    Baltimore School of Massage and Anne Arundel
      Community College
    Baltimore, Maryland
Will Parks—Acupressure Massage Integration
    Connecticut Center for Massage Therapy
    Newington, Connecticut
Dale Perry—Lymphatic Facilitation
    CNW School of Massage
    Albany, New York
    Brenneke School (Cortiva)
    Seattle, Washington
Beverly Schoenberger—Polarity Therapy Licensed
    Psychotherapist and Physical Therapist
    Newington, Connecticut

Paula Stone—Reflexology
    The Stone Institute
    St. Charles, Missouri
    The reflexology section in Chapter 18 Contemporary
      Massage and Bodywork is adapted from her
      book, *Therapeutic Reflexology* (2011).
Xie Ling Welch—Qi Gong for Self-Care
    Qi Gong Instructor and Licensed Massage Therapist
    Oak Park, Illinois

Video

Christopher Alvarado
Joli Behr-Cook
Dr. S. C. Benanti
Bobbe Berman
Danielle Bianchi
Annette Chamness
Larry Clemmons
Maria Durban Cooper
Cheryl Coutts
Christopher Coutts
Jennifer van Dam
Selene DelValle
Caleb Edmond
Julie Favaro
Wayne Hussey
Theresa Cecylija Leszczynski
Connie Love
John Magruder
Jeff Mann
Abby Nickerson
Will Parks
Dale Perry
Patricia Vater
Xie Ling Welch

REVIEWERS

Elizabeth Aerts, BS, MBA, NCTMB
Co-Director
The School of Integrative Therapies
Holmdel, New Jersey

Bernice Bicknase, AAS, BS
Program Chair, Therapeutic Massage
Ivy Tech Community College Northeast
Fort Wayne, Indiana

Monique Blake, MS
Program Coordinator, Massage Therapy
Keiser Career College
Miami Lakes, Florida

Mary C. Capozzi, MS, RN, LMT, NCBTMB
Coordinator, Therapeutic Massage
Finger Lakes Community College
Canandaigua, New York

Ellen M. Caravati, BA, LMT
Massage Therapy Program Coordinator
Keiser University
Daytona Beach, Florida

Richard Ceroni, PhD, MA, M.Ed, LMT, LICDC
Dean of Education
Carnegie Institute of Integrative Medicine
Suffield, Ohio

Jennifer M. DiBlasio, AST, ACMT, CHT
Assistant Director
Career Training Academy
New Kensington, Pennsylvania

Lorena M. Haynes, BS, LMT
Instructor
Westside Tech—OCPS
Winter Garden, Florida

Charles C. Houston Jr., B.msc, LMT, LMTI, MMP
Founder/Director
Amarillo Massage Therapy Institute
Amarillo, Texas

Tom Johnston, MEd, LMP, BMHHP
Director
BodyMind Academy
Kirkland, Washington

JeraiLyn Jones, CMT, CSCS
Director of Education
Lakeside School of Massage Therapy
Milwaukee, Wisconsin

Mary McCluskey, MA
Director
Wisconsin School of Massage Therapy
Germantown, Wisconsin

Karen Murphy, LMT
Instructor/Massage Therapist
Lourdes Institute of Wholistic Studies
Collingswood, New Jersey

Andrea Robins, MS
Instructor
Keiser University
Daytona Beach, Florida

Karla Ross, AA, AS, LMT
Instructor
Exceptional Massage Institute
Hot Springs, Arkansas

Pamela Shelline, LMT
Director
Massage Therapy Academy
St. George, Utah

Victoria Jordan Stone, MA, NCMT
Academic Director
Blue Ridge School of Massage & Yoga
Blacksburg, Virginia

Efthimios Vlahos, CMT, MBA
Program Coordinator, Massage Therapy
Northwestern College
Chicago, Illinois

Janet Waid, LMBT, NCTMBT
Instructor, Therapeutic Massage
Carteret Community College
Morehead City, North Carolina

A Commitment to Accuracy

As a student embarking in healthcare you probably already know how critically important it is to be precise in your work. Clients and co-workers will be counting on you to avoid errors on a daily basis. Likewise, we owe it to you—the reader—to ensure accuracy in this book. We have gone to great lengths to verify that the information provided in *Pearson's Massage Therapy: Blending Art with Science* is complete and correct.

To this end, here are the steps we have taken:

1. *Editorial Review*   No fewer than 12 content experts have read each chapter for accuracy. In addition, some members of our developmental team were specifically assigned to focus on the precision of each illustration that appears in the book.
2. *Accurate Ancillaries*   The teaching and learning ancillaries are often as important to instruction as the textbook itself. Therefore, we took steps to ensure accuracy and consistency of these components by reviewing every ancillary component. The author and editorial team studied every PowerPoint slide and online course frame to ensure the context was correct and relevant to each lesson.

While our intent and actions have been directed at creating an error-free text, we have established a process for correcting any mistakes that may have slipped past our editors. Pearson takes this issue seriously and therefore welcomes any and all feedback that you can provide along the lines of helping us enhance the accuracy of this text. If you identify any errors that need to be corrected in a subsequent printing, please send them to:

Pearson Health Editorial
Massage Therapy Corrections
One Lake Street
Upper Saddle River, NJ 07458

Thank you for helping Pearson reach its goal of providing the most accurate textbooks available.

Massage Practice Sequences

Contents

PART 2   KNOWLEDGE FOR PLANNING MASSAGE SESSIONS   251

Chapter 7   Effects of Massage   252

PART 4   ADJUNCT THERAPIES AND SPECIAL APPLICATIONS   463

Chapter 16   Hydrotherapy and Temperature Therapies   464

Chapter 17   Spa Applications   484

Chapter 18   Contemporary Massage and Bodywork   518

APPENDICES

Fast Track to Success

Before you begin, we encourage you to read this brief section to help you get off to a great start in your studies and test-taking.

STUDY TIPS

Knowing your own learning style is a key to success in school. Are you primarily a visual, auditory, or kinesthetic learner? Do you learn best alone or in a study group? Do you study better in the morning or at night? Do you have a learning disability, and if so, have you gotten help to learn compensation techniques? Develop a learning strategy that works best for you, and take responsibility for using it in school and beyond.

Big Picture versus Details

Research indicates that learners fall into two camps: "right brained" learners who process information by focusing on the big picture and relationships between ideas; and "left brained" learners who process information in a sequential step-by-step fashion focusing on details. Each style of learning has strengths and drawbacks. For example, right-brain learners can miss important details, while left-brain learners may get so bogged down in details that they miss the big picture. Be aware of your natural style, but incorporate methods that help you get both the big picture as well as the details.

Better Study Habits

Here are some simple things you can do to improve your study habits:

- Understand the learning outcomes for a class, and keep your attention on material that helps you achieve them. Be selective and focused.

- Read assigned material before a lecture so that you are not hearing about the subject for the first time in class. The lecture will sink in more deeply if you are already somewhat familiar with terminology and concepts presented. You will be less likely to get lost in class.

- Underline, highlight, and write in the margins of reading material to identify important terms and concepts. Be selective in finding the most important ideas. Mark passages directly related to topics from classes. Don't highlight too much.

- Pick out key terms and write out their definitions. Identify related concepts and subtopics.

- Become familiar with the features in your textbooks. The table of contents, figures, tables, appendix, glossary, and index provide valuable information, and help you find what you are looking for more quickly.

- Within 24 hours after a class, review and rewrite your class notes. Write summaries of major topics in your own words, noting where ideas covered in class are found in your textbooks.

- If you learn best by hearing (auditory learner), ask permission to tape lectures so that you are not distracted from what the teacher is saying by taking notes. Replay the tapes after class, and then make notes of the most important ideas.

- If you learn best by doing (kinesthetic learner), write out concepts and definitions, draw pictures and diagrams, and outline chapters in your textbooks. Do things like handle bones of the skeleton when learning anatomy, palpate muscles as you memorize their locations and attachments, and combine doing massage techniques with memorizing their effects.

- In study groups, explain basic concepts to each other, ask each other questions, and discuss important topics. Listen to what others have to say, and also practice saying your ideas out loud to others. This helps you clarify your thoughts.

- Use study guides and supplemental materials that come with your textbooks.

Take Time

Set aside enough time to read, discuss, think about, and test yourself on material you are learning. The more you review the material and interact with it in different ways, the better your grasp of it will be. A general rule is to study 3 hours for every hour you are in class. Finally, tell the instructor or a counselor if you are getting lost or behind in class. Be open to suggestions and to trying new learning methods.

Remember the old adage "you can lead a horse to water, but you can't force him to drink." The school and teachers are responsible for setting up a good learning environment, but you must do your part for learning to take place.

TAKING TESTS

Written examinations are a fact of life in school and in attaining certification and licensing. Some people find exams a positive experience. They enjoy testing their knowledge, and approach them like game shows on TV. Others find exams anxiety provoking and decidedly unpleasant. Following some simple guidelines can maximize the chances that your test results will truly reflect what you have learned.

Get Focused

First, arrive early and get organized and settled into your seat. Get out your pencil and other items you will need for the test. Put your other things away and out of sight so that you have a clear space to work and think. Do whatever works for you to calm down, focus, and concentrate; for example, quiet sitting or deep breathing.

If you get distracted easily, find a quiet place in the room away from doors and windows. Sit in the front row near a wall if possible. Ask the monitor if you can wear earplugs to muffle distracting sounds.

Understand the Test

Read and understand the test directions before you start. Ask the monitor for an explanation of directions you do not understand. Quickly look over the entire test to see how long it is and what types of questions are on it, so that you can plan your time.

Read each question carefully before answering. Reading too quickly can cause you to miss important words. Be sure you fully understand what the question is asking.

Don't panic if you have a momentary lapse of memory. If you draw a blank on a question, skip over it, and go back to it later. Don't be disturbed if others finish before you do. Focus on what you are doing and take the time allowed to finish. If you have extra time, check over your answers to catch careless mistakes, or reread and improve essay answers.

Answer Questions Thoughtfully

ESSAY QUESTIONS   First, determine what level of knowledge the question requires. Action words like *list*, *define*, *compare*, *analyze*, and *explain* tell you how to approach your answer. Outline your answer on a scratch sheet to organize your thoughts and identify important points.

Do not write everything you remember about the topic. Be sure that your answer addresses the specific question asked. Be concise and direct in your answer. Don't ramble. Write legibly, and in complete sentences. Use good grammar and correct spelling. Come back to your answer later if you have time to recheck for accuracy, completeness, clarity, and to correct grammatical and spelling errors.

If you run out of time, quickly outline an answer. Providing some information is better than leaving the question blank.

OBJECTIVE TEST QUESTIONS   The most common objective test questions are multiple choice, true/false, and matching. Answer the questions in order, marking the ones you are not sure of in the margin. Do not spend too much time on any one question. Give it your best guess and move on. You can go back to it later if you have time.

Watch out for negative wording such as *not* or *least*, "double negatives," and qualifying words like *always*, *seldom*, *never*, *most*, *best*, *largest*. Read each question thoroughly for full understanding of what it says.

Multiple-choice questions are designed so that only one choice is correct. A good strategy is to find the correct answer by the process of elimination of the incorrect ones. Grammatical inconsistencies may tip you off to the right answer or to a wrong one. Read the question and your choice together to make sure it makes grammatical sense.

True/false questions need to be read very carefully. One incorrect detail makes the whole statement false. If a sentence has two parts (a compound sentence), both parts need to be true for the whole question to be true.

For matching questions, use one column as your reference. For each item in that column, go through all items in the second column until you find a match. Match all the ones you are sure of first, and then go back to match the others with your best guess.

Do not change your answers without good reason. First "guesses" tend to be better than "second guessing." If you are not guessing, but have a good reason to change your mind, go ahead and change an answer.

YOUR RESOURCE FOR LEARNING

Pearson's Massage Therapy: Blending Art with Science is intended to be your resource for learning. Every feature is designed to lead you to success in laying the foundations for your career in massage therapy. By keeping your career goals in sight, you can find motivation to do what it takes to get the most out of your time in school.

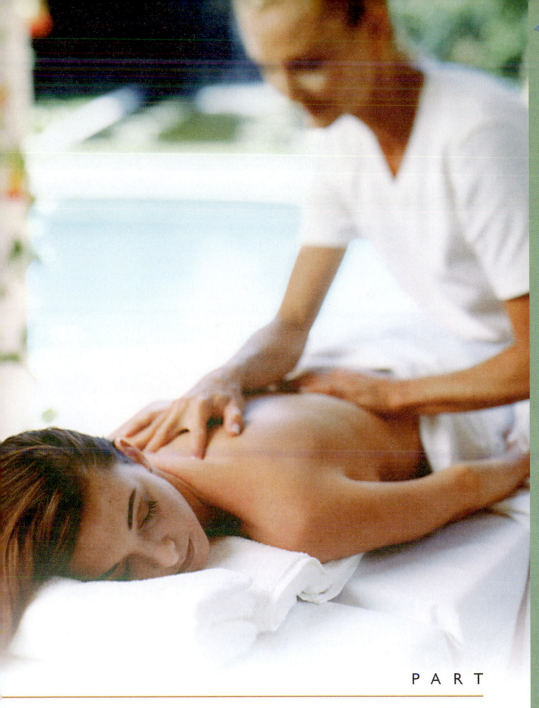

PART

1

Foundations

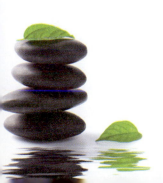

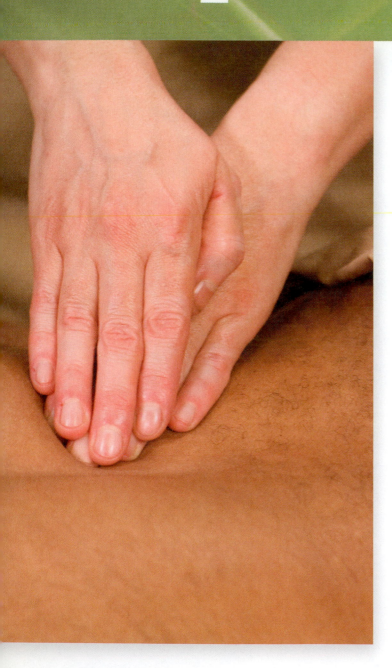

CHAPTER 1

The Massage Therapy Profession

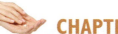

CHAPTER OUTLINE

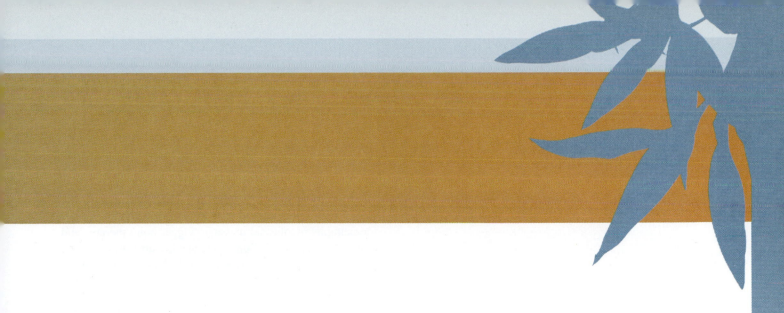

 ## LEARNING OUTCOMES

After studying this chapter, you will have information to:

1. Define massage therapy.
2. Explain the scope of massage therapy using the Wellness Massage Pyramid.
3. Identify trends related to massage therapy.
4. Summarize the variety of career opportunities for massage therapists.
5. Describe the unique knowledge base of massage therapy.
6. Discuss education standards for massage therapists.
7. Describe the types of credentials available to massage therapists.
8. Distinguish among various kinds of professional organizations.
9. Identify major sources of information about massage therapy.
10. Describe the state of massage therapy research.

 ## KEY TERMS

Accreditation 12

Complementary and alternative medicine (CAM) 5

Continuing education (CE) 13

Credentials 13

Ethical standards 19

Health care settings 8

Home visit practice 9

Integrative medicine center 8

Massage 4

Massage therapy 4

National certification 13

Occupational licensing 14

Personal care settings 7

Private practice settings 9

Professional associations 16

Sports, fitness, and recreation settings 7

Wellness Massage Pyramid (WMP) 4

Wellness profession 5

MASSAGE *in* ACTION

On your DVD, explore:

- A Variety of Workplaces for Massage Therapists
- The Wellness Massage Pyramid
- Licensing and Credentials
- Organizations
- Research
- Ethics

THE JOURNEY

Welcome! You have begun the journey to becoming a successful massage therapist. The next several months will be a period of transformation as you learn to be a competent and caring professional. Your education will be a holistic experience as you physically master massage techniques, mentally absorb the science and theory of massage therapy, and practice the social skills needed for good relationships with clients. You will exercise your memory, develop reasoning skills, and internalize the principles of ethical behavior. You will learn about employment opportunities and how to start and maintain your own massage therapy practice.

The first step in this journey is to survey the landscape of massage therapy, that is, to get the big picture of the career that you have chosen. That means understanding what massage therapy is, its broad scope as a wellness profession, trends related to its use, and where massage therapists work. The next step is to understand the nuts and bolts of the massage therapy profession, such as educational, certification, and licensing requirements, how research aids knowledge, and the organizations and publications available to the massage therapist.

MASSAGE DEFINED

Massage is the intentional and systematic manipulation of the soft tissues of the body to enhance health and healing. Massage is performed with or without lubricating substances such as oil and lotion. Joint movements and stretching are commonly performed as part of massage. Adjunct modalities within the scope of massage include the use of hot and cold packs and hydrotherapy in the form of whirlpool bath, sauna, and steam room.

Simple hand tools are sometimes used to apply pressure during massage, as are machines that mimic massage techniques. However, massage is primarily manual therapy, that is, it is performed by hand. It is the person-to-person touch essential to massage that gives it a unique healing potential.

The most common system of massage in North America and Europe is traditional Western massage, sometimes called *Swedish massage*. Western massage is based on an understanding of anatomy, physiology, pathology, and other biosciences. The seven technique categories of Western massage are effleurage, petrissage, tapotement, friction, vibration, touch without movement, and joint movements. Western massage techniques are applied to improve overall functioning of the body systems, to enhance healing, and for relaxation of body and mind.

Other Western systems of soft tissue manipulation include specialized manual techniques to affect specific body systems, for example, myofascial massage, trigger point therapy, and lymphatic facilitation. Some massage therapy systems have developed alternative theories of how the body works, in addition to Western sciences, for example, reflexology and polarity therapy.

Massage and bodywork traditions are found all over the globe. In addition to Western massage, major traditions include folk and native practices from different areas of the world, Ayurvedic massage from India, Asian bodywork therapies based in Chinese medicine, and eclectic forms that combine theory and techniques from several systems.

Massage therapy is a general term used to describe all of the different systems of soft tissue manipulation. *Bodywork* is a term coined in the late twentieth century to encompass a wide variety of manual therapies including massage, movement integration, structural integration, and energy balancing. The terms *massage* and *bodywork* are often used together to describe the occupational field of massage therapy, as in National Certification for Therapeutic Massage & Bodywork. Appendix A on page A-1 is a guide to 25 different forms of massage and bodywork, including their origins, techniques, theories, and websites for further information.

WELLNESS PROFESSION

Massage therapists apply massage and related modalities to help clients on their quest for high-level wellness. This includes massage therapy for stress reduction, for treatment and recovery from illness and injuries, as a simple healthy pleasure, and for many other purposes. The broad scope of the field is evident in the **Wellness Massage Pyramid (WMP)** in Figure 1.1■.

The WMP illustrates the major goals of massage therapy and its many applications. The goal at the top is high-level wellness, a condition of optimal physical, emotional, intellectual, spiritual, social, and vocational well-being. The concept of wellness is holistic at its core, encompassing the whole person.

The three levels at the base of the pyramid address *deficiency* needs related to illness and injury. These include applications of massage therapy for treatment of, recovery from, and prevention of illness and injury. Satisfying those needs brings one to the *neutral zone*, which is the old definition of health as the absence of disease.

Next in the WMP are the *growth* levels. These include massage therapy applications for health maintenance, personal growth, and enjoyment of life to its fullest—all aiming

FIGURE 1.1
Wellness Massage Pyramid.

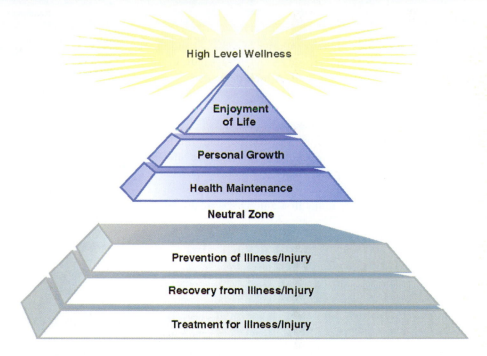

toward a state of high-level wellness. The upper part of the pyramid encompasses massage therapy for purposes such as optimal body system functioning, developing greater awareness of the inner self, feeling integrated in body and mind, and enjoying the healthy pleasure of caring touch.

Massage therapy is sometimes referred to as a **complementary and alternative medicine (CAM)** therapy. CAM therapies are healing systems or modalities generally outside of mainstream allopathic medicine, for example, herbal remedies, acupuncture, naturopathic medicine, biofeedback, and music therapy. The White House Commission on CAM Policy (2002) cited therapeutic massage, bodywork, and somatic movement therapies as a major CAM domain (www.whccamp.hhs.gov). Massage therapy as a CAM domain generally refers to applications of massage at the base of the WMP.

In its fullest sense, massage therapy is best thought of as a **wellness profession**, since the work of massage therapists spans the entire wellness massage paradigm. Because of its broad scope, there are a wide variety of career opportunities for massage therapy practitioners. These include developing general practices, or more narrow specializations such as in personal care, sports and fitness, or health care. Some massage therapists focus on a particular client group, such as the elderly, athletes, people with cancer, children, or other special populations. Over time, massage and bodywork practitioners learn new skills, deepen their knowledge, take advanced training, and change work settings. Because it is a wellness profession, a career in massage therapy opens many opportunities for satisfying individual interests, talents, and strengths.

CRITICAL THINKING

Think about your current state of well-being. Note where improvements can be made and formulate some wellness goals for yourself. Now determine how massage might fit into a plan to meet those goals.

1. Consider the broad scope of wellness including physical, emotional, intellectual, spiritual, social, and vocational well-being.
2. Use the Wellness Massage Pyramid to identify areas of personal deficiency (e.g., illness or inury) and areas for personal growth.

3. Explain how massage might fit into a plan to help you meet your personal wellness goals.

4. Compare the benefits you might expect from massage to others in the class. Notice how each person's needs and desires are unique.

TRENDS

Surveys reveal trends in the popularity of massage and the reasons people seek it out. Several recent surveys indicate an increased use of massage overall. A high percentage of the increase in the use of massage was in spas and as a CAM therapy for various ailments and injuries.

The Spa Association (SPAA) surveyed more than 3,500 spas about their services and reported their findings in the 2004 State of the Industry Report. Massage was offered at 97 percent of the spas responding and generated the largest amount of money compared with any other spa service. ("Study shows massage ranks first among spa treatments," *Hands-On* 2004.)

A 2007 consumer survey of 1,008 adults living in the continental United States examined who was receiving massage and identified some of the factors that motivate people to get massage. The survey was commissioned by the American Massage Therapy Association® and conducted by the CARAVAN® Opinion Research Corporation. It found that of people who had had massage in the past 5 years, 30 percent reported the reason as pain management, injury rehabilitation, migraine headache control, or overall wellness. Only 22 percent reported having massage for simple relaxation, and just 13 percent indicated that massage was a "special indulgence." It also found that more women had had a massage in the past 5 years (43 percent) than men (25 percent). Respondents between the ages of 45 to 64 who had received massage in the past year had an average of 7 sessions, while those aged 18 to 44 averaged 5 sessions for the year. See Figure 1.2■ for survey results.

The annual National Health Interview Survey (NHIS) conducted by the National Center for Complementary and Alternative Medicine (NCCAM) and the National Center for Health Statistics gathered information in 2003 about the use of alternative and complementary therapies in the United States, including massage therapy (NCCAM *Newsletter*

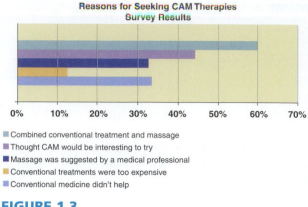

Reasons for Seeking CAM Therapies
Survey Results

- Combined conventional treatment and massage
- Thought CAM would be interesting to try
- Massage was suggested by a medical professional
- Conventional treatments were too expensive
- Conventional medicine didn't help

FIGURE 1.3

Data from the annual National Health Interview Survey (NHIS) conducted by National Center for Complementary and Alternative Medicine (NCCAM) and the National Center for Health Statistics.

2004). Some of the most popular CAM therapies mentioned included acupuncture, chiropractic, naturopathy, biofeedback, energy healing, homeopathy, yoga, tai chi, qi gong, and massage therapy. Massage was cited by respondents as the ninth most used CAM therapy with 5 percent of the 39,000 adults surveyed reporting having received massage in the past year. See Figure 1.3■ for the reasons people choose massage for CAM therapy. General findings were that women were more likely than men to use CAM, that CAM use increased with age and education level, and that those who had been hospitalized in the past year were more likely to turn to CAM.

The American Hospital Association (AHA) survey of the use of CAM therapies in U.S. hospitals sheds light on the use of massage in mainstream health care. The survey of 1,007 hospitals revealed that 82 percent of the hospitals reporting use of CAM therapies had incorporated massage into hospital care. Of those offering massage, 74 percent use it for stress management in patients, 69 percent for stress relief in hospital staff, 59 percent for cancer patients, and 55 percent for pregnant women. Relief of stress and pain were cited most often as the reasons for the use of massage.

The surveys discussed here point to a trend of increased desire for and use of massage therapy for a variety of reasons and in a variety of settings. The use of massage in spas for relaxation and rejuvenation and its use as a CAM therapy are particularly evident in recent surveys. It is not surprising then that according to the U.S. Department of Labor, employment for massage therapists is expected to increase 20 percent from 2006 to 2016, faster than the average for all occupations (American Massage Therapy Association, 2008).

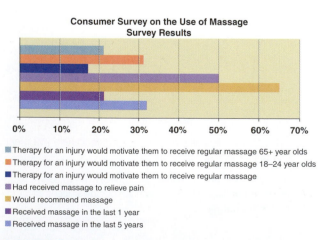

Consumer Survey on the Use of Massage
Survey Results

- Therapy for an injury would motivate them to receive regular massage 65+ year olds
- Therapy for an injury would motivate them to receive regular massage 18–24 year olds
- Therapy for an injury would motivate them to receive regular massage
- Had received massage to relieve pain
- Would recommend massage
- Received massage in the last 1 year
- Received massage in the last 5 years

FIGURE 1.2

Data from 2007 Massage Therapy Consumer Survey Fact Sheet, American Massage Therapy Association®.

TYPICAL WORK SETTINGS

Massage therapists work in a variety of settings, reflecting the broad range of the benefits of massage. Four categories of typical work settings include personal care; sports, fitness, and recreation; health care; and private practice. Table 1.1■ lists examples of places where massage therapists typically work. Appendix B on page A-8 is a guide to personal care providers and health care professionals who interact with massage therapists in these work settings and are mentioned throughout this textbook.

Personal Care

Personal care settings focus on personal grooming, relaxation, and rejuvenation. They include beauty salons and barbershops, and day, destination, and specialty spas. In these settings, massage is just one of several services offered. Chapter 17, Spa Applications describes several of the services a massage therapist working in a spa might perform after receiving additional training, such as aromatherapy, body wraps, exfoliations, and stone massage.

Beauty salons and barbershops cater to consumers' needs related to hair, nails, and skin care. These establishments are found in storefronts, shopping malls, department stores, hotels, and other commercial spaces. Cosmetologists, beauticians, barbers, and estheticians are licensed professionals providing services in these businesses. Massage may be part of their services within their scope of practice; for example, cosmetologists are usually permitted by law to perform facials and pedicures that include massage. In this setting, massage therapists usually offer full body massage for relaxation.

Spas also offer a variety of personal care services. Spas are defined by the International SPA Association (ISPA) as "entities devoted to enhancing overall well-being through a variety of professional services that encourage renewal of mind, body and spirit." Seven kinds of spas recognized by ISPA include club spa, cruise ship spa, day spa, destination spa, medical spa, mineral spring spa, and resort/hotel spa. The ISPA motto summarizes the intent of the spa experience as to "relax, reflect, revitalize, and rejoice" (www.experienceispa.com).

Day spas offer many of the same services as beauty salons and barbershops, plus special services such as herbal wraps, different kinds of hydrotherapy (e.g., whirlpool, sauna, steam room), mud baths, mineral baths, exercise facilities, and therapeutic massage and bodywork. See Figure 1.4■. Patrons come for one or more services, staying a short time or the entire day. Massage therapists are sometimes trained to perform services in addition to massage, for example, herbal wraps.

Destination spas are places with overnight accommodations, which immerse guests in a healthy environment. Services include fitness activities, nutritious meals, lifestyle education, and the day spa services listed earlier, including massage.

Other types of spas are distinguished either by focus or location. For example, club spas are fitness facilities that also offer spa services. Medical spas integrate spa services with conventional and complementary therapies for healing mind and body. Cruise ship spas are located aboard cruise ships, and mineral spring spas at mineral and hot springs. Resort and hotel spas cater to business and vacation travelers staying at their establishments. The range of services offered in different spas varies, but their common purpose is renewal and rejuvenation through personal care. Massage is an integral part of the modern spa scene.

Sports, Fitness, and Recreation

Sports, fitness, and recreation settings are facilities whose main purpose is to provide opportunities for physical

TABLE 1.1 Typical Work Settings for Massage Therapists			
Personal Care	**Sports, Fitness, and Recreation**	**Health Care**	**Private Practice— Self-employed**
• Beauty salon and barbershop	• Nonprofit community center	• Conventional health care center	• Massage therapy office or clinic
• Spa	• Commercial health club	*Medical office or clinic*	• Storefront business
Club spa	• Specialty exercise studio	*Hospice service*	• Home-based practice
Cruise ship spa	• Sports club or team	*Hospital*	• Home visit practice
Day spa		*Nursing home*	• On-site chair massage
Destination spa		• Integrative medical center	
Medical spa		*Integrative medical clinic*	
Mineral spring spa		*Sports medicine clinic*	
Resort/hotel spa		*Medical spa*	
		Wellness center	
		• Alternative health care center	
		Chiropractic office	
		Naturopathic clinic	
		Chinese medicine clinic	

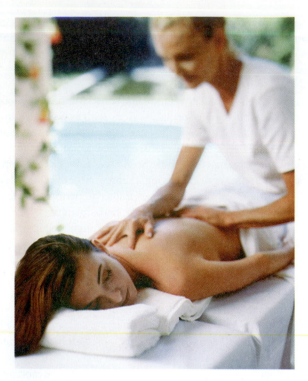

FIGURE 1.4

Personal care setting.

exercise and sports, but that also provide support services such as massage. These include nonprofit community centers such as the YMCA, commercial health clubs, and specialty exercise studios such as yoga centers. Some massage therapists work with professional or amateur sports teams at their own training facilities and on the road. See Figure 1.5■.

Massage is offered in these settings as an adjunct to fitness and sport training regimens. Massage therapists interact with other health professionals working in these facilities,

including coaches, personal trainers, exercise physiologists, and athletic trainers. The focus of massage here is to help clients achieve their fitness goals, improve athletic performance, and enhance healing from minor injuries.

Health Care

Health care settings are places where patients are treated for illnesses and injuries. They include conventional Western medical facilities such as doctors' offices and clinics, hospitals, hospice facilities, nursing homes, and rehabilitation centers. Integrative medical settings offer both conventional and complementary and alternative healing methods as options, based on the greatest potential benefit for the patient. Health care also includes alternative medicine settings such as chiropractic clinics, naturopathic offices, and Chinese medicine and acupuncture clinics.

In conventional health care settings, massage therapists work in conjunction with doctors, nurses, physical therapists, and other health care professionals within the tradition of Western medicine. Hospital-based massage is a specialty in which massage is integrated into the regular hospital setting, such as in the pediatric ward, cancer unit, or cardiac care (Figure 1.6■). For more information visit the Hospital-Based Massage Network (www.hbmn.com).

Conventional health care centers may take an integrative approach by having alternative healing practitioners, including massage therapists, available to patients. An **integrative medicine center** goes one step further by offering a team approach between a variety of Western medical health care providers, traditional and indigenous healers, and CAM practitioners in a collaborative effort. Massage therapists in these settings are an integral part of a health care team.

Integrative medical settings take different forms. In sports medicine centers, massage therapists team up with physical therapists and athletic trainers for rehabilitation of athletic injuries and improvement of sports performance. In

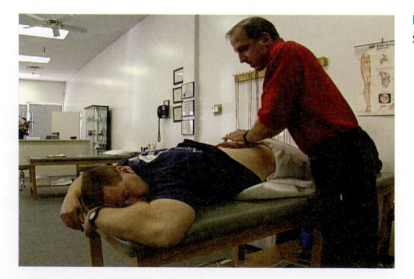

FIGURE 1.5

Sports, fitness, recreation setting.

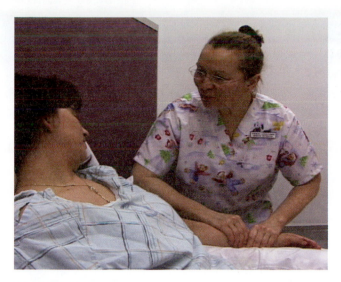

FIGURE 1.6
Health care setting.

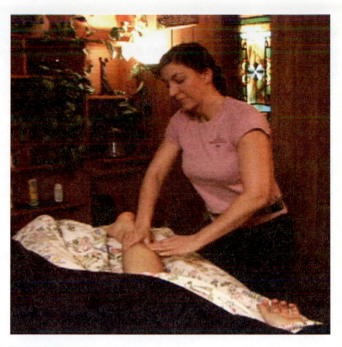

FIGURE 1.7
Private practice setting.

medical spas, conventional and complementary therapies are available in a spa environment. Wellness centers connected to hospitals offer fitness activities, rehabilitation programs, massage therapy, and classroom instruction in preventing disease and developing a healthy lifestyle.

Chiropractors hire massage therapists to work with their patients in conjunction with regular chiropractic treatment. Massage may be given before or after a chiropractic adjustment or at a different time as part of an overall treatment plan. Chiropractors also lease space to massage therapists to whom they refer patients for ongoing massage for prevention of problems and general well-being.

Naturopathic physicians often refer patients for massage as part of a treatment strategy. They also hire massage therapists to work in their clinics, or they may lease space to massage therapists so that they are on-site at the naturopathic office.

Chinese medicine clinics hire practitioners skilled in Western massage and Asian bodywork therapy. Asian bodywork systems that complement traditional healing practices such as acupuncture and herbs include tuina, amma, shiatsu, acupressure, and Jin Shin Do®.

Private Practice

Private practice settings are the most varied. Massage therapists in private practice are self-employed and develop their businesses to suit their own interests and talents and to respond to current consumer demands.

The most common private practice setting is the one-room massage office, or massage clinic with two or more rooms, in an office building. A storefront massage business might be on a commercial street, in a shopping mall, or airport. A dedicated massage room can be set aside in a residence for a home-based practice where not prohibited by zoning laws (Figure 1.7■). Clients come to the massage therapist's space for appointments in these settings.

An alternative is for the massage therapist to travel to the client's home, sometimes called a **home visit practice**. There the massage therapist creates a setting for massage in an appropriate space provided by the client. The home visit practice is convenient for busy working clients and the homebound elderly and disabled.

With the invention of the special massage chair, settings for massage have expanded to the workplace and various public places. Seated massage settings have been created in such places as parks, inside grocery or department stores, and at trade shows and conferences. The traveling or *on-site massage practice* can be set up temporarily in a small space using portable equipment suitable for the situation.

Many massage therapists develop eclectic practices, for example, combining an office practice with making home visits or part-time employment at a spa or chiropractic office. Specialized or advanced training may be required to work in certain settings, but the examples described earlier portray the broad and diverse range of career opportunities for massage therapists in today's world.

BECOMING A MASSAGE THERAPY PROFESSIONAL

Massage therapists contribute to the overall health and well-being of their clients and their communities. As the benefits of massage therapy become better appreciated and the

PRACTICAL APPLICATION

Prepare an informal survey of the availability of massage in your community and the varieties of career opportunities for massage therapists there.

1. Make a list of the places in your community where massage is available.
2. Look at the types of settings, for example, personal care, sports and fitness, health care, and private practice.
3. Indicate the name and address of the business, and what type of massage they offer. Note the environment, for example, if massage is one of many services offered like at a spa, or is unique like chair massage at a health food store, or a separate massage office.
4. Divide the list according to how close the places are to where you live. Are they within a half-mile, one mile, more than one mile?
5. Comment on the accessibility of massage in your community and the potential for career opportunities for massage therapists there.

demand for massage therapy grows, there are corresponding expectations that massage therapists become increasingly professional. That means being better educated, having valid credentials, adhering to a code of ethics, and generally being held to a higher standard. Massage therapy is considered an emerging profession in that some of the hallmarks of a mature profession are still in development.

The benchmarks of mature professions include having a unique body of knowledge and skills, and intensive entry-level education. It also includes continuing education throughout a career and valid credentials. The theoretical and scientific information underlying a profession develops through experience, as well as scholarship and research, and is published in professional journals. Professionals form associations that sup-

CASE FOR STUDY

Sarah and Finding the Right Massage

Sarah has read a lot about the benefits of receiving massage and has decided to try it for herself. She sees massage advertised in different places in her community and wonders where the best place to go for massage would be for her. Sarah has been feeling stressed out lately and somewhat sore from her new fitness program. She has a few health problems like mild asthma and allergies. She has a busy schedule and values convenience highly, but also wants a high-quality massage experience.

Question:

How should Sarah go about finding the right place to receive massage for herself?

Things to consider:

- What might Sarah's initial goals be for her massage session?
- What might her priorities be in terms of location and setting?
- What types of settings might she explore for a massage that meets her current needs?

Where might Sarah go for massage in your community?

Using the information from the preceding Practical Application exercise in this chapter, determine the two best places for Sarah to go for massage in your community. (Assume she lives near you.)

_____

_____

_____

port their members, set standards, represent the profession to the public, and promote professional interests.

Ethical codes and standards of practice describe expectations of excellence and good conduct. They are the foundations of self-determination and self-regulation for a profession. The overall focus of all professions is commitment to service and the good of humanity. This latter commitment sets professions apart from other businesses and occupations. The public trust afforded to professionals is based on an expectation of honesty, integrity, and selfless service.

All of the benchmarks mentioned earlier set the stage for acceptance by other professionals and recognition by the general public. The professionalizing of massage therapy has occurred at a steady pace since the 1980s. Box 1.1● summarizes the foundational characteristics of a profession.

Since organizations have such a significant role in professions, it is important to know the major organizations in the profession you have chosen. They are typically known by their acronyms or initials, and the "alphabet soup" of organizations can be confusing. Use Table 1.2■ as a reference for the organizations mentioned in this chapter. Some of the important aspects of professionalism in massage therapy today are explored in the following paragraphs.

BODY OF KNOWLEDGE AND SKILLS

The body of knowledge and skills that define the massage therapy profession is unique in many respects, while sharing some things with other professions. The uniqueness of massage therapy lies in the primacy of touch and soft tissue manipulation in its skill base and the broad range of applica-

| BOX 1.1 | Characteristics of a Profession |

- Specialized knowledge and skills
- Intensive entry-level education
- Accreditation
- Continuing education
- Valid credentials
  - National certification
  - Specialty certification
  - Occupational licensing
- Professional associations
- Ethical codes and standards of practice
- Acceptance among other professionals
- Recognition by the general public
- Commitment to public service and the good of humanity

tions throughout the entire Wellness Massage Pyramid. The knowledge base for massage therapy, although occasionally borrowing from other professions, is uniquely focused on the use of soft tissue manipulation to improve the well-being of recipients. The profession is rooted in the tradition of natural healing and maintains a holistic and wellness perspective.

Examples of shared knowledge are the sciences of anatomy, physiology, and pathology that are basic to all health professions. Concepts such as the therapeutic relationship and related ethical principles are common to professions with one-on-one interaction with clients and patients. The communication skills involved in health history taking and documentation are also required in other professions.

TABLE 1.2	Guide to Major Massage Therapy Organizations in the United States*	
Acronym	Name	Type
ABMP	Associated Massage & Bodywork Professionals	Member Organization
AMTA	American Massage Therapy Association (Professional and school membership)	Professional Association
AOBTA	American Organization for Bodywork Therapies of Asia (Professional and school membership)	Specialty Association
COMTA	Commission on Massage Therapy Accreditation (USDE recognized)	School Accreditation
IMSTAC	Integrative Massage and Somatic Therapies Accreditation Council (ABMP affiliate)	School Accreditation
FSMTB	Federation of State Massage Therapy Boards	Licensing Boards, Licensing Exam
MSA	Massage School Alliance (ABMP affiliate)	School Membership
MTF	Massage Therapy Foundation	Research, Education, Outreach
NCBTMB	National Certification Board for Therapeutic Massage and Bodywork	National Certification, Licensing Exams

*Many other massage therapy organizations have been founded to serve the profession, and many others can be found in countries outside of the United States. This is a sample of the largest and most influential organizations in the United States in 2010.

Massage skills are part of the scope of other professionals (e.g., estheticians, physical therapists, athletic trainers). However, soft tissue manipulation is only a small part of other professions, while it is the defining modality for massage therapists. Massage therapists apply massage through the entire range of wellness applications as depicted in the Wellness Massage Pyramid (WMP)—from treatment, recovery, and prevention of illness and injury to health maintenance, personal growth, and enjoyment of life.

This unique body of knowledge is found in the increasing number of textbooks and journals written specifically for massage therapists. It is also reflected in massage therapy program curriculum standards, core competencies, job analyses, and licensing examinations for massage therapists.

EDUCATION

Entry-level education lays the foundation of knowledge and skills needed to perform massage therapy competently. The curriculum typically includes basic massage and bodywork techniques; sciences of anatomy, physiology, kinesiology, and pathology; assessment skills; client communication skills; hygiene and safety; professional standards, ethics and law; and business practices. Basic massage techniques and their applications are learned in hands-on classes (Figure 1.8■).

The Commission on Massage Therapy Accreditation (COMTA) has identified core competencies for massage therapists. Competencies define education in terms of what a practitioner can actually do, rather than just having completed a number of hours in certain subjects. COMTA competencies for entry level massage therapy programs include plan and organize an effective massage and bodywork session, perform massage therapy for therapeutic benefit, develop and implement a self-care strategy, develop ethical relationships with clients, develop a strategy for a suc-

cessful practice, and identify strategies for professional development. A more extensive list of standards can be found on the COMTA website (www.comta.org).

Most massage therapy programs are offered in private vocational schools and community colleges, and award a diploma or certificate, associate degree, or, in a few cases, an academic bachelor's degree. The general standard for length of entry level programs varies from 500–1,000 clock hours. The Commission on Massage Therapy Accreditation (COMTA) requires 600 clock hours of classroom instruction.

Massage programs in the United States are required to be approved by the state government agency that oversees vocational, academic, or other school programs. This ensures minimal standards of operation. In other countries, a provincial or national education agency typically approves school programs. For example, in Canada, education is a responsibility of the individual provinces.

Massage schools, and massage programs within larger institutions such as community colleges, may seek additional recognition through **accreditation**. Accreditation is awarded by a nongovernmental organization whose mission is to uphold high educational standards. Accreditation organizations develop evaluation criteria and conduct peer evaluations to confirm that their standards are met. For example, the Integrative Massage and Somatic Therapies Accreditation Council (IMSTAC), a division of Associated Massage and Bodywork Professionals (ABMP), is a body that sets standards for massage programs.

The U.S. Department of Education publishes a list of nationally recognized nonprofit accrediting commissions determined by their criteria to be reliable. Some USDE recognized accrediting bodies that accredit massage programs include the Accrediting Bureau of Health Education Schools (ABHES), Accrediting Commission for Career Schools and Colleges of Technology (ACCSCT), and the National Accrediting Commission of Cosmetology Arts and Sciences (NACCAS). The

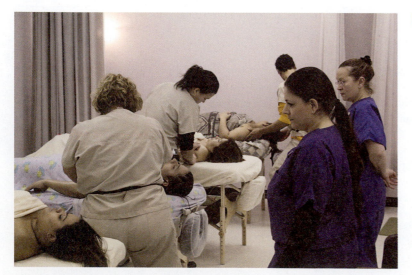

FIGURE 1.8

Hands-on class in a massage therapy program.

Commission on Massage Therapy Accreditation (COMTA) is the only accrediting agency focused exclusively on massage therapy programs and recognized by the USDE. A complete list of USDE recognized accrediting agencies can be found on the USDE website (www.ed.gov).

Massage schools and programs may also join member organizations that provide forums for discussion of education related issues, publications, liability insurance, and other resources. Do not confuse membership in these organizations with accreditation. The Massage School Alliance, affiliated with ABMP, is an example. AMTA has a school member category for massage programs.

Continuing Education

Continuing education (CE) is education beyond entry-level training. Continuing education keeps massage therapy professionals up-to-date and offers the opportunity to gain a higher level of knowledge and skills. A certain number of hours of continuing education are generally required for occupational license and certification renewals, and by some membership organizations.

Continuing education is provided by massage schools, individual teachers, and professional associations. CE providers may be required to be approved for license or certification renewal. The National Certification Board for Therapeutic Massage and Bodywork has a list of their Approved CE Providers and the criteria for approval on their website (www.ncbtmb.org). If your state or local government licenses massage therapists, check with them for their approved providers of continuing education.

CREDENTIALS

Credentials testify to the accomplishments of the person holding them. They are a method for the general public, other professionals, and employers to evaluate a person's background in a given field. Credentials are awarded by a school,

organization, or government agency to a person meeting their criteria for the credential. Using the language of credentials properly is important as massage therapists take their place in the larger world of health professionals. Presenting credentials honestly is a basic ethical principle. Four types of credentials available to massage therapists are a school diploma or certificate, national certification, specialty certification, and occupational licensing.

School Diploma

A school diploma or certificate is a statement that a person has graduated or successfully completed a course of study. It is the piece of paper hung on the wall to show the public the education a massage therapist has had. It designates the school name, location, course of study, number of hours completed, and date of graduation, and is signed by school officials (Figure 1.9■). A *transcript* is a more detailed record of a student's performance while in school, including specific subjects studied, grades, and attendance, in addition to the information on the diploma. An original transcript carrying the school seal is usually required for official purposes such as obtaining a license to practice.

National Certification

National certification is a term usually reserved for a credential given by a nongovernmental nonprofit organization that attests to a person's competency in a given profession. It involves qualifying by virtue of education and/or experience, and passing a written examination and/or performance evaluation based on an objective analysis of job requirements. Those certified agree to abide by a specific code of ethics. National certification is renewed periodically, which usually requires a certain amount of continuing education. It is sometimes referred to as *board certification*.

How does one know if a national certification credential is based on accepted standards and will be respected by other professionals? The National Commission for Certifying Agencies (NCAA) accredits certifying programs that

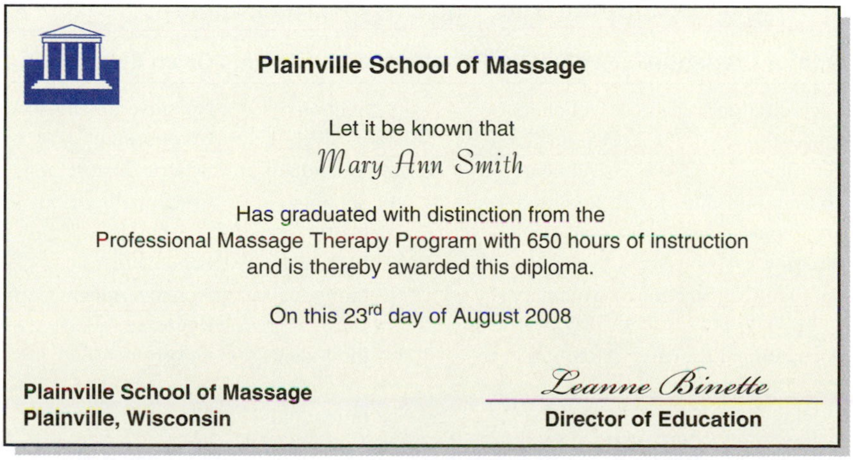

FIGURE 1.9

Diploma or certificate is proof of education completed.

Plainville School of Massage

Let it be known that

Mary Ann Smith

Has graduated with distinction from the
Professional Massage Therapy Program with 650 hours of instruction
and is thereby awarded this diploma.

On this 23rd day of August 2008

Plainville School of Massage
Plainville, Wisconsin

Leanne Binette
Director of Education

comply with their standards. Many certification programs in the health professions seek NCCA recognition. A list of NCCA accredited programs can be found on their website (www.noca.org/ncca/accredorg.htm). Two NCCA accredited programs apply to massage and bodywork practitioners.

The National Certification Board for Therapeutic Massage and Bodywork (NCBTMB) is an organization that offers recognized credentials for massage therapists. It currently offers two credentials: Nationally Certified in Therapeutic Massage and Bodywork (NCTMB), and Nationally Certified in Therapeutic Massage (NCTM). Eligibility criteria and content outlines for their exams can be found on their website (www.ncbtmb.org).

The National Certification Commission for Acupuncture and Oriental Medicine (NCCAOM) offers a credential called Diplomate in Asian Bodywork Therapy (Dipl. A.B.T.–NCCOAM). Information about this certification and others in oriental medicine, acupuncture, and Chinese herbology can be found on their website (www.nccaom.org).

Specialty Certification

To be certified in a specific massage and bodywork system (e.g., polarity therapy, reflexology, or shiatsu) involves some combination of education, skill development, internship, written and performance tests, ethical code, continuing education, and/or periodic renewal. Specialty certifications can be as rigorous as a 1,000 clock-hour program with internship and written and performance exams, or as minimal as a weekend workshop. Therefore, determining what a specialty certification really means requires some information about who is offering it and what is involved in getting it.

Since massage therapy is an emerging profession, and retains some entrepreneurial aspects, the terms *certification* and *certified* are sometimes used with ambiguity. For example, a course of study is sometimes called a *certification program* when it would be more correctly referred to as a *certificate program* for which a *certificate of completion* is given. In established professions, the term *certification* is more commonly reserved for credentials with more exten-

sive education, examinations, continuing education, and renewal.

Some massage and bodywork systems are protected by trademark, and the name is registered with the U.S. Patent and Trademark Office. These systems use the registered trademark symbol ®. Practitioners may not use a trademarked name to describe their work unless certified by their organization or properly authorized to do so. Examples are Jin Shin Do® (www.jinshindo.org), Rolfing® (www.rolf.org), and Bonnie Prudden Myotherapy® (www.bonnieprudden.com).

Occupational Licensing

When deemed in the public interest, governments may choose to regulate a profession. A growing number of governments are licensing massage therapists. The main purposes of **occupational licensing** are consumer protection and the assurance of a minimal level of competence of practitioners. However, in the case of massage, an underlying motivation may also be to weed out practitioners using massage as a cover for prostitution.

In the United States, occupational licensing is done at the state level. In some unlicensed states, jurisdictions like big cities or counties may choose to license massage therapists. In Canada, occupational licenses are administered at the provincial level, and in some other countries at the federal or national level of government.

Occupational licensing is permission granted to qualified practitioners to accept compensation for massage in a specific governmental jurisdiction. Licenses are awarded by the government agency that regulates professions in the jurisdiction. It is required to practice, unlike the national or specialty certifications described earlier which are voluntary. Table 1.3■ compares and contrasts diplomas, national certification, occupational licensing, specialty certification, and accreditation.

The details vary, but massage licenses typically require being a certain age (usually 18 years old), having a minimum level of general education (usually a high school

TABLE 1.3	Guide to Credentials in Massage Therapy			
Type of Credential	Voluntary/Required	Given To	Given By	Purpose
Accreditation	Voluntary	School	Nongovernment Accreditation Commission	Testify that school meets commission standards
Certificate	Voluntary	Individuals	Schools/Instructors	Proof of education completed
Continuing Education Approval	Required	Schools/Instructors	Credentialing Body	Approval of education programs for credential renewal
Diploma	Voluntary	Individuals	Schools/Instructors	Proof of education completed
National Certification	Voluntary	Individuals	Nongovernment Certification Board	Attest to competency in the profession
Occupational License	Required	Individuals	Government	Permission to practice in jurisdiction
Specialty Certification	Voluntary	Individuals	Nongovernment Organization/Instructor	Attest to competency in specialization

FIGURE 1.10

States that require licensing or certification. (Graphic provided by Associated Bodywork & Massage Professionals.)

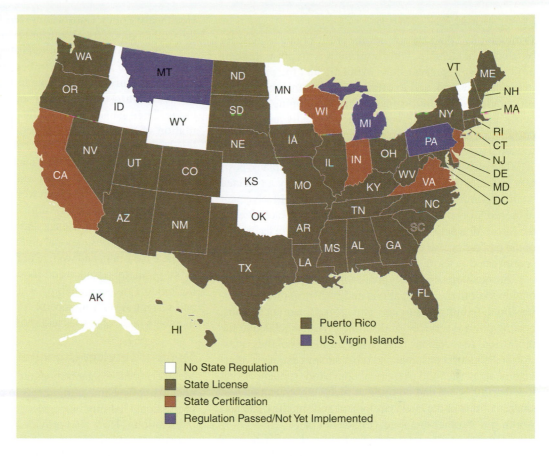

Puerto Rico

US. Virgin Islands

☐ No State Regulation

■ State License

■ State Certification

■ Regulation Passed/Not Yet Implemented

diploma), completing massage therapy education of a defined length (usually from 500–1,000 clock hours), passing a designated written and/or practical test, having no criminal record, abiding by a code of conduct, and paying fees. People practicing without a license are subject to fines, and, in some cases, criminal prosecution.

A few states have created their own licensing exams. Most states, however, accept one or more of the standardized exams developed to test minimum competency. The most widely used exams are the NCTMB and NCTM exams mentioned earlier, and the Massage & Bodywork Licensing Examination (MBLEx) developed by the Federation of State Massage Therapy Boards.

Occupational licensing may be called certification or registration in some jurisdictions. Variations of licensing include a form of government regulation called *registration*, in which only those meeting certain requirements can call themselves massage therapists, but other practitioners are not prohibited from working.

In the United States today, 42 states plus the District of Columbia regulate massage therapists, and licensing bills are pending in several other states. Figure 1.10■ shows the states that require licensing or certification. The most current information on licensing can be found at professional organizations' websites, such as the sites sponsored by the AMTA and ABMP.

The Federation of State Massage Therapy Boards (FSMTB) was established in 2005 to facilitate communication among boards that regulate massage therapy in the United States. Its mission is "to support its Member Boards in their work to ensure that the practice of massage therapy is provided to the public in a safe and effective manner." FSMTB concerns include standardizing license requirements and promoting portability of massage licenses from state to state.

A different type of license called an *establishment license* might also be required for a massage practice at a specific location. This is a business license to operate a commercial space where customers come for massage. Also for public protection, establishment licenses typically require revealing the business ownership, a certain level of hygiene and safety, posting services and prices, and that all practitioners in the establishment have the required occupational licenses.

ORGANIZATIONS

Massage and bodywork practitioners have formed several organizations to address their needs and promote the profession. They can be categorized as general membership organizations and specialty organizations. General membership organizations welcome practitioners of different forms of massage and bodywork, and can be further categorized into professional associations and member services organizations. Specialty associations are composed of practitioners of a particular style of bodywork such as polarity therapists, or those who work in a particular setting like the nurse massage therapists.

Professional Associations

Professional associations are nonprofit organizations run by elected leadership, whose mission is to promote their profession, to represent their members and the profession in the larger world, and to offer services to members. They set standards for the profession by developing codes of ethics and standards of practice. They typically have an IRS designation as 501(c)(6) corporations, that is, nonprofit professional association.

The mission of the association, its goals and plans, position statements, and services are determined by an elected board and implemented by volunteers and staff. Involvement in the work of committees, special projects, and activities of the association help develop the present and future leadership of the profession. All the money generated by the association is reinvested in its mission.

Association services typically include providing information via official publications and websites, offering professional liability insurance and group insurance plans, hosting referral services, and selling products related to the profession. Associations raise public awareness of the profession and conduct consumer and other surveys to collect information about the field. At annual conventions, members get together for board and committee meetings, education sessions, exhibits of the latest equipment and supplies, and networking with other members (Figure 1.11■).

Governments consult with professional associations as representatives of the profession in developing legislation such as licensing and establishment laws. They also turn to associations when seeking participants in studies and policy development. For example, professional associations participated in preparing the report of the White House Commission on Complementary and Alternative Medicine Policy (2002) (www.whccamp.hhs.gov/finalreport.html).

Organizations also look to professional associations for participation in multidisciplinary projects. An example of this is the participation of massage organizations in the Integrated Healthcare Policy Consortium (IHPC) (http://ihpc.info) of the Collaboration for Healthcare Renewal Foundation.

Some professional associations have local chapters to address the needs of members in a particular state or other local jurisdiction. Chapters provide opportunities for leadership development and networking closer to home. They are important in the United States where regulation of massage therapy occurs at the state and local levels.

The American Massage Therapy Association (AMTA), founded in 1943, is the oldest and largest professional association for massage and bodywork therapists in the United States (www.amtamassage.org). Its mission is "to develop and advance the art, science and practice of massage therapy in a caring, professional and ethical manner in order to promote the health and welfare of humanity." Its core purpose is "to promote, advance and provide innovative thinking in the field of massage therapy while facilitating, supporting and serving AMTA members." It currently has over 58,000 members in 27 countries and chapters in all 50 states.

Member Services Organizations

Member services organizations are general membership organizations whose major mission is to provide benefits such as professional liability insurance, group health insurance, and publications. They also provide information of interest to their members in newsletters and on websites. These organizations may also act to protect the interests of members, for example, related to licensing and legislation. They differ from professional associations in that they may be for-profit businesses, and if so, the owner sets policy and determines the direction of the organization. They typically do not hold conventions nor have elected leadership.

The Associated Bodywork and Massage Professionals (ABMP), founded in 1987, is the largest member services organization for massage and bodywork practitioners in the United States, with over 65,000 members (www.abmp.com).

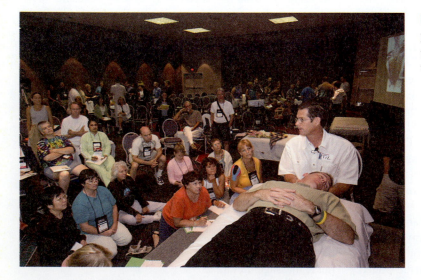

FIGURE 1.11

Professional association conventions provide opportunities for networking with other massage therapists.

PRACTICAL APPLICATION

Explore student membership in a major professional organization. Use the organization's website and promotional materials for information.

1. Write a brief description listing the specific benefits offered with student membership.

2. Discuss with a classmate or study partner the potential value to you of joining a professional organization while still a student.

3. Answer the question: How might student membership in a major professional organization give me a head start in my career?

Its goal is "to provide massage, bodywork, skin care and somatic therapies practitioners with professional services, information, and public and regulatory advocacy. ABMP is devoted to promoting ethical practices, protecting the rights of practitioners, and educating the public regarding the benefits of massage and bodywork."

Specialty Associations

Massage therapy, like many other professions, can be divided into subgroups of practitioners with special knowledge and skills. They may focus on a particular form of massage and bodywork, a specific population of clients, or in a particular setting. Specialty groups often form their own associations to address their unique needs and interests. They offer members many of the same benefits as general membership organizations. The following are examples of different types of specialty associations for massage and bodywork practitioners.

The American Organization of Bodywork Therapies of Asia (AOBTA) is a professional association founded in 1989. It represents over 1,400 practitioners of forms of bodywork based in traditional Chinese medicine developed in China, Japan, Korea, and other Asian countries (www.aobta.org). It has some state chapters.

The American Polarity Therapy Association (APTA) was founded in 1984 as an educational and charitable nonprofit organization (www.polaritytherapy.org). Its members include practitioners, teachers, and students of Polarity Therapy as developed by Randolph Stone. It promotes practitioner standards, approves education programs, sponsors education events, and publishes a newsletter and other materials.

The Rolf Institute® of Structural Integration was established in 1971 as an educational and scientific nonprofit organization (www.rolf.org). Its purpose is to promote a form of myofascial bodywork called Rolfing®, provide quality training programs in Rolfing®, certify Rolfing® practitioners, provide continuing education, and promote research and public awareness of the value of Rolfing®.

The International Association of Infant Massage (IAIM®) was formed in 1980 and incorporated in 1986. The IAIM® mission is "to promote nurturing touch and communication through training, education, and research so that parents, caregivers, and children are loved, valued, and respected throughout the world community." The organization trains and certifies Certified Infant Massage Instructors (CIMI®) who in turn teach parents and caregivers to massage their babies.

ROB

REALITY CHECK

ANITA: Remembering all of the massage organizations and credentials seems impossible. I'm not even sure why it's important. I just want to get a job doing massage after graduation.

ROB: There's a difference between seeing massage therapy as a job and thinking about it as a career. A career in massage therapy opens the door to a future doing meaningful work and options for any number of jobs or a private practice. The organizations and credentials related to massage therapy may seem confusing at first, but over time you'll become familiar with them. You'll read about them in publications for massage therapists, and you may want to join an organization as a student member. And building a résumé includes decisions about what organizations to join and what credentials you need for your dream job. Knowing all that's available to you as a massage therapist will help you make better choices.

The National Association of Nurse Massage Therapists (NANMT), established in 1987, is a nonprofit organization for nurses who are also trained in some form of massage and bodywork, and work in health care settings. Their basic philosophy includes a respect for holistic healing, practices grounded in nursing theory, and the need to balance high-tech medicine with personalized touch-based therapies. One of their goals is to compile research related to massage in health care, and implement findings into practice.

Notice that most of the organizations described were founded in the late twentieth century, when the field of massage and bodywork experienced a period of growth and expansion. Many other specialty organizations have been formed since that time. They can be located on the Internet.

SCHOLARSHIP AND PUBLICATIONS

Scholarship in therapeutic massage and bodywork has been increasing in volume and quality over the past 25 years. Vehicles for this information have evolved from a few self-published manuals in the 1970s to a variety of well-documented and illustrated texts published by major publishing houses today.

The depth of scientific knowledge in anatomy, physiology, kinesiology, and pathology required by today's practitioners has spawned a number of books written specifically for massage and bodywork practitioners. Authors with extensive academic backgrounds in human sciences, who are also massage therapists, have provided a depth of knowledge absent in the past. The same can be said for the areas of pharmacology, psychology, and professional ethics.

As the profession of massage therapy matures, and experienced practitioners become teachers and authors, the understanding of massage therapy theory and principles deepens. In addition, massage therapists who have come from more established professions have enriched massage therapy scholarship. Nurses, physical therapists, physical and health educators, athletic trainers, psychologists, pharmacologists, and other professionals who have come into the field have helped transform massage theory and practice in a number of areas.

For example, information from other professions related to things such as the therapeutic relationship, assessment skills, effects of medications, documentation, and ethics have been integrated into the massage therapy knowledge base. The result is a more developed body of knowledge for massage therapists.

A variety of publications disseminate information about massage and bodywork to practitioners and the general public. The *Massage Therapy Journal* is the official publication of the AMTA, and ABMP publishes *Massage & Bodywork*. Although intended for a general audience, *Massage* magazine also provides information about the massage and bodywork

profession. *Massage Today* is a monthly publication in newspaper format that contains news about the field, as well as informative articles on a variety of related subjects.

Peer-reviewed publications that report research related to massage therapy are *The Journal of Bodywork and Movement Therapies* and the free online journal *International Journal of Therapeutic Massage & Bodywork* (IJTMB) sponsored by the Massage Therapy Foundation. Peer review is a more rigorous process than editorial review used by most trade magazines. Peer reviewed means that a panel of massage therapists with expertise in the subject of an article evaluates the article for accuracy, reviews any research for validity, and approves the article for publication.

RESEARCH

A research base for massage therapy is developing gradually. Scientific studies about massage therapy are now conducted primarily within more established health professions and in connection with universities and hospitals. The result is an emphasis on clinical applications of massage, with less attention to applications at the top of the Wellness Massage Pyramid, such as fitness and personal growth.

Two obstacles to massage therapy research are lack of an academic infrastructure to support it and inadequate funding. Vocational schools and community colleges, where most massage therapy education takes place, do not ordinarily have the resources to conduct research. Neither do they have faculty with advanced training in experimental design and statistics to conduct the studies. The limited number of peer reviewed research journals specifically for massage therapy means that reports of massage research are scattered among journals from other health professions.

There are, however, some developments to advance research in the profession. The Massage Therapy Foundation was founded in 1990 to promote massage therapy research. It funds studies and maintains a database of massage therapy research on its website (www.massagetherapy foundation.org). The MTF published a report called the *Massage Therapy Research Agenda* in 1999. The report calls for greater research literacy among massage therapists; more funding for studies about the safety and efficacy of massage, physiological and other mechanisms of massage, massage in a wellness paradigm; and studies about the therapeutic massage profession.

The Touch Research Institute (TRI) at the University of Miami, School of Medicine was founded by director Tiffany Field, MD, in 1992. It was the first center in the world devoted to the study of the use of touch and massage in the treatment of various ailments. Its website (www.miami.edu/touch-research.html) has information about many studies sponsored by TRI.

ETHICAL STANDARDS

Knowledge of ethics and ethical behavior are essential competencies for massage therapists. There is a growing body of literature about ethical behavior in the profession.

Ethical standards in massage therapy are reflected in the codes of ethics and standards of practice of professional organizations. The National Certification Board for Therapeutic Massage and Bodywork (NCBTMB) requires certificants to abide by their code and standards and to have continuing education in professional ethics as a condition of renewal. Professional organizations also have disciplinary procedures for censoring members not in compliance with their ethical standards. Further discussion of professional ethics can be found in Chapter 5, Ethics and the Therapeutic Relationship, on page 94 and Chapter 23, Business Ethics, on page 648.

RECOGNITION BY THE PUBLIC AND HEALTH PROFESSIONALS

Evidence of public acceptance of massage therapy is found in the many positive articles appearing in newsstand magazines and health and fitness publications. Massage therapy is also a popular service at spas and health clubs.

Consumer surveys confirm the growing acceptance of massage therapy by the general public. Annual AMTA consumer surveys conducted between 2003 and 2008 found that an average of 21 percent of adult Americans received massage at least once a year. An average of 32 percent of those surveyed received a massage in the previous five years. Women (45 percent) reported receiving massage more than men (21 percent). Spas now appear to be the most popular place to get a massage. The public seeks massage for stress relief, pain management, injury rehabilitation, headache relief, and overall health and wellness (AMTA *Massage Therapy Industry Fact Sheet* 2009).

Two stereotypes that have negatively affected the level of public acceptance of massage therapy in the past are diminishing. These are the association of massage with prostitution and with quackery and pseudoscience. As massage therapists achieve greater degrees of professionalism, these stereotypes will continue to decrease in the future.

Recognition from Other Professionals

There is ample evidence of the recognition of the massage therapy profession by the government and by other professionals. For example, manual therapies, including massage, were included in a report on alternative medicine to the National Institutes of Health (NIH) in 1992. The White House Commission on Complementary and Alternative Medicine Policy (WHCCAMP) cited therapeutic massage, body work, and somatic movement therapies as a major CAM domain in its Final Report (2002).

More doctors and healthcare providers are recommending massage therapy to their patients than in the past. In a 2008 survey, 13 percent of respondents reported discussing massage therapy with their healthcare providers, with 57 percent of those indicating that their doctor strongly recommended or encouraged them to get massage. And 69 percent of massage therapists reported receiving referrals from health care professionals (AMTA *Massage Therapy Industry Fact Sheet* 2009).

Representatives of the massage therapy profession have been asked to participate in a variety of professional activities. For example, an AMTA representative was appointed in 2003 to the CPT® Committee of the American Medical Association. CPT®, or Current Procedural Code, lists the code for official reporting of medical services and procedures. Massage therapy is also represented on the Academic Consortium for Complementary and Alternative Health Care (ACCAHC).

The formal activities cited earlier, along with countless referrals and inclusion in integrative health care settings, attests to the growing acceptance of massage therapy and massage therapists as professionals.

CRITICAL THINKING

Think about the effect that negative stereotypes have had on the acceptance of the massage therapy profession by the general public and by other health professionals.

1. Identify those stereotypes.

2. Write a brief explanation of why you think the stereotypes developed and why they still exist.
3. What factors related to massage therapy as an emerging profession are likely to lessen negative stereotypes about massage?

CASE FOR STUDY

Jim and Explaining Massage Therapy as a Profession

Jim enrolled in a massage therapy program after high school to learn a marketable skill so he could eventually have his own business. He liked to work with his hands and was interested in health and fitness. He had received massage while recovering from a sports injury and thought he would like to be a massage therapist. He saw many career opportunities for his future in massage therapy. Jim's old high school friends could not understand the attraction of massage therapy as a career, nor did they think one had to go to school to learn something that seemed so simple.

Question:

What can Jim tell his friends to explain the profession of massage therapy to them and its growing importance as a health practice?

Things to consider:

- What can he say about the growing acceptance of massage by the general public and other health professionals?
- How can he explain the extent of his education and the skills he is learning?

- What other occupations or professions might he compare to being a massage therapist?
- What can he point out about the credentials he is working toward having?
- How might he describe professional associations he may join or has joined?
- What publications can he show them to illustrate what massage therapy is all about?
- How would mentioning massage therapy research help explain the profession and its place in health and healing?

What three things could Jim focus on to best explain the massage therapy profession to his friends?

1. _____

2. _____

3. _____

CHAPTER HIGHLIGHTS

- The journey to becoming a successful massage therapist is a holistic experience requiring development of physical, mental, and social skills.
  - The first step on the journey is to survey the landscape to get the big picture of massage therapy as a career choice.
- Massage is the intentional and systematic manipulation of the soft tissues of the body to enhance health and healing.
  - Massage and bodywork is a term often used to describe the occupational field of massage therapy.
- Massage is performed with or without oil and may include joint movements and stretches, as well as hydrotherapy.
- Massage is primarily a manual therapy, and the person-to-person touch essential to massage gives it a unique healing potential.
- The Wellness Massage Pyramid (WMP) illustrates the broad scope of massage therapy. In this schematic, the goal for the client is achieving high-level wellness.

  - The three base levels of the pyramid include deficiency needs related to treatment, recovery from, and prevention of illness and injury. Satisfying these needs gets one to the neutral zone.
  - Above the base levels are growth levels related to health maintenance, personal growth, and enjoyment of life.
- As wellness professionals, massage therapists work within the entire wellness massage paradigm, although individuals may focus on a specific level of the WMP or with a certain client population.
- Recent surveys reveal a trend in increasing popularity of massage at spas and as a CAM therapy.
  - In hospital settings massage is used for stress reduction in patients and staff, for pregnant women, and for pain management.
- Typical work settings for massage therapists include:
  - Personal care (e.g., beauty salons and spas)
  - Sports, fitness, and recreation (e.g., health clubs, exercise centers, sports teams)

- ○ Health care (e.g., conventional Western medical centers, integrative health care centers, chiropractic offices, naturopathic centers, and Chinese medicine clinics)
- ○ Private practice (e.g., commercial office or storefront, home visit practice, and on-site business)
- Massage therapists often develop eclectic practices working in a variety of settings.
- Massage therapy, a modern profession with a tradition as old as time, has evolved into a wellness profession, with corresponding expectations that massage therapists be increasingly professional.
- Massage therapy is an emerging profession that has achieved some of the benchmarks of a mature profession.
- The body of knowledge and skills that defines the massage therapy profession is unique in many respects, while sharing some things with other professions.
  - ○ The uniqueness of massage therapy lies in the primacy of touch and soft tissue manipulation in its skill base, and the broad range of applications throughout the entire Wellness Massage Pyramid.
  - ○ The profession is rooted in the tradition of natural healing and maintains a holistic and wellness perspective.
- Curriculum standards for entry-level education in massage therapy range from 500–1,000 clock hours of instruction and include the knowledge and skills required for competency in the field.
- Accreditation is a voluntary, nongovernmental process for massage schools and programs that ensures compliance with established standards.
  - ○ The U.S. Department of Education recognizes agencies that accredit massage programs and meet their standards.
- Continuing education beyond initial training is often required for renewal of certifications, licenses, and by some general membership organizations.
- Four types of credentials available to massage therapists include a school diploma or certificate, national certification, specialty certification, and occupational licensing.
  - ○ A diploma or certificate is evidence of having completed a particular course of study.
  - ○ National certification is a nongovernmental voluntary credential that shows competency in the field.
  - ○ Specialty certification attests to education and competency in a specific form of massage and bodywork.
  - ○ An occupational license is a permission to practice in a certain jurisdiction, and massage therapy is regulated in 42 states plus Washington, DC, in the United States and some provinces in Canada.
- Massage therapists have founded a number of professional organizations that include general membership organizations (i.e., professional associations and membership services organizations) and specialty associations.
- Scholarship in therapeutic massage and bodywork has been growing in volume and quality over the past 25 years.
  - ○ An increasing number of textbooks and journals have been published specifically for massage therapists.
  - ○ Professionals from other fields, who are also massage therapists, have enriched the scholarship in the field.
- The Massage Therapy Foundation, established in 1990, has developed a research agenda and provides a research database and electronic peer-reviewed research journal on its website.
- Ethical standards for the profession are embodied in codes of ethics and standards of practice developed by professional associations.
- Many accomplishments in the massage therapy profession in recent years have led to greater acceptance by the general public and recognition by other health professionals.

EXAM REVIEW

Key Terms

Match the following key terms to their descriptions. For additional study, look up the key terms in the Interactive Glossary on page G-1 and note other terms that compare or contrast with them.

_____ 1. Accreditation
_____ 2. Complementary and alternative medicine (CAM)
_____ 3. Continuing education (CE)
_____ 4. Credentials
_____ 5. Ethical standards
_____ 6. Health care settings
_____ 7. Home visit practice
_____ 8. Integrative medicine center
_____ 9. Massage
_____ 10. Massage therapy
_____ 11. National certification
_____ 12. Occupational licensing
_____ 13. Personal care settings
_____ 14. Private practice settings
_____ 15. Profession associations
_____ 16. Sports, fitness, and recreation settings
_____ 17. Wellness Massage Pyramid (WMP)
_____ 18. Wellness profession

a. Awarded by a school, organization, or government agency to a person meeting their criteria
b. Offers a team approach to healing including a variety of conventional health care providers, traditional healers, and CAM practitioners in a collaborative effort
c. Awarded to a school or program by a nongovernmental organization whose mission is to uphold high educational standards
d. General term used to describe the many systems of soft tissue manipulation
e. Provides consumer protection and the assurance of a minimal level of competence of practitioners
f. Education beyond entry-level training
g. Healing systems or modalities generally outside of mainstream allopathic medicine
h. Can be a one- or two-room office space, a storefront in a mall or airport, or a dedicated room in a residence
i. The massage therapist travels to the client's home to perform massage therapy
j. Focus on personal grooming, relaxation, and rejuvenation, and include beauty salons, barbershops, and spas
k. Illustrates the major goals of massage therapy and its many applications
l. Reflected in the codes of ethics and standards of practice of professional organizations
m. Nonprofit organizations run by elected leadership, whose mission is to promote their profession, to represent their members and the profession in the larger world, and to offer services to members
n. Facilities whose main purpose is to provide opportunities for physical exercise and sports, but that also provide support services such as massage
o. Term that reflects the broad scope of the massage therapy profession
p. Credential given by a nongovernmental nonprofit organization that attests to a person's competency in a given profession
q. Intentional and systematic manipulation of the soft tissues of the body to enhance health and healing
r. Places where patients are treated for illnesses and injuries

Memory Workout

To test your memory of the main concepts in this chapter, complete the following sentences by circling the most correct answer from the two choices provided.

1. Massage is the (intuitive and orderly) (intentional and systematic) manipulation of the soft tissues of the body.
2. Massage is primarily a (manual) (digital) therapy, meaning it is performed by hand.
3. There are (seven) (nine) technique categories of Western massage.
4. The occupational field of massage therapy is often called (professional) (therapeutic) massage and bodywork.
5. Because the work of massage therapists spans the entire Wellness Massage Pyramid, massage therapy is best thought of as a (wellness) (medical) profession.
6. Spas with overnight accommodations, which immerse guests in a healthy environment, are referred to as (day) (destination) spas.
7. The focus of massage therapy in (sports) (personal care) settings is to help clients achieve their fitness goals, improve sports performance, and enhance healing from minor injuries.
8. In (conventional) (integrative) health care settings, both allopathic and CAM therapies are available.
9. Massage therapists in private practice are (self-employed) (employees).
10. The term *profession* is used to describe an occupation with a higher level of (ethical standards) (potential income).
11. A specific number of hours of (continuing) (entry level) education is often required for renewal of occupational licenses, certifications, and membership in some professional organizations.
12. A diploma or certificate is a statement of (registration) (completion) of a course of study.
13. The main purpose of occupational licensing is (massage therapist) (consumer) protection.
14. (Alternative) (Specialty) associations are formed by practitioners who focus on a particular form of massage and bodywork.
15. Two stereotypes that have negatively affected massage therapists in the past and that are (increasing) (diminishing) today are the association of massage with quackery and prostitution.
16. Ethical standards in massage therapy are reflected in the (standards of practice) (membership requirements) developed by professional associations.

Test Prep

The following multiple-choice questions will help to prepare you for future school and professional exams.

1. Which of the following is not within the scope of massage therapy as practiced in the United States?
   a. Soft tissue manipulation
   b. Joint movements
   c. Spinal adjustments
   d. Use of hot packs
2. Which of the following would appear nearest the top of the Wellness Massage Pyramid?
   a. Prevention of illness
   b. Enjoyment of life
   c. Recovery from illness
   d. Neutral zone
3. Herbal remedies, acupuncture, music therapy, and massage therapy are considered:
   a. Allopathic medicine
   b. Mainstream medicine
   c. Conventional medicine
   d. Complementary and alternative medicine
4. "Enhancing overall well-being through a variety of professional services that encourage renewal of mind, body and spirit" is the main focus of which type of setting?
   a. Health club
   b. Naturopathic physician office
   c. Spa
   d. Private practice
5. Health care settings that use a collaborative approach to healing by including a variety of Western medical health care providers, traditional and indigenous healers, and/or CAM practitioners, are referred to as:
   a. Integrative
   b. Comprehensive
   c. Conventional
   d. Alternative
6. Facilities connected to hospitals that offer fitness activities, rehabilitation programs, massage therapy, and classroom instruction in developing a healthy lifestyle are called:
   a. Sports medicine centers
   b. Medical spas
   c. Wellness centers
   d. Chiropractic offices
7. A massage practice in which seated massage is given on special massage chairs at the workplace or at events such as health fairs is called:
   a. Home visit practice
   b. On-site practice
   c. Sports massage practice
   d. Integrative practice

8. Combining a massage office with some home visits and part-time employment at a spa or chiropractic office is called:
   a. Environmental practice
   b. Ecological practice
   c. Eclectic practice
   d. Eccentric practice

9. A specific position of employment is called a(n):
   a. Occupation
   b. Profession
   c. Job
   d. Calling

10. Which of the following statements about massage therapy today is *not* true?
    a. It is rooted in the tradition of natural healing.
    b. It is narrowly focused on medical applications.
    c. It maintains a wellness perspective.
    d. It is holistic at its core.

11. Recognition given to a school by a nongovernmental organization for upholding high educational standards is called:
    a. Accreditation
    b. Certification
    c. Licensing
    d. Approval

12. A detailed record of a student's performance while in school is called a:
    a. Diploma
    b. Certificate
    c. Resume
    d. Transcript

13. A credential given by a nongovernmental nonprofit organization that attests to a person's competency in a given profession is called:
    a. Specialty certification
    b. National certification
    c. Accreditation
    d. Licensing

14. In the United States, what level of government typically regulates professions such as massage therapy by issuing occupational licenses?
    a. Town
    b. County
    c. State
    d. Federal

15. Nonprofit organizations run by elected leadership, whose mission is to promote their profession, to represent their members and the profession in the larger world, and to offer services to members are called:
    a. Professional associations
    b. Member services organizations
    c. Specialty associations
    d. Certification boards

16. The growing acceptance of massage therapy by the general public is confirmed in:
    a. Hospital surveys
    b. Licensing laws
    c. Consumer surveys
    d. Government reports

Video Challenge

Watch the appropriate segment of the video on your DVD and then answer the following questions.

The Massage Therapy Profession

The Wellness Massage Pyramid
1. Give examples from the video of massage therapists working at different levels of the Wellness Massage Pyramid.

A Variety of Workplaces for Massage Therapists
2. Can you see yourself working in any of the settings shown in the video? Which settings appeal to you the most and why?

Licensing and Credentials
3. What credentials are available to massage therapists as shown in the video?

Comprehension Exercises

The following short answer questions test your knowledge and understanding of chapter topics and provide practice in written communication skills. Explain in two to four complete sentences.

1. Define massage therapy. What are its essential characteristics? What is its intent?
2. Describe the variety of settings in which massage therapists work today. Discuss which settings are best suited for your interests and talents as you currently see them.
3. Who licenses massage therapists and why? What are the pros and cons of occupational licensing for massage therapists? What are the penalties for practicing without a license?

For Greater Understanding

The following exercises are designed to take you from the realm of theory into the real world. They will help give you a deeper understanding of the subjects covered in this chapter. Action words are underlined to emphasize the variety of activities presented to address different learning styles and to encourage deeper thinking.

1. Interview a successful massage therapist, and describe his or her practice in terms of the types of clients served and the setting in which the therapist works. Write a report, and present it to a study partner or to a class.
2. Find the most recent massage therapy industry information reported by a professional organization. Analyze the data to see what it says about the massage therapy profession and the acceptance of massage therapy by the general public and other health professionals. The information is based upon what factual sources? Discuss the implications of the findings with the class.
3. Attend a state, regional, or national convention sponsored by a professional association for massage therapists. Take advantage of all of the opportunities offered at the event including education, networking, massage equipment and supplies vendors, and organizational meetings. Report to the class about your experience.

2 The History of Massage as a Vocation

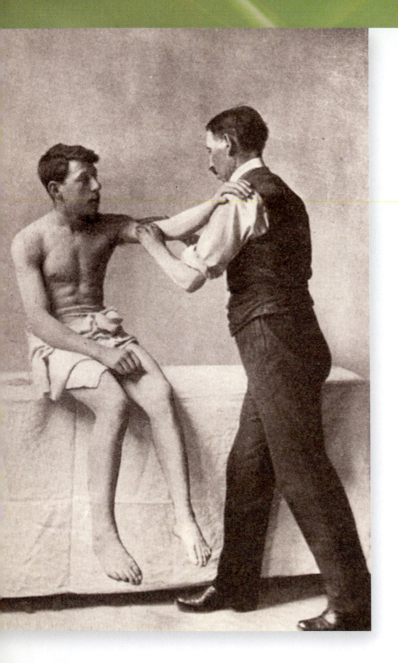

CHAPTER HIGHLIGHTS

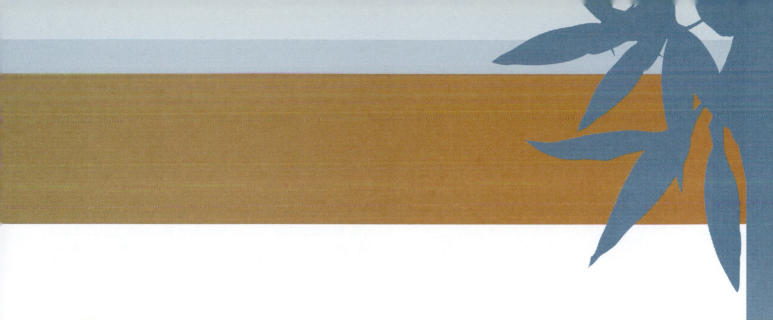

LEARNING OUTCOMES

After studying this chapter, you will have information to:

1. Trace the history of massage related to personal care services.

2. Describe the use of massage for athletes from ancient times to the present.

3. Explain how massage has been used over the centuries in Western medicine.

4. Identify aspects of today's massage therapy that can be traced to the natural healing philosophy.

5. Name important figures in the history of massage and describe their contributions.

6. Discuss factors leading to the revival of massage as a popular health practice in the 1970s.

7. Describe important developments in the massage profession in recent decades.

KEY TERMS

Aleiptes *31*

Ammashi *28*

Bath attendant *30*

Health service operator *33*

Massage operator *31*

Masseurs/Masseuses *31*

Medical gymnast *36*

Rubbers *31*

Sobardoras *33*

Trained masseuses *35*

MASSAGE *in* ACTION

On your DVD, explore the history of:

- Personal Care
- Sports and Fitness
- Health Care
- Natural Healing
- Massage Therapy 1970–1980s

HISTORY OF A VOCATION

The term *vocation* means the work a person has chosen to do for his or her livelihood, especially one for which the individual has talent or is drawn to. It comes from the Latin *vocare,* to call, and refers to the concept of having "a calling" to a particular type of work. Over the centuries, many have been called or have chosen to be massage practitioners.

Like other vocations, massage therapy has its own history. Massage practitioners of the past include servants and slaves, tribal and village healers, rubbers and masseurs, doctors and nurses, medical gymnasts, natural healers, Swedish masseuses, and 1960s hippies. Today's massage therapists are the latest in the line of countless massage practitioners that have gone before. Each generation received knowledge and skills from its predecessors and shaped the future for those who followed.

The history of massage as a vocation looks at several different aspects of the work, for example, who went into the occupation, how they were trained, what types of skills and knowledge they had, their work conditions, and their status in society. This history describes differences in various times and locations, how situations changed over the years, and what factors influenced the work of massage practitioners. It offers a better understanding of today's environment and the outlook for massage therapists in the future.

There are four major branches of the history of massage as a vocation. They roughly parallel today's work settings: personal grooming and rejuvenation, sports and fitness, health care, and natural healing. A few examples from this vast history offer an appreciation for the experiences of massage practitioners in the past.

PERSONAL GROOMING AND REJUVENATION

Massage has been part of personal care from time immemorial. As people groomed themselves by bathing, cleaning and cutting their hair, and trimming their nails, the pleasurable and rejuvenating effects of rubbing their skin were obvious. People in dry climates learned to rub vegetable and mineral oil on their skin to keep it moistened and healthy. This practice would have been natural for mothers caring for infants and children, those caring for the frail and elderly, and people grooming themselves and family members.

In ancient civilizations, it was often slaves or domestic servants who provided personal care services, including massage, in the private sphere or home. These servants had low social status, were uneducated, and learned their skills from family members or others performing massage.

In ancient Greece, friction and rubbing with oil was a daily practice. The ancient historian, Plutarch, reports that Alexander the Great (356–323 BCE) traveled with a personal attendant who rubbed him and prepared his bath. Other nobles of that time also "used fragrant ointment when they went to their inunction [application of skin moisturizer] and bath, and they carried about with them rubbers (triptai), and chamberlains" (Johnson 1866, pp. 4–5).

In ancient India, royalty and nonroyalty alike enjoyed a similar practice. The Greek geographer Strabo (63 BCE– 24 CE) described how Indian royalty rubbed their skin with staves or flat sticks, "and they polished their bodies smooth by ebony staves." He also mentions that the king received foreign ambassadors while being rubbed, and "there are four rubbers standing by."

In the 1800s, the British used the English word *shampooing* to describe massage practices seen in India, China, and the Middle East. The word is thought by some to come from the Sanskrit word transliterated as *tshampua* meaning body manipulation. Shampooing was a full-body experience that often involved a hot, soapy bath, followed by a form of bodywork involving percussion and friction massage, joint cracking, and applying scented oils or perfume. It was said to give "ineffable happiness and energy" and that "the Indian ladies seldom pass a day without being thus shampooed by their slaves" (Taylor 1900, p. 40).

In China in the 1800s, barbers set up shop in markets and parks offering grooming services and a type of bodywork (Figure 2.1■). Patrons sat on stools while the barbers cut hair, shaved or trimmed beards, cut nails, cleaned ears, or gave a percussive type of massage. As itinerant tradesmen, these Chinese barbers also were part street performers who played "a thousand tricks to please and amuse their customers, to whom and the surrounding audience they tell their gossiping stories" (M'Lean c.1914).

The blind masseurs or **ammashi** of Japan have their own unique story. In the 1800s, the government of Japan decreed that the occupation of ammashi (amma = traditional Japanese massage; shi = practitioner) be reserved for blind persons as a welfare measure. As a result, government programs for training ammashi were created, and blind amma practitioners were licensed and enjoyed public respect. See Figure 2.2■. These blind ammashi walked the streets announcing their presence: "Formerly they used to blow a small flute as they went about, and people used to call them in as they heard the sounds" (Joya 1958). It is said that at the outbreak of World War II in the 1940s, 90 percent of the ammashi in Japan were blind. After the war, blind ammashi were found mainly in rural districts.

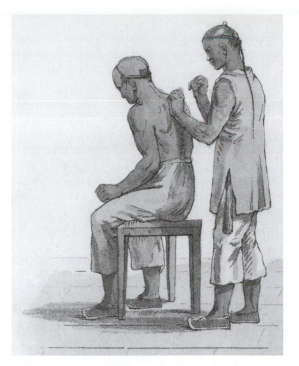

FIGURE 2.1

Chinese barber performing a form of percussion on a seated patron in China in the 1790s.

From *Picturesque Representations of the Dress and Manners of the Chinese* by Thomas M'Lean, published in 1814.

Public Baths

Public bathhouses are community centers for personal hygiene, grooming services, pleasure and rejuvenation, and social interaction. They are found all over the world. In the past, they were sometimes operated by the government, as in ancient Rome, but most were commercial bathhouses. Today, massage continues to be an integral part of the public bath tradition in its latest form, day and destination spas.

Ancient Greece and Rome, ancient China and Japan, Medieval Europe, and the Middle East all had public baths.

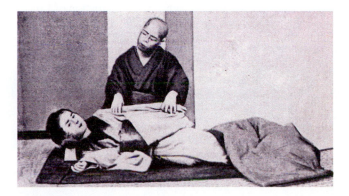

FIGURE 2.2

Blind Japanese masseur or ammashi, c.1880.

(From *The Art of Massage* by Kellogg 1895.)

In times and places where individual homes did not have indoor plumbing, public baths provided bathing and grooming facilities and services, as well as community gathering places.

The Roman bath is the prototype public bath in Western civilization. These bathhouses provided by the state were built all over the Roman Empire, which extended from Asia Minor in the East to the British Isles in the west (27 BCE–476 CE). In addition to exercise courts, warm rooms (tepidarium), steam rooms (caldarium), and a cold pool (frigidarium), there were spaces for bodywork. The massage providers would have been slaves or servants to individuals, or possibly slaves or employees of the state that operated the bath.

After the fall of the Roman Empire, public baths remained popular in Medieval Europe until the sixteenth century when the spread of communicable diseases and promiscuous behavior made common bathing undesirable. A woodcut from the sixteenth century shows a person receiving a back rub in the corner of a public bath (Haggard 1932). See Figure 2.3■.

The Turkish bath, also called a *hammam,* based on the Roman prototype, became popular in the Middle East and reached Europe in the 1800s. After bathing, and perhaps a haircut and a shave, patrons received a vigorous type of bodywork from a practitioner called a *telltack.* It involved gripping and pressing the muscles, stretching, and cracking the joints (Johnson 1866). The telltack would have learned his trade

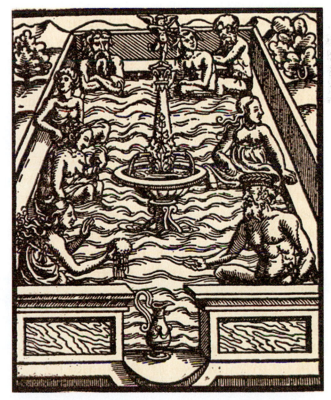

FIGURE 2.3

Massage at medieval public bath, sixteenth century.

(From *The Lame, the Halt, and the Blind* by Haggard 1932.)

by informal apprenticeship and was unlikely to have had anything other than a practical knowledge of human anatomy learned on the job. The Turkish bath was popular in the cities of Europe and North America through the first half of the twentieth century and is still found in the Middle East.

The Chinese bathhouse tradition appears very similar in nature to those found elsewhere. An example can be seen in a Chinese film called *Shower* in English. The film is set in a late twentieth-century Chinese bathhouse that is slated to be torn down to make way for modern buildings. Local men come to the bathhouse to take hot baths and showers, sleep on cots, listen to music, get their hair and nails trimmed, gossip, play board games, hold cricket fights, and drink tea—the Chinese version of the Turkish bath. The bathhouse owner serves as bath attendant and massage practitioner. A brief massage scene shows a patron lying on a bench and the bathhouse owner applying percussion techniques such as slapping and cupping with open hands. A little later he resets a patron's shoulder that had gone out of joint (Zhang 2000).

The occupational designation of **bath attendant** stems from ancient traditions of servants or attendants giving a rubdown, or rubbing in scented oils, after a bath. This low-skilled friction and rubbing hardly equates with the more highly skilled massage that evolved for health and healing. Nevertheless, bath attendants were misleadingly equated with massage therapists in government occupational codes until the 1980s. Bath attendants at a late nineteenth-century European spa are shown in Figure 2.4■.

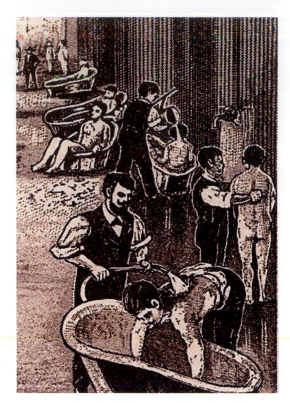

FIGURE 2.4

Bath attendants, c.1890.

(From *The Natural Method of Healing,* Vol. 2, Bilz Sanitorium in Germany, 1898.)

Salons and Spas

In the early 1900s, women went to salons or parlors for personal care services. *Beauty culture* was the term used for the art and science of grooming women's hair and nails, applying makeup or cosmetics, and other beauty treatments to enhance appearance. Massage for rejuvenation, reducing, and bust development were part of beauty culture in the early twentieth century.

In large urban areas in the United States, upscale salons such as Elizabeth Arden and Helena Rubenstein enjoyed downtown locations, while smaller beauty salons (also known as beauty parlors and beauty shops) dotted local neighborhoods. Specialists in hair, skin, and nail grooming learned their trade in vocational schools and became licensed as beauticians or cosmetologists in most states. In their scope of practice, massage was largely limited to the head, neck and shoulders, hands and arms up to the elbow, and feet and lower leg up to the knee (Livingston and Maroni 1945). These were superficial massage applications done during personal grooming at the salon. The first U.S. licenses for barbers and beauticians appeared around 1900.

Full body massage remained part of the beauty culture scene and was offered in salons for relaxation and rejuvenation. Swedish massage, an amalgamation of Ling's medical gymnastics (or Swedish movement cure) and

PRACTICAL APPLICATION

Find some historical objects or pictures that you could use for decoration or conversation pieces in your future office. Old massage machines, oil and liniment bottles, books, drawings, and photos can spark the interest of people who see them. Having one or more historical objects around can also offer you a special depth of connection to your chosen field.

Mezger's massage, became the signature massage of salons. By the 1930–1940s, colleges of Swedish massage were training **masseurs** (men) and **masseuses** (women) to work in a variety of places, including personal care settings. See Figure 2.5■.

Graduate masseuse or graduate masseur was the title for a practitioner trained in a school, as opposed to someone who learned massage by apprenticeship or on the job, and served as a kind of credential. Careers as graduate masseuses were extolled in college catalogs. Massage students had courses in anatomy and physiology, dietetics, hydrotherapy, light therapy, electrotherapy, and massage (College of Swedish Massage *Catalogue* c.1939).

Swedish masseuses were also trained in *reducing massage,* a form of massage erroneously thought to help women slim down. Swedish masseuses at reducing salons offered reducing massage, as well as nutritional advice, exercise, and steam room and steam cabinets. Many masseuses also taught exercise classes. Breast massage was advertised as developing "firmness and plumpness of the bust" (Benjamin 2001, 2002).

Several well-respected massage programs in the 1930–1940s were correspondence courses. The knowledge base was learned through the mail, followed by a week of more intensive training at the school to learn the physical skills. This arrangement, called distance learning today, was ideal for people who did not live in big cities where schools were readily available. Most people still lived in small towns prior to World War II, and transportation was difficult.

These correspondence courses gave people who did not live in big cities the opportunity to receive massage training.

Massage technician or **massage operator** was considered a good career option in the 1930–1940s for those wanting to develop a private practice—much like today. Although graduate masseurs and masseuses formed professional associations, such as the American Association of Masseurs and Masseuses established in 1943, they did not seek licensing in most states.

Over sixty years later, day spas and full service salons continue to offer personal grooming services, and some modern establishments are incorporating hydrotherapy facilities such as those found in European spas. Swedish massage and other forms of massage therapy continue to be provided in these settings by graduate, and in most states, licensed massage therapists.

SPORTS AND FITNESS

From ancient Greek times, massage has been associated with sports and fitness. The Greek gymnasia were places where freeborn citizens went to train their bodies and minds. Athletes were rubbed with oil by practitioners called **aleiptes,** "whose business it was to anoint the wrestlers before and after they exercised, and took care to keep them sound and in good complexion" (Graham 1902, p. 19). The last part of the gymnasium exercises was called *apotherapeia,* or a routine for recovery. Its purpose was ridding the body of waste products and preventing fatigue. It consisted of bathing, friction, and inunction or applying oil (Graham 1902, p. 28).

Paidotribes in ancient Greece were like the trainers in Western sports many centuries later. They were often former athletes and served in many capacities, including coach, nutritionist, masseur, physiotherapist, and hygienist. Although the paidotribes were self-taught or trained by apprenticeship, they would have been exposed to theories about diet, exercise, muscle physiology, and therapies of Greek medicine (Johnson 1866).

Rubbers and Athletic Masseurs

When amateur sports gained popularity in the eighteenth to nineteenth centuries, the rubdown after a bath was a mainstay of the care of athletes. It consisted of rubbing and friction of the limbs. It was performed by the trainers themselves, but also by specialists called **rubbers.** Rubbers were unschooled massage practitioners who might have been athletes themselves who had a knack for rubbing. They learned their skills on the job or from other rubbers. When describing the treatment for sore shins, trainer and early Olympic track coach Michael Murphy noted, "If the runner has the services of a trainer and rubber he will be properly cared for" (1914, p. 161).

As in the Greek gymnasium, athletic facilities such as the YMCA and sports centers also had pools, showers, and

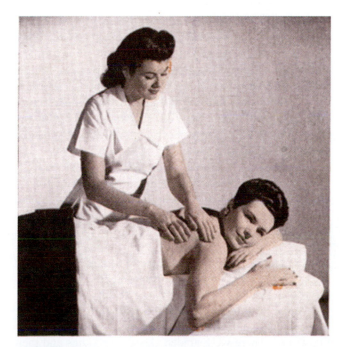

FIGURE 2.5

Swedish masseuse, c.1925.

(From *The College of Swedish Massage Catalogue,* Chicago, 1939.)

steam rooms. The bath attendant was a familiar figure there who might also be skilled in a rubdown-style massage. In 1902, a trainer named Pollard commented that "in all cases vigorous rubbing should follow the use of water; a bath attendant who knows something about massage is invaluable, for how to rub down a man or a horse is an art" (p. 21).

Early twentieth-century trainers were multitalented and helped athletes with sports skills, conditioning, motivation, and injury rehabilitation. Many had been athletes themselves, and were drawn to training, or had "good hands" and became masseurs. In professional sports such as boxing, and club sports like track and field, athletic masseurs were either self-taught or apprenticed. Their knowledge of anatomy consisted of what they learned around the gym. A trainer-masseur from the early 1900s named Harry Andrews is shown in Figure 2.6■.

The specialty of massage for athletes became more sophisticated in the mid-twentieth century. Although many trainers had learned through experience on the athletic field, others were starting to be trained in colleges and universities. The term *athletic masseur* was used to indicate a higher level of training and knowledge than that of the rubbers of the past.

In the 1930–1940s, some athletic masseurs were graduates of colleges of Swedish massage. Working with athletes and professional sports teams was one of the career paths for graduate masseurs. Others were trained in physical education programs in colleges and universities, where they learned basic sciences, musculoskeletal anatomy, kinesiology, sports injuries, and other sport sciences—as well as massage applications for athletes.

This affiliation with physical education departments in colleges eventually led to a separate profession for athletic trainers. The National Athletic Training Association (NATA) was formed in 1950. Athletic trainers soon dropped massage as used in training athletes in the past and patterned their new profession on physical therapy, focusing almost exclusively on injuries.

For about 20 years, the old skills of the athletic masseurs were not available to college and professional athletes in the United States except where the old-school rubbers and athletic masseurs continued their work. This was not the case in many European countries, where the tradition of athletic massage remained strong.

Then in the 1970s in the United States, within the emerging profession of massage therapy, the tradition now called *sports massage* was revived. Athletes who had been turned on to massage as a training aid because of the success of European athletes sought specialists in this old art. The knowledge and skills of massage for athletes had fallen out of the realm of the modern professions of coach and athletic trainer, and so it made sense that massage specialists with an affinity for athletics would respond to the call.

Trained massage therapists, like the graduate masseurs and masseuses before them, already had knowledge of muscular anatomy and physiology, and highly developed hands-on skills. Work with athletes, or sports massage, continues to be a specialty for massage therapists.

Fitness/Health Service Operators and Expert Masseuses

In the first half of the twentieth century, masseurs and masseuses worked in athletic clubs, private gymnasia, and YMCAs providing massage for health and fitness buffs. As early as 1915, a rub down by a bath attendant was an established part of the routine at the YMCA. R. Tait McKenzie described a workout at the Y as a mixture of Swedish and German gymnastics and games, "ending with a bath and a rub down" (1915, p. 170).

Commercial health clubs for office workers and businessmen were popping up in cities across America. A December 1917 advertisement for Postl health club in Chicago featured a photo of 14 trainers and masseurs who have "adequate experience and know the laws of health through long service with us." (See Figure 2.7■.) They promised to give "physical and mental health, strength, and vigor," and "steal your weak stomach and tired nerves, sending you away vibrating with glowing health and ambition."

An ad for Burke's Gymnasium from 1932 boasted "the finest and most completely equipped health institution in San Francisco." There were graded classes for ladies and their children, handball and tennis courts, and acrobatics for girls. The ladies' Turkish bath, with its cabinet baths, blanket sweats, hot room, and steam room, offered a course of baths

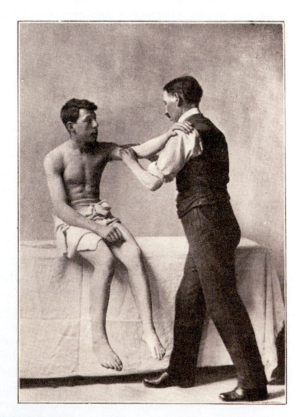

FIGURE 2.6

Athletic masseur, Harry Andrews c.1900.

(From *Massage and Training* by Andrews, 1910.)

FIGURE 2.7

Masseurs and trainers from the Postl heath club in Chicago.

(From a "Physical Training for the Tired Business Man," ad in *Chicago Tribune Pictorial Weekly*, December 9, 1917.)

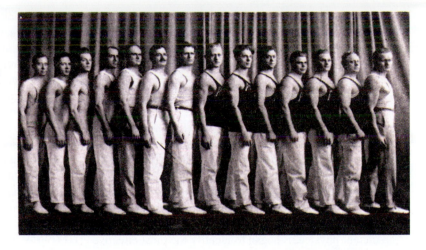

and reducing treatments. It was under the management of "expert masseuses."

By 1943, 274 YMCAs in the United States were operating health service departments that offered massage. The scope and methods of these YMCA massage operators was described by Frierwood in 1953: "The technician uses massage, baths (shower, steam, electricity cabinet), ultraviolet irradiation (artificial and natural sunlight), infrared (heat), instruction in relaxation and in some cases directed exercises. The adult members secure a relief from tensions, gain a sense of well-being, give attention to personal fitness and develop habits designed to build and maintain optimum health and physical efficiency throughout the lifespan" (p. 21).

The **health service operator** was trained in the familiar cluster of natural health and healing methods sometimes called physical therapeutics or physiotherapy. These were massage, hydrotherapy, electrotherapy, light, relaxation techniques, and exercise. The goals however were not medical, but focused on health, fitness, and general well-being.

Health service operators and masseurs were trained in YMCA colleges in physical education departments, as well as in colleges of Swedish massage. The Dayton YMCA in Ohio established a School of Health Service and Massage in 1937. A professional association called the Health Service Operators Society was established in 1942 "to combat the abuses of commercial bathhouses and the unethical conduct of 'cure-all' agents in the health field" (Williams 1943, p. 30). The association was active through the 1950s.

Health clubs today have adopted the YMCA format of exercise, hydrotherapy (steam room, sauna, whirlpool) and massage. It is the same format as the ancient Greek gymnasium.

HEALTH CARE

In its broadest sense, health care encompasses all of the arts and sciences of healing. Rubbing, friction, and pressing of the soft tissues have been a mainstay of health care across time and place. In primitive cultures, massage was performed in the treatment of a variety of ailments by shamans and traditional healers, as well as family members. It was often the domain of women.

Captain James Cook, on an expedition to Tahiti in the 1770s, gives a firsthand account of how the mother and sisters of a native named Tu used massage to treat "rheumatick pain" in his hip and leg. Cook relates, "I was desired to lay down in the midst of them, then as many as could get around me began to squeeze me with both hands from head to foot, but more especially the parts where the pain was, till they made my bones crack and a perfect Mummy of my flesh. . . . I found immediate relief from the operation. They gave me another rubbing down before I went to bed" (Thomas 2003, p. 342). These women were not "professionals" in the sense of having an occupation, but performed massage as part of everyday family care skills.

On the other hand, traditional Hispanic healers called **sobardoras** are trained by apprenticeship to use massage in treating ailments of those in the community who call on their services. They also use ritual, herbal remedies and bone-setting manipulation techniques in their work. Sobardoras are part of the healing tradition of *curanderas,* who combine folk traditions from Spain and Mexico. It is believed that curanderas inherit their power to heal, although an individual may be called to healing and given the *don,* translated as "gift." These traditional healers are professional-like in the sense that they feel called to the work, go through a long apprenticeship, and it becomes their occupation in the community (Perrone, Stockel, and Krueger 1989).

Western Medicine

The history of modern medicine begins in ancient Greece with Hippocrates (450–377 BCE). The writings attributed to Hippocrates began a shift away from magic, ritual, and superstition in healing practices. Hippocratic writings emphasized observation, logic, diagnosis and treatment, and relationship to the patient. The Greek physician observed symptoms, related those symptoms to the internal and external environment, and prescribed therapy in accordance with nature as he understood it.

Physicians trained in the Hippocratic methods were taught rubbing and frictions: "The physician must be experienced in many things, but assuredly also in rubbing; for things that have the same name have not the same effects. For rubbing can bind a joint which is too loose, and loosen a joint that is too rigid. Hard rubbing binds; soft rubbing loosens; much rubbing causes parts to waste; moderate rubbing makes them grow" (Hippocrates, "Peri Arthron" quoted in Graham 1902, p. 21). The implication is that practitioners must be skilled in different rubbing techniques to elicit different effects.

Those in ancient Greece who specialized in rubbing were called *triptai.* Massage and bodywork was called the *anatriptic art.* Anatriptic meant to "rub up" or toward the body's center, presumably when rubbing the arms and legs.

Ancient physicians began to identify the most effective soft tissue technique applications for various conditions. For example, Hippocrates advises "to rub the shoulder gently and smoothly" after resetting a dislocated shoulder. Celsus (25 BCE–50 CE), a Roman physician, said to stroke "the chest with a gentle hand" for a cough, and use "soft and long continued rubbing of the affected part" for a spasm. Galen (130–230 CE) advised physicians to warm the body with moderate rubbing with a linen cloth before applying oil and compressing tissues, and that "one should first rub quietly, and afterwards gradually increasing it, push the strength of the friction so far as evidently to compress the flesh but not to bruise it" (Johnson 1866, pp. 12–19). Obviously, skilled massage applications took more knowledge and skill than mere rubbing.

The more recent tradition called medical rubbing began to emerge in eighteenth to nineteenth century Europe. Douglas Graham's *A Treatise on Massage* (1902) devoted two chapters to the history of massage and names several physicians who used soft tissue manipulation in medical treatments during this and earlier periods. One of these was Dr. J. B. Zabludowski of Berlin, Germany, shown in Figure 2.8■ performing massage of the ankle, c.1910.

Much earlier, in 1780, a well-known French professor of clinical medicine named Simon Andre Tissot, wrote about massage and exercise called *gymnastique medicinale et chirurgicalein.* An English physician named William Balfour published a book on the subject in 1819. Other English physicians of the time, such as the surgeon Mr. Grosvenor of Oxford, developed medical rubbing systems. In 1859, Mr. Beveridge of Edinburgh published a pamphlet called, "The cure of disease by manipulation, commonly called medical rubbing."

But medical rubbing did not catch on at the time in mainstream English medicine, "and from that time to this [1866] rubbing has been left almost wholly in the hands of unprofessional persons . . . some of whom used simple rubbing . . . while others employed various kinds of liniments and ointments" (Johnson 1866, p. 8). By the end of the nineteenth century, the practice of medical rubbing would evolve into a budding profession for trained masseurs and masseuses.

TRAINED MASSEUSES

About a century ago, the word *massage* replaced *medical rubbing* to describe the treatment of illness and injury with soft tissue manipulation. The French had developed soft tissue manipulation skills they called *massage,* and the term was later popularized by Johann Mezger, a physician from Amsterdam. The word *massage* stuck as the generic term for soft tissue manipulation and is used to this day. The terms *massotherapy* and *manual therapeutics,* once used to describe skilled massage, are not used anymore.

Johann Mezger (1838–1909) developed a system of soft tissue manipulation that is the basis for today's traditional Western massage. Using French terminology, Mezger called the work massage, and its practitioners, masseurs and masseuses. He categorized massage techniques as effleurage, petrissage, friction, and tapotement; vibration was added later. The place where massage was given was called a parlor or salon. Mezger's massage became popular throughout Europe and North America.

Although a number of physicians championed massage as a treatment modality, most assigned the actual massage work to assistants. Some training schools for nurses gave general instruction in massage. Graham thought that *manipulators,* or massage practitioners, should have "a natural tact, talent, and liking for massage, with soft elastic, and strong hands and physical endurance sufficient to use them,

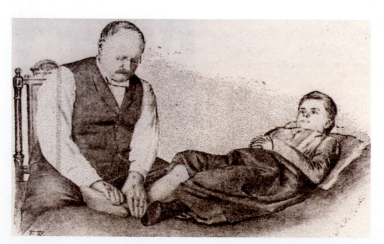

FIGURE 2.8

Dr. J. B. Zabludowski of Berlin, Germany, performs massage of the ankle, c.1910.

(From *Zabludowski's Technik der Massage* by Eiger 1911.)

together with abundance of time, patience, and skill acquired by long and intelligent experience" (1902, p. 52).

That there were many untrained massage practitioners is mentioned in textbooks from the early 1900s. Graham lamented that "it is not to be wondered at that many a shrewd, superannuated auntie, and others who are out of a job, having learned the meaning of the word massage, immediately have it printed on their card and continue their 'rubbin,' just as they have always done" (Graham 1902, pp. 51–52).

On the other hand, **trained masseuses** took courses of study in private schools and hospital programs. *A Manual for Students of Massage* written by Mary Anna Ellison (1909) outlines a typical turn-of-the-century massage curriculum. After an overview of anatomy, topics include massage techniques, how to give a general massage, vibration treatment, Schott treatment for heart disease, treatment for locomotor ataxia, Weir-Mitchell treatment for neurasthenia, and the Swedish system of medical gymnastics, which was considered a specialty.

Trained masseuses were valued by the doctors who employed them. Weir Mitchell, who developed the famous Rest Cure, found many benefits from massage itself and valued observations about his patients by "practiced manipulators." He found that "their daily familiarity with every detail of the color and firmness of the tissues is often of great use to me" (Mitchell 1877).

The level of professionalism expected of trained masseuses is evidenced by the "hints to masseuses" given by Ellison. She admonishes students to cease treatment "if you have real cause for believing that it or your personality is in any way prejudicial," and to concentrate their attention on the patient "having her mind full of healthfulness and hope regarding . . . her work" (p. 138). A list of *don'ts* include "don't discuss the doctor's methods with the patient, and don't mention the names of other patients in conversation" (pp. 143–144). Other hints are listed in Figure 2.9■ and offer good advice 100 years later, particularly Ellison's comment: "One thing I am assured of—that is, the absolute necessity for a masseuse . . . to keep her mind in as well-balanced condition as possible, and during her treatment to concentrate her attention (as fully as circumstances permit) on the patient and her needs, not necessarily speaking much, but having her mind full of healthfulness and hope as regards the ultimate issue of her work. She follows up *mentally,* as it were, the results she is trying to achieve *manually.*" The Society of Trained Masseuses was formed in England in 1894 to raise professional standards for massage specialists working in the medical field.

As mainstream health care developed in the United States through the twentieth century, massage became a minor modality within the scope of other professions such as

FIGURE 2.9

Hints for Masseuses.

(From *A Manual for Students of Massage* by Ellison 1909.)

Hints for Masseuses, c. 1909

- ❧ Don't take a case without medical permission, at least, if not supervision. Fatal results have sometimes followed massage of unsuitable cases.
- ❧ Don't discuss the doctor's methods with the patient, and don't mention the names of other patients in conversation.
- ❧ Don't talk scandal to your patients, and, on the other hand, avoid shop talk.
- ❧ Don't speak as if you were the one competent masseuse to be had.
- ❧ Don't undertake more cases than you have energy and vitality for, or both you and the patients will suffer.
- ❧ Don't accept any stimulants at a patient's house.
- ❧ Don't abuse any confidence reposed in you, or publish abroad private matters that come to your knowledge.
- ❧ Don't continue your attendance a day longer than is necessary, or if you see that massage is not providing beneficial results.
- ❧ Don't forget that you have come on business, and don't give the impression that massage is an act of condescension on your part.
- ❧ Don't neglect to study your patient's individuality, and if you can in any way rest her mind as well as her body, do so.
- ❧ Don't give the servants more trouble than you can help, whilst maintaining your position with dignity.
- ❧ Don't allow a patient to experience the discomfort of feeling your breath.
- ❧ Don't wear rings or bracelets.
- ❧ Don't sweep the patient's skin with your sleeve or any part of your dress.

CRITICAL THINKING

Analyze the "Hints to Masseuses" made in 1909 by Mary Anna Ellison listed in Figure 2.9.

1. What do the hints reveal about masseuses of one hundred years ago?

2. Which ones are still applicable today?
3. What do they tell you about the historical development of ethics for massage therapists?

nursing and physical therapy. The occupation of masseuse and masseur never rose to the level of a separate profession within institutionalized medicine. Massage specialists were relegated to natural healing settings and deemed "alternative." That is why although massage therapy has a long tradition as a healing agent, massage is considered an alternative therapy in today's health care system.

MEDICAL GYMNASTS

A separate but related tradition of bodywork was known variously as medical gymnastics, mechanotherapy, and physical therapeutics. This was the curing of diseases through movement, that is, active and passive exercises. Although the Swede, Pehr Henrik Ling (1776–1839) is perhaps the most famous individual who developed a system of medical gymnastics, others preceded him. In the sixteenth century, Mercurialis wrote "De Arte Gymnastica" or the science of bodily exercise, including movements for the cure of diseases. An English physician, Thomas Fuller, published "Medicina Gymnastica" in 1704, and a French physician, Clement Tissot, wrote "Gymnastique Medicinale" in 1781.

Ling's system was comprehensive and included educational gymnastics for building strong healthy bodies, military gymnastics for hand-to-hand and small weapons combat, and medical gymnastics for treating diseases. Ling based his exercises on knowledge of anatomy and physiology as he understood them and so is credited with putting the practice on a rational or scientific basis. Physical educators, physical therapists, and massage therapists all consider Ling a "father" of their profession.

The Swedish system of medical gymnastics was considered an alternative therapy. While allopathic medicine relied on drugs and surgery as its major modalities, Ling's system was an alternative for treating a variety of chronic diseases from asthma to spinal curvature to headaches. In its heyday, before strict medical licensing, movement cure practitioners were considered primary health care providers and accepted patients for diagnosis and treatment (Roth 1851). Many were also MDs, but there were many lay practitioners too.

One of Ling's greatest contributions was the development of **medical gymnast** as an occupation. Whereas others wrote books and taught individual students, Ling founded a school

that gained international fame and trained thousands of practitioners from all over the world in his system. His school, the Royal Gymnastic Central Institute, was established in 1813 in Stockholm. It was open to men and women, and the curriculum included anatomy, physiology, pathology, hygiene, diagnosis, principles of the movement treatment, and the use of exercises for general and local development (Nissen 1920).

Graduates of Ling's program, and spin-off programs in the United States and Europe, found employment as physical education teachers in the schools (educational gymnastics), and as medical gymnasts at Swedish movement cure institutions. In places such as the Swedish Cure Institute in New York, founded by Dr. George Taylor, medical gymnasts led patients through active movements and applied passive movements or soft tissue manipulations. Medical gymnasts assisting a patient through a movement prescription are shown in Figure 2.10■.

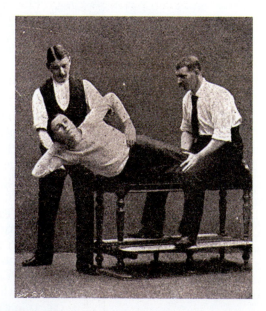

FIGURE 2.10

Medical gymnasts assist patient in performing movements, 1909.

(From *Handbook of Medical and Orthopedic Gymnastics* by Wide 1909.)

By the late nineteenth century, medical gymnasts adopted Mezger's system of massage as a compliment to Ling's system. Eventually, Ling's and Mezger's systems of bodywork were so identified together that they became known in the United States as Swedish massage.

Many colleges that adopted the Swedish system for physical education classes also began training physical educators in the tradition of Ling. The location of these training programs within colleges influenced the direction of the development of the athletic training and physical therapy professions.

Physical therapy began to form as a separate profession around World War I when practitioners, called *reconstruction aides,* were trained to help rehabilitate wounded soldiers. Many reconstruction aides were trained in departments of physical education in colleges, where they learned to apply corrective exercise and massage. In fact, up to World War II, a prerequisite for many physical therapy (also called physiotherapy) programs was a degree in physical education. A photograph of a corner of the general massage department of an army hospital in the 1920s shows soldiers receiving massage in chairs as well as on tables (Figure 2.11■).

Physical therapists formed their first professional association in 1921, the American Women's Physical Therapeutic Association. The name was changed in the 1940s to the American Physical Therapy Association. Occupational licensing for physical therapists in the 1940–1950s anchored the profession to mainstream medicine. Today, physical therapists have their own associations and training programs at the bachelor and master degree levels.

The distinction between massage therapists working in medical settings and physical therapy professionals was not crystal clear in the 1940–1950s. Many physical therapists had been initially trained in colleges of Swedish massage where Ling's work was also taught. In fact, the American Association of Masseurs and Masseuses (AAMM), founded in 1943, changed its name to the American Massage & Therapy Association in 1958 to reflect that some of its members identified themselves as massage practitioners and some as physical therapists.

By the 1960s, those who wanted to work in medical settings were grandfathered into physical therapy licenses. The professions of physical therapy and massage therapy were now going their separate ways. As the distinction between the professions became clearer, the "&" was dropped from the AM&TA, and it became the American Massage Therapy Association (AMTA) in 1983.

NATURAL HEALING AND DRUGLESS DOCTORS

The natural healing movement began in the late 1800s. Natural healing practitioners rejected the allopathic methods of drugs and surgery, and instead used natural remedies to treat ailments. They were known as the *drugless doctors.* They relied on medicinal herbs, mineral waters, hydrotherapy, colonic irrigation, therapeutic massage and movement, hypnosis, meditation, and electrotherapy. They promoted healthy practices such as rest, exercise, good nutrition, deep breathing of fresh air, sunbathing, singing, and laughter. Many were vegetarians. They recognized that true health is a matter of body, mind, and spirit.

Fundamental to the natural healing philosophy is a belief in the innate healing power of nature, or "the inherent restorative power for health that resides in every organism" (Erz c.1924). The job of the natural healing practitioner is to facilitate that natural process and avoid "heroic" or intrusive methods. Preventing illness and promoting healthful natural living were also essential to this philosophy. The natural healing movement was a precursor to today's wellness movement and spawned the profession of naturopathic physician.

Naturopaths, the drugless healers, had begun to organize their profession in 1902 with the founding of the Naturopathic Society of America. It was reorganized as the American Naturopathic Association (ANA) in 1919. *The Naturopath,* a magazine focused on the "interests of all schools of drugless healing," and "the Art of Natural Living," also "devotes itself especially to the defense of the individual drugless practitioner persecuted by the Medical and Osteopathic Trust" (advertisement 1925). Today, the profession of naturopathic physician is licensed in 14 of the 50 states in the United States.

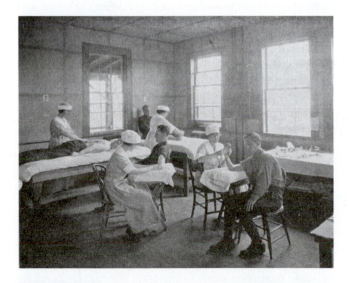

FIGURE 2.11

A corner of the general massage section of an army hospital from Sampson's book, *A Practice of Physiotherapy,* published in 1926.

Massage in the Natural Healing Tradition

Massage and the Swedish movements were important natural healing methods. Dr. P. Puderbach, director of the Brooklyn School for Massage and Physiotherapy and author of *The*

Massage Operator, wrote that massage "has taken its rank as the equal of other sanative [healing] methods, and thus we see in the Massage that is applied correctly by experienced hands, a powerful means for the rejuvenation of mankind, the beautification of the human body, the alleviation of innumerable weaknesses, and the cure of many diseases that have been the curse of humanity (1925, p. 7)."

Dr. Puderbach's school trained massage specialists to work in natural healing environments. Figure 2.12■ shows an operator massaging the shoulders and using a heat lamp or radiant rays. These lamps were used to relax muscles and increase local circulation, "producing the most favorable conditions for effective massage" (Puderbach 1925, p. 7).

Several well-known natural healing centers appeared at the turn of the century in the form of country resorts. Benedict Lust (1872–1945), a German immigrant, was considered a "father" of naturopathy. Lust operated two such places called Yungborn in Butler, New Jersey, and Tangerine, Florida. Yungborn in New Jersey, established in 1896, was billed as the "original nature cure resort and recreation home," and "the parent institution of naturopathy in America." An advertisement for Yungborn lists massage, Swedish movements, and mechanotherapy as some of many treatments available at the nature resort.

Perhaps the most famous natural healing center was the Battle Creek Sanitarium in Michigan run by J. Harvey Kellogg

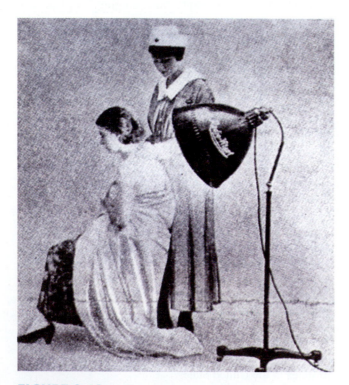

FIGURE 2.12

Masseuse performs massage of the shoulder under heat lamp, c.1925.

(From *The Massage Operator* by Puderbach 1925.)

(1852–1943). Kellogg, who is widely known for Kellogg cereals, had a great interest in health and nutrition and was especially interested in massage. He wrote a classic on the subject titled *The Art of Massage: Its Physiological Effects and Therapeutic Applications* (1895). The manual was intended for medical and nursing students, but also became a standard text for masseurs and masseuses. Kellogg employed 10 to 20 masseurs and masseuses at the "San" at any one time.

Kellogg numbered the descriptions of different massage techniques and applications so that physicians could prescribe the exact methods they wanted the massage practitioner to perform on an individual patient. But the experienced masseur and masseuse were also expected to modify the application for each case and not follow the written prescription "slavishly."

Kellogg makes reference to the work of Ling in the preface to *The Art of Massage* (1895). He states that "it is rare that the most perfect results can be obtained without supplementing the treatment by massage with a judiciously conducted course of gymnastics" (p. v). He suggests that a translation of Ling's work on medical gymnastics "ought to be in the hands of every masseur" (p. vi). So just as medical gymnasts at that time were adopting massage to complement their work, masseurs and masseuses were adopting the Swedish movements as a natural complement to massage.

A popular version of natural healing was promoted by Bernarr Macfadden (1868–1955), which he called *physical culture.* Macfadden opened physical culture resorts, and a Physical Culture Training School in Chicago that graduated "doctors" of hydropathy, kinesitherapy, and physcultopathy. Physcultopathists were essentially medical gymnasts trained in Macfadden's school. This is an early example of an entrepreneurial enterprise in massage therapy (Armstrong and Armstrong 1991).

Today's massage therapy profession is a direct outgrowth of this natural healing tradition. This is evident in the affinity of massage therapists for natural healing methods, in the adoption of the wellness model to define our scope, and in our identity as an alternative or CAM therapy. Issues related to differences in philosophy and the mistrust of mainstream medicine, as well as the push for freedom of choice in medical treatment, stem from this history.

The first convention of the American Association of Masseurs and Masseuses in 1946 included a lecture on zone therapy (i.e., reflexology) by Eunice Ingham, massage and multitherapy by John Granger, an equipment demonstration by a representative of the Therm-Aire Corporation, and a talk on "cradepathy." Their first president, Clark Cottrell, said about this event, "I am sure we are on the right track to the natural methods of healing" (Benjamin 1986).

It is important to understand this connection to the natural healing tradition as the profession of massage therapy interfaces with mainstream medicine in the twenty-first century. This history is especially important to remember as massage therapists work to maintain their integrity while they find their place in integrative medical settings. The fundamental identity of massage therapy as a natural healing agent is a primary strength it brings to integrative health care today.

MASSAGE THERAPY REVIVED IN THE UNITED STATES

The 1950s were a dark time for the massage profession in the United States. Physical therapists and athletic trainers were developing their own professions and were being educated in colleges and universities. Most of the old colleges of Swedish massage were closing. Mainstream America considered natural healing the province of "health nuts" or akin to quackery, and massage was being used blatantly as a cover for prostitution. "Massage parlor" had become permanently associated with houses of ill repute.

During this time, massage was kept alive by natural healers working out of their homes, in private practice, and at places like the YMCAs. Their only organized presence in the 1950s was in the American Massage & Therapy Association, formerly the American Association of Masseurs and Masseuses. In 1958, they had dropped "masseurs and masseuses" in their name partly because those terms were deemed obsolete and in disrepute. The AM&TA had a few hundred members at that time and quietly developed educational standards, a code of ethics, and a credential called the "registered massage therapist." They would later be the locus of the revival of the massage therapy profession in the 1980s.

Beginning in the 1960s and through the 1970s, there were several different happenings in American society that led to the revival of the massage profession. Two related movements based in California that reintroduced massage as a valuable health practice were the Human Potential Movement and the Counterculture Movement. Forms of bodywork that emerged from the Human Potential Movement included Rolfing®, the Trager® approach, and the Feldenkrais Method®. These became trademarked therapies, and practitioners continue to be trained and certified by their organizations.

A simplified form of massage was developed at the Esalen Institute in Big Sur, California. Called Esalen massage, it incorporated simple Western massage techniques and emphasized sensual aspects using scented oils, candle lighting, incense, and "new age" music. Draping of the body was optional. Its purpose was to help the giver and receiver alike get in touch with their senses. At first, Esalen massage was adopted as a tool for personal growth and learned in meditation and self-improvement centers. It was associated with the "hippie" counterculture.

Some of the hippies who performed Esalen massage recognized its potential for health and healing and wanted to do the work for their livelihood. Some of those joined the natural healers in the AM&TA, giving the organization and the profession an influx of people and new energy. Mistrust of "establishment" health care, openness to non-Western health and healing practices, ambivalence toward regulation, and awareness of the psychological and spiritual aspects of massage are some of the values that they reinforced in the field.

Other factors that contributed to a revival of massage therapy in the 1970s were an interest in Eastern philosophies and health practices, particularly from India, China, and Japan. Yogis founded ashrams in the United States that promoted ancient Indian health practices such as meditation, deep breathing, vegetarianism, and massage. Trade with China was reopened in the 1970s, leading to exchange of information about medical practices such as acupuncture and *tuina*. Shiatsu and amma practitioners from Japan came to the United States and trained people in their arts.

A new fitness craze called "aerobics" also emerged in the 1970s. Ordinary people began taking aerobic exercise classes and jogging and running in local fun runs and marathons. And the success of European athletes revived an interest in sports massage in the United States for massage for athletes. The wellness movement gained ground in the field of health and physical education. It urged people to take responsibility for their own well-being and emphasized a holistic approach for body, mind, and spirit.

REALITY CHECK

BARBARA

SHANNON: A newspaper article I read a few days ago featured a local spa and called the massage therapist working there a "masseuse." I know the writer had good intentions since he talked about the benefits of massage, but calling her a masseuse sounded like she worked in a red light district. Don't people know the difference?

BARBARA: Masseuse is just an old term used decades ago to describe women who did Swedish massage. Some people haven't caught up with changing times, and still call massage therapists "masseuses." And they confuse "masseuse" with "masseur" which is even worse. "Masseur" is the correct term for a male. A good approach might be to contact this writer and politely educate him about how using the term "masseuse" effects massage therapists negatively by its current association with prostitution, and that the correct term today is "massage therapist" for both men and women. We can be proud of our heritage as masseurs and masseuses, but still ask others to use the more correct name today.

All these factors led to consumer demand for massage therapy and to the establishment of vocational schools to train massage practitioners. New schools of massage based on the holistic and wellness perspective appeared in the early 1980s. The ranks of massage therapists and bodyworkers swelled, as did membership in professional organizations.

MASSAGE THERAPISTS AND BODYWORKERS

In the 1970s, massage therapy was largely unregulated, entrepreneurial, and alternative. Only a few states regulated massage in the 1970s, notably Ohio, Oregon, Washington, Florida, and North Dakota.

Many who became massage therapists at that time were looking for a second career, an alternative to corporate life, and/or a more holistic approach to health care. Many were escaping what they considered soulless overregulated professions, and were drawn to the independent, nonstandardized field of massage and bodywork.

The term *massage* was still tainted, and so the term *massage therapy* was adopted to distinguish legitimate massage from massage as a cover for prostitution. It was also accepted as the designation of choice for the field as a whole, including traditional Western massage and other forms of manual therapy. Some practitioners who had been trained in distinct forms of manipulation (e.g., Rolfing® and Polarity Therapy), and who did not wish to be associated with massage, coined the term *bodywork* to describe the larger occupational field.

Unlike physical therapists and athletic trainers, practitioners of the manipulative arts are not in agreement on one name for the profession. This ambivalence is seen in the various names of organizations such as the American Massage Therapy Association (AMTA), the Associated Massage Bodywork Professionals (ABMP), and the National Certification Board for Therapeutic Massage and Bodywork (NCBTMB). Most however, use various combinations of *massage* and/or *bodywork* with or without references to therapy. *Somatic therapy* (i.e., body therapy) is a less used term for the field as a whole.

Regardless of what the practitioners were called, more and more consumers were looking for massage and bodywork services. And the benefits of massage touted by practitioners and their organizations were beginning to be accepted by the general public. Graduates of massage programs in the 1980s opened private practices that attracted a diverse population of clients (Figure 2.13■). The momentum for massage that began in the 1970s carried over into the 1980s and beyond to the present time.

Some indication of the growth of the profession can be seen in the steady increase in the number of members in professional organizations. In 1960, the AMTA had 359 mem-

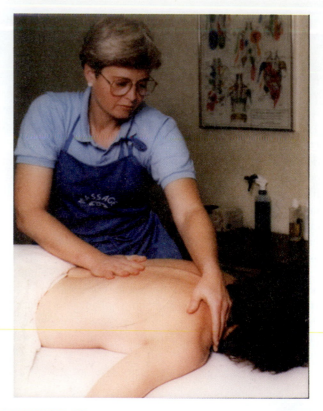

FIGURE 2.13

Massage therapist, c.1985.

(From an ad for Wellspring Massage Therapy in Villa Park, Illinois. Author's private photo collection.)

bers; 1,051 members in 1970; 1,405 in 1980; 3,183 in 1985 (National Historian's Report, 1987). AMTA has grown to over 58,000 members in 2009. AMBP, founded in the 1980s, has over 65,000 members today.

Professional challenges during the 20-year period 1980–2000 ranged from winning the respect of the general public to gaining acceptance as health professionals by the health care community to establishing educational and competency standards. Appropriate dress, draping standards, and the ethics of the therapeutic relationship were hashed out in professional publications and meetings.

Many of the benchmarks of a profession listed in Box 1.1 in Chapter 1, on page 11, have been achieved in the last few decades. The early 1990s were particularly busy with the first National Certification Examination for Therapeutic Massage and Bodywork, the incorporation of the Massage Therapy Foundation, the founding of the Touch Research Institute at the University of Miami, and the establishment of the Office of Alternative Medicine at the U.S. National Institutes of Health. The Commission on Massage Therapy Accreditation (COMTA) received U.S. Department of Education recognition in 2002. The number of states licensing or certifying massage therapists has grown from about six in 1985 to 44 plus the

CASE FOR STUDY

Alex and Researching Historical Background for a Legislative Issue

Alex, a massage therapist, is on the law and legislation committee of a professional organization that is preparing comments on a change in the definitions and scope of practice sections of the massage therapy licensing law. His task is to provide historical background on the issues involved.

Question:

Where would Alex look for relevant historical information that would provide broader understanding of the issues his committee is investigating?

Things to consider:

- History of the passage of the licensing law and amendments made over the years.
- Definitions and scope of practice statements in current and old versions of the licensing law in question, as well as similar laws in other states.

- Identification of issues that have risen over the years related to definition and scope of practice; note individuals and organizations involved.
- Definitions and scope of practice statements in current and old versions of licensing laws for cosmetologists, estheticians, physical therapists, and other relevant occupations.
- Historical relationships among professionals who use massage within their scope, for example, cosmetologists, physical therapists, and athletic trainers; focus on similarities and differences; local issues; and organizations and people involved.
- Advances in the massage therapy profession throughout recent history, including advances in education and research.

Important historical information you have learned about massage laws in your geographic area:

_____

_____

_____

District of Columbia in 2009 with licensing laws working their way through the legislative process in several states today.

Unified Profession

The trend in the early twenty-first century is toward a more unified profession of massage therapy. Although there are notable exceptions, most massage and bodywork practitioners find common ground in entry-level educational standards, licensing requirements, and national certification. They are comfortable with diversity, and just as medical gymnasts of the nineteenth century embraced the new massage treatment, massage therapists today combine different systems of soft tissue manipulation.

Many of the image problems of the past have been resolved with the creation of recognized credentials identifying legitimate massage practitioners and the adoption of codes of ethics. Some states, such as Illinois, prohibit the use of the word *massage* by anyone except licensed massage therapists.

The profession is becoming more standardized as more massage therapists enter the field through educational pro-

grams that meet accreditation and licensing requirements instead of through trademarked systems. Many techniques and approaches that were originally trademarked in the 1970–1980s have been absorbed into massage therapy in generic form. For example, myofascial massage, trigger point therapy, and various styles of shiatsu were originally introduced in trademarked systems, but are now integrated into many basic massage therapy programs.

There has been some discussion of splitting the field into levels or tiers, thereby distinguishing between so-called relaxation massage and medical massage. The intent of this proposal is to resolve issues related to minimum education standards. Perhaps this is a reflection of the historical tension between medical and natural healing models, and the use of massage for personal care. A better option might be to hold fast to the wellness model and embrace the whole scope of the field as outlined in the Wellness Massage Pyramid. Educational standards could be resolved by adopting entry-level standards for everyone, with additional knowledge and skills needed for those working in specialty areas or specific settings. This is an issue to resolve in the years to come.

CHAPTER HIGHLIGHTS

- Over the centuries, many have been called or have chosen to be massage practitioners; their stories form the history of massage as a vocation.
- The four major branches of this history are (1) massage for personal grooming and rejuvenation, (2) sports and fitness, (3) health care, and (4) natural healing.
- In ancient civilizations, domestic servants and slaves performed many personal care services, including helping with bathing, rubdowns, and applying scented oils.
- In China in the 1800s, street barbers performed a type of seated massage, and in Japan at the same time, blind masseurs called ammashi traveled the streets blowing a flute to attract customers.
- Massage has been available in public bathhouses all over the world. The occupational designation of bath attendant stems from this ancient tradition.
- In the early 1900s, massage was part of personal care services called beauty culture.
  - A limited use of superficial massage continues in the scope of practice of barbers and cosmetologists, who began to be licensed around 1900.
  - Full body massage for rejuvenation and reducing and breast massage were performed by Swedish masseuses in the 1920–1940s in beauty culture settings.
  - Practitioners trained in schools were called graduate masseuses and masseurs.
- Massage for athletes has a long tradition.
  - Massage with oil by aleiptes and paidotribes was part of the routine at the ancient Greek gymnasium.
  - Bath attendants and rubbers provided massage to amateur athletes in the eighteenth to nineteenth centuries in Europe and North America.
  - In the twentieth century, athletic masseurs were trained in schools.
  - By 1950, athletic trainers had developed their own profession specializing in sports injuries, and athletic massage in America largely died out.
  - Sports massage was revived in the United States in the 1970s within the growing profession of massage therapy.
- In the early twentieth century, masseurs and masseuses provided massage in health clubs in American cities.
  - Health service operators and masseurs offered massage and related services in YMCAs.
  - The Health Service Operators Society was established in 1942.
- Massage has been used for healing from time immemorial by families and tribal and community healers.
  - At the beginning of Western medicine, massage was used by Greek and Roman physicians.
- Some European physicians of the eighteenth to nineteenth centuries utilized soft tissue manipulation in medical treatment.
  - American physicians of the early twentieth century prescribed Mezger's massage to be performed on patients by assistants.
  - The occupation of trained masseuse was formed as a greater level of skill and professionalism was required to work with patients.
- Practitioners of Ling's system of medical gymnastics applied active and passive movements to treat various chronic diseases.
  - Ling founded a school in Stockholm, Sweden, in 1813 to train educational and medical gymnasts.
  - Medical gymnasts, also known as movement cure practitioners, were alternative medical providers in the late nineteenth century. They eventually adopted Mezger's massage into their work, which then became known in America as Swedish massage.
- By the 1950s, a separate profession of physical therapy was formed for physiotherapists working in mainstream medical settings.
  - The American Women's Physical Therapeutic Association was founded in 1921.
  - Swedish massage practitioners working within a natural healing framework founded the American Association of Masseurs and Masseuses in 1943, changed to the American Massage & Therapy Association in 1958, and known as the American Massage Therapy Association today.
- Massage was an important part of natural healing systems of the late nineteenth and early twentieth centuries.
  - Naturopaths, or drugless healers, began to organize their profession in 1902 with the founding of the Naturopathic Society of America.
  - Massage operators were trained in schools to work in natural healing resorts.
  - In 1895, Kellogg wrote *The Art of Massage,* which became a classic massage textbook.
  - A popular version of natural healing called physical culture, with practitioners called physcultopathists, was promoted by Bernarr Macfadden.
- Today's massage therapists are part of the natural healing tradition as evidenced in their attraction to natural healing methods, adoption of the wellness model, identity as a CAM profession, mistrust of mainstream medicine, and champions of choice in medical treatment.
- An understanding of the tradition of massage within natural healing is important to massage therapists as they find their places today in integrative medical settings.

- The use of massage in the United States declined in the 1950s. It was revived in the 1970s through a variety of factors, including the Human Potential Movement and counterculture, which spawned Esalen massage, general interest in Asian health practices, a physical fitness movement, and the use of massage by elite athletes.
- An increased number of people seeking massage therapy, and the founding of new massage training

schools, helped increase the number of massage practitioners in the 1980s.
  - The 1980–1990s were a period of growth and the professionalizing of massage therapy.
- In the early twenty-first century, massage therapy has become a more unified profession comfortable with diversity in approaches and moving toward generally recognized standards.

EXAM REVIEW

Key Terms

Match the following key terms to their descriptions. For additional study, look up the key terms in the Interactive Glossary on page G-1 and note other terms that compare or contrast with them.

_____ 1. Aleiptes
_____ 2. Ammashi
_____ 3. Bath attendant
_____ 4. Health service operator
_____ 5. Massage operator
_____ 6. Masseurs/Masseuses
_____ 7. Medical gymnast
_____ 8. Rubbers
_____ 9. Sobardoras
_____ 10. Trained masseuses

a. Specialists who rubbed and frictioned athletes in the early twentieth century
b. Terms for male and female massage therapists in the mid-twentieth century
c. Traditional Hispanic healers trained to use massage for treating ailments of those in their communities
d. Those who rubbed athletes with oil in ancient Greek gymnasia
e. Women massage therapists who studied in private schools and hospital programs in the early part of the twentieth century
f. Blind masseurs of Japan
g. Term for massage therapist in the natural healing tradition in the 1920s
h. Occupation stemming from the ancient traditions of servants or attendants giving a rubdown, or rubbing in scented oils, after a bath.
i. Worked in YMCAs in the early twentieth century offering physical therapeutics or physiotherapy and focused on health, fitness, and general well-being
j. Practitioners trained in the system of bodywork developed by Pehr Henrik Ling of Sweden in the nineteenth century.

Memory Workout

To test your memory of the main concepts in this chapter, complete the following sentences by circling the most correct answer from the two choices provided.

1. The four major branches of the history of massage as a vocation roughly parallel today's (approaches to bodywork) (work settings).

2. A British delegation to China in the 1790s described street (barbers) (performers), who offered grooming services, including a form of seated bodywork.
3. (Deaf) (Blind) masseurs of Japan walked the streets announcing their presence by playing a small flute.
4. The occupational designation of (rubbers) (bath attendant) stems from ancient traditions of servants or

other assistants giving a rubdown, or rubbing scented oils into the skin after a bath.

5. As early as 1915, (a rubdown) (medical rubbing) by a bath attendant was an established part of the routine at the YMCA.

6. Traditional Hispanic healers called (sobardoras) (curanderas), specialize in massage to treat a variety of ailments.

7. In the eighteenth century, the general name for soft tissue manipulation as used in medical settings was (medical rubbing) (medical massage).

8. The Society of Trained Masseuses was formed in (United States) (England) in (1894) (1943) to raise professional standards for massage specialists working in the medical field.

9. In the 1950s, massage was being used as a cover for prostitution in the United States, and the term massage (parlor) (establishment) had become permanently associated with houses of ill repute.

10. In the 1970s, a movement in the field of health and physical education encouraged people to take responsibility for their own well-being and emphasized a holistic approach to health. This was known as the (human potential) (wellness) movement.

Test Prep

The following multiple-choice questions will help to prepare you for future school and professional exams.

1. In ancient civilizations, who typically provided personal care services like grooming and bathing in the home?
   a. Well-paid employees
   b. A class of priests and priestesses
   c. Slaves and domestic servants
   d. Older family members

2. The name used by the British to describe a practice from India that involved a hot soapy bath, followed by a form of bodywork involving percussion and friction massage, joint cracking, and applying scented oils or perfume is:
   a. Anatriptic art
   b. Shampooing
   c. Padshah's bath
   d. Ammashi

3. The prototype public bath in Western civilization and forerunner of today's day spa is the:
   a. Greek gymnasium
   b. Roman bath
   c. Mineral bath
   d. Beauty salon

4. Women massage practitioners working in beauty and reducing salons in the early 1900s were typically called:
   a. Manipulators
   b. Health service operators
   c. Swedish masseurs
   d. Swedish masseuses

5. In the 1940s, massage practitioners who worked with athletes and who were well trained in the massage field were typically called:
   a. Athletic masseurs
   b. Paidotribes
   c. Rubbers
   d. Bath attendants

6. In the United States in the late 1800s, Ling's medical gymnastics used to treat chronic diseases was known as:
   a. Physical culture
   b. Mechno-manipulation
   c. Swedish massage
   d. Swedish movement cure

7. The person who developed a system of soft tissue manipulation in the 1800s that is the basis for today's traditional Western massage is:
   a. Pehr H. Ling of Sweden
   b. Johann Mezger of Amsterdam
   c. J. Harvey Kellogg of United States
   d. Douglas Graham of the United States

8. In the United States in the 1970s, a simplified form of massage was developed in California that incorporated simple western massage techniques and emphasized sensual aspects using scented oils, candle lighting, incense, and "new age" music. It was called:
   a. Swedish massage
   b. Esalen massage
   c. Shampooing
   d. Anatriptic art

Video Challenge

Watch the appropriate segment of the video on your DVD and then answer the following questions.

History of Massage as a Vocation

1. Identify the various settings in which massage practitioners of the past worked, giving examples from the video.
2. Describe the dress of massage practitioners of the past as shown in the video. Explain how their dress, even though outdated today, shows a sense of professionalism.
3. Look closely at the photos of massage shown in the video. Do you notice anything that would probably be done differently today, for example, draping or techniques? Is there anything that would be done exactly the same today?

Comprehension Exercises

The following short answer questions test your knowledge and understanding of chapter topics and provide practice in written communication skills. Explain in two to four complete sentences.

1. Name the four branches of the history of massage as a vocation. Give examples of settings today that correspond to these historical branches.
2. Briefly trace the history of sports massage, and identify the names used over the centuries for massage practitioners specializing in working with athletes.
3. What do the terms *massage parlor* and *masseuse* mean in the context of the history of massage?

For Greater Understanding

The following exercises are designed to take you from the realm of theory into the real world. They will help give you a deeper understanding of the subjects covered in this chapter. Action words are underlined to emphasize the variety of activities presented to address different learning styles and to encourage deeper thinking.

1. <u>Imagine</u> that you are walking around a village in ancient China, and <u>describe</u> the different forms of massage and bodywork that you might see there. <u>Repeat</u> for the cities and towns of ancient Rome, Medieval Europe, 1880 Europe, and then 1920, 1950, and 1990 United States. <u>Note</u> that at any one time and place, massage and bodywork can be found in a number of settings and performed by practitioners with different backgrounds.
2. <u>Visit</u> a day or destination spa, and <u>note</u> the services on the menu. <u>Receive a massage</u> or other spa services if possible. <u>Compare and contrast</u> your experience to bath houses and natural healing resorts of the past. <u>Report</u> your findings to the class.
3. <u>Locate</u> a historical facility in your community where massage has been available for a long time or was offered in the past (e.g., old YMCA, Turkish bath, athletic club, beauty salon, resort, mineral spring spa). <u>Look</u> for an ad for the facility from the past, especially one that mentions massage. <u>Share</u> your discovery with the class. (Variation: <u>Report</u> on a place you visited on vacation that had historical connections to massage.)

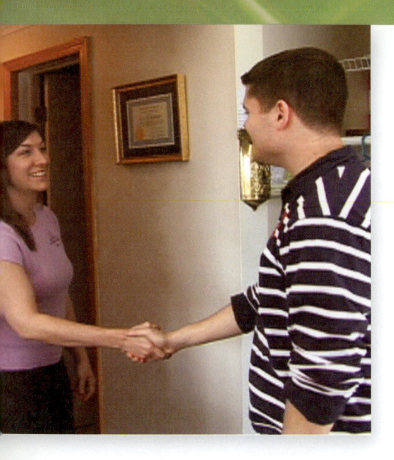

CHAPTER

3 Professional and Personal Development

CHAPTER OUTLINE

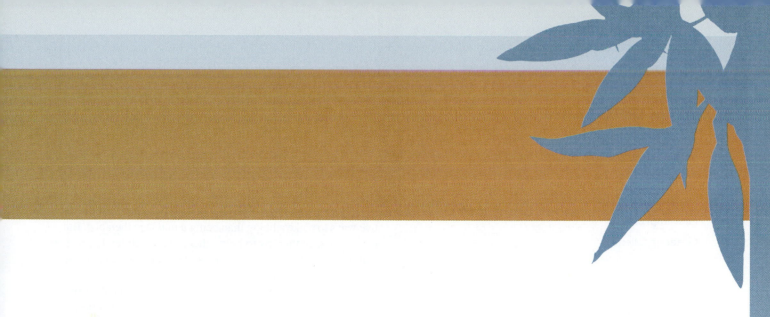

LEARNING OUTCOMES

After studying this chapter, you will have information to:

1. Describe the importance of personal growth for professional development.
2. Understand *service* as an important value for massage therapists.
3. Develop a strong work ethic.
4. Look and behave professionally.
5. Develop intellectual skills and concentration.
6. Develop greater emotional intelligence.
7. Use basic courtesy and good manners.
8. Communicate well and be a good listener.
9. Resolve conflicts peacefully and positively.
10. Present yourself to the public with confidence.

KEY TERMS

Body language *62*

Compassion *57*

Concentration *54*

Conflict resolution *60*

Critical thinking *53*

Emotional intelligence *56*

Ethics *52*

Intellectual skills *53*

Intuition *55*

Listening *64*

Problem solving *54*

Professional boundaries *51*

Professional image *49*

Service *48*

Social skills *58*

Work ethic *48*

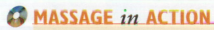

MASSAGE *in* ACTION

On your DVD, explore:

- Professional Dress, Posture, and Speech
- Image Detractors
- Professional Boundaries
- Emotional Intelligence
- First Impressions
- Greeting Clients

PROFESSIONALISM IN MASSAGE THERAPY

Becoming a successful massage therapist is a journey of transformation. Part of that journey is learning to be a professional. What is professionalism? It is more than knowing the Latin names of muscles and bones and performing massage techniques skillfully.

> Professionalism is a state of mind, a way of "being," "knowing," and "doing" that sets you apart from others. It gives you direction to how you look, behave, think, and act. It brings together who you are as a person, what you value, how you treat other people, what you contribute in the workplace, and how seriously you take your job. . . . To *be* a professional, you must *feel like* a professional. (Makely 2005, pp. xiv–xv)

Feeling like a professional comes from the inside, but it manifests in the image you present by your appearance and behavior. Likewise, by presenting a professional image, you cultivate feeling like a professional. When you finally become a professional, the inside and outside are totally in sync, and your professional presence is genuine.

Attitude is the sum of how a person presents him- or herself to the world—a way of acting, thinking, and feeling. To have a professional attitude is to embody all that it means to be a professional.

Becoming a professional massage therapist inevitably involves change and personal growth. Some of the key growth areas are dedication to service, developing a strong work ethic, establishing a professional image, cultivating intellectual skills, improving concentration, developing intuition, and nurturing emotional intelligence. Social and communications skills are essential to a massage therapist.

Service

The essence of the massage therapy profession is serving others. Dedication to **service** means that we hold clients' well-being above our own desire for money, power, and worldly recognition. It means that the primary motivation for being massage therapists is to help people achieve their personal wellness goals.

Dedication to service helps keep priorities in order. It focuses attention on the well-being of our clients rather than on us. It guides our way and offers a higher and more satisfying motivation than merely making money. It spurs us to being the best that we can be. It provides a moral compass for ethical decision making.

There are much easier, more prestigious, and more lucrative ways to make a living than being a massage therapist. But using massage therapy to help others live healthier, happier, and more stress-free lives provides great satisfaction to those who chose this work.

Many start on the road to becoming a massage therapist for other reasons. But those who stay and find satisfaction in their work realize that the ultimate motivation is to be of service to those who come to us for massage.

Work Ethic

A strong work ethic provides a firm foundation for all other aspects of professionalism. **Work ethic** is described as "positioning your job as a high priority in your life and making sound decisions about how you approach your work" (Makely 2005, p. 5). It means taking your work seriously, staying focused, and applying yourself to doing a good job.

A strong work ethic is reflected in good attendance and punctuality, reliability and accountability, positive attitude and enthusiasm, and taking responsibility for doing the highest quality work of which you are capable. It starts when you are a student and carries on into your professional life. It is a trait that employers value highly and an essential characteristic for success in private practice.

Good attendance means showing up when expected or when scheduled, and punctuality means showing up on time. Punctuality also entails getting to school or work early enough that you are settled in and ready to go when the class starts or when the client arrives. Running in late or at the last minute prevents you from preparing, centering, and focusing yourself. It shows disrespect for your classmates, teachers, and clients.

Reliability is a related trait that means people can depend on you to do what you say you are going to do, when you are supposed to do it. If you are reliable, people will have trust and confidence in you. Accountability means that you accept responsibility for your actions, and do not make excuses for repeated mistakes. You apologize sincerely for and correct mistakes that you have made.

A positive attitude and enthusiasm shows in how you speak about your work and the energy you put into it. The word *enthusiasm* comes from the Greek language and means possessed or inspired by the gods. If you have enthusiasm, you exhibit keen interest and eagerness for your work. You value it and look forward to studying, practicing, and learning more about it.

With a strong work ethic, you take responsibility for doing your highest quality work every time. Regardless of

PRACTICAL APPLICATION

Analyze your own work ethic as reflected in your behavior so far in massage school and your attitude toward class work and homework. Concentrate on attendance, punctuality, behavior in class, and getting assignments in on time, as well as good attitude and enthusiasm.

1. Do you see areas for improvement?
2. Can you pick out three things you can start doing today that show a commitment to your massage training and enthusiasm for massage therapy?
3. How will that help you in your career as a massage therapist?

---

whatever else is going on in your life, you strive for quality in your work. You exhibit competence in applying the knowledge and skills of your profession for the good of your clients.

PROFESSIONAL IMAGE

Your appearance reflects your inner state of professionalism. A **professional image** makes a favorable impression on your clients, and identifies you as someone they can have confidence in and trust. Your appearance should be clean, neat, modest, and appropriate for the setting in which you work. Establishing a professional presence involves attention to dress, grooming, posture, and language.

Dress

The way you dress sets the tone of your relationship with clients—respectful, nonsexual, and trusting. It also helps set boundaries by saying to the client that this is a professional relationship. Remember that as a professional massage therapist you are not dressing to impress your friends or attract a romantic date (Figure 3.1 ■).

Many massage therapists adopt a uniform look such as loose pants and polo shirt, hospital scrubs, sports clothes, or martial arts outfit. A spa might have a required uniform such as a smock with the company logo. With a little thought and creativity, you can find work clothes that are attractive, practical, and express who you are as a professional.

Some guidelines for professional dress are:

- Have work clothes that are separate from your everyday clothes.
- Choose clothes that are conservative and modest.
- Choose clothes that can be cleaned easily.
- Wear clothes that allow the freedom of movement you need for your work.
- Wear clothes appropriate for your work setting and in compliance with your employer's dress code.
- Wear closed-toed shoes, or other coverings that enclose the feet (e.g., socks with sandals).
- Keep clothes clean, neat, and odor-free.

Some generally accepted *don'ts* for professional dress are:

- Don't wear tops that show cleavage or breast tissue (e.g., low-cut tops or sleeveless shirts with large armholes).
- Don't wear tops with large or long sleeves that may touch the client.
- Don't wear pants that are tight or provocative (e.g., show the navel).
- Don't wear short shorts or short skirts.
- Don't wear denim jeans, either long or short.
- Don't wear sandals without socks or go barefoot.
- Don't wear T-shirts with advertising or sayings that may be offensive.

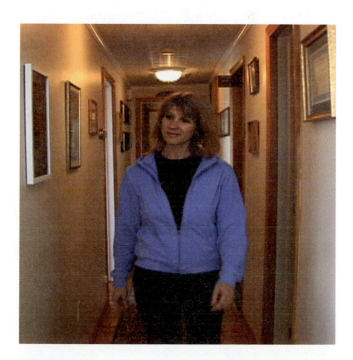

FIGURE 3.1

Your appearance reflects your professionalism.

- Don't wear jewelry that is likely to touch the client, (e.g., dangling necklaces and rings). Rings can also be unsanitary if dirt and skin cells collect around and underneath them.
- Don't wear clothing that suggests a social setting rather than a professional setting.

An employer may have a mandatory dress code. Ask about it in your job interview so you are clear about what is expected. Most dress codes identify acceptable and unacceptable attire and indicate whether a uniform is required. They specify rules about jewelry and body decoration such as tattoos and body piercings.

Grooming

Grooming is an important part of appearance that includes nails, hair, and skin. Your hands, the instruments of massage, should receive special attention. Keep fingernails clean and short, that is, below the line of the fingertips. If you hold up the palm of your hand and look at the fingers, the fingernails should not be visible. Keep cuticles neat and trimmed.

Rough spots on the hands can be softened and cracks prevented with the application of healing lotions and creams. Since you will be washing your hands frequently, it is important to use soap with lotion added and to dry your hands thoroughly to prevent chapping. Chapped hands with cracked skin provide an entry point for germs and can feel rough on the client's body.

Use face makeup conservatively. Applying makeup to enhance appearance in a professional setting is appropriate. Being "made-up" to make a trendy statement or as you might for a date or social event is not appropriate.

Body piercing and tattoos may be all right if within the norms acceptable to your employer and clients. Cover any tattoo that you think might be offensive to clients. Consider removing potentially offensive tattoos that you might have had done before your professional life as a massage therapist.

Wash your hair regularly using unscented or lightly scented products. Adopt a hairstyle that prevents the hair from falling forward when bent over or from touching the client in any way. Men with facial hair should keep it clean and trimmed.

Body odor can be a problem in a profession such as massage that involves physical activity and close contact with clients. Always use an underarm deodorant. Those who do not shave under the arms should be aware that hair retains sweat, and that unpleasant odor develops faster there than on shaved areas. If necessary, wash under the arms during the day, and change your shirt after a few massage sessions.

Breath odor is another potential trouble spot. If you like to eat spicy foods or smoke, adopt strategies to eliminate the resulting odor. Breath mints can be effective for normal instances of "stale breath." Smokers must also consider the smell of smoke on their hands, clothes, and hair. Nonsmokers are more sensitive to cigarette and cigar smoke, so they can often smell odors that smokers cannot. Remember that when working around your client's head and face, he or she will be very aware of the smell of your hands. Here is a summary of guidelines for good grooming:

- Keep nails trimmed and manicured below the tips of the fingers; avoid nail polish.
- Keep hair clean and in a style that prevents it from touching the client.
- Keep skin on hands healthy and soft.
- Take precautions to prevent offensive body odor.
- Take precautions to prevent offensive breath odor.
- Keep areas around body piercing jewelry clean.

Posture

Good posture is not only healthy, it also enhances your professional presence. Keep your back and neck in good alignment, head up, and muscles relaxed. Good posture should feel balanced and uplifting. Avoid slouching, leaning, tilting, and other poor postural habits. By correcting poor postural habits, you set a good example for clients. Chapter 12, Body Mechanics, Table Skills, and Application

CRITICAL THINKING

Visit three different places where massage therapists work, and evaluate the level of professionalism you see there.

1. Report your findings to the class or study group, noting specific details of dress, grooming, posture, speech, and image detractors on which you base your evaluation.

2. Compare what you see in different settings, and notice whether there is more than one way to look and be professional.

3. Determine which elements you find essential to presenting a professional image and those that are a matter of choice.

Guidelines, on page 366 outlines the elements of good sitting and standing posture in greater detail.

Image Detractors

Needless to say, annoying habits detract from a professional image. Nervous habits such as finger tapping, nail biting, knuckle cracking, leg bouncing, and hair twirling are best left to private moments. Other detractors include noisy jewelry, chewing gum, smoking, eating, or drinking in a client's presence.

PROFESSIONAL BOUNDARIES

Boundaries communicate limits or borders that define personal and professional space. They are the fences we place around ourselves to preserve our integrity as individuals. Good boundaries allow two individuals to meet with integrity and without violation of the other's space, but close enough to make connection.

Professional boundaries clarify the nature of the therapeutic relationship and help us to differentiate the roles of massage therapist and client. Such boundaries communicate to the client that the relationship is professional, not personal, and define ethical behavior for both parties. It is the responsibility of massage therapists to establish and maintain professional boundaries in their practices through their communications with clients.

> Boundaries are the heart of how we protect ourselves and our clients. A boundary is like a protective circle drawn around ourselves and our clients; it defines what goes on within that circle and the ways practitioners will and will not treat each other. (McIntosh 1999, p. 25)

There are five types of boundaries according to Benjamin and Sohnen-Moe (2003): (1) physical, (2) emotional, (3) intellectual, (4) sexual, and (5) energetic. Setting appropriate professional boundaries in these five areas is a matter of ethics as well as social propriety.

How far we sit or stand from each other sets physical boundaries for personal space. Invading people's space by getting too close to them can make them nervous and uncomfortable. Clothes also serve as physical boundaries, as does draping during a massage session. Physical boundaries limit where and when it is appropriate to touch a client and vice versa. Leaving the room when clients are dressing and undressing gives them personal space and preserves their boundaries.

The physical space for massage, that is, office and massage room, should be free of personal property such as family photos or collections of objects. If practicing in a home, segregate the reception area, bathroom, and massage room from personal and family space as much as possible, especially from bedrooms.

Emotional boundaries limit disclosure about feelings. Since massage therapists are not professionals in psychology, too much emotional disclosure on the client's part may cross the line of a massage therapist's scope of practice. Emotional disclosure by the massage therapist may turn the tables in the therapeutic relationship by seeming to call for help from the client.

Intellectual boundaries demand respect for other people's beliefs and restrict forcing our beliefs and opinions on others. For example, some massage therapists who are health conscious may try to indoctrinate their clients regarding their eating habits, for example about their belief in vegetarianism. This is not only an intellectual boundary violation, but also a scope-of-practice problem.

Sexual boundaries in a professional relationship are absolute. They protect both massage therapists and clients. Sexual boundary violations by massage therapists are unethical and illegal.

Energetic boundaries are less obvious; for example, not letting a client's bad mood or "negative energy" affect your state of being. Clients who seek massage are frequently stressed out and carry a lot of nervous energy. Helping clients disperse this energy without permeating the massage therapist's boundaries is an important self-care consideration.

Professional boundaries are also defined by routine office procedures and policies. These include policies for clients arriving late for sessions, not showing up for appointments, standards of hygiene, and payment due dates. Communicating policies clearly reduces misunderstanding and increases satisfaction when expectations are met.

Keeping good professional boundaries is a key factor in maintaining ethical massage therapy practices. Common boundary violations are discussed further on page 103 in Chapter 5, Ethics and the Therapeutic Relationship.

ETHICS FOR THE MASSAGE STUDENT

Ethics is the study of the nature of moral behavior, of right and wrong. It examines choices for behavior and uses a decision-making process to determine the degree of morality of certain actions.

Ethics have a positive aspect related to *what to do,* and a negative aspect related to *what not to do.* Common values upon which ethical choices are made include honesty, integrity, compassion, quality care, respect for persons, privacy and confidentiality, abiding by law, keeping professional ethical standards, and doing no harm.

Professional ethics looks at common ethical situations that arise within a specific occupation such as massage therapy. Codes of ethical behavior and standards of practice are developed by professional associations as the collective standard for the profession. Chapter 5, Ethics and the Therapeutic Relationship, on page 92 is devoted to ethics for massage therapists. In addition, Chapter 23, Business Ethics, on page 648

CRITICAL THINKING

We have many professional relationships in our lives, for example, doctors, dentists, lawyers, teachers, school administrators, and more. We also have relationships with service providers such as hairstylists, personal trainers, and car mechanics.

Choose one such person in your life and analyze your relationship with him or her. Write a short essay answering the following questions:

1. What is your role and the other person's role in the relationship?
2. What boundaries can you identify in the relationship?
3. How were those boundaries established? Are they implicit or explicit?
4. How do the established boundaries enhance the relationship? Do you think there are adequate boundaries, or would you feel more comfortable if the boundaries were clearer?

Now, consider your relationship with practice clients. Write out a plan for establishing professional boundaries with them. Include physical, emotional, intellectual, sexual, and energetic boundaries. Continue your essay by answering the following questions:

1. What professional boundaries will you establish as a student of massage with your practice clients?
2. What are some polite but clear methods you can employ to communicate those boundaries effectively?
3. Explain why such boundaries are important to practice now while you are still in training to be a massage therapist.

discusses ethical behavior in the operation of a massage therapy practice.

Massage therapy students have their own unique circumstances that require ethical consideration. Some are the same for all students, but others are unique to massage therapy students. The standards for massage students listed below are a good a start to learning professional ethics as graduate massage therapists.

Standards for massage students include:

Professionalism

1. Dress professionally for school.
2. Practice good hygiene.
3. Bring equipment and supplies needed for class.
4. Avoid offensive language and behavior with classmates.
5. Come to class on time and sober.

Class Work

6. Meet or exceed attendance requirements.
7. Put your best efforts into class, homework, and tests.
8. Devote adequate time to study and practice.
9. Present your own work in class, homework, and on tests (do not plagiarize or cheat).

Relationship with Classmates

10. Respect all classmates regardless of gender, ethnic background, religious tradition, sexual orientation, disability, or other distinguishing characteristic.
11. Respect the powerful effects of a relationship based on touch.

12. Refrain from a sexual relationship with a classmate until after graduation.
13. Take precautions to prevent the spread of disease in school.
14. Keep personal information about classmates confidential.
15. Practice informed consent with classmates.

Professional Boundaries

16. Change clothes modestly during hands-on classes.
17. Practice proper draping in class.
18. Keep good professional boundaries when practicing on family and friends.
19. Never engage in sexual behavior in the context of practicing massage therapy.

Relationship with the School

20. Treat your teachers and school administrators with respect.
21. Abide by school policies.
22. Represent your school professionally at public events.
23. Take care of school equipment and use it safely.

INTELLECTUAL SKILLS

Massage therapy is performed with the head, heart, and hands. **Intellectual skills,** or thinking skills, play an important part in being a professional massage therapist. From learning about the human body to planning massage sessions to making ethical decisions, the ability to use your head is essential.

Intellectual or cognitive skills can be thought of as having six levels (Bloom 1956). The first level is *knowledge* of terms, concepts, principles, facts, and methods. At this level the massage therapist can recall or remember things such as the names of bones or different massage techniques. The second level is *comprehension,* in which he or she can reorganize, paraphrase, or explain the material beyond mere recall. For example, the therapist can describe in his or her own words how a synovial joint works, or why a specific massage technique has a certain effect.

The third level is *application,* in which knowledge is used in real-life situations. For example, when giving a massage for stress reduction, the massage therapist uses principles learned previously, such as using long flowing strokes and avoiding stimulating techniques such as tapotement. The fourth level is *analysis,* or breaking down a communication or situation into its parts and identifying specific elements, relationships among parts, patterns, and overall organization. Analysis is an important skill in assessing a problem a client is having or in considering an ethical question.

The fifth level is *synthesis* or putting together the pieces to create a whole, or arrive at a solution. For example, after an analysis of a problem presented by a client, a massage therapist takes all that he or she knows about massage therapy and creates a session plan to achieve certain goals. The sixth level is *evaluation,* for example, judging to what extent a certain massage application was successful in achieving session goals. These last three levels (analysis, synthesis, and evaluation) are the foundations of goal-oriented session planning explained in Chapter 10, Goal-Oriented Planning and Documentation, on page 314. The six levels of intellectual skills are summarized in Table 3.1■.

Higher Level Thinking

There will be many situations in your career that call for higher level thinking. Two types of higher level thinking useful to massage therapists are critical thinking and problem solving, as well as related applications such as planning sessions for clients and making ethical choices. Higher level thinking involves all six levels of intellectual skills described earlier.

CRITICAL THINKING

Critical thinking helps you get at the truth and avoid being deceived. A childhood learning specialist noted that "Noncritical thinkers accept far too much at face value. They may be more concrete and have trouble looking beneath the surface, analyzing and evaluating that which is more than meets the eye" (Levine 2002, p. 203). Noncritical thinkers tend to be naïve and gullible. Levine cautions though about going too far and becoming cynical, doubting everything and trusting nothing. Asking pertinent questions to discover the truth is a sign of healthy skepticism.

Critical thinking weighs reasons to believe against reasons to doubt. It looks for objective evidence, confirmation of claims, errors, distortions, false information, and exaggerations. It looks beneath the surface for authenticity and honesty. It takes into consideration the thinker's own prejudices and beliefs, which is an exercise in self-reflection.

Critical thinking is bolstered by communicating the thought process to another person. In explaining their thinking, people clarify their ideas and test their logic and conclusions. Listening to others can add information, opinions, and provide valuable insights from another perspective.

An example of critical thinking about a product being sold involves a series of questions:

- What are the claims about this product?
- Is there any objective evidence for the claims?
- How good is that evidence?
- Who is presenting the claims, and do they have a personal stake (e.g., monetary interest) in the situation?
- What do others say about this product?
- What is the basis for their thinking?
- Have I used the product, and do the claims ring true given my experience?
- Is there anything that might influence my perception of the product; for example, knowledge of similar products or attractive packaging?
- Do I have likes or dislikes, prejudices or beliefs that might influence my evaluation?
- What is the level of risk involved in believing or not believing the claims?
- If I buy the product, how will I benefit from it, and do I really need it?

TABLE 3.1	Six Levels of Intellectual Skills	
Level	Intellectual Skill	Description
1	Knowledge	Recall or remember terms, concepts, principles, facts, and methods.
2	Comprehension	Reorganize, paraphrase, or explain the material beyond mere recall.
3	Application	Use information in real-life situations.
4	Analysis	Break down a communication or situation into its parts, and identify specific elements, relationships among parts, patterns, and overall organization.
5	Synthesis	Put together the pieces to create a whole, or a solution.
6	Evaluation	Form a judgment; determine the worth, value, or quality.

Critical thinking is important to massage therapists in situations such as spending money on equipment and supplies and deciding whether to believe a claim made for massage or other healing practice. It is useful in choosing continuing education in a particular form of massage therapy and for evaluating a contract for a business partnership. Important issues in the profession call for critical thinking, such as whether to support a certain provision in a licensing law or a position taken by a professional association. Critical thinking is a good habit for a mature professional.

PROBLEM SOLVING

Problem solving in its various forms is a systematic approach to finding a solution to a problem using critical thinking skills. The starting point for problem solving is some issue, question, or dilemma for which there are response options. Time and effort are taken to gather the information needed to make an informed choice or formulate a solution. Gathering information involves listing the facts, soliciting opinions, understanding the history of the situation, and recalling similar situations. Decisions made in similar circumstances, and their results, are important to note. Information gathered is then analyzed and evaluated, and finally a choice or decision made.

A significant aspect of problem solving is self-reflection as found in critical thinking. Things that may color your thinking, such as fears, prejudices, habits, past experiences, and feelings, are taken into consideration in a conscious way. This is not to negate them, but to put them into the equation with other information. Self-reflection promotes greater objectivity.

Evaluation involves weighing the pros and cons of choices for action, or clarifying the priority of values involved. The conclusion or final choice of action is based on some criteria such as highest values (ethical decisions), legal considerations, good business principles, or meeting client goals (goal-oriented session planning).

Systematic problem solving leads to better decisions because the process helps avoid common pitfalls like jumping to conclusions, narrow thinking, and lack of clarity about reasons for choices. It allows thoughtful consideration of complex situations. Critical thinking and problem-solving skills are summarized in Table 3.2■.

The basic elements of problem solving are found in its specific applications. For example, goal-oriented session planning described in Chapter 10, Goal-Oriented Planning and Documentation, on page 314, and ethical decision making described in Chapter 5, Ethics and the Therapeutic Relationship, on page 97 are variations on the basic process of problem solving.

Concentration

Concentration is the ability to sustain attention on something for a period of time. *Attention span* is the length of time a person can concentrate before becoming distracted. Concentration is a mental skill that can be developed with practice.

The ability to concentrate is important to massage therapists for several reasons. For students, it makes learning easier and attending classes more productive. You can hear what the teacher is saying in class, pay attention to details, and make connections between facts and concepts. You can attain a greater depth of understanding.

Massage therapists are more present while talking to clients and during massage sessions if they focus their attention. An aware client can feel when the massage therapist's mind is wandering, much the same way you can tell if someone in front of you is not listening to what you are saying. A wandering mind interferes with the essential connection or presence with a client.

Details also tend to get lost if the mind is jumping from one thing to another. For example, it takes time to absorb sensations from your hands and interpret them as you perform massage techniques. If your mind is not present, even if your hands are working, a lot of information will be lost.

Letting the mind wander in activities such as daydreaming, ruminating about the past, worrying, or looking forward

TABLE 3.2	Higher Level Thinking Skills Used in Massage Therapy
Critical Thinking	• Process for discovering the truth and avoiding deception. • Weigh reasons to believe against reasons to doubt. • Look for objective evidence, confirmation of claims, errors, distortions, false information, and exaggerations. • Look beneath the surface for authenticity and honesty. • Take into consideration the thinker's own prejudices and beliefs, which is an exercise in self-reflection.
Problem Solving	• Systematic approach to finding a solution to a problem using critical thinking skills. • Starting point is an issue, question, or dilemma for which there are choices for responding. • Information needed to make an informed choice or formulate a solution is gathered. • List the facts, solicit opinions, understand the history of the situation, and recall similar situations. • Information gathered is analyzed and evaluated, and finally a choice or decision is made. • Solution based on some criteria such as highest values (ethical decisions), legal considerations, good business principles, or meeting client goals (goal-oriented session planning).

to a future event is a barrier to good concentration. Being easily distracted by sights and sounds in the environment shortens the attention span. The mind goes off somewhere and is not paying attention to the task at hand.

IMPROVING CONCENTRATION

Concentration can be improved through minimizing attention disruptors, single-tasking, creating a more distraction-free environment, and practicing focusing the mind through meditation techniques.

Stressful situations, lack of sleep, illness, and overuse of stimulants such as caffeine can temporarily disrupt the ability to concentrate. Conversely, relaxation techniques, getting enough sleep, taking care of health problems, and proper nutrition improve the ability to concentrate. Recreation activities and light entertainment can offer a break from work, helping to calm and focus the mind. As mentioned previously, massage itself is known to improve mental alertness and focused attention.

Single-tasking, or doing one thing at a time, is a prerequisite for concentration. Its antithesis, *mult-tasking,* or doing more than one thing at a time, is a modern stress producer. Watching television while trying to study, reading e-mail while on the phone, and planning a grocery list in your mind while doing massage, are examples of multitasking. The quality of one or both activities suffers as a result of split attention. Single-tasking is a practice in concentration.

Simple uncluttered space minimizes visual distracters. Silence, "white noise," or quiet background music also help concentration. Students can cut down distracters by sitting in the front of the classroom and eliminating behavior such as eating and drinking, doodling, and talking during class time. Electronic devices are perhaps the biggest distracters of modern times. During periods of concentration, turn off all electronic appliances such as cell phones, pagers, and personal digital assistants. Being constantly interrupted breaks concentration.

Massage therapists create distraction-free environments for themselves and their clients. Dim lights, soft music, and minimal talking allow concentration on the massage itself. Using meditation to increase your powers of concentration is discussed in Chapter 4, Physical Skills, Fitness, and Self-Care for the Massage Therapist, on page 83.

INTUITION

Intuition is defined as "a direct perception of the truth, independent of any rational process . . . [it] lets us see and respond to our environment without calling rational problem-solving into play. There is an organic knowing at work." Intuition is related to *instinct,* which has been called "the hardware of intuition" (McCormick and McCormick 1997, p. 99). Our instincts help guide us through complex situations without having to stop and think everything through.

Instincts come in handy when we are faced with unfamiliar situations, don't have all the facts, or have to act quickly. "Trust your instincts" is good advice when safety is involved. The terms *common sense* and *horse sense* have this same connotation, (i.e., knowing through an inner voice). Intuition is like a sixth sense. People with developed intuition can sense things, or have hunches about things they cannot fully explain.

Intuition has its place in the practice of massage therapy. Massage therapists who work intuitively are not thinking through every move they make. Their hands "know" where to go and what to do. These are called *intelligent hands,* as if the hands themselves were doing the work disconnected from the brain.

Of course, just because the brain is not consciously thinking doesn't mean it is not involved. All the stored knowledge and experience are available in the brain and working on an unconscious level as skills are performed. If something doesn't seem right according to intuition, the thinking brain becomes engaged to do rational problem solving as the situation requires.

A case can be made for the value of adding intuition to the massage therapist's tool chest of knowledge and skills. Intuition is developed by quieting the mind and letting go of conscious thinking. When a student is first learning massage techniques, he or she thinks about every move, but after a while and with practice, the mind can loosen its grip and intuition be given more rein. Such a massage is felt by the receiver as smooth and effortless.

EMOTIONAL INTELLIGENCE

Emotional intelligence is the "heart" in the familiar triumvirate—head, heart, and hands. Emotional skills work hand-in-hand with intellectual and physical skills for full maturity as a massage therapy professional.

Neuroscientists are exploring the complex connections between the limbic structures of the brain, which are the seat of emotions, and the neocortex, or thinking brain. It turns out that rather than being totally independent, these two "minds" interact continuously. The head and heart work together for best results:

> In a sense we have two brains, two minds—and two different kinds of intelligence: rational and emotional. How we do in life is determined by both. . . . Indeed, intellect cannot work its best without emotional intelligence. . . . The new paradigm urges us to harmonize head and heart. (Goleman 1995, pp. 28–29)

Emotional intelligence is defined in Goleman (1995) by a set of skills related to five domains:

1. Knowing one's emotions
2. Managing emotions
3. Motivating oneself

4. Recognizing emotions in others

5. Handling relationships

Emotional skills are important in laying the foundation for success, for example, maintaining a positive outlook, building healthy relationships with clients, dealing with conflict, and making good decisions. They are essential for success in school and building thriving practices afterwards.

Like mental IQ, everyone is born with brain circuitry that provides a starting point for emotional intelligence. And like thinking skills, emotional skills are first learned in childhood and developed throughout a lifetime.

Self-Awareness

The keystone of emotional intelligence is self-awareness, that is, recognizing a feeling as it happens and its accompanying emotion or impulse to act. Understanding the difference between a feeling and an emotion is a good starting point for self-awareness.

Although these are often equated, there is a subtle difference between *feelings* and *emotions*. The verb *feel* comes from an old English word related to sensation and perception, while *emotion* comes from an old French word related to movement and behavior. "Emotions are the outward expressions we use to either display or disguise an underlying feeling, matching or masking our inner state" (McCormick and McCormick 1997, p. 84). People described as *emotional* freely display their feelings outwardly.

There is no agreement about which emotions are primary. However, some common emotions and their variations can be identified: enjoyment (happiness, joy, amusement, sensual pleasure, satisfaction); love (friendliness, kindness, devotion, adoration, infatuation, selfless love or *agape*); surprise (shock, astonishment, amazement, wonder); anger (outrage, resentment, annoyance, irritability, hatred, violence); sadness (grief, sorrow, loneliness, self-pity, depression); fear (anxiety, nervousness, dread, fright, phobia, panic); disgust (contempt, distain, scorn, aversion, revulsion); shame (guilt, embarrassment, remorse, humiliation, regret, contrition). Figure 3.2■ depicts the broad range of emotions of which humans are capable.

Temperament is a term for a person's basic disposition, or tendency toward certain moods or emotions. Extremes of temperament can be a negative factor in being a massage therapist. For example, being excessively shy or sad can interfere with developing a practice. Being excessively bold can result in poor judgment about behavior toward clients. Recognizing our basic temperament and learning to improve aspects that interfere with our life and work is part of developing emotional intelligence. An added incentive to become more self-aware is that the more we understand ourselves, the more we'll understand and have empathy for clients.

Naming our moods and emotions is an empowering step. Naming requires the ability to pause and look at emotion from the thinking brain. Humans have a unique capability of self-reflection that allows us to look at ourselves with some outside perspective. This provides the separation necessary to recognize the difference between emotions and our reactions to them. Naming emotions lays the foundation for identifying their causes and learning to manage them.

Managing Emotions

Once there is self-awareness, managing emotions becomes possible. Managing emotions involves learning to handle emotions so they are healthy expressions of our feelings and appropriate for the setting. This means recognizing them and responding in ways that benefit self and others. A balance must be struck between suppressing emotions and letting them get out of control.

Two examples of managing emotions related to being a massage therapist are dealing with annoyance with a client and continuing to work while feeling sad about a recent loss. In the first instance, being direct with the client about the cause of annoyance (e.g., habitual lateness) is appropriate, whereas allowing feelings of anger to fester is not. In the second instance, something simple like having fresh flowers in the room may cheer you up, while ruminating about your situation would not help.

A basic aspect of managing emotions is controlling impulses. Emotion is by definition an impulse to action. Being overcome with emotion can short circuit the rational brain, leading to actions regretted later. Anger management

Enjoyment	Love	Compassion	Surprise	Sadness	Fear	Disgust	Shame	Anger
Happiness	Friendliness	Empathy	Shock	Grief	Anxiety	Contempt	Guilt	Outrage
Joy	Kindness	Sympathy	Astonishment	Sorrow	Nervousness	Disdain	Embarrassment	Resentment
Amusement	Devotion	Pity	Amazement	Loneliness	Dread	Scorn	Remorse	Annoyance
Sensual Pleasure	Adoration		Wonder	Self-Pity	Fright	Aversion	Humiliation	Irritability
Satisfaction	Infatuation				Phobia	Revulsion	Regret	Hatred
	Selfless Love				Panic		Contrition	

FIGURE 3.2

The broad range of human emotions.

is an example of learning impulse control. Strategies include walking away, counting to 10, and taking a cooling-off period. Chronic anxiety may be managed by learning relaxation and mind-calming techniques.

Delayed gratification is also possible when a person has impulse control. That means resisting an impulse today for a greater reward at a later date. The ability to delay gratification is a sign of maturity and makes many things possible, such as staying with an exercise routine, studying for classes, saving money for a new massage table, or responding ethically to a client.

Motivating Yourself

Two useful skills for self-motivation are nurturing an optimistic outlook and learning to get into the flow of peak performance. Taking responsibility for cultivating these abilities is part of emotional intelligence.

Optimism is a known contributor to success in school, sports, and even healing. Being optimistic means expecting that things will turn out all right in the end, despite setbacks and difficulties. An optimistic attitude helps a person persevere when the going gets rough. Being pessimistic, or expecting failure, leads to giving up when there are bumps in the road.

Optimism may be part of inborn temperament; however, a positive outlook can be nurtured. It is related to what psychologists call *self-efficacy,* the belief that you have the skills to meet the challenges you will face. A sense of self-efficacy can be nurtured by challenging yourself within your current abilities and building on those abilities by making the challenges progressively more advanced. Once a person knows this principle, he or she can work on developing a sense of self-efficacy, and, therefore, a sense of optimism.

Flow, or being in the *zone,* refers to a state of complete harmony during peak performance. There is a fluidity, sense of ease, and mastery that makes the performance a joyful experience. Performers get lost in the action as they become totally absorbed in what they are doing. Flow is a state that can be accessed. It involves quieting and focusing the mind on the task at hand and experiencing the sheer joy of the activity. It occurs most easily when the activity is challenging, but not too hard. Flow can be experienced in learning something new, practicing a skill, or during a challenge such as a test. Flow is thwarted by worry, boredom, or too much thinking.

Recognizing Emotions in Others

Empathy, or recognizing emotions in others, is an important social skill for massage therapists. It is essential for good communications with clients and developing effective therapeutic relationships. It is the basis for creating rapport and is the root of caring.

The ability to read someone else's emotions is based primarily on nonverbal cues. It means noticing things such as tone of voice, facial expression, and gestures, and then matching emotions accurately to what is observed. Reading emotions can be very subtle, that is, interpreting *how* things are said, not

just the words that are said. For example, a person with empathy can detect underlying sadness, anger, or anxiety in a client's words or actions. Empathy is emotional attunement with clients.

Empathy does not mean taking on someone else's pain as your own. It differs from *sympathy,* which is defined as a relationship in which whatever affects one person correspondingly affects the other, and *pity,* which is feeling sorrow for someone else's misfortune. Sympathy and pity result from a lack of emotional boundaries with others and can lead to burnout for practitioners in the caring professions.

Compassion takes empathy one step further. **Compassion** is the "deep awareness of the suffering of another coupled with the wish to relieve it" (American Heritage Dictionary, 2000). Compassion combines empathy with a dedication to service to others. Compassion within the context of the massage therapy profession means the wish to relieve the suffering of others with the work of our hands.

Handling Relationships

The fifth domain of emotional intelligence is handling interpersonal relationships. The fundamental relationship between a massage therapist and client is called the *therapeutic relationship.* Elements of a healthy therapeutic relationship include clarity about the nature of the relationship, understanding of individual roles within the relationship, and establishing clear boundaries related to roles.

For the massage therapist, it means taking responsibility for the relationship and being honest, trustworthy, and ethical. For the client, it involves confidence in the therapist's abilities, trust and respect for the therapist, and satisfaction with the service provided. The massage therapist takes the lead in resolving conflict, responding to a client's anxiety or anger, and keeping good professional boundaries.

Examples of situations calling for skill in interpersonal relationships include resolving a misunderstanding about a cancellation policy, counseling a client with a body odor problem, or showing concern for a grieving client. Massage therapists might also have to respond to clients who use offensive language, come for massage under the influence of alcohol, or make romantic or sexual advances. The therapeutic relationship is discussed further in Chapter 5, Ethics and the Therapeutic Relationship, on page 100.

SOCIAL SKILLS

Massage therapy practices are built and maintained upon a foundation of good social skills, resulting in successful relationships. These include relationships with clients, other health professionals, and people encountered in a place of employment or while managing a private practice. Massage therapy is a person-to-person profession, and even the most skillful massage techniques cannot make up for poor people skills. Social skills are essential abilities for massage therapists.

Social skills encompass behaviors between people that promote harmony, understanding, and connection, while peacefully solving problems like disagreements, misunderstandings, and reconciliation after harm done. The primary goal of social skills is building good relationships. The social skills described in this chapter are specific to massage therapists and the situations they encounter daily.

Courtesy and Good Manners

Courtesy and good manners are behaviors that are expected in social situations, such as saying "please" and "thank you," listening when someone is speaking to you, and introducing newcomers to a group. Courteous behavior shows respect for others and exhibits thoughtfulness about their feelings, comfort, and safety. It is essential for client satisfaction and good customer service.

The unwritten rules of good manners vary in different societies and in specific situations, and change over time. Today, good manners include turning off audible signals on cell phones and other electronic devices in places where silence is appreciated, such as theaters, classrooms, and massage rooms. Good manners also include not having personal conversations on the phone when clients are present.

Good manners in school show respect for teachers, classmates, and yourself. Disturbing class by talking when the teacher is talking, eating during class, letting a cell phone ring, fidgeting, and leaving a mess where you were working are examples of bad manners in school.

Courteous, respectful language goes along with good manners. Use of offensive slang, crude sayings, and angry or demeaning words are especially out of place in school and professional settings.

While good manners open the door to good professional relationships, bad manners can slam the door shut. People have certain expectations about how they will be treated, and showing disrespect can evoke feelings of anger, disappointment, or annoyance. Having good manners is a sign of emotional intelligence and thoughtfulness.

Because what is considered good manners varies by culture and changes over time, professionals working in diverse environments become very aware of their behavior toward others. Business is particularly sensitive to this as it expands into a global marketplace. Professionals remain aware and flexible, adapting to times and circumstances to support building good relationships.

Courtesy and good manners can become second nature, but awareness and practice are prerequisites. Many of the social and professional skills described in this chapter are considered good manners and are expected of trained professionals.

First Impressions

It is a truism that you only get one chance to make a first impression. When you greet clients, potential employers, and others for the first time, they get an immediate impression of your professionalism.

Whenever we walk into a room, our clothing, manners, and mannerisms are on display. Others assess our self-confidence and our ability to present ourselves based on 60 seconds of information. Each of us has our own signature of professional presence—an indelible statement that we make the instant we show up. (Bixler and Dugan 2001, p. 7)

Because massage therapy is based on touch and close contact, it is especially important to establish good rapport right away, as well as confidence, trust, and a certain comfort level. In addition to projecting a professional image as described earlier in this chapter, the manner of greeting is also part of a first impression.

Greeting a First-Time Client

The elements of greeting a client are to make eye contact, say the person's name, introduce yourself, shake hands, and give further directions. In the therapeutic relationship, the massage therapist is in charge, so it is her or his responsibility to take the initiative in greeting and helping the client feel comfortable.

Ten minutes before a client is expected, check your dress and grooming. Clean and organize your office space to make sure it projects a professional image. Review the available client information. If possible, greet the client in a reception area.

When the client arrives, stand up, make friendly eye contact, and smile. Really look at the person to gauge his or her state of being and comfort level. Does the individual seem happy or sad, in pain, nervous, shy, or tired? Your assessment of the client for planning the massage session starts now. Then say the client's name to continue to make a connection and introduce yourself. Say, for example, "Hello Dennis, my name is Debra and I will be your massage therapist today." You would have learned the client's name from checking the appointment book. Now shake hands, and invite the client to sit down (Figure 3.3■). All this takes place in a matter of seconds.

The handshake is the first time you touch your client so it is especially important in establishing good rapport. Try not to reach over a barrier, like a desk or counter, when you shake hands. Extend your hand to the client first. Meet the client's grip palm to palm with good quality contact as you would during the massage. Squeeze firmly, but not too hard, for about 3 seconds and then release the hand. A general rule is to meet the other person's force, and squeeze more gently if the person is weak or injured.

Avoid the "bone crusher," "limp noodle," and "two-finger wiggle" handshake styles. Variations of the handshake include the "handshake sandwich" with your two hands around the client's one hand, which may be perceived as overpowering or patronizing; and the handshake with the left hand on the other person's forearm or shoulder, which is more intimate. Do not use these variations, or perhaps use them only later in the relationship as a comforting gesture in special circumstances. If a person is missing the right hand, or has a pros-

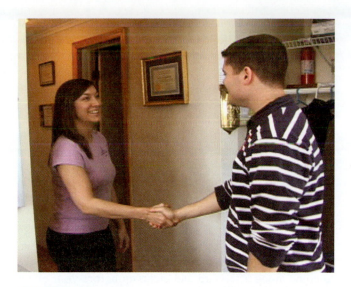

FIGURE 3.3

Greet a first-time client with a firm handshake.

thetic arm, extend your left hand instead. The handshake should not feel rushed, but also should not linger too long, suggesting familiarity.

Hugs are a gesture used frequently in American society and may be appropriate in certain situations. However, when establishing professional boundaries, the handshake is a clearer statement of the business nature of the relationship and is safer for first-time clients. Use your judgment about hugs before or after subsequent appointments. Do not feel that you must hug a client to appear friendly or caring. Hug only if you have clear professional boundaries with a particular client, if you want to express particular affection for some specific reason, if it is acceptable to the client, and if it fits your personality. Remember that hugs may seem invasive to certain clients.

There are cultural differences in what is considered acceptable for greetings. For example, in some Asian and Middle Eastern countries, direct eye contact shows disrespect. Or touching at any time outside of the massage may seem too intimate. These are judgment calls that will become easier with more awareness and experience.

After the handshake, a client needs direction about what to do next. It could be, "please sit down while we go over your goals for the session," or "let's take a moment to go over your health history," or whatever you would like the client to do next. Be clear in your direction when pointing to a chair, or leading the client to the massage room. Clients receiving massage for the first time will need more guidance and assurance.

Introductions

Making introductions is a basic social skill used during the regular business day and at meetings or conferences. Introductions help people feel comfortable and welcome, as well as transmit useful social information. They are an essential networking tool.

The golden rule of introductions is to mention the name of the most honored person first. Other considerations are rank, gender, and age. If people are of equal rank, the woman's name is mentioned first. In a professional practice, the client is always the most honored person, but in other situations, determining the most honored is a judgment call.

The first person's name is followed by a phrase like, "I'd like you to meet [second person's name]," or simply, "This is [second person's name]." If possible, follow up the second person's name with a comment containing information about one or the other person. Ideally the comment would be something to further identify a person, or acknowledge his or her relationship to the situation. Say, for example, "John is a massage therapist at the Marian Hospital Integrative Health Care Center," or "Deidre works with me at the Rejuvenation Spa in Centerville," or "Kristin is going to the workshop on sports massage next month." This opens the door to further conversation and a sense of connection.

Here are some examples of brief introductions:

"Mary, I'd like you to meet Bill. Bill has a massage therapy practice in Milwaukee specializing in orthopedic massage. Mary is in from Minneapolis."

"Dr. Hernandez, this is Jerry Black, a massage therapist. Jerry has a question about a possible contraindication for one of his clients. Would you mind talking to him about it?"

"Dylan Smith, I'd like you to meet Reuben Jones. You two have something in common as fellow reflexologists."

Name tags that are worn prominently and can be read clearly are valuable social devices. Wear yours so that others can readily identify you, call you by name, and introduce you to other people more easily. If you work in a clinic or spa with other employees, a name tag identifies you to clients. Name tags worn at conferences facilitate networking.

There are times when introductions are not necessary. For example, if other massage therapists or clients are in the reception area, you would not ordinarily be expected to introduce everyone to everyone else as you would in a social situation. Your business is with your client, and no other introductions are expected.

Conflict Resolution

Conflicts can arise in any relationship. Conflicts occur when personalities or styles clash, or when people trying to work together have different goals or expectations. Differences of perception, belief, opinion, values, or understanding of facts can cause strife and disharmony. Conflicts often manifest as arguments, disappointment, anger, annoyance, or frustration. They involve two or more people at odds with one another.

Conflict resolution means resolving conflicts amicably and begins with a conscious desire to do so. It involves setting aside competitiveness and the need to win, and focusing on goals rather than obstacles. Five basic approaches to dealing with conflict (Cole 1994) are:

1. *Collaboration*—Taking the time to find a solution together is the way to go when building a long-term

relationship, when goals are too important for compromise, or when you need to work together for the greater good.

2. *Force*—Demanding that your way be followed is only acceptable in an emergency, when the stakes are high and the relationship nonessential, or when a higher principle is at stake and you have the power to enforce your will.

3. *Avoidance*—Not acknowledging a conflict is risky because unresolved conflicts seem to grow worse rather than go away. Avoidance may be all right if it is a temporary situation, and the issue is minor.

4. *Accommodation*—Letting the other person have his or her way is best when keeping harmony in the relationship is most important, when the issue is more important to the other person than to you, when you cannot win, or when you realize that you are wrong.

5. *Compromise*—Both people adjusting their original positions works best when a quick resolution is the goal, when the problem is temporary, or when a complete solution is impossible after much negotiation.

The approach that is most appropriate for a given situation depends on the importance of two factors: (1) Concern for others versus concern for your own needs and desires, and (2) importance of the relationship. Box 3.1● explains when each approach is most appropriate.

Minor conflicts occur all the time in therapeutic relationships with clients. Because the relationship is of such high importance, accommodation and collaboration are the usual modes of resolution, followed in order by compromise, avoidance, and force. Force would rarely be used and only in cases of emergency.

An example of a midlevel conflict is a client who misses an appointment once and does not want to pay the cancellation fee. If keeping the client is important, then accommodation may be the answer; that is, waiving the fee for this time. Avoidance, or not bringing the issue up, is a bad idea since it does not call attention to the policy, and the client may think that it is unimportant. If the client misses again, then the stakes are higher, and you might want to insist on charging the cancellation fee.

Another example is a conflict with a fellow massage therapist who shares a massage room with you at a clinic. She always leaves the massage room messy, and you have to come along afterward and clean up before your client arrives. Given that the relationship and your needs are both important, as well as the principle of the situation, your best choice is an attempt at collaboration. That would involve confronting the other person with the facts as you see them and asking her to be more conscientious about cleaning up. You may be surprised to find out that she thought other workers at the spa or clinic were supposed to clean up, or maybe she has to rush out to another job and forgets about cleaning up. Collaboration involves listening and coming to agreement on a solution.

Major conflicts are uncommon but do happen occasionally. There may also be unethical situations such as a client who wants to date you, or expects treatment outside of your scope of practice, or asks for sexual favors. For this type of conflict, insistence on ethical behavior is the only way to go.

Tips for successful conflict resolution include:

- Being respectful in language and demeanor
- Keeping a positive attitude
- Looking for the win-win situation
- Finding a way for everyone to save face
- Staying open to options
- Being a good listener
- Finding common goals

Resolution barriers are:

- Needing to win
- Taking things personally
- Letting hostility fester
- Giving orders

Phrases such as "you must," "you should," and "you have to" are sure to rankle the other person. Remember that conflicts are inevitable among people working together. Approach conflict resolution as an opportunity to practice your social skills rather than as a chore to be avoided.

BOX 3.1	Choosing the Best Conflict Resolution Approach	
Method of Conflict Resolution	**Relationship Importance**	**Need or Desire to Win**
Collaborate	Very High	Equal
Accommodate	Very High	Low
Compromise	High	Moderate
Avoid	Low	Low
Force	Low	High

Special Situations

When building long-term relationships:	Collaborate
When you need their support to reach goals:	Collaborate
When harmony is more important than the issue:	Accommodate
When you realize you are wrong:	Accommodate
When you cannot win:	Accommodate
When time is short:	Compromise
When an issue has low importance:	Compromise
When the conflict is a one-time thing:	Avoid
When the conflict is trivial:	Avoid
When you need to act fast in an emergency:	Force
When the issue is ethical or legal:	Force

CASE FOR STUDY

Elise and a Conflict in Appointment Times

Elise has a steady client who recently changed jobs and is now on a different schedule. The times he prefers for massage appointments are now outside of Elise's regular hours. She sees clients from 10:00AM–4:00PM on Tuesday–Saturday. Elise would like to keep the client, but needs to resolve this conflict in their schedules.

Question:

Can Elise find a satisfactory appointment time for this steady client?

Things to consider:

- How important is it for Elise to continue with this client?
- How much outside of her regular hours would the new appointment time have to be?
- Does he have time for appointments outside of his "preferred" times?
- How flexible is he willing to be?
- How firm do her work hours need to be?
- Does she have family or other obligations that limit her availability?
- How willing is each person to compromise? Accommodate the other? Collaborate to find a solution?
- Is there a point at which dissolving the relationship is the only option?

Write examples of different scenarios for resolving this conflict.

1. **Accommodation:** _____ _____

2. **Compromise:** _____ _____

3. **Collaboration:** _____ _____

COMMUNICATION SKILLS

Communication skills facilitate information exchange between people, and include verbal (i.e., speech and writing) and nonverbal (i.e., body language and facial expression) methods. Good communication avoids misunderstanding, confusion, and lack of clarity that can produce social friction. Social and communication skills are polished through awareness, learning, experience, and practice.

Verbal Skills

Speech or verbal communication is the primary medium of delivery during telephone calls and for important tasks such as greeting and interviewing clients, explaining policies and procedures, networking with other health professionals, and giving presentations. The delivery of the spoken word in verbal communication can sometimes be more important than the content. It is estimated that in a spoken message, body language accounts for 55 percent of the communication, voice for 38 percent, and the words for 7 percent (Cole 2002).

A good general rule is to speak with moderate speed in a calm, steady, strong voice. Vary the energy, rhythm, and inflection to make the delivery more interesting. Articulate clearly and avoid mumbling. Try to modulate accents unfamiliar to listeners.

Talk more slowly to people who have a different native language than the one you are speaking. Learn a few key words in the language of your regular clients; for example, words for *hello, pressure, pain, turn over,* and *good-bye.* If speaking a language that is not your own, be more conscious of using your voice quality, hand gestures, and body language to clarify your meaning.

When speaking to persons with hearing challenges, face them directly so they can read your lips. Speak slowly with good articulation, but do not exaggerate your words. Turn up the volume on your speech a little, but do not shout, especially to a person wearing a hearing aid. Learn some sign language if you work in a situation where you have regular clients who are hearing impaired.

Voice quality is also important. Lower pitched voices sound more confident and competent. Avoid seeming harsh or being overly loud or soft. Be aware that your tone of voice can type you; for example, a whining, nasal voice sounds like a complainer; a high-pitched, quavering voice sounds nervous; a breathy, slow voice sounds seductive. To add volume and richness to your voice, breathe deeply and relax your neck muscles and vocal cords. Your voice should come from the diaphragm rather than the throat (Cole 2002).

Poor speech habits include using sounds like "uh" as space fillers, constantly clearing the throat, pausing too long between words, and speaking too fast. Ending sentences with a high inflection, as in asking a question, sounds uncertain and unconfident.

Avoid street slang and use good grammar. Call adult females "women" and adult males "men." Do not use terms of familiarity such as "sweetie," "dear," "doll," or "dude" when talking to clients. Also avoid overly formal language and use of technical terms that clients might not understand. It is not appropriate to "show off" by using anatomical terms unfamiliar to the general public. For example, the term *thigh* will do just as well as *femur* in most cases. Using anatomical terms when educating the client about what you are doing is acceptable if done in moderation and the client is able to understand what you are saying.

Speech is a product of experience and habit and can be improved with practice. Become aware of your speech and develop speaking habits that enhance your verbal communications with clients and other social contacts.

TELEPHONE USE

Telephones and answering machines are essential communication tools for massage therapy practices. Clients usually call via telephone for their first appointments, so it is important to have good phone skills. Use the good speech habits as described earlier in this chapter.

Chances are that in private practice, a prospective client's first encounter with you will be via an answering machine. Script your answering machine message to be clear and concise. For example: "Hello. You have reached Green Fields Massage Therapy. I am unable to take your call at this time. Please leave a short message including your name and telephone number, and I will return your call as soon as possible. Please wait for the beep to record your message." Re-record your message until you are satisfied that it sounds open, inviting, and professional.

When answering your telephone, visualize a prospective client at the other end. In other words, be friendly and relaxed (Figure 3.4■). If you feel hurried or stressed, pause and take a deep breath to calm yourself down before you answer. Identify yourself right away. For example: "Hello. This is Thomas Alter of Green Fields Massage Therapy. How may I help you?"

Here are some other tips for telephone use:

- Have a phone line dedicated to your practice.
- Do not make client calls on a cell phone while driving or in public places.
- Do not accept other incoming calls (e.g., call waiting) when on the phone for business.
- Turn off ringers and cell phones when in a massage session.
- Do not interrupt a massage session to answer a phone call.
- Avoid distractions or multitasking while on the phone.
- Smile while on the phone. It can project a friendly impression.

Return calls promptly within 24 hours, if possible. If you will be unavailable to return calls for more than a day, change your message to alert callers when you will return their calls. This shows that you are reachable and reliable.

Body Language

Body language speaks volumes. Your posture, how close you stand to others, hand gestures, eye contact, and facial expression communicate your mood, interest, and even respect for a person you are talking to. As a massage therapist, knowing some of the common meanings of body language can help you project the meaning that you want and also understand others better.

Good upright, aligned posture commands respect and confidence. On the other hand, slouching, tilting, looking around, and a drooping head can communicate disinterest, evasion, or boredom.

The comfortable distance between people who are talking varies somewhat with culture. Be aware of your own comfort level and how it might differ from a client's preferred distance. Moving closer can indicate an interest in the subject, friendliness, or just difficulty hearing. Moving uncomfortably close is a type of physical boundary violation.

REALITY CHECK

MARIA

DAVID: I'm really shy around strangers and don't have a lot of confidence in my social skills. I never seem to know what to say. I'd rather just do the massage and not have to talk to anyone. How can I learn to relate professionally to clients when I don't know where to start?

MARIA: What you say and how you treat clients sets the stage for the massage experience itself. It won't matter how good your massage skills are if you don't have good people skills. Acknowledging your current limitations is a good first step. That's self-awareness. Now try observing people you think have the confidence and social skills you want to develop. What is it exactly that gives them that image? Notice their body language and the actual words that they use. Develop a professional persona in your mind's eye—the person you want to be. Try using that persona when you're in the role of massage therapist—like playing a part in a drama. Ask a friend to role-play meeting new clients with you to practice being your professional self. Remember that you are not being someone different from who you are. You are just being yourself in your new professional role.

FIGURE 3.4

Be friendly and relaxed when talking on the phone to clients.

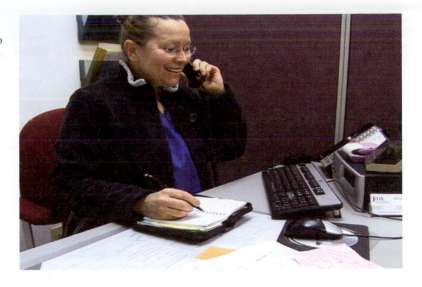

Arms crossed in front convey a sense of protection or distancing, while arms uncrossed and relaxed convey openness. Legs crossed can project the same sense as crossed arms. Hands on the hips signal impatience or anger. Fidgeting or habits such as tapping a pencil or doodling project boredom, nervousness, or distraction.

Hand gestures are particularly communicative. In some cultures people seem to "talk with their hands" as they accentuate the meaning of their words with gestures. Putting a hand over the heart area or placing a hand lightly on another person's arm expresses sympathy and is a way of "reaching out" or making a connection. On the other hand, putting a hand out in front with palm facing the other person implies "stop" or "wait a minute." A common gesture to avoid is finger pointing, which seems accusatory and scolding.

Eye contact is extremely important. Looking at someone when you are speaking or being spoken to makes an essential connection. Knowing when to break eye contact is also important. Staring, looking too intently or too long, can be uncomfortable to a recipient. Break eye contact every so often and then come back. Looking away or around the room when someone is speaking to you is taken as a sign of disrespect or dismissal.

The eyes can also communicate such things as friendliness, concern, annoyance, anger, pleasure, confusion, questioning, flirting, and seduction. Eyes communicate best along with other aspects of facial expression. The massage therapist in Figure 3.5■ displays openness to the client through body language and a friendly smile. Having an expression that is hard to decipher, the so-called "poker face," might be useful in some circumstances, but tends to make people distrustful and uncomfortable.

The smile is perhaps the most universally recognizable sign of friendliness. A warm smile when greeting someone is welcoming. But beware—a genuine smile is hard to fake.

Remember that body language is only one piece of the communication puzzle. It is part of the whole communica-

FIGURE 3.5

Relaxed posture and a friendly smile communicate an open and welcoming attitude toward clients.

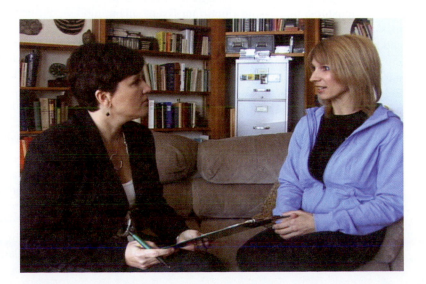

PRACTICAL APPLICATION

Situations in which the words, voice quality, and body language are not in sync can lead to miscommunication. When this happens, one or both parties may feel uncomfortable, misunderstand what is being communicated, or even look for a way to end the conversation. This awkward, out-of-sync interaction is the kind of communication you want to avoid having with your massage clients.

With a study partner, role-play situations in which what is intended to be communicated does not match the voice quality, inflection, or body language used. For example, try greeting a client with arms folded and frowning. Next, try playing a client who claims to feel fine and have no pain, while the body language clearly portrays discomfort, pain, or unease. Then correct the out-of-sync elements to communicate your message clearly. Switch roles with your partner a few times and be creative.

For a variation, try role-playing using different types of eye contact. Include not looking at the other person, staring too long without a break, or looking around the room. Switch roles.

1. What can you learn about a client from voice quality and body language? Can you learn even more than his or her words alone convey?
2. What messages might you inadvertently communicate to a client through your body language? How might you ensure that your communication is clear?
3. What degree of eye contact is the most comfortable? What does your study partner communicate by having little or no eye contact with you when you are conversing?

---

tion package, along with facial expression, voice quality, words, and the general situation. People's personal habits (e.g., they might always fold their arms) must also be taken into consideration. The better you know someone, the easier it is to "read" him or her. Piece all the parts together to understand the full meaning being projected by a person's body language.

Listening

Listening involves taking in and trying to understand what someone else is communicating to you. "I hear you" is a familiar expression that means "I understand (or empathize with) what you just said."

Listening is an essential communication skill for building relationships, discussing important issues, planning massage sessions, solving problems, resolving conflicts, and negotiating contracts. It also plays a big part in learning and critical thinking. Listening allows you to gather information, understand others better, and take in new ideas. Being a good listener begins with the intention to hear what others are really saying and overcoming poor listening habits.

Poor listening habits include letting the mind wander and formulating replies while others are speaking. Other bad habits are interrupting speakers, tuning out different points of view, jumping to conclusions, finishing people's sentences for them, and talking while others are speaking. People also tend to hear what they want to hear and tune out what they don't want to deal with. Do not try to talk over environmental noise such as street sounds or music playing in the background. Background noise interferes with hearing someone else's words.

Really listening involves focusing on what a speaker is saying (the words), feeling, and meaning. Know that people sometimes have trouble expressing in words what they mean. The Chinese character for *listen* consists of four characters: the heart, the mind, the ears, and the eyes (Cole 2002).

When "listening" for feelings, pay attention to how the words are said, that is, inflection and voice quality. Watch body language and facial expressions as well. Listening for feelings is important for developing *empathy,* or recognizing emotions in others, as discussed earlier in this chapter in the section on emotional intelligence.

Listening for the context is also important for understanding what someone is really trying to say. Getting the full picture helps you respond appropriately. Listen for what is not being said, and ask questions to "fill in the blanks." Summarize what you think you heard and check out your accuracy. This is an important interviewing skill, as discussed later in this chapter.

AFFIRMATIVE LISTENING

This type of listening involves letting the speaker know that you are paying attention. This is accomplished by occasional verbal cues and body language. These affirming cues by the listener include nodding, saying "uh-huh" or "I see" or "yes," and repeating a word or key phrase or idea. Body language such as leaning slightly forward toward the speaker and orienting your body to face the speaker also indicates attention. Eye contact, too, is important (Cole 2002).

Affirmative listening allows someone to say all that they have to say without interruption. However, active listening is good for promoting true understanding of someone's ideas and feelings and is an important communication skill for massage therapists.

ACTIVE LISTENING

Active listeners become more engaged in the communication process by reflecting back to the speaker what they think was said. This is not done by parroting the words exactly, but by paraphrasing or restating the words to clarify their meaning. Reflective listening is useful because "by paraphrasing their views, you give talkers a chance to reflect on what they just said, to make sure that's what they mean, maybe even to change what they think or feel after hearing it again" (Booher 1994, p. 151).

These lead-in phrases are useful for active listening:

"You seem to be saying . . ."

"If I understand you correctly, you're saying . . ."

"Let me see if I get where you're coming from. You think that . . ."

"Am I hearing this right? You think . . ."

"Help me sort this out. You feel that . . ."

Notice that some lead-ins refer to the factual meaning of what was said and some are geared toward the feelings behind the words. They are statements, not questions. By paraphrasing, you are neither agreeing nor disagreeing with what was said. You are just checking out the meaning.

Five guidelines for reflective (active) listening are (Cole 1994, p p. 158–159):

1. When several points are made, summarize the one that you want to focus on. This will help you keep the conversation pointed in the direction you want to take.
2. When several emotions are expressed, reflect the final one, as this is usually the most accurate.
3. Keep your reflective listening restatement short in order to keep the focus on the speaker.
4. Only reflect what's there—don't start guessing.
5. Wait out thoughtful silences.

Active listening is useful for drawing out information, understanding new ideas, being clear about statements, and clarifying your understanding. It can also be used in conflict situations to defuse emotion (yours or the speaker's), allow the speaker to express the emotions underlying his or her words, and show empathy. Cole suggests not using reflective listening if you don't like or respect the speaker. This avoids the possibility of unintentionally displaying your negative feelings. Also, do not use reflective listening as a substitute for stating your own thoughts and feelings on a subject.

Presentations

Massage therapists make presentations in a variety of informal and formal ways. One-to-one, informal presentations include explaining policies and procedures to new clients and showing clients self-massage techniques to use at home. More formal presentations may include talking to local community groups about the benefits of massage, or to a governing body in favor of or opposing legislation that affects massage therapists. Explaining, demonstrating, and persuading are useful communication skills in these situations.

Since presentations are essentially teaching opportunities, the audience receiving the presentation can be thought of as a group of learners. Include as many facets of learning as you can, for example, auditory, visual, and kinesthetic elements.

The first rule in making presentations is to know your goals. Why are you making the presentation? What do you expect to gain from it? Second is to know the audience and their expectations. Knowing the audience includes understanding their level of knowledge and experience with what you are presenting. Knowing their expectations helps you plan your presentation to meet their goals as well as yours. Then organize and plan what you want to say.

Explanations are verbal descriptions telling the what, how and/or why of something. For routine tasks such as explaining policies and procedures to new clients, develop a loose script with an opening statement, points to emphasize, and an ending such as "Do you have any questions?" Use props such as a copy of the policies that you can read together. Give yourself a time limit and stick to it.

It might be useful to explain to clients why you are using particular techniques to address their goals for a massage session. For example, you might explain that "Given that our goal today is to reduce your postexercise soreness, I'll be doing a lot more stroking, kneading, and stretching to improve circulation and elongate those tight muscles. I'll be paying more attention to your legs since that's where you're feeling the soreness most." Do not explain more than the client needs to know, and gear the explanation to his or her current knowledge of the human body and experience with massage. Anatomy charts and models are handy props for reinforcing verbal explanations of what is happening in the body during massage.

Demonstrations involve showing an audience how something is done or how something works by actually performing the action while giving a verbal description or explanation. Demonstrations enhance learning by giving the audience the opportunity to watch actions that would take many words to describe. A demonstration is worth ten thousand words. For example, demonstrating self-massage or stretching techniques to clients is more effective than verbal explanations alone. Performing massage techniques while explaining the effects of massage adds a valuable component when making a presentation to a community group or other health professionals.

When doing a demonstration, keep things simple. Avoid the urge to expound on everything you know about a topic, or things that you find interesting. Tell your audience what you will show and why it is important to them, followed by a step-by-step explanation as you perform the actual demonstration. Allow for questions from the audience either during or after the demonstration.

The room setup is particularly important for demonstrations because the audience needs to see what you are doing. Be aware of how far away they are from you and their angle of viewing. For larger groups, having a video camera that can project the demonstration onto a screen is useful.

The art of persuasion comes into play when you are trying to convince an audience to behave a certain way, take a specific course of action, agree on a particular solution to a problem, or accept a certain fact or belief. For example, you might persuade a client to allow you to massage a tight area even though it will be uncomfortable at first, or persuade legislators to vote for a massage licensing bill, or convince an audience that getting massage regularly is a good idea.

The first concern in persuasion is establishing credibility, trust, and confidence in you, the persuader. Informing the audience of your training and experience is useful, as is presenting a confident and professional appearance.

An organized presentation of ideas is next. The four steps in a persuasive presentation (Booher 1994) are:

1. Get the audience's attention.
2. Present the conclusion, action, or decision that you are looking for and its key benefits.
3. Build your case in detail.
4. Call for a specific action or decision.

To build your case, establish a need or goal, and then show how your plan can meet it. Anticipate objections, and answer them in your presentation. Clear thinking is persuasive in itself. Avoid being too pushy or demanding. Invite others to your way of thinking.

A word of caution is in order here. Persuading clients to accept a certain approach to their therapeutic goals or to allow you to perform specific techniques when they would really rather not, is more coercion than persuasion and is considered unethical. In Chapter 5, Ethics and the Therapeutic Relationship, on page 107, the idea of *informed consent* is explained as a way of giving clients choice while presenting your case.

All presentations should end with an opportunity for the audience to ask questions for clarification. For a client, you might say "Was that clear?" "Do you have any questions?" For a formal presentation, you might invite questions during the talk, or leave time for a short question and answer period at the end.

Written Communication

Written communication is a statement of who you are and a reflection of your level of professionalism. There is a greater likelihood that you will be listened to and understood, and your goals achieved, if your written correspondence is well formatted, grammatically correct, neat, and clearly stated.

Memos, e-mails, and business letters are the most common types of written correspondence for massage therapists and demand basic writing skills such as correct spelling, punctuation, and grammar. Simple sentence construction, clear organization of thought, and brevity are hallmarks of good business correspondence.

MEMOS

Memos are informal notes used to communicate information in short form to clients, coworkers, and colleagues. They dispense with some of the formalities of the business letter, but can retain a professional look by being printed on business stationary. All the elements of a memo are important, especially the date, which is often overlooked. The block format makes skimming the memo content easier for the recipient.

Memos are appropriate for short notes, unofficial business, and other informal correspondence. Note that memos are still business correspondence and should project a professional image using professional language. The memo format and an example are found in Figure 3.6■.

E-MAIL

E-mail is essentially an electronic memo. The e-mail format varies with the computer program used, but usually contains all the elements of a standard memo. E-mail is becoming the preferred method of correspondence in both personal and professional settings. Delivery is fast, inexpensive, and e-mail is easy to respond to. However, there are some pitfalls to watch out for when using e-mail for business purposes.

First is your e-mail address. Have separate personal and professional e-mail addresses if possible. Use a professional-sounding address, such as your own formal name or the name of your practice (e.g., jonesmassagetherapy@email.com). Avoid abbreviations and trendy e-mail jargon. Leave out "emoticons" for more professional correspondence, for example, smiley face :) sad face :(or perplexed :/. Remember that using all capital letters is like SHOUTING at the recipient—never do it.

State your message concisely and clearly. People are being overwhelmed by the volume of e-mails they receive, and the messages you send are more likely to be read if they are short. Always put an informative title in the subject line. Use a phone call, paper memo, or letter if the message is

FIGURE 3.6

Memo format and example.

MEMO

Date

To
From
Subject

Main message (1–3 sentences)
Closing (1–2 sentences)

Signature/Initials

Example

MEMO

October 22, 2010

To: Jose Rodriquez
From: Timothy Kim, Massage Therapist
Re: Presentation at Rotary Club Meeting

Hello Jose—This is a note to confirm that I will give a 30-minute presentation on the benefits of massage at the Rotary Club luncheon on November 15, 2007, at 12:00 noon at the Bebop Café in Brenton. I understand that you will have a microphone and overhead projector available for my use.
Thank you again for the invitation to speak to the club.

Jim

---

lengthy. Memos and letters can be faxed if speed of delivery is desirable.

BUSINESS LETTER

Formal business letters are used for official correspondence with government agencies, insurance companies, vendors, employers, and clients. When corresponding for the first time with other health professionals, use the business letter format. They are also preferred for legal matters. The formal business letter format, and the use of official stationary, lends a more serious tone to a document.

Business letters have more identification and introductory information than memos and usually longer paragraphs. There are several different acceptable formats, and it is advisable to choose one to use for your practice and stick to it (Hahn 2003). The basic business letter format in Figure 3.7■ uses a modified block style, that is, aligned with the left-hand margin.

WRITTEN CORRESPONDENCE GUIDELINES

Remember that business correspondence has a different function than social correspondence and is more formal. Some general guidelines for written correspondence related to a massage therapy practice are:

- Choose the appropriate format for the correspondence (memo, e-mail, or letter).
- Use official printed stationary for memos and letters.
- Type business correspondence; memos may be written or printed legibly.
- Use correct grammar, punctuation, and spelling.
- Keep sentences simple and organization logical.
- Use a more formal tone, and avoid slang and jargon.
- Do not put anything in writing that you would not like to see in a court of law.
- Keep a file of all of your written correspondence in chronological order.

Business/Practice Name
Address/P. O. Box
City, State, Zip Code
Phone/E-Mail

Date: Month-Day-Year

Recipient Name
Address/ P. O. Box
City, State, Zip Code

Dear [Title] First name, middle initial, last name:

Introductory paragraph

Middle paragraph

Closing paragraph

Sincerely,

Signature

Printed name, title

Example

Anita Davis, Licensed Massage Therapist
1234 Box Street
Everytown, CA. 44444
(123) 456-7890 / adavis@email.com

June 14, 2010

Mineral Water Spa
567 South Street
Watertown, CA. 44445

Dear Ms. Edie Giacomo:

Thank you for the opportunity of interviewing for the position of full-time massage therapist at the Mineral Water Spa last Wednesday. I enjoyed seeing your facility and meeting other spa staff members. I was impressed by the level of professionalism and care for guests that I saw there.

I have enclosed the additional information you requested. This includes a copy of my license to practice massage therapy, my massage school transcript, and a list of my continuing education for the past five years.

Please let me know if you need anything else for your review of my credentials. I would welcome the opportunity to be a massage therapist at the Mineral Water Spa.

Sincerely,

Anita Davis

Anita Davis, Licensed Massage Therapist

FIGURE 3.7

Business letter format and example.

CHAPTER HIGHLIGHTS

- The journey to becoming a professional massage therapist involves personal growth and change.
- To have a professional attitude is to embody a professional way of acting, thinking, and feeling.
- Dedication to service means that the client's well-being is held above the massage therapist's own desire for money, power, and worldly recognition. This provides a moral compass for ethical decision making and the motivation to be the best that you can be.
- Having a good work ethic means giving work a high priority in your life and is reflected in good attendance, punctuality, reliability, accountability, positive attitude, and enthusiasm.
- Projecting a professional image means dress that is modest, clean, and allows freedom of movement, and good personal grooming, posture, and speech.
- Professional boundaries clarify the nature of the therapeutic relationship, and the roles of both massage therapist and client.
  - Five types of professional boundaries are (1) physical, (2) emotional, (3) intellectual, (4) sexual, and (5) energetic.
- Keeping good professional boundaries is a key factor in maintaining ethical massage therapy practices.
- Ethical standards for massage students lay the foundation for ethical practice after graduation and include the areas of professionalism, class work, relationship with classmates, professional boundaries, and relationship with the school.
- Intellectual skills needed by massage therapists span the range from knowledge to comprehension, application, analysis, synthesis, and evaluation. Higher level thinking skills include critical thinking and systematic problem solving.
- The ability to concentrate makes studying more productive and performing massage better focused.
  - Concentration is improved through minimizing attention disruptors, single-tasking, creating a more distraction free environment, and learning to focus the mind.
- Intuition is direct perception of the truth without using rational problem solving and is useful for performing smooth, effortless massage.
- Emotional intelligence is defined by self-awareness, managing emotions, self-motivation, recognizing emotions in others, and handling relationships. It is essential for developing healthy and ethical therapeutic relationships with clients.
- Good social and communication skills are essential for success as a massage therapist.
  - Social skills promote harmony and connection between people, and resolve disagreements and misunderstandings.
  - Verbal and nonverbal communication skills facilitate the exchange of information and are polished through awareness, learning, experience, and practice.
- Courtesy and good manners are the foundation of customer service.
  - What is considered good manners varies by culture and can change over time.
- First impressions are important to establish rapport with new clients.
- Greeting clients involves making eye contact, saying the person's name, introducing yourself, shaking hands, and giving further directions.
  - The handshake is the first time you touch your client so it is important to have good, firm contact.
  - Use good judgment in hugging clients to maintain professional boundaries and avoid violating the client's comfort level.
- Introductions help people feel comfortable and welcome, as well as transmit useful social information.
  - In introducing two people, say the most honored person's name first.
- Five basic approaches to conflict resolution are (1) collaboration, (2) accommodation, (3) compromise, (4) avoidance, and (5) force.
  - Choose the best approach to any specific conflict, taking into consideration the priority of your own needs versus the other person's needs and the importance of the relationship. Try for a win-win resolution.
- Verbal communication is improved through practice.
  - Speak in a calm, steady, strong voice; vary energy, rhythm, and inflection to make delivery interesting; articulate clearly and avoid mumbling.
- Telephones and answering machines are essential communication tools.
  - Use a clear and concise answering machine message, and return calls within 24 hours.
  - Turn off ringers and cell phones when in a massage session.
  - Avoid distractions and multitasking while on the phone.
- Body language speaks volumes.
  - Use good upright, aligned posture and avoid slouching, tilting, and a drooping head.
  - Use welcoming and friendly posture and gestures; communicate with your eyes and smile.
- Being a good listener begins with the intention to hear what others are really saying and to overcome poor listening habits.
  - Focus on what the speaker is saying (words), feeling, and meaning. Avoid letting the mind wander and formulating replies while others are speaking.

- Affirmative listening lets the speaker know that you are paying attention through verbal cues and body language.
- In active listening, you reflect back to the speaker in your own words what you think he or she said.
- Massage therapists make presentations in a variety of informal and formal ways to both individuals and groups.
  - Know your goals and your audience, and then organize and plan what you want to say.
  - Explanations are verbal descriptions telling the what, how, and/or why of something.
  - Use loose scripts and props for routine explanations to clients.
- Demonstrations involve showing an audience how something is done or how something works by performing the action while giving a verbal description.
  - Keep descriptions clear and simple, and be sure the audience can see the demonstration well.

- In making persuasive presentations, first establish your credibility, then get the audience's attention, present your point and build your case for it, and call for action.
  - Always provide an opportunity for listeners to ask questions.
- Written correspondence reflects your level of professionalism.
  - Use correct spelling, punctuation, and grammar, as well as simple sentence construction and brevity.
  - Memos and business letters are written in a more formal tone on printed stationary using the correct format.
  - E-mail is an electronic memo and follows rules of any other business correspondence.
  - Keep a file of all written correspondence in chronological order.

EXAM REVIEW

Key Terms

Match the following key terms to their descriptions. For additional study, look up the key terms in the Interactive Glossary on page G-1 and note other terms that compare or contrast with them.

_____ 1. Body language
_____ 2. Compassion
_____ 3. Concentration
_____ 4. Conflict resolution
_____ 5. Critical thinking
_____ 6. Emotional intelligence
_____ 7. Ethics
_____ 8. Intellectual skills
_____ 9. Intuition
_____ 10. Listening
_____ 11. Problem solving
_____ 12. Professional boundaries
_____ 13. Professional image
_____ 14. Service
_____ 15. Social skills
_____ 16. Work ethic

a. Primary motivation is to help others
b. Taking your work seriously, staying focused, and applying yourself to doing a good job
c. Attention to dress, grooming, posture, and language
d. Sets limits or borders that define personal and professional space
e. The study of moral behavior, of right and wrong
f. Thinking or cognitive skills
g. Type of higher-level thinking that helps you get at the truth and avoid being deceived
h. The ability to sustain attention on something for a period of time
i. Set of skills important for self-awareness, self-motivation, and building healthy relationships with clients
j. Deep awareness of the suffering of another coupled with the wish to relieve it
k. A direct perception of the truth, independent of any rational process
l. Behaviors that promote harmony, understanding, and connection, while peacefully solving problems such as disagreements, misunderstandings, and reconciliation after harm done
m. Posture, hand gestures, eye contact, facial expression
n. Trying to understand what someone else is communicating to you.
o. Resolving differences amicably
p. Systematic approach to finding a solution to a problem using critical thinking skills

Memory Workout

To test your memory of the main concepts in this chapter, complete the following sentences by circling the most correct answer from the two choices provided.

1. Dedication to (service) (self-development) offers a higher and more satisfying motivation than merely making money, and provides a moral compass for ethical decision making.
2. (Accountability) (Reliability) means that people can count on you to do what you say you are going to do, when you say you will do it.
3. Have work clothes that are (separate from) (similar to) your everyday clothes.
4. (A work ethic) (Boundaries) communicate(s) limits that define personal and professional space.
5. Intuition is a direct perception of the truth, independent of any (thought) (meditation) process.
6. Recognizing a feeling in oneself and its accompanying impulse to act as it happens is called (self-awareness) (self-motivation).
7. Good (intellectual) (social skills) promote harmony, understanding, and connection between people.
8. A general rule when shaking hands is to (match) (exceed) the other person's force
9. Wearing name tags at professional conferences facilitates (networking) (listening).
10. The delivery of the spoken word is usually more important than (content) (voice quality).
11. (Lower) (Higher) pitched voices sound more confident and competent.
12. Good upright, aligned posture commands respect and (compassion) (confidence).
13. Poor listening habits include letting the mind wander and formulating (replies) (interruptions) while others are speaking.
14. Presentations are essentially (teaching) (motivational) opportunities.
15. Business correspondence has a different function than personal correspondence and is more (legal) (formal).

Test Prep

The following multiple choice questions will help to prepare you for future school and professional exams.

1. Taking your work seriously, staying focused, and applying yourself to getting the job done right is known as having a good:
   a. Service orientation
   b. Punctuality
   c. Work ethic
   d. Sense of ethics
2. Which of the following is considered professional dress?
   a. Short shorts
   b. Denim jeans
   c. Closed-toe shoes
   d. Dangling jewelry
3. Nervous habits such as finger tapping, nail biting, knuckle cracking, leg bouncing, and hair twirling can be:
   a. Stress reducers
   b. Image detractors
   c. Image enhancers
   d. Grooming problems
4. Using knowledge in real life situations is an example of intellectual skill at the following level:
   a. Comprehension
   b. Application
   c. Analysis
   d. Synthesis
5. What type of higher level thinking weighs reasons to believe something against reasons to doubt it?
   a. Logical thinking
   b. Problem solving
   c. Clinical reasoning
   d. Critical thinking
6. Which of the following does *not* improve the ability to concentrate?
   a. Single-tasking
   b. Multitasking
   c. Meditation
   d. Distraction-free environment
7. A deep awareness of the suffering of others coupled with a desire to relieve it is called:
   a. Empathy
   b. Sympathy
   c. Compassion
   d. Appreciation
8. Which of the following directions for greeting a first time client is not correct?
   a. Make eye contact
   b. Offer your hand to shake
   c. Wait for the client to speak before introducing yourself
   d. Smile

9. When introducing two people, whose name is said first?
   a. The oldest
   b. The youngest
   c. The most honored
   d. The woman's

10. In terms of body language, arms crossed in front of the body can convey a sense of:
    a. Protection and distancing
    b. Welcome and openness
    c. Confidence and trust
    d. Friendliness and invitation

11. The type of listening that lets a speaker know that you are paying attention is:
    a. Attentive listening
    b. Distracted listening
    c. Active listening
    d. Affirmative listening

12. What type of conflict resolution is most appropriate when building long-term relationships, or when you need to work together with someone for the greater good?
    a. Force
    b. Collaboration
    c. Accommodation
    d. Compromise

13. Which of the following statements about phone use in your private practice is *not* good advice?
    a. Try to return phone calls within 24 hours.
    b. Keep phone ringers on low volume during massage sessions.
    c. Do not interrupt a massage session to answer the phone.
    d. Do not interrupt a phone call with a client to answer another call, for example, with call waiting.

14. The first rule in making presentations is to know:
    a. How much time you have
    b. Your goals
    c. Your audience
    d. The room setup

15. The most appropriate form of written correspondence for official business is:
    a. A memo
    b. An e-mail
    c. A brief note
    d. A business letter

Video Challenge

Watch the appropriate segment of the video on your DVD and then answer the following questions.

Professional and Personal Development

Professionalism
1. What do the massage therapists interviewed in the video say about clothes and projecting a professional image?
2. What advice do the massage therapists give about greeting clients?
3. Which of the image detractors discussed in the video do you recognize in yourself?

Emotional Intelligence
1. Identify ways that the massage therapists interviewed in the video show a high level of emotional intelligence. How is that important to a successful massage therapy practice?
2. What do the facial expressions of massage therapists in the video convey to their clients? What similarities do you see in the massage therapists' expressions? Do you see any differences?
3. What do the massage therapists in the video say about establishing good relationships with their clients?

Social and Communication Skills
1. Review the scenes in the video in which massage therapists are greeting clients. Identify ways that professionalism, competence, and confidence are communicated.
2. In what ways do the massage therapists in the video create professional boundaries with their clients? Comment on the different kinds of boundaries established.
3. What principles of good communication do you see in video scenes showing client interviews? How do the massage therapists create a sense of openness to encourage client response?

Comprehension Exercises

The following short answer questions test your knowledge and understanding of chapter topics and provide practice in written communication skills. Explain in two to four complete sentences.

1. What are some important elements of a good work ethic? Why is this important for success in school and as a future massage therapist?

2. What are professional boundaries? Give some examples of physical, emotional, and intellectual boundaries with clients.

3. In addition to words, what are you listening for when talking to clients? What is the difference between affirmative and active listening?

For Greater Understanding

The following exercises are designed to take you from the realm of theory into the real world. They will help give you a deeper understanding of the subjects covered in this chapter. Action words are underlined to emphasize the variety of activities presented to address different learning styles and to encourage deeper thinking.

1. <u>Choose</u> a dilemma related to massage therapy for an exercise in critical thinking; for example, whether you should buy a certain a product (e.g., type of oil, table, or massage tool); or take a certain elective class; or spend time and money on a particular certification program; or support a proposed licensing provision (e.g., hours of continuing education for license renewal). <u>Analyze</u> the situation listing pertinent questions, <u>evaluate</u> the situation, and <u>decide</u> on a course of action. What influenced your final decision?

2. <u>Create and practice</u> a routine for greeting regular clients to make them feel welcome, comfortable, and confident in you. Take into consideration your body language, voice quality, and words. Have a study partner help you develop this professional "persona." (Variation: <u>Videotape</u> your greeting and <u>analyze</u> it with classmates. <u>Modify</u> it as needed to project what you want.)

3. <u>Practice</u> affirmative and active listening with a partner. <u>Listen</u> to how his or her day went yesterday, and at first simply nod and give affirmative signals that you are listening. Then <u>practice</u> active listening by <u>reflecting back</u> what you thought the person said for clarification.

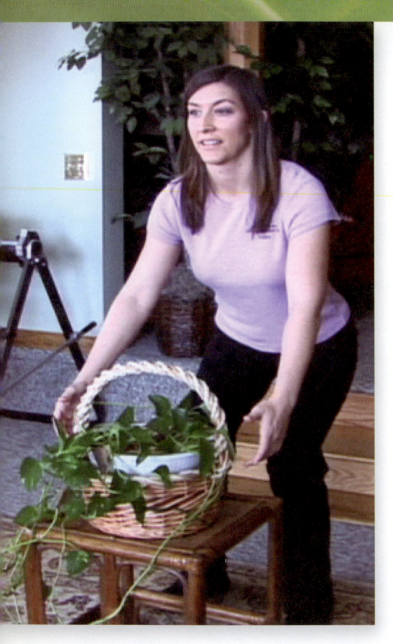

 CHAPTER OUTLINE

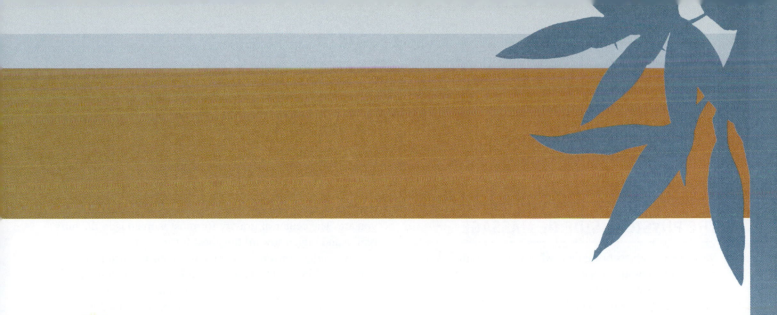

LEARNING OUTCOMES

After studying this chapter, you will have information to:

1. Develop good body awareness.
2. Describe the elements of skilled touch needed by massage therapists.
3. Summarize the basic elements of physical fitness.
4. Evaluate your overall level of physical fitness.
5. Explain how body-mind practices develop coordination.

6. Improve concentration through meditation.
7. Plan a personal stress-management strategy.
8. Create a time-management plan.
9. Describe the basics of good nutrition.
10. Develop a holistic self-care program.

KEY TERMS

THE PHYSICAL SIDE OF MASSAGE

Massage therapists bring their whole selves to their work—body, mind, emotions, and spirit. They need the intellectual, emotional, social, and communication skills described in Chapter 3, Professional and Personal Development. But perhaps most fundamental are the physical abilities and fitness that allows them to apply massage skillfully and continue to perform massage day after day. Developing physical skills and fitness is an important part of being a massage student, and implementing a self-care plan lays the foundation for years of success in the profession.

Massage is performed with the whole body, not just the hands and arms. Being a massage therapist requires a certain level of body awareness, touch skills, and physical fitness. Self-care practices related to the physical body not only develop the physical conditioning necessary to perform massage, but also help prevent repetitive strain injuries that can cut short a career in massage therapy.

BODY AWARENESS

Learning physical skills begins with body awareness. **Body awareness** is the ability to sense where your body is in space while at rest and in motion and to coordinate movement with mind. It entails an integration of body and mind so that a person exists as an embodied being.

People who lack body awareness have difficulty following instructions for good body mechanics and for performing techniques because they are not "in their bodies." There is a disconnect between body and mind, as expressed in this James Joyce quote from *Dubliners:* "Mr. Duffy lived a short distance from his body."

Body awareness is one of the beneficial effects of receiving massage and bodywork, and it is a wellness goal for clients. Body awareness is also essential for learning massage techniques and skillful implementation of massage sessions. Athletes and dancers, artists and craftsmen, musicians, and others who use their bodies in their work and leisure pursuits develop good body awareness over time. It is an awareness that can be developed through movement exercises. It can only be learned by actually performing movements and paying attention to how they feel.

Being centered and grounded are two basic concepts related to body awareness. **Center** has a physical and psychological dimension and refers to a focal point or point of organization from which being and movement occur. Its opposite is being scattered, off balance, and moving from the periphery. Being centered refers to finding your center and staying there while you move about.

Center of gravity is a biomechanical concept indicating the point at which body weight is equally balanced in all directions. Think of the point at which your body is balanced from top to bottom, front to back, and left to right. Your exact center of gravity depends on your body shape and how tall you are. The center of gravity for most women is in the hip region and higher toward the chest for most men.

A similar concept of center is found in Eastern practices. In Chinese, the center is called the *dan tian* (pronounced *dan tyen*) located about 1.5 inches below the navel and one third of the way from front to back. In Japanese, it is called *hara*. The hara is not only a place of physical centering, but a point of organization on many levels. This center is "a state of unity in which effective action, emotional balance, mental alertness, and spiritual vision are in a harmonious balance. When we are centered our actions are coherent with what we care about" (Heckler 1997, p. 96). You can begin to find this centered state by learning to move from the physical center.

The tai chi stance and walk are simple exercises that give you a sense of moving from the center. They can also be the foundation of learning good body mechanics for applying massage therapy. Figures 4.1■ and 4.2■ describe these useful exercises for developing good body awareness.

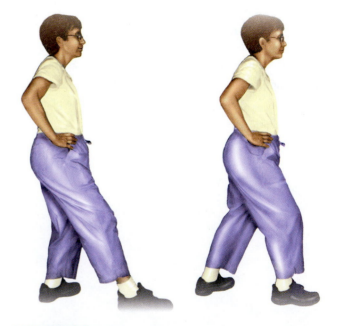

FIGURE 4.1

Tai chi stance with front foot pointing straight ahead and back foot at 45° angle, heels in line, and feet shoulder width apart. Shift weight back and forth feeling the movement from the hara or center.

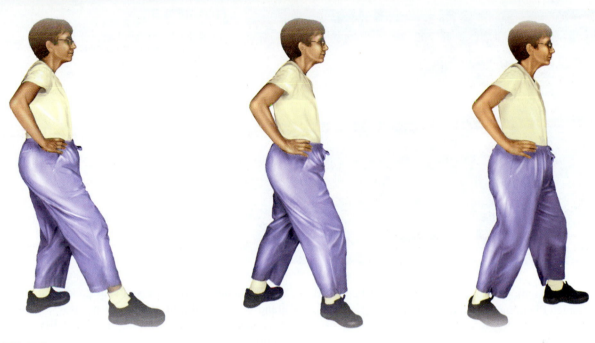

FIGURE 4.2

Tai chi walk along straight line. From tai chi stance, shift weight to the back leg and turn the front foot 45° degrees outward. Then shift weight to front leg while bringing the back leg to the front along the straight line; the new front leg receives the weight. Shift weight back and repeat the walk. Keeping hands near the hara helps you feel the movement from the center.

Ground refers to the firmness of the earth. The act of grounding refers to establishing a conn6ection or being rooted to the earth through the legs and feet. The meaning can be extended to having a stable base and connection to a foundation whether standing or sitting. This idea becomes important as you learn to move from and use the power of your legs in performing massage. The energy of the movement comes up from the ground through the legs, into the center, and then into the upper body. This concept will be explored further in Chapter 12, Body Mechanics, Table Skills, and Application Guidelines.

SKILLED TOUCH

Since touch is the basis of massage, **skilled touch** is essential for success as a massage therapist. Skilled touch has four dimensions important to massage therapists:

1. Contact
2. Qualities of touch
3. Communication
4. Palpation

Contact refers to the sense presence of the massage therapist's hands on the client's body. When contact is good, the client feels a full, confident, deliberate, and warm connection with the massage therapist (Figure 4.3■). Poor contact feels tentative, hesitant, unsure, fearful, or distracted.

Qualities of touch are related to contact and vary from soft and gentle to hard and rough. Human beings are capable of many nuances in quality of touch, and massage therapists become more conscious of how they are touching their clients and what is an appropriate quality to use in a given situation. For example, athletes often prefer a firmer, deeper, and more vigorous massage, while a person who is ill requires a gentler touch.

Communication through touch is achieved by the contact and different qualities of touch applied during massage, or before or after the session when greeting or saying good-bye to a client. Be conscious of what you might be communicating when you touch your clients. Caring and openness are examples of what can be communicated through touch. Touch during massage should be caring, but never personal, sexual, or aggressive.

Respect for your clients' boundaries is a significant aspect of skilled touch. Know what is off limits for everyone (e.g., touching genitals), and for each individual client (e.g., ticklish feet or an old injury site). Obtaining informed consent for permission to touch is an important communication skill discussed in Chapter 5, Ethics and the Therapeutic Relationship on page 107.

Palpation is sensing information about the client through touch and by the feel of tissues and movement at joints. Palpatory literacy involves the ability to locate specific anatomical structures and detect normal and abnormal conditions. The nature and importance of palpation skills in

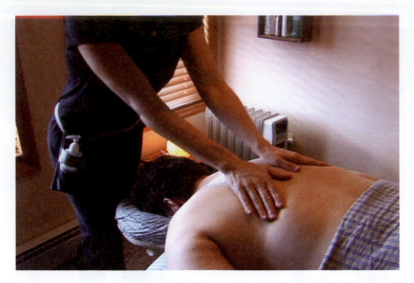

FIGURE 4.3

Good contact feels full, confident, and deliberate, and establishes a warm connection between massage therapist and client.

goal-oriented planning is discussed further in Chapter 10, Goal-Oriented Planning and Documentation.

PHYSICAL FITNESS

In addition to being good role models for their clients, having a good level of physical fitness allows massage therapists to work without undue stress and strain. Learning the fundamentals of fitness is also good for better understanding the health of clients. Basic fitness includes cardiovascular function, strength, flexibility, and body composition.

Testing by a fitness professional using the latest methods will give the most accurate results. However, the simple tests described in the following sections offer a general fitness profile and demonstrate the concepts involved. Elements of a physical fitness profile are shown in Figure 4.4■.

FIGURE 4.4

Physical fitness profile form.

Name _____   Date _____

♥ **Cardiovascular Fitness**

Resting Heart Rate (RHR)   _____

Blood Pressure (BP)   _____ / _____

| Cardiovascular Endurance | poor | fair | good | excellent |

🏋 **Muscular Strength/Endurance**

| Abdominal/Sit-Ups | poor | fair | good | excellent |
| Upper Body/Push-Ups | poor | fair | good | excellent |

() **Flexibility**

| Sit and Reach | poor | fair | good | excellent |

△ **Body Composition**

| Body Mass Index (BMI) | underweight (less than 19) | healthy (19-24.5) | overweight (25-29.9) | obese (30+) |

Waist Measurement (inches)*   _____

Note: Fitness test results tables can be found in books like *Fitness for Dummies* by S. Schlosberg and L. Neporent (Wiley Publishing).

*Waist measurement as an indication of healthy body composition is discussed in *You on a diet: The owner's manual for waist management* by M. F. Riozen and M.C. Oz (Free Press). Recommended is 32.5 inches or less for a woman and 35 inches or less for a man.

Cardiovascular Fitness

A basic cardiovascular (CV) fitness profile includes resting heart rate, blood pressure, and cardiovascular endurance. Measurements of these three aspects of CV fitness give an indication of how efficient and strong the heart is, and the level of stress on the blood vessels and the system as a whole.

Take your resting heart rate (RHR) either at the wrist below base of the thumb, or on the anterior neck (carotid artery). The best time to measure your RHR is in the morning just after waking up and before any activity. As an alternative, sit still for 10 minutes and then find your pulse with your index and middle fingers, not the thumb. Count the number of beats for 1 minute (or number of beats per 15 seconds × 4). Normal resting heart rate is 60–80 beats per minute.

Blood pressure (BP) is measured with a device called a sphygmomanometer or blood pressure machine. Blood pressure readings have two numbers, (e.g., 120/80). The first or top number is the *diastolic pressure,* that is, the pressure of the blood on the vessels when the heart contracts. The second number is the *systolic pressure,* that is, the pressure on the blood vessels between beats. Anyone with BP over 140/90 is considered hypertensive and should see a doctor about it. High blood pressure puts stress on blood vessels and can lead to stroke and other serious health problems.

Cardiovascular endurance refers to the heart's capacity to keep up with a certain workload and its ability to recover afterwards. A simple test to demonstrate this concept is the 3-minute step test. This test is performed by stepping on and off a 12-inch-high bench for 3 minutes and then immediately checking your heart rate (HR) (Figure 4.5■). Check the HR again at 1-minute intervals to see when it starts to drop back to the RHR. The lower the HR after the exercise, and the faster the recovery, the better the CV endurance is.

Good CV endurance increases the capacity to work longer without fatigue and offers protection against heart disease. Cardiovascular endurance is improved by participating in exercises like walking, running, or cycling for at least 30 minutes 5 days per week. The activity should be vigorous enough to get the heart rate elevated and the body sweating, but not so high that you cannot carry on a conversation. The better the CV endurance, the more effort it will take to feel like you're working hard.

Muscular Strength and Endurance

Overall muscular strength and endurance is developed naturally as the time spent performing massage gradually increases. However, by increasing muscular fitness beyond what is needed to perform massage, less of the muscles' total capacity is used up when working, so there is less stress and fatigue at the end of the day.

Muscular strength refers to a muscle's ability to move a maximum amount of resistance once, while *muscular endurance* indicates the capacity to move against resistance for a number of repetitions over time. Strength and endurance are related since the stronger a muscle is the less hard it has to work to complete a task. Simple tests for muscular endurance include the number of push-ups or squats you can

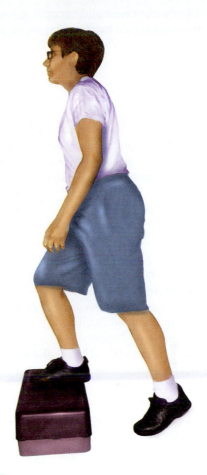

FIGURE 4.5

Step test for cardiovascular endurance.

do, or the number of sit-ups in one minute (Figure 4.6■). These tests taken together evaluate the major muscle groups of the body.

In addition to strength in large muscle groups, massage therapists benefit from having exceptional strength in the shoulders, arms, wrists, and hands. Resistance exercises for

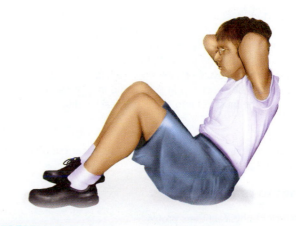

FIGURE 4.6

One minute sit-up test for abdominal muscle strength and endurance.

the upper body can help build strength in those important areas. Use of resistance bands offers a convenient way to increase strength in muscles used most in massage.

Flexibility

Flexibility is the ability to flex or the possible range of movement at joints. Range of motion at each joint can be measured precisely using an instrument called a goniometer, which works like a protractor used in geometry. Normal range of motion for major joints is described on page 213 in Chapter 6, Anatomy and Physiology, Pathology, and Kinesiology.

A simple test for overall body flexibility is the sit-and-reach test, which is really a test of lower back, hamstring, and shoulder flexibility. Sit with the bottoms of your feet flat against a stair or low box. With no warm-up tries, reach forward as far as you can toward your toes and hold the position (Figure 4.7■). Note how far you reach, that is, how far short of your toes or past your toes your fingers extend. For good flexibility, you should be able to reach past your toes.

Flexibility is maintained by regular stretching. Getting into the habit of stretching everyday and between client appointments can protect you from tight, shortened muscles. A regular stretching routine should include stretches for the legs and hips, arms and shoulders, wrists and hands. Figures 4.8■ shows a variety of stretching techniques for massage therapists to address the shoulders, arms, and hands.

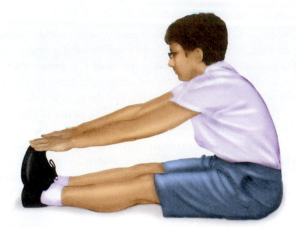

FIGURE 4.7

Sit and reach test for overall flexibility.

Body Composition

Body composition refers to your body-fat percentage; that is, how much of your body is composed of fat tissue in comparison to other tissues (muscle, bones, organs, etc). It is a general indication of health and a signal for health risk factors. Tests like skin-fold calipers, underwater weighing, bioelectrical impedance analysis (BIA), and other methods have been developed to measure body composition with varying levels of accuracy.

The BMI (body mass index) is a method that compares your height and weight to come up with an index number

---

CASE FOR STUDY

Robin and Getting into Shape for Massage

Robin started massage school about 2 months ago and is now noticing that she has difficulty getting through technique classes without feeling extremely tired and sore. She always thought of herself as being in good shape, but now realizes that doing physical work such as massage might require a higher fitness level. She knows that to be successful in school and in a massage practice afterwards, she must get into better physical condition.

Question:

What can Robin do to get into better physical condition for doing massage?

Things to consider:

- Current physical fitness profile.
- Areas (e.g., muscles, joints) that feel stressed after practicing massage.

- Current types and level of exercise (e.g., CV, strength, flexibility).
- Quality of body mechanics while practicing massage techniques.
- Related health practices:
  ○ Amount of sleep each night.
  ○ Eating habits.
  ○ 3Rs (rest, relaxation, recreation)
- Areas for improvement
- Possibilities for fitness activities

Now put yourself in Robin's place. What three things can you do to improve your physical fitness for performing massage?

1. _____

2. _____

3. _____

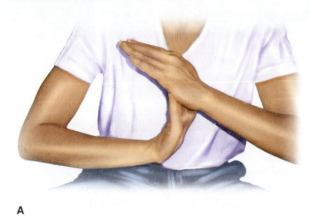

A

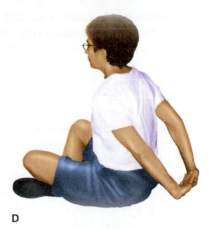

D

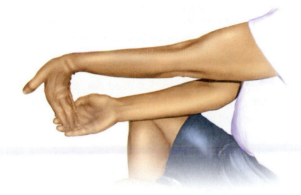

B

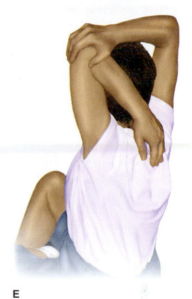

E

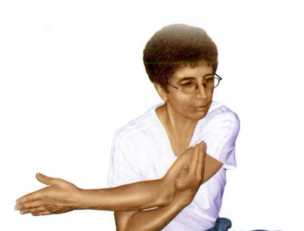

C

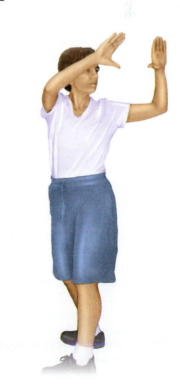

F

FIGURE 4.8

A. Palm stretch by hyperextending the fingers.
B. Forearm and palm stretch by hyperextending the wrist.
C. Shoulder stretch by horizontal flexion of arm.
D. Shoulder and pectoral muscles stretch by reaching behind.
E. Triceps and side stretch with arm overhead.
F. Shoulder and torso stretch by twisting and looking behind.

to determine your weight status. Some BMI calculations also factor in chest and waist measurements. BMI is not as accurate a measurement as the more technical methods mentioned above, but offers a general indication of healthy body composition and is used here for demonstration purposes. Knowing your BMI can help you make informed decisions about your diet and exercise habits.

A simple BMI calculation is: weight ÷ (height in inches × height in inches) × 705. BMI categories are underweight (less than 18.5), healthy (18.5–24.9), overweight (25–29.9), and obese (30 or greater) (National Heart, Lung, and Blood Institute). Visit the National Heart, Lung, and Blood Institute website (www.nhlbisupport.com/bmi/bmicalc.htm) for a quick calculation of your BMI.

Body type and shape are determined by heredity and affect body composition. But genetic predisposition can be managed with a program of good nutrition and exercise. It is important to maintain a BMI that allows for the level of endurance necessary for activity as a massage therapist.

SELF-CARE PRACTICES

It can be a challenge to balance family and friends plus work and school while training to become a massage therapist. It takes a comprehensive, realistic plan. **Self-care** is a term used by massage therapists to describe how they take care of their own well-being while they fulfill their career goals and are of service to clients.

Body-Mind Practices

Some physical exercises do not fit neatly into the strength, flexibility, and cardio fitness categories described above. Yet they are useful for improving various aspects of physical fitness with the added benefit of developing coordination, body awareness, and concentration. And they are performed in a way that promotes relaxation. These can be thought of as **body-mind practices** or "any type of exercise that requires a conscious effort to link how [what] you are feeling to what your body is doing" (Schlosberg 2005, p. 14).

Body-mind practices popular today include yoga, tai chi, qi gong, and Pilates. Although the first three practices stem from larger systems of philosophy and health practices in India and China, they can be found today adapted and simplified for Westerners. It is not necessary to know or accept the entire philosophical context to benefit from the exercises themselves.

Yoga is an ancient practice from India that concentrates on holding various postures thought to balance energy as understood in Ayurveda, and which improve bodily strength, flexibility, and body awareness. Yoga also includes meditation and breathing exercises.

The Chinese developed exercises to stimulate the flow of life energy or Qi (also *chi*). *Qi gong* [chi-*gong*] literally means *energy exercises* and focuses on the mind, posture,

breathing, and movement. Qi gong is a very useful supplement to Asian bodywork therapy since it has the same goal, which is to improve the flow of Qi in the body's energy channels (Chuen, 1991). Chapter 19, Eastern Bodywork, offer examples of yoga and qi gong exercises.

Tai chi [ti-*chi*], another ancient practice from China, was originally based on martial arts. Tai chi involves movements that promote balance, coordination, control, and strength. The movements are performed alone or in movement routines called forms. The quality of movement in the popular Yang style is slow and flowing. Tai chi stances and locomotion, weight transfer, and quality of movement are ideal for learning good body mechanics for performing massage.

Pilates [pih-*lah*-teez] is a modern system of exercise developed by Joseph Pilates, who created the movements to treat injured dancers. Pilates emphasizes the body's core; that is, the abdominal muscles, upper and lower back, and hips and thighs. The exercises focus on using good alignment and strengthening muscles used for good posture (Figure 4.9■). Pilates is eclectic, borrowing from yoga, ballet, and standard strengthening exercises. Its uniqueness and benefit lies in its concentration on core muscles, good posture, and correct form. It increases body awareness and control as it promotes good body mechanics.

There are many styles or spin-offs of these systems of exercise. Doing a little homework and critical thinking about them will help you choose one or a combination of practices appropriate for your wellness goals.

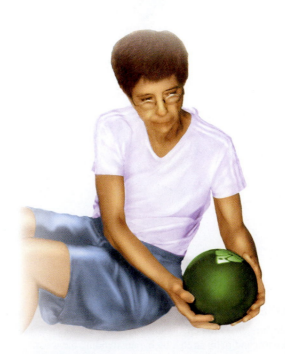

FIGURE 4.9

Pilates exercises strengthen the body's core muscles.

Meditation

Meditation techniques are designed to quiet the mind and enhance the ability to pay focused attention. The essence of modern meditation techniques is choosing something like a word or object to place attention on, and when the mind wanders as it invariably does, bringing it back to the object of attention. It is that simple—and that difficult—since the mind likes to wander.

Learning focused attention is like trying to teach a puppy to sit and stay. You place the puppy into a sitting position and tell him to stay. He stays for a few seconds, then sees something interesting and wanders off. You gently bring him back to the same spot, sit him down, and tell him to stay. This routine is repeated again and again, and gradually his ability to stay improves. Similarly, a person's concentration ability improves with meditation practice.

A good posture for practicing meditation is seated in a comfortable chair or cross-legged on a cushion. Keep the back upright and in alignment, and let the hands rest on the thighs. If in a chair, feet are flat on the floor. Meditation can be practiced with the eyes closed or open slightly (soft eyes) looking 6–10 feet ahead. Good meditation posture is demonstrated in Figure 4.10■.

The surroundings should be quiet and free of distractions. Although meditation can be practiced at any time, many find the early morning or late evening more conducive for calming the mind. Set aside 10–30 minutes daily for best results. Consistency is important for developing concentration ability over time.

A simple form of meditation is called *peaceful abiding*. The object of attention in peaceful abiding is the breath. "In peaceful abiding, we ground our mind in the present moment. We place our mind on the breath and keep it there" (Mipham 2003, p. 24). By having a focal or reference point like the breath, we can better detect when concentration is broken, and bring it back as we practice focused attention. The end result is a clear, focused, uncluttered mind.

Another form of meditation is called *quiet sitting*. This is the practice of taking time to calm your mind, collect your thoughts, and center yourself. It is taking a break from the distractions of life and sitting quietly for a moment. The idea

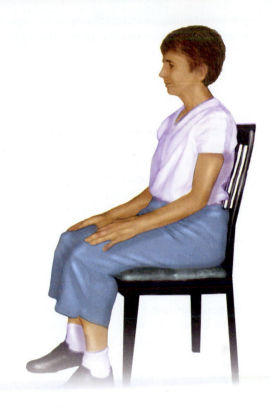

FIGURE 4.10

A good posture for practicing meditation is seated in a chair with the back upright and in alignment, the hands resting on the knees, feet flat on the floor, with soft eyes looking 6–10 feet ahead.

is to find a comfortable place to sit, close your eyes, and calm your breathing and your thoughts. Keep your thoughts centered on this quiet moment, and let go of unnecessary thinking. After a few moments, resume activity keeping the calmness you have created (Simpkins and Simpkins, 2000).

In *active meditation*, an activity like walking, knitting, or even doing the dishes can be used as a practice for focusing the mind. The point here is to focus on thoughts relevant to what you are doing, and let go of unrelated thoughts. If your mind drifts into other thoughts, gently bring it back to the task at hand. By raising awareness of when the mind

PRACTICAL APPLICATION

Practice some form of sitting meditation for 10–15 minutes every day for 2 weeks. Evaluate how regular meditation affects you and your experience with learning massage.

1. What method of meditation most appeals to you?
2. Can you find a regular time and place for meditation?
3. Does it become easier with practice to minimize distracting thoughts?
4. Can you focus better in class and with practice clients at home?

is wandering and learning to bring it back to the object of attention, you are increasing your ability to concentrate.

Athletes try to improve their powers of concentration for better sports performance. Zen practices like kyudo (archery), flower arranging, and tea ceremony are ancient forms of active meditation. Eventually, massage itself becomes an active meditation in the sense that you are concentrating on what you are doing without distraction.

Many massage therapists do a variation on quiet sitting before going in to a massage session. They take a few moments to stand outside the door to the massage room and collect and focus their thoughts. This prepares them to be present and to give the massage session focused attention.

Stress-Control Strategies

Massage therapists appreciate the major role that stress can play in undermining health and fitness. Students are under special circumstances that increase the stress in their lives, and therefore need **stress-control strategies** to help maintain good health. Good stress-control habits developed while in school can continue throughout your life.

Consequences of stress overload for students include problems like inability to pay attention in class (distraction), poor attendance and lateness, test anxiety, and chronic emotional upset. Stress-control plans include strategies like good time management, adequate rest and relaxation, and anxiety reduction techniques including massage.

Poor time management is perhaps the biggest stress producer for students. Developing a good time management plan as described later in this chapter is the cornerstone of a stress-control strategy.

Adequate rest, relaxation, and recreation are essential stress-control strategies. Getting 7–9 hours of sleep per night and having at least 30 minutes of "downtime" or quiet time per day are good goals. Recreation (think of *re-creation*) activities offer a break from work and revive the spirit. The three R's should be scheduled into your time management plan.

Massage therapists, who are looked to as experts in stress reduction, accumulate a number of different methods to promote relaxation. These include relaxation audiotapes or CDs, physical practices like yoga and tai chi, meditation and quiet sitting, and massage itself. The more students practice relaxation techniques, the better able and more credible they will be when helping clients who come to them to reduce the stress in their lives.

Time Management

Time management involves planning a workable schedule. It is a matter of priorities, which means making time for what matters most and letting go of the rest. A common mistake of students is to try to fit school into an already crowded schedule. Being rushed or late, eating on the run, cramming for classes and exams, and suffering from sleep deprivation are symptoms of poor time management. You have to *make* time for what you value most.

So the first step in time management is to identify goals and priorities for the time under consideration. That could

REALITY CHECK

LUTHER

CHERISE: I know cardiovascular fitness is important, but I'm not the marathon runner type. And I don't have the time or money to join a gym. Isn't there something simple I can do to get more fit?

LUTHER: Running really isn't necessary. Walking at least 30 minutes 5 days a week will get you on the road to cardiovascular fitness. That doesn't mean a stroll, but a moderate to fast-paced walk. Your breathing will be a little faster and you may sweat a little if you are moving at a good pace. You can combine your walks with your stress-management strategy. Either walk by yourself for some alone time, or walk with a friend for some relaxing social time. You also can include the time spent walking to and from the bus or train in your total for the day, or you might try taking a walk at lunchtime. Fifteen minutes twice a day would also count. After a few weeks of walking, you'll see a boost in your fitness level.

be for a week, a month, a year. It might be defined by your life at the moment, such as the time you are in school or for the semester. If priorities are not clear, it is difficult to make good choices about the use of time. Students who start with school as a top priority are more likely to produce a time management plan that leads to success.

Plotting out a weekly schedule is the next step toward getting your use of time under control. The time management chart in Figure 4.11■ is an example of planning adequate time for regular activities.

A time management plan for students includes the following: work, school (classes and homework/practice), commuting, regular appointments and meetings, family time, sleeping, eating, rest/relaxation, and recreation. A good rule of thumb is to plan 60–75 percent of your time and leave 25–40 percent for unplanned or spontaneous activities. Working while attending school tends to decrease "spontaneous" time, but may be manageable for a short period.

A good time management tip is to identify *time wasters* and eliminate them from your life. A time waster would be something that does not contribute to your high-priority goals. Delayed gratification and learning to say "no" to yourself, with sights on a higher goal, are important signs of emotional maturity.

Reserve your prime time for high-priority tasks. For example, plan to study when you are most awake and full of energy. Also figure in adequate travel time between scheduled

Time Period September – December (Fall Semester)			Class Time: 24 hrs		Study/Practice Time: 20 hrs	
Time	**Monday**	**Tuesday**	**Wednesday**	**Thursday**	**Friday**	**Saturday**	**Sunday**
5:00 am	sleep	sleep	sleep	sleep	sleep	sleep	sleep
6:00	sleep	sleep	sleep	sleep	sleep	sleep	sleep
7:00	up & eat	up & eat	up & eat	up & eat	up & eat	up & eat	sleep
8:00	travel	travel	travel	travel	travel	travel	up & eat
9:00	class	class	class	class	work	work	recreation
10:00	class	class	class	class	work	work	recreation
11:00	class	class	class	class	work	work	recreation
12 noon	lunch	lunch	lunch	lunch	work	work	lunch
1:00 pm	class	class	class	clinic	lunch	lunch	study/practice
2:00	class	class	class	clinic	work	study/practice	study/practice
3:00	class	class	class	clinic	work	study/practice	study/practice
4:00	travel	travel	travel	travel	work	study/practice	study/practice
5:00	dinner	dinner	dinner	dinner	work	study/practice	dinner
6:00	work	study/practice	work	read/study	dinner	dinner	read/study
7:00	work	study/practice	work	read/study	recreation	recreation	read/study
8:00	work	study/practice	work	read/study	recreation	recreation	recreation
9:00	read/study	study/practice	read/study	read/study	recreation	recreation	recreation
10:00	relax/meditation	relax/meditation	relax/meditation	relax/meditation	recreation	recreation	relax/meditation
11:00	sleep	sleep	sleep	sleep	sleep	sleep	sleep

FIGURE 4.11

Sample time management planning chart for a massage student.

events. For example, list 7:30AM—leave for school, as well as 8:30AM—anatomy class begins.

Plan enough time for homework and practicing massage skills. For each hour of lecture class allot 2–3 hours of study time. Practice massage as required in your program for at least 4–6 hours per week outside of class time. Practice is not only for doing your homework and honing your massage skills, but also for building the strength and stamina to make a living as a massage therapist after graduation. By graduation, you should be comfortably performing the number of hours of massage (class plus practice time) that you are aiming for in your practice start-up.

Get in the habit of using a daily or weekly planner to keep track of regular and special appointments, events, and deadlines. Check your schedule at the beginning of each month, week, and day for an overview of the time period. Refer to your planner when making appointments so that you don't double schedule a time period.

Good time management while at school will naturally spill over into postgraduate employment and private practices. Build good habits in school that will serve you well afterwards.

Nutrition

Nutrition refers to the intake of food and drink to nourish the body and mind. Eating healthy food in appropriate amounts lays the foundation for all round well-being. Nutrition and physical activity go hand-in-hand in maintaining a healthy lifestyle. Their essential relationship is reflected in the United

CRITICAL THINKING

Analyze the level of stress in your life. Develop a strategy for minimizing harmful stressors and for including more stress-reducing activities.

1. What are the biggest stress-producing aspects of your life right now?
2. Which stressors are under your control and which are outside of your control?

3. Do you have adequate time for rest, relaxation, and recreation?
4. Can better time management help manage your stress level?

States Department of Agriculture (USDA) Food Guide Pyramid shown in Figure 4.12■. This newest food guide published in 2005 depicts a figure running up the side of the pyramid as a visual reminder of the need for physical activity for a balanced nutritional picture.

Giving nutritional advice to others is not within the scope of massage therapy, but healthy eating is an important aspect of self-care for everyone. A basic knowledge of nutrition provides a starting place for learning more about choosing the right foods and developing good eating habits.

Nutrients are substances in food used by the body to generate energy and to promote normal growth, maintenance, and repair. Six major categories of nutrients are carbohydrates, lipids, proteins, vitamins, minerals, and water. Broadly speaking, carbohydrates are composed of sugars and starches, lipids are fats, and proteins are amino acids found in fish, meat, seeds, nuts and legumes. Vitamins are organic nutrients and minerals are inorganic substances that the body needs in small amounts. Water is especially important since about 50–60 percent of a healthy adult's body weight is water, and fluid balance is essential for many physiological processes. (Marieb, 2009)

Food is the familiar form of plant and animal products that we eat to obtain nutrients. When planning meals, it is easier to think in terms of food groups to include in different amounts. The USDA Food Guide Pyramid identifies 6 food groups as grains, vegetables, fruits, oils, milk, and meat and beans. Different foods contain a variety of nutrients in combination. For example, vegetables contain carbohydrates, water, vitamins, and minerals. Fish and legumes typically contain protein, lipids, vitamins, and minerals. Table 4.1■ identifies some of the major nutrients found in different foods.

Calories measure the energy value of food. The number of calories in a particular food is a measurement of how much energy that food can produce when used in the body. For example, 2 tablespoons of almond butter contains about 190 calories, while 8 fluid ounces of orange juice provides about 110 calories. Some foods are "empty calories," that is, they add to the total calories consumed per day, but have no or little nutritional value.

The number of calories needed per day varies for different people depending on their gender, age, height, activity level, and other health factors. For example, if you are 30 years old, female, 5′6″ tall, and engage in 30–60 minutes of physical activity per day, your energy needs are about 2200 calories per day. If you are a 25 year old male, 5′11″ tall, and engage in moderate exercise, your energy needs are about 2800 calories per day (www.MyPyramid.gov).

If you consume more calories than you use each day, you gain weight. If you consume fewer calories than you need each day, you lose weight. To maintain your ideal weight, the number of calories you consume each day should match the number you use for energy. Charts have been developed that show ideal weight for people of different ages. Body Mass Index (BMI), as described earlier in this chapter, is also a method of determining if you are underweight, normal, overweight, or obese.

The United States government has developed a program to help people reach and maintain their ideal weight, while eating a nutritionally balanced diet. It is based on U.S. Dietary Guidelines and can be found on-line at www.MyPyramid.gov. The program helps you to determine your ideal weight and to plan healthy meals. MyPyramid worksheets include suggestions for amounts of food to eat from different food groups (grains, vegetables, fruits, milk, meat and beans), and space for tracking what you actually eat each day.

The U.S. Department of Health and Human Services publishes information on healthy eating in several different documents. *Dietary Guidelines for Americans,* 2005 and *Toolkit for Health Professionals* are examples that can be found at www.health.gov/dietaryguidelines.

Practicing good nutrition and maintaining a healthy weight are important for massage therapists. Performing massage and keeping a full schedule of appointments are easier if you are in optimal physical condition. In addition, being a good role model for clients is an important aspect of being in a health profession.

HOLISTIC SELF-CARE PLAN

A **holistic self-care plan** includes those activities that support your development as a massage therapist and that minimize factors that lead to illness and injury. It means having a plan for physical, mental, and emotional health and fitness, and avoiding undue stress and burnout. Even though self-care plans are as unique as the individuals involved, they have some common elements.

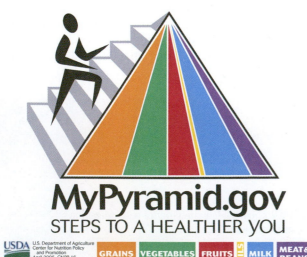

FIGURE 4.12

USDA Food Guide Pyramid.

TABLE 4.1   Basic Food Groups and Their Major Nutrients

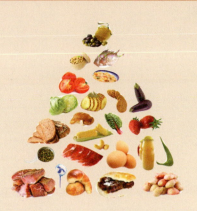

GROUP	EXAMPLES	NUTRIENTS *Supplied by all in food group*	NUTRIENTS *Supplied by some in food group*
Fruits	Apples, bananas, grapes, oranges, pears, kiwi, pomegranate, mango, tomatoes	Carbohydrate Water	Vitamins: A, C, folic acid Minerals: Iron, potassium Fiber
Vegetables	Broccoli, leafy greens, eggplant, green beans, peas, lettuce, potatoes, sweet potatoes, squash	Carbohydrate Water	Vitamins: A, C, E, K, B vitamins except B_{12} Minerals: Calcium, magnesium, iodine, manganese, phosphorus Fiber
Grain products	Breads, cereals, pasta, crackers, tortillas, cookies *Sources*: wheat, oats, rice, quinoa, spelt, amaranth (whole grains are best)	Carbohydrate Protein Vitamins: Thiamin (B_1), niacin	Water Fiber Minerals: Iron, magnesium, selenium
Dairy products	Milk, cheese, yogurt, kefir, ice cream *Sources*: cow, goat, or sheep's milk	Protein Fat Vitamins: Riboflavin, B_{12} Minerals: Calcium, phosphorus Water	Carbohydrate Vitamins: A, D
Meat and vegetarian protein sources	Beef, poultry, fish, eggs, seeds, nuts, soybeans, tofu, legumes (beans)	Protein Vitamins: Niacin, B_6 Minerals: Iron, zinc	Carbohydrate Fat Vitamins: B_{12} thiamin (B_1) Water Fiber

Self-care plans include healthy nutrition, physical fitness, rejuvenation, and stress control. Good body mechanics while performing massage is essential to prevent injury and increase longevity as a massage therapist. Quiet sitting or some other form of meditation helps maintain mental alertness and emotional calm. Taking time for recovery, rest, and relaxation prevents burnout. Good time management is the foundation of putting it all together and making it happen.

Keeping a journal or logbook, especially while putting a self-care plan into place, can help track progress and identify aspects that need to be strengthened. Figure 4.13■ is an example of a page from a journal for tracking a holistic self-care plan.

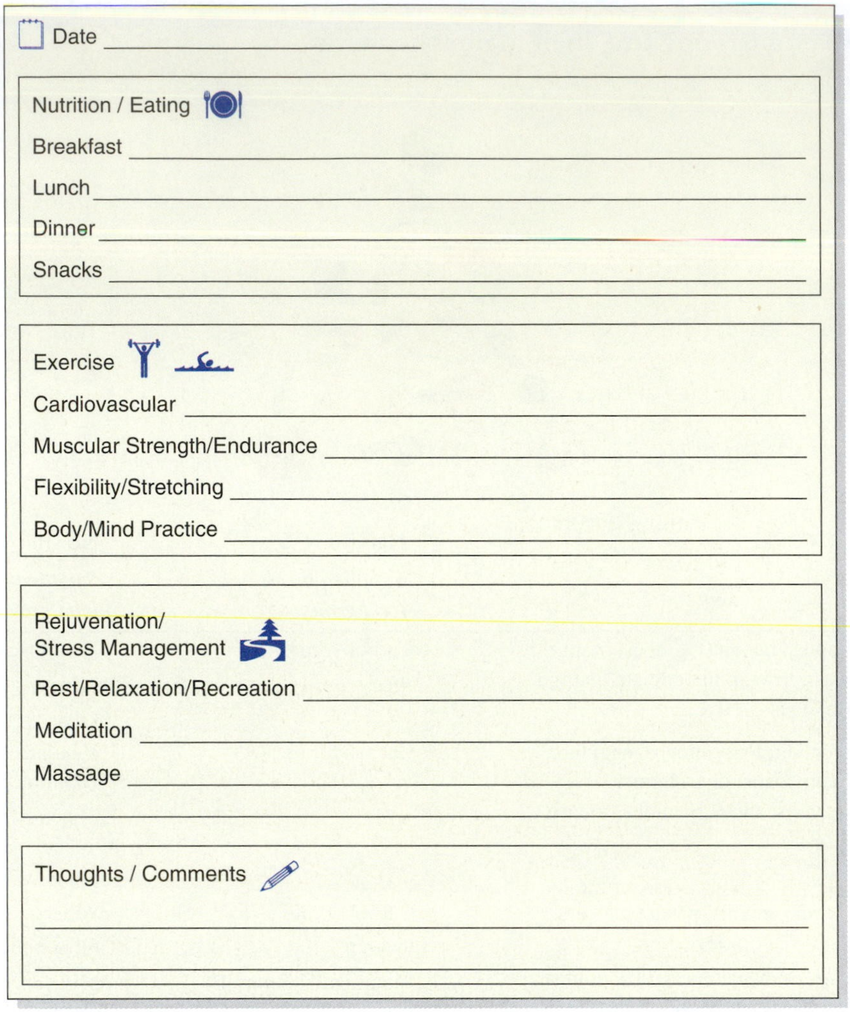

Date _____

Nutrition / Eating 🍽

Breakfast _____

Lunch _____

Dinner _____

Snacks _____

Exercise 🏋 🏊

Cardiovascular _____

Muscular Strength/Endurance _____

Flexibility/Stretching _____

Body/Mind Practice _____

Rejuvenation/
Stress Management 🌲

Rest/Relaxation/Recreation _____

Meditation _____

Massage _____

Thoughts / Comments ✏

_____

_____

FIGURE 4.13

Sample daily log for holistic self-care plan.

CHAPTER HIGHLIGHTS

- Being a massage therapist requires having good body awareness.
  - Body awareness is the ability to sense where your body is in space while at rest and in motion and to coordinate movement with mind.
  - Being centered and grounded are two important aspects of body awareness.
- Skilled touch has four dimensions important to massage therapists: contact, qualities of touch, communication, and palpation.
  - *Contact* refers to the sense presence of the massage therapist's hands on the client's body.
  - *Qualities of touch* are related to contact and vary from soft and gentle to hard and rough.
  - Caring and openness are examples of what can be *communicated* through touch.

- *Palpation* is sensing information about the client through touch and by the feel tissues and movement at joints.
- Physical fitness includes cardiovascular health, muscular strength and endurance, flexibility, and body composition.
  - A basic cardiovascular (CV) fitness profile includes resting heart rate, blood pressure, and cardiovascular endurance.
  - *Muscular strength* refers to a muscle's ability to move a maximum amount of resistance once, while *muscular endurance* indicates the capacity to move against resistance for a number of repetitions over time.
  - Flexibility is the "ability to flex" or the possible range of movement at joints.

- ○ Body composition can be measured using the Body Mass Index (BMI) to determine if you are underweight, normal, overweight, or obese.
- Self-care is taking care of your own well-being while fulfilling family, work, and school responsibilities.
- Body–mind practices such as yoga, tai chi, qi gong, and Pilates develop coordination, body awareness, and concentration.
- Meditation techniques are designed to quiet the mind and enhance the ability to pay focused attention; methods include peaceful abiding and quiet sitting.
- Stress-control strategies include the 3 Rs: adequate rest, relaxation, and recreation; help prevent overload and burnout.
- Time management involves planning a workable schedule; includes setting priorities and eliminating time wasters.

- ○ Plotting out a weekly schedule, and using a daily or weekly planner to keep track of regular and special appointments, events, and deadlines helps get your use of time under control.
- Nutrition refers to the intake of food and drink to nourish the body and mind; includes concepts of nutrients, food groups, and calories.
  - ○ Good nutrition and healthy weight result from balanced eating habits and adequate physical activity.
  - ○ The U.S. government publishes dietary guidelines and sponsors a healthy eating program at www.MyPyramid.gov.
- A holistic self-care plan encompasses the many aspects of well-being, including the physical, mental, emotional, and social.
  - ○ Keeping a self-care log or journal tracks progress and is motivating.

EXAM REVIEW

Key Terms

Match the following key terms to their descriptions. For additional study, look up the key terms in the Interactive Glossary on page G-1 and note other terms that compare or contrast with them.

_____ 1. Body awareness
_____ 2. Body-mind practices
_____ 3. Center
_____ 4. Communication
_____ 5. Contact
_____ 6. Ground
_____ 7. Holistic self-care plan
_____ 8. Nutrition
_____ 9. Palpation
_____ 10. Qualities of touch
_____ 11. Self-care
_____ 12. Skilled touch
_____ 13. Stress-control strategy
_____ 14. Time management

a. The firmness of the earth; having a stable base and connection to a foundation whether standing or sitting
b. The basis of massage; skill in physical contact with clients
c. Related to contact and varies from soft and gentle to hard and rough
d. Taking care of your own well-being
e. Planning a workable schedule
f. The ability to sense where your body is in space while at rest and in motion and to coordinate movement with mind
g. Exercises that require a conscious effort to link what you are feeling to what your body is doing
h. Includes good time management, adequate rest and relaxation, and anxiety reduction techniques
i. Achieved by the contact and different qualities of touch applied during massage
j. Includes all activities that support your development as a massage therapist and minimize factors that lead to illness and injury
k. A focal point or point of organization from which being and movement occur
l. The intake of food and drink to nourish the body and mind
m. Sensing information about the client through touch and by the feel of tissues and movement at joints
n. The sense presence of the massage therapist's hands on the client's body

Memory Workout

To test your memory of the main concepts in this chapter, complete the following sentences by circling the most correct answer from the two choices provided.

1. Knowing where your body is in (space) (time) while it is at rest or in motion is called body awareness.
2. Establishing a connection to the earth through the legs and feet is called being (centered) (grounded).
3. A basic cardiovascular fitness profile includes (regular) (resting) heart rate (RHR).
4. Flexibility is maintained by regular (walking) (stretching).
5. Sensing information about the client through touch and by the feel of tissues and movement at joints is referred to as (intuition) (palpation).
6. (Body–mind) (Cardiovascular) practices such as yoga and tai chi help improve coordination, body-awareness, and concentration.
7. A good meditation posture is sitting in a chair with your back upright and hands resting on the (thighs) (knees).
8. The three Rs of (stress-control) (time management) strategy are rest, relaxation, and recreation.
9. Carbohydrates are composed of sugars and (starches) (fats).
10. In developing a time management schedule, a good rule of thumb is to leave (25–40) (5–20) percent of your time for unplanned or spontaneous activities.

Test Prep

The following multiple choice questions will help to prepare you for future school and professional exams.

1. The point of organization in your body from which being and movement occur is referred to as your:
   a. Body awareness
   b. Physical fitness
   c. Ground
   d. Center
2. The sense of presence of the massage therapist's hands on the client's body during massage should feel:
   a. Deliberate and nervous
   b. Confident and warm
   c. Hesitant and fearful
   d. Full and unsure
3. The capacity to move against resistance for a number of repetitions over time is called:
   a. Cardiovascular endurance
   b. Muscular strength
   c. Muscular endurance
   d. Grounding
4. Palpatory literacy involves the ability to:
   a. Locate specific anatomical structures
   b. Detect normal tissue conditions
   c. Feel abnormal tissue conditions
   d. All of the above
5. The essence of modern meditation techniques is choosing something like a word or object to place attention on, and when the mind wanders, to:
   a. Bring it back to the object of attention
   b. Let it wander
   c. See where it takes you
   d. Change the object of attention
6. Grains, vegetables, fruits, oils, milk, and meat and beans are the basic:
   a. Nutrient categories
   b. Empty calorie sources
   c. Food groups
   d. Amino acids
7. Organic nutrients that the body needs in small amounts are called:
   a. Carbohydrates
   b. Vitamins
   c. Minerals
   d. Sodium
8. Body-mind exercises require a conscious effort to link what your body is doing to:
   a. Verbal instructions
   b. Written instructions
   c. Role models
   d. What you are feeling inside
9. A self-care plan that includes goals for physical, mental, and emotional well-being is called:
   a. Fitness
   b. Focused
   c. Nutritional
   d. Holistic
10. Planning a workable schedule for good time management is a matter of:
    a. Setting priorities
    b. Instant gratification
    c. Finding time wasters
    d. Luck

Video Challenge

Watch the appropriate segment of the video on your DVD and then answer the following questions.

Physical Skills, Fitness, and Self-Care for the Massage Therapist

Holistic Self-Care Plan

1. What methods of developing physical fitness are shown in the video? How do they compare with your physical fitness activities?

2. Identify the different methods of stress control and relaxation shown in the video. How do they compare with your stress-control strategy?

3. What aspects of time management are mentioned in the video? How can you improve time management in your life?

Comprehension Exercises

The following short answer questions test your knowledge and understanding of chapter topics and provide practice in written communication skills. Explain in two to four complete sentences.

1. Define centering and grounding. Why are these concepts important for massage therapists?

2. Describe the basic components of physical fitness. Give an example of how each component can be evaluated.

3. Explain what the Body Mass Index (BMI) measures. What is your BMI score and what does it mean?

For Greater Understanding

The following exercises are designed to take you from the realm of theory into the real world. They will help give you a deeper understanding of the subjects covered in this chapter. Action words are underlined to emphasize the variety of activities presented to address different learning styles and to encourage deeper thinking.

1. Evaluate your level of physical fitness, and fill out the Physical Fitness Profile Form in Figure 4.4 on page 78. Identify your areas of strength and weakness, and set some physical fitness goals.

2. Fill out a time management chart for the rest of this semester or the next. Use the chart in Figure 4.11 on page 85 as an example. Discuss your plan with a study group or classmate, and evaluate it according to the priorities you set for yourself. Note how well it supports your success in the massage school program.

3. For at least 2 weeks, keep a daily log of your self-care activities. Use the form in Figure 4.13 on page 88. Use your increased awareness of holistic self-care to build good habits for a healthier life.

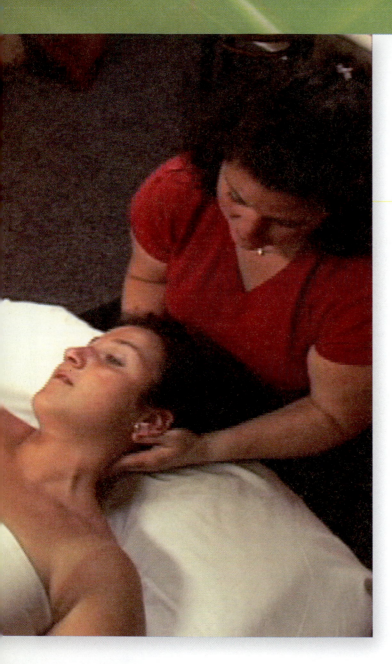

 CHAPTER OUTLINE

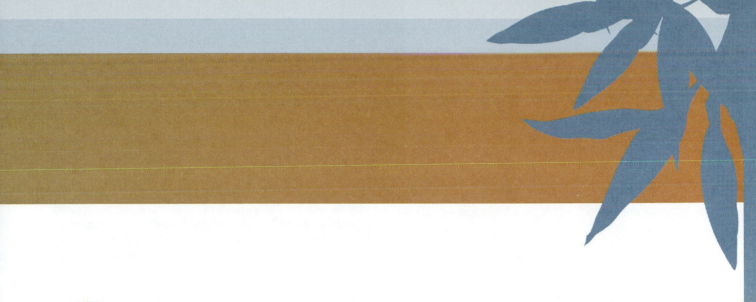

 ## LEARNING OUTCOMES

After studying this chapter, you will have information to:

1. Explain values, rights, and duties as the basis of ethics.
2. Describe ethical standards for massage therapists.
3. Understand the consequences of unethical behavior.
4. Use a decision-making model to address ethical questions.
5. Establish appropriate roles in the therapeutic relationship.
6. Avoid all levels of sexual misconduct.
7. Obtain informed voluntary consent when appropriate.
8. Stop inappropriate client behavior using the intervention model.
9. Stay within the scope of practice of massage therapy.
10. Keep client information confidential.

 ## KEY TERMS

Boundary crossing 103
Codes of ethics 96
Confidentiality 112
Defense mechanisms 102
Dual relationship 103
Duties 95
Ethical decision-making model 98
Ethical dilemmas 98

Ethical judgment 100
Ethical questions 98
Ethics 94
Informed voluntary consent 107
Intervention model 108
Personal boundary 103
Personal temptations 98
Power differential 101

Professional ethics 94
Rights 95
Scope of practice 110
Sexual misconduct 106
Standards of practice 96
Therapeutic relationship 100
Transference 102
Values 94

⊙ MASSAGE *in* ACTION

On your DVD, explore:

- The Ethical Decision-Making Model
- Ethical Judgment
- Roles and Responsibilities
- Informed Voluntary Consent
- Intervention Model

OVERVIEW

Being a mature massage therapist goes beyond having good hands-on skills. Employers and clients expect their massage therapists to behave with honesty and integrity and to uphold the ethical standards of their profession. Clients especially want the people who touch them to be trustworthy and to act in their clients' best interests. But knowing the right thing to do in different situations can be challenging, especially in professional relationships based on touch. The roles and responsibilities are very different from more familiar relationships with family and friends and in other types of work.

The study of ethics, specifically ethics for massage therapists, complements the physical, intellectual, and social skills needed by well-rounded professionals. Understanding the nature of ethics sets the stage for examining ethical standards for massage therapists.

NATURE OF ETHICS

Ethics is the study of moral behavior; that is, determining the *right* thing to do in a specific situation. Ethical behavior conforms to certain values such as honesty and fairness, upholds human rights such as privacy and safety, and reflects the duties inherent in being in a position of power. Ethical codes and standards translate moral values into guidelines for daily living.

Laws are sometimes enacted by governments to enforce ethical behavior. These laws are passed for the protection of the public. However, many behaviors considered unethical are perfectly legal. For example, gossiping about a client may not land you in jail, but it is considered unethical.

Professional ethics is the study of moral behavior relative to a specific occupation such as massage therapist. Because massage therapy falls into the categories of service, helping, and therapeutic professions, standards of behavior are high. Although the first rule is "to do no harm," professional standards also take into consideration what is best therapeutically for the client.

Such standards specify those behaviors which have proven counter-therapeutic and are therefore considered unacceptable by the professional community. In other words, sets of ethical guidelines *encourage* behavior that is most effective therapeutically and *discourage* behavior that is ineffective or therapeutically harmful. (Taylor 1995, p. 5)

Professional organizations develop codes of ethics and standards of practice to clarify the values of the group and serve as references for ethical decision making. These documents contain the collective wisdom of the profession regarding ethical behavior among its members. "Establishing an ethical code is an exercise in self-reflection and clarification of values for those who write, review, and approve such documents" (Taylor 1995, p. 233). See Appendix D on page A-12 for the National Certification Board for Therapeutic Massage and Bodywork (NCBTMB) Code of Ethics and Standards of Practice.

Business ethics concern the commercial aspects of being a massage therapist and the treatment of clients as consumers. Business ethics encompass the areas of advertising, payment policies and procedures, keeping proper licenses, and other business matters. It can be thought of as that part of professional ethics that has to do with having a private practice. Chapter 23, Business Ethics, on page 648 specifically focuses on ethical issues in running a business.

VALUES, RIGHTS, AND DUTIES

Ethical principles are founded on the values, rights, and duties deemed important in society. Professionals apply these factors in determining acceptable conduct in the practice of their work.

Values

Values are principles, traits, or qualities considered worthwhile or desirable. Ethical codes and standards are developed to protect the values that give meaning and direction to the profession. For example, the standard that massage therapists represent their qualifications truthfully stems from the value of *honesty.*

Values that have come to the forefront in the massage and bodywork profession include *compassion,* or the wish to relieve suffering, and *selfless service,* or giving clients' well-being top priority. For example, "refuse any gifts or benefits intended to influence a referral, decision, or treatment that are purely for personal gain and not for the good of the client" (NCBTMB 2008).

Honesty is speaking the truth and avoiding deception, while *integrity* is living up to our values consistently. Being *trustworthy* includes being reliable, honest, and principled.

Equality, fairness, and *nondiscrimination* entail treating others with equal respect and not playing favorites. *Unconditional regard for others* calls for being nonjudgmental and giving our best efforts to everyone regardless of who they are. An item in the NCBTMB Code of Ethics (2008) directs massage therapists "to respect the inherent worth of all persons."

For every positive value, there is an opposite or negative, which is often the thing that catches our attention. People have inner voices or consciences that tell them that something is wrong. For example, you might have an uncomfortable feeling when talking about one of your clients to a friend. Knowing about the principle of *confidentiality* helps you sort out which actions are ethical and which are not.

A better sense of important values can be cultivated by study and discussion. Some values, like honesty, are widely recognized and deeply ingrained. But how these values are applied in a specific profession may not be so obvious at first, like applying the concept of honesty to making health claims for the benefits of massage therapy.

Values provide a moral compass to point the way when we are lost or confused. Having an awareness of the values held by the profession is a prerequisite for making ethical decisions as massage therapists.

Rights

Rights also come into play when discussing ethical behavior. **Rights** are claims to certain treatment or protection from certain treatment. Rights are expected to be honored by others and enforced by standards or laws if necessary. For example, clients have a right to privacy, which is the basis for draping practices and confidentiality policies. They also have a right to freedom from violations such as sexual misconduct. Client rights that play an important part in ethical standards for massage therapists are the rights to privacy, self-determination, and safety.

The client's *right to privacy* is the root of several ethical standards. Draping procedures and the practice of leaving the room while clients are undressing preserve their privacy. Prohibitions against revealing information about clients to others, or *confidentiality,* also protects their privacy. Confidentiality rights related to medical records are protected by law through the Health Information Portability and Accountability Act (HIPAA). HIPAA is discussed in greater detail later in the chapter.

The client's *right to self-determination,* also called *autonomy,* affirms that clients should have the opportunity to make informed choices about what happens to them. Self-determination is protected by standards about massage therapists obtaining informed voluntary consent from clients to perform certain massage techniques or to work in certain body areas. Another is "the client's right to refuse, modify, or terminate treatment regardless of prior consent given" (NCBTMB 2008).

The client's *right to safety* is the basis of hygiene standards and regulations. Clients have a right to expect cleanliness and a germ-free environment in a massage room, as well as that tables and other equipment be in good repair. Also related is the standard that massage therapists "provide only those services which they are qualified to perform" (NCBTMB 2008).

In recent years, the consumer rights movement has led to a crackdown on deceptive business practices and the enactment of a number of consumer protection laws. How these relate to massage therapists is discussed in Chapter 23, Business Ethics.

Massage therapists have rights, too; for example, the right to fair compensation for their work and the right to a safe environment. They have the right to create and enforce policies for their practices. The NCBTMB Code of Ethics recognizes the right "to refuse to treat any person or part of the body for just and reasonable cause."

Duties

Duties or *responsibilities* are obligations to act in a particular way. Duties arise out of being in a certain position in relationship to others or as the result of some action. Massage therapists have duties related to their clients, colleagues, coworkers, employers, and others. Duties reflect moral bonds that are generally recognized in a society and deeply felt as obligations or things that we "ought to" do by individuals. They are intricately related to the values and rights discussed earlier.

A basic duty of massage therapists is to maintain professional boundaries that clarify and preserve the roles inherent in the therapeutic relationship. It is the massage therapist's responsibility to establish good boundaries regardless of what the client wants. This potential dilemma is discussed later in the chapter.

Duties can arise out of the rights of others; that is, if individuals have a right to something, and a massage therapist is in a position to influence what happens to them, then that massage therapist has a duty to protect those rights. For example, given that clients have a right to a safe environment when receiving massage, massage therapists have a duty to keep their spaces clean and remove potential safety hazards.

Duties related to being a health professional include *nonmaleficence* (refraining from harming anyone), *beneficence* (doing good for those in our care), *fidelity* (keeping promises—explicit or implicit), and *veracity* (telling the truth). Causing harm or wrong to someone else calls for *reparations,* while *gratitude* is due when someone is good to us (Purtilo 1993).

Just as with values and rights, there is no finite list of duties for massage therapists. However, the concept of duties is useful when discussing ethical behavior for two reasons. First, duties have the weight of moral obligations. Second, when values, rights, and duties are in conflict, creating an ethical dilemma, critical thinking about such a situation calls for consideration of all sides of the issue, including the duties involved. Table 5.1 ■ lists many of the foundation values, rights, and duties on which ethical principles are based.

TABLE 5.1	The Basis of Ethical Principles for Massage Therapists	
Values	**Rights**	**Duties**
Compassion	**Client**	Beneficence
Equality	Personal respect	Avoid harm
Fairness	Privacy	Professional
Honesty	Self-determination	boundaries
Integrity	Safety	Gratitude
Nondiscrimination	Fair treatment	Veracity
Selfless service	Honest advertising	Reparation
Unconditional regard	Best effort of massage	Fidelity
for others	therapist	Trustworthy
	Massage Therapist	
	Fair compensation	
	Respect	
	Safe environment	
	Practice policies	

found in a need to feel loved and accepted, a need to be right, a lack of assertiveness, or even sloppy bookkeeping. Unexamined personal issues may also trip you up in the therapeutic relationship, for example, transference and countertransference, in which negative or positive feelings toward someone in their pasts are brought into the therapeutic relationship by either the client or therapist. Transference and countertransference are discussed in greater detail later in this chapter.

Self-care in all facets of life lessens vulnerability to unethical behavior. Wellness in the physical, mental, emotional, social, spiritual, and financial realms is a foundation for clear, ethical thinking. Even good time management plays a role, since caregiver burnout can lead to poor judgment when making decisions.

Lack of skill in ethical decision making also leaves one vulnerable. Knowing standards and possessing the ability to apply them in specific situations are very different. It is also harder to think clearly when in the midst of difficult or emotional circumstances. Practicing the steps in ethical decision making in simpler situations is good preparation for the more difficult and complex issues that come up. The process of ethical decision making is explained in more detail in a following section.

VULNERABILITY TO UNETHICAL BEHAVIOR

Almost everyone considers him- or herself a moral, ethical person. However, if people are honest with themselves, everyone can think of instances when they didn't live up to ethical standards, or, in retrospect, would have acted differently (i.e., more ethically) in a given situation. Admitting our human vulnerability and making a conscious commitment to be ethical massage therapists is the first step on the path to building ethical practices.

The next step is to learn about ethical standards in the profession and take them seriously. Ignorance of ethical standards leaves one vulnerable to unethical behavior. Codes of ethics and standards of practice are documents that open the door to discussion of ethical issues in the profession. They should be familiar to all massage and bodywork practitioners. Codes of ethics and standards of practice are discussed further in the next section.

A key principle for behaving ethically is to hold your client's well-being above your personal gain. This principle is sometimes expressed as "selfless service." This does not mean that you work for free, since you have a right to make a living as a massage therapist. It means that when making decisions that might affect your clients' well-being, you do nothing that has the potential to cause them harm, even if for you it means a loss of money, power, or other desirable gain. For example, you do not expose your clients to illness by dragging yourself to work when you are contagious with the flu.

For personal ethical development, it is important to know your weaknesses as well as your strengths. Issues related to money, power, and sex are the usual culprits in unethical decisions. But less obvious roots of unethical behavior might be

ETHICAL CODES AND STANDARDS

Most major professional organizations for massage therapists have published codes of ethics, and some have developed standards of practice. **Codes of ethics** are usually stated in broad terms as general principles that reflect commonly held values. **Standards of practice** are longer, more detailed documents that go into specifics in interpreting ethical principles. These documents can be found on organization websites.

Ethical codes and standards are the products of the collective thinking of a group of professionals. They take into consideration the traditional values and recognized clients' rights related to the profession. These ethics documents are updated from time to time to reflect current issues and new awareness. As ethical understanding evolves, so do the documents that codify the latest thinking on the subject.

Professional organizations organize and display their codes of ethics differently. Some go into more detail than others in a combined codes/standards document. However, the values and clients' rights contained in the codes are very similar. The summary of ethical principles for massage therapists found in Box 5.1● is based on the major common themes from current massage therapy organization codes of ethics.

The summary of ethical principles is a good overview for discussing ethics for entry-level massage therapists. Some items present general principles that can be expanded (e.g., "Give your best effort to each client"), and others describe specific behavior (e.g., "Refrain from alcohol and recreational drugs when performing massage") to give more pointed guidance to students. This list can be used along with other codes and standards in ethical decision making.

BOX 5.1	Summary of Ethical Principles for Massage Therapists

Massage Therapist

1. Give your best effort to each client.
2. Hold your clients' well-being above your own personal gain.
3. Present a professional image.
4. Present your credentials honestly.
5. Perform only those services for which you are trained and qualified.
6. Stay within your legal scope of practice.
7. Refrain from alcohol and recreational drugs when performing massage.
8. Keep licenses to practice massage therapy current.
9. Stay up-to-date in your field by continued education.

Therapeutic Relationship

10. Set clear professional boundaries with clients.
11. Treat all clients equally with courtesy and respect.
12. Honor your clients' physical, intellectual, and emotional boundaries.
13. Practice good draping skills for client privacy and comfort.
14. Get clients' informed voluntary consent for all massage therapy performed and for touching sensitive body areas.
15. Do not perform massage when it is contraindicated for a client.
16. Acknowledge your limitations, and refer clients to other health care professionals as appropriate.
17. Keep your professional and social lives separate.
18. Do not engage in sexual activities with clients, or sexualize a massage session in any way.
19. Keep your clients' information confidential.

Business Practices

20. Do not make claims for massage therapy that are not true or that you cannot reasonably defend.
21. Do not sell or recommend health products or services outside of your area of expertise.
22. Develop written policies about time and money, and make sure clients understand them.
23. Keep the massage room, equipment, and yourself sanitary.
24. Do not solicit tips.
25. Keep accurate client and financial records.
26. Abide by all local and state laws related to your practice.

Based on the codes of ethics of major massage therapy organizations (American Massage Therapy Association—AMTA; American Organization for Bodywork Therapies of Asia—AOBTA; Associated Bodywork and Massage Professionals—ABMP, National Certification Board for Therapeutic Massage & Bodywork—NCBTMB).

Professional ethics are the province of associations, which adopt codes of behavior related to the practice of the profession. These are enforced within the group, usually by disciplinary action against members who violate the accepted code of behavior. Disciplinary actions for ethical code violations generally range from letters of reprimand, to probation, to suspension of membership for a period of time, to cancellation of membership in the organization. The decision usually follows a hearing in which the accused is given the opportunity to defend him- or herself. This enforcement of values within the group is referred to as *self-regulation* within a profession.

Laws, on the other hand, are passed by governmental bodies at the local, state, and federal levels to protect the public from harm or to ensure fair practices. Laws are usually only passed when there is a compelling public reason. Violations of law are determined by a judge or by trial and are punishable by fines, community service, or time in jail.

Some of the ethical principles recognized by professional associations have been given the force of law. An example is the federal HIPAA privacy law that ensures confidentiality of medical records. This law lifts the ethical principle of confidentiality to a legal status and specifies what that means under federal law.

In addition, laws licensing massage therapists usually have sections dealing with ethical issues. For example, the Illinois Massage Licensing Act, Section 45 Grounds for Discipline prohibits "advertising in a false, deceptive, or misleading manner," and "making any misrepresentation for the purpose of obtaining a license." If convicted of an offense, a massage therapist licensed in Illinois can be assessed a fine, be put on probation, or have his or her license suspended or revoked. Disciplinary actions are matters of public record. Currently 42 states plus Washington, DC, in the United States have similar provisions for regulating massage therapists. Whereas violations of association codes of ethics can result in censure by the organization a person belongs to, violations of the law can lead to losing a license, paying fines, and/or spending time in jail.

Another connection between professional ethics and law is found in legal cases where the standard of behavior is based on the accepted practices in the profession. An example would be a massage therapist who is being sued for injury to a client during a massage session. If by professional standards the massage therapist should have known about a contraindication for the massage technique used, or if it was outside of the therapist's scope of practice, then the judgment may be in favor of the person making the complaint. In other words, the judge may use a recognized professional standard to decide a case when no specific law pertains to the situation.

ETHICS AND LAW

Ethics and law are related but are not the same. Both ethics and law are based on values, rights, and duties recognized by a community, but they are enacted and enforced in different ways by different entities.

ETHICAL DECISION MAKING

Massage therapists make ethical decisions every day. Most are small, uncomplicated issues such as keeping client records secure, staying within the scope of practice, and giving their

CRITICAL THINKING

Examine a code of ethics or standards of practice document for massage and bodywork therapists. Analyze the underlying values, rights, and duties for each item.

1. Do some values, rights, or duties appear more than others?

2. Are there any relationships among these values, rights, and duties?
3. What does your analysis say about the ethical principles most important to massage therapists?

---

best effort to each client. Other situations can be complex and pose a dilemma about the best way to act. The ethical decision-making model explained below provides a step-by-step method of sorting out the answers to ethical questions and dilemmas.

Ethical Questions and Dilemmas

Ethical issues are most often framed like questions; for example, "Is it ethical to. . . .? **Ethical questions** are frequently followed by qualifiers; for example, "Is it ethical to (do something), if (this is the situation)? Many ethical questions can be answered by reviewing a code of ethics or standards of practice to find the profession's view of the subject. However, as in all complex human interactions, the variables of the situation can influence a decision and make it a judgment call.

It is important to distinguish between ethical questions and legal questions. As mentioned before, something may be quite legal, but unethical by professional standards. However, if something is illegal, it is automatically unethical since an all encompassing ethical principle is to abide by all local, state, and federal laws related to the practice of massage.

Ethical dilemmas occur "when two or more principles are in conflict, and regardless of your choice, something of

value is compromised" (Benjamin and Sohnen-Moe 2003, p. 9). Put another way, no matter what you do, some harm will result or some good not happen. The ethical dilemma is in selecting the lesser harm or greater good.

Ethical dilemmas are in a different league than **personal temptations** to act unethically. For example, it may be a personal temptation to mix your social and professional lives, and that may be a personal dilemma ("What am I going to do?"), but it is not an ethical dilemma ("What is the most ethical action to take?"). Those are two different questions.

Temptations often involve time and/or money. Working when sick, skimping on hygiene, not completing session notes, constantly arriving late for appointments, and keeping a client who should be referred to another health professional are all personal temptations. These should take a backseat to doing what is best for the client.

The Ethical Decision-Making Model

The **ethical decision-making model** is a step-by-step process of thinking through an ethical question or ethical dilemma. It involves critical thinking, since you are analyzing the situation, and taking into consideration your own motivations and biases. Both external standards, like codes of ethics and laws, and internal standards, like your own sense of right and

---

PRACTICAL APPLICATION

An important way to learn ethical behavior and how to navigate ethical issues is by observing others who model ethical conduct. Interview a practicing massage therapist about his or her most memorable ethical issue or dilemma. Listen not only to the massage therapist's narrative, but also observe the body language while this person describes his or her ethical decision and its consequences.

Questions to consider:

1. What was the ethical question?
2. What were the most important factors in the situation?
3. What were the consequences of the therapist's actions?
4. Do you think this massage therapist handled the issue appropriately and made the best ethical decision? Why?

BOX 5.2	Ethical Decision Making Model

Step 1 Define the ethical question or ethical dilemma.
"Is it ethical to . . . (do something), if . . . (if this is the situation)?"
"Is it more ethical to . . . (do something), or to . . . (do something else)?"

Step 2 Determine if this is also a legal issue.
Consumer protection laws
Privacy laws (e.g., HIPAA)
Licensing laws
Other laws (e.g., zoning)

Step 3 Identify values, rights, and professional standards that apply.
What values or rights are involved?
Is this situation mentioned in a code of ethics or standards of practice?
Does an employer policy apply to the situation?

Step 4 List the people who might be affected by the outcome of the decision.

Step 5 List alternative courses of action.

Step 6 Identify the most important values, rights, standards, and other considerations.
Is there an overriding principle that applies (e.g., do no harm, selfless service, abide by laws)?

Step 7 Identify your own motivations or interest in the outcome, and any personal temptations.

Step 8 Consider advice from others.
Consult colleagues or former teachers or an association
Consult coworkers or work supervisors
Consult a professional supervisor

Step 9 Select the course of action that maintains the highest values, or that results in the greatest good with the least harm. Do the right thing.

Step 10 Evaluate the consequences of your decision, and learn from your experience.

wrong, play a part. It is essentially a problem-solving process for an ethical situation.

A 10-step ethical decision-making model is summarized in Box 5.2•. Although the model is listed in steps, implying a linear sequential process, it is best thought of as a logical process that proceeds in an orderly manner. Information may be gathered, and steps revisited, at any time. For Step 9, selecting the course of action, it is useful to review the information gathered in Steps 1 through 8 in order to have a full picture of the situation.

The first step in ethical decision making is to define the ethical question or ethical dilemma. Remember that some choices are not ethical questions if no moral principle is involved. It might simply be a business decision or choice between two plans of action. Frame the situation by filling in the blanks: "Is it ethical to . . . (do something), if . . . (this is the situation)?" or "Is it more ethical to . . . (do something), or to . . . (do something else)?"

Next, determine if this is also a legal issue. Some situations are covered by consumer protection, privacy, licensing, zoning, or other laws. The overriding principle of abiding by local, state, and federal law may apply.

Identify the values, rights, and professional standards relevant to the situation. For example, is it a matter of honesty, integrity, beneficence, fairness, or privacy? Look through the professional code of ethics and standards of practice for massage therapists to see if the ethical question is covered. If the situation is not specifically mentioned, is there a relevant principle, value, or right that can be applied in this case?

List the people who might be affected by the decision. They might include yourself, the client, the client's family or friends, your family and friends, coworkers, employers, or landlords. Remember that actions can have ripple effects.

List alternative courses of action. Include all possibilities even if you reject them later, since they may suggest new approaches you had not thought of at first. Consider creative solutions to the problem that preserve important values or rights.

Identify the most important values, rights, standards, and other considerations. This is especially important in ethical dilemmas where competing values or rights are at stake. An overriding principle, such as "do no harm" or "abide by the law," may apply.

Before you choose an action, identify your own motivations or interest in the outcome. Look at your personal temptations related to time, money, power, or social advantage. Remember the overriding principle to "hold the client's well-being above your own personal gain."

Consult with others to get a more objective view of the situation, generate more options for actions, and check your own biases and temptations. Sometimes just talking it through with someone else can help you see things more clearly. People familiar with professional ethics and who have experience in the field are especially good to consult. They may have dealt with similar problems in the past and can help you sort out alternatives.

In the end, you have to decide what to do. Base your choice on the action you think will maintain the highest values, or that will result in the greatest good with the least harm. Then do the right thing. Knowing what to do and actually doing it are two different things. Get emotional support if you need it.

Finally, learn from the outcome. The end result will help you judge whether your decision was the best. Analyze the consequences of your decision. Did it uphold the values or rights as you thought it would? Was there something you didn't take into consideration that you should have? Were there any surprises? Would you do it differently next time?

Learn from your successes and your mistakes. You will get better at making ethical decisions with experience. Examples of ethical decision making related to the therapeutic relationship are discussed later in the chapter.

CASE FOR STUDY

Twila and the Flu

Twila works as a part-time massage therapist at a day spa. She woke up on Tuesday feeling weak and sick to her stomach. She was running a mild fever. Several people in her family had the flu over the past week, and she thought she might be coming down with it, too. Twila is a responsible person and did not want to miss the four massage appointments scheduled for the day. She also did not want to lose the income if she stayed home from work.

Question:

Is it ethical for Twila to take some over-the-counter medicine to reduce her symptoms and help her get through her massage appointments?

Things to consider:

- Is this situation covered in a code of ethics or standards of practice for massage therapists?

- What is Twila's responsibility to her clients in terms of their health and safety?
- Who might be affected by Twila's decision?
- What are the "worst case" and "best case" scenarios?
- What are her alternative courses of action?
- What would her supervisor advise her to do?
- What are the most important considerations in this situation?
- What decision would result in the greatest good with the least harm?

Your Reasoning and Conclusions:

_____

_____

_____

_____

DEVELOPMENT OF ETHICAL JUDGMENT

The development of **ethical judgment,** that is, consistency in making good ethical decisions, is a lifelong process. Just being aware that decisions might have ethical consequences is important. Ethical behavior is strengthened by continued learning, including learning from successes and mistakes. Ethical judgment improves with critical thinking and evaluating results.

Codes of ethics can be framed and hung in offices to show a commitment to ethics in a practice. Keeping a code of ethics and standards of practice for massage therapists on file for reference makes it easier to consult when an issue arises.

Some licensing laws and certification programs require continuing education in ethics for renewal. Classes in ethics are offered through massage schools and by professional associations. Classes in ethics for health professionals and business ethics classes offer a wider perspective on the subject.

Networking with other massage therapists in professional associations increases awareness of ethical issues that come up in practices and consequences of certain actions. Reading professional journals helps massage therapists keep up-to-date on the latest thinking about ethical issues. Reports on individual cases dealing with ethics can be instructive.

Clinical supervision involves consultation about different issues that come up in the therapeutic relationship. It is done in a formal setting with a specially trained supervisor. Clinical supervision is an idea borrowed from mental health

professionals that is catching on in the massage and bodywork community. Supervision sessions are an opportunity for massage therapists to process what is happening in their practices and their experiences with clients.

Group supervision of practitioners in similar circumstances can be especially useful. "In a group setting clinical supervision undertakes 4 functions: (1) addressing the relationship issues that arise between clients and practitioners; (2) functioning as a support group for the participants; (3) serving as a forum for didactic instruction on important psychological concepts (such as projection, transference, countertransference); and (4) training the participants in supervisory skills so that they feel confident continuing this helpful type of coaching by themselves at a later date without a supervisor" (Benjamin and Sohnen-Moe 2003, p. 243).

Good ethical judgment comes with learning and experience. Mistakes will most likely happen along the way. There might be errors in judgment or lapses of moral behavior. The important thing is to make a commitment to ethical behavior as a massage therapist, learn from successes and failures, and re-energize your ethical sense from time to time throughout your career.

THE THERAPEUTIC RELATIONSHIP

The **therapeutic relationship** begins when a client seeks greater well-being through massage from a particular massage therapist, and the massage therapist agrees to provide that service. It is a special relationship based on specific roles and responsibilities.

In nonmedical settings such as spas and health clubs, the relationship is *therapeutic* in a more general sense in that the goals are the improved health and well-being of the client. In clinical settings, the therapeutic relationship may be part of the treatment itself and a key to the healing process. "The most healing aspect of a series or course of massage therapy sessions, especially in the longer term, can be the relationship between client and therapist. The massage therapist can facilitate this through building a trusting relationship by being non-judgmental, reliable, and supportive" (Greene and Goodrich-Dunn 2004, p. 17).

Therapeutic relationships are very different from social relationships (e.g., between friends) and have a deeper dimension than simple business transactions. The therapeutic relationship in massage therapy is more intimate and personal than relationships in most commercial settings because clients are seeking help for their personal well-being from a service based on touch.

The intimacy in massage therapy is *physical* since it involves caring touch; *emotional,* as feelings of support and closeness develop; and *verbal* because there is disclosure of personal information. However, the appropriate intimacy in the therapeutic relationship is one-way.

> Practitioners physically touch their clients, allow them to disclose thoughts and feelings, and offer both verbal and physical support. The therapeutic relationship's function is not for the clients to do the same for the practitioner. (Benjamin and Sohnen-Moe 2003, p. 112)

There is also an inherent **power differential** between massage therapists and their clients in therapeutic relationships. That is, massage therapists have more power in the relationships by virtue of their training and experience, and by their being in a position of authority (Figure 5.1■). It is similar to other familiar relationships such as teacher–student, boss–employee, and nurse–patient. "Even if the massage therapist does not want or seek out power, clients still ascribe power to the therapist because power *is an intrinsic element in the therapist–client relationship*" (Greene and Goodrich-Dunn 2004, p. 13).

> Our clients come to us in pain or in need of help. Just by showing up at our offices, they make themselves vulnerable. They are hurting, and we are the authority. Even though they may not be conscious of it, we can become a doctor/parent figure in their eyes. Our responsibility is to meet that vulnerability with respect and kindness. (McIntosh 2005, p. 17)

The massage therapist, therefore, has a fiduciary responsibility in the therapeutic relationship. Fiduciary is a legal term used to describe a relationship in which person A has

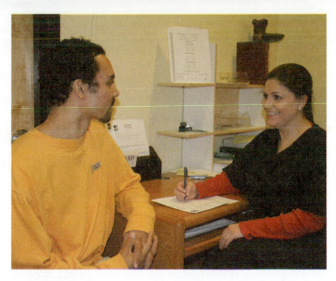

FIGURE 5.1

There is an inherent power differential between massage therapists and their clients.

placed a special trust in person B, who is then obligated to watch out for person A's best interests. In other words, the client puts a special trust in the massage therapist, who is then obligated to look out for the client's best interests.

There are both explicit and implicit agreements in the therapeutic relationship. Explicit agreements are spoken or written, and include things such as pricing information, payment policies, cancellation policies, and the type of massage and bodywork provided. Implicit agreements are those commonly understood for this type of relationship, which may be unspoken and unwritten. These include being on time, doing no harm, acting in the best interest of the client, keeping client information confidential, providing a safe environment, and staying within the scope of practice.

When a client comes for massage, there is an implicit understanding that the massage therapist is upholding the standards of the profession. These standards are found in codes of ethics and standards of practice documents that outline what is expected of competent and ethical massage therapists.

As in any relationship, human interactions in the therapeutic relationship can be influenced by psychological factors. Massage therapists can learn to recognize those factors at work in their relationships with clients. In addition to improving the quality of their therapeutic relationships, awareness of the potential influence of psychological factors can help massage therapists make better ethical choices. Two factors with great potential to influence therapeutic relationships are transference and countertransference.

Transference and Countertransference

Transference occurs when a client transfers negative or positive feelings toward someone from his or her past into the therapeutic relationship. The feelings transferred would typically be about an authority figure such as a parent, teacher, or other person important to the client when he or she was growing up. Transference has been called "a kind of spell generated by one's own psyche," with the result that the client "cannot see the therapist and/or the therapy as they actually are" (Greene and Goodrich-Dunn 2004, p. 55).

A client who is experiencing *positive transference* projects good feelings toward the massage therapist. Positive transference can contribute to the therapeutic relationship by opening the door to acceptance, cooperation, and trust.

However, positive transference can also blind the client. For example, the client might place the massage therapist on a pedestal, thinking the therapist to be more knowledgeable than he or she actually is, or try too hard to please the therapist, or be overly submissive. A client in positive transference might give inappropriate gifts, or want to step over the line into a social or romantic relationship. The danger in positive transference is the temptation for massage therapists to relax professional boundaries, or to lose sight of who they (the massage therapists) really are.

Negative transference, or the projection of negative or bad feelings into the therapeutic relationship, can cause more obvious problems. A client thinking that the massage therapist doesn't like her, feeling like she just can't please the massage therapist, trying to argue with the massage therapist, or thinking that the massage therapist doesn't know what he or she is doing, all work against the massage therapy itself. If it is a case of transference, these negative thoughts and feelings have nothing to do with the reality of the situation with the massage therapist, but have been transferred from another relationship in the past.

Because massage therapists are not trained as psychotherapists, cases of positive and negative transference may be hard for them to identify. Suspect transference if you are uncomfortable with a client's behavior and you can say to yourself, "Her reaction doesn't make sense," or "This is not about me," or "This is not about this therapeutic relationship." When going through an ethical decision-making process as described earlier in the chapter, take the possibility of transference into consideration.

The best strategy when faced with a client's transference is to maintain your objectivity through critical thinking and getting someone else's viewpoint. Do not try to analyze your client's behavior, which is outside of your scope of practice. Keep good professional boundaries.

Countertransference occurs when massage therapists transfer positive or negative feelings toward others from their pasts into the therapeutic relationship. In this case, the massage therapists are under a "spell," and do not see the clients or the therapeutic situations as they really are. Trying too hard to please clients, relaxing professional boundaries against better judgment, and feeling more knowledgeable or powerful than they really are exemplify countertransference by massage therapists.

Being grounded in your role as a massage therapist, and in your own thoughts and feelings, helps minimize the effects of countertransference. Because it is an unconscious response, however, countertransference is difficult to detect in ourselves. Personal awareness, peer advice, and professional supervision can help sort out issues of transference and countertransference.

Defense Mechanisms

Defense mechanisms are behaviors or thoughts that help us cope with unwanted feelings such as fear, anxiety, guilt, and anger. Both massage therapists and clients bring their defense mechanisms into the therapeutic relationship. These defenses can be amplified when receiving bodywork. Common defense mechanisms are projection, denial, repression, displacement, and resistance. Although there are subtle differences in these mechanisms, their common purpose is to protect the psyche from unwanted feelings.

Projection occurs when someone imputes to someone else a behavior that they themselves are doing, or a feeling that they are having. For example, a massage therapist who is attracted to a client might suppress that feeling within him- or herself, and instead perceive the client as seductive. Or a client may think of a massage therapist as a "know it all" instead of acknowledging his or her own feelings of superiority.

Denial is blocking out the existence of an unwanted feeling or refusing to recognize the reality of a situation. For example, a massage therapist may not recognize that a valued client is taking advantage of him or her by frequently canceling at the last minute. Fear of losing the client may create a situation of denial. Or because of fear, a client may be unwilling to admit to him- or herself the pain he or she is feeling, and therefore not give useful feedback about pressure during a massage session.

Repression involves burying unwanted feelings, for example, by erasing them from conscious memory or not allowing them to be felt. Repressed feelings can cause anxiety and depression unless and until they surface and are resolved. Either the massage therapist or client may have repressed feelings from past events or trauma.

Displacement is reacting to a feeling generated by a person or situation by acting out toward someone else or in different situation. For example, bringing anger from something that happened at home or in your private life into the workplace is displacement. You're angry with your best friend, and you take it out on a coworker—that is displacement.

Resistance occurs when a client refuses to cooperate or fails to participate in plans for his or her well-being. Resistance is usually unconscious and can take many forms, such as being unable to relax during a massage, missing appointments, or forgetting suggestions for self-massage at home. Resistance would be something that comes up with regular clients, or those coming for a series of massage sessions as treatment for a condition.

The resistance might have nothing to do with the massage therapist, but could be due to some other factor, such as failure to commit to the therapeutic process. It is not massage therapists' place to judge their clients' behavior, but just noticing resistance and bringing up observations with clients can be enough to bring it to a conscious level for resolution.

Defense mechanisms can cause problems in therapeutic relationships because they tend to deflect attention from the reality of a situation. The key is not to eliminate them (a near impossible task because they are habitual behaviors), but to recognize them when they surface and minimize their negative impact. Seeing through defense mechanisms can help massage therapists build healthier therapeutic relationships and avoid unethical behavior.

ROLES AND BOUNDARIES

Both massage therapists and clients have specific roles to play in the therapeutic relationship. The massage therapists' general role is to apply their training and experience within their scope and standards of practice to help clients meet their health goals. The clients' general role is to provide relevant information, participate cooperatively in massage therapy sessions, abide by policies and procedures, and pay the fees.

Professional boundaries maintain these roles within therapeutic relationships. As explained in detail in Chapter 3, Professional and Personal Development, on page 51, these include physical, emotional, intellectual, sexual, and energetic limits on what will and will not happen between the massage therapist and client. It is the massage therapist's responsibility to create the framework that defines these boundaries, for example, with policies, rules, procedures, and the whole massage environment into which clients walk. Practical aspects of maintaining professional boundaries are discussed further in sections on dual relationships, sexual misconduct, and scope of practice found later in this chapter.

In addition to professional boundaries, massage therapists and clients have personal boundaries that must be respected. A **personal boundary** is a limit established by a person to maintain his or her own integrity, comfort, or well-being. For example, a client may ask a massage therapist not to touch his feet or not to use oil with a fragrance. Or a massage therapist may prefer handshakes to hugs or refuse to use petroleum-based oil. These are legitimate personal boundaries.

The NCBTMB Code of Ethics (see Appendix D, Code of Ethics and Standards of Practice, on page A-12) directs massage therapists to "respect the client's boundaries with regard to privacy, disclosure, exposure, emotional expression, beliefs, and the client's reasonable expectations of professional behavior. Practitioners will respect the client's autonomy." That includes the client's right to set personal boundaries.

"Stepping over the line," or boundary crossings and violations, can be ethical matters if they harm the therapeutic relationship or the individuals involved. A **boundary crossing** has been defined as "a transgression that may or may not be experienced as harmful," while a *boundary violation* "is a harmful transgression of a boundary" (Benjamin and Sohnen-Moe 2003, p. 39). So whether a boundary transgression is a crossing or a violation is a matter of degree and a matter of consequences. If a boundary crossing is not experienced as harmful, then it does not rise to the level of a violation, although it can be problematic. Boundary crossings can be annoying, intrusive, hurtful, or just uncomfortable. For example, a client answering a cell phone during a massage session might be annoying. A massage therapist may ask a client a question that seems intrusive or too personal. Or a client may be uncomfortable with a massage therapist massaging her neck but says nothing about it. These are examples of boundary crossings but probably not violations.

Violations leave one with a sense of being *violated,* a much stronger feeling than just feeling annoyed or uncomfortable. Integrity is compromised in some way, and the agreement within the therapeutic relationship is broken. Examples of boundary violations include a client who learns that the massage therapist talked to someone else about his or her medical condition without permission; a massage therapist whose client calls him or her at home to ask for a date; or a massage therapist touching a part of the body he or she was asked not to touch or for which there is an implicit agreement to avoid, such as a woman's breasts.

All professional and personal boundary violations are unethical, since some harm has been done. Even unintentional harm is still harm and may have adverse consequences. At minimum, there will be negative consequences to the therapeutic relationship, and there may also be personal, professional, employment, or legal repercussions.

According to McIntosh (2005), the majority of client complaints about massage therapists fall into two general categories of boundary violations: (1) blurring professional and social roles, and (2) going beyond their expertise and training.

DUAL RELATIONSHIPS

A **dual relationship** means that in addition to the therapeutic relationship, there are other social or professional connections between a client and a massage therapist. This applies to clients who are also family members, friends, coworkers, neighbors, fellow organization members, service providers such as accountants and plumbers, or any other additional relationship.

In some cases a dual relationship can enhance a therapeutic relationship. This works if the two people involved are emotionally mature and able to keep their roles in different situations separate. For example, the familiarity between friends can give the massage therapist greater insight into what the client-friend is experiencing. However, a friend who becomes a client would have to agree to the role of a client during massage sessions and be comfortable with the appropriate professional boundaries set for that time. The same would apply to the massage therapist, who would have to set aside his or her own needs and wants and keep to a professional role during the massage time.

In reality, most dual relationships have problematic dimensions. Issues are magnified if the power differential between the client and massage therapist varies in different situations. For example, in a client–neighbor dual relationship, the massage therapist holds a power role during massage sessions, but is an equal outside of the sessions. Or in a client–family member situation, family dynamics may come into play and affect the therapeutic relationship.

Financial or economic arrangements outside of the massage therapy relationship have their own potential problems. Two common scenarios involve bartering and employment. Bartering for services, such as accounting or website design, can be a mutually beneficial arrangement as long as both parties feel that they are getting a fair deal and follow through on their agreement. The exchange might be hour for hour, or session for session, regardless of time involved. Or for an accountant, it might be six massage sessions for doing the massage therapist's taxes for the year. A verbal contract for bartering needs to be crystal clear to avoid someone feeling taken advantage of. Exchanging invoices for services can reduce the potential for misunderstandings.

Being a massage therapist to a boss or an employee also calls for very clear boundaries, since the power differential changes with the different roles. In the boss–client scenario, the boss is in a position of authority in the workplace, while during massage therapy, the practitioner is in charge. As long as both people can accept their roles in the different situations, the arrangement can work. However, it can become awkward if something happens that crosses boundaries, such as your boss asking you for information about your coworker while he or she is getting a massage.

Perhaps the most difficult lines to draw are those about socializing with clients. Degrees of socializing range from a cup of tea before a massage session, to meeting for coffee outside of the massage setting, to belonging to the same club or organization, to attending events together. Ethical issues that might come up during socializing are failing to protect other clients' confidentiality and offering too much self-disclosure about the massage therapist's personal life.

As mentioned previously, when people known in social settings become clients, strong professional boundaries can minimize problems. However, when a current client initiates a social invitation, a massage therapist must take into consideration the possibility of transference and consequences for the therapeutic relationship. The risk may outweigh any benefits, and romantic or sexual socializing would be unethical, as is explained in more detail later in this chapter. A massage therapist whose personal social circle is heavily populated by clients is taking advantage of his or her practice for the wrong reasons. It is obvious that the variety of dual relationships is endless, and each one needs to be thought through carefully.

Evaluating Dual Relationships

For a massage therapist, deciding whether to enter into a dual relationship with a client, or to continue one already established, requires evaluating the potential benefits and risks. As the person in authority in the therapeutic relationship, it is the massage therapist's responsibility to make decisions in the best interest of the client. It is unethical to enter into or continue a dual relationship if there is high potential of harm to either party or if the therapeutic relationship will be compromised.

One factor for consideration is the nature of the relationships involved. Are there conflicting power differentials? Do they involve money, friendship, love? Are they of short or long duration? Another factor is the maturity of the people involved. Are they good at keeping boundaries and cooperative in respecting limits? Do both parties understand the complexities involved? Experience says that both people involved must agree to the arrangement, understand the potential pitfalls, and be willing to end the dual relationship if necessary.

Motivations for entering into the dual relationship need to be scrutinized. Does one party benefit at the possible expense of the other? Is there a possibility of transference or countertransference clouding the reality of the situation? Professional standards can help in certain situations, for example, the special case of sexual relationships, which is discussed in the next section.

The potential effects of the dual relationship on the therapeutic relationship are important to consider. Can both parties maintain their respective roles as massage therapist and client in relation to massage sessions?

"Worst case" and "best case" exercises are useful for making decisions about dual relationships. For example, a best-case scenario for a dual relationship in which the massage therapist hires a mechanic/client to repair his or her car is that the car gets fixed satisfactorily, and the therapeutic relationship continues unaffected. A worst-case scenario might be that the mechanic damages the engine and refuses to make fair compensation. Negative feelings from that scenario are likely to affect the therapeutic relationship, and possibly damage it beyond repair. The question to ask is this: Is hiring the client worth the risk, or can someone else do the job just as well without the complicating factor?

A good question for a massage therapist to ask him- or herself is, "If this dual relationship does not work out . . . am I willing to lose this person as a client? Or, am I willing to lose this person as a beautician (or accountant, friend, etc.)? Am I willing to jeopardize my other job (or membership in an organization, etc.)?" It is important not to underestimate the possible consequences of the dual relationship, but to enter into such relationships with thoughtfulness and clear vision. This is another case where discussing the situation with someone familiar with the complexities of dual relationships would be useful, for example, with a colleague, supervisor, or other professional.

REALITY CHECK

DENISE

YOLANDA: I find it hard to stick to boundaries in my relationships with clients. I'm just an outgoing person who wants to be friends with people. A client asked me out for coffee the other day because we're both interested in environmental issues. If I didn't already have other plans, I might have gone. How do you handle this kind of situation?

DENISE: I really try to keep my professional and personal lives separate. I've learned from experience that socializing with clients isn't best for my practice or my social life either. When clients walk in the door, I focus on meeting their needs and goals within massage therapy. It's true that sometimes you pass up the opportunity to know some really interesting people better, but keeping good boundaries helps me stay clear about what I am doing here as a massage therapist. And I've found plenty of other friends outside of my professional life. Think of a polite way to refuse this kind of invitation like "Thank you for asking, but this isn't a good time."

SEXUAL RELATIONSHIPS

There are two general scenarios for professional relationships involving sexual partners. One is when a current client wants to become romantically or sexually involved with the massage therapist (and vice versa), and the other is when a current spouse or romantic friend becomes a client. These are two very different situations with different ethical considerations.

First of all, it should be noted that sexual activity with a client is strictly prohibited by professional standards and by massage therapist licensing laws. The NCBTMB Code of Ethics states that massage and bodywork practitioners should "refrain, under all circumstances, from initiating or engaging in any sexual conduct, sexual activities, or sexualizing behavior involving a client, even if the client attempts to sexualize the relationship."

That means no dating or even socializing with clients who have romantic intentions. The power differential in the therapeutic relationship and the possibility of transference or other psychological factors having an influence make it unethical to enter into such a relationship. It can be dangerous emotionally for one or both parties and distorts the therapeutic relationship.

The NCBTMB Standards of Practice, however, offers a solution for special cases that would minimize the dangers involved (see Appendix D, Code of Ethics and Standards of Practice on page A-13). It states that the massage practitioner should "refrain from participating in a sexual relationship or sexual conduct with a client, whether consensual or otherwise, from the beginning of the client/therapist relationship and for a minimum of six months after the termination of the client-therapist relationship." It also makes allowances for pre-existing relationships. The general ethical principle

CASE FOR STUDY

Rebecca and the Movie Invitation

Rebecca graduated from massage school and got a job at a local health club working part time. She likes to exercise and stay fit, so the setting was perfect for her. Dan comes to the health club to work out several times a week and gets a massage regularly. He enjoys Rebecca's massage, so lately he has been going to her exclusively. They are both single and like each other. Dan asked her to go with him to a movie they both wanted to see.

Question:

Is it ethical for Rebecca to go with Dan to the movie?

Things to consider:

- Does the health club have a policy about staff dating members?
- Is this situation covered in a code of ethics or standards of practice for massage therapists?

- Who might be affected by this decision?
- What are the "worst case" and "best case" scenarios?
- What are alternative courses of action?
- What are the most important considerations in this situation?
- What might Rebecca's motivation be for accepting the invitation? Declining it?
- What would a former teacher advise Rebecca to do?
- What decision would maintain the highest standards?

Your Reasoning and Conclusions:

_____

_____

_____

_____

is to end the therapeutic relationship and wait for a period of time before beginning the romantic/sexual relationship. Waiting clearly separates the roles in time and provides perspective on the situation.

Developing a romantic relationship with someone special, who just happens to be a former client, can be perfectly ethical. However, dating a current client or regularly dating former clients is clearly considered unethical by professional standards.

If someone who is *already* a spouse, significant other, boyfriend or girlfriend, or a romantic or sexual partner later becomes a client, clear boundaries are a must. In addition to power issues coming into the therapeutic relationship, there is the potential for the association of massage therapy with sexual activity. During time set aside for massage therapy, there is no place whatsoever for sexual activity.

Engaging in sexual behavior during a time set aside for massage therapy, and especially on a massage table or in a space set aside for massage practice, is confusing on many levels even if the person is a spouse. Why? For the massage therapist, his or her professional role strictly prohibits sexual activity with a client, and so the situation is a blurring of roles. For the client–spouse, the association is made between massage therapy and sex, so he or she may feel uneasy, often unconsciously, about what his or her partner-therapist is doing with other clients. A clear separation of massage therapy and sexual activity in time and space is the only workable approach.

SEXUAL MISCONDUCT

Sexual misconduct involves any sexualizing of the relationship between a massage therapist and a current client. Sexual misconduct can occur before, after, or during a massage session and can be perpetrated by the massage therapist or by the client.

Forms of sexual misconduct range from those involving speech and body language to inappropriate touch to sexual contact to sexual assault. Box 5.3● lists categories and examples of sexual misconduct encountered in massage practices.

The degree of severity of sexual misconduct ranges from relatively minor to very severe. How serious the offense is depends on the intentions of the initiator, the experience of the victim, whether physical contact is involved, and the resulting physical or psychological harm.

The most common forms of sexual misconduct involve flirting, suggestive comments about a person's body or appearance, and off-color jokes or innuendo. Discussion of the sexual performance, preferences, or problems of either party sexualizes the situation. Seductive behavior is an open invitation to misconduct.

Sexual misconduct by a massage therapist also includes exposing clients' genitals or women's breasts. Good draping technique can prevent accidental exposure. Watching a client undress or dress, except in cases of advanced age or disability when assistance is needed, is also inappropriate. Respecting a client's privacy is essential.

BOX 5.3   Forms of Sexual Misconduct

Categories of sexual misconduct that grow progressively more serious:

- No touch involved: suggestive speech and body language
- Inappropriate touch involved
- Direct sexual contact
- Sexual assault

Examples of sexual misconduct of clients and massage therapists that grow progressively more serious:

Client

Flirting
Use of slang or crude words referring to the genitalia
Jokes with sexual content or innuendo
Talk about personal sexual experiences or problems
Seductive speech
Exposes his or her genitalia; woman exposes her breasts
Asks for sexual favors

⇓

Touches the massage therapist on thigh or buttocks seductively
Stimulates him- or herself sexually during massage

⇓

Assaults the massage therapist sexually; rape

Massage Therapist

Flirting
Use of slang or crude words referring to the genitalia
Jokes with sexual content or innuendo
Talk about personal sexual experiences or problems
Seductive speech
Exposes client through improper draping
Watches client dress or undress
Sexual fantasies about a client

⇓

Touches sensitive areas (e.g., upper thigh) without informed consent
Positions or braces the client using face or front of pelvis
Uses chest, head, face, lips, hair, pelvis, or breasts to massage a client

Outside of massage session

Dating or romantic socializing with a client
Sexual activity outside of massage setting

During massage session

Touches client's genitals or nipples
Fails to intervene when client sexually stimulates him- or herself
Stimulates him- or herself sexually during massage
Sexually stimulates client during massage

⇓

Assaults the client sexually; rape

Because of the physical contact involved, misconduct related to touch is especially harmful. Inappropriate touch by a massage therapist is a gross violation of the therapeutic relationship. Guidelines for appropriate touch include:

- Use only hands, forearms, elbows, and feet to massage a client.
- Never use the chest, head, face, lips, hair, pelvis, or breasts to massage a client.
- Use only knees, shoulders, lateral hip, and lower leg for bracing or stabilizing.
- Never use the face or front of the pelvis for bracing or stabilizing.
- Never massage in the nipple or genital areas.
- Never touch any part of your body to the client's genital area.
- Get informed consent to massage high on the thigh, around breast tissue, the buttocks, anywhere near the genitals, and on the abdomen.

(Adapted from the *Report of the Sexual Abuse Task Force of the AMTA Council of Schools,* January 1991)

Informed Voluntary Consent

Informed voluntary consent is a process used by massage therapists to get the client's permission to touch areas that may have sexual associations (e.g., high on the thigh, buttocks, abdomen), or areas out of the scope of general care (e.g., ear canal, nasal passages, mouth, anal canal, and breast tissue). For some areas, the NCBTMB Standards of Practice further require *written* consent and that the treatment be part of a plan of care (Standard VI: Prevention of Sexual Misconduct).

The words used to describe this process tell the story of its key elements. It is *informed* in that the client receives information about the proposed action and the reasons for it. It is *voluntary* in that the client freely agrees to the proposal. Finally, there is *consent* or permission by the client who exercises his or her right to self-determination.

The process of informed voluntary consent has five parts. First, the massage therapist informs the client about the nature and duration of the proposed action, that is, the body part to be touched, the technique to be used, or other relevant factors. Second, the massage therapist gives reasons for the proposed action. Third, the massage therapist describes what the client should expect. Fourth, the massage therapist gives the client the option to say no, either before beginning or at any time during the application. Fifth, the massage therapist explicitly asks permission to touch the area. This process is summarized in Box 5.4●.

For areas that are generally within the scope of a regular massage, but that may have sexual associations, verbal consent is usually adequate. Informed voluntary consent in these cases may be simple. For example, to an athlete complaining of tight thigh muscles, you might say, "I'd like to work the tendons to the muscles in your thighs closer to their points of insertion. That's a little higher than you're used to me working. But it should help those muscles loosen up better. I'll

---

BOX 5.4   Informed Voluntary Consent

Obtain permission to touch areas with sexual association (e.g., buttocks, inner thigh) and areas outside of the norm for massage (e.g., nasal passages, mouth). Touching the genitals is never allowed even with consent.

Step 1 Inform the client about the nature and duration of the proposed action; for example, the body part to be massaged, the massage techniques to be used, the amount of time involved.

Step 2 Explain the reasons for the proposed action; for example, the goals and therapeutic benefits expected.

Step 3 Describe what the client should expect to feel.

Step 4 Invite the client to agree to the goals and methods for the proposed action; the client has complete freedom to accept or reject the proposed action, or any part of it, before the massage is applied or anytime during the application.

Step 5 Ask permission to touch the area, and to begin the massage application; client signs written consent if applicable.*

*Written consent is advised for all massage treatments involving nasal passages, mouth, ear canal, anal canal, and women's breasts.

---

adjust the drape to make sure you're covered. The inner thigh can be sensitive so it may feel a little strange to you. If it gets uncomfortable at any time, just let me know. Is that all right with you? Shall I go ahead and start?" If the client says yes, remain aware of nonverbal communication such as facial expression and muscle tightening that may signal discomfort. That could also signal "no" or "I changed my mind."

For body areas out of the general scope of massage, the ethical requirements are stricter. Special training is necessary to enter body orifices like the nose, mouth, and anus, and to massage the breasts. In addition, written consent must be obtained. Massage techniques for these areas are not usually taught in entry-level programs in the United States, or may be advanced treatments taught in longer, medically oriented programs. Working in these areas may also be outside of a massage therapist's legal scope of practice under his or her license.

The NCBTMB Standards of Practice require that massage treatments in these sensitive areas be performed within a *plan of care*. That means that there should be a medical reason for the special massage techniques, and the massage is part of an overall treatment plan. This also implies that other medical professionals may be aware of the massage treatment. The standards stop short of requiring a prescription from a doctor. However, such a prescription would validate the therapeutic necessity of the procedure and provide justification if needed. There are legal as well as ethical issues to consider.

Sexual Misconduct by a Client

Although the vast majority of clients respect the professional nature of massage therapy, massage therapists should be prepared to handle sexual misconduct by a client.

This is a matter of safety as well as ethics for the massage therapist.

The importance of establishing a professional setting and boundaries cannot be emphasized enough. If the massage therapist is fuzzy about his or her boundaries, the client will also be unclear about where to draw the line on behaviors like flirting, jokes, and more overt sexual behavior.

Depending on where you work (e.g., spa, health club, clinic, office at home), and the amount of confusion in your city, town, or local area about the difference between legitimate massage and sexual massage, you may want to be more explicit about your standing. For example, when making appointments, you may want to state up-front, "You understand that this is therapeutic and not sexual massage." Or you may wish to highlight a similar statement in the policy document that clients sign at their first appointment.

Client misconduct on any of the levels shown in Box 5.3● should be addressed with directness and assertiveness. A client intent on sexualizing the massage will often begin testing the waters with minor misconduct such as flirting and then escalate the sexual behavior over time. Stopping the misconduct early will clearly draw the boundary of acceptable behavior.

Minor misconduct can be addressed by clarifying boundaries. For example, "Seth, this is a professional setting. Please don't tell a joke like that again." Or "Barbara, I appreciate the invitation, but I am declining because socializing like that with clients can lead to problems in our relationship here." Or "Ricardo, you understand that as your massage therapist, I cannot go on a date with you. It is against our professional standards." If the client is mature and respects your professionalism, then that should be enough.

Clients looking for sexual gratification might come right out and ask for it. They might use euphemisms such as "Do you give a *full* massage?" (with a vocal emphasis on *full*). Or "Do you give the 'happy ending'?" If that comes up before the massage, an assertive statement about your professional standards will usually send the client looking somewhere else. If it happens during the session, use the intervention model explained in the next section.

A client, either male or female, may become sexually aroused during a massage session with no prior intention of that happening. This might occur either in a cross-gender or same-gender session. While there is no exact formula for dealing with the situation, there are some guidelines to consider.

One possibility is that a technique that the massage therapist is performing, the body area he or she is massaging, or a combination of the two is causing an arousal response. If this is the case, changing the technique, tempo, or area being massaged can interrupt the process and the arousal may subside. Whether to talk to the client about the incident is a judgment call. It may be an opportunity to explain that sexual arousal can be a short-lived physiological response, and it need not be interpreted as deliberate or improper. However, it should be avoided if possible, interrupted if it occurs, and never acted on during massage therapy.

If a man has a partial or full erection during a massage session, it may or may not be necessary to intervene. If he shows no signs of embarrassment or sexual intent, it may be an innocent physiological response as described previously, and no formal intervention is necessary at that time. If he acts uncomfortable or embarrassed, even though he has not behaved inappropriately in any way, it is best to talk to him about it and assure him that you understand the physiological response involved. However, if he has made suggestive comments or other sexual overtures, touches himself, or asks you to touch him inappropriately, then you are ethically obligated to intervene and stop the session.

More extreme forms of sexual misconduct may also be illegal. Cases of assault, battery, gross indecency, and threatening behavior by clients should be reported to the local police. Massage therapists who have been victims of illegal client misconduct have been known to take their clients to court. This helps protect massage therapists and others in the community from becoming future victims of the perpetrator.

Intervention Model

The **intervention model** is a useful tool to address misconduct or suspected misconduct by clients. A seven-step approach is presented in Box 5.5●. For minor misconduct, an abbreviated version of the model may be all that is necessary. For more severe misconduct, all seven steps are recommended.

First, stop the massage session or interrupt the behavior, using assertive verbal and body language. Assertive behavior signals that you are competent and in charge. If misconduct occurs during a massage session, remove your hands from the client's body and step away from the table. You want the client's full attention. Address the client calmly but firmly by name, and make a statement about why you are intervening. For example, say something like, "Peter, we need to talk about what just happened." Or "Vanessa, I'd like to talk about what you just said."

Next, describe the behavior you are concerned about. Be as specific as possible. For example: "That was the second time your hand brushed my leg. It seems to be intentional." Or "You keep removing the drape and exposing yourself." Or "You continue talking about your sexual relationship with your husband."

Ask the client to clarify his or her behavior, if appropriate. For example: "Are you trying to sexualize this massage?"

BOX 5.5   Intervention Model—Response to Client Misconduct

Step 1 Stop the session using assertive behavior.
Step 2 Describe the behavior you are concerned about.
Step 3 Ask the client to clarify the behavior.
Step 4 Restate your intent and professional boundaries.
Step 5 Evaluate the client's response.
Step 6 Continue or discontinue the session as appropriate.
Step 7 Document the situation and discuss it with a trusted colleague.*

*Assault, battery, gross indecency, and threatening behavior should also be reported to the local police.

PRACTICAL APPLICATION

The following client situations involve setting professional boundaries. With a friend or study partner, practice what you would say in these situations to maintain professional boundaries.

Responding to a client who:

- Invites you out for social time
- You want to hire to do your taxes
- Is habitually late
- Talks through the whole massage session

- Asks about another client's health
- Tells off-color or ethnic jokes or uses profanity

1. How did you feel during each role-playing exercise?
2. Was your verbal and nonverbal communication about your professional boundaries clear?
3. How could you modify what you said to make it clearer?
4. What are some other boundary-setting situations in which it would be useful to rehearse your response?

Or "Are you looking for professional help with your sexual problems with your spouse?"

Restating your intent and professional boundaries may be all that is needed to get things back on track. For example, you can state, "This is a nonsexual massage, and you must stay draped at all times." Or "Sexual problems are outside of the scope of massage therapy, and I am not a psychotherapist. Please keep the conversation related to massage." Or "Touching me that way is not all right with me. Please stop."

Then evaluate the client's response. If you believe that the client will keep the reinforced boundaries, and you are comfortable and feel safe, you may continue the massage. If the client repeats the misconduct, or, in spite of what he or she says, you still feel uncomfortable or unsafe, you should terminate the session. Trust your intuition. This is a judgment call. You have a right to a professional, safe, and comfortable environment.

If you are in a public facility such as a spa or clinic, you are less vulnerable to misconduct. If you have a private practice in an office or in your home, or are at a client's home or in a hotel, you are more vulnerable. Have an emergency plan in place including contacts, phone numbers, and an escape route. If you fear for your safety, leave the office or house and go somewhere people can help you.

Finally, document your experience either in the client's file or in a separate incident report file. Remember that clients have a right to see their personal files, and anything written in them should be descriptive (not interpretive) and professional. Other massage therapists who are scheduled with the client will appreciate knowing about what happened.

In terms of self-care, massage therapists who have experienced an incident of sexual misconduct by a client, especially one involving the intervention model, should talk about it with a trusted friend, colleague, or supervisor. Talking helps a person analyze and process the situation, which may have been upsetting. Getting it out in the open also helps to objectify the incident and use it as a learning experience.

RELATIONSHIPS IN SCHOOL

Massage therapy students have the potential for dual relationships with classmates, teachers and administrators, practice clients, and clients in student clinics and at outreach sites. Each of these situations deserves some careful thought. While some of these ideas were introduced in Chapter 3, Professional and Personal Development, they are discussed more fully here.

Classmates often get to know one another well during the course of a massage program. Relationships among classmates have some similarities to relationships with clients. Although these are not therapeutic relationships by a strict definition, they are special relationships based on giving and receiving massage and involve knowledge of personal information about the people in class. Classmates become somewhat vulnerable to one another, and a level of trust is established. Friendships also develop among classmates, and these are dual relationships with their own dimensions. Being a student of massage therapy is very different from other vocational and academic programs because of the intimate contact inherent in the learning situation.

There are implicit agreements among classmates involving confidentiality, trust, and respect just like in the therapeutic relationship. Box 5.6● lists some of the important ethical aspects of relationships among classmates. It is a matter of integrity that ethical principles related to the therapeutic relationship carry over into massage school classmate relationships.

As in any school setting, friendships and socializing between students and teachers or school staff is a double-edged sword. Learning may be enhanced through informal interactions; on the other hand, the inherent power differential can cause problems similar to problems in dual relationships between clients and massage therapists. In this case, students are in a position of lesser power. It is the teacher's or staff member's responsibility to maintain appropriate social boundaries with students. Students can also recognize and avoid problems by limiting such socializing to official school events and group activities.

BOX 5.6	Ethical Principles Regarding Relationships with Classmates

To promote trust, respect, and harmony, and to avoid unethical behavior, classmates agree to:

1. Treat all classmates with equal respect, and avoid cliques and exclusive social groups during class time.
2. Keep personal information, including medical information, about classmates confidential, and refrain from gossiping about classmates with other classmates and with family and friends.
3. Respect classmates' privacy and modesty in hands-on technique classes while dressing and undressing, and by using proper draping.
4. Practice massage therapy techniques with care and attention to classmates' well-being, and respond promptly to their feedback about pressure, pain, and other concerns.
5. Observe precautions and contraindications with classmates regardless of a technique assignment, and consult with the teacher for necessary modifications to practice with a specific classmate.
6. Use informed voluntary consent as with any client.
7. Seriously consider the possible impact of transference and other psychological factors in relationships with classmates, and refrain from a sexual relationship with a classmate until after graduation.
8. Report to school personnel about personally experienced or suspected cases of unethical behavior, especially inappropriate touching, intentional nudity, and other sexual misconduct of classmates during class time and practice sessions outside of class.
9. Do not ask or expect a classmate to lie, cheat, or cover up unethical behavior for another classmate.

Another dual relationship situation occurs when students become massage therapy clients of teachers. These relationships can be problematic, especially for the teacher-massage therapist who may have conflicting roles in the two settings. The positive and negative aspects of such a relationship need to be weighed before entering into it.

It is helpful to remember that after graduation, the relationships between graduates and teachers and school staff are more equal. Waiting to develop other relationships with teachers and school staff is much safer after graduation. It is wise to know and obey school policies about dual relationships between teachers and students.

A third type of dual relationship encountered by students is with family and friends who agree to be practice clients. Thinking of these people as special kinds of clients, rather than as "practice dummies" or "guinea pigs" will help students understand how they should be treated. Practice clients should receive all the respect and care due to paying clients in the future. Practice time offers the opportunity to learn how to maintain professional boundaries and to internalize professional standards. Your practice clients will appreciate and respect the level of professionalism that you show during practice sessions.

Finally, providing massage therapy to the general public at outreach sites and in student clinics is usually a student's first encounter with "real" clients. Even though students may not be paid for these services since the experience is part of their education, these are real clients in every sense of the term, and all professional standards apply.

SCOPE OF PRACTICE

Massage therapists are required by their ethical standards and by law to stay within their scope of practice. **Scope of practice** means the range of methods and techniques used in a profession or by a professional, which may also include their intention in performing them (e.g., relaxation or treatment of a medical condition). Scope of practice is defined by professional organizations and licensing laws, often in their official definitions of massage therapy.

The scope of practice for massage therapists generally includes various soft tissue manipulation techniques, joint movements, and hydrotherapy. Different systems or modalities fall under the general scope of massage therapy, for example, trigger point therapy, polarity therapy, and lymphatic massage. A more broadly defined scope of practice might also include massage with mechanical and electronic devices, energy bodywork, relaxation techniques, and physical exercises.

The scope of massage therapy as taught in the United States today does not include "chiropractic adjustments" of the spine and other joints. It also excludes psychotherapy, nutrition, and methods designated exclusively for other professions by law (e.g., skin care by estheticians). Scope of practice can change over time; for example, colon therapy (colonics) was once within the scope of Swedish massage, but is now a separate profession.

A massage therapist's personal scope of practice is limited ethically by the extent of his or her training, that is, massage therapists "will provide only those services which they are qualified to perform" (NCBTMB Code of Ethics 2008). For example, it would be unethical to accept clients for physical rehabilitation if a massage therapist's training was primarily relaxation oriented.

Scope of practice in any particular state, province, or country is defined by licensing or other laws. Massage therapists are prohibited from diagnosing medical conditions. For example, according to the Illinois licensing law, the purpose of massage is "to enhance the general health and well-being of the mind and body of the recipient" and "does not include the diagnosis of a specific pathology" (Illinois Massage Licensing Act [225 ILCS 57/] 2003). Even if massage therapists are well trained in a certain method, it might be outside of their legal scope of practice under their particular licensing law.

In its grounds for discipline, the Illinois Massage Licensing Act includes "practicing or offering to practice beyond the scope permitted by law or accepting and performing professional responsibilities which the licensee knows or has reason to know that he or she is not competent to perform" (Section 45). Massage therapists could face probation or lose their massage licenses if it is determined that they are practicing beyond their scope.

It is noteworthy that massage is within the legal scope of practice of several other licensed professions. Nurses, physical therapists, and athletic trainers typically use a limited amount of massage as part of the scope of their work. Cosmetologists and barbers are allowed to use massage during facials, manicures, and pedicures. However, the title *massage therapist* is usually restricted to those with professional training and credentials in massage therapy.

Some massage therapists are trained and licensed in more than one profession, for example, nurse–massage therapists. Other common professional combinations are massage therapist and chiropractor, athletic trainer, physical therapist, physical therapy assistant, psychotherapist, colon therapist, esthetician, or cosmetologist. Individuals with more than one license need to keep good boundaries about which "hat" they are wearing (i.e., which role they are playing) in a specific setting or with a specific client. When working under a license, a professional must keep within that particular license's legal scope of practice.

Staying in Bounds

To stay within their scope of practice, massage therapists need to understand two things. First, the legal scope for massage therapy in the specific jurisdiction, and second, the personal scope dictated by their training and experience. Keep a copy of the licensing law under which you practice handy for reference. Read the definition of massage therapy or scope of practice section carefully to understand what is allowed and not allowed under the law in your area.

Do not give advice to clients in areas outside of that scope, and refer clients to the appropriate professionals when their goals or conditions are outside of your scope. Three areas that massage therapists need to be especially clear about are their limits related to treating clients with musculoskeletal injuries and other pathologies, giving nutritional advice, and psychotherapy.

When clients come for massage with physical complaints such as pain or limited movement, it is the massage therapist's responsibility to determine if massage is indicated or contraindicated. Remember that the first principle is to "do no harm." Always ask clients if they have seen medical providers for diagnoses of their complaints. A medical diagnosis can tell you whether massage might do some good, or whether it should be avoided.

For undiagnosed musculoskeletal injuries accompanied by severe pain, deformity, or acute inflammation (redness, swelling, pain), it is best to refer clients to their health care providers or to an emergency room for evaluation. Symptoms for other pathologies that might be detected by massage therapists include skin diseases such as cancerous moles, tumors, and misaligned vertebrae or ribs.

Do not verbally speculate about what you think is going on, especially using medical terms. While it is acceptable to observe things like swelling, redness, limited movement, or a client's level of pain, it is inadvisable to use diagnostic terms like *second-degree sprain, plantar fasciitis,* or *cancer.* Putting a label on a set of symptoms is considered diagnosis, and medical diagnosis is not within the scope of practice of massage therapists.

When clients' needs are within the scope of massage therapy, but not within your personal scope, refer clients to another massage therapist who does have the appropriate training and experience. Remember that you can widen your personal scope by getting advanced training and certifications.

Giving nutritional advice, including suggestions about food supplements such as vitamins is outside of the scope of massage therapy. It may be tempting to share with clients your personal beliefs and practices in the area of nutrition. But remember that to clients, you are a person of authority, and they may take what you say as expert advice. Do not say things like "You should try this . . ." or, "Take two of these each day, and your joints will feel better."

You could use a qualifier like, "You might want to ask your doctor about . . . ," or "You might want to read the research about . . . ," or "Other clients have reported good results with . . . ," to point them in a direction that you think might be helpful. You can also share information such as an article or pamphlet, but avoid seeming like you are telling a client to do something specific outside of your area of expertise.

Massage therapists sometimes increase their incomes by selling food supplements or other products. It is unethical to pressure massage clients to buy anything you are selling, especially if it has the appearance of a prescription.

Mental and emotional wellness is another area in which scope of practice is important to define. When does listening to clients' emotional problems, which may also relate to their physical stresses and illnesses, step over the line of scope of practice? Or as Deane Juhan puts it in the Foreword to *Beyond Technique: The Hidden Dimensions of Bodywork,* what is the difference between "practicing professional psychology and the responsible handling of a range of psychological issues that are likely to emerge in the course of any bodywork practice?" (Kisch 1998).

The massage therapist's role is to provide massage, which is fundamentally a hands-on therapy. As clients relax during massage and let down their defenses, buried emotions may surface. In the course of a massage session, massage therapists may provide emotional support, listen to a client's concerns, or just be there when a client becomes emotional during a session.

The proper approach is to be supportive while not becoming too involved or trying to help the client resolve his or her feelings by talking. When discussing the client's emotional or mental issues becomes the focus of massage sessions, or the client looks to the massage therapist to resolve psychological issues, the scope of practice has been exceeded. Boundaries must be drawn "between intelligent, compassionate support on the part of the bodyworker and the recognition of the need for further discussion, clarification, and possible referral to various other forms of therapy" (Juhan in Kisch 1998).

Similar to not diagnosing physical pathologies, massage therapists should not diagnose psychological pathologies such as posttraumatic stress disorder, depression, bipolar disorder, disassociation, and psychotic episodes. These are specific medical diagnoses. Massage therapists can, however, recognize symptoms and refer clients to mental health professionals when appropriate.

CASE FOR STUDY

Samantha and the Nutritional Supplements

Samantha is a massage therapist who works in a spa and has built a regular clientele among the spa customers. She has a side business selling nutritional supplements, some of which are advertised as aids to losing weight. Sara, one of Samantha's regulars, is overweight and has expressed an interest in finding a good weight-loss plan.

Question:

Is it ethical for Samantha to mention the nutritional supplements and offer to sell them to Sara?

Things to consider:

- Does selling nutritional supplements fall under Samantha's scope of practice as a massage therapist?
- Are there different roles for Samantha as massage therapist and Samantha as sales representative for the supplements?
- How does the power differential in the therapeutic relationship impact this situation?
- Does the spa have a policy about staff selling their own products?

- Is this situation covered in a code of ethics or standards of practice for massage therapists?
- Is there potential for causing harm? For doing good?
- What are alternative courses of action?
- What are the most important considerations in this situation?
- What might Samantha's motivation be for selling the product to Sara?
- What would a former teacher advise Samantha to do?
- What decision would maintain the highest standards?

Your Reasoning and Conclusions:

_____

_____

_____

_____

Some forms of bodywork (e.g., Hakomi and Rosen Method) are specifically designed to help clients resolve psychological issues. These certified practitioners are highly trained in their approaches, and mental and emotional problems are within their scope of practice.

Education and Home Care

It is outside of the scope of practice of massage therapists to give prescriptions, sometimes abbreviated *Rx*. *Prescription* is a medical concept that implies a command on the part of the person making the prescription. Rx implies "do this" or "take this medication" and is sometimes called an "order." Prescriptions are written instructions that patients take to the pharmacy or to another health care professional. Doctors typically prescribe medications and sometimes physical therapy or even massage therapy. Prescriptions are given by doctors for medical conditions and may be paid for by insurance companies.

Massage therapists, on the other hand, provide information and education. They make suggestions to clients about home care for conditions within their scope of practice. For example, a massage therapist might show a client a self-massage technique for recovery after running, or a stretch to help relax and elongate a certain muscle group. Therapists may suggest an ointment for stiff joints or taking advantage of the whirlpool at the health club. Massage thera-

pists do not give prescriptions for topical applications or anything taken internally.

This careful use of words is very important for clarity about scope of practice. Massage therapists do not prescribe, but do offer information, education, and suggestions for home care.

CONFIDENTIALITY AND HIPAA

Confidentiality is an implicit agreement between massage therapist and client, that is, there is an understanding and trust that the massage therapist will not reveal personal or medical information about the client to others without the client's permission. This principle is based on the client's right to privacy.

Confidential information includes what is written on health history forms, what is discussed in massage sessions, and observations about the physical, mental, and emotional health of the client. Even mentioning to someone else that a certain person is a client can be considered a breach of confidentiality. It is unethical to use people's names in advertising without their permission, especially celebrities or people prominent in the community. Gossiping about a client's personal life is a serious breach of trust.

The NCBTMB Code of Ethics states that practitioners must "safeguard the confidentiality of all client informa-

CASE FOR STUDY

Jason and His Former Teammates

Jason has accepted some of his former teammates from high school as massage clients. They have kept in touch over the years and get together periodically to watch basketball games. One of these clients, Bill, is a very sociable person. During every appointment, Bill wants to talk to Jason about what's going on with the others. Bill knows some of them come for massage and that Jason has probably seen them more recently than he has.

Question:

Is it ethical for Jason to discuss his other clients with Bill?

Things to consider:

- Is this situation covered in a code of ethics or standards of practice for massage therapists?
- What is Jason's responsibility to his other clients in regards to confidentiality?
- What aspects of this dual relationship are problematic?

- Who might be affected by Jason talking to Bill about other clients during massage sessions?
- What if he just listened to what Bill had to say?
- What are the "worst case" and "best case" scenarios?
- What are alternative courses of action?
- What are the most important considerations in this situation?
- What might Jason's motivation be for talking about their mutual friends to Bill?
- What would a former teacher advise Jason to do?
- What decision would maintain the highest standards?

Your Reasoning and Conclusions:

_____

_____

_____

_____

tion, unless disclosure is required by law, court order, or is absolutely necessary for the protection of the public." In some states, licensed massage therapists may have responsibility for reporting cases of abuse of minors and the elderly.

In 1996, the U.S. Congress passed the Health Insurance Portability and Accountability Act (HIPAA) to protect the privacy of medical records. HIPAA requires health care providers to inform patients/clients about their privacy rights and how their information will be used. Providers must get permission in writing to contact insurance companies and other third parties interested in the health records.

Providers must implement procedures to ensure the confidentiality of records, and train employees to comply. In an office or clinic with more than one employee, a person must be designated as responsible for seeing that privacy policies are followed.

Patients/clients have the right to see their records and obtain copies upon request. They may ask for corrections to records if they find mistakes.

Patient/client records must be secured, and only those who need to see them should have access. For example, hard copies of records should be kept in locked files,

PRACTICAL APPLICATION

It is the responsibility of massage therapists to protect their clients' rights to confidentiality, privacy, and safety. The following three activities explore ways that you might protect clients' rights in your practice.

1. Develop a written statement of policies and procedures related to confidentiality of client information. Include elements required by HIPAA rules for clinical and office situations. Visit the HIPAA website (www.hhs.gov/ocr/hipaa) for details on the applicable rules.
2. Research the legal responsibility of licensed massage therapists in your state to report suspected cases of child,

spousal, or elder abuse. Discuss your ethical responsibility in these cases. Identify the agencies to which these reports would be made. How does the principle of confidentiality relate to these situations?

3. Research how and to whom to report a massage therapist whom you suspect is doing something unethical. When is it appropriate to make such accusations? What steps do you take to ensure that you approach the situation ethically and protect yourself legally? After you've developed your answers in writing, discuss them with a group of classmates or a study partner.

preferably in isolated records rooms, and electronic files should be protected by passwords on office computers. Patients/clients must give written consent for the use and disclosure of information for treatment, billing, and other health care operations.

Client records in a massage therapy office may or may not fall under HIPAA. More clinically or medically oriented practices, especially those that keep records electronically and that take insurance payments, are more clearly subject to

HIPAA requirements. In any case, HIPAA offers practical guidelines for ensuring client confidentiality, and massage therapists are encouraged to follow them.

HIPAA is administered by the U.S. Department of Health & Human Services (DHHS), and enforcement and complaints are handled by the DHHS Office of Civil Rights (OCR). Information about HIPAA can be found on the HHS website (www.hhs.gov/ocr/hipaa).

CHAPTER HIGHLIGHTS

- Ethics is the study of moral behavior; that is, determining the "right" thing to do in a specific situation.
  - Professional ethics is the study of moral behavior relative to a specific occupation such as massage therapist.
  - Business ethics concern the commercial aspects of a massage practice.
- Values, rights, and duties provide the foundation for ethical principles.
  - Values are principles, traits, or qualities considered worthwhile that serve as a moral compass.
  - Rights are claims to certain treatment or protection from certain treatment.
  - Duties are obligations to act in a particular way.
- Building ethical practices starts with acknowledging human vulnerability to unethical behavior. This vulnerability can be minimized by making a commitment to ethical practices and learning about ethical standards in the profession.
- A key ethical principle is selfless service or holding your client's well-being above your own personal gain.
- Two overriding ethical principles are *do no harm* and *obey the law.*
- Professional organizations develop codes of ethics and standards of practice that are updated periodically to reflect current thinking in the field related to ethics.
  - Ethical standards are enforced within organizations through disciplinary action against members who violate the standards.
- Some ethical principles are given the force of local, state, or federal law.
  - Violators of laws can be fined, lose their licenses, or end up in jail.
- Ethical questions can be framed in this way: "Is it ethical to . . . (do something), if . . . (this is the situation)?"

- An ethical dilemma occurs when two values or rights conflict.
  - Personal temptations to act unethically should not be confused with true ethical questions or dilemmas.
- The ethical decision-making model is a step-by-step process of thinking through an ethical question or dilemma. It involves critical thinking, making ethical choices, and analyzing the consequences of the final decision.
- Development of ethical judgment is facilitated through having professional standards ready for reference, continuing education classes, professional networking, and clinical supervision.
- The therapeutic relationship between a massage therapist and client is based on specific roles and responsibilities.
  - There is an inherent power differential between massage therapists and their clients, with the massage therapist in the position of authority and trust.
  - Massage therapists have a fiduciary responsibility to act in the client's best interests.
  - The therapeutic relationship involves both explicit and implicit agreements, and the massage therapist is expected to uphold the standards of the profession.
- Psychological factors can influence the therapeutic relationship.
  - Transference and countertransference.
  - Defense mechanisms such as projection, denial, repression, displacement, and resistance.
  - Being aware of these psychological factors and their impact helps build healthier therapeutic relationships and avoid unethical behavior.
- It is the massage therapist's responsibility to ensure that professional and personal boundaries are respected.

- ○ Boundary crossings may be annoying or uncomfortable.
- ○ Boundary violations are crossings that cause harm.
- Dual relationships between massage therapists and clients should be avoided or entered into only after evaluating the potential benefits and risks. They can work only if both parties are emotionally mature and able to maintain appropriate roles in the therapeutic relationship.
- When an already established sexual partner becomes a client, it is important to enforce professional boundaries during massage sessions.
- Sexualizing the relationship with a current client is highly unethical. Professional standards require ending the therapeutic relationship and waiting for a period of time before beginning a sexual relationship with a former client.
- Sexual misconduct ranges in severity from relatively minor to severe, and includes flirting, suggestive comments, jokes, discussing sex, seductive behavior, inappropriate touching, and sexual contact.
- Use the intervention model to deal with suspected sexual misconduct by a client.
  - ○ The intervention model includes interrupting the behavior, describing it, asking for clarification, restating your nonsexual intent, evaluating the client's response, and deciding whether to continue the session or to end it.
  - ○ Afterward, the massage therapist documents the incident in writing, and for self-care, discusses it with a friend or colleague.
- ○ Illegal misconduct by clients should be reported to the local police.
- Informed voluntary consent is used to get a client's permission to touch him or her in certain areas.
  - ○ Five parts of informed voluntary consent are informing, explaining, describing, agreeing, and consenting.
- Relationships in school include those with classmates, teachers and administrators, practice clients, and student clinic clients. Ethical principles related to the therapeutic relationship may carry over into these relationships as well.
- The scope of practice of massage therapists is defined by professional organizations and by law.
  - ○ Massage therapists' personal scope of practice is limited by their training and experience.
  - ○ Massage therapists should know their legal scope of practice, and stay within that scope.
  - ○ Three areas to be especially clear about are limits on treating clients with illness and injuries, giving nutritional advice, and psychotherapy.
  - ○ Massage therapists do not give prescriptions (Rx) to clients, but do provide information, education, and suggestions for home care.
- Massage therapists are bound to keep client information confidential. Confidentiality is expected unless disclosure is required by law or necessary to protect the public.
  - ○ HIPAA was enacted in 1996 to protect the privacy of medical records.

EXAM REVIEW

Key Terms

Match the following key terms to their descriptions. For additional study, look up the key terms in the Interactive Glossary on page G-1 and note other terms that compare or contrast with them.

_____ 1. Boundary crossing
_____ 2. Codes of ethics
_____ 3. Confidentiality
_____ 4. Defense mechanisms
_____ 5. Dual relationship
_____ 6. Duties
_____ 7. Ethical decision-making model
_____ 8. Ethical dilemmas
_____ 9. Ethical judgment
_____ 10. Ethical questions
_____ 11. Ethics
_____ 12. Informed voluntary consent
_____ 13. Intervention model
_____ 14. Personal boundary
_____ 15. Personal temptations
_____ 16. Power differential
_____ 17. Professional ethics
_____ 18. Rights
_____ 19. Scope of practice
_____ 20. Sexual misconduct
_____ 21. Standards of practice
_____ 22. Therapeutic relationship
_____ 23. Transference
_____ 24. Values

a. The study of moral behavior; determining the *right* thing to do in a specific situation
b. Principles, traits, or qualities considered worthwhile or desirable
c. Claims to certain treatment or protection from certain treatment enforced by standards or laws
d. The study of moral behavior relative to a specific occupation
e. Way of framing an ethical situation
f. List of general principles that reflect commonly held values in a profession
g. Urge to act in a way that is unethical for your own personal gain
h. Defined by specific roles assumed by the massage therapist and the client
i. Obligations to act in a particular way
j. Documents that go into detail in interpreting ethical principles
k. Differences of perceived power within a professional relationship
l. Occurs when a client injects negative or positive feelings toward someone from his or her past into the therapeutic relationship
m. When two or more principles are in conflict, and regardless of your choice, something of value is compromised
n. Step-by-step process of thinking through an ethical question or ethical dilemma
o. Behaviors or thoughts that help us cope with unwanted feelings like fear, anxiety, guilt, and anger
p. Stepping over personal or professional limits within the therapeutic relationship
q. Other connections between a client and a massage therapist in addition to the therapeutic relationship
r. Consistency in making good ethical decisions
s. A process used to get the client's permission to touch areas that may have sexual associations, or areas out of the scope of general care
t. A limit established by a person to maintain his or her own integrity, comfort, or well-being
u. Tool to address misconduct or suspected misconduct by clients
v. Implicit agreement that the massage therapist will not reveal personal or medical information about the client to others without the client's permission.
w. Range of methods and techniques used by a professional; may be legally defined
x. Sexualizing of the relationship between a massage therapist and a current client

Memory Workout

To test your memory of the main concepts in this chapter, complete the following sentences by circling the most correct answer from the two choices provided.

1. Ethics is the study of (moral) (social) behavior.
2. Speaking the truth and avoiding deception is called (honesty) (integrity).
3. The principle of *confidentiality* stems from a client's right to (fairness) (privacy).
4. That clients get to make informed choices about what happens to them is based on their right to (safety) (self-determination).
5. Issues related to money, sex, and (respect) (power) are the usual culprits in unethical decisions.
6. The ethical decision-making model is an (intuitive) (orderly) process of thinking through an ethical question or dilemma.
7. Before making a final ethical decision, examine your own (motivation) (logic), or interest in the outcome.
8. Ethical (supervision) (judgment) refers to developing consistency in making good ethical decisions.
9. Consulting with others about an ethical issue offers a more (knowledgeable) (objective) view of the situation.
10. Clinical supervision is done in a(n) (informal) (formal) setting with a specially trained supervisor.
11. The therapeutic relationship is a special relationship based on specific (roles and responsibilities) (rules and regulations).
12. Failure or refusal of a client to cooperate in the therapeutic process is called (denial) (resistance).
13. A limit established to maintain a person's own integrity, comfort, or well-being is called a (professional) (personal) boundary.
14. Bartering for services can be (mutually) (morally) beneficial if both parties feel that they are getting a fair deal.
15. Sexual activity with a client is strictly (prohibited) (discouraged) by professional standards.
16. When massaging areas outside of the general scope of massage (e.g., inside the mouth), a plan of care and (verbal) (written) consent is required.
17. After an intervention with a client related to sexual misconduct, (document the incident in writing) (report incident to licensing board).
18. Time with (paying) (practice) clients offers the opportunity to learn early about how to maintain good professional boundaries.
19. To stay within their scope of practice, massage therapists need to understand the (legal) (professional) scope in their governmental jurisdiction.
20. When discussing a client's emotional issues becomes the focus of sessions, the massage therapist's scope of practice has been (exceeded) (achieved).
21. Client information may be ethically disclosed if required by law, or is absolutely necessary for public (safety) (information).
22. According to HIPAA Rules, medical records must be kept confidential, and only those who (want) (need) to see them should have access.

Test Prep

The following multiple-choice questions will help to prepare you for future school and professional exams.

1. Values are:
   a. Principles, traits, or qualities considered worthwhile
   b. Claims to certain treatment or to protection from certain treatment
   c. Obligations to act in a certain way
   d. Moral bonds with society
2. Integrity means:
   a. Telling the truth
   b. Keeping your promises
   c. Living up to your values consistently
   d. Learning from your mistakes
3. Unconditional regard for others calls for giving our best efforts to everyone and being:
   a. Honest
   b. Critical
   c. Judgmental
   d. Nonjudgmental
4. In contrast to a code of ethics, standards of practice are:
   a. Shorter
   b. More general
   c. More detailed
   d. Stated in broad terms
5. How do professional organizations typically enforce ethical standards?
   a. Criminal prosecution
   b. Disciplinary action such as probation or revoking membership
   c. Jail time
   d. Filing lawsuits
6. An ethical dilemma occurs when:
   a. Values, rights, or ethical principles are in conflict.
   b. An overriding ethical principle is violated.
   c. There is personal temptation to act unethically.
   d. An ethical question is unclear.

7. Which of the following is the *least* important consideration in making an ethical decision?
   a. Determining what will maintain the highest values
   b. Judging what will result in the greatest good overall
   c. Judging what will result in the least harm overall
   d. Determining what will produce the best monetary outcome for myself

8. Which of the following is an important reason to discuss an ethical situation with a colleague?
   a. To get a more objective view of the situation
   b. To generate more options for action
   c. To check my own biases and temptations
   d. All of the above

9. Which of the following statements about the power differential in the therapeutic relationship is correct?
   a. The power in the therapeutic relationship is equal between adults.
   b. Clients have greater power in the therapeutic relationship since they are paying for the massage.
   c. Massage therapists have greater power by virtue of their perceived authority.
   d. Power is not an important factor in the therapeutic relationship.

10. Behaviors or thoughts that help us cope with unwanted feelings such as fear, guilt, and anger are called:
    a. Offense mechanisms
    b. Defense mechanisms
    c. Boundary crossings
    d. Self-disclosure

11. When a massage therapist transfers positive or negative feelings about someone in his or her past into the therapeutic relationship, it is called:
    a. Countertransference
    b. Repression
    c. Projection
    d. Denial

12. A boundary transgression experienced as harmful is called a:
    a. Boundary collapse
    b. Boundary violation
    c. Boundary crossing
    d. Faulty boundary

13. Which of the following factors is *least* important in determining the potential success of a dual relationship with a client?
    a. The emotional maturity of each person
    b. The ability of each person to maintain their proper role in the therapeutic relationship
    c. The power differential within the relationship outside of the therapeutic relationship
    d. How often you socialize outside of the therapeutic relationship

14. Before massaging an area that may cause the client embarrassment or discomfort, the following procedure should always be followed:
    a. Informed voluntary consent
    b. Intervention
    c. Informed intervention
    d. Written consent

15. What is the most ethical response for a massage therapy student to give to a student clinic client who asks him/her out for a dinner date?
    a. "Call me later this week when I am not working in the student clinic."
    b. "Yes, but don't let anyone here know about it."
    c. "Yes, but only as friends."
    d. "No thank you. I prefer to keep my social and professional lives separate."

16. Which of the following is an example of a massage therapist who has clearly exceeded his or her scope of practice?
    a. One who refers a client to another health professional for a condition beyond her training
    b. One who gives advice about taking certain vitamins to improve a client's health
    c. One who listens to a client's concern about her situation at work
    d. One who instructs a client on how to give herself self-massage for home care between appointments

Video Challenge

Watch the appropriate segment of the video on your DVD and then answer the following questions.

Ethics and the Therapeutic Relationship

The Ethical Decision-Making Model

1. What everyday ethical situations are mentioned in this video segment?
2. How did the massage therapist in the video handle the situation of a client who asked her out on a date?
3. What ethical decision-making steps are presented in the video?

Informed Voluntary Consent

4. Locate the situation involving informed voluntary consent depicted in the video. Identify the essential aspects of informed voluntary consent that are illustrated.

Intervention Model

5. What steps in the intervention model are outlined in the video? Give examples of sexual misconduct by clients that may call for using the intervention model.

Comprehension Exercises

The following short answer questions test your knowledge and understanding of chapter topics and provide practice in written communication skills. Explain in two to four complete sentences.

1. Contrast codes of ethics and the law. What are they based on? Who develops them? How are they enforced?

2. Explain how a therapeutic relationship is different from a social relationship. Include the concept of *power differential* in your explanation.
3. Explain the process of *informed voluntary consent.* When is it used?

For Greater Understanding

The following exercises are designed to take you from the realm of theory into the real world. They will help give you a deeper understanding of the subjects covered in this chapter. Action words are underlined to emphasize the variety of activities presented to address different learning styles and to encourage deeper thinking.

1. Locate an article about ethics in a professional journal for massage therapists. What ethical question or ethical dilemma is addressed? What values, rights, or duties are involved? What factors were considered in decision-making? What did you learn from the situation presented?

2. Examine the massage licensing law in your state or a neighboring state for the section on ethics and discipline. What is the defined scope of practice for massage therapists? What ethical principles are reinforced in the law? What are the consequences for violations of the law?
3. Discuss in small groups or with a study partner, any boundary issues that you are having with practice clients. Define the problem, and discuss how you are currently handling the issue, and how you might approach it better in the future.

6 Anatomy & Physiology, Pathology, and Kinesiology

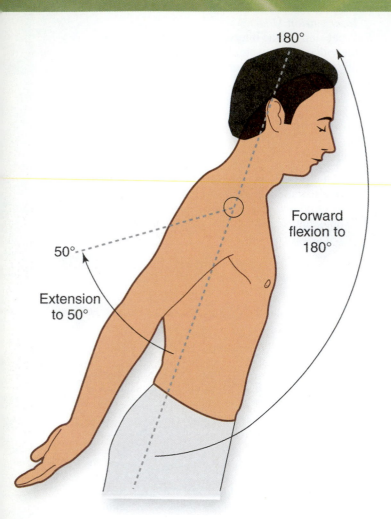

180°

Forward flexion to 180°

50°

Extension to 50°

CHAPTER OUTLINE

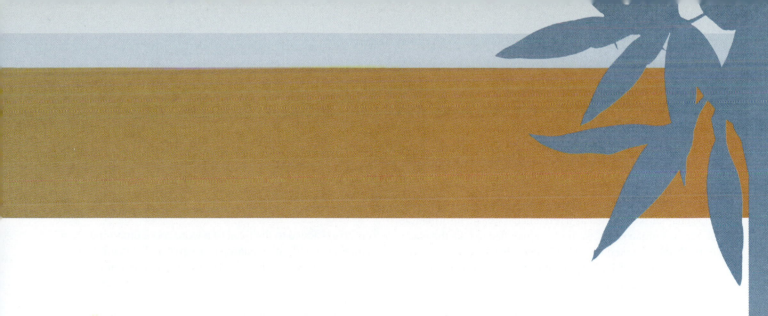

LEARNING OUTCOMES

After studying this chapter, you will have information to:

1. Interpret common medical terms.

2. Explain the general organization of the human body.

3. Describe anatomical positions, locations, body planes, and cavities.

4. Use directional terms in relation to the human body.

5. Describe the function and organs of each body system.

6. Describe common pathologies for each body system.

7. Discuss the massage implications for common pathologies.

8. Describe the structure and normal range of motion at major joints.

9. Identify the attachments and actions of major muscles.

10. Describe good postural alignment and the primary muscles involved in maintaining it.

KEY TERMS

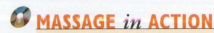

MASSAGE *in* ACTION

On your DVD, explore:
- Gait Analysis

OVERVIEW

This chapter is designed as a reference for basic information about the human sciences. It is not intended to take the place of textbooks devoted to these sciences, but to serve as a convenient review of basic information when discussing the effects of massage, contraindications, clinical applications, and massage techniques. Information that has special significance in massage therapy is noted as a *Massage Connection.*

The chapter begins with medical terminology, which is the language of health professionals. It then looks at the organization of the body as a whole, and at each body system in an overview format. It includes the kinesiology detail important to massage therapists and concludes with an extensive, illustrated table of the attachments, actions, and nerves of the muscles of the body.

Common pathologies for each body system are listed along with brief descriptions and their massage implications. These are not exhaustive lists, and given the overview nature of this chapter, the massage implications presented are very general. They serve as examples of considerations when confronted with a client with a particular pathology.

Implications for pathologies are limited to general contraindication, local contraindication, cautions, and medical emergency. Since massage applications vary widely, a definitive statement about massage implications is difficult at best. Unless stated otherwise, *massage* refers here to standard Western massage which includes a variety of techniques designed to improve circulation and promote general and muscular relaxation. In real-life situations, each case and each massage application needs to be examined thoroughly and judged on its unique merits. Students are advised to consult one of the references listed for this chapter in Appendix H, References and Additional Resources, on page A-65 for further information. The human sciences are a career-long area of continuing education for massage therapists.

MEDICAL TERMINOLOGY

Understanding medical terminology and becoming proficient in using it correctly begins with learning the word parts, or components, that form the terms. These word parts are prefixes, word roots/combining forms, and suffixes. For instance, the prefix *mal-* (bad) and the word root *format* (a shaping) plus the suffix *–ion* (process) produces the term *malformation,* meaning the process of being deformed or badly shaped.

Once you learn the word parts, you have a logical system for interpreting what an unfamiliar term means and for

speaking and writing in a language used by others in the health professions. The most efficient way of understanding a medical term is to read the term from the end of the word (suffix) back to the beginning (prefix) and then look at the word root. For example, the term *pericarditis* can be translated as inflammation (*-itis*) surrounding (*peri-*) the heart (*cardi/o*).

Prefixes

A prefix is added to the front of a word root/combining form to alter or modify its meaning or to give additional information, such as the location of an organ, the number of parts, or the frequency of an action. For example, the prefix *bi-* means two, and the term *bilateral* means having two sides. The prefix *dys-* means difficult, and the term *dyspnea* means difficult breathing. Not all medical terms have prefixes. Table 6.1■ lists common prefixes.

Word Roots/Combining Forms

The main part of the word is the word root, which provides the general meaning of the word. For instance, *cardi* means heart, as in the term *cardiac,* and tells us which body system is being discussed. *Cis* means to cut, as in the term *incision,* and tells us the action being taken. Sometimes more than one word root can form a term. For instance, *osteoarthritis* is formed from two word roots, *oste* meaning *bone,* and *arthr* meaning *joints.* Adding the suffix *–itis,* which means *inflammation,* gives us the meaning of the term: inflammation of bone at the joints.

The combining form is simply the word root combined with a vowel, which makes it easier to pronounce long medical terms. Most often this is the vowel *o* used between two word roots (oste/o arthr -itis) or between a word root and a suffix (cardi/o -logy). Table 6.2■ lists common word roots and their combining vowel.

Suffixes

A component added to the end of a word, a suffix adds additional meaning to the term, such as condition, disease, or procedure. Every medical term has a suffix. Generally it is added to a word root; however, it can also be added to a prefix without a word root. For example, the term *prognosis,* which means the prediction of the course of disease and recovery, is formed from the prefix *pro-,* meaning *before,* and the suffix *–gnosis,* meaning *knowledge.* If a suffix begins with a vowel, the combining vowel of the word root is dropped. Table 6.3■ lists common suffixes.

Singular and Plural Endings

Forming the singular and plural versions of many medical terms follows the rules of the originating languages of the terms, which are Greek and Latin. For example, the heart has a left atrium and a right atrium. When we speak of two, however, we say *atria,* not *atriums.* Other words, such as *virus,* form their plurals using English rules, making the

TABLE 6.1	Common Prefixes		
Prefix	**Meaning**	**Example**	**Definition**
a-	Without, away from	Aphasia	Without speech
an-	Without	Anoxia	Without oxygen
ante-	Before, in front of	Antepartum	Before birth
anti-	Against	Antibiotic	Against life
auto-	Self	Autograft	A graft from one's own body
bi-	Two	Bilateral	two sides
brady-	Slow	Bradycardia	Slow heartbeat
circum-	Around	Circumduction	Joint movement around a circle
contra-	Against, opposite	Contraindicated	Not indicated
di-	Two	Diplegic	Paralysis of two extremities
dia-	Through	Dialysis	Procedure that removes uric acid from circulating blood
dis-	Separate, apart from	Dislocation	A part is away from its normal position in the body
dys-	Painful, difficult	Dysfunction	Difficult or painful function
ecto-	Outer, outside	Ectoderm	Outer layer of cells
endo-	Within, inner	Endoderm	Inner layer of cells
eu-	Good, normal	Eupnea	Normal breathing
ex-	Out, away from	Extention	Move away from
extra-	Outside, beyond	Extraocular	Outside the eye
hemi-	Half	Hemiplegia	Paralysis of one side or half of the body
hetero-	Different	Heterograft	A graft from another person's body
homo-	Same	Homozygous	Having two identical genes
hydro-	Water	Hydrotherapy	Water treatment
hyper-	Over, above	Hypertrophy	Overdevelopment
hypo-	Under, below	Hypoglossal	Under the tongue
in-	In, into, not	Insomnia	Condition of not being able to sleep
infra-	Under, beneath, below	Infraspinatus	Muscle under the spine of the scapula
inter-	Among, between	Intervertebral	Between the vertebrae
intra-	Within, inside	Intravenous	Within a vein
macro-	Large	Macrocephalic	Having a large head
meta-	Beyond, over, between	Metacarpals	Pertaining to the bones beyond the wrist
micro-	Small	Microcephalic	Having a small head
mono-	One	Monoplegia	Paralysis of one extremity
multi-	Many	Multipara	More than one birth
neo-	New	Neonate	Newborn
pan-	All	Pancarditis	Inflammation of all the heart
para-	Beside, beyond, near	Paraspinal	Alongside the spine
per-	Through	Percutaneous	Through the skin
peri-	Around	Pericardial	Around the heart
poly-	Many	Polyuria	Large amounts of urine
post-	After	Postpartum	After birth
pre-	Before, in front of	Prefrontal	In front of the frontal bones
quad-	Four	Quadriplegia	Paralysis of all four extremities
retro-	Backward, behind	Retrograde	Movement in a backward direction
semi-	Partial, half	Semiconscious	Partially conscious
sub-	Below, under	Subcutaneous	Under the skin
super-	Above, upper, excess	Superficial	Pertaining to the surface
supra-	Above	Supraspinatus	Muscle above the spine of the scapula
tachy-	Rapid, fast	Tachycardia	Fast heartbeat
trans-	Through, across	Transdermal	Through the skin
tri-	Three	Triceps	Muscle with three heads
ultra-	Beyond, excess	Ultrasound	Beyond sound
uni-	One	Unilateral	One side

TABLE 6.2 Common Root Words and Combining Forms

Root Word/Combining Form	Meaning	Example	Definition
abdomin/o	Abdomen	Abdominopelvic	Abdominal and pelvic regions of the body
aden/o	Gland	Adenopathy	Gland disease
arteri/o	Artery	Arteritis	Inflammation of an artery
arthr/o	Joint	Arthroplasty	Surgical repair of a joint
carcin/o	Cancer	Carcinoma	Cancerous tumor
cardi/o	Heart	Cardiopulmonary	Pertaining to the heart and lungs
cephal/o	Head	Cephalic	Pertaining to the head
chem/o	Chemical	Chemotherapy	Treatment with chemicals
cis/o	To cut	Incision	Process of cutting into
cost/o	Rib	Intercostals	Pertaining to between the ribs
crani/o	Skull	Craniotomy	Incision into the skull
dermat/o	Skin	Dermatology	Study of the skin
enter/o	Small intestines	Enteric	Pertaining to the small intestines
gastr/o	Stomach	Gastric	Pertaining to the stomach
gynec/o	Female	Gynecology	Study of females
hemat/o	Blood	Hematology	Study of the blood
hydr/o	Water	Hydrotherapy	Treatment with water
immun/o	Immune	Immunology	Study of immunity
laryng/o	Voice box	Laryngeal	Pertaining to the voice box
mamm/o	Mammary gland, breast	Mammography	Process of obtaining images of the breast
my/o	Muscle	Myoma	Tumor containing muscle tissue
nephr/o	Kidney	Nephrology	Study of the kidneys
neur/o	Nerve	Neural	Pertaining to a nerve
ophthalm/o	Eye	Ophthalmic	Pertaining to the eye
oste/o	Bone	Osteoporosis	Condition that results in reduction of bone mass
ot/o	Ear	Otic	Pertaining to the ear
path/o	Disease	Pathology	Study of disease
ped/o	Foot, child	Pedal	Pertaining to the foot
phleb/o	Vein	Phlebitis	Inflammation of the vein
psych/o	Mind	Psychology	Study of the mind
pulmon/o	Lung	Pulmonary	Pertaining to the lungs
rhin/o	Nose	Rhinoplasty	Surgical repair of the nose
therm/o	Heat	Thermotherapy	Treatment with heat
thorac/o	Chest	Thoracoplasty	Surgical repair of the chest
ur/o	Urine, urinary tract	Urology	Study of the urinary tract
ven/i, ven/o	Vein	Venipuncture	To pierce a vein with a needle
vertebr/o	Spine, vertebra	Vertebral	Pertaining to a vertebra

TABLE 6.3	Common Suffixes		
Suffix	**Meaning**	**Example**	**Definition**
-algia	Pain	Neuralgia	Nerve pain
-cele	Hernia, protrusion	Cystocele	Protrusion of the bladder into the vagina
-cise	Cut	Excise	To cut out
-cyte	Cell	Hemocyte	Blood cell
-dynia	Pain	Cardiodynia	Heart pain
-ectomy	Surgical removal	Appendectomy	Surgical removal of the appendix
-gen	That which produces	Mutagen	That which produces mutations
-genesis	Produces, generates	Osteogenesis	Producing bone
-genic	Producing	Carcinogenic	Producing cancer
-gram	To record	Electrocardiogram	Record of heart's activity
-graph	Instrument for recording	Electrocardiograph	Instrument for recording the heart's electrical activity
-ia	State, condition	Hemiplegia	Condition of being half paralyzed
-ism	State of	Hypothyroidism	State of low thyroid
-itis	Inflammation	Cellulitis	Inflammation of cells
-logist	One who studies	Cardiologist	One who studies the heart
-logy	Study of	Cardiology	Study of the heart
-lysis	Destruction	Osteolysis	Bone destruction
-megaly	Enlargement, large	Cardiomegaly	Enlarged heart
-meter	Process of measuring	Audiometer	Instrument to measure hearing
-ectomy	Surgical removal	Gastrectomy	Surgical removal of the stomach
-ology	Study of	Hematology	Study of the blood
-oma	Tumor, mass	Carcinoma	Cancerous tumor
-osis	Abnormal condition	Lordosis	Abnormal curvature of the lumbar spine
-ostomy	Surgically create an opening	Colostomy	Surgically create an opening for the colon through the abdominal wall
-pathy	Disease	Myopathy	Muscle disease
-penia	Lack of, deficiency	Osteopenia	Lack of Bone
-plasia	Development, growth	Dysplasia	Abnormal development
-plasty	Surgical repair	Dermatoplasty	Surgical repair of the skin
-rrhage	Excessive, abnormal flow	Hemorrhage	Excessive bleeding
-rrhea	Discharge, flow	Rhinorrhea	Discharge from the nose
-sclerosis	Hardening	Arteriosclerosis	Hardening of an artery
-scopy	Process of viewing or examining	Orthoscopy	Viewing the eye through an orthoscope
-stenosis	Narrowing	Angiostenosis	Narrowing of a vessel
-therapy	Treatment	Hydrotherapy	Treatment with water
-thermy	Heat	Hydrothermy	Treatment using heated water
-trophy	Development, nourishment	Hypertrophy	Excessive development

plural of virus *viruses*. Table 6.4■ illustrates how to form the singular and plural endings of some common medical terms.

Abbreviations and Symbols

Abbreviations and symbols are commonly used in medical records to save time and space. They can be confusing, however, and incorrect use of an abbreviation can cause serious problems in documents and records. If unsure, it is better to spell out the word rather than use an abbreviation or symbol. Never make up your own abbreviations or symbols. See Table 6.5■ for a list of common abbreviations and symbols that massage therapy professionals will find helpful. For greater ease of use, highlight terms used most often in your practice and keep the list handy when you are writing or reading notes. Consult a medical dictionary for a complete list of medical abbreviations and symbols.

TABLE 6.4 Common Singular and Plural Endings

Words Ending In	Singular	Plural
-a	Vertebra	Vertebrae
-ax	Thorax	Thoraces
-ex or -ix	Appendix	Appendices
-is	Metastasis	Metastases
-ma	Sarcoma	Sarcomata
-nx	Phalanx	Phalanges
-on	Ganglion	Ganglia
-us	Nucleus	Nuclei
-um	Ovum	Ova
-y	Biopsy	Biopsies

TABLE 6.5 Common Abbreviations and Symbols Used by Massage Therapists

Abbreviation/Symbol	Meaning	Abbreviation/Symbol	Meaning
General			
ASAP	As soon as possible	pre	Before
@	At	Δ	Change
Cl, CL	Client	c/o	Complains of
CI, contra	Contraindication	CSTx	Continue same treatment
DOB	Date of birth	crep	Crepitus
Dx	Diagnosis	DOI	Date of injury
DKA	Did not keep appointment	↓	Decrease, down
Hx	History	DDD	Degenerative disk disease
HW	Homework	DJD	Degenerative joint disease
LTG	Long-term goal	ed	Edema
MT	Massage therapist	/	Elevation
MTx	Massage therapy session	=	Equals, is
meds	Medications	xs	Excessive
N/A	Not applicable	FT	Fibrous tissue
Ø	NO, none	HA	Headache
#	Number	HOH	Hearing impaired (hard of hearing)
Rx	Prescription	HBP	High blood pressure, hypertension
rec	Recommendation	tens, ≡ HT	Hypertonic, tense muscle
rpt	Reported	→	Leading to, resulting in
STG	Short-term goal	↔	Lengthened, longer than normal
Sx	Symptoms	L	Light, low, mild
X	Times, repetitions	LBP	Low back pain
Tx	Treatment, therapy	mob	Mobility
unk	Unknown	mod	Moderate
w/	With	N	Normal
w/o	Without	≈	Numbness, tingling
Descriptions, Symptoms		•	Pain
Abn	Abnormal	P & B	Pain and burning
ADL	Activities of daily living	POM	Pain on motion
adh, X	Adhesion	1°	Primary
post	After	2°	Secondary, due to
&, +	And	sev	Severe
~	Approximate	>-<	Shortened, shorter than normal
BA	Backache	SD	Sleep disturbance

TABLE 6.5 Common Abbreviations and Symbols Used by Massage Therapists

Abbreviation/Symbol	Meaning	Abbreviation/Symbol	Meaning
STI	Soft tissue injury	gastroc	Gastrocnemius
SP, ≈	Spasm, cramping	gluts	Gluteal muscles
st	Stiffness	hams	Hamstrings
INFLAM, ⇔	Inflammation	ITB, IT band	Iliotibial band
TeP, ∞	Tender point	lats	Latissimus dorsi
TP, TrP, ꜱ	Trigger point	lev scap	Levator scapulae
↑	Up, increase	LB	Low back
VGH	Very good health	L, L1-5	Lumbar, lumbar vertebrae
Massage and Related Techniques		mm	Muscles
AAS	Active assisted stretching	pecs	Pectoralis muscles
AROM	Active range of motion	PSIS	Posterior superior iliac spine
ACU	Acupuncture, acupressure	QL	Quadratus lumborum
aroma	Aromatherapy	quads	Quadriceps femoris
CP	Cold packs	rhomb	Rhomboid muscles
CTM	Connective tissue massage	scal	Scalene muscles
CST	Craniosacral therapy	ST	Soft tissue
XFF	Cross fiber friction	SCM	Sternocleidomastoid muscles
DT	Deep tissue	SI	Sacroilia
DP	Direct pressure	T, T1-12	Thoracic, thoracic vertebrae
eff	Effleurage	TFL	Tensor fascia latae
EW	Energy work	TMJ	Temporomandibular joint
Ex	Exercise (active movement)	traps	Trapezius muscles
Fx	Friction	**Locations, Directions, Movement**	
FBM	Full body massage	abd	Abduction
FBRM	Full body relaxation massage	add	Adduction
HP	Hot packs	ant	Anterior
hydro	Hydrotherapy	ⒷⓁ Ⓑ	Bilateral, both
ICES	Ice, compression, elevation, support	circ	Circumduction
MLD	Manual lymph drainage	dep	Depression (e.g., scapula)
M	Massage	DF	Dorsiflexion
MET	Muscle energy technique	ele	Elevation
MFR	Myofascial release	ever	Eversion
NMT	Neuromuscular therapy	ext	Extension
palp	Palpation	ext	External
PB	Paraffin bath	flex	Flexion
PROM	Passive range of motion	int	Internal
pet	Petrissage	inv	Inversion
PR	Positional release	lat	Lateral
PNF	Proprioceptive neuromuscular facilitation	lat flex	Lateral flexion
RI	Reciprocal inhibition	L	Left
reflex	Reflexology	med	Medial
SFT	Soft tissue mobilization	PF	Plantarflexion
SCS	Strain, counterstrain	post	Posterior
str	Stretching	pro	Pronation
SwM	Swedish massage	prox	Proximal
T&R	Tense and relax	ROM	Range of motion
Anatomical Terms		AROM	Active range of motion
abs	Abdominals	PROM	Passive range of motion
ACL	Anterior crutiate ligament	RROM	Resisted range of motion
ASIS	Anterior superior iliac spine	rot	Rotation
C, C1-7	Cervical, cervical vertebrae	Ⓡ	Right
CT	Connective tissue	SB	Sidebending
delt	Deltoid	sup	Supination
ES	Erector spinae	WNL	Within normal limits

ORGANIZATION OF THE BODY

Adipose (ADD-ih-pohs) tissue
Body
Bone
Cardiac (CAR-dee-ak) muscle
Cartilage (CAR-tih-lij)
Cell
Cell Membrane
Connective tissue
Cytoplasm (SIGH-to-plazm)
Epithelial (ep-ih-THEE-lee-al) tissue
Fascia (FASH-ee-ah)
Ligaments
Nervous tissue
Nucleus
Organs
Skeletal (SKELL- eh-tal) muscle
Smooth muscle
Tendons
Tissues

The human body consists of cells, tissues, organs, and systems. **Cells** come together to form tissues, **tissues** come together to form organs, and **organs** work together to form systems. All the **body systems** together form the whole organism—the human body (Figure 6.1■).

Cells
- Basic unit of all living organisms.
- Make up all tissues and organs in the body.
- Specialize to perform specific functions, such as respiration, metabolism, reproduction, muscle contraction, etc.
- Basic components are cell membrane, cytoplasm, nucleus with chromosomes; specialized cells form specific tissues.

Tissues
- Form when like cells group together to perform one activity, e.g., muscle cells combine to form muscle tissue.
- There are four types of tissue in the human body:
  1. Muscle tissue—produces movement through contraction and shortening; forms one of three basic types of muscles: skeletal muscle, smooth muscle, or cardiac muscle.
  2. Epithelial tissue—found throughout the body as lining for internal organs and also forms the outer skin or epidermis.
  3. Connective tissue—supports and protects the body structures; adipose tissue or fat, dermis, fascia, ligaments, tendons, bone, and cartilage are connective tissues.
  4. Nervous tissue—forms a network of nerves throughout the body, allowing conduction of electrical impulses between the brain and the rest of the body.

Organs
- Composed of different types of tissue that work as a unit to perform specific functions; *example:* the stomach contains muscle fibers, nervous tissue, and epithelial tissue, all of which allow it to contract and mix food with digestive juices.

Systems
- Composed of several organs working together to perform certain functions; *example:* Digestive System—mouth, stomach, esophagus, liver, pancreas, small intestine, and colon work together to ingest, digest, and absorb food.

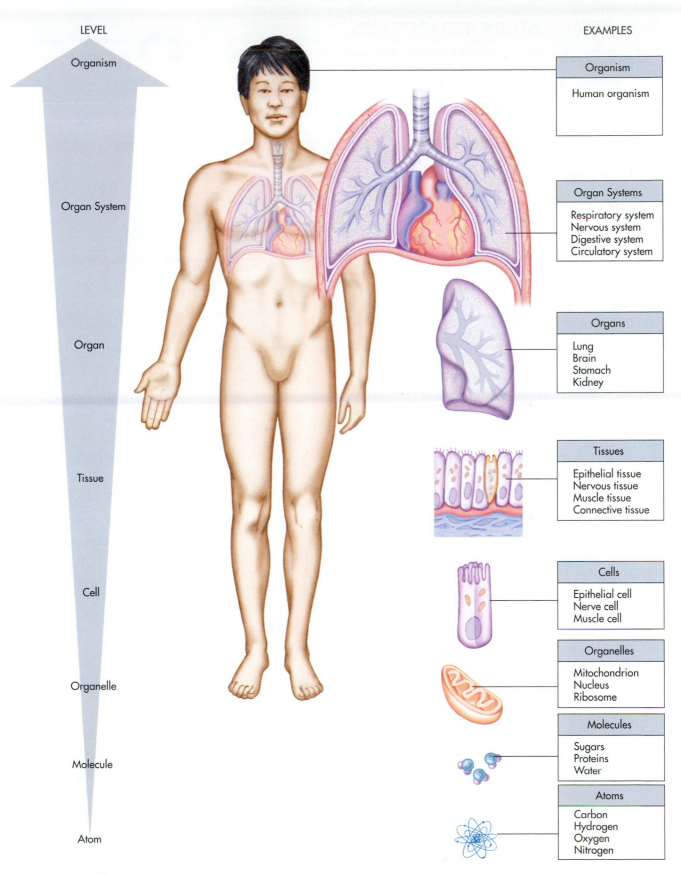

FIGURE 6.1

Levels of organization of the human body.

ANATOMICAL POSITION AND LOCATIONS

Abdominopelvic (ab-dom-ih-noh-PELL-vik) cavity
Anatomical position
Cavities
Coronal (kor-RONE-al) plane
Cranial (KRAY-nee-al) cavity
Direction
Dorsal (DOR-sal) cavity
Diaphragm (DYE-ah -fram)
Pericardial (pair-ih-CAR-dee-al) cavity
Planes
Pleural (PLOO-ral) cavity
Regions
Sagittal (SAJ-ih-tal) plane
Spinal cavity
Thoracic (tho-RASS-ik) cavity
Transverse (trans-VERS) plane
Ventral (VEN-tral) cavity

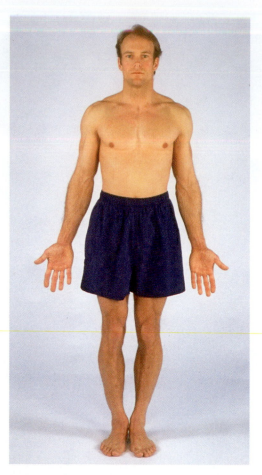

FIGURE 6.2

The anatomical position.

To provide uniformity, the **anatomical position** is used when describing the positions and relationships of structures in the human body. In the anatomical position, a person is standing erect with arms at the sides, legs together, toes pointing forward, palms of the hands facing forward, and the head is centered with eyes looking straight ahead (Figure 6.2■). For descriptive purposes, left and right are from the subject's not the examiner's perspective.

In addition to anatomical position, there are other reference systems for describing the body. They are direction, planes, cavities, and regions.

Direction

Directional terms describe the positions or locations of organs or body structures relative to one another. Using these terms helps health care professionals to be specific in discussing or charting the locations of symptoms, complaints, and injuries. Figure 6.3■ illustrates directional terms. Commonly used directional terms are listed and described in Table 6.6■. Figure 6.4■ shows supine and prone positions.

FIGURE 6.3

Front (anterior) and side (lateral) views of the body illustrating directional terms.

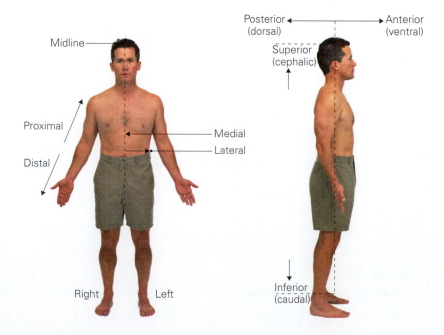

TABLE 6.6	Directional Terms	
Term	Description	Example
Anterior	Toward the front; the front side of the body; ventral	The kneecap is on the anterior side of the leg.
Distal	Located farther away from the point of attachment to the torso (for upper and lower extremities)	The wrist is distal to the elbow.
Inferior	Lower; below another structure; caudal	The stomach is inferior to the heart.
Lateral	Toward the side; away from the midline of the body	The hip is lateral to the spine.
Medial	Toward the midline of the body	The eye is medial to the ear.
Posterior	Toward the back; the back side of the body; dorsal	The Achilles' tendon is located on the posterior side of the lower leg.
Prone	Horizontal and facing downward position (Figure 6.4A)	Adjust the face cradle for comfort when the client is in the prone position on the massage table.
Proximal	Located nearer the point of attachment to the torso (for upper and lower extremities)	The thigh is proximal to the ankle.
Superior	Closer to the head or upper part of the body; cephalic	The neck is superior to the shoulders.
Supine	Horizontal and facing upward position (Figure 6.4B)	Abdominal massage is applied with the client lying in the supine position.

Body Planes

Imagining the body bisected at different angles into planes or flat surfaces allows us to use specific language in describing the body and its parts (Figure 6.5■). The three body planes are:

1. Sagittal plane—also called the *median plane;* runs vertically (lengthwise) from front to back, dividing the body or any of its parts into right and left sides.
2. Frontal plane—also called the *coronal plane;* runs vertically, dividing the body into anterior (front) and posterior (back) portions.
3. Transverse plane—also called the *horizontal plane;* a crosswise plane that runs parallel to the ground (horizontally), dividing the body into upper (superior) and lower (inferior) parts.

Body Cavities

The body has many cavities or open spaces that contain the internal organs. Cavities are either ventral (anterior) or dorsal (posterior). Major subdivisions include the thoracic, pleural, pericardial, abdominopelvic, cranial, and spinal cavities. Figure 6.6■ shows the major body cavities and their subdivisions.

Ventral cavity
● Larger of the two cavities.
● Extends from neck to pelvis.

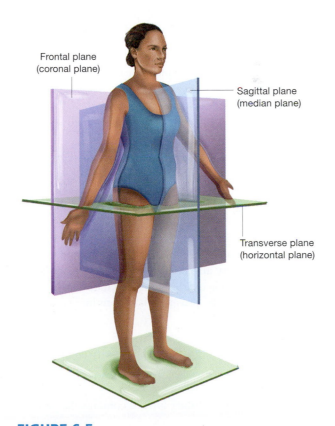

Frontal plane (coronal plane)

Sagittal plane (median plane)

Transverse plane (horizontal plane)

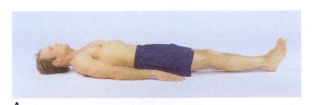

A

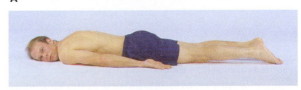

B

FIGURE 6.4

A. The supine position. B. The prone position.

FIGURE 6.5

The planes of the body.

FIGURE 6.6

Major body cavities.

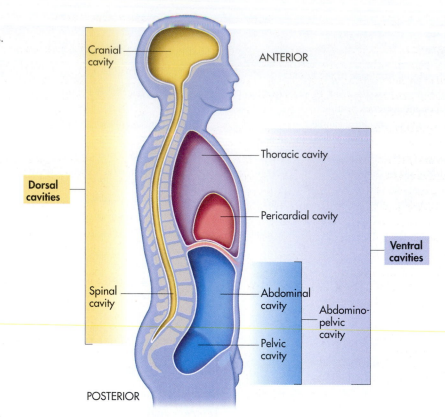

- Contains the heart and organs of respiration, digestion, elimination, and reproduction.
- Divided into two parts, the thoracic cavity and abdominopelvic cavity, by the diaphragm, a respiratory muscle.

Thoracic cavity
- Contains the lungs in the pleural cavities and the heart in the pericardial cavity.
- Other organs include the esophagus, trachea, thymus, large blood vessels, and nerves.

Abdomino-pelvic cavity
- Divided into two sections, the abdominal cavity and the pelvic cavity.
- The abdominal cavity contains stomach, spleen, liver, gallbladder, pancreas, and portions of the small intestine and colon.
- The pelvic cavity contains urinary bladder, ureters, urethra, and portions of the small intestine and colon.
- The pelvic cavity also contains reproductive organs. In the female: uterus, ovaries, fallopian tubes, and the vagina; in the male: prostate gland, seminal vesicles, part of the vas deferens.

Dorsal cavity
- Divided into two parts, the cranial cavity and the spinal cavity.

Cranial cavity
- The upper portion of the cavity, it contains the brain.

Spinal cavity
- Also called the *vertebral canal,* it houses the spinal cord.

Abdominal Region Quadrants

The abdominal region can be divided into four areas or *quadrants* for ease of locating and palpating internal organs (Figure 6.7■). The quadrants are:

Right upper quadrant (RUQ)
- Contains right lobe of liver, gallbladder, part of the pancreas, right kidney, and part of the small and large intestines.

Left upper quadrant (LUQ)
- Contains left lobe of liver, spleen, stomach, most of the pancreas, left kidney, part of the small and large intestines.

Right lower quadrant (RLQ)
- Contains part of the small and large intestines, appendix, right ureter, and in the female, the right ovary and fallopian tube.

Left lower quadrant (LLQ)
- Contains part of the small and large intestines, left ureter, and in the female, the left ovary and fallopian tube.

Some organs, such as the urinary bladder, the uterus in the female, and the prostate gland in the male, fall half in the right quadrant and half in the left quadrant, and are referred to as *midline organs* or as being located in the *midline* of the body. Table 6.7■ gives examples of additional body region terms that signify body locations to health care professionals.

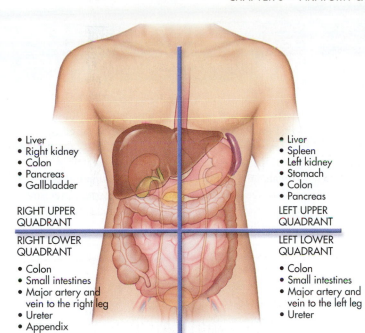

FIGURE 6.7
The four quadrants of the abdomen with related organs and structures.

• Liver
• Right kidney
• Colon
• Pancreas
• Gallbladder

RIGHT UPPER QUADRANT

RIGHT LOWER QUADRANT

• Colon
• Small intestines
• Major artery and vein to the right leg
• Ureter
• Appendix

• Liver
• Spleen
• Left kidney
• Stomach
• Colon
• Pancreas

LEFT UPPER QUADRANT

LEFT LOWER QUADRANT

• Colon
• Small intestines
• Major artery and vein to the left leg
• Ureter

MIDLINE AREA
• Aorta
• Pancreas
• Small intestines
• Bladder
• Spine

INTEGUMENTARY SYSTEM

Apocrine (APP-oh-krin) glands

Basal (BAY-sal) layer

Collagen (KOL-ah-jen) fibers

Corium (KOH-ree-um)

Dermis (DER-mis)

Epidermis (ep-ih-DER-mis)

Hair

Integumentary (in-teg-you-MEN-tah-ree) system

Keratin (KAIR-ah-tin)

Lipocytes (LIP-oh-sights)

Melanin (MEL-ah-nin)

Nails

Sebaceous (see-BAY-shus) glands

Sebum (SEE-bum)

Sensory receptors

Skin

Subcutaneous layer (sub-kyoo-TAY-nee-us)

Sweat glands

TABLE 6.7	**Body Region Terms and Their Locations**		
Term	**Location**	**Term**	**Location**
Antebrachial	Forearm	Lumbar	Lower back
Antecubital	Depressed area at the bend of the elbow	Nasal	Nose
Axillary	Armpit	Oral	Mouth
Brachial	Upper arm	Orbital	Eye area
Buccal	Cheek	Patellar	Knee
Carpal	Wrist	Pedal	Foot
Cervical	Neck	Plantar	Sole of foot
Costal	Ribs	Pubic	Genital region
Cubital	Elbow	Sacral	Sacrum of spinal column
Deltoid	Deltoid muscle area	Scapular	Shoulder blade area
Digital	Fingers	Sterna	Breastbone area
Facial	Face area	Thoracic	Chest
Femoral	Upper inner thigh	Vertebral	Vertebrae of spinal column
Gluteal	Buttocks		

TABLE 6.8	Integumentary System Abbreviations
Abbreviation	**Meaning**
BCC	Basal cell carcinoma
BX, bx	Biopsy
Decub	Decubitus ulcer
Der, Derm	Dermatology
ID	Intradermal
MM	Malignant melanoma
SCC	Squamous cell carcinoma
SLE	Systemic lupus erythematosus
Subcu, SC, sc, subq	Subcutaneous
UV	Ultraviolet

MASSAGE CONNECTION

The sense of touch is at the heart of the experience for both giver and receiver of massage. The massage therapist touches the client skillfully to evoke particular effects. Touch receptors in the skin allow the massage therapist to detect the condition of the tissues and locate anatomical structures (i.e., palpation skills). The client feels touch sensations such as heat, pressure, pleasure, and pain. Figure 6.8■ illustrates some of the possibilities for touch sensations.

The integumentary system protects the body by forming a two-way barrier of skin over internal body structures, helps to regulate body temperature, contains millions of sensory receptors, and secretes perspiration to cool the body and sebum to lubricate the skin. It consists of the skin, which is the largest organ in the body, and its accessory structures: sweat glands, sebaceous glands, hair and nails. See Table 6.8■ for abbreviations that relate to the integumentary system. See Table 6.9■ at the end of this section for common pathologies of the skin and their massage implications.

Functions of the Integumentary System

Protection

- Forms a protective two-way barrier over internal body structures.
- Keeps disease-causing agents (bacteria, viruses, pollution) and harmful chemicalfrom entering the body.
- Prevents body fluids from escaping the body.
- Protects internal organs and structures from harmful ultraviolet rays through the production of melanin.

Regulation

- Regulates body temperature.
  - Evaporation of sweat and dilation of superficial blood vessels in the skin cool the body.
  - Constriction of superficial blood vessels warms the body.
  - Continuous layer of fat under the skin acts as insulation.

Sensory reception

- Millions of nerve endings (sensory receptors) that detect temperature, pain, touch, and pressure are located in the middle layer of the skin and send messages of sensations to the spinal cord and brain.

Secretion

- Sweat glands help the body maintain its internal temperature by secreting perspiration (sweat), which cools the body as it evaporates.
- Sebaceous glands secrete oil or sebum that lubricate the skin.

FIGURE 6.8

Common touch sensations.

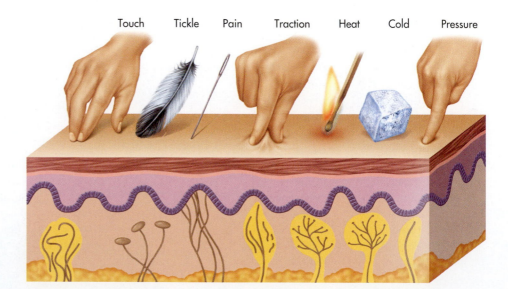

Layers of the Skin

Epidermis

- Thin outer membrane layer composed of squamous epithelial cells.
  - Flat and scalelike, these cells are arranged in overlapping layers.
- Blood supply to epidermis comes from the deeper layers of skin.
- Basal layer is deepest layer within the epidermis, with cells continually growing and multiplying, and pushing old dead cells toward outer layer.
- As basal layer cells shrink and die, they become filled with a hard protein called keratin, which allows the skin to act as a barrier to infection and make it waterproof.
- Basal layer produces melanin, a pigment responsible for the color of one's skin.
- Melanin also helps to protect the skin against damage from the ultraviolet rays of the sun.

Dermis

- Middle layer of the skin; also called the *corium.*
- Living tissue with good blood supply.
- Composed of connective tissue and collagen fibers.
- Contains hair follicles, sweat glands, sebaceous glands, blood vessels, lymph vessels, sensory receptors, nerve fibers, and muscle fibers.

Subcutaneous layer

- Third and deepest layer of skin is formed of fat cells called lipocytes.
- Protects the deeper tissues of the body and acts as insulation for heat and cold.

The three layers of the skin are shown in Figure 6.9■. Chapter 7, Effects of Massage, discusses the effects of massage on the integumentary system on page 262.

Accessory Organs

The accessory organs of the skin, including hair, nails, sweat glands, and sebaceous glands, are located within the dermis (see Figure 6.9).

Hair

- Hair fibers are composed of the protein keratin.
- Deep cells in the hair root force older keratinized cells to move upward, forming the hair shaft, which grows toward the skin surface within the hair follicle.
- Melanin gives hair its color.
- Sebaceous glands release sebum directly into the hair follicle.

Nails

- Formed of a flat plate of keratin called the nail body that covers the ends of fingers and toes, and is connected to the tissue underneath by the nail bed (Figure 6.10■).
- Grow from the nail root, found at the base of the nail, and protected and covered by soft tissue called the cuticle.

Sweat glands

- Located in the dermis, about two million sweat glands are found throughout the body.
- Sweat travels to the surface of the skin in a sweat duct, opening into a sweat pore.
- Secrete sweat or perspiration through sweat pores, which helps to cool the body and rid it of waste.
- Most sweat is colorless and odorless, except for that produced by sweat glands called apocrine glands found in the pubic and underarm areas; these glands secrete a thicker sweat that produces an odor when it comes in contact with bacteria on the skin.

Sebaceous glands

- Found in the dermis, these glands secrete sebum, an oily substance that lubricates the hair and skin.

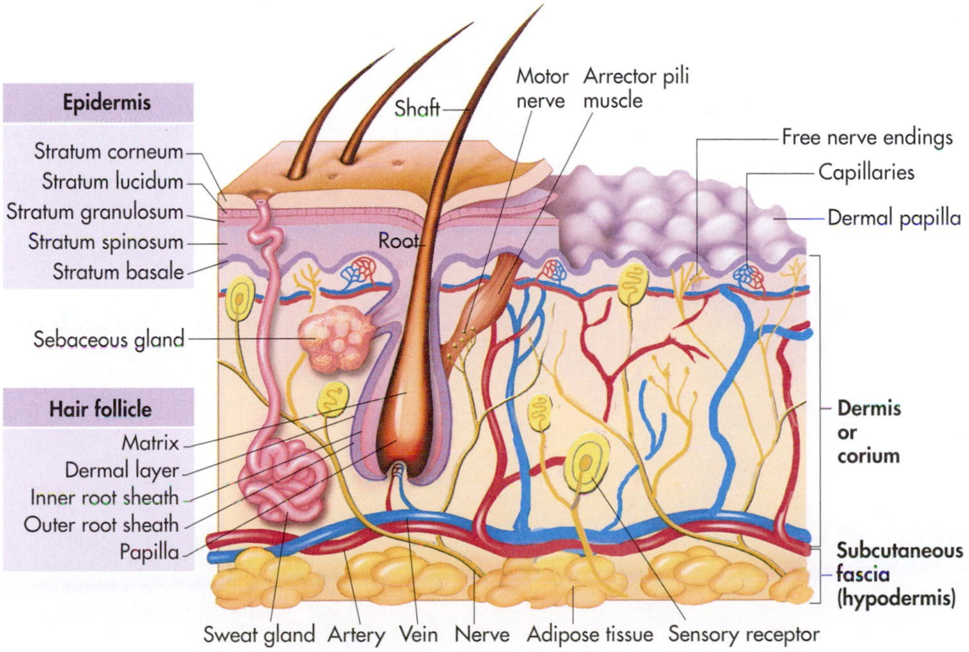

FIGURE 6.9

The three layers of the skin and the accessory organs: sweat gland, sebaceous gland, and hair.

Epidermis

Stratum corneum
Stratum lucidum
Stratum granulosum
Stratum spinosum
Stratum basale

Sebaceous gland

Hair follicle

Matrix
Dermal layer
Inner root sheath
Outer root sheath
Papilla

Shaft
Motor nerve
Arrector pili muscle
Root

Free nerve endings
Capillaries
Dermal papilla

Dermis or corium

Subcutaneous fascia (hypodermis)

Sweat gland   Artery   Vein   Nerve   Adipose tissue   Sensory receptor

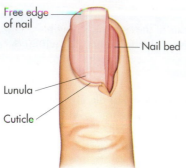
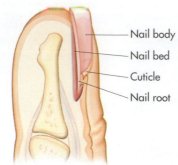

Free edge of nail

Nail bed

Lunula

Cuticle

Nail body

Nail bed

Cuticle

Nail root

FIGURE 6.10

External and internal structures of the fingernail.

- Such secretions, controlled by the endocrine system, increase during adolescence and decrease with aging.

Skin Signs

Skin signs are tactile and visual evidence of disease or injury to the skin. Figure 6.11■ shows common skin signs.

Wounds and Tissue Repair

Wounds are injuries to the skin that result in breaks in the skin and tissue damage. Types of wounds include lacera-

MASSAGE CONNECTION

Massage therapists evaluate skin signs to determine if massage is contraindicated. Local or general contraindications may apply if the underlying condition would be worsened or spread to other parts of the body with the application of massage techniques.

FIGURE 6.11

Skin signs can be seen, felt, or measured. They are evidence of illness or a disorder.

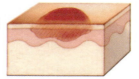

A macule is a discolored spot on the skin; freckle

A pustule is a small, elevated, circumscribed lesion of the skin that is filled with pus; varicella (chickenpox)

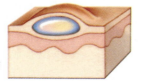
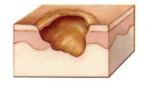

A wheal is a localized, evanescent elevation of the skin that is often accompanied by itching; uticaria

An erosion or ulcer is an eating or gnawing away of tissue; decubitus ulcer

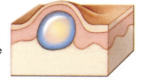

A papule is a solid, circumscribed, elevated area on the skin; pimple

A crust is a dry, serous or seropurulent, brown, yellow, red, or green exudation that is seen in secondary lesions; eczema

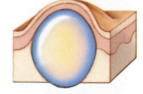

A nodule is a larger papule; acne vulgaris

A scale is a thin, dry flake of cornified epithelial cells such as psoriasis

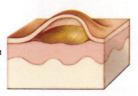
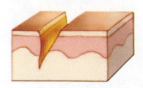

A vesicle is a small fluid filled sac; blister. A bulla is a large vesicle

A fissure is a crack-like sore or slit that extends through the epidermis into the dermis; athlete's foot

tions (rips and tears), incisions (cuts), and excoriations (scratches).

Tissue/wound repair has three phases: inflammation, regeneration, and remodeling. Chapter 7, Effects of Mas-sage, on page 259 discusses the role of massage in tissue repair and related contraindications. Figure 7.1 on page 260 shows the three phases of the tissue/wound repair process.

TABLE 6.9	Common Pathologies of the Integumentary System	
Disease/Disorder	Description	Massage Implications
Acne (ACK-nee)	Inflammatory condition of the sebaceous glands and hair follicles that results in pimples, whiteheads, blackheads, and cysts (Figure 6.12■)	Local contraindication

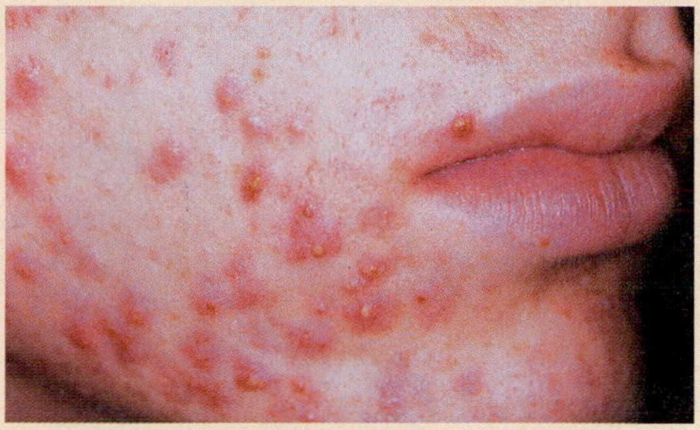

FIGURE 6.12

Acne.

Courtesy of Jason L. Smith, MD.

Acrochordon (ak-ro-KOR-don)	Small outgrowth of epidermal and dermal tissue; also called skin tags (Figure 6.13■)	None

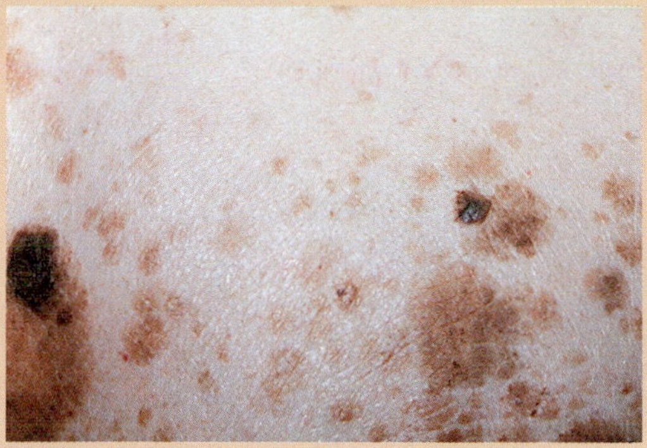

FIGURE 6.13

Acrochordon (skin tags).

Courtesy of Jason L. Smith, MD.

Basal cell carcinoma (BCC)	Slow-growing, cancerous tumor of the basal cell layer of the epidermis; common type of cancer arising on sun-exposed skin (Figure 6.14■)	Local contraindication

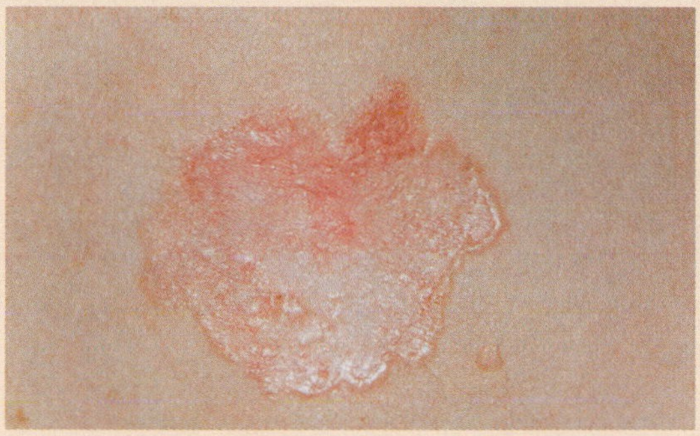

FIGURE 6.14

Basal cell carcinoma.

Courtesy of Jason L. Smith, MD.

TABLE 6.9	Common Pathologies of the Integumentary System (continued)	
Disease/Disorder	Description	Massage Implications
Burns	Injury to tissue by heat, fire, chemicals, radiation First-degree: red, swollen, painful epidermis; no blisters or scars Second-degree: blistered, painful epidermis; damage extends into the dermis; scarring may occur Third-degree: pale or charred skin with exposed underlying fat tissue; damage extends through skin layer and into underlying tissues; infection and fluid loss can be life threatening; skin grafts usually required and scarring will occur	Local contraindication
Carbuncle (CAR-bung-kl)	Cluster of boils; infection of the subcutaneous tissue	Local contraindication
Cellulitis (sell-you-LYE-tis)	Acute infection and inflammation of the skin (Figure 6.15■)	General contraindication

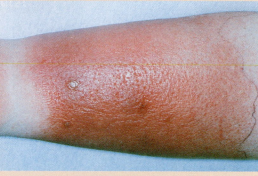

FIGURE 6.15

Cellulitis.

Courtesy of Jason L. Smith, MD.

Dermatitis (der-mah-TYE-tis)	Inflammation of the skin; contact with the poison ivy plant is a common cause (Figure 6.16■)	Local contraindication

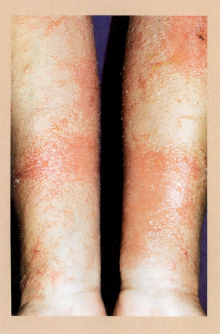

FIGURE 6.16

Dermatitis.

Courtesy of Jason L. Smith, MD.

TABLE 6.9	Common Pathologies of the Integumentary System (continued)	
Disease/Disorder	Description	Massage Implications
Eczema (EK-zeh-mah)	Inflammation of the epidermis with red, itchy lesions	Local contraindication
Folliculitis	Inflammation of hair follicle with pustules (Figure 6.17■)	Local contraindication

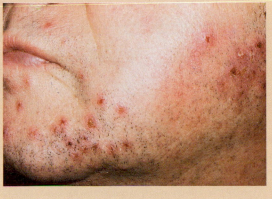

FIGURE 6.17

Folliculitis.

Courtesy of Jason L. Smith, MD.

Furuncle (FOO-rung-kl)	Bacterial infection of a hair follicle with redness, pain, and swelling; a boil	Local contraindication
Gangrene (GANG-green)	Tissue necrosis (death) usually due to deficient blood supply	Medical emergency
Herpes	Small, painful blisters caused by herpes virus (Figure 6.18■)	Local contraindication

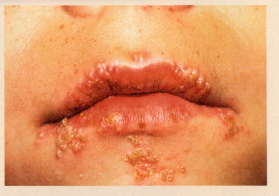

FIGURE 6.18

Herpes labialis.

Courtesy of Jason L. Smith, MD.

Kaposi's sarcoma (KAP-oh-seez sar KOH-mah)	Form of skin cancer frequently seen in AIDS patients; brownish-purple papules spread from the skin and metastasize to internal organs (see Figure 6.81 on page 187)	Local contraindication
Malignant melanoma (MM) (mah-LIG-nant mel-a- NOH-ma)	Form of skin cancer that can quickly metastasize and spread to internal organs; shows as a mole that changes size and color, bleeds and itches, with irregular border (Figure 6.19■)	Local contraindication

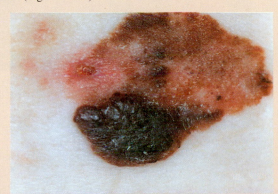

FIGURE 6.19

Melanoma.

Courtesy of Jason L. Smith, MD.

TABLE 6.9	Common Pathologies of the Integumentary System (continued)	
Disease/Disorder	**Description**	**Massage Implications**
Nevus (mole)	Pigmented, elevated spot above the surface of the skin (Figure 6.20■)	None

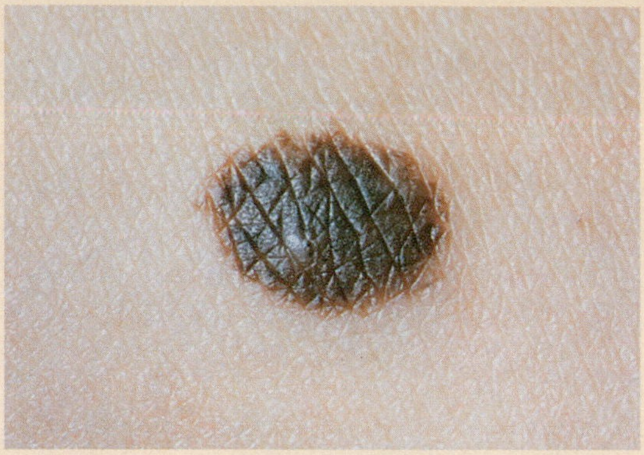

FIGURE 6.20

Nevus (mole).

Courtesy of Jason L. Smith, MD.

Psoriasis (soh-RYE-ah-sis)	Chronic inflammatory condition with crusty, red lesions with silvery scales that form patches with circular borders (Figure 6.21■)	Local contraindication in acute outbreak

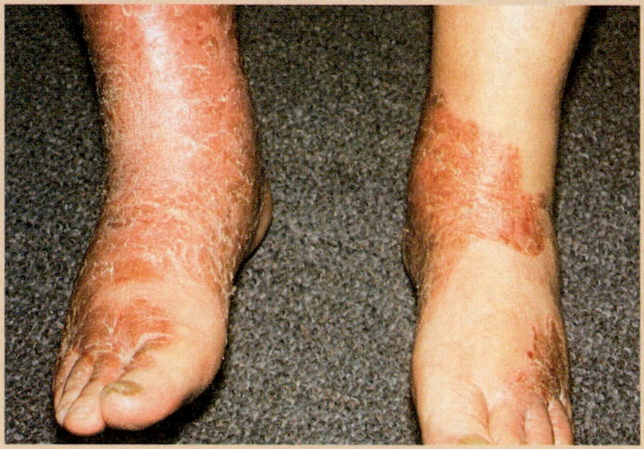

FIGURE 6.21

Psoriasis.

Courtesy of Jason L. Smith, MD.

Purpura (PER-pew-rah)	Hemorrhages into the skin due to fragile blood vessels; commonly seen in elderly people (Figure 6.22■)	Use light pressure

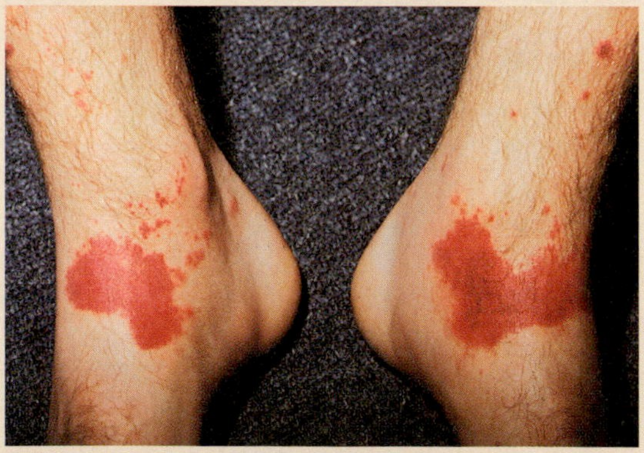

FIGURE 6.22

Purpura.

Courtesy of Jason L. Smith, MD.

Rubella (roo-BELL-ah)	Contagious viral skin infection with rash and fever; commonly called *German measles*	General contraindication
Sebaceous cyst (see-BAY-shus SIST)	Lump under skin surface filled with sebum or oil from a blocked sebaceous gland duct	Local contraindication
Scabies	Contagious skin disease with itching, blisters, and pustules; caused by a mite	General contraindication
Shingles (SHING-lz)	Rash and pain that erupt along nerve paths of the body; caused by the same virus as chicken pox (see Figure 6.59 on page 170)	General contraindication in acute stage

TABLE 6.9	Common Pathologies of the Integumentary System (continued)	
Disease/Disorder	**Description**	**Massage Implications**
Squamous cell carcinoma (SCC) (SKWAY-mus sell kar-sih-NOH-ma)	Epidermal cancer that can infiltrate underlying tissue but does not generally metastasize; crusted nodule that ulcerates and bleeds (Figure 6.23■)	Local contraindication

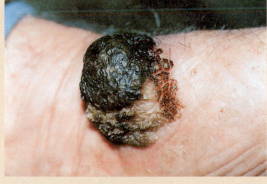

FIGURE 6.23

Squamous cell carcinoma.

Courtesy of Jason L. Smith, MD.

Tinea (TIN-ee-ah)	Fungal skin disease with itchy, scaly lesions; painful raw rash; commonly called *ringworm* (Figure 6.24■)	Local contraindication

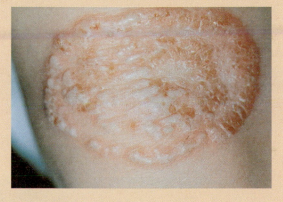

FIGURE 6.24

Tinea, commonly called ringworm.

Courtesy of Jason L. Smith, MD.

Tinea capitis (TIN-ee-ah CAP-it-is)	Fungal infection of the scalp; commonly called *ringworm*	Local contraindication
Tinea pedis (TIN-ee-ah PED-is)	Fungal infection of the foot; commonly called *athlete's foot*	Local contraindication
Urticaria (er-tih-KAY-ree-ah)	Skin eruption of pale reddish wheals with severe itching; also called *hives;* often associated with stress or food or drug allergies (Figure 6.25■)	General contraindication in acute phase; local contraindication in subacute phase

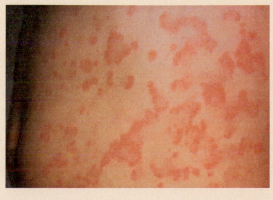

FIGURE 6.25

Urticaria, commonly called hives.

Courtesy of Jason L. Smith, MD.

TABLE 6.9   **Common Pathologies of the Integumentary System (continued)**

Disease/Disorder	Description	Massage Implications
Varicella (VAIR-ih-chell-a)	Contagious viral skin infection; commonly called *chicken pox* (Figure 6.26■)	General contraindication

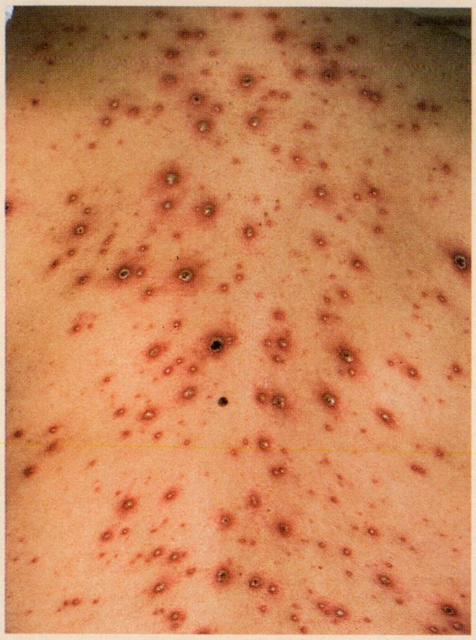

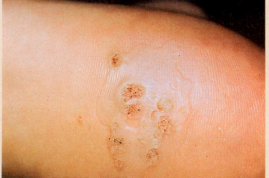

FIGURE 6.26

Varicella, commonly called chicken pox.

Courtesy of Jason L. Smith, MD.

Disease/Disorder	Description	Massage Implications
Vitiligo (vit-ill-EYE-go)	Lack of pigment in areas of the skin causing milky-white appearance	None
Wart	Benign growth with rough surface caused by a virus; a plantar wart forms on a pressure-bearing area of the body, often the sole of foot (Figure 6.27■)	Local contraindication

FIGURE 6.27

Plantar wart.

Courtesy of Jason L. Smith, MD.

SKELETAL SYSTEM

Appendicular skeleton (app-en-DIK-yoo-lar)

Axial skeleton (AK-see-al)

Bones

Bursa (BER-sah)

Cancellous bone (CAN-sell-us)

Cartilage (CAR-tih-lij)

Cartilaginous (car-tih-LAJ-ih-nus) joints

Compact bone

Diaphysis (dye-AFF-ih-sis)

Epiphysis (eh-PIF-ih-sis)

Fibrous (FYE-bruss) joints

Joints

Ligaments (LIG-ah-ments)

Medullary cavity (MED-you-lair-ee)

Periosteum (pair-ee-AH-stee-um)

Ribs

Spine

Sternum (STER-num)

Synovial (sin-OH-vee-al) joints

Tendons

Vertebrae (VER-teh-bray)

The 206 bones of the skeletal system serve as the body's frame, or skeleton, and protect vital organs, store minerals,

and, along with the muscular system, allow for movement. The skeletal system is divided into two main groups of bones: the *axial skeleton,* which consists of 80 bones from the axis of the body, including the skull, spine, ribs, and sternum, and the *appendicular skeleton,* consisting of the remaining 126 bones, including the extremities, and shoulder and pelvic girdles (Figure 6.28■). Cartilage, tendons, ligaments, and joints are additional parts of the skeletal system. See Table 6.10■ for abbreviations that relate to the skeletal system. See Table 6.14■ at the end of this section for common pathologies of the skeletal system and their massage implications.

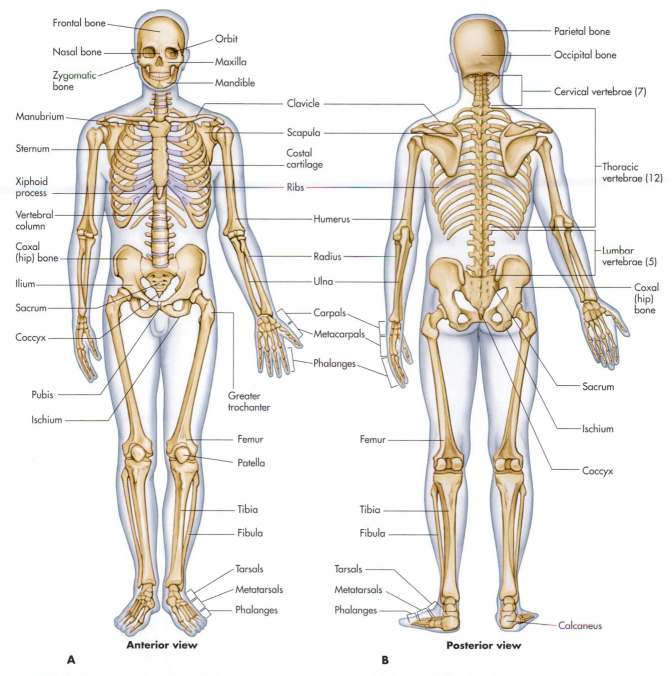

Anterior view

A

Posterior view

B

FIGURE 6.28

The human skeleton, anterior and posterior views.

TABLE 6.10 Skeletal System Abbreviations

Abbreviation	Meaning	Abbreviation	Meaning
AE	Above elbow	LLE	Left lower extremity
AK	Above knee	LUE	Left upper extremity
BE	Below elbow	OA	Osteoarthritis
BK	Below knee	Orth, ortho	Orthopedics
C1, C2, etc.	First cervical vertebra, second cervical vertebra, etc.	RA	Rheumatoid arthritis
		RLE	Right lower extremity
CDH	Congenital dislocation of the hip	RUE	Right upper extremity
CTS	Carpal tunnel syndrome	T1, T2, etc.	First thoracic vertebra, second thoracic vertebra, etc.
DJD	Degenerative joint disease		
FX, Fx	Fracture	THR	Total hip replacement
L1, L2, etc.	First lumbar vertebra, second lumbar vertebra, etc.	TKR	Total knee replacement
		TMJ	Temporomandibular joint
LAT, lat	Lateral	TX, tx	Traction, treatment
LE	Lower extremity	UE	Upper extremity

Parts and Functions of the Skeletal System

Bones

- Two types of bone tissue: compact and spongy.
- Provide support and framework for the body and protect internal organs.
- Play an important role in formation of red blood cells within the bone marrow.
- Store mineral salts, calcium, phosphorus.
- Provide areas for the attachment of skeletal muscles.
- Help make movement possible through articulation.

Cartilage

- Dense connective tissue that forms part of the adult skeleton and the major portion of the embryonic skeleton.
- Forms a flexible and cushioning connection between bones; can withstand tensing, flexing, and pressure.

Tendons

- Cordlike connective tissue that attaches muscles to bone.

Ligaments

- Tough bands that connect the ends of bones, joining them together to facilitate motion in joints.

Joints

- Places where two bones connect and allow movement; also called an *articulation* (Figure 6.29■).
- Protected by cartilage and lubricated by synovial fluid, which is released from a small sac called the *bursa* commonly found in elbow, knee, and shoulder joints.

Classification of Bones

Bones are classified according to six common shapes: long, short, flat, irregular, sesamoid, and sutural or wormian. Figure 6.30■ shows different shapes of bones.

FIGURE 6.29

Typical joint (knee).

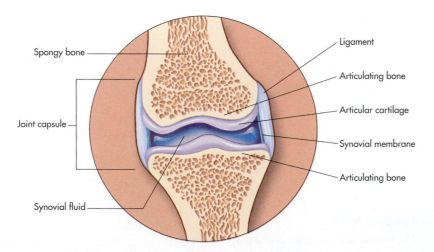

Spongy bone

Joint capsule

Synovial fluid

Ligament

Articulating bone

Articular cartilage

Synovial membrane

Articulating bone

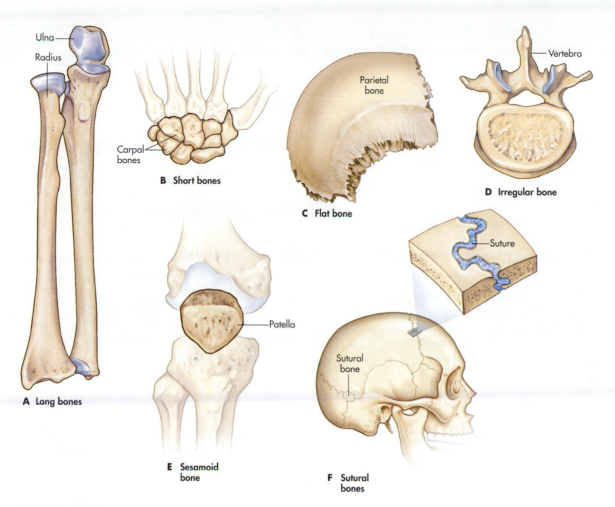

FIGURE 6.30

Classification of bones by shape.

Long bones
- Longer than they are wide; found mainly in arms and legs; *example:* humerus (arm), femur (thigh).

Short bones
- Equal sized in width and length; found mainly in wrists and ankles; *example:* tarsals (ankle), carpals (wrist).

Flat bones
- Thinner and platelike in shape; can be flat or curved; *example:* scapula (shoulder blade), ribs.

Irregular bones
- Odd-shaped bones that connect to other bones; *example:* vertebrae, hip bones.

Sesamoid bones
- Special type of short bone; forms within tendons; *example:* patella (kneecap).

Sutural bones
- Located at suture lines between the bones of the skull.

Structure of Bones

Long bones, such as the femur, have most of the components found in all bones (Figure 6.31■).

Epiphysis
- Ends of a developing bone.

Periosteum
- Tough, fibrous connective tissue forming the covering of bones; contains blood vessels that transport blood and nutrientsinto the bone and bone cells; acts as anchor points for ligaments and tendons.

Diaphysis
- Hollow shaft of a long bone

Medullary cavity
- Narrow canal within the diaphysis; storage area for yellow bone marrow, which is mainly fat cells.

Compact bone
- Strong, dense, hard tissue composing the shaft of long bones and the outer layer of other bones.

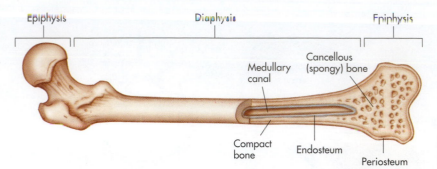

FIGURE 6.31

Features found in a long bone.

Cancellous bone

- Spongy appearance is due to irregular holes in the bone tissue that provides space for red bone marrow, which produces red blood cells, and also makes bones lighter in weight; also called *spongy bone*.

Bones have both projections (bumps) called *processes,* which serve as points of attachment for muscles, ligaments, and tendons (Figure 6.32■), and depressions (grooves), which serve as pathways for nerves and blood vessels. Table 6.11■ lists and describes these bone surface structures.

Axial Skeleton

The bones of the axial skeleton form the central axis for the entire body. They protect many internal organs, such as the lungs and heart. Refer to Figure 6.28 to see the all the bones of the axial skeleton in relation to the appendicular skeleton.

TABLE 6.11	Bone Surface Structures
Bone Projections/Processes	**Description**
Head	Large, smooth ball-shaped end on a long bone, sometimes separated from the shaft of the bone by a narrow area called the *neck*
Condyle (KON-dile)	Smooth, rounded part at the end of a bone
Epicondyle (ep-ih-KON-dile)	Projection located on or above a condyle
Trochanter (tro-KAN-ter)	Large, rough process for the attachment of a muscle
Tubercle (TOO-ber-kl)	Small, rough process for the attachment of tendons and muscles
Tuberosity (too-ber-OSS-ih-tee)	Large, rough process for the attachment of tendons and muscles
Spine	Sharp, pointed projection
Crest	Narrow ridge of bone
Bone Depressions/Openings	
Sinus (SIGH-nus)	Hollow cavity within a bone
Meatus	Tube or canal-like passageway through a bone
Foramen (for-AY-men)	Smooth round or oval opening for nerves, blood vessels, and ligaments
Fossa (FOSS-ah)	Groove or shallow depression on the surface of a bone
Fissure (FISH-er)	Narrow, slitlike opening

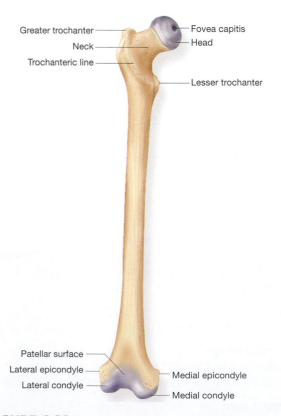

FIGURE 6.32

Bony process of the femur bone.

Figure 6.33■ shows the divisions of the vertebral column, which houses the spinal cord. Figure 6.34■ shows the structures of the thoracic cage. Figure 6.35■ shows the bones of the skull. Table 6.12■ describes the bones of the axial skeleton.

Appendicular Skeleton

The appendicular skeleton is composed of the bones of the upper and lower extremities (limbs) and the pectoral and pelvic girdles, which attach the limbs to the axial skeleton. Refer to Figure 6.28 to see the all the bones of the appendicular skeleton in relation to the axial skeleton. Figure 6.36■ shows the

FIGURE 6.33

Divisions of the vertebral column.

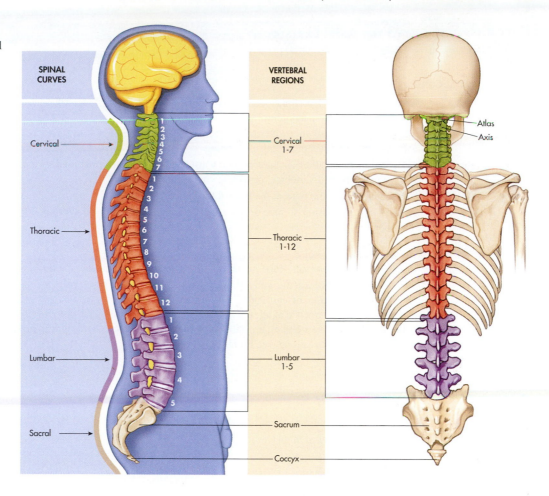

bones of the pectoral girdle and upper extremity. Figure 6.37■ shows the bones of the pelvic girdle and lower extremity. Table 6.13■ describes the bones of the appendicular skeleton.

Types of Joints

Joints are classified according to their structure and the type of movement they permit (Figure 6.38■).

Fibrous joints

- Produce no movement because there is no joint cavity; also called *synarthrotic joints.*
- Subcategories: suture (*example:* interlocking bones of the cranium); syndesmosis (*example:* distal ends of tibia and fibula).

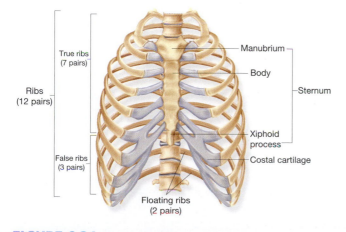

FIGURE 6.34

Structures of the thoracic cage.

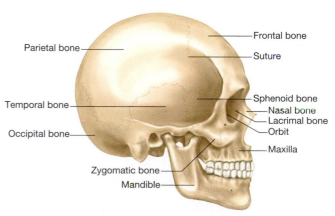

FIGURE 6.35

Bones of the skull.

TABLE 6.12 Bones of the Axial Skeleton

Bone(s)	Description
Vertebral/Spinal Column	
Cervical vertebrae	Vertebrae in the neck region (7); an intervertebral disc formed of fibrocartilage lies between each pair of vertebrae, providing cushioning
Thoracic vertebrae	Vertebrae in the chest area with ribs attached (12); an intervertebral disc formed of fibrocartilage lies between each pair of vertebrae, providing cushioning
Lumbar vertebrae	Vertebrae in the small of the back around waist level (5); an intervertebral disc formed of fibrocartilage lies between each pair of vertebrae, providing cushioning
Sacrum (SAY-crum)	Triangular-shaped flat bone at the base of the vertebral column (1)
Coccyx (COCK-six)	Formed from the fusion of three to five small vertebrae attached to the sacrum; considered to be the human "tailbone" (1)
Thoracic Cage	
Sternum (STER-num)	Flat bone that is the result of the fusion of three bones: the *manubrium,* the *body,* and the *xiphoid process*
Ribs	Twelve pairs of ribs form the walls of the thoracic cage; the first seven pairs are called *true ribs* and are attached to the sternum by cartilage; the next five pairs are called *false ribs* and attach indirectly to the sternum or are not attached at all; the last two pairs of false ribs, which are attached only to the vertebral column and not to the sternum, are called *floating ribs;* the spaces between the ribs are filled with intercostals muscles that aid in breathing (see Figure 6.121 on page 277)
Skull	
Cranial Bones	
Frontal bone	Forehead (1)
Parietal bone	Upper sides of cranium and roof of the skull (2)
Occipital bone (ock-SIP-eh-tal)	Back and base of the skull (1)
Temporal bone (TEM-por-al)	Sides and base of cranium (2)
Sphenoid bone (SFEE-noyd)	Spans the width of the skull, forms part of the floor of the cranial cavity, and sides of the eye orbits; butterfly shaped (1)
Ethmoid bone (ETH-moyd)	Irregularly shaped; forms part of the eye orbit, nose, and floor of the cranium
Facial Bones	
Lacrimal bone (LACK-rim-al)	Inner corner of each eye (2)
Nasal bone	Form part of nasal septum and support the bridge of the nose (2)
Maxilla (mack-SIH-lah)	Upper jaw (1)
Mandible (MAN-dih-bl)	Lower jawbone; this is the only movable bone of the skull (1)
Zygomatic bone (zeye-go-MAT-ik)	Cheekbones (2)
Vomer bone (VOH-mer)	Base of nasal septum (1)
Palatine bone (PAL-ah-tine)	Forms the hard palate of the mouth and floor of the nose (1)
Hyoid bone (HIGH-oyd)	Not technically part of the skull, but closely related to the temporal and mandible bones; suspended in the mid-neck region above the larynx; acts as movable base for the tongue and an attachment point for neck muscles that raise and lower the larynx, allowing speaking and swallowing

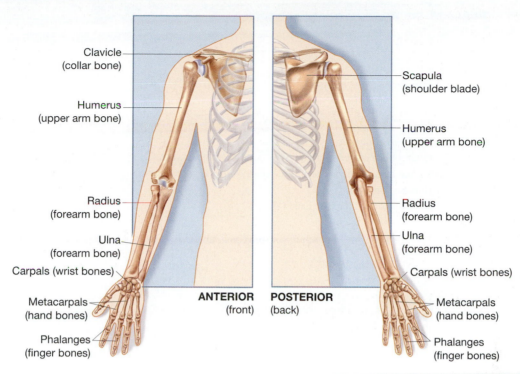

FIGURE 6.36

Bones of the pectoral girdle and upper extremity.

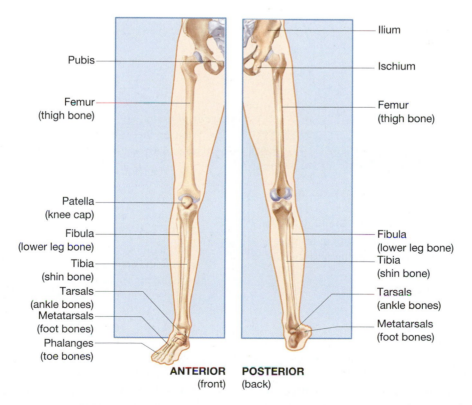

FIGURE 6.37

Bones of the pelvic girdle and lower extremity.

TABLE 6.13   Bones of the Appendicular Skeleton

Bone(s)	Description
Pectoral Girdle	
Clavicle (CLAV-ih-kl)	Collarbone (2)
Scapula (SKAP-yoo-lah)	Shoulder blade (2)
Upper Extremity	
Humerus (HYOO-mer-us)	Upper arm bone (2)
Radius (RAY-dee-us)	Lateral bone of the forearm (thumb side of lower arm) (2)
Ulna (UHL-nah)	Medial bone of the forearm (little finger side of lower arm) (2)
Carpals (CAR-pals)	Bones of the wrist (16)
Metacarpals (met-ah-CAR-pals)	Bones in the palm of the hand (10)
Phalanges (fah-LAN-jeez)	Finger bones; three in each finger (proximal, middle, and distal) and two in each thumb (proximal and distal) (28)
Pelvic Girdle	
Ilium (ILL-ee-um)	Part of the pelvis (2)
Ischium (ISS-kee-um)	Part of the pelvis (2)
Pubis (PYOO-bis)	Part of the pelvis (2)
Lower Extremity	
Femur (FEE-mer)	Thigh bone; strongest and heaviest bone in the body (2)
Patella (pah-TELL-ah)	Kneecap (2)
Tibia (TIB-ee-ah)	Shin bone (2)
Fibula (FIB-yoo-lah)	Thin long bone in lateral side of lower leg; forms the outer part of the ankle (2)
Tarsals (TAHR-sals)	Ankle and heel bones (14)
Metatarsals (met-ah-CAR-pals)	Form the sole of the foot (10)
Phalanges (fah-LAN-jeez)	Toe bones; three in each toe and two in the big toe (28)

MASSAGE CONNECTION

The structure of a joint determines the type of movement possible there. Massage therapists keep this in mind when applying joint movements. Abnormalities in joint structure due to a congenital condition, disease, or injury are taken into consideration during massage applications.

Cartilaginous joints

- Permits very slight movement; also called *amphiarthrotic joints.*
- Subcategories: synchondrosis (*example:* between rib 1 and the sternum); symphyses (*example:* intervertebral discs and adjacent vertebrae); symphysis (*example:* public symphysis).

Synovial joints

- Joint cavities are lined with synovial membranes and filled with synovial fluid; most joints are this type; also called *diarthrotic joints* (Figure 6.39■).
- Subcategories: multiaxial (*example:* shoulder); uniaxial (*example:* elbow); biaxial (*example:* intercarpal hand joints).
- Provide free movement in many directions; *examples:*
  ○ Pivot joints—rotate; found in neck and forearm.
  ○ Ball and socket joints—all types of movement including rotation; found in hips and shoulders.
  ○ Hinge joints—open and close; found in knees and elbows.
  ○ Gliding joints—slide back and forth; found in wrists and ankles.
  ○ Saddle joints—rock up and down and side to side; found in base of thumb.
  ○ Condyloid joints—movement from one plane to another; found in the knuckles.
  ○ Ellipsoidal joints—provided two axes of movement through the same bone; found in the wrist.

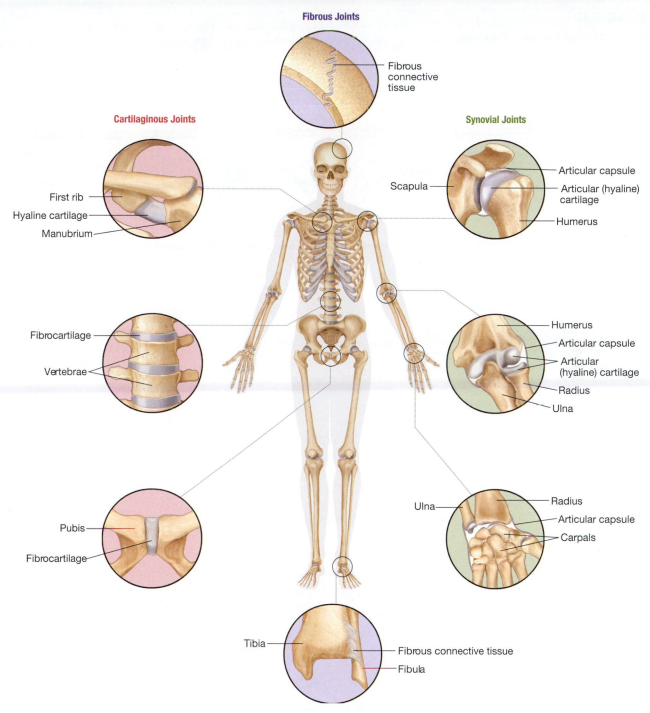

FIGURE 6.38

Types of joints.

Skeletal Alignment

Proper skeletal alignment while standing, sitting, and moving facilitates ease of motion and minimal strain on joints and muscles. Chronic misalignment can cause muscle strain, injury, and pain. Standing alignment is evaluated using anatomical landmarks. Posture analysis is discussed on page 324 in Chapter 10, Goal-Oriented Planning and Documentation. Also see a body chart for standing posture assessment in Figure 10.4 on page 325.

MASSAGE CONNECTION

Massage therapists observe clients' skeletal alignment as part of an informal assessment or of a formal posture analysis. Misalignment in standing posture offers clues to areas of muscle shortening or weakness.

FIGURE 6.39

Structure of the synovial joint of the knee.

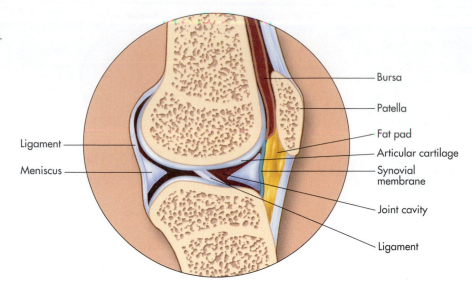

Bursa

Patella

Fat pad

Articular cartilage

Synovial membrane

Joint cavity

Ligament

Ligament

Meniscus

TABLE 6.14	Common Pathologies of the Skeletal System	
Disease/Disorder	Description	Massage Implications
Ankylosing spondylitis (ang-kih-LOH-sing spon-dih-LYE-tis)	Inflammatory spinal condition with stiffening and eventual fusion of the vertebrae	Indicated in subacute phase in conjunction with health care team; contraindicated during inflammatory phase
Arthritis	Inflammation of a joint	Indicated in subacute phase; contraindicated during acute inflammation
Bunion (BUN-yun)	Inflammation of the bursa of the big toe	Local contraindication
Bursitis	Inflammation of a bursa	Local contraindication
Carpal tunnel syndrome (CTS) (CAR-pal TUN-el)	Compression of the nerve as it passes between the bones and ligaments of the wrist causing pain (Figure 6.40■)	Indicated for treatment; contraindicated during acute inflammation
Dislocation	Displacement of a bone from a joint	Contraindicated until after reduction; indicated when condition of affected tissues allow

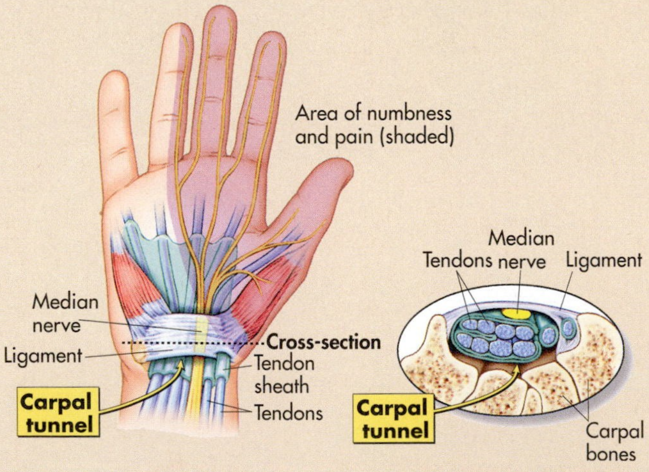

Area of numbness and pain (shaded)

Median nerve

Ligament

Carpal tunnel

Cross-section

Tendon sheath

Tendons

Median Tendons nerve   Ligament

Carpal tunnel

Carpal bones

FIGURE 6.40

Anatomy of carpal tunnel syndrome.

TABLE 6.14	Common Pathologies of the Skeletal System (continued)	
Disease/Disorder	Description	Massage Implications
Fracture (FX, Fx)	Broken bone; classified based on external appearance, site of fracture, and nature of crack or break in the bone; (Figure 6.41■) *examples of types of fractures:* Closed: simple fracture; internal; no break in the skin Open: compound fracture; bone projects through the skin; risk of infection or hemorrhage Comminuted: part of the bone is shattered into fragments Transverse: shaft of the bone is broken across its longitudinal access Greenstick: one side of the bone shaft is broken, the other side is bent; usually occurs in young children Spiral: fracture is spread along the length of the bone; can be caused by a twisting injury Colle's: common type of wrist fracture Compression: fractures of the vertebrae caused by severe stress or force	Local contraindication during early stages of healing; indicated for surrounding soft tissues in later stages of healing; limit movement of surrounding joints until completely healed.

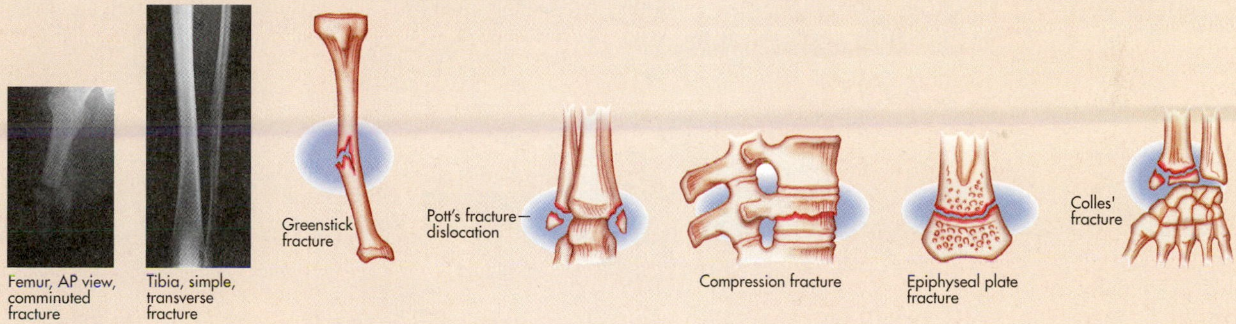

Femur, AP view, comminuted fracture
Tibia, simple, transverse fracture
Greenstick fracture
Pott's fracture—dislocation
Compression fracture
Epiphyseal plate fracture
Colles' fracture

FIGURE 6.41

Various types of fractures.

Ganglion cyst	Fluid-filled synovial sacks found on joint capsules and tendons	Local contraindication
Gout (GOWT)	Inflammation of the joints caused by excessive uric acid in the body	General contraindication
Kyphosis (ki-FOH-sis)	Abnormal outward curvature of the thoracic spine; also referred to as *humpback* (Figure 6.42A■)	Position client comfortably with bolsters; light pressure with suspected osteoporosis

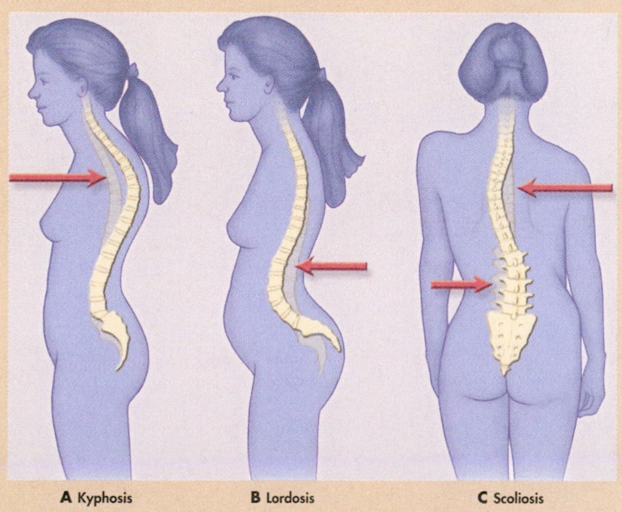

A Kyphosis   B Lordosis   C Scoliosis

FIGURE 6.42

Spinal misalignments. A. Kyphosis. B. Lordosis. C. Scoliosis.

TABLE 6.14 Common Pathologies of the Skeletal System (continued)

Disease/Disorder	Description	Massage Implications
Lordosis (lor-DOH-sis)	Abnormal forward curvature of the lumbar spine; also called *swayback* (Figure 6.42B)	Indicated for shortened, tight lower back muscles
Myeloma (my-ah-LOH-mah)	Malignant tumor of the bone marrow	Health care provider permission advised
Osteoarthritis (oss-tee-oh-ar-THRY-tis)	Degeneration of bones and joint due to arthritis; can result in bone rubbing against bone in joints	Indicated for treatment; contraindicated during acute inflammation
Osteogenic sarcoma (oss-tee-oh-GIN-ik sark-OH-ma)	Common type of bone cancer	Health care provider permission advised
Osteomalacia (oss-tee-oh-mah-LAY-she-ah)	Softening of the bones due to calcium deficiency	Light pressure only
Osteomyelitis	Infection of the bone and bone marrow causing inflammation	General contraindication
Osteoporosis (oss-tee-oh-por-ROH-sis)	Loss of bone density and thinning of bone tissue; often results in fractures; seen most commonly in postmenopausal women (Figure 6.43■)	Light pressure and gentle stretching only

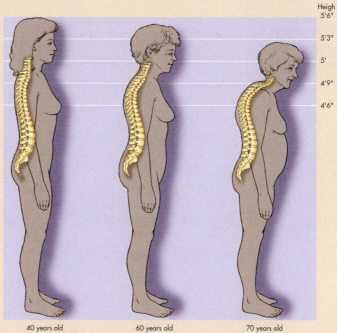

FIGURE 6.43

Spinal changes caused by osteoporosis.

40 years old   60 years old   70 years old

Paget's (PAH-jets) disease	Metabolic disease of the bone causing bone destruction and deformity; often seen in older people	Light pressure and gentle stretching only

TABLE 6.14 Common Pathologies of the Skeletal System (continued)

Disease/Disorder	Description	Massage Implications
Rheumatoid arthritis (ROO-maah-toyd ar-THRY-tis)	Autoimmune disorder with inflammation of joints, swelling, stiffness, and pain; can result in deformities of the hand and other parts of the body (Figure 6.44■)	Light massage indicated for treatment; contraindicated during acute inflammation

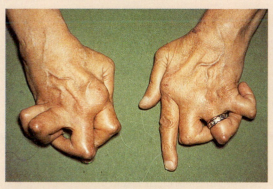

FIGURE 6.44
Contractures of rheumatoid arthritis.

Disease/Disorder	Description	Massage Implications
Rickets (RIK-ets)	Deficiency in calcium and vitamin D in early childhood resulting in bone deformities, particularly bowed legs	Light massage only
Ruptured intervertebral disk	Herniation or protrusion of a disk between two vertebrae; also called *herniated disk* or *slipped disk*	Local contraindication; position client comfortably with bolsters
Scoliosis (skoh-lee-OH-sis)	Abnormal lateral curvature of the spine; often appears during adolescence (see Figure 6.42C)	Light massage to tolerance; ice massage for muscle spasms
Spinal stenosis (ste-NOH-sis)	Narrowing of the spinal canal causing pressure on the spinal cord and surrounding nerves	Light massage to tolerance
Spondylosis (spon-dih-LOH-sis)	Degenerative condition of the vertebral column; osteoarthritis of the spine	Light massage to tolerance
Sprain	Damage to the ligaments surrounding a joint due to overstretching	Local contraindication in inflammatory phase; lymphatic facilitation to reduce swelling; massage to tolerance in surrounding musculature in subacute phase; limit movements at affected joint.
Whiplash	Injury to the bones in the cervical area of the spine due to violent movement backward and forward of the head and neck; often due to sudden impact of auto accidents	Contraindication in acute phase; massage indicated during scar formation and remodeling

MUSCULAR SYSTEM

Cardiac muscle

Fascia (FASH-ee-ah)

Fascicles (FAS-ih-culs)

Involuntary muscle

Motor Unit

Muscle fiber

Muscles

Myofibril (my-uh-FIGH-brul)

Reciprocal inhibition

Sarcomere (SAR-ka-meer)

Skeletal muscle

Smooth muscle

Tendons

Voluntary muscle

The muscular system provides the mechanism for movement of the body and locomotion from one place to another. It functions in close coordination with the skeletal and nervous systems. In addition to causing movement, muscles help the body maintain posture and stability (holding bones together and keeping joints stable), and produce heat. There are three major types of muscles: skeletal, smooth, and cardiac, which are classified as to their function and appearance. Table 6.15■ lists abbreviations that relate to the muscular system. See Table 6.17■ at the end of this section for common pathologies of the muscular system and their massage implications.

TABLE 6.15	Muscular System Abbreviations
Abbreviation	Meaning
DTR	Deep tendon reflex
IM	Intramuscular
MD	Muscular dystrophy

Parts and Functions of the Muscular System

Muscles

- Cause movement of the body, maintain posture and stability, control openings of the digestive tract, produce heat.
- Comprise almost 42 percent of a person's normal body weight.
- Consist of a group of fibers held together by connective tissue and enclosed in a sheath of fascia.
- Contain blood and lymphatic vessels that supply nutrients and oxygen, and remove metabolic wastes.
- Receive nerve impulses to produce movement, and store glycogen to use as fuel.
- Divided into three major types: skeletal, cardiac, and smooth muscles (Figure 6.46■).

Skeletal muscles

- Attached directly or indirectly to bones and overlap joints.
- Composed of a group of fibers wrapped in layers of fibrous connective tissues called *fascia* that narrow and form tendons at the ends of the muscle; these tendons anchor muscles to bones (Figure 6.45■)
- Fascial sheaths in muscles include the endomysium around individual muscle fibers, the perimysium that bundles muscle fibers together into fascicles, and the epimysium that wraps the fascicles and gives a muscle its characteristic shape (Figure 6.45).

- Composed of three parts:
  - Body—main portion.
  - Origin—fixed attachment of a muscle to a bone.
  - Insertion—attachment point on the bone that moves.
- Produce different kinds of voluntary body movement through rapid contraction, extension, and elasticity.
- Have a striped or striated appearance (Figure 6.46A■); also called *striated muscle*
- Stimulated by motor neurons of the nervous system.

Cardiac muscles

- Comprise the wall of the heart; also called the *myocardium.*
- Produce involuntary contractions that cause the heart to pump blood out of its chambers and through the blood vessels.
- Have a striated appearance (Figure 6.46B).

Smooth muscles

- Responsible for the involuntary muscle actions of the internal organs, such as pushing food through the digestive system, constricting or dilating a blood vessel, and uterine contractions.
- Mostly found in the organs of the digestive, respiratory, urinary, and vascular systems, and certain muscles of the eye and skin; also called *visceral muscle*
- Appearance is smooth, with no striations (Figure 6.46C).

Tendons

- Bands of connective tissue that anchor muscles to bones.

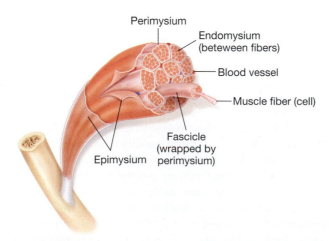

FIGURE 6.45

A skeletal muscle is composed of a group of fibers held together by connective tissue called fascia.

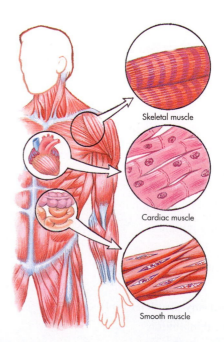

FIGURE 6.46

Three types of muscle. A. Skeletal. B. Cardiac. C. Smooth.

MASSAGE CONNECTION

Massage therapists palpate individual muscles wrapped in the fascia of the epimysium. Restrictions or adhesions between any of the fascial sheaths related to a muscle can result in the muscle not functioning properly. Some massage techniques, such as kneading and broadening, mechanically separate fascial tissues that are sticking together. Specialized myofascial massage techniques are designed specifically to release deep fascial restrictions in the musculature.

Skeletal Muscle and Contraction

Skeletal muscles are made up of bundles of muscle fibers. Each muscle fiber contains functional units called myofibrils. Each myofibril is a chain of contractile units called sarcomeres (Figure 6.47A■). It is action within the sarcomeres that causes muscle contraction (Figure 6.47B).

Skeletal muscle
- A bundle of muscle fibers with a characteristic shape that causes skeletal movement, e.g., biceps.

Muscle fiber
- A multi-nucleus cell made up of myofibrils bundled together.
- Plasma membrane around the bundle of myofibrils is called the *sarcolemma*.

Myofibril
- Chain of contractile units called *sarcomeres*.

Sacromere
- Made up of threadlike structures called myofilaments.
  - Thick myofilaments = myosin.
  - Thin myofilament = actin.
  - Bare zone between actin filaments.
  - Z lines separate sarcomere units and give the striated appearance to skeletal muscle.

Muscle contraction
- Occurs from shortening of the sarcomeres.
- Actin and myosin myofilaments slide toward each other.
- A molecule called adenosine triphosphate (ATP) provides energy for the formation of crossbridges that cause muscle contraction.

Functional properties of muscle
- *Excitability* or the ability to respond to a stimulus.
- *Contractibility* or the ability to shorten forcibly when adequately stimulated.
- *Extensibility* or ability to be stretched.
- *Elasticity* or ability to resume resting length after a stretch.

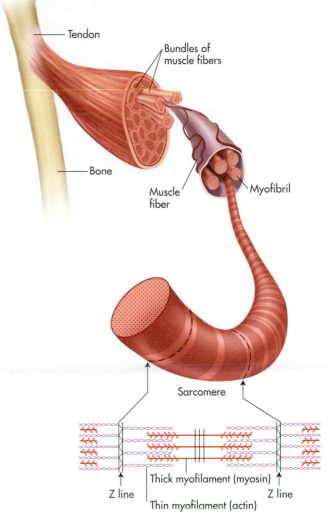

A MUSCLE SEGMENT WITH SARCOMERE

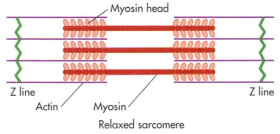

B SARCOMERE

FIGURE 6.47

A. Muscle segment with sarcomere. B. Relaxed and contracted sarcomeres.

Motor unit
- A *motor unit* includes a motor neuron and all of the muscle fibers attached to it (Figure 6.48■).
- *Motor neurons* reside in the spinal column and their *axons* extend to the muscle.
- Axons branch into *axon terminals* each of which joins a different muscle fiber at the *neuromuscular junction*.

FIGURE 6.48

Motor unit.

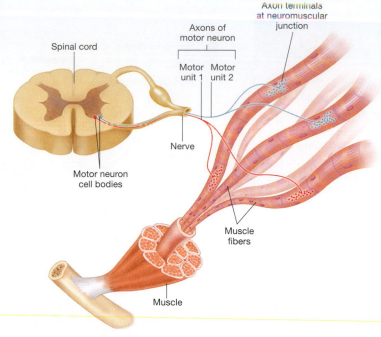

- There is a gap or *synaptic cleft* between the nerve endings and the muscle fibers.
- Axons transmit nerve impulses that cause a neurotransmitter called acetylcholine (ACh) to be released into the synaptic cleft.
- ACh sets off a chain of events that leads to a muscle contraction.

Reciprocal inhibition

- When a muscle contracts, its opposing muscle (antagonist) relaxes slightly to allow the desired movement to occur. This reflex mechanism is called reciprocal inhibition.

Skeletal Muscle Structure

Muscle fiber bundles called fascicles are arranged in different patterns to produce the different shapes of individual skeletal muscles (Figure 6.49■). See Table 6.16■ for descriptions and examples of fascicle patterns.

MASSAGE CONNECTION

Massage techniques are sometimes applied to specific muscles and muscle groups in relation to the arrangement of muscle fibers. For example, techniques may run parallel to the fiber arrangement (e.g., muscle stripping) or at an angle to fiber arrangement (e.g., cross-fiber friction).

Skeletal Muscles: General Locations

There are hundreds of skeletal muscles in the human body. Figure 6.50■ shows the anterior and posterior views of the major skeletal muscles. Specific skeletal muscles of different parts of the body are shown in Figures 6.116 through 6.139 in the kinesiology section of this chapter.

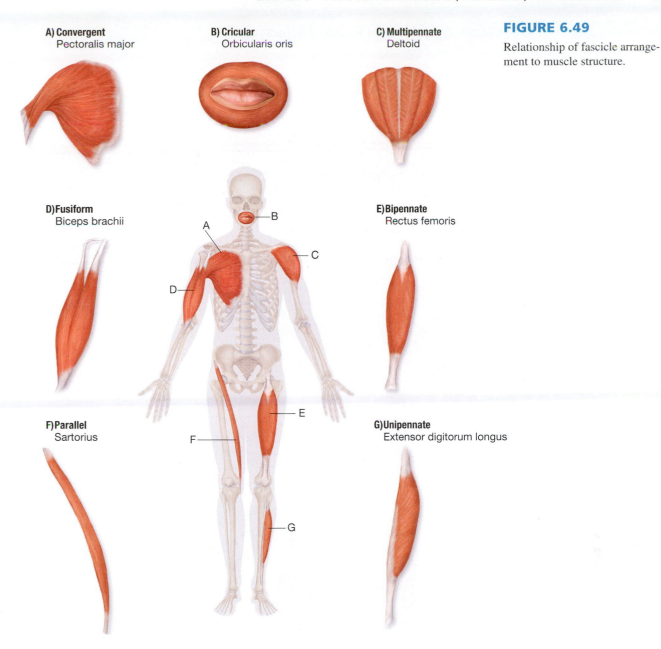

A) Convergent
Pectoralis major

B) Cricular
Orbicularis oris

C) Multipennate
Deltoid

D) Fusiform
Biceps brachii

E) Bipennate
Rectus femoris

F) Parallel
Sartorius

G) Unipennate
Extensor digitorum longus

FIGURE 6.49

Relationship of fascicle arrangement to muscle structure.

TABLE 6.16	Fascicle Patterns	
Fascicle Pattern	**Description**	**Example(s)**
Convergent	Fascicles converge toward a single insertion tendon; muscles are triangular or fan-shaped	Pectoralis major Latissimus dorsi
Fusiform	Spindle-shaped muscle with an expanded muscle belly; modification of parallel pattern	Biceps brachii
Parallel	Fascicles run parallel to the long axis of the muscle	Sartorius
Circular	Fascicles are in concentric rings	Orbicularis oris
Pennate	Fascicles are in a "feather" pattern with short fascicles running obliquely into a central tendon	
Multipennate	Fascicles insert from several different sides	Deltoid
Bipennate	Fascicles insert on both sides	Rectus femoris
Unipennate	Fascicles insert on one side only	Extensor digitorum longus

Major Muscles and Related Structures

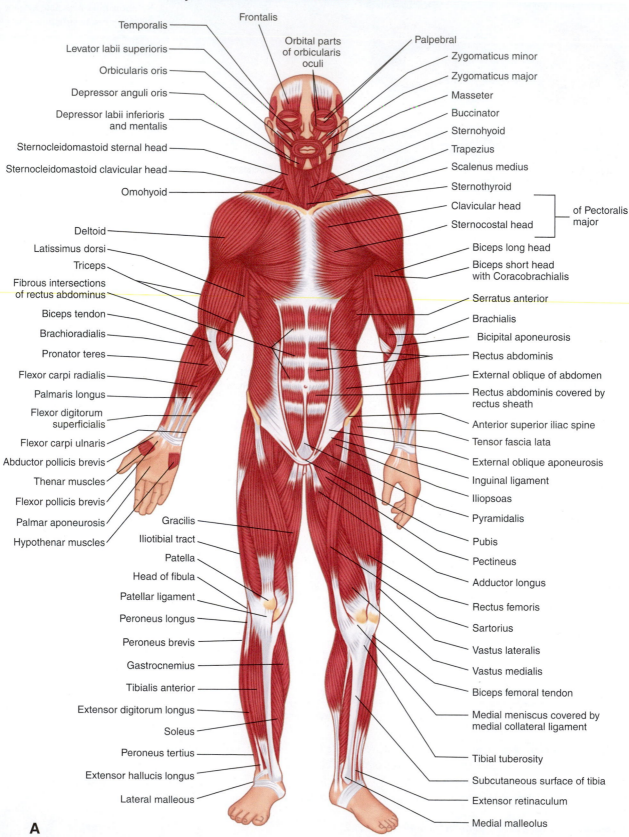

Temporalis
Frontalis
Levator labii superioris
Orbital parts of orbicularis oculi
Palpebral
Orbicularis oris
Zygomaticus minor
Depressor anguli oris
Zygomaticus major
Depressor labii inferioris and mentalis
Masseter
Buccinator
Sternocleidomastoid sternal head
Sternohyoid
Sternocleidomastoid clavicular head
Trapezius
Omohyoid
Scalenus medius
Sternothyroid
Deltoid
Clavicular head
Sternocostal head
of Pectoralis major
Latissimus dorsi
Triceps
Biceps long head
Fibrous intersections of rectus abdominus
Biceps short head with Coracobrachialis
Biceps tendon
Serratus anterior
Brachioradialis
Brachialis
Pronator teres
Bicipital aponeurosis
Flexor carpi radialis
Rectus abdominis
Palmaris longus
External oblique of abdomen
Flexor digitorum superficialis
Rectus abdominis covered by rectus sheath
Flexor carpi ulnaris
Anterior superior iliac spine
Abductor pollicis brevis
Tensor fascia lata
Thenar muscles
External oblique aponeurosis
Flexor pollicis brevis
Inguinal ligament
Palmar aponeurosis
Iliopsoas
Hypothenar muscles
Gracilis
Pyramidalis
Iliotibial tract
Pubis
Patella
Pectineus
Head of fibula
Adductor longus
Patellar ligament
Rectus femoris
Peroneus longus
Sartorius
Peroneus brevis
Vastus lateralis
Gastrocnemius
Vastus medialis
Tibialis anterior
Biceps femoral tendon
Extensor digitorum longus
Medial meniscus covered by medial collateral ligament
Soleus
Peroneus tertius
Tibial tuberosity
Extensor hallucis longus
Subcutaneous surface of tibia
Lateral malleous
Extensor retinaculum
Medial malleolus

A

FIGURE 6.50

A. Anterior view of major skeletal muscles.

Major Muscles and Related Structures

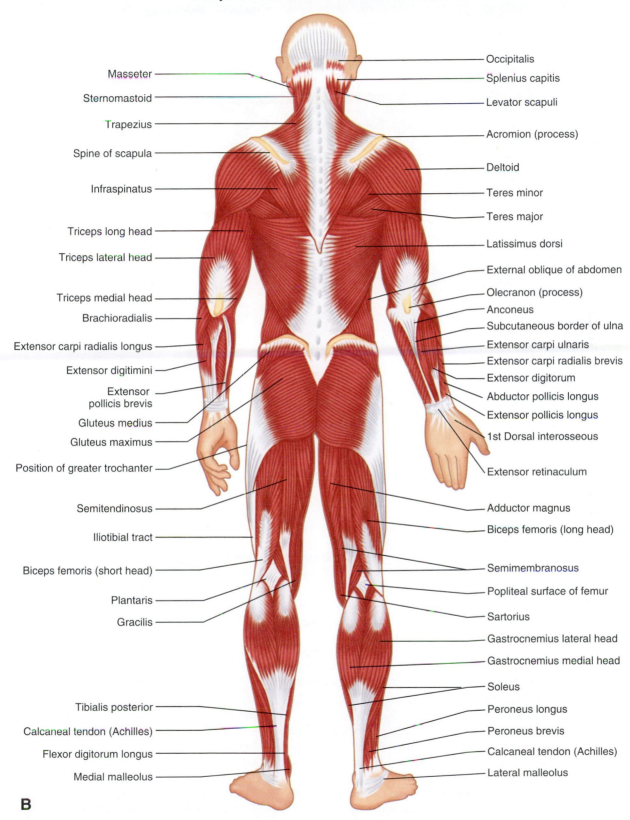

Masseter

Sternomastoid

Trapezius

Spine of scapula

Infraspinatus

Triceps long head

Triceps lateral head

Triceps medial head

Brachioradialis

Extensor carpi radialis longus

Extensor digitimini

Extensor pollicis brevis

Gluteus medius

Gluteus maximus

Position of greater trochanter

Semitendinosus

Iliotibial tract

Biceps femoris (short head)

Plantaris

Gracilis

Tibialis posterior

Calcaneal tendon (Achilles)

Flexor digitorum longus

Medial malleolus

Occipitalis

Splenius capitis

Levator scapuli

Acromion (process)

Deltoid

Teres minor

Teres major

Latissimus dorsi

External oblique of abdomen

Olecranon (process)

Anconeus

Subcutaneous border of ulna

Extensor carpi ulnaris

Extensor carpi radialis brevis

Extensor digitorum

Abductor pollicis longus

Extensor pollicis longus

1st Dorsal interosseous

Extensor retinaculum

Adductor magnus

Biceps femoris (long head)

Semimembranosus

Popliteal surface of femur

Sartorius

Gastrocnemius lateral head

Gastrocnemius medial head

Soleus

Peroneus longus

Peroneus brevis

Calcaneal tendon (Achilles)

Lateral malleolus

B

FIGURE 6.50

B. Posterior view of major skeletal muscles.

TABLE 6.17	Common Pathologies of the Muscular System	
Disease/Disorder	Description	Massage Implications
Adhesion	Binding between layers of fascial tissue	Fascial massage techniques indicated for treatment
Atrophy (AT-rah-fee)	Loss of muscle mass and strength due to the immobility and the disuse of muscles over a long period of time	Massage indicated for treatment
Contracture (kon-TRACK-chur)	Abnormal shortening of muscle fibers, tendons, and/or fascia, resulting in difficulty stretching the muscle	Massage indicated for treatment
Fibromyalgia (figh-broh-my-AL-jee-ah)	Chronic condition with widespread pain and aching in the muscles and soft tissue and debilitating fatigue; Figure 6.51■ shows the 18 tender points on the body that are affected by the syndrome	Massage to tolerance indicated for treatment

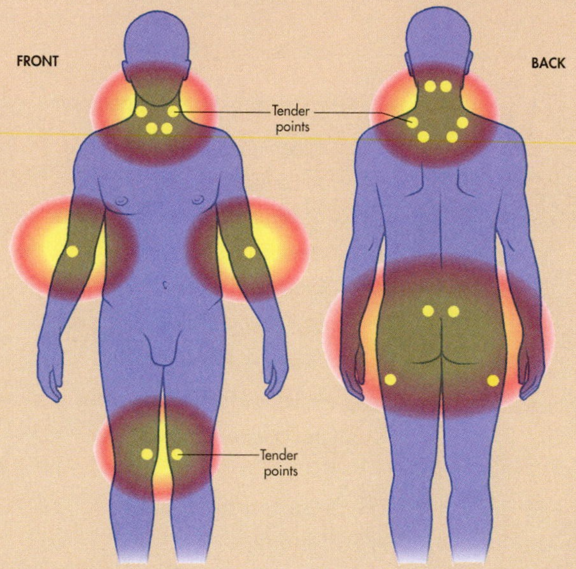

FIGURE 6.51

The 18 tender points on the body that are affected by fibromyalgia.

Hernia	Tear in a muscle wall that allows an organ to protrude from the body	Local contraindication
Lateral epicondylitis (ep-ih-kon-dih-LYE-tis)	Inflammation of the muscle attachment to the lateral epicondyle of the elbow; also called *tennis elbow*	Deep transverse friction over lesion indicated with ice therapy; ice massage indicated
Muscular dystrophy (MD) (MUSS-kew-ler DIS-troh-fee)	Group of chronic, genetic diseases causing progressive muscular degeneration and weakness resulting in atrophied muscles	Massage indicated as part of comprehensive health care treatment
Myasthenia gravis (my-ass-THEE-nee-ah GRAV-iss)	Neuromuscular disease involving both the muscular and nervous systems; characterized by increasing muscle weakness leading to complete paralysis	Massage indicated as part of comprehensive health care treatment
Paralysis	Partial or total loss of the ability of voluntary muscles to move	Massage indicated as part of comprehensive health care treatment
Repetitive motion disorder	Damage to tendons, muscles, joints, and/or nerves due to repetitive movements for long periods of time	Indicated for treatment, especially trigger point therapy
Scar tissue	Randomly arranged collagen fibers laid down over an injury site in muscles and tendons.	Deep transverse friction indicated for treatment along with stretching and cryotherapy
Shin splints	Pain in the muscles and surrounding tissues of the anterior lower leg; a common running- or exercise-related injury	Local contraindication during acute phase; massage, especially muscle stripping, indicated for treatment along with stretching and cryotherapy

TABLE 6.17	Common Pathologies of the Muscular System (continued)	
Disease/Disorder	Description	Massage Implications
Spasm	Sudden and violent contraction of a muscle for a period of time; also called *cramp*	Manual techniques indicated to relieve spasm along with cryotherapy
Strains	Injury or tears in muscles and tendons	Local contraindication in inflammatory phase; lymphatic facilitation to reduce swelling; massage to tolerance in surrounding musculature in subacute phase; deep transverse friction to lesion site in remodeling phase; limit movements at affected joint.
Tendinitis (TEN-din-aye-tis)	Inflammation of a tendon usually after excessive repetitive movements	Local contraindication during acute phase; deep transverse friction indicated for treatment along with ice massage and cryotherapy
Tetanus	Often fatal bacterial disease characterized by painful muscle spasms, including "locking" of the jaw (*lockjaw*) that prevents the mouth from opening	Medical emergency

NERVOUS SYSTEM

Autonomic (aw-toh-NOM-ik) nervous system

Axon (AK-son)

Brain stem

Brain

Central nervous system

Cerebellum (ser-eh-BELL-um)

Cerebrum (SER-eh-brum)

Cranial nerves (KRAY-nee-al)

Dendrites (DEN-drights)

Diencephalon (dye-en-SEFF-ah-lon)

Efferent fibers (EFF-er-ent)

Medulla oblongata (meh-DULL-ah ob-long-GAH-tah)

Midbrain

Nerves

Nervous tissue

Neurons (NOO-ronz)

Parasympathetic division (pair-ah-sim-pah-THET-ik)

Peripheral nervous system (per-IF-er-al)

Pons

Somatic nerves

Spinal cord

Spinal nerves

Sympathetic division (sim-pah-THET-ic)

The task of the nervous system is to coordinate and control all the activities of the body. It receives information from internal and external sensory receptors, and acts on that information to carry out muscular and glandular functions to satisfy the needs of the body. Composed of nervous tissue, the nervous system is subdivided into the central nervous system (CNS), the peripheral nervous system (PNS), and the autonomic nervous system (ANS). See Figure 6.52■. The CNS is made up of the brain and spinal cord; the PNS consists of cranial and spinal nerves; and the ANS, which is considered to be a part of the PNS, is composed of efferent fibers from cranial and spinal nerves, and is responsible for keeping the body in a state of homeostasis. Table 6.18■ lists abbreviations that relate to the nervous system. Table 6.19■ at the end of this section lists common pathologies of the nervous system and their massage implications.

Parts and Functions of the Nervous System

Nerve tissue

- Consists of two types of cells: neurons, which are individual nerve cells that conduct electrical impulses in response to a stimulus, and neuroglial cells, which form supportive tissue for the neurons.
- Three main types of neurons are motor neurons, sensory neurons, and interneurons.
- Motor neurons control most of the body's functions, such as muscular contractions and secretions from glands and organs; they have three main parts: dendrites, a nerve cell body that contains the nucleus, and an axon (Figure 6.53■).
  - Dendrites are multiple-branched projections that *receive* electrical impulses.
  - The axon is a singular long projection that *sends* an electrical impulse toward its destination—the dendrites of another neuron or the targeted organ itself.
  - The synaptic cleft is the gap between the axon of one neuron and the dendrites of the next neuron; a chemical called a neurotransmitter assists the electrical impulse to jump from one neuron to another.
- Sensory neurons are attached to sensor receptors and transmit impulses to the cell body and the CNS, which

FIGURE 6.52

The nervous system. The central nervous system (CNS) consists of the brain and spinal cord. The peripheral nervous system (PNS) consists of peripheral nerves.

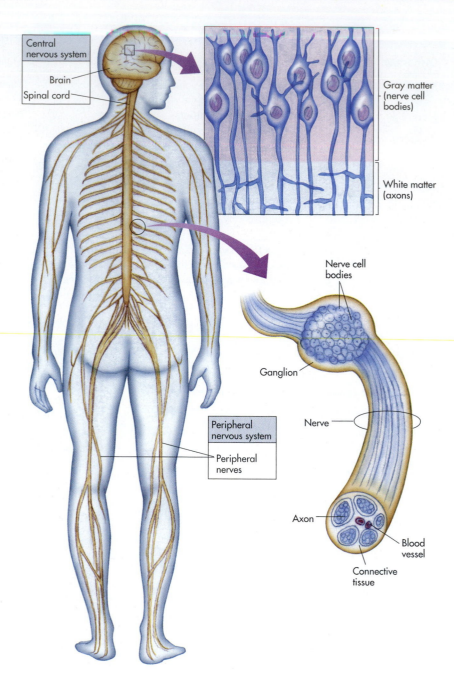

TABLE 6.18	Nervous System Abbreviations
Abbreviation	**Meaning**
ANS	Autonomic nervous system
CNS	Central nervous system
CSF	Cerebrospinal fluid
CVA	Cerebrovascular accident
CVD	Cerebrovascular disease
HA	Headache
ICP	Intracranial pressure
PNS	Peripheral nervous system

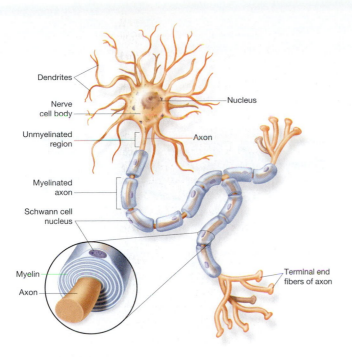

FIGURE 6.53

The structure of a neuron, showing dendrites, nerve cell body, and axon.

then stimulates motor neurons in response, causing movement.
- Different in structure than motor neurons and lacking dendrites, sensory neurons process and transmit information with peripheral processes, which somewhat resemble axons.
- Interneurons are located within the CNS and mediate impulses between the motor and sensory neurons.

Nerves

- A nerve fiber is generally an axon from a motor neuron or a peripheral process from a sensory neuron covered in a protective membrane called a sheath.
- A nerve is composed of bundles of nerve fibers, located outside the brain and spinal cord, connecting different parts of the body.
  - Afferent (sensory) nerves transmit messages *to* the CNS; efferent (motor) nerves transmit messages *from* the CNS.
- Nerve tracts are groups of nerve fibers within the CNS that have the same origin, function, and termination.

Central nervous system (CNS)

- Composed of the brain and spinal cord, the CNS receives impulses from all over the body, processes the information, and then responds with an appropriate action.
  - The action can be at the conscious or unconscious level, depending on the source of the sensory stimulus.

- Encased and protected by three layers of connective tissue membranes called the meninges.
- Has four interconnected cavities in the brain called ventricles, which are contiguous with the central canal of the spinal cord, containing cerebrospinal fluid (CSF), a clear liquid that cushions and protects the brain and spinal cord from damage, as well as nourishing them with oxygen and glucose.
- Consists of both gray and white matter; gray matter is unsheathed cell bodies and dendrites; white matter is nerve fibers sheathed in myelin, a fatty, insulating substance.

Brain

- Coordinates most body activities and governs sensory perceptions, thought, memory, judgment, and emotions; different parts of the brain control different body functions such as temperature regulation, breathing, and blood pressure.
- The four sections of the brain (Figure 6.54■) are:
  1. Cerebrum—processes thoughts, judgment, memory, problem solving, and language; divided into left and right halves called cerebral hemispheres; each hemisphere has four lobes:
     - Frontal lobe—controls motor function, personality, and speech.
     - Parietal lobe—receives and interprets nerve impulses from sensory receptors; interprets language.
     - Occipital lobe—controls vision.
     - Temporal lobe—controls hearing and smell.
  2. Diencephalon—contains the thalamus and the hypothalamus.
     - Thalamus—relays impulses from the eyes, ears, and skin to the cerebrum; controls pain perception.
     - Hypothalamus—link between the nervous and endocrine systems; controls the autonomic nervous system; acts as endocrine organ secreting hormones RH (releasing hormone) and IH (inhibiting hormone) to regulate the anterior pituitary gland; releases hormones ADH and oxytocin to posterior pituitary gland; affects body temperature, appetite, sleep, sexual desire, emotions, circulation, and digestion; also see endocrine system on page 170.
  3. Cerebellum—coordinates voluntary body movement; helps to maintain balance and equilibrium.
  4. Brain stem—comprises the midbrain, pons, and medulla oblongata.
     - Midbrain—pathway for impulses conducted between the brain and spinal cord.
     - Pons—connects the cerebellum to the rest of the brain.
     - Medulla oblongata—connects the brain to the spinal cord; regulates respiration, heart rate, temperature, and blood pressure; controls swal-

FIGURE 6.54

The sections of the brain.

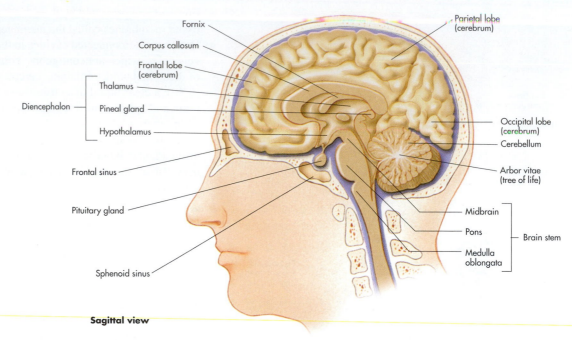

Fornix

Corpus callosum

Frontal lobe (cerebrum)

Thalamus

Diencephalon — Pineal gland

Hypothalamus

Frontal sinus

Pituitary gland

Sphenoid sinus

Parietal lobe (cerebrum)

Occipital lobe (cerebrum)

Cerebellum

Arbor vitae (tree of life)

Midbrain

Pons — Brain stem

Medulla oblongata

Sagittal view

lowing, coughing, and sneezing; here is where nerve tracts cross from one side of the brain to control actions on the other side of the body (right side of the brain controls the left side of the body and vice versa).

Spinal cord
- Provides a pathway for impulses traveling to and from the brain; also performs as a reflex center for nerve impulses that do not need to pass through the brain.
- Consists of a column of nervous tissue extending from the medulla oblongata of the brain down to the second lumbar vertebra (L_2) within the vertebral column.

Peripheral nervous system (PNS)
- Connects the central nervous system to organs of the body, including sensory organs such as eyes and ears, muscles, blood vessels, and glands.
- Composed of a network of nerves branching throughout the body from the brain and spinal cord; 12 pairs of cranial nerves attach to the brain, mainly at the medulla oblongata; 31 pairs of spinal nerves connect to the spinal cord; and one pair (a right and a left) exits between each pair of vertebrae.

Cranial nerves
- Provide sensory input and motor control; arranged symmetrically, there are 12 on each side of the brain; their names reflect the area or function they impact:
  - Olfactory (I)—responsible for sense of smell.
  - Optic (II)—responsible for vision.
  - Oculomotor (III)—conducts motor impulses for eye muscle and pupil.
  - Trochlear (IV)—controls the eye's oblique muscles.

- Trigeminal (V)—provides sensory input from the face and top of the head; controls muscles for chewing.
- Abducens (VI)—controls eyeball muscle.
- Facial (VII)—controls muscles of the face and scalp, salivary glands, lacrimal glands of the eye; sense of taste from the tongue.
- Vestibulocochlear (VIII)—influences equilibrium and hearing.
- Glossopharyngeal (IX)—provides for taste; regulates swallowing and saliva production.
- Vagus (X)—controls muscles of the pharynx, larynx, thoracic and abdominal organs.
- Accessory (XI)—controls neck and shoulder muscles.
- Hypoglossal (XII)—controls tongue muscles.

Spinal nerves
- Distributed along the length of the spinal cord, providing two-way communication between the spinal column and parts of the arms, legs, neck, and trunk of the body.
- The 31 pairs are grouped according to the portion of the spinal column from which they originate (Figure 6.55■).
  - Eight pairs of cervical nerves (C1-C8).
  - Twelve pairs of thoracic nerves (T1-12).
  - Five pairs of lumbar nerves (L1-L5).
  - Five pairs of sacral nerves (S1-S5).
  - One pair of coccygeal nerves.

Somatic nerves
- Nerves of the peripheral nervous system serving the skin and skeletal muscles.

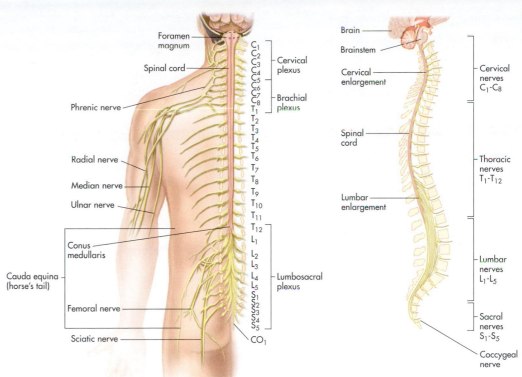

FIGURE 6.55
The 31 pairs of spinal nerves.

- Responsible for voluntary activities of the body, such as sending information to the brain about touch, temperature, and pain gathered from sensory receptors in the skin; also carry motor commands to skeletal muscles.
- Complex networks of nerves called plexus are found in the limbs. Figure 6.56■ shows the brachial plexus, lumbar plexus, and sacral plexus.

Autonomic nervous system (ANS)
- Responsible for involuntary functions of the body such as sweating, secretions from glands, gastrointestinal activity, arterial blood pressure, smooth muscle tissue, respiratory functions, the heart's electrical activity, and other bodily functions.
- Divided into two subsystems: the sympathetic and the parasympathetic; these two divisions act in tandem on the same organs but cause opposite effects, thus counterbalancing each other's actions and keeping the body in a state of homeostasis.

Sympathetic division
- Controls the "fight or flight" response in times of stress and danger, stimulating organs and mobilizing needed energy.
- Raises blood pressure and heart rate; increases blood supply to skeletal muscles; dilates the pupils of the eyes and bronchioles (improving vision and oxygenation); slows down gastrointestinal activity; stimulates glycogenolysis (breakdown of glycogen to glucose) in the liver and lipolysis (breakdown of fat) in the adipose tissue.

Para-sympathetic division
- Responsible for the "downtime" between stressful situations, when the body needs to rest and renew energy reserves; activation results in the "relaxation response."
- Lowers blood pressure and heart rate; contracts the pupils and bronchioles; diverts blood back to the gastrointestinal organs.

MASSAGE CONNECTION

Pressure directly over a nerve or nerve plexus that is unprotected by layers of muscle is contraindicated. These are endangerment sites.

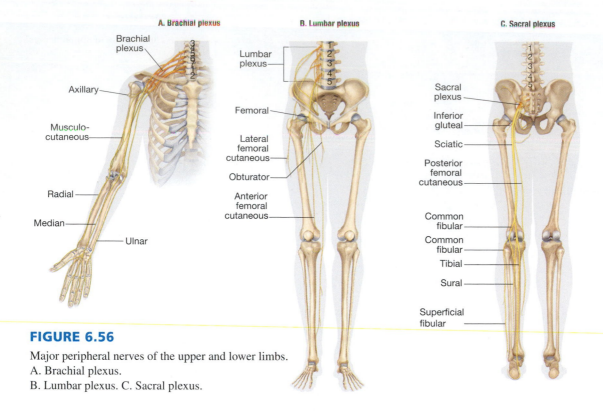

FIGURE 6.56

Major peripheral nerves of the upper and lower limbs.
A. Brachial plexus.
B. Lumbar plexus. C. Sacral plexus.

TABLE 6.19	Common Pathologies of the Nervous System	
Disease/Disorder	Description	Massage Implications
Alzheimer's disease (ALTS-high-merz)	Progressive, degenerative disease of the brain consisting of dementia, memory loss, impairment to speech, gait, and other cognitive functions	Indication for gentle massage along with comprehensive health care treatment
Amyotrophic lateral sclerosis (ALS) (ah-my-oh-TROFF-ik LAT-er-al skleh-ROH-sis	Degeneration of motor neurons at the spinal cord causing muscular weakness and atrophy, cause unknown; also called *motor neuron disease* or *Lou Gehrig's disease,* after the baseball player who died from the disease	Indication for massage along with comprehensive health care treatment
Bell's palsy	Inflammation of the facial nerve resulting in temporary paralysis of one side of the face; recovery usually occurs within weeks or months (Figure 6.57■)	Indication for massage of face and neck muscles in postinflammation phase

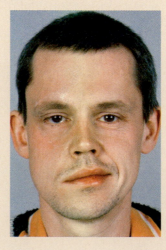

FIGURE 6.57

Man with Bell's palsy.

TABLE 6.19	Common Pathologies of the Nervous System (continued)	
Disease/Disorder	**Description**	**Massage Implications**
Brain tumor	Cranial tumor either benign or malignant	Indication for massage along with comprehensive health care treatment for cancer
Cerebral palsy (CP) (ser-REE-bral PAWL-zee)	Brain damage causing motor and posture dysfunctions; result of defect, trauma, or oxygen deprivation at birth	Indication for massage along with comprehensive health care treatment
Cerebrovascular accident (CVA) (ser-eh-broh-VASS-kyoo-lar)	Death of brain tissue resulting from a lack of blood and oxygen in the brain; can be caused by an arterial clot (embolus) that blocks the flow of blood to the brain or a hemorrhage in the brain; also called *stroke* (Figure 6.58■)	Medical emergency; indication for massage during rehabilitation

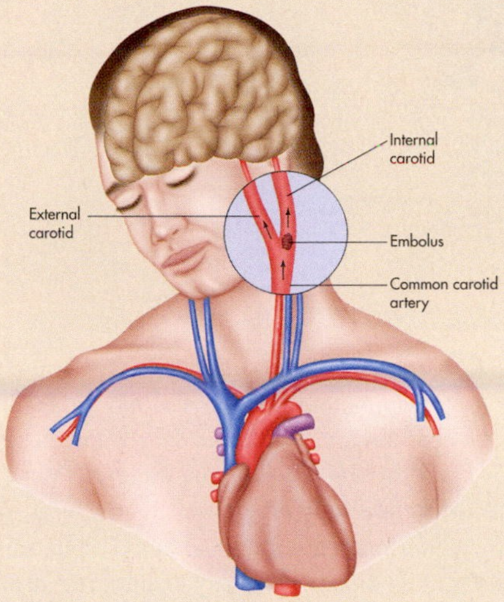

FIGURE 6.58

Arterial clot (embolus) blocks the flow of blood to the brain.

Concussion (kon-KUSH-un)	Injury to the brain caused by a blow or impact; loss of consciousness, dizziness, vomiting, and shock can result	Medical emergency
Epilepsy (EP-ih-lep-see)	Neurological disorder caused by interference in the brain's electrical impulses resulting in episodic seizures; convulsions, muscle spasms, and loss of consciousness can occur	Contraindication for massage if uncontrolled; caution: review first aid for seizures
Guillain-Barré syndrome (GHEE-yan bah-RAY)	Condition in which the myelin sheaths covering peripheral nerves are destroyed, resulting in loss of sensation and muscle control beginning at the legs and continuing up the body; paralysis can occur	Indication for massage in rehabilitation
Headaches	Moderate or intense pain in the head; may be episodic or chronic; types of headache include: Migraine—generally pain is experienced on one side of the head behind the eye Tension—squeezing or pressing pain on both sides of the head and sometimes the facial area Cluster—excruciating pain behind the eyes or in the temples may occur over 2 to 3 months, often at night Posttraumatic—symptoms similar to migraine or tension headaches due to a head or neck injury	Migraine, cluster, or posttraumatic—general contraindication Tension—Indication for massage, including trigger point therapy
Meningitis	Bacterial or viral infection of the meninges that surround the brain and spinal cord; can be fatal if untreated	Medical emergency
Multiple sclerosis (MS) (MULL-tih-pl skleh-ROH-sis)	Chronic autoimmune disease affecting the brain and spinal cord; the body attacks and destroys the myelin sheaths surrounding brain and spinal cord nerves	Indication for massage when in subacute stage; caution: do not overstimulate, avoid heat, and use only light pressure if sensation is diminished

TABLE 6.19   Common Pathologies of the Nervous System (continued)

Disease/Disorder	Description	Massage Implications
Neuralgia (noo-RAL-jee-ah)	Intense pain caused by irritation or injury to a nerve	General contraindication
Parkinson's disease (PARK-in-sons)	Chronic disorder of the nervous system resulting in tremors, muscular weakness, rigidity, and a shuffling gait	Indication for massage along with comprehensive health care treatment
Sciatica	Pain along the large sciatic nerve that runs from the lower back down the back of each leg; often caused by pressure on the nerve from a herniated (slipped) disk	Contraindication if source of pain undiagnosed; indication for massage if muscle tension/spasm contributing to pain
Shingles	Painful rash erupting along a sensory nerve path (Figure 6.59■)	General contraindication

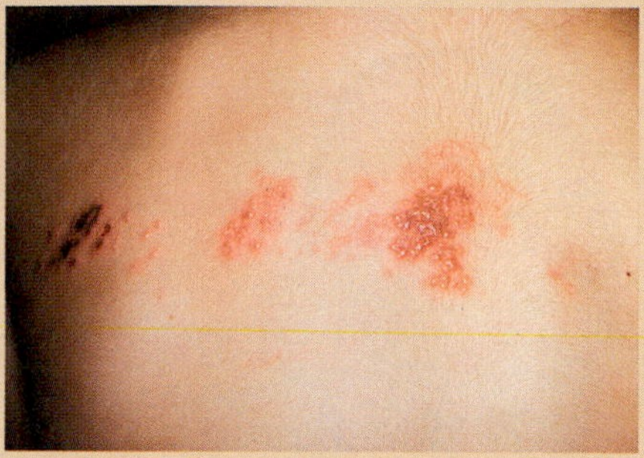

FIGURE 6.59

Skin rash associated with shingles.

Disease/Disorder	Description	Massage Implications
Spinal cord injury (SCI)	Damage to the spinal cord due to trauma; can result in paralysis of certain areas of the body; paraplegia refers to paralysis from the waist down; quadriplegia refers to paralysis from the shoulders down	General contraindication in acute phase of injury; indication for massage as part of rehabilitation
Transient ischemic attack (TIA) (TRAN-shent iss-KEM-ik)	Temporary interference with blood and oxygen supply to the brain; also called *ministroke;* may lead to true stroke	Medical emergency

ENDOCRINE SYSTEM

Adrenal (ad-REE-nal) glands

Endocrine (EN-doh-krin) system

Homeostasis (hoe-me-oh-STAY-sis)

Hormones (HOR-mohnz)

Hypothalamus (high-poh-THAL-ah-mus)

Pancreas (PAN-kree-ass)

Parathyroid (pair-ah-THIGH-royd) glands

Pineal (pih-NEAL) gland

Pituitary (pih-TOO-ih-tair-ee) gland

Thymus (THIGH-mus) gland

Thyroid (THIGH-royd) gland

The endocrine system consists of a group of glands and the hormones they secrete. Hormones are chemical messengers sent from glands to target organs or cells via the circulatory system. Hormones regulate many body activities such as growth, development, water and mineral balance, metabolism, immune system responses, and sexual function. The goal of the endocrine system is to keep the body in a state of homeostasis—a stable environment—by controlling the activity level of its tissues and organs.

The nervous system plays an important role in the endocrine system. The hypothalamus, a region of the lower central part of the brain that regulates automatic body responses, is the link between the two systems (Figure 6.54). Nerve cells in the hypothalamus control the pituitary gland, one of the most far-reaching and influential glands. See page 165 for more information about the hypothalamus.

The major glands of the endocrine system are the pituitary, pineal, thyroid, thymus, parathyroid, pancreas, adrenals, ovaries (in the female), and testes (in the male). See Figure 6.60■. Table 6.20■ lists abbreviations that relate to the endocrine system. Table 6.21■ at the end of this section lists common pathologies of the endocrine system and their massage implications.

Glands, Functions, and Hormones of the Endocrine System

Pituitary gland

- Called the "master gland" because its secretions regulate all of the other endocrine glands; it is subject to control by the chemical secretions of the hypothalamus.
- Small, bean-shaped gland located near the base of the brain; attached to the hypothalamus by the infundibulum stalk (see Figure 6.60).
- Divided into two sections: the anterior lobe and the posterior lobe.

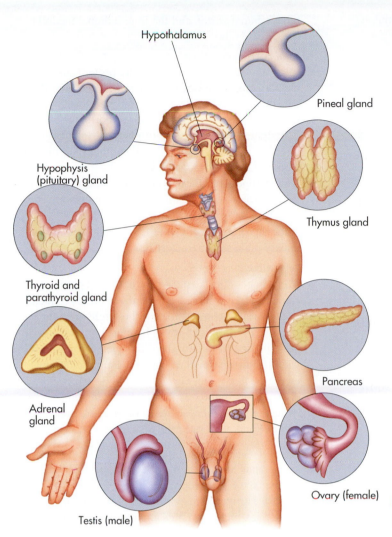

FIGURE 6.60

Primary glands of the endocrine system.

Anterior lobe secretions

- Growth hormone (GH)—stimulates cells to increase in size and divide promoting growth of bones, muscles, and other organs in the body.
- Thyroid-stimulating hormone (TSH)—regulates thyroid gland function; stimulates production of thyroxine (T₄) and triiodothyronine (T₃), which influence metabolism.
- Adrenocorticotropin hormone (ACTH)—regulates adrenal cortex function.

- Prolactin (PRL)—stimulates milk production in the mammary glands after childbirth.
- Follicle-stimulating hormone (FSH)—influences the male and female gonads; responsible for development of ova in ovaries and sperm in testes; stimulates estrogen secretion in the ovaries.
- Luteinizing hormone (LH)—influences the male and female gonads; stimulates sex hormone secretion in males and females.

TABLE 6.20	Endocrine System Abbreviations		
Abbreviation	Meaning	Abbreviation	Meaning
ACTH	Adrenocorticotropin hormone	MSH	Melanocyte-stimulating hormone
ADH	Antidiuretic hormone	NIDDM	Non-insulin-dependent diabetes mellitus
BMR	Basal metabolic rate	PRL	Prolactin
FBS	Fasting blood sugar	PTH	Parathyroid hormone
FSH	Follicle-stimulating hormone	RAI	Radioactive iodine
GH	Growth hormone	T₃	Triiodothyronine
GTT	Glucose tolerance test	T₄	Thyroxine
IDDM	Insulin-dependent diabetes mellitus	TFT	Thyroid function test
LH	Luteinizing hormone	TSH	Thyroid-stimulating hormone

- Melanocyte-stimulating hormone (MSH)—stimulates the production of melanin, which controls skin pigmentation.

Posterior lobe secretions

- Antidiuretic hormone (ADH)—responsible for water reabsorption by the kidney tubules; also called *vasopressin.*
- Oxytocin—stimulates uterine contractions during childbirth and the release of milk from the mammary glands.

Pineal gland

- Small gland located in the thalamus region of the brain (see Figure 6.60).
- Secretes melatonin—helps with sleep and plays a role in the body's circadian rhythm (sleep-wake cycle).
- Secretes serotonin—a neurotransmitter; low levels of this hormone are frequently linked with mental depression.

Thyroid gland

- Butterfly-shaped gland with two lobes, one on either side of the trachea in the neck (see Figure 6.60).
- Secretes thyroxine (T_4)—essential to the maintenance and regulation of the basal metabolic rate (BMR); influences both physical and mental growth and development.
- Secretes triiodothyronine (T_3)—influences the BMR.
- Secretes calcitonin—influences bone and calcium metabolism.

Thymus gland

- Located in the mediastinal cavity just above the heart; composed of two lobes, right and left (see Figure 6.60).
- Plays an important role in the immune system as well as the endocrine system.
- Secretes thymosin—important for the development of the immune system in the newborn and throughout childhood; essential for the development of T cells (thymic lymphocytes).

Parathyroid gland

- Four small glands located on the posterior side of the thyroid gland (see Figure 6.60).
- Secretes parathyroid hormone (PTH)—regulates the amount of calcium and phosphorus in the blood.

Pancreas

- Located along the lower portion of the stomach (see Figure 6.60), it is the only organ that has both exocrine and endocrine functions; the exocrine portion releases digestive enzymes; the endocrine portion (also called *islets of Langerhans*) produces two hormones that have opposite effects.
- Secretes insulin—stimulates cells in the body to take in glucose from the blood, lowering the body's blood sugar level.
- Secretes glucagon—stimulates the liver to release glucose, thus raising the body's blood sugar level.

Adrenal glands

- Two triangle-shaped glands each one located above one of the kidneys; composed of two sections, the outer adrenal cortex and the inner adrenal medulla (see Figure 6.60).

Adrenal cortex secretions

- Cortisol—regulates carbohydrate, protein, and fat metabolism; increases blood sugar levels; provides anti-inflammatory effect; a steroid hormone.
- Corticosterone—contributes to the normal use of carbohydrates, the absorption of glucose, and has an effect on the potassium (K) and sodium (Na) metabolism; a steroid hormone.
- Aldosterone—regulates water and electrolyte balance.
- Testosterone—responsible for development of secondary male sex characteristics.
- Androsterone—responsible for development of secondary male sex characteristics.

Adrenal medulla secretions

- Dopamine—dilates arteries so that blood pressure and cardiac output is increased; increases urine production.
- Epinephrine—responsible for the "fight or flight" response; responds to stress by causing vasoconstriction, dilation of the pupils of the eyes, decreased salivation, slowing down of gastrointestinal functions, increased heart rate, elevated blood pressure and dilated bronchial tubes; also called *adrenaline.*
- Norepinephrine—causes vasoconstriction, higher blood pressure and heart rate, and increased glucose levels.

Ovaries

- Two glands located in the abdominopelvic area of the female (see Figure 6.60).
- Secrete estrogen—responsible for the female secondary sex characteristics and regulation of the menstrual cycle.
- Secrete progesterone—prepares the uterine environment for pregnancy.

Testes

- Two oval-shaped glands located in the scrotum of the male (see Figure 6.60).
- Secrete testosterone—responsible for the male secondary sex characteristics and sperm production.

MASSAGE CONNECTION

Chronic stress causes prolonged stimulation of the adrenal glands which secrete hormones involved in the "flight or fight" response. This chronic emergency state can result in stress-related health problems, such as indigestion, high blood pressure, abnormal blood sugar, and chronic anxiety. Relaxation massage stimulates the parasympathetic nervous system, which diminishes signals to the adrenal glands, thus reducing the release of stress-related hormones.

TABLE 6.21	Common Pathologies of the Endocrine System	
Disease/Disorder	Description	Massage Implications
Acromegaly (ak-roh-MEG-ah-lee)	Condition that results in elongation and enlargement of the bones of the head and extremities in adults, a result of hypersecretion of growth hormone (GH) in the pituitary gland; also called gigantism	Caution: adjust massage for abnormal body structure
Addison's disease	Condition caused by hyposecretion of adrenocortical hormone (cortisol); increased pigmentation of the skin, weakness, and weight loss may occur	Indication for relaxation massage to tolerance
Adenocarcinoma (ad-eh-no-car-sih-NO-mah)	Cancerous tumor in an endocrine gland that is able to produce the hormones secreted by that gland; a cause of some hypersecretion pathologies	General contraindication
Cushing's syndrome	Condition that results from hypersecretion of cortisol in the adrenal cortex; may be caused by an adrenal gland tumor; symptoms can include upper body obesity, round face, easy bruising, osteoporosis, fatigue, high blood pressure, high blood sugar (Figure 6.61■)	Indication for relaxation massage to tolerance

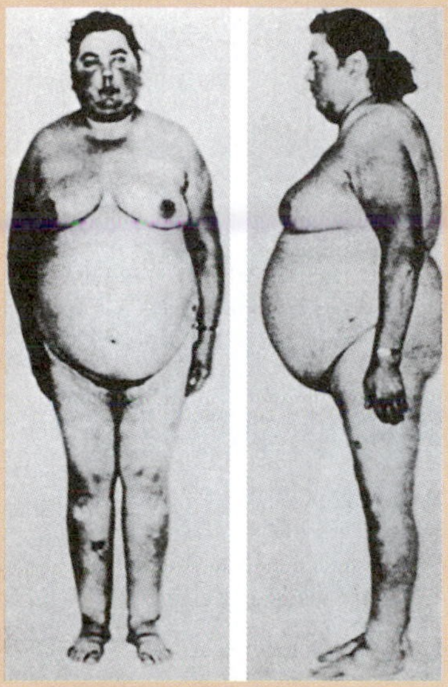

FIGURE 6.61

A patient with Cushing's syndrome.

Diabetes insipidus (DI) (dye-ah-BEE-teez in-SIP-ih-dus)	Disorder caused by inadequate secretion of antidiuretic hormone (ADH) by the posterior lobe of the pituitary gland	Caution: massage only if condition is stable with health care treatment
Diabetes mellitus (DM) (MELL-ih-tis)	Chronic disorder of carbohydrate metabolism in which the pancreas does not produce enough insulin or the body does not properly use the hormone, resulting in hyperglycemia (excessive sugar in the blood) and glycosuria (sugar in the urine); Type 1 diabetes mellitus (IDDM) requires that the patient take daily injections of insulin; Type 2 (NIDDM) patients may not need to take insulin	Cautions: massage only if condition is stable with health care treatment; contraindications to watch for include numbness, poor circulation, and kidney failure.
Dwarfism (DWARF-izm)	Condition of being abnormally short in height; can be caused by hyposecretion of growth hormone (GH)	Caution: adjust massage for abnormal body structure

TABLE 6.21   **Common Pathologies of the Endocrine System (continued)**

Disease/Disorder	Description	Massage Implications
Goiter (GOY-ter)	Enlargement of the thyroid gland; some types of goiter can be caused by untreated hypothyroidism; simple (endemic) goiter is caused by a deficiency of iodine in the diet (Figure 6.62■)	General contraindication while thyroid is enlarged

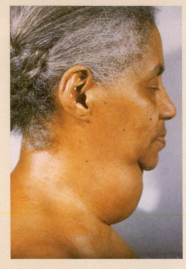

FIGURE 6.62

Patient with endemic goiter.

Grave's disease	Condition resulting from hypersecretion of thyroid hormones T_3 and T_4 of the thyroid gland; symptoms include goiter and exophthalmos (excessive protrusion of the eyeballs) (Figure 6.63■); also called *hyperthyroidism*	Indication for relaxation massage for stress-related symptoms

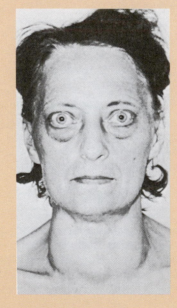

FIGURE 6.63

Patient with exophthalmos, a sign of Grave's disease (hyperthyroidism).

Hashimoto's disease (hash-ee-MOH-tohz)	Chronic form of thyroiditis resulting in hyposecretion of thyroid hormones T_3 and T_4	Indicated in comprehensive health care treatment plan
Hirsutism (HER-soot-izm)	Condition of having an excessive amount of body hair; generally used to describe females having the adult male pattern of hair growth; often due to an imbalance of hormones	None
Hypoparathyroidism (HIGH-poh-pair-ah-THIGH-royd-izm)	Condition resulting from hyposecretion of PTH in the parathyroid gland; can result in tetany (tonic muscular contractions/intermittent cramp)	Indicated in comprehensive health care treatment plan

TABLE 6.21 Common Pathologies of the Endocrine System (continued)

Disease/Disorder	Description	Massage Implications
Hypothyroidism (high-poh-THIGH-royd-izm)	Condition caused by deficient thyroid gland secretions of thyroid hormones T_3 and T_4, resulting in lowered basal metabolism rate, dry skin, slow pulse, low blood pressure, sluggishness, and goiter	Indicated in comprehensive health care treatment plan
Myxedema (miks-eh-DEE-mah)	Condition resulting from hyposecretion of thyroid hormones T_3 and T_4 in the thyroid gland; anemia, slow speech, enlarged tongue and facial features, edema of the skin, drowsiness, and mental apathy can result (Figure 6.64■)	Indicated in comprehensive health care treatment plan

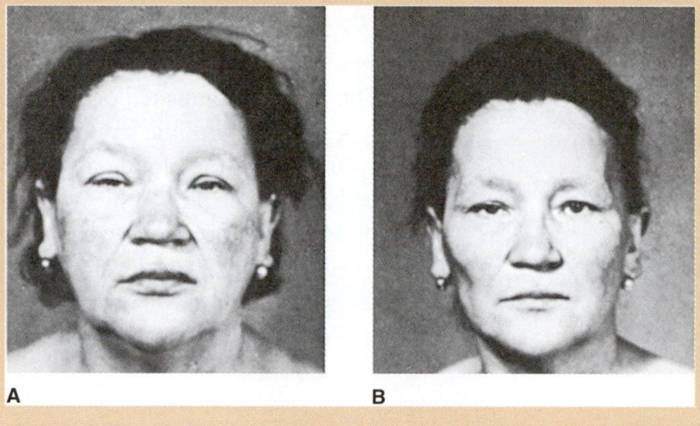

FIGURE 6.64

A. Patient with myxedema. B. Same patient after being treated with thyroid hormones for 3 months.

Thyrotoxicosis (thigh-roh-toks-ih-KOH-sis)	Overproduction of the thyroid hormones T_3 and T_4 in the thyroid gland, resulting in rapid heart action, tremors, enlarged thyroid gland, exophthalmos, and weight loss	Indicated in comprehensive health care treatment plan

CARDIOVASULAR SYSTEM

Arteries (AR-te-reez))

Arteriole (ar-TEE-ree-ohl)

Atria (AT-tree-ah)

Blood

Blood vessels

Capillaries (CAP-ih-lair-eez)

Cardiovascular (car-dee-oh-VAS-kew-lar)

Diastolic (dye-ah-STOL-ik)

Endocardium (en-doh-CAR-dee-um)

Heart

Myocardium (my-oh-CAR-dee-um)

Pericardium (pair-ih-CAR-dee-um)

Systolic (sis-TOL-ik)

Ventricles (VEN-trik-lz)

The cardiovascular system, also called the *circulatory system,* supplies oxygenated and nutrient-rich blood to the body's tissues, thereby delivering a constant flow of oxygen and nutrients to every cell, while also carrying away waste prod- ucts, such as carbon dioxide. The main organs of the cardio- vascular system are the heart, a muscular organ that pumps the blood; the blood vessels, such as arteries, veins, and cap- illaries; and the blood. Table 6.22■ lists abbreviations that

TABLE 6.22 Cardiovascular System Abbreviations

Abbreviation	Meaning
AF	Atrial fibrillation
AS	Arteriosclerosis
BP	Blood pressure
bpm	Beats per minute
cath	Catheterization
CP	Chest pain
CV	Cardiovascular
ECG, EKG	Electrocardiogram
ECHO	Echocardiogram
HTN	Hypertension
IV	Intravenous
P	Pulse
Vfib	Ventricular fibrillation

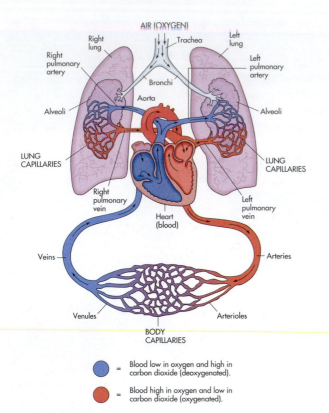

FIGURE 6.65

Overview of the cardiovascular system.

relate to the cardiovascular system. Table 6.23■ at the end of this section lists common pathologies of the cardiovascular system and their massage implications.

Parts and Functions of the Cardiovascular System

Heart

- Hollow, muscular pump with four chambers (cavities) that circulates blood throughout the body (Figure 6.65■).

○ Pulmonary circulation, between the heart and lungs, transports deoxygenated blood to the lungs to get oxygen, then back to the heart.

○ Systemic circulation takes oxygenated blood away from the heart to the tissues and cells of the body, then back to the heart.

- Located in the mediastinum slightly to the left of the center of the chest cavity (Figure 6.66■).
- Weighs about 9 ounces and is the size of a human fist; pumps about 4,000 gallons of blood each day.
- Cardiac muscle is controlled by the autonomic nervous system.

Layers

- The heart is composed of three layers (Figure 6.67■):
  ○ Endocardium: the smooth, thin inner lining reduces friction as the blood passes through the heart chamber.
  ○ Myocardium: the muscular middle layer; contraction of this layer develops the pressure required to pump blood through the blood vessels.
  ○ Pericardium: outer membranelike sac surrounding the heart.

Chambers

- The four chambers of the heart are the right and left upper chambers called *atria* and the right and left lower chambers called *ventricles* (see Figure 6.67).
- The two atria receive blood from various parts of the body; the two ventricles pump blood to different areas of the body.

Valves

- Valves are located at the entrance and exits of each ventricle; by opening and closing, they control the direction of the flow of blood within the heart (see Figure 6.67).

Conduction system

- Special tissue within the heart (the sinoatrial node, also called the *pacemaker*), regulated by the auto-

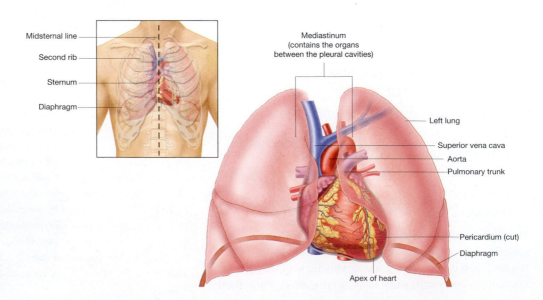

FIGURE 6.66

Location of the heart within the mediastinum of the chest cavity.

FIGURE 6.67

Internal view of the heart showing the layers, chambers, and valves.

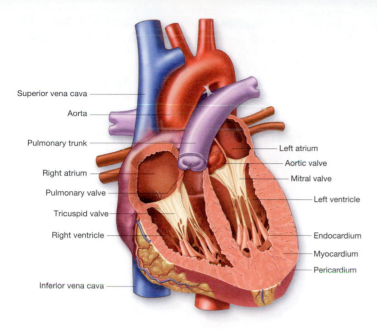

Superior vena cava
Aorta
Pulmonary trunk
Right atrium
Pulmonary valve
Tricuspid valve
Right ventricle
Inferior vena cava

Left atrium
Aortic valve
Mitral valve
Left ventricle
Endocardium
Myocardium
Pericardium

nomic nervous system, sends electrical impulses that stimulate different areas of the heart to contract in the proper order.

Blood vessels

- Responsible for forming pathways that carry blood from the heart to all cells of the body and then back again.

Arteries

- System of vessels that carries blood away from the heart (Figure 6.68■):
  - The pulmonary artery carries deoxygenated blood from the right ventricle to the lungs.
  - The aorta, the largest artery, carries oxygenated blood to all the body systems.
  - Coronary arteries branch out from the aorta and provide blood to the heart muscle.
  - The smallest sized arteries (arterioles) deliver blood to the capillaries.
- Artery walls can expand (during contraction of the heart) or relax (between beats of the heart)
- All arteries have a pulse that reflect the rate of the heart; Figure 6.69■ shows some of the places on the body where the pulse can be felt.

Veins

- Thin-walled vessels that transport blood from peripheral tissues and the lungs back to the heart (Figure 6.70■).
- Valves prevent the backflow of blood.
- More superficial than arteries, veins are the vessels used to remove blood for analysis or to administer intravenous (IV) medications.

Capillaries

- Tiny blood vessels with thin, single-celled walls that allow the exchange of oxygen and nutrients into the

tissues, and the removal of accumulated waste and carbon dioxide.

Blood

- Fluid form of connective tissue responsible for three functions:
  1. Transports oxygen from the lungs, nutrients and fat cells from the digestive system, and hormones from the endocrine system to all the cells in the body.
  2. Regulates pH (levels of acidity or alkalinity) and electrolytes to keep within normal levels for proper cell functioning; also regulates body temperature and fluid balance of the body.
  3. Protects the body from invasion and infection by pathogens, such as bacteria and viruses.
- Composed of plasma and formed elements:
  - Plasma, a straw-colored liquid, is about 90 percent water; nutrients, salts, hormones, enzymes, fats, proteins, oxygen, and other substances are transported to the body's cells in plasma.
  - Formed elements include red blood cells (erythrocytes), white blood cells (leukocytes), and platelets (thrombocytes).
  - Red blood cells transport oxygen from the lungs to the cells in the body; they also help transport carbon dioxide from the cells to the lungs for elimination.
  - White blood cells help the body fight infection and foreign invaders.
  - Platelets are responsible for blood's ability to form a clot, thus preventing blood loss.
- Deoxygenated blood flows through the heart to the lungs, where it receives oxygen, then back to the heart, then out to the body tissues and organs via the aorta (Figure 6.71■).

FIGURE 6.68

Major arteries of the body.

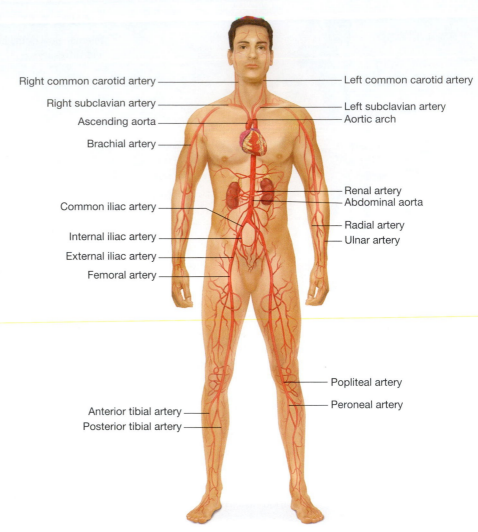

Right common carotid artery —
Right subclavian artery —
Ascending aorta —
Brachial artery —

— Left common carotid artery
— Left subclavian artery
— Aortic arch

Common iliac artery —

— Renal artery
— Abdominal aorta

Internal iliac artery —

— Radial artery
— Ulnar artery

External iliac artery —
Femoral artery —

— Popliteal artery
— Peroneal artery

Anterior tibial artery —
Posterior tibial artery —

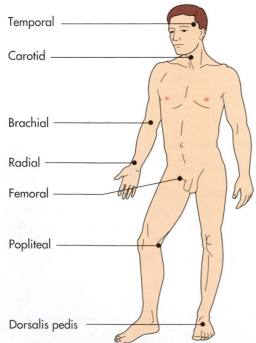

Temporal —
Carotid —
Brachial —
Radial —
Femoral —
Popliteal —
Dorsalis pedis —

FIGURE 6.69

Primary pulse points of the body.

Blood pressure

- Measurement of the force exerted by blood against the wall of a blood vessel.
- Normal BP range for adults is 90/60 to 140/90, with 120/80 considered optimum.
- The first number is the systolic pressure (recorded during ventricular contraction), and the second number is the diastolic pressure (recorded during ventricular relaxation).

MASSAGE CONNECTION

Circulatory massage temporarily lowers blood pressure slightly as local circulation in body tissues increases, much the same as during physical exercise. Blood pressure too low can cause lightheadedness or fainting. Clients with low blood pressure should be advised to get up slowly after lying on the massage table for some time. See *orthostatic hypotension* in Table 6.23, Common Pathologies of the Cardiovascular System, on page 182.

FIGURE 6.70

Major veins of the body.

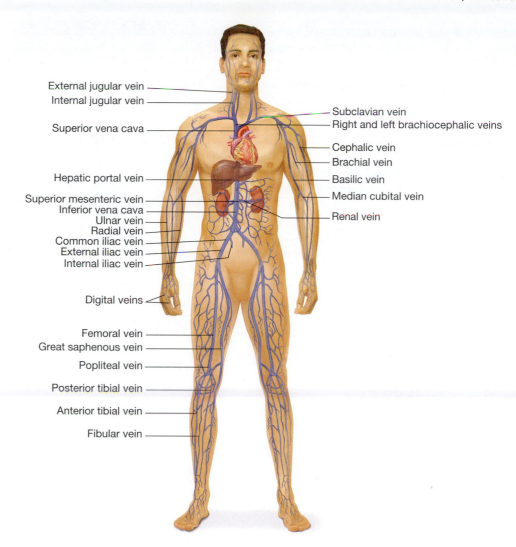

External jugular vein
Internal jugular vein
Superior vena cava
Hepatic portal vein
Superior mesenteric vein
Inferior vena cava
Ulnar vein
Radial vein
Common iliac vein
External iliac vein
Internal iliac vein
Digital veins
Femoral vein
Great saphenous vein
Popliteal vein
Posterior tibial vein
Anterior tibial vein
Fibular vein

Subclavian vein
Right and left brachiocephalic veins
Cephalic vein
Brachial vein
Basilic vein
Median cubital vein
Renal vein

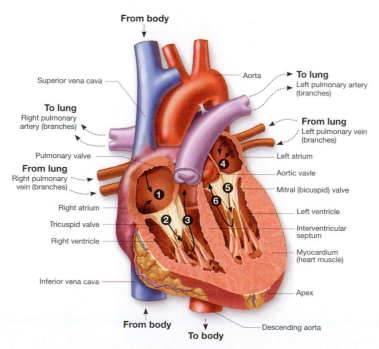

From body

Superior vena cava

To lung
Right pulmonary artery (branches)

Pulmonary valve

From lung
Right pulmonary vein (branches)

Right atrium

Tricuspid valve

Right ventricle

Inferior vena cava

From body

To body

Aorta

To lung
Left pulmonary artery (branches)

From lung
Left pulmonary vein (branches)

Left atrium
Aortic vavle
Mitral (bicuspid) valve
Left ventricle
Interventricular septum
Myocardium (heart muscle)

Apex

Descending aorta

FIGURE 6.71

The path of blood through the chambers of the heart.

TABLE 6.23	Common Pathologies of the Cardiovascular System	
Disease/Disorder	Description	Massage Implications
Anemia	Deficiency in the number of circulating red blood cells in the blood	None
Aneurysm (AN-yoo-rizm)	Weakness in an artery wall that causes a widening of the artery and a sac to form; common sites include the abdominal aorta and the cerebral arteries	General contraindication
Angina pectoris (an-JYE-nah PECK-tor-is)	Severe chest pain with the sensation of constriction around the heart; caused by restricted blood flow to the heart due to diseased blood vessels; often referred to as *angina*	General contraindication
Angioma (an-jee-OH-ma)	Tumor consisting of blood vessels; usually benign	Local contraindication
Arrhythmia (ah-RITH-mee-ah)	Irregularity in the heartbeat; also called *dysrhythmia*	Caution: light massage only; shorten sessions; ask about medications
Arteriosclerosis (ar-tee-ree-oh-skleh-ROE-sis)	Hardening, thickening, and loss of elasticity of the walls of the arteries generally due to atherosclerosis (Figure 6.72■)	Caution: avoid massage to lateral neck; ask about medications

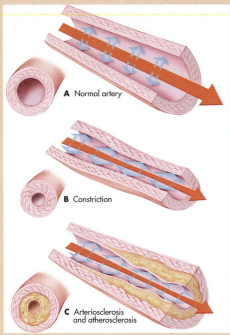

FIGURE 6.72

Blood vessels. A. Normal artery. B. Constriction. C. Arterosclerosis and atherosclerosis.

Arteritis (ar-ter-EYE-tis)	Inflammation of an artery	General contraindication

TABLE 6.23   **Common Pathologies of the Cardiovascular System**   (continued)

Disease/Disorder	Description	Massage Implications
Atherosclerosis (ath-er-oh-skleh-ROH-sis)	Buildup of fatty substances (cholesterol and triglycerides) on the inner walls of arteries; most common form of arteriosclerosis (see Figure 6.72)	Caution: avoid massage to lateral neck; ask about medications
Bradycardia (brad-ee-CAR-dee-ah)	Abnormally slow heartbeat (under 60 beats per minute)	None
Cardiac arrest	Stopping of all heart activity	Medical emergency
Cardiomyopathy (CMP) (car-dee-oh-my-OP-ah-thee)	Disease of the myocardium (heart muscle) that causes deterioration of the muscle and its ability to pump	Caution: light massage only; shorten sessions
Congestive heart failure (CHF) (kon-JESS-tiv)	Condition that can affect the right or left side of the heart; left-side failure leads to pulmonary edema; right side failure causes systemic edema; symptoms include fatigue and difficulty breathing (Figure 6.73■)	Caution: light massage only; shorten sessions

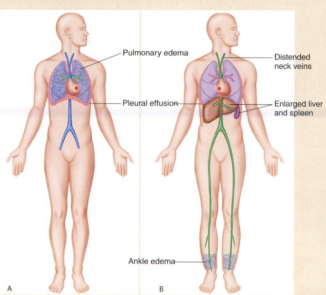

FIGURE 6.73

A. Left-sided congestive heart failure.
B. Right-sided congestive heart failure.

Coronary artery disease (CAD) (KOR-ah-nair-ee)	Narrowing or blockage of the coronary arteries causing insufficient blood supply to the heart; can cause angina pectoris and myocardial infarction (heart attack) (Figure 6.74■)	General contraindication

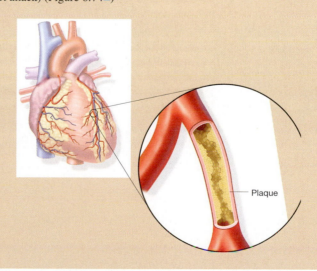

FIGURE 6.74

Formation of plaque within a coronary artery can lead to coronary artery disease.

TABLE 6.23 Common Pathologies of the Cardiovascular System (continued)

Disease/Disorder	Description	Massage Implications
Deep vein thrombosis (DVT)	Inflammation of a vein with blood clotting; major signs are pain, heat, redness, swelling, pitting edema	Medical emergency
Embolism (EM-boh-lizm)	Obstruction of a blood vessel by a blood clot or foreign substance	Medical emergency
Endocarditis (en-doh-car-DYE-tis)	Inflammation of the membrane lining the heart	General contraindication
Fibrillation (fih-brill-AY-shun)	Serious form of arrhythmia with abnormal quivering or contractions of heart fibers; can result in cardiac arrest and death	Medical emergency
Flutter	Type of arrhythmia in which the atria or ventricles contract too rapidly but in a regular pattern	Caution: light massage only; shorten sessions; ask about medications
Hemophilia (hee-moh-FILL-ee-ah)	Genetically transmitted blood disease in which blood-clotting time is prolonged due to the lack of a vital clotting factor; almost exclusively a disease of males	Caution for mild cases; contraindication for severe cases
Hypertension (HTN) (high-per-TEN-shun)	Persistently high blood pressure that can damage the blood vessels and the heart	Caution for mild cases; contraindication for severe or untreated case; ask about medications
Hypotension (high-poh-TEN-shun	Decreased blood pressure that can occur due to shock, infection, anemia, cancer, or as death approaches	Caution: check for underlying contraindications
Ischemia (is-KEYH-mee-ah)	Local and temporary deficiency of blood supply due to an obstruction in the circulation	Indicated for treatment unless otherwise contraindicated
Leukemia (loo-KEE-mee-ah)	Cancer of the white blood cells	Caution: massage to level of tolerance
Murmur (MUR-mur)	Soft blowing or rasping sound heard during auscultation (use of a stethoscope to hear sounds within the body)	Caution for mild cases; contraindication for severe cases
Myocardial infarction (MI) (my-oh-CAR-dee-al in-FARC-shun	Condition resulting from the partial or total closing of one or more coronary arteries; can result in death; also called *heart attack*	Medical emergency
Orthostatic hypotension	Condition resulting in sudden drop in blood pressure when changing position from sitting or lying down to standing up.	Caution when getting off a massage table or chair
Peripheral vascular disease (PVD)	Abnormal condition affecting blood vessels outside the heart, such as in the legs; pain, numbness, and loss of circulation and pulses may be symptoms	Indication for treatment under health care provider
Phlebitis (fleh-BYE-tis)	Inflammation of a vein	General contraindication
Reynaud's phenomenon (ray-NOZ)	Disorder of the blood vessels of the fingers and toes due to oxygen deficiency; cold, emotional stress, or smoking can cause blood vessels in the digits to narrow producing pallor, cyanosis (blue/gray color of the skin), pain, or a burning feeling	Indication for treatment under health care provider
Rheumatic heart disease (roo-MAT-ik)	Disease of the heart valves due to having had rheumatic fever	Caution for mild cases; contraindication for severe cases
Septicemia (sep-tih-SEE-mee-ah)	Condition in which bacteria or their toxins are in the blood; also called *blood poisoning*	Medical emergency

TABLE 6.23	Common Pathologies of the Cardiovascular System (continued)	
Disease/Disorder	Description	Massage Implications
Shock	Disruption of oxygen supply to the tissues and return of blood to the heart; see Figure 6.75■ for symptoms of a person in shock	Medical emergency

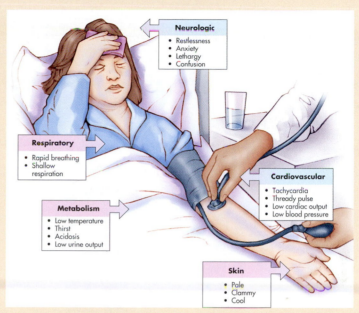

FIGURE 6.75

Symptoms of a patient in shock.

Spider veins	Superficial dense network of veins (Figure 6.76■)	Local caution: light massage only

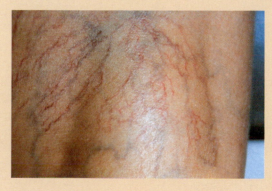

FIGURE 6.76

Spider veins. Courtesy of Jason L. Smith, MD.

Tachycardia (tak-ee-CAR-dee-ah)	Abnormally fast heartbeat (over 100 beats per minute)	Indication for treatment under health care provider
Thrombophlebitis (throm-boh-fleh-BYE-tis)	Inflammation and clotting of blood within a vein (Figure 6.77■) (also see *deep vein thrombosis*)	General contraindication

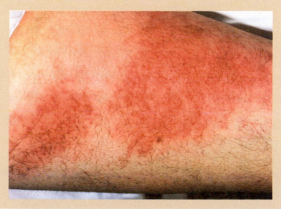

FIGURE 6.77

Thrombophlebitis. Courtesy of Jason L. Smith, MD.

TABLE 6.23   Common Pathologies of the Cardiovascular System   (continued)

Disease/Disorder	Description	Massage Implications
Thrombus (THROM-bus)	Blood clot within a blood vessel	General contraindication
Varicose veins (VAIR-ih-kos)	Swelling and distention of veins usually occurring in the lower legs; caused by blood pooling within the veins due to decreased, stagnated blood flow (Figure 6.78■)	Caution: use light broad pressure only over the area affected; contraindication if clotting suspected

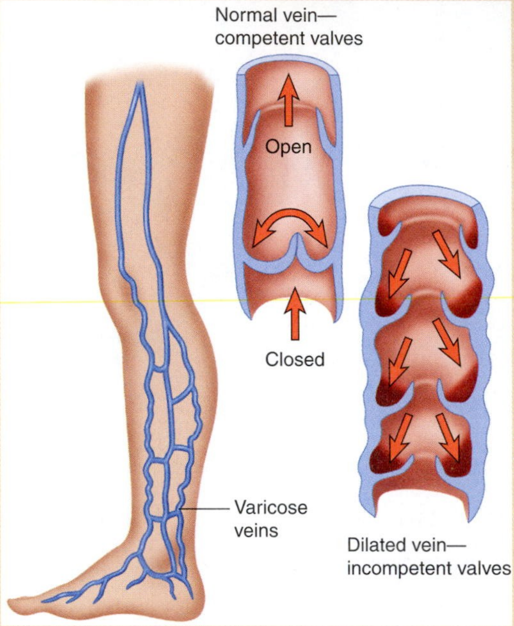

FIGURE 6.78

Development of varicose veins.

LYMPHATIC SYSTEM

Antigen (AN-tih-jen)

Immune system

Lymph (LIMF) vessels

Lymphatic (lim-FAT-ik) ducts

Lymphatic system

Spleen

T cells

Thymus (THIGH-mus) gland

Tonsils (TON-sulls)

The main work of the lymphatic system is to transport excess fluid, proteins, and organic substances from body tissues back to the circulatory (cardiovascular) system. Thus, while it is a system unto itself composed of a network of lymph vessels, the lymphatic system functions in conjunction with the cardiovascular system (Figure 6.79■). The lymphatic system is also part of the immune system, which defends the body against pathogens and other foreign invaders, and also removes the body's own cells that have become diseased. Because the work of the lymphatic system and the immune system are so closely enmeshed, the immune system is briefly discussed at the end of this section. Lymphatic vessels, lymphatic ducts, lymphatic nodes, the spleen, the thymus gland, and the tonsils are the components of the lymphatic system. Table 6.24■ lists abbreviations that relate to the lymphatic system. Table 6.25■ at the end of this section lists common pathologies of the lymphatic system and their massage implications.

Parts and Functions of the Lymphatic System

Lymphatic vessels
- Form an extensive network throughout the body for the purpose of transporting *lymph* (Figure 6.80■).
  - Vessels include the lymph capillaries or I/T vessels, collector vessels, and transport vessels.

TABLE 6.24   Lymphatic System Abbreviations

Abbreviation	Meaning
HIV	Human immunodeficiency virus
mono	Mononucleosis
NHL	Non-Hodgkin's lymphoma
NK	Natural killer cells
PCP	*Pneumocystis carinii* pneumonia

FIGURE 6.79

The lymphatic system functions in conjunction with the cardiovascular system. Lymphatic vessels pick up excess tissue fluid, purify it in the lymph nodes, then return it to the circulatory system.

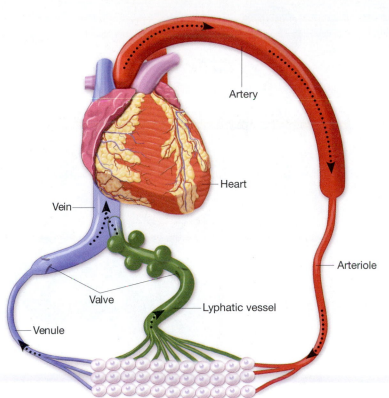

Artery

Heart

Vein

Valve

Venule

Arteriole

Lyphatic vessel

Cells in the body tissues

○ Lymph, a clear liquid that is mostly water, is primarily composed of fluid from blood plasma that has seeped out of capillary walls into body tissue; also called *lymphatic fluid.*

● Serve as one-way vessels sending lymph from the tissues toward the thoracic cavity and eventually draining into either the *right lymphatic duct* or the *thoracic duct* (see Figure 18.15 on page 530)

Lymphatic ducts
● The right lymphatic duct, the smaller of the two, drains the right arm and the right side of the neck and chest, then empties into the right subclavian vein.
● The thoracic duct drains lymph from the rest of the body, then empties into the left subclavian vein.

Lymph nodes
● Small organs composed of lymphatic tissue that act as a filtration system to destroy pathogens and remove cell debris; also called *lymph glands.*
● Found along the lymphatic vessels, with concentrations in several regions of the body, such as the cervical, axillary, inguinal, pelvic, abdominal, and thoracic areas (see Figure 18.15 on page 530 and Figure 18.19 on page 532)

Accessory Organs
Spleen
● Found in the upper left quadrant of the abdomen (see Figure 6.80).

● Serves as a reservoir for blood; destroys old red blood cells; filters microorganisms from the body.

Thymus gland
● Found in the upper portion of the mediastinum (see Figure 6.80).
● Forms antibodies and the development of the immune response in infants and children; manufactures infection-fighting T cells.

Tonsils
● A collection of lymphatic tissue found on each side of the throat (see Figure 6.80).

MASSAGE CONNECTION

A specialized form of massage called lymphatic facilitation improves lymphatic system circulation by increasing the uptake of interstitial fluid at the lymphatic capillaries and facilitating its movement toward the thoracic ducts. A more detailed discussion of the lymphatic system related to lymphatic facilitation techniques can be found in Chapter 18, Contemporary Massage and Bodywork, on page 529.

FIGURE 6.80

Lymphatic vessels, tonsils, lymph nodes, thymus, spleen, and an expanded view of a lymph node.

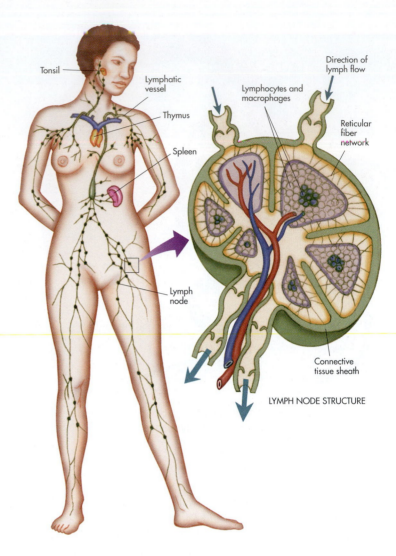

Immune System

The immune system is dependent on many of the tissues and organs of the lymphatic system in its work to identify and protect the body from abnormal cells, foreign substances, and pathogens that have entered the body.

Natural defenses of the body

- Intact skin.
- Secretions, such as tears and mucus.
- White blood cells.
- Body chemicals, such as hormones and enzymes.
- Antibodies.

Immune response

- How the body reacts to and protects itself from a foreign substance:
  - ○ Foreign substances display proteins that are different from a person's natural proteins; these proteins, called antigens, instigate the immune response.
  - ○ In response to the antigen, the body produces antibodies, also protein substances, that neutralize or destroy the foreign substance that produced the antigen.

- Two types of immune responses: humoral immunity (also called *antibody-mediated immunity*) and cellular immunity (also called *cell-mediated immunity*).
  - ○ In humoral immunity, the body produces plasma lymphocytes (B cells) in response to the presence of an antigen and the formation of antibodies; major defense against bacterial infections.
  - ○ In cellular immunity, lymphocytes (T cells) are produced in response to injury; NK (natural killer) cells are produced to attack and destroy foreign cells, cancer cells, and virus-infected cells; major defense against viruses, fungi, cancerous tumors, and some bacteria.

MASSAGE CONNECTION

Research provides evidence that massage improves the body's immune response. See page 267 in Chapter 7, Effects of Massage, for more information.

TABLE 6.25   Common Pathologies of the Lymphatic and Immune Systems

Disease/Disorder	Description	Massage Implications
Acquired immunodeficiency syndrome (AIDS) (im-you-noh-dee-FIH-shen-see)	Disease involving a defect in the cell-mediated immunity system; syndrome of opportunistic infections occur in the final stages of infection with the human immunodeficiency virus (HIV), which reduces the body's ability to fight infection	Indication for treatment under health care supervision; cautions: massage to tolerance, practice heightened hygiene, check for contraindications, ask about medications
AIDS-related complex (ARC)	Complex of symptoms that occur in the early stage of AIDS; symptoms include weight loss, fatigue, skin rash, and anorexia	Indication for treatment under health care supervision; cautions: massage to tolerance, practice heightened hygiene, check for contraindications, ask about medications
Allergy (AL-er-jee)	Abnormally strong immune response to a common substance in the environment; the immune system causes tissue damage as it fights a perceived threat to the body that actually would be harmless; also called *hypersensitivity*	Caution: eliminate allergy triggers; use hypoallergenic oil or lotion; be careful about strong fragrances and smells in the room
Autoimmune disorders	Conditions in which the body's immune system becomes defective and produces antibodies against itself; examples include systemic lupus erythematosus (SLE), multiple sclerosis, rheumatoid arthritis, myasthenia gravis, and scleroderma	Caution: check contraindications for specific diseases; general contraindication in active phase of the disease
Elephantiasis (el-eh-fan-TYE-as-sis)	Disease caused by the parasite (*Wuchereria bancrofti*) that blocks lymph nodes, causing swelling usually in the legs and genitalia	Indication for treatment as part of health care along with medication
Hodgkin's disease (HD)	Cancer of the lymphatic system; also called *Hodgkin's lymphoma*	Light massage only as part of comprehensive health care treatment.
Kaposi's sarcoma (KS) (KAP-oh-seez sar-KOH-mah)	Form of skin cancer often seen in people with AIDS; brownish-purple papules spread from the skin and metastasize to internal organs (Figure 6.81■)	Local contraindication; also see AIDS

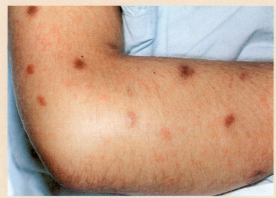

FIGURE 6.81

Papules on the arm of a patient with Kaposi's sarcoma. Courtesy of Jason L. Smith, MD.

Disease/Disorder	Description	Massage Implications
Lymphadenitis (lim-fad-en-EYE-tis)	Inflammation of the lymph nodes; also called *swollen glands*	General contraindication
Lymphangioma (limf-an-GEE-oh-ma)	Benign mass of lymphatic vessels	Local contraindication

TABLE 6.25   Common Pathologies of the Lymphatic and Immune Systems (continued)

Disease/Disorder	Description	Massage Implications
Lymphedema (limf-eh-DEE-mah)	Excessive amounts of fluid in the body tissues (edema) in the extremities due to lymph flow obstruction in the lymphatic vessels (Figure 6.82■)	Manual lymphatic drainage indicated within comprehensive care with Complete Decongestive Therapy (CDT); other massage contraindicated

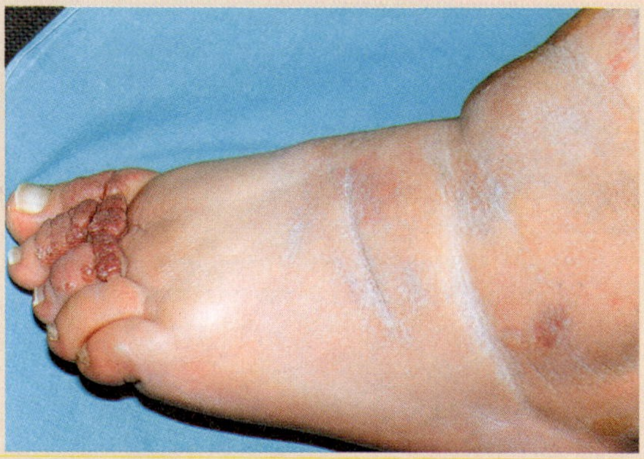

FIGURE 6.82

Chronic lymphedema. Courtesy of Jason L. Smith, MD.

Disease/Disorder	Description	Massage Implications
Lymphoma (lim-FOH-ma)	Malignant tumor of the lymph nodes and tissues	General contraindication
Mononucleosis (mono) (mon-oh-nook-lee-OH-sis)	Acute infectious disease with a large number of abnormal lymphocytes; caused by the Epstein-Barr virus; abnormal liver function and spleen enlargement may be present	General contraindication
Non-Hodgkin's lymphoma	Malignant, solid tumors of the lymphoid tissue	General contraindication
Sarcoidosis (sar-koyd-OH-sis)	Inflammatory disease of the lymph system; lesions may appear in the lymph nodes, liver, skin, lungs, spleen, eyes, and small bones of the hands and feet	General contraindication
Splenomegaly (splee-noh-MEG-ah-lee)	Enlargement of the spleen	General contraindication
Thymoma (thigh-MOH-mah)	Malignant tumor of the thymus gland	General contraindication

RESPIRATORY SYSTEM

Bronchial (BRONG-key-al) tubes

Diaphragm (DYE-ah-fram)

Intercostal (in-ter-COS-tal) muscles

Larynx (LAIR-inks)

Lungs

Nose

Pharynx (FAIR-inks)

Respiration

Respiratory system

Trachea (TRAY-kee-ah)

The respiratory system brings air and its oxygen into the lungs (inhalation), and expels the carbon dioxide (CO_2) that is a by-product of the body's use of the oxygen (exhalation). This process is called *respiration*. The organs of the respiratory system include the nose, pharynx, larynx, trachea, bronchi, and lungs (Figure 6.83■). Accessory organs are the diaphragm and the intercostal muscles. Table 6.26■ lists abbreviations that relate to the respiratory system. Table 6.27■ at the end of this section lists common pathologies of the respiratory system and their massage implications.

Parts and Functions of the Respiratory System

Nose

- Rigid structure in the center of the face made of cartilage and bone that is the beginning of the upper airway.
- External entrance to the nose is the anterior nares (nostrils) through which air is inhaled into the body (Figure 6.84■).
- Behind the nose is the nasal cavity, which is divided down the center by the nasal septum, made of cartilage; each of the two nasal cavities contains vestibular, olfactory, and respiratory regions.

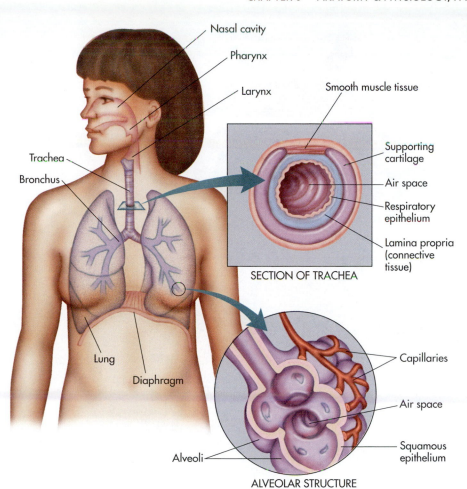

FIGURE 6.83
The respiratory system.

- ○ Vestibular region: lined with mucous membrane and cilia (fine hairs) that filter out dirt, pollen, and foreign particles before they can enter the lungs.
- ○ Olfactory region: located on the roof of the nasal cavity, this area is responsible for the sense of smell, which is related to the sense of taste.

- ○ Respiratory region: warms inhaled air to body temperature and moistens it so that the airways and lungs do not dry out.
- Paranasal sinuses (air-filled cavities) are located in the skull and connect with the nasal cavity through small passageways; they are lined with membranes that secrete mucus and drain into the nose; the sinuses contribute to sound production and give resonance to the voice (Figure 6.85■).

Pharynx

- Also called the *throat,* it is about 5 inches long and receives the inhaled air from the nose, as well as food and liquids ingested from the mouth.
  - ○ At the end of the pharynx, food and liquids are diverted into the esophagus and air enters the trachea.
- Divided into three sections, nasopharynx (upper), oropharynx (middle), and laryngopharynx (lower) (see Figure 6.84).
  - ○ Nasopharynx contains the pharyngeal tonsils (also called *adenoids*) that help keep pathogens from entering the body; the opening of the eustachian tube, which connects to the middle ear, is also found here.

TABLE 6.26	Respiratory System Abbreviations
Abbreviation	**Meaning**
ARDS	Acute respiratory distress syndrome
CO_2	Carbon dioxide
CPR	Cardiopulmonary resuscitation
CXR	Chest x-ray
ENT	Ear, nose, and throat
O_2	Oxygen
R	Respiration
RDS	Respiratory distress syndrome
SARS	Severe acute respiratory syndrome
SOB	Shortness of breath
TPR	Temperature, pulse, and respiration
URI	Upper respiratory infection

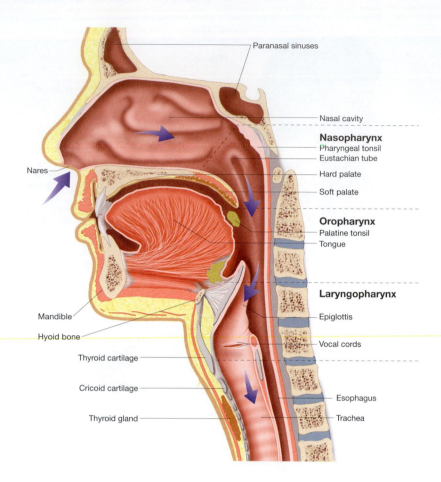

FIGURE 6.84

Internal structure of the upper respiratory system showing the nasal cavity, pharynx, larynx, and trachea.

○ Oropharynx contains the palatine and lingual tonsils.

○ Laryngopharynx houses the larynx.

Larynx

• Muscular structure, composed of cartilage plates bound by ligaments and muscles, that contains the vocal cords; also called the *voice box* (see Figure 6.84).

• Vocal cords are folds of tissue membranes that vibrate as air passes through the glottis (the opening between the two vocal cords), thus producing sound.

• Sitting above the glottis is the epiglottis, a flap of cartilaginous tissue that covers the larynx and trachea during swallowing, and directs the food and liquid traveling down the pharynx into the esophagus, thus preventing them from being inhaled into the lungs.

• The largest cartilage plate forms what is called the *Adam's apple;* usually larger in males, it contributes to the deeper male voice.

Trachea

• Passageway for air extending from the pharynx and larynx down to the main bronchial tubes; about 4 inches long; also called the *windpipe.*

• Composed of smooth muscle and rings of cartilage; lined with mucous membrane and cilia.

• Cleanses, warms, and moisturizes air on its way to the lungs.

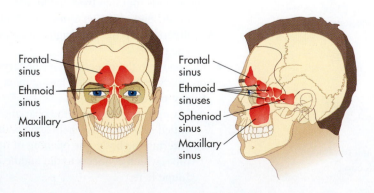

FIGURE 6.85

Paranasal sinuses.

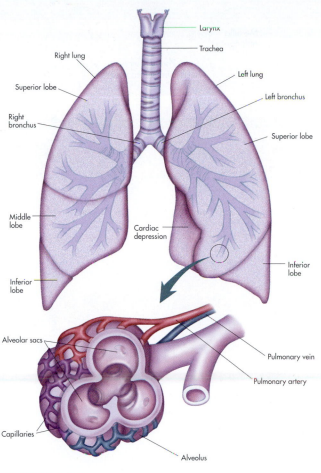

FIGURE 6.86

The bronchial tree with an expanded view of an alveolus and the pulmonary blood vessels.

Bronchi

- The trachea divides at its distal end into the left and right bronchi, which are a further passageway for moving air into the lungs.
- Each bronchus enters one of the lungs at a depression called the hilum, and, like an upside down tree, branches repeatedly into narrower and narrower branches called bronchioles; this is also called the *bronchial tree* (Figure 6.86).
- The bronchioles end at the alveoli, small air sacs that support a network of capillaries; it is here that the exchange of oxygen and carbon dioxide take place.
  - Alveoli are similar to small balloons that inflate and deflate as air moves in and out; there are about 150 million in each lung (see Figure 6.86■).

Lungs

- Two large, conical-shaped organs located in the chest on either side of the mediastinum and protected from damage by the ribs (Figure 6.87■); they are gray colored, porous, spongy in texture, and highly elastic; protected by a double membrane called the pleura that forms a sac around each lung, which is referred to as the pleural cavity.
  - Serous fluid lies between the layers of the pleura, providing lubrication that reduces friction as the lungs expand and contract.
- The right lung has three lobes, called upper, middle, and lower; the left lung has two lobes, upper and lower.
- The lungs have three important functions:
  1. Supply oxygen to the body.
  2. Remove wastes and toxins.
  3. Defend against invasive foreign matter.

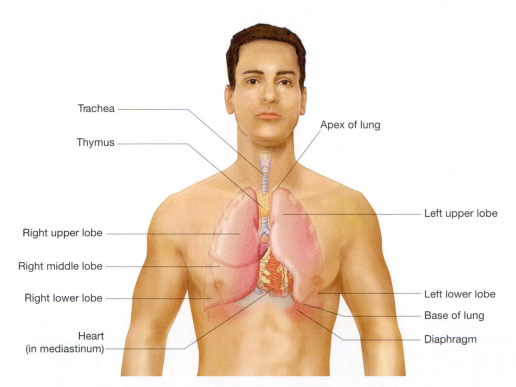

FIGURE 6.87

Position of the lungs within the chest cavity.

Accessory Organs

Diaphragm

- The muscle separating the abdomen from the thoracic (chest) cavity.
- When the diaphragm contracts and moves downward, it changes the balance between the level of atmospheric pressure and the level of pressure within the chest cavity, and causes air to flow into the lungs (inhalation); when the diaphragm relaxes, the chest cavity becomes smaller, changing the balance in pressure and resulting in air flowing out of the lungs (exhalation) (Figure 6.88■).
- This process, breathing, is controlled by an area of the brain called the medulla oblongata; the diaphragm is told what to do (contract, relax) by a signal that travels from the brain along the phrenic nerve.

Intercostal muscles

- Muscles located between the ribs that assist in inhalation by raising the rib cage to allow further expansion of the chest cavity; they assist in exhalation by relaxing.

MASSAGE CONNECTION

Muscle tension in the upper body is sometimes related to habitual chest breathing, that is, relying on shoulder muscles to elevate the rib cage for inhalation rather than using the diaphragm. Massage therapists can address the muscle tension in the shoulders with massage, plus instruct the client on proper diaphragmatic breathing.

MASSAGE CONNECTION

Chest breathing is sometimes related to feelings of anxiety or panic. Relaxation from massage can relieve anxiety and encourage deep diaphragmatic breathing. Clients with habitual chest breathing patterns can learn to breathe more deeply during massage sessions.

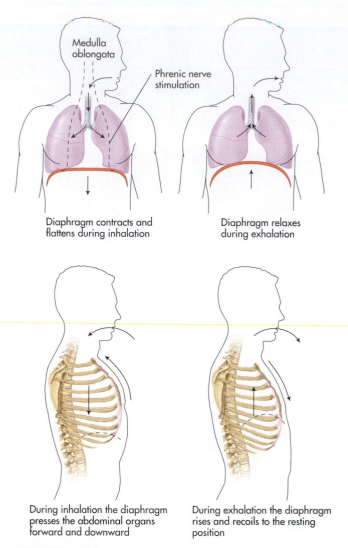

Diaphragm contracts and flattens during inhalation

Diaphragm relaxes during exhalation

During inhalation the diaphragm presses the abdominal organs forward and downward

During exhalation the diaphragm rises and recoils to the resting position

FIGURE 6.88

The breathing process.

TABLE 6.27	Common Pathologies of the Respiratory System	
Disease/Disorder	Description	Massage Implications
Asthma (AZ-mah)	Chronic inflammatory disease in which allergens or other substances cause swelling in the bronchial tubes or lining of the trachea; symptoms include coughing, wheezing, and dyspnea (difficult breathing) (Figure 6.89■)	Indication for massage, especially of muscles of respiration

Normal bronchiole

Constricted bronchiole

Asthma attack

Contracted smooth muscle

Mucous membrane

Smooth muscle

Swollen mucous membrane

Excessive mucus secretion

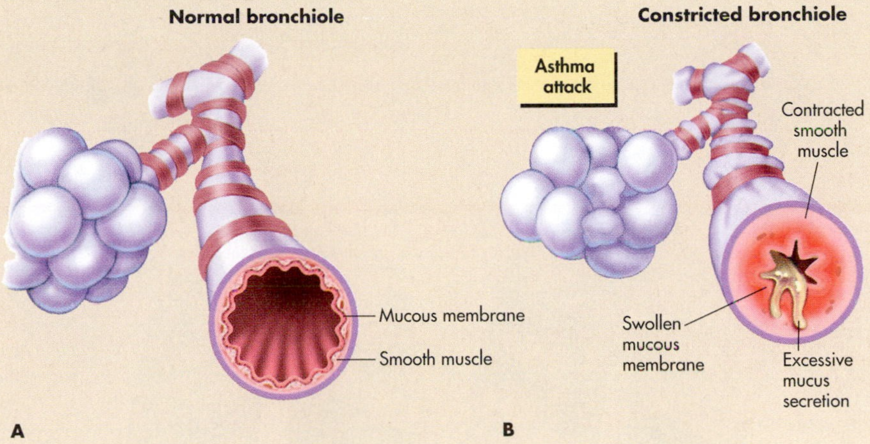

FIGURE 6.89

A. Normal bronchiole. B. Changes to bronchiole during an asthma attack.   **A**   **B**

Bronchitis (brong-KIGH-tis)	Inflammation of a bronchus; symptoms include chest pains, dyspnea, chronic cough	Contraindication in acute phase with fever; caution in subacute phase, consider semireclining positioning
Bronchogenic carcinoma (brong-koh-JEN-ik car-sin-OH-mah)	Malignant tumor originating in the bronchi; also called *lung cancer;* often associated with a history of cigarette smoking	Indicated as part of comprehensive treatment for cancer.
Chronic obstructive pulmonary disease (COPD)	Progressive, chronic group of pulmonary conditions, such as emphysema and chronic bronchitis, with obstruction of air through the airways	Indication for massage, especially of muscles of respiration
Common cold	Viral infection that causes nasal congestion, cough, and sore throat	Contraindicated with fever; caution in later stages of illness, massage to tolerance; lymphatic facilitation indicated to relieve congestion
Croup (KROOP)	Acute respiratory condition with a barking type of cough; generally found in infants and children	General contraindication

TABLE 6.27   **Common Pathologies of the Respiratory System (continued)**

Disease/Disorder	Description	Massage Implications
Emphysema (em-fih-SEE-mah)	Chronic, progressive disease in which the walls of the alveoli are destroyed, resulting in fewer air sacs to assist in respiration; shortness of breath, difficulty in breathing, coughing, and wheezing are symptoms; often caused by cigarette smoking (Figure 6.90■)	Indication for massage, especially of muscles of respiration

Normal lung   Emphysema

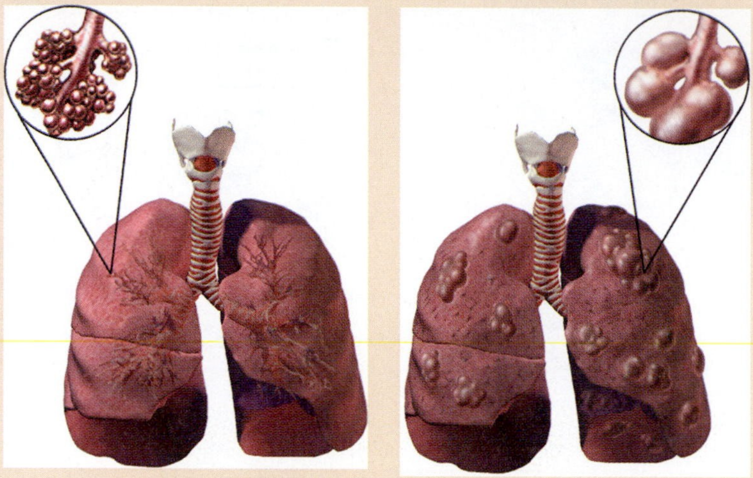

FIGURE 6.90

Normal lung and one with emphysema.

Disease/Disorder	Description	Massage Implications
Influenza (in-floo-EN-za)	Viral infection of the respiratory system; symptoms include fever, body aches, headache, chills, and fatigue; commonly called the *flu*	General contraindication
Pertussis (per-TUH-sis)	Infectious bacterial disease of the upper respiratory system; due to the sound made when coughing, it is commonly called *whooping cough*	General contraindication
Pleurisy (PLOOR-ih-see)	Inflammation of the pleural membranes with sharp chest pain upon inhalation	Contraindication in acute phase; indicated in subacute phase, especially muscles of respiration
Pneumonia (new-MOH-nee-ah)	Bacterial or viral infection of the lung; symptoms include inflammation, chest pain, fluid in lung, fever, and cough	General contraindication
Pulmonary edema (PULL-mon-air-ee eh-DEE-mah)	The retention of excessive amounts of fluid in the lung tissue; symptoms include dyspnea	General contraindication
Pulmonary fibrosis (fi-BROH-sis)	Formation of scar tissue in the lungs that causes difficulty in the expansion of the lungs, thus difficulty taking in enough oxygen	Indication for massage, especially of muscles of respiration
Sinusitis	Inflammation of a sinus	Contraindication in acute phase; caution in later stages of illness, massage to tolerance; lymphatic facilitation indicated to relieve congestion
Tonsillitis (ton-sull-EYE-tis)	Bacterial or viral infection of the tonsils; symptoms include inflammation, difficulty swallowing, and pain in the throat; the pharynx and the larynx can be infected in the same manner; laryngitis causes hoarseness and aphonia (no voice)	General contraindication
Tuberculosis (TB) (too-ber-kyoo-LOH-sis)	Highly infectious bacterial infection that commonly affects the respiratory system; causes inflammation and calcification in the lungs; characterized by coughing up of blood, tissue, and bacteria	General contraindication with active infection; afterward massage indicated as part of treatment, especially muscles of respiration

DIGESTIVE SYSTEM

Anus (AY-nus)

Digestion

Elimination

Esophagus (eh-SOFF-ah-gus)

Gallbladder

Gastrointestinal (gas-troh-in-TESS-tih-nal) tract

Large intestine

Liver

Oral cavity

Pancreas (PAN-kree-ass)

Pharynx (FAIR-inks)

Salivary (SAL-ih-vair-ee) glands

Small intestine

Stomach

Teeth

TABLE 6.28	Digestive System Abbreviations
Abbreviation	**Meaning**
ac	Before meals
BM	Bowel movement
BS	Bowel sounds
FOBT	Fecal occult blood test
GB	Gallbladder
GI	Gastrointestinal
HAV	Hepatitis A virus
HBV	Hepatitis B virus
HCV	Hepatitis C virus
HSV-1	Herpes simplex virus type 1
n&v	Nausea and vomiting
pc	After meals
PO	By mouth

The digestive system takes food into the body (ingestion), breaks it down into small molecules (digestion), gets nutrients into the blood stream (absorption), and removes the leftover waste products (elimination). The major structure of the digestive system is a long muscular tube, called the alimentary canal or gastrointestinal tract. This tract runs through the center of the body. It begins at the mouth, where food and drink enter the system, and ends at the anus, where waste matter (feces) leaves the body. During the process of food moving through the tract, juices are produced to assist in digestion and the absorption of nutrients.

Structures of the digestive system include the oral cavity, pharynx, esophagus, stomach, small intestine, and large intestine. Accessory organs include the salivary glands, gallbladder, liver, and pancreas (Figure 6.91■). Each is attached to the gastrointestinal tract by a duct. Table 6.28■ lists abbreviations that relate to the digestive system. Table 6.29■ at the end of this section lists common pathologies of the digestive system and their massage implications.

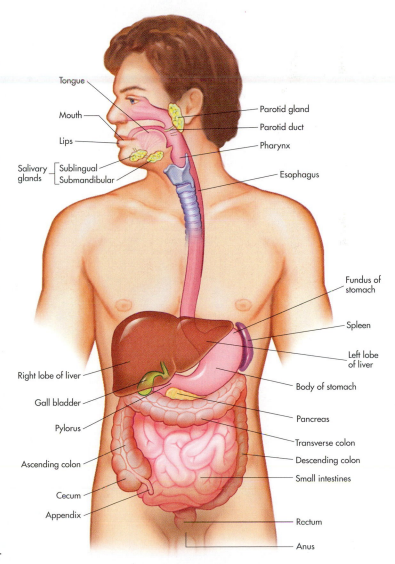

FIGURE 6.91

The digestive system.

Parts and Functions of the Digestive System

Oral cavity

- Consists of the mouth, the teeth, and the salivary glands; it is lined with mucous membrane.
- Digestion begins when food enters the mouth and is masticated (chewed) by the teeth; the salivary glands secrete saliva to moisten and begin the chemical breakdown of the food.
- The chewing action plus the saliva and the actions of the tongue form the food into a bolus (ball), which can then be swallowed (Figure 6.92■).

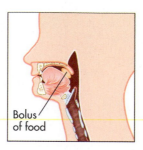

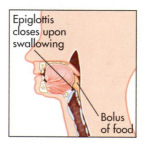

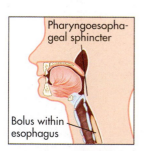

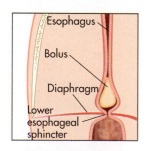

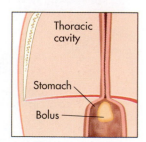

FIGURE 6.92

The movement of a bolus of food from the mouth, down the esophagus, and to the stomach.

Mouth

- The cavity formed by the palate (roof of the mouth), the lips and cheeks on the sides, and the tongue on the floor of the mouth.
- The palate is subdivided into the hard palate, the bony anterior portion, and the soft palate, the flexible posterior portion.
  - At the posterior end of the soft palate sits a piece of dangling tissue called the uvula; it separates the oral cavity from the pharynx and aids in swallowing by guiding food toward the pharynx and preventing it from backing up into the nose.
- The tongue is skeletal muscle covered in mucous membrane and attached to the underlying tissue by a membrane called the lingual frenulum.
  - The tongue senses temperature, texture, and taste of food, manipulates the food in the mouth while chewing, and aids in swallowing.
  - Taste buds, which distinguish bitter, sweet, sour, and salty flavors, and papillae (elevations) are located on the tongue's surface.

Teeth

- Two sets of teeth have been formed by the age of 21 in most people: the 20 deciduous teeth, also called *baby teeth* or *milk teeth,* which are replaced, starting at the age of six, with the 32 permanent teeth.
- The crown of a tooth, composed of the pulp cavity, a thick layer of dentin, and then covered in a layer of hard enamel, is the part above the gum line; the root of a tooth, composed of the root canal filled with blood vessels, nerves, and lymph vessels, lies below the gum line.
  - The root is held in place in a bony socket of the jaw by cementum, a layer of bone covering the surface of the root, and small periodontal ligaments.
- Mastication of the food by the teeth is the first step in digestion.
  - Incisors and cuspids (canines) in the front of the mouth bite into, tear, and cut food into small pieces.
  - Bicuspids and molars in the back of the mouth grind and crush food into smaller, finer pieces.

Pharynx

- The beginning of the tube leading to the stomach, it lies posterior to the mouth; used by both the respiratory and digestive systems (see Figure 6.91).
- Swallowed food and drink pass through the pharynx into the esophagus by muscular contractions.
- The epiglottis covers the trachea to prevent food from entering the respiratory system.

Esophagus

- Muscular tube, running from the pharynx through the chest cavity and into the abdominal cavity, which empties food into the stomach (see Figure 6.91).
- Wavelike, muscular contractions called *peristalsis* propel food through the esophagus and the rest of the gastrointestinal tract.

Stomach

- Saclike, muscular organ that collects food and begins the process of digestion (Figure 6.93).
- Upper region of the stomach is called the *fundus,* the main portion is called the *body,* and the lower region is the *antrum.*
- *Rugae* are folds in the lining of the stomach that stretch when the stomach fills with food.
- Hydrochloric acid and other gastric juices convert food into a semiliquid state called *chime,* which then passes into the small intestine.
- At the antrum, a valve called the *pyloric sphincter,* regulates the passage of chime into the small intestine.

Small intestine

- Located between the pyloric sphincter and the large intestine; the longest part of the gastrointestinal tract, approximately 20 feet by 1 inch in diameter (see Figure 6.91).
- Divided into three sections: duodenum, jejunum, and ileum
  - Duodenum: the first 10–12 inches, it extends from the pyloric sphincter to the jejunum; digestion is completed here as the chime mixes with digestive juices from the pancreas and gallbladder.
  - Jejunum: about 8 feet long, it extends from the duodenum to the ileum.
  - Ileum: about 12 feet long, it connects to the large intestine with a sphincter called the *ileocecal valve.*
- Major site of digestion and absorption of nutrients from food
  - Nutrients are absorbed into small capillaries that line the walls of the small intestine and transmitted to body cells through the circulatory system.

Large intestine

- Approximately 5 feet long and 2.5 inches in diameter, extending from the ileocecal valve to the anus (see Figure 6.91).

- Divided into the cecum, the colon, the rectum, and the anus:
  - Cecum: saclike area in the first 2–3 inches of the large intestine with the appendix, a small appendage with no known function, attached to it.
  - Colon: the major portion of the large intestine; consists of the ascending colon, transverse colon, descending colon, and sigmoid colon; the sigmoid colon ends at the rectum.
  - Rectum: stores feces (solid waste that is left after digestion and absorption); leads into the anus.
  - Anus: Controlled by the anal sphincter, which is composed of rings of involuntary muscles that control the evacuation of feces (defecation or bowel movement).
- Peristalsis continues in the large intestine, slowly moving fecal matter to the rectum.
- Minor site of continuing digestion and absorption and water reabsorption.
- Bacteria in the large intestine contribute to the breakdown of indigestible materials and produce B complex vitamins and most of the Vitamin K needed for proper blood clotting
- The waste products of the digestive process are stored and compacted in the rectum, then eliminated from the body through the anus.

Accessory Organs

Salivary glands

- Three pair of glands located in the mouth: the parotid (located on either side of the face), the submandibular (located on the floor of the mouth), and the sublingual (located below the tongue) (see Figure 6.91).
- Stimulated to produce saliva, a liquid that contains amylase, an enzyme that helps to break down carbohydrates, by the sight, smell, thought, or taste of food.
- Saliva moistens and begins the chemical breakdown of food to form a bolus, chewed food that is ready to be swallowed (see Figure 6.92).

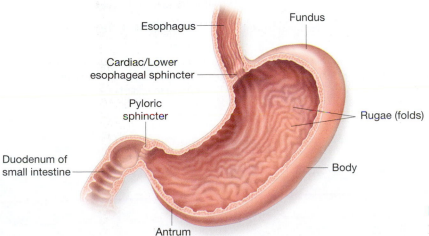

FIGURE 6.93

Regions and internal structures of the stomach.

Liver

- Large glandular organ that weighs about 3.5 pounds; located in the upper right part of the abdomen (see Figure 6.91).
- Plays an important role in the metabolism of carbohydrates, fats, and proteins.
- Manufactures:
  - Bile: a digestive juice important for the digestion of fats and lipids.
  - Fibrinogen and prothrombin: coagulants essential for blood clotting.
  - Heparin: anticoagulant that prevents the clotting of blood.
  - Blood proteins: albumin and gamma globulin.
- Detoxifies potentially harmful substances in the body such as drugs and alcohol; stores iron and vitamins B_{12}, A, D, E, and K.

Gallbladder

- Membranous sac attached to the liver where excess bile produced in the liver is stored and concentrated (see Figure 6.91).
- During the digestion process, bile is sent to the duodenum when needed to emulsify fat in the chyme.

Pancreas

- An endocrine gland that produces the hormones insulin and glucagon, the pancreas also produces two important substances for digestion—buffers and pancreatic enzymes (see Figure 6.91).
  - Buffers neutralize acidic chime that has just left the stomach.
  - Pancreatic enzymes chemically digest carbohydrates, fats, and proteins.

TABLE 6.29	Common Pathologies of the Digestive System	
Disease/Disorder	Description	Massage Implications
Anorexia (an-oh-REK-see-ah)	Loss of appetite that can accompany other conditions; anorexia nervosa is an eating disorder involving refusal to eat	Indicated as part of comprehensive treatment
Appendicitis (ah-pen-dih-SIGH-tis)	Inflammation of the appendix, an organ with no known function located in the lower right part of the abdomen and attached to the first part of the colon; surgical removal is the usual treatment	Medical emergency
Bulimia (buh-LEE-mee-ah)	Eating disorder characterized by binge eating and then purging with the use of laxatives and vomiting	Indicated as part of comprehensive treatment
Cholecystitis (koh-lee-sis-TYE-tis)	Inflammation of the gallbladder often caused by gallstones in the gallbladder or bile duct	General contraindication
Cirrhosis (sih-ROH-sis)	Chronic disease of the liver causing liver dysfunction	Indicated in comprehensive health care treatment; contraindicated in advanced stages
Colorectal cancer (kohl-oh-REK-tall)	Cancers of the colon (large intestine) often beginning in benign polyps in the lining of the intestine; second-leading cause of cancer deaths in the United States (lung cancer is the first)	Indicated as part of comprehensive health care treatment for cancer; abdominal massage contraindicated
Constipation (kon-stih-PAY-shun)	Difficult or infrequent defecation	Indicated for treatment
Crohn's disease (KROHNZ)	Chronic inflammatory bowel disease affecting the ileum and/or colon; also called *regional ileitis*	Contraindication for abdominal massage
Diarrhea (dye-ah-REE-ah)	Passing of frequent watery bowel movements; usually accompanies gastrointestinal disorders	Abdominal massage contraindicated; caution: check for contraindications related to underlying condition

TABLE 6.29 Common Pathologies of the Digestive System (continued)

Disease/Disorder	Description	Massage Implications
Diverticulitis (dye-ver-tik-yoo-LYE-tis)	Inflammation of a diverticulum (an outpouching of the gut) in the intestinal tract, frequently in the colon; often the result of food becoming trapped within the pouch and not being eliminated (Figure 6.94■)	General contraindication in acute inflammatory phase; contraindication for abdominal massage

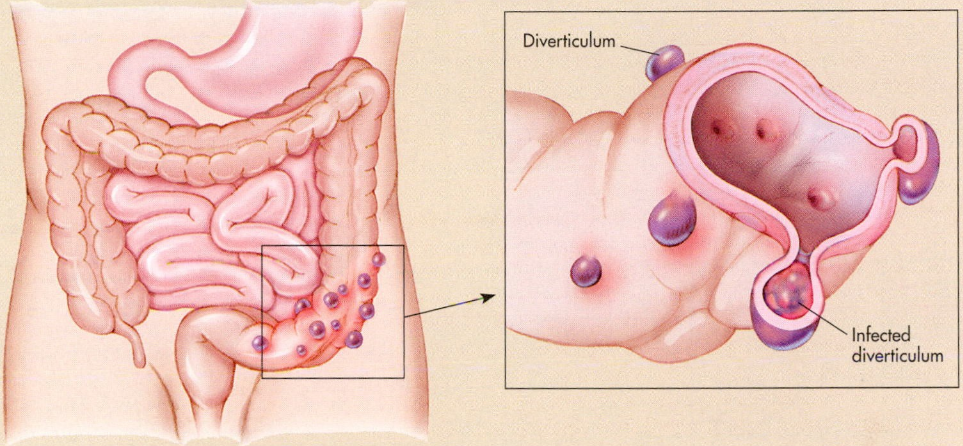

FIGURE 6.94

Diverticulitis.

Disease/Disorder	Description	Massage Implications
Diverticulosis (dye-ver-tik-yoo-LOW-sis)	Condition of having diverticula in the intestinal tract, which increases the possibility of one or more becoming inflamed, leading to diverticulitis	Contraindication for abdominal massage
Dyspepsia (dis-PEP-see-ah)	Indigestion	Contraindication for abdominal massage
Enteritis (en-ter-EYE-tis)	Inflammation of the small intestine	General contraindication
Esophageal stricture (eh-soff-ah-JEE-al STRIK-chur)	Narrowing of the esophagus, making it difficult to swallow foods and fluids	None
Gastritis (gas-TRY-tis)	Inflammation of the stomach; symptoms include pain, tenderness, nausea, and vomiting	General contraindication
Gastroenteritis (gas-troh-en-ter-EYE-tis)	Inflammation of the stomach and small intestine	General contraindication
Gastroesophageal reflux disease (GERD) (gas-troh-ee-sof-ah-GEE-all REE-fluks)	Inflammation and pain caused by stomach acid backing up into the esophagus; commonly called by its acronym *GERD*; also called *reflux esophagitis*	Contraindication for abdominal massage
Hemorrhoids (HEM-oh-roydz)	Varicose veins in the rectum	None
Hepatitis (hep-ah-TYE-tis)	Inflammation of the liver generally due to a viral infection	Medical emergency

TABLE 6.29   Common Pathologies of the Digestive System (continued)

Disease/Disorder	Description	Massage Implications
Hiatal hernia (high-AY-tal HER-nee-ah)	Abnormal protrusion (hernia) of the upper portion of the stomach into the chest cavity through an opening of the diaphragm called the esophageal hiatus; gastroesophageal reflux disease is a common symptom (Figure 6.95A■)	Contraindication for abdominal massage

A Hiatal hernia

Esophagus
Diaphragm
Stomach
Herniation of the stomach through the hiatal opening

B Inguinal hernia

Small intestine
Inguinal ligament
Direct inguinal hernia

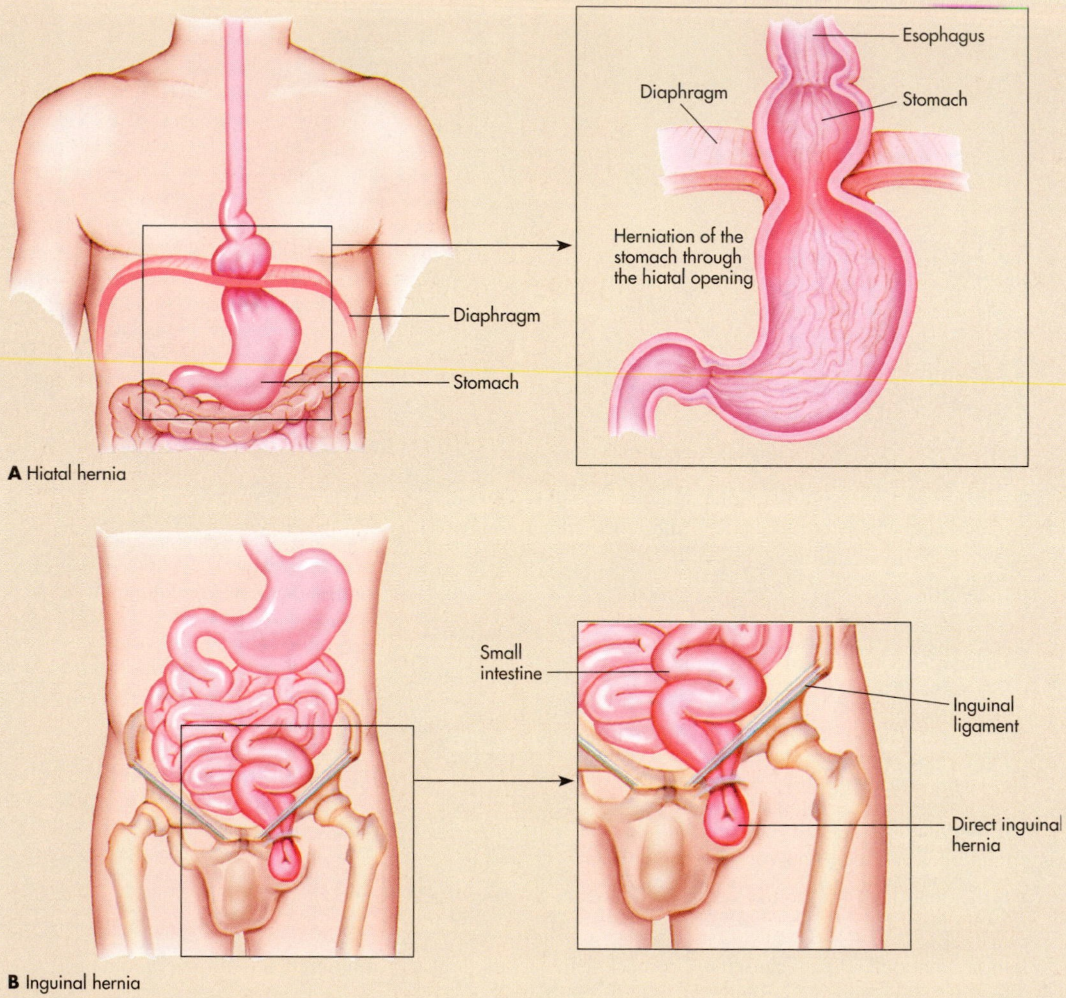

FIGURE 6.95
A. Hiatal hernia.
B. Inguinal hernia.

Disease/Disorder	Description	Massage Implications
Inflammatory bowel disease (IBD)	Chronic inflammatory condition with multiple ulcers forming on the mucous membrane of the colon; also called *ulcerative colitis*	Contraindication for abdominal massage
Inguinal hernia (ING-gwih-nal)	Abnormal protrusion (hernia) of a portion of the small intestines into the inguinal area (groin) through a weak spot in the abdominal wall that becomes a hole; surgical repair may be necessary (Figure 6.95B)	Contraindication for abdominal massage
Irritable bowel syndrome (IBS)	Disturbance in intestinal function from unknown causes; may cause changes in bowel function and abdominal pain; also called *spastic colon*	Contraindication for abdominal massage
Pancreatic cancer (pan-kree-AT-ik)	Cancer of the pancreas usually arising from the exocrine glands; vague, nonspecific symptoms (abdominal and/or back pain, loss of appetite, weight loss, bloating, diarrhea, jaundice) contribute to diagnosis only in the more advanced stages leading to a high mortality rate	Indicated in comprehensive treatment for cancer

TABLE 6.29	Common Pathologies of the Digestive System (continued)	
Disease/Disorder	Description	Massage Implications
Peptic ulcer disease (PUD) PEP-tik ULL-sir)	Ulcer occurring in the lining of the lower esophagus, stomach, or duodenum; thought to be caused by gastric acids; symptoms include pain, nausea, vomiting, and weight loss	Contraindication for abdominal massage
Polyps	Small tumors attached to the mucous membrane of the colon (large intestine); may be benign, precancerous, or the site of cancer	Contraindication for abdominal massage if precancerous or cancerous
Pyrosis (pie-ROW-sis)	Painful burning sensation generally caused by stomach acid splashing up into the esophagus; also called *heartburn*	Contraindication for abdominal massage
Volvulus (VOL-vyoo-lus)	Painful condition in which the bowel twists upon itself causing an obstruction; generally requires immediate surgery	Medical emergency

URINARY SYSTEM

Electrolytes (ee-LEK-troh-lites)

Kidneys

pH level

Ureters (yoo-REE-ters)

Urethra (yoo-REE-thrah)

Urinary (YOO-rih-nair-ee)bladder

Urine (YOO-rin)

The urinary system makes urine, filters and removes waste products, adjusts water and electrolyte levels, and maintains the correct pH level, thus maintaining a stable internal environment for the body. The organs of the urinary system include the kidneys, which manufacture urine; ureters, which transport urine from the kidneys to the urinary bladder, an organ that temporarily stores urine; and the urethra, the passageway of urine out of the body (Figure 6.96■). Table 6.30■ lists abbreviations that relate to the urinary system. Table 6.31■ at the end of this section lists common pathologies of the urinary system and their massage implications.

Parts and Functions of the Urinary System

Kidneys

- Functions:
  - Filter waste substances from the blood.
  - Produce urine, a transparent yellow fluid, to carry these waste products out of the body.

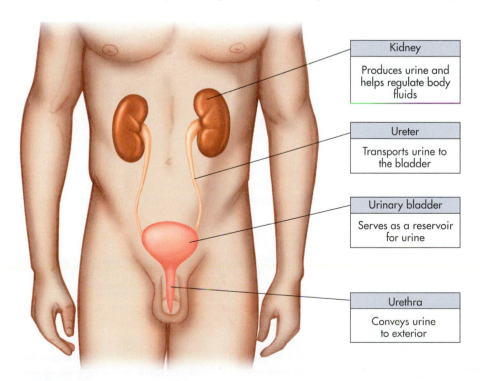

Kidney
Produces urine and helps regulate body fluids

Ureter
Transports urine to the bladder

Urinary bladder
Serves as a reservoir for urine

Urethra
Conveys urine to exterior

FIGURE 6.96

The urinary system.

TABLE 6.30	Urinary System Abbreviations
Abbreviation	Meaning
ARF	Acute renal failure
CAPD	Continuous ambulatory peritoneal dialysis
cath	Catheterization
Cl	Chloride
CRF	Chronic renal failure
ESRD	End-stage renal disease
GU	Genitourinary
HD	Hemodialysis
H_2O	Water
I&O	Intake and output
IPD	Intermittent peritoneal dialysis
K^+	Potassium
KUB	Kidney, ureter, bladder
mL	Milliliter
Na^+	Sodium
pH	Acidity or alkalinity of urine
U/A, UA	Urinalysis
UC	Urine culture

○ Help the body maintain fluid balance (homeostasis) by allowing reabsorption of water and some electrolytes back into the blood.

○ Maintain the body's correct pH level, keeping it neither too acidic nor too alkaline.

- The kidneys are the primary organs of the urinary system; two bean-shaped structures located in the lumbar region of the back above the waist and flanking the vertebral column.

- Each kidney is encapsulated in layers of connective membrane, fatty tissue for protection, and fibrous tissue that helps anchor the kidney to surrounding structures.

- The renal artery, delivering waste-filled blood to the kidney, and the renal vein, returning cleansed blood to the general circulation, enter and leave the kidney at a notch in its edge called the hilum (Figure 6.97■).

- The hilum of the kidney is also the site where the ureter connects with the renal pelvis, a saclike area that collects urine as it is formed (Figure 6.97).

- The cortex, the shell-like outer layer of the kidney, contains arteries, veins, convoluted tubules, and glomerular capsules.

- The medulla, the inner area of the kidney, contains renal pyramids that connect with the renal pelvis.

- The filtration of wastes from the blood takes place in the over one million microscopic nephrons in each kidney.

- Each nephron consists of the renal corpuscle, which filters the blood, and the renal tubule, which carries away the water and waste removed from the blood (Figure 6.97).

○ The renal corpuscle contains the glomerulus, a ball of capillaries, surrounded by a protective structure

called Bowman's capsule (also called a glomerular capsule); this attaches to the proximal convoluted tubule, which becomes the loop of Henley, and then the distal convoluted tubule, which opens into a collecting tubule, and then connects to the ureter (Figure 6.97).

Ureters

- Narrow, muscular tube that carries urine down from the renal pelvis of each of the two kidneys to the urinary bladder (see Figure 6.96).
  ○ Lined by mucous membrane; 10 to 12 inches long and about one-quarter of an inch wide

Urinary bladder

- Elastic, muscular sac that receives urine from the ureters, stores it, and excretes it by urination through the urethra (see Figure 6.96).

- Located in the pelvic cavity; consists of smooth muscle tissue lined with mucous membrane that contains rugae (folds) that allow it to stretch when full of urine.

- After collecting a quantity of urine, *involuntary* muscle action causes the bladder to contract and the internal sphincter to relax; *voluntary* muscle action allows the external sphincter to open at the appropriate time and urination or emptying of the bladder occurs as the urine flows through the urethra.

Urethra

- Mucous-membrane lined tubular canal extending from the urinary bladder to the urinary meatus, the external opening through which urine flows out of the body.
  ○ In males, the urethra is about 8 inches long and serves an additional purpose—as a pathway for semen to leave the body (Figure 6.98A■); in females, the urethra is about 1.5 inches long and functions solely as an outlet for urine (Figure 6.98B).

Urine

When waste products are removed from the blood by the nephrons within the kidneys, other substances such as water, electrolytes, and nutrients are removed as well; however, they need to be returned to the blood. This process, which produces urine in its final form ready to be eliminated, consists of three stages: filtration, reabsorption, and secretion.

MASSAGE CONNECTION

The kidneys are situated against the dorsal body wall, and extend from about T-12 to L-3 vertebrae. They are partially protected by the ribs (Figure 6.99■). Because the kidneys are relatively close to the surface when the client is prone, they are an endangerment site. Do not apply heavy percussion techniques over this area.

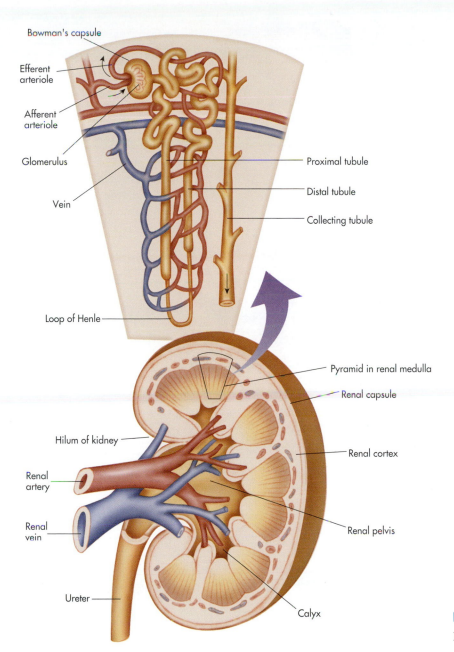

Bowman's capsule

Efferent arteriole

Afferent arteriole

Glomerulus

Vein

Loop of Henle

Proximal tubule

Distal tubule

Collecting tubule

Pyramid in renal medulla

Renal capsule

Hilum of kidney

Renal artery

Renal vein

Ureter

Renal cortex

Renal pelvis

Calyx

FIGURE 6.97

Kidney with an expanded view of a nephron.

1. Filtration—occurs in the renal corpuscle as the pressure of blood flowing through the glomerulus forces filtered material from the blood through the wall of Bowman's capsule and into the renal tubules. This fluid, called the glomerular filtrate, is composed of water, electrolytes, nutrients, and waste substances.

2. Reabsorption—the glomerular filtrate passes through the four sections of the tubule (proximal tubule, loop of Henle, distal tubule, collecting tubule), during which water (up to 99 percent) and many of the dissolved substances (electrolytes and nutrients) are reabsorbed into capillaries surrounding the renal tubes and then re-enter the circulating blood.

3. Secretion—special cells of the renal tubules secrete ammonia, uric acid, and other waste materials into the renal tubule, supplementing the initial glomerular filtration. This is the final stage of urine production; urine passes through the kidneys into the ureters and then into the urinary bladder for storage.

MASSAGE CONNECTION

The urinary bladder is located in the lower abdomen. During abdominal massage, pressure applied to the lower abdomen may cause discomfort if the bladder is full.

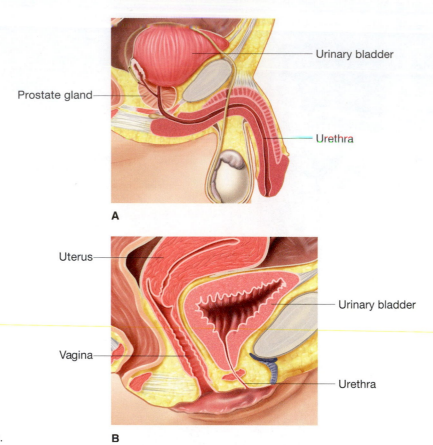

A

FIGURE 6.98

A. The male urethra. B. The female urethra.

B

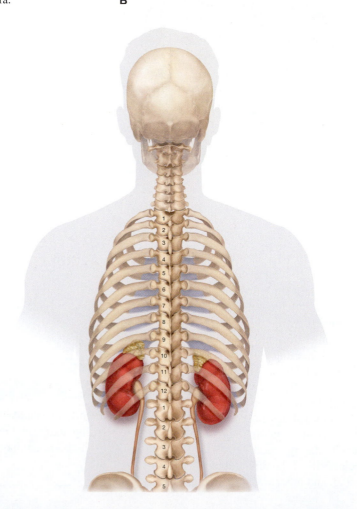

FIGURE 6.99

Location of the kidneys—posterior view.

TABLE 6.31	Common Pathologies of the Urinary System	
Disease/Disorder	Description	Massage Implications
Cystitis (sis-TYE-tis)	Inflammation and irritation of the bladder often caused by bacterial infection; more common in women	General contraindication in acute phase; local contraindication in post–acute phase until infection is completely gone
Glomerulonephritis (gloh-mair-yoo-loh-neh-FRYE-tis)	Inflammation of the kidney (primarily the glomerulus) following prior infection elsewhere in the body; results in protein in the urine, edema, hypertension, and symptoms of infection; may be acute or chronic	General contraindication for circulatory massage
Kidney stones	Deposits of calculi (mineral salts) in the kidneys that can lead to irritation and/or blocked urine flow if they become lodged in the ureter (Figure 6.100■)	General contraindication in acute phase

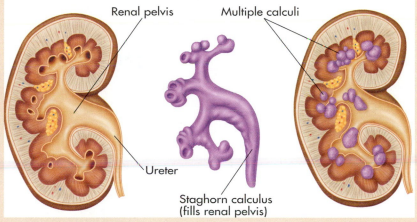

Renal pelvis   Multiple calculi

Ureter

Staghorn calculus
(fills renal pelvis)

FIGURE 6.100
Urinary calculi (kidney stones).

Polycystic kidney disease (PKD) (POL-ee-sis-tik)	Formation of multiple noncancerous cysts within the kidneys, leading to destruction of kidney tissue, uremia, and high blood pressure	General contraindication for circulatory massage
Pyelonephritis (pye-eh-loh-neh-FRYE-tis)	Infection of the kidney and renal pelvis; may be acute or chronic; permanent kidney damage can occur if not treated with antibiotics (Figure 6.101■)	General contraindication for circulatory massage

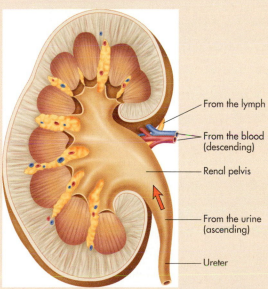

From the lymph

From the blood
(descending)

Renal pelvis

From the urine
(ascending)

Ureter

FIGURE 6.101
Routes of infection for pyelonephritis.

TABLE 6.31	Common Pathologies of the Urinary System (continued)	
Disease/Disorder	Description	Massage Implications
Renal failure	Condition in which the kidneys are unable to clear the blood of urea and other waste products, which can become toxic; may be acute or chronic; uremia is the terminal stage of renal failure	General contraindication for circulatory massage
Urinary incontinence	Leakage of urine frequently caused by age-related weakening of the urethral sphincter muscles	Contraindication for abdominal massage
Urinary tract infection (UTI)	Infection, usually bacterial, of any organ of the urinary system; more common in women	General contraindication in acute phase; local contraindication in post–acute phase until infection is completely gone

FEMALE REPRODUCTIVE SYSTEM

Breasts

Fallopian (fah-LOH-pee-an) tubes

Fetus (FEE-tus)

Ova (OH-vah)

Ovaries (OH-vah-reez)

Pregnancy (PREG-nan-see)

Sex hormones

Uterus (YOO-ter-us)

Vagina (vah-JIGH-nah)

Vulva (VULL-vah)

The function of the female reproductive system is to perpetuate the species through sexual (germ cell) reproduction. Its organs secrete sex hormones, produce ova (female reproductive cells, or eggs), provide a location for fertilization to take place and a fetus to grow during pregnancy, and provide nourishment to the newborn. The organs of the female reproductive system in the pelvic area include two ovaries, two fallopian tubes, a uterus, a vagina, and a vulva. Women's breasts are also considered part of the reproductive system (Figure 6.102■). Table 6.32■ lists abbreviations that relate to the female reproductive system. Table 6.33■ at the end of this section lists common pathologies of the female reproduction system and their massage implications.

Parts and Functions of the Female Reproductive System

A side view of the position of the female reproductive organs in relation to other pelvic structures appears in Figure 6.103■.
Uterus
- Muscular hollow organ with three major functions:
  ○ Site of monthly discharge of blood (menses).
  ○ Provides a place for the development of the fetus during pregnancy.
  ○ Contracts rhythmically during labor to help expel the fetus.

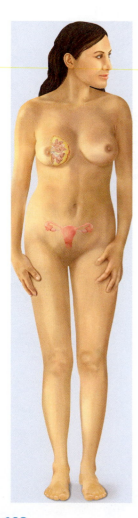

FIGURE 6.102

Female reproductive system.

- Located in the center of the pelvic cavity between the bladder and the rectum, it is held in position by several ligaments.
- Three sections of the uterus are the fundus (upper portion), which lies between where the fallopian tubes

TABLE 6.32	Female Reproductive System Abbreviations
Abbreviation	**Meaning**
AB	Abortion
CS, C-section	Cesarean section
D&C	Dilation and curettage
ERT	Estrogen replacement therapy
FTND	Full-term, normal delivery
GYN, gyn	Gynecology
HPV	Human papilloma virus
HRT	Hormone replacement therapy
LMP	Last menstrual period
OB	Obstetrics
OCPs	Oral contraceptive pills
PAP	Papanicolaou test
TSS	Toxic shock syndrome

connect to the uterus; the corpus (central portion); and the cervix (lower portion or neck), which opens into the vagina (Figure 6.104■).

- The myometrium is the thick muscular wall of the uterus; its contractions help to propel the fetus through the birth canal at delivery.
- The endometrium is the blood-rich inner lining of the uterine wall; in response to monthly hormonal changes, it either prepares to receive a fertilized ovum, which implants in the endometrium and receives fetal nourishment and protection throughout the pregnancy; or, if

pregnancy is not established, the endometrium sloughs off, resulting in menstruation (menstrual period).
  - A female's first menstruation (usually occurring in the early teenage years) is called menarche; the ending of a female's childbearing and menstruating years is called menopause (usually between the ages of 40 and 50).

Fallopian tubes

- Serve as ducts that move the ovum from the ovary to the uterus (after ovulation) and also convey sperm from the uterus (after sexual intercourse) toward the ovaries.
- Extend laterally from either side of the uterus near each ovary; each ends in a funnel-shaped opening called the ostium, which is surrounded by fimbriae (see Figure 6.104).
- The fimbriae (fingerlike structures) help to propel the ovum into the tube where it moves toward the uterus; fertilization (conception) occurs if the ovum becomes impregnated by sperm while in the tube.

Ovaries

- Produce ova (eggs) and female sex hormones.
- Small, almond-shaped glands located on either side of the uterus (see Figure 6.104).
- Follicle-stimulating hormone (FSH) and luteinizing hormone (LH) are secreted from the pituitary gland approximately every 28 days; they stimulate the maturation of ovum and trigger ovulation.
  - During ovulation one ovary releases an ovum, which is propelled into the fallopian tube, where it

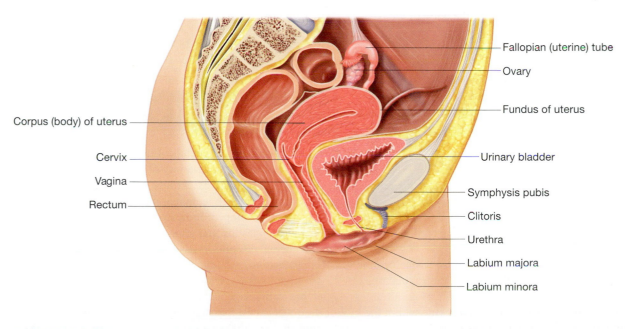

FIGURE 6.103

A side view of the position of the female reproductive organs in relation to other pelvic structures.

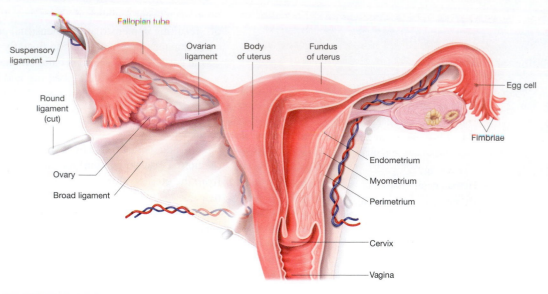

FIGURE 6.104

The uterus and its relationship to the cervix, fallopian tubes, ovaries, and vagina.

may or may not be fertilized, and then into the uterus.

- Estrogen and progesterone, the principal female sex hormones, are produced by the ovaries
- They stimulate the endometrium to be prepared to receive a fertilized ovum; they also promote the growth and development of the female secondary sex characteristics.

Vagina

- Muscular tube lined with mucous membrane that has three main functions:
  - Allows for the passage out of the body of menstrual blood.
  - Receives the male penis and semen during intercourse (copulation).
  - Serves as the birth canal through which the infant leaves the woman's body.
- Extends from the cervix of the uterus to the outside of the body; situated between the bladder and rectum (see Figure 6.104).

Vulva

- Consists of a group of organs that make up the female external genitalia:
  - Mons pubis—triangular-shaped pad of fatty tissue over the symphysis pubis that is covered with hair after puberty.
  - Labia majora—two folds of adipose tissue forming liplike structures on either side of the vaginal opening.
  - Labia minora—two thin folds of tissue within the labia majora enclosing the vestibule.
  - Vestibule—the cleft between the labia minora containing the urethra, the vagina, and the two

Bartholin's glands, which secrete lubricating mucus during intercourse.
  - Clitoris—small organ containing sensitive erectile tissue that corresponds to the male penis.
- The perineum, a muscular sheet of tissue, forms the pelvic floor; located between the vulva and the anus.

Breasts

- Two exterior mammary glands that produce milk (lactation) to nourish the newborn.
- Lying in front of the pectoral muscles, they are composed of 15 to 20 glandular tissue lobes separated by connective tissue.

MASSAGE CONNECTION

Breast massage is a specialization applied for general breast health and for a variety of therapeutic goals. Women's breasts are essentially complex glandular structures for which technical massage applications have been developed. Indications for breast massage include congestion and tenderness, drainage problems and edema, discomfort associated with pregnancy and breastfeeding, and scarring from surgery or cancer treatment. Massage therapists need specialized training in breast massage techniques and related ethical considerations. Breast massage requires written informed consent, and may be outside the legal scope of massage in some jurisdictions.

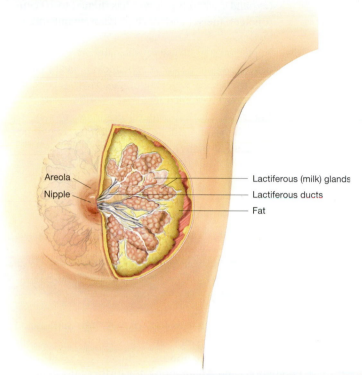

FIGURE 6.105

The breast, showing external and internal features.

- Milk is produced by the lactiferous glands; it is carried to the nipple by the lactiferous ducts (Figure 6.105■).
  - The areola is the pigmented area surrounding each nipple that contains the lactiferous glands.
- Prolactin, produced by the pituitary gland, is the major hormone involved in milk production.

Pregnancy

Pregnancy is the period of time from conception to birth during which the fetus grows and develops in the mother's uterus, also called the *womb*. Figure 6.106■ shows the position of the fetus in a full-term pregnancy.

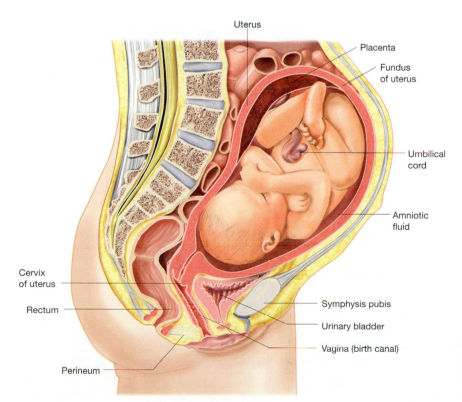

FIGURE 6.106

Full-term pregnancy. Position of the fetus and structures associated with pregnancy are shown.

Gestation

- The gestation or normal length of time for a pregnancy is 40 weeks.
- From the fertilized egg's implantation in the uterus until the end of the eighth week, it is called an embryo; during this time all the major organs and body systems are formed.
- From the ninth week until birth, it is called a fetus, and the organs mature and begin to function.
- Two membranous sacs, the amnion (filled with amniotic fluid) and the chorion, surround and protect the fetus.
- Present only during pregnancy, the placenta is a spongy structure that forms in the uterus joining fetus to mother and providing nourishment and a common blood supply; also called the *afterbirth*.
    - The umbilical cord attaches the fetus to the placenta.
    - Secretes chorionic gonadotropin hormone—helps to keep the pregnancy ongoing; also secretes estrogen and progesterone.

Labor and delivery

- The stages of labor:
    - Dilation stage—contractions of the uterine muscles; fetal pressure on the cervix causing it to dilate (expand); when the cervix has dilated to 10 centimeters, the second stage of labor, expulsion, begins.
    - Expulsion stage—usually the baby presents head first, called crowning; when the buttocks appear first, it is called a breech presentation; this part of labor ends with delivery of the infant.
    - Placental stage—the uterus continues to contract after the infant is delivered in order to expel the placenta through the birth canal.

MASSAGE CONNECTION

Massage for pregnant women requires training related to contraindications and cautions, positioning, and specific goals. See page 588 in Chapter 20, Special Populations and Adaptations, for further information about this application.

TABLE 6.33 **Common Pathologies of the Female Reproductive System**

Disease/Disorder	Description	Massage Implications
Breast cancer	Malignant tumor of the breast	Indication for relaxation massage within comprehensive treatment for cancer
Cervical cancer (SER-vih-kal)	Malignant growth in the cervix sometimes caused by the human papilloma virus (HPV), a sexually transmitted virus	Indication for relaxation massage within comprehensive treatment for cancer
Dysmenorrhea (dis-men-oh-REE-ah)	Painful cramping associated with menstruation	General contraindication during painful cramping
Endometrial cancer	Cancer of the endometrial lining of the uterus	Indication for relaxation massage within comprehensive treatment for cancer
Fibrocystic breast disease (figh-bro-SIS-tik)	Benign cysts form in the breast	None
Fibroid tumor (FIGH-broyd)	Benign, fibrous growth often occurring in the uterus	None
Mastitis (mas-TYE-tis)	Inflammation of the breast	General contraindication in acute stage
Menorrhagia (men-oh-RAY-jee-ah)	Excessive bleeding during the menstrual period	General contraindication during menstruation
Ovarian cancer (oh-VAY-ree-an)	Cancer of the ovary	Indication for relaxation massage within comprehensive treatment for cancer
Ovarian cyst	Cyst or multiple cysts that develops in the ovary; can rupture and cause pain and bleeding	Local contraindication for abdominal massage
Pelvic inflammatory disease (PID) (PEL-vik in-FLAM-mah-toh-ree)	Inflammation of the female reproductive organs, generally bacterial in nature	General contraindication

TABLE 6.33	Common Pathologies of the Female Reproductive System (continued)	
Disease/Disorder	Description	Massage Implications
Preeclampsia (pre-eh-KLAMP-see-ah)	Toxemia of pregnancy resulting in hypertension, headaches, and edema; can lead to the more dangerous eclampsia, causing seizures and coma	Medical emergency
Premenstrual syndrome (PMS) (pre-MEN-stroo-al)	Condition that affects some females 1 to 2 weeks before the beginning of menstruation; symptoms include abdominal bloating, breast swelling with pain, edema, headache, backache, constipation, depression, anxiety, and other unpleasant effects	Indication for relaxation massage
Prolapsed uterus	Fallen uterus that can cause the cervix to protrude through the vaginal opening	Contraindication for abdominal massage

Sexually transmitted diseases can occur in men, women, and children, and be passed by sexual contact or from mother to child. To avoid repetition, they are discussed in the male reproductive section.

MALE REPRODUCTIVE SYSTEM

Bulbourethral (buhl-boh-yoo-REE-thral) glands

Epididymis (ep-ih-DID-ih-mis)

Penis (PEE-nis)

Prostate (PROSS-tayt) gland

Scrotum (SKROH-tum)

Semen (SEE-men)

Seminal vesicles (SEM-ih-nal VESS-ih-kls)

Sperm cells

Testes (TESS-teez)

Urethra (yoo-REE-thrah)

Vas deferens (VAS DEF-er-enz)

The function of the male reproductive system is to secrete the male hormones, and produce and deliver to the female reproductive tract the sperm cells necessary to fertilize the ovum, thus perpetuating the species. Its organs include the external organs of reproduction: the scrotum and the penis, and the internal organs: the testes, the epididymis, the urethra, the vas deferens, and glands such as the bulbourethral, prostate, and seminal vesicles (Figure 6.107■). Table 6.34■ lists abbreviations that relate to the male reproductive system. Table 6.35■ at the end of this section lists common pathologies of the male reproductive system and their massage implications.

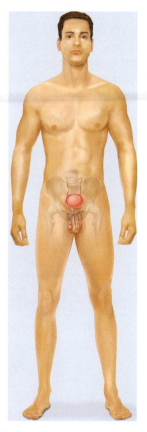

FIGURE 6.107

Male reproductive system.

Parts and Functions of the Male Reproductive System

A side view of the position of the male reproductive organs in relation to other pelvic structures appears in Figure 6.108■.

EXTERNAL ORGANS

The scrotum and the penis are the external organs of male reproduction.

Scrotum

- Pouchlike structure located behind the penis; divided into two sacs, each housing one of the testes and its connecting tube, the epididymus.
- The muscular tissue of the scrotum contracts when exposed to cold, bringing the testes closer to the warmth of the body; this protects the viability of the sperm cells.

TABLE 6.34	Male Reproductive System Abbreviations
Abbreviation	Meaning
ED	Erectile dysfunction
GC	Gonorrhea
GU	Genitourinary
VD	Venereal disease

Penis

- Composed of erectile tissue encased in skin, the penis is the male organ of copulation—it delivers sperm-rich semen into the female's vagina; also contains the orifice through which urine is eliminated.
- The glans penis is the soft tip of the organ; it is protected by the prepuce or foreskin (see Figure 6.108).
  - A surgical procedure called circumcision removes the foreskin; this is done for religious, cultural, or medical reasons.
- The urethra runs through the penis from the urinary bladder to the urinary meatus (the external opening); both urine and semen flow through the urethra.

INTERNAL ORGANS

The testes, epididymis, vas deferens, seminal vesicles, prostate and bulbourethral glands, and urethra are the internal organs of the male reproductive system (see Figure 6.108).

Testes

- Contained in the scrotum, the two testes produce sperm; also called *testicles*.
- The process, called spermatogenesis, occurs within the seminiferous tubules that make up the interior of the testes.
- Testosterone, the male sex hormone, also is produced by the testes; it is responsible for the development of the male reproductive organs, sperm, and secondary sex characteristics.

Epididymis

- Serves as the location for sperm maturation and storage until it is ready to be sent into the vas deferens.
- Coiled, elongated tubule that sits on top of each of the testes.

Vas deferens

- Duct that carries sperm from each epididymis into the pelvic cavity where it eventually empties into the urethra.

Seminal vesicles

- Secrete a glucose-rich liquid that nourishes the sperm; this fluid plus the sperm make up semen, the fluid that is ejaculated during sexual intercourse.
- Two small glands located at the base of the urinary bladder and connected to the vas deferens just before it empties into the urethra.

Prostate gland

- Secretes an alkaline fluid that helps keep sperm alive by neutralizing the pH of the urethra and vagina.

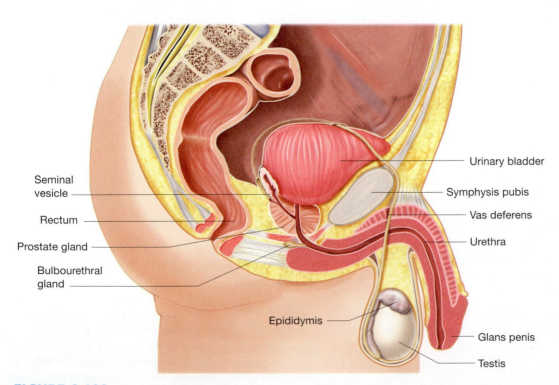

FIGURE 6.108

A side view of the position of the male reproductive organs in relation to other pelvic structures.

TABLE 6.35	Common Pathologies of the Male Reproductive System	
Disease/Disorder	Description	Massage Implications
Benign prostatic hypertrophy (BPH) (bee-NINE pross-TAT-ik high-PER-troh-fee)	Enlargement of the prostate gland; common in men over 50 years of age	None
Chlamydia (klah-MID-ee-ah)	Sexually transmitted bacterial infection causing genital inflammation; can cause pelvic inflammatory disease in females and lead to infertility	General contraindication during acute infection
Genital herpes (JEN-ih-tal HER-peez)	Sexually transmitted viral infection causing blisters in genital region	General contraindication during flare-up
Genital warts (JEN-ih-tal)	Growth of warts on the genitals of both males and females; can lead to cancer of the cervix in women; caused by the sexual transmission of the human papilloma virus (HPV)	None
Gonorrhea (gon-oh-REE-ah)	Sexually transmitted bacterial infection of the mucous membranes of either sex	General contraindication during acute infection
Priapism (pri-ah-pizm)	Long-lasting and painful erection due to pathological causes, not sexual arousal	General contraindication
Prostate cancer (PROSS-tayt)	Generally a slow-growing cancer that frequently occurs in males after the age of 50	Indication for relaxation massage within comprehensive treatment for cancer
Sexually transmitted disease (STD)	Disease acquired through sexual intercourse; formerly called venereal disease (VD)	General contraindication during acute infection
Syphilis (SIF-ih-lis)	Sexually transmitted bacterial infection; eventually fatal if not treated	General contraindication during acute infection
Testicular carcinoma (tes-TIK-yoo-lar)	Cancer of one or both testicles	Indication for relaxation massage within comprehensive treatment for cancer

- Located below the urinary bladder and surrounding the urethra.

Bulbourethral glands
- Produce a mucuslike lubricant that joins with the semen to become part of the ejaculate.
- Two small glands lie on either side of the urethra below the prostate gland.

Urethra
- Runs through the center of the penis and transmits urine and semen out of the body.

MASSAGE CONNECTION

A nonsexual erection of the penis may occur during massage due to increased blood flow to the area. If any erection occurs, a massage therapist must evaluate the situation to determine whether there is sexual intent or not. If sexualizing the massage is suspected, the massage therapist must intervene and stop the massage. See the Intervention Model on page 108 of Chapter 5, Ethics and the Therapeutic Relationship.

KINESIOLOGY

Kinesiology is the study of human movement. Kinesiology looks at the combined action of the muscular, skeletal, and nervous systems that result in movements such as picking up objects, walking, and breathing. Knowledge of joints, muscle attachments and actions is an essential part of kinesiology.

Movement at Joints—General Terminology

The bony structure of a joint and the action of the muscles crossing it determine the movement possible at that joint. Some common movements are shown in Figure 6.109■. Box 6.1 lists the terminology used to describe joint movements.

Range of Motion (ROM)

Range of motion refers to the direction and distance a joint can move to its full potential. Each joint has a normal range of motion that is expressed in degrees from neutral. Measurement of range of motion is done with an instrument called a goniometer (i.e., an instrument that measures angles from the axis of the joint; see Figure 10.3 on page 324). The normal ranges of motion for major joints are shown in Figure 6.110■.

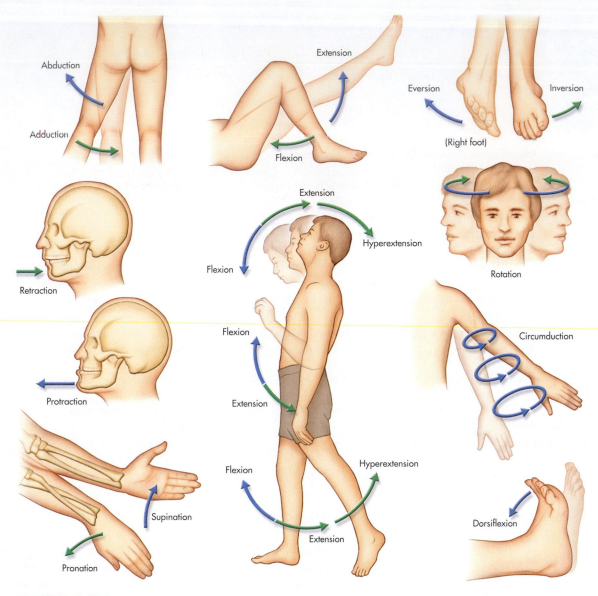

FIGURE 6.109

Classification of joint movements.

BOX 6.1	Joint Movement Terminology		
Flexion	• Bending at a joint; angle decreases.	Depression	• Lowering a body part; downward movement.
Extension	• Straightening a joint; angle increases		
Lateral Flexion	• Bending away from the midline.	Dorsiflexion	• Flexion of the foot at the ankle.
Abduction	• Movement away from the midline of the body.	Plantarflexion	• Extension of the foot at the ankle.
		Supination	• Turning the palm or foot upward.
Adduction	• Movement toward the midline of the body.	Rotation	• Movement around a central axis.
Medial Rotation	• Internal rotation; rotation inward.	Pronation	• Turning the palm or foot downward.
Lateral Rotation	• External rotation; rotation outward.	Eversion	• Turning the foot bottom toward the midline; supination.
Circumduction	• Movement in a circle around a central point.	Inversion	• Turning the foot bottom away from the midline; pronation.
Protraction	• Movement away from the center.		
Retraction	• Movement toward the center.	Anterior Tilt	• Rotation of the pelvis forward.
Elevation	• Raising a body part; upward movement.	Posterior Tilt	• Rotation of the pelvis backward.

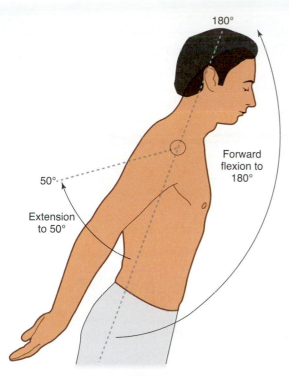

A. Flexion and extension of the shoulders.

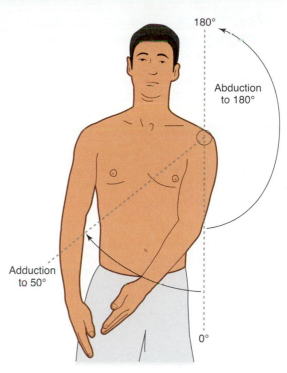

B. Abduction and adduction of the shoulder.

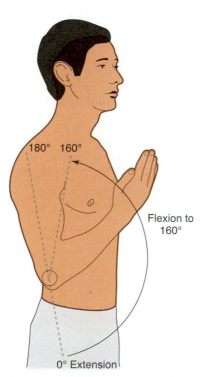

C. Flexion and extension of the elbow.

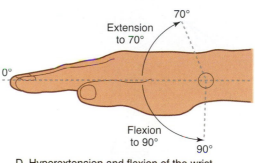

D. Hyperextension and flexion of the wrist.

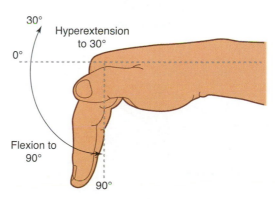

E. Flexion and extension of the fingers.

FIGURE 6.110

Normal range of motion at major joints.

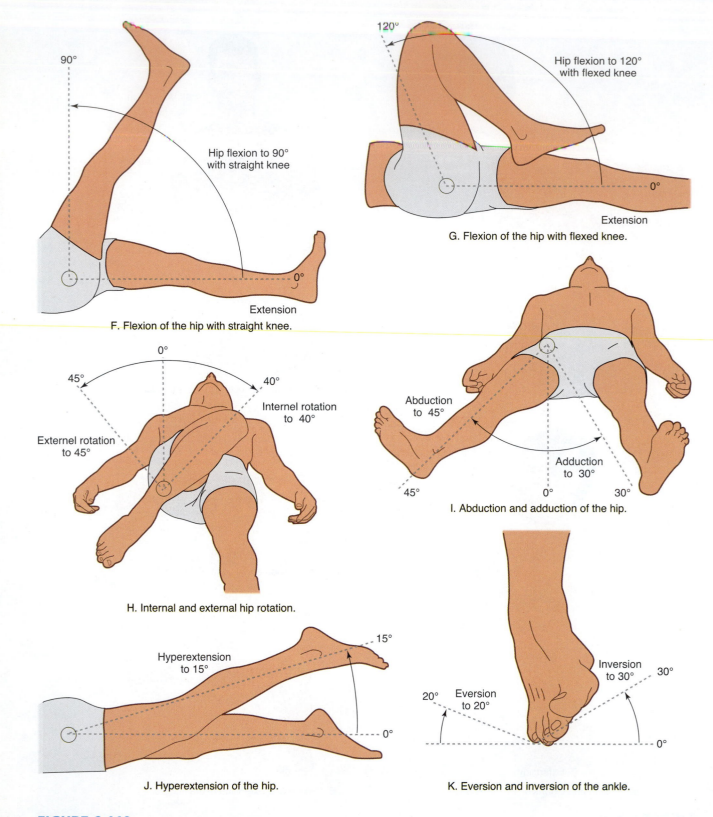

90°

Hip flexion to 90°
with straight knee

0°

Extension

F. Flexion of the hip with straight knee.

120°

Hip flexion to 120°
with flexed knee

0°

Extension

G. Flexion of the hip with flexed knee.

0°

45°   40°

Internel rotation
to 40°

External rotation
to 45°

H. Internal and external hip rotation.

Abduction
to 45°

Adduction
to 30°

45°   0°   30°

I. Abduction and adduction of the hip.

15°

Hyperextension
to 15°

0°

J. Hyperextension of the hip.

Inversion
to 30°   30°

20°   Eversion
to 20°

0°

K. Eversion and inversion of the ankle.

FIGURE 6.110

continued

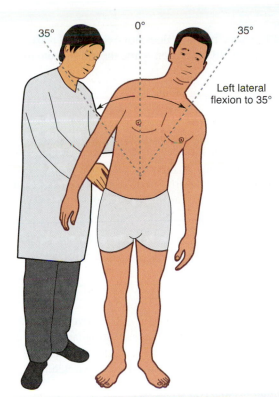

L. Lateral flexion of the spine.

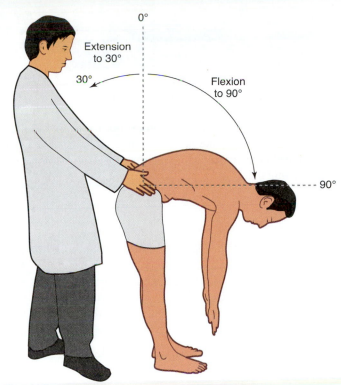

M. Forward flexion of the spine.

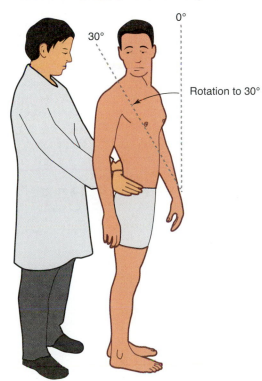

N. Rotation of the spine.

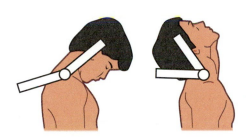

O. Neck extension and flexion.

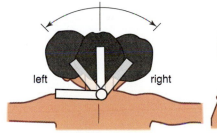

P. Neck lateral bending.

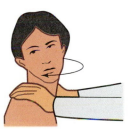

Q. Neck rotation

FIGURE 6.110

continued

MASSAGE CONNECTION

Knowledge of normal range of motion at each joint is useful when applying joint mobilizing and stretching techniques, which are always kept within the normal range. Going outside of the normal range can cause injury. ROM evaluation can identify abnormal joints, or muscle shortening that can be addressed with massage therapy.

Types of Muscle Contractions

Muscle contractions affect the body in different ways. Some contractions result in movement, others do not. Some contractions occur as a muscle shortens, others occur while it lengthens. The types of muscle contraction are isotonic, isometric, concentric, and eccentric.

Isotonic
- Muscle contraction that results in muscle shortening and movement.

Isometric
- Muscle contraction performed against a stable resistance; muscle remains the same length; does not result in movement.

Concentric
- Muscle contraction that overcomes a resistance and results in muscle shortening and movement.

Eccentric
- Muscle contraction that does not overcome a resistance and results in tension while the muscle lengthens.

Proprioceptors

Proprioceptors are sensory organs embedded in tendons and muscles that detect the amount of stretch or tension that is occurring. This information is used to make the proper adjustments to maintain balance and normal posture and to protect the associated structures from injury. Proprioceptors consist of muscle spindles and Golgi tendon organs.

Muscle spindles
- Located within the muscle belly between muscle fibers (Figure 6.111■).
- Sense change in muscle length.
- Play a dual role as receptor and motor effector in a reflex arc called the gamma loop.
- When muscles lengthen rapidly, or are overstretched, gamma afferents in the spindle are stimulated, causing a protective contraction of the muscle; stretch reflex.
- Protect muscles from injury due to overstretching.

Golgi tendon organs (GTO)
- Located in muscle tendons and musculotendinous junctions (Figure 6.112■).
- Sense tension in the muscle.
- Respond to excessive increased tension by inhibiting contraction; inverse stretch reflex or tendon reflex.
- Protect tendons from tearing due to excessive muscle tension.

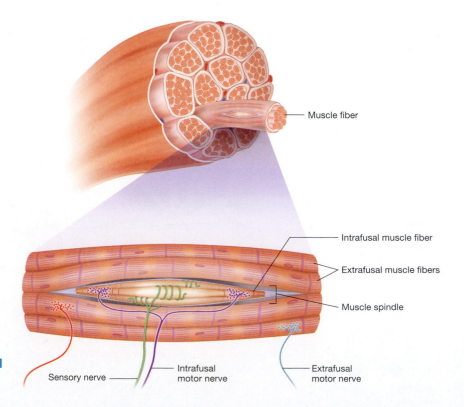

FIGURE 6.111
Muscle spindles.

Muscle fiber

Intrafusal muscle fiber

Extrafusal muscle fibers

Muscle spindle

Extrafusal motor nerve

Intrafusal motor nerve

Sensory nerve

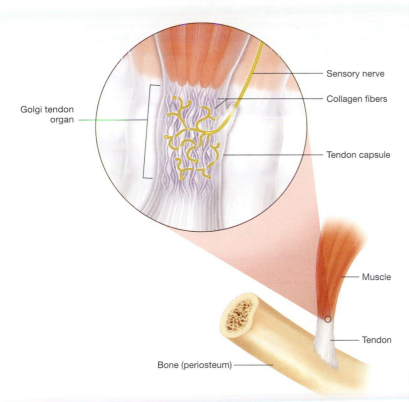

FIGURE 6.112

Golgi tendon organs.

MASSAGE CONNECTION

Knowledge of proprioceptors guides the application of certain massage techniques. For example, stretches are applied slowly and steadily to avoid stimulating the muscle spindles, which would elicit a protective contraction or stretch reflex. A technique for relieving muscle spasms called *approximation* uses the Golgi tendon organ response. To apply approximation to a muscle in spasm (e.g., gastrocnemius), the ends of the muscle belly are pushed toward each other rapidly, stretching the tendons and causing the Golgi proprioceptors to fire, which signals the muscle to relax (inverse stretch reflex).

Biomechanics of Movement

Biomechanics is the study of movement in living organisms. The body moves through a system of levers created by the muscular and skeletal systems. Figure 6.113■ shows 1st-, 2nd-, and 3rd-Class lever systems.

1st-Class lever system
- The fulcrum is located between the force and the resistance.

2nd-Class lever system
- The fulcrum is at one end of the bar, the force is applied at the other end, and the resistance is in between.

3rd-Class lever system
- The fulcrum is at one end, the resistance is at the other end, and the force is applied between them. Most of the large muscles of the body cause movement as part of Class 3 levers.

Flexion at the elbow as a 3rd-Class lever system is illustrated in Figure 6.114■. Note:

- Upper and lower arm bones act as the bars.
- The elbow is the *fulcrum.*
- *Force* or input effort is applied at the point of insertion of the biceps brachii.
- The *resistance* or load moved is the weight held in the hand.

Biomechanical Analysis

Biomechanical analysis of movement requires understanding the anatomical structures involved (muscles and bones), as well as mechanical principles (levers). Massage therapists use this knowledge in certain massage applications (e.g., joint movements), and in assessing a client's movement patterns that may be causing muscle overload and imbalance.

Gait Analysis

Gait analysis examines biomechanics while walking or running. Assessment of a client's gait can reveal deviations from normal that may be causing muscle overload or imbalance. See page 326 in Chapter 10, Goal-Oriented Planning and Documentation, for further discussion of gait analysis. Figure 10.7 on page 326 shows normal walking gait, and Table 10.1 on page 327 lists common causes of walking gait deviations.

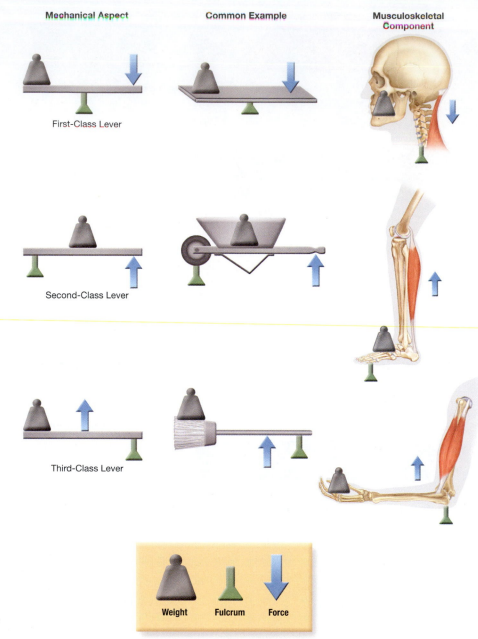

Mechanical Aspect   **Common Example**   **Musculoskeletal Component**

First-Class Lever

Second-Class Lever

Third-Class Lever

| Weight | Fulcrum | Force |

FIGURE 6.113

1st-Class, 2nd-Class, and 3rd-Class lever systems.

MASSAGE CONNECTION

Massage therapists practice good body mechanics while performing massage to enhance technique applications and help avoid overload, overwork, and injury.

Postural and Phasic Muscles

Muscles can be categorized as postural and phasic. **Postural muscles** are stabilizers that support the body against gravity. They tend to shorten and tighten under strain and are over-worked if upright posture is unbalanced. **Phasic muscles** are movers that cause movement against gravity. They tend to weaken when postural muscles are shortened.

MAJOR POSTURAL MUSCLES

- ***Upper Body***
  Neck extensors
  Sternocleidomastoid (SCM)
  Scalenes
  Levator scapulae
  Trapezius
  Lattisimus dorsi
  Pectoralis

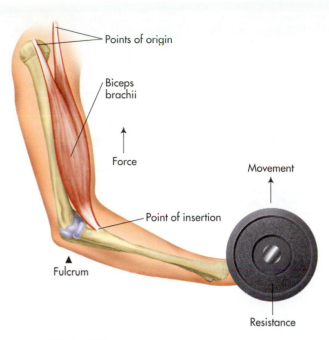

FIGURE 6.114

Flexion at the elbow as a 3rd-Class lever system.

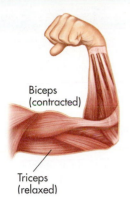

FIGURE 6.115

Coordination of muscles to perform movement.

MASSAGE CONNECTION

Poor upright alignment causes overwork in postural muscles. Look for muscle tension and trigger points in postural muscles if your assessment of a client's posture reveals misalignment. Learn about posture evaluation on page 324 in Chapter 10, Goal-Oriented Planning and Documentation. Figure 10.4 on page 325 shows a body chart for standing posture assessment.

- *Torso*
  Erector spinae group
  Quadratus lumborum
  Abdominal muscles
- *Lower Body*
  Psoas
  Piriformis
  Adductors
  Rectus femoris
  Hamstrings (medial)
  Tensor fascia lata
  Gastrocnemius
  Soleus

MAJOR PHASIC MUSCLES

- *Upper Body*
  Neck flexors
  Deltoid
  Biceps brachii
  Triceps brachii
  Brachioradialis
- *Lower Body*
  Gluteus maximus
  Quadriceps group
  Hamstrings
  Tibialis anterior

ROLES OF MUSCLES IN MOVEMENT

Body movement requires coordination between the contraction of one muscle or muscle group, and the simultaneous relaxation of opposing muscles (Figure 6.115■). When

explaining muscle movement, the following terms are used to describe the roles of the muscles involved.

Agonist   Muscle that is the primary mover in a particular movement produced by its contraction; also called *prime mover*.

Synergist   Muscle that acts with another muscle to produce movement.

Antagonist   Muscle that opposes, or counteracts, the action of another muscle.

MUSCLE ATTACHMENTS, ACTIONS, AND NERVES

The origins, insertions, actions, and nerves of the muscles of the body are shown in Table 6.36■.

MASSAGE CONNECTION

When using reciprocal inhibition to enhance a stretch, it is essential to identify the antagonist to the targeted muscle. Contracting the antagonist prior to the stretch will cause the targeted muscle to relax and to be stretched more effectively.

TABLE 6.36 Muscles of the Body: Their Attachments, Actions, and Nerves

Muscles of the Spine

- Found along the spine from the sacrum to the occiput
- Attach to the spine
- Move the spine

Erector Spinae Group
(part of the *paraspinal muscles*)

Location: Most superficial of the spinal muscles
(See Figure 6.116■)

Spinalis *Subgroups* capitis, cervicis, thoracis	*Origin:* Spinous processes of the upper lumbar, lower thoracic, and C-7 vertebrae, ligmentum nuchae *Insertion:* Spinous processes of the upper thoracic and cervical vertebrae (except C-1) *Action:* Bilaterally extends the spine; flexes the spine laterally to one side *Nerve:* Dorsal spinal nerves
Longissimus *Subgroups* capitis, cervicis, thoracis	*Origin:* Transverse processes of the upper 5 thoracic vertebrae and common tendon (thoracis) *Insertion:* Transverse processes of thoracic vertebrae and lower 9 ribs *Action:* Bilaterally extends the spine; flexes the spine laterally to one side *Nerve:* Dorsal spinal nerves
Illiocostalis *Subgroups* cervicis, thoracis, lumborum	*Origin:* Posterior ribs 1–12 and common tendon (cervicis) *Insertion:* Transverse processes of lumbar vertebrae 1–3 and posterior surface of ribs 6–12 *Action:* Bilaterally extends the spine; flexes the spine laterally to one side *Nerve:* Dorsal spinal nerves

Transversospinalis Group
(part of the *paraspinal muscles*)

Location: Deep to the erector spinae
(See Figure 6.117■)

Multifidi	*Origin:* Sacrum and transverse processes of lumber through cervical vertebrae *Insertion:* Spinous processes of lumbar vertebrae through second cervical vertebrae; span 2–4 vertebrae *Action:* Extends the spine; rotates the spine to one side *Nerve:* Dorsal spinal nerves
Rotatores *Subgroups* longus, brevis	*Origin:* Sacrum and transverse processes of lumber through cervical vertebrae *Insertion:* Spinous processes of lumbar vertebrae through second cervical vertebrae; span 1–2 vertebrae *Action:* Extends the spine; rotates the spine to one side *Nerve:* Dorsal spinal nerves
Semispinalis *Subgroups* capitis, cervicis, thoracis	*Origin:* Transverse processes of thoracic vertebrae and articular processes of lower cervical vertebrae *Insertion:* Spinous processes of upper thoracic, cervicals (except C-1) and superior nuchal line of occiput *Action:* Extends the spine and head *Nerve:* Dorsal spinal nerves

TABLE 6.36	Muscles of the Body: Their Attachments, Actions, and Nerves (continued)

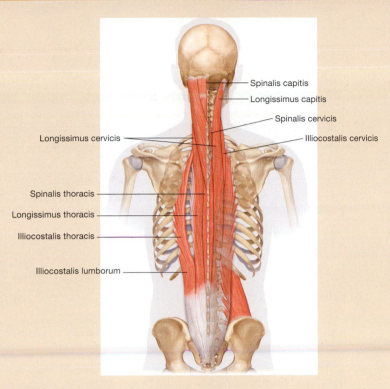

FIGURE 6.116

Erector spinae muscles.

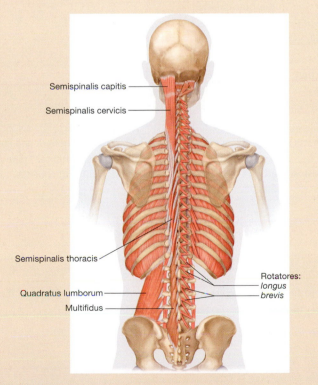

FIGURE 6.117

A. Transversospinalis muscles. B. Semipinalis.

TABLE 6.36	Muscles of the Body: Their Attachments, Actions, and Nerves (continued)
Splenius Muscles	
Location: Along the posterior neck, deep to the trapezius (See Figure 6.118)	
Splenius capitis	*Origin:* Nuchal ligament processes of C-7 to T-3
	Insertion: Mastoid process, lateral nuchal line
	Action: Extends the neck and head; rotates the head to the same side; laterally flexes the neck and head
	Nerve: Branches of cervical dorsal nerves
Splenius cervicis	*Origin:* Spinous processes of T-3 to T-6
	Insertion: Transverse processes of upper cervical vertebrae
	Action: Extends the neck and head; rotates the head to the same side; laterally flexes the neck and head
	Nerve: Branches of cervical dorsal nerves
Suboccipital Muscles	
Location: Deep under the occiput (See Figure 6.119)	
Rectus capitis posterior major	*Origin:* Spinous process of C-2 (axis)
	Insertion: Inferior nuchal line
	Action: Extend the head; rotate the head to the same side
	Nerve: Suboccipital
Rectus capitis posterior minor	*Origin:* Posterior tubercle of C-1 (atlas)
	Insertion: Inferior nuchal line
	Action: Extend the head
	Nerve: Suboccipital
Oblique capitis superior	*Origin:* Transverse process of C-1 (atlas)
	Insertion: Inferior nuchal line
	Action: Extend the head; laterally flexes the head
	Nerve: Suboccipital
Oblique capitis inferior	*Origin:* Spinous process of C-2 (axis)
	Insertion: Transverse process of C-1 (atlas)
	Action: Rotate the head to the same side
	Nerve: Suboccipital
Related Structures	
Supraspinous ligament	Connects spinous processes from C-7 to L-5; provides strength and stability
Nuchal ligament	Attaches the occipital bone of the skull to all cervical vertebrae spinous processes; stabilizes the neck and provides muscle attachment sites
Muscles of the Thorax	
• Found on the back and in abdominal regions • Attach to the spine and rib cage • Move the torso	
Quadratus lumborum (See Figure 6.117)	*Origin:* Posterior iliac crest, iliolumbar ligament
	Insertion: Transverse processes of L-1 to L-4, and the last rib
	Action: Elevates the pelvis, laterally flexes the spine, extends the spine
	Nerve: Branches of the first lumber and twelfth thoracic

TABLE 6.36   **Muscles of the Body: Their Attachments, Actions, and Nerves (continued)**

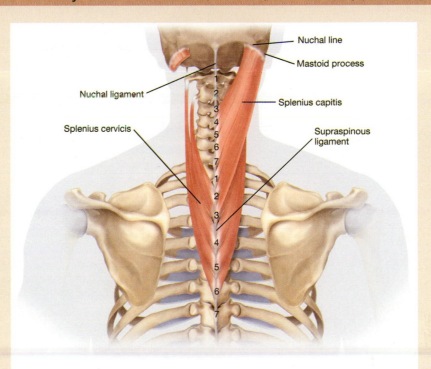

FIGURE 6.118

Splenius capitus and cervicis.

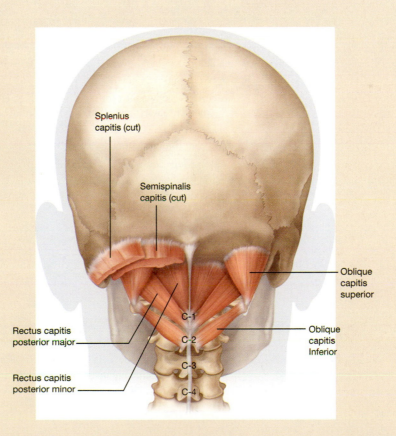

FIGURE 6.119

Suboccipital muscles.

TABLE 6.36	Muscles of the Body: Their Attachments, Actions, and Nerves (continued)
Abdominal Muscles (See Figure 6.120)	
Rectus abdominus	*Origin:* Pubic crest, pubic symphysis
	Insertion: Cartilage of ribs 5–7 and xiphoid process
	Action: Flexes the spine and compresses the abdomen
	Nerve: Branches of thoracic nerves
External oblique	*Origin:* Ribs 5–12
	Insertion: Anterior iliac crest, and abdominal aponeurosis to the linea alba
	Action: Bilaterally flexes the spine, compresses the abdomen, assists in deep exhalation; unilaterally laterally flexes the spine to the same side, rotates the spine to the opposite side
	Nerve: Branches of the intercostals
Internal oblique	*Origin:* Lateral inguinal ligament, iliac crest, thoracolumbar fascia
	Insertion: Cartilage of ribs 8–12 linea alba, and xiphoid process of sternum
	Action: Bilaterally flexes the spine, compresses the abdomen, assists in deep exhalation; laterally flexes the spine to the same side, rotates the spine to the same side
	Nerve: Branches of the intercostals
Transverse abdominis	*Origin:* Lateral inguinal ligament, iliac crest, thoracolumber fascia; cartilage of ribs 7–12
	Insertion: Linea alba and pubis
	Action: Compresses the abdomen
	Nerve: Branches of the intercostals
Muscles of Breathing (See Figure 6.121)	
Diaphragm	*Origin:* Inner surface of ribs 1–6, upper 3 lumbar vertebrae, inner part of xiphoid process
	Insertion: Central tendon
	Action: Draws down the central tendon of the diaphragm, increases the volume of the thoracic cavity; major muscle of respiration
	Nerve: Phrenic
External intercostals	*Origin:* Inferior border of the rib above
	Insertion: Superior border of the rib below
	Action: Draw the ventral part of the ribs upward, increase space in thoracic cavity; assists in inhalation
	Nerve: Intercostal
Internal intercostals	*Origin:* Inferior border of the rib above
	Insertion: Superior border of the rib below
	Action: Draw the ventral part of the ribs downward, decrease space in thoracic cavity; assists in exhalation
	Nerve: Intercostal
Related Structures	
Thoracolumbar aponeurosis	A broad flat diamond-shaped tendon on the back that stretches from the sacrum and posterior iliac crest to the lower thoracic vertebrae; provides anchor for several muscles
Linea alba (white line)	Connective tissue structure that runs down the midline of the abdomen; formed by the fusion of the aponeuroses of the abdominal muscles

TABLE 6.36	Muscles of the Body: Their Attachments, Actions, and Nerves (continued)

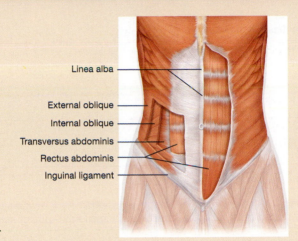

FIGURE 6.120

Abdominal muscles.

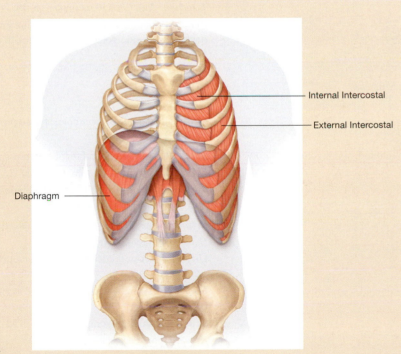

FIGURE 6.121

Muscles of breathing.

TABLE 6.36   Muscles of the Body: Their Attachments, Actions, and Nerves (continued)

Muscles of the Neck
- Found between the shoulders and the head
- Attached to the spine, skull, and clavicle
- Move the neck and head

Posterior Neck Muscles
- See muscles of the cervical spine
  Erector spinae
  Transversospinalis
  Splenius
  Suboccipitals

Lateral Neck Muscles
(See Figure 6.122)

Sternocleidomastoid (SCM)	*Origin:* Sternal head—top of manubrium; clavicular head—medial third of clavicle
	Insertion: Mastoid process; lateral half of superior nuchal line
	Action: Unilateral: laterally flexes head to same side, rotates head to opposite side; bilateral: flexes head, assistant in inhalation
	Nerve: Cranial nerve 11
Scalenes	*Origins:* Anterior: transverse processes of C-3 to C-6 (anterior tubercles); Medius: Transverse processes of C-1 to C-7 (posterior tubercles); Posterior: transverse processes of C-5 to C-7 (posterior tubercles)
Subgroups anterior, middle, posterior	*Insertion:* Anterior and medius: first rib; Posterior: second rib
	Action: Bilateral: elevate the ribs during inhalation; unilateral: laterally flex neck to same side, rotate head and neck to opposite side, flex the neck (anterior)
	Nerve: Cervical plexus

Anterior Neck Muscles
(See Figure 6.123)

Suprahyoids	*Origin:* Underside of mandible, styloid process
Subgroups	*Insertion:* Hyoid bone
Geniohyoid, mylohyoid, stylohyoid	*Action:* Elevate hyoid and tongue; depress mandible
	Nerve: Hypoglossal, mylohyoid, facial
Digastric	*Origin:* Mastoid process through tendinous sling on hyoid bone
	Insertion: Inferior border of mandible
	Action: Depresses the mandible, elevates the hyoid, retracts mandible
	Nerve: Mylohyoid, facial
Infrahyoids	*Origin:* Superior border of scapula (omothyroid); manubrium (sternohyoid and sternothyroid)
Subgroups	
Omohyoid, sternohyoid, sternothyroid	*Insertion:* Hyoid bone (omohyoid and sternohyoid; thyroid cartilage (sternothyroid)
	Action: Depresses hyoid bone and thyroid cartilage
	Nerve: Upper cervical
Longus capitis	*Origin:* Transverse processes of C-3 to C-5
	Insertion: Occipital bone
	Action: Unilateral: laterally flexes the neck; Bilateral: flexes the neck
	Nerve: Anterior rami
Longus colli	*Origin:* Transverse processes of C-3 to C-5, vertebral bodies of C-5 to T-3 (anterior)
	Insertion: Anterior tubercle of C-1, transverse processes of C-5 to C-6, vertebral bodies C-2 to C-4
	Action: Unilateral: rotates the head, laterally flexes the neck; Bilateral: flexes the neck
	Nerve: Anterior rami

TABLE 6.36	Muscles of the Body: Their Attachments, Actions, and Nerves (continued)

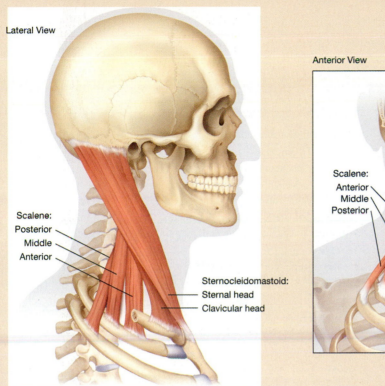

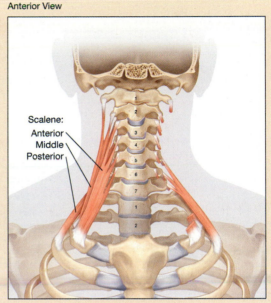

FIGURE 6.122

A. Posterior/lateral neck muscles. B. Scalenes.

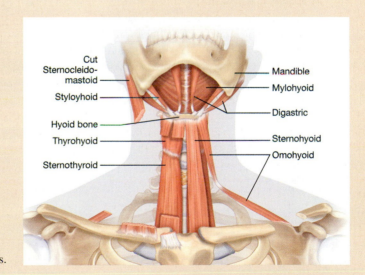

FIGURE 6.123

Anterior neck muscles.

TABLE 6.36   Muscles of the Body: Their Attachments, Actions, and Nerves (continued)

Muscles of the Head and Face

- Found on the head and face
- Attach to the skull and facial fascia and musculature
- Move the jaw and facial structures
  (See Figure 6.124)

Masseter	*Origin:* Zygomatic arch
	Insertion: Angle and ramus of mandible
	Action: Elevates mandible
	Nerve: Trigeminal
Pterygoids	*Origin:* Sphenoid bone (both)
Subgroups medial, lateral	*Insertion:* Mandible angle and ramus (medial); condylar process of mandible and TM joint capsule (lateral)
	Action: Unilateral: lateral movement of the mandible; Bilateral: elevates and protracts the mandible (medial), depresses and protracts the mandible (lateral)
	Nerve: Cranial Nerve 5
Temporalis	*Origin:* Temporal fossa and fascia
	Insertion: Coronoid process of mandible
	Action: Elevates and retracts the mandible
	Nerve: Trigeninal

Facial Expression or Mimetic Muscles
(See Figure 6.125)

Frontalis	*Origin:* Galea aponeurotica
	Insertion: Skin over the eyebrows
	Action: Raises the eyebrows and wrinkles the forehead
	Nerve: Facial
Occipitalis	*Origin:* Galea aponeurotica
	Insertion: Superior nuchal line of the occiput
	Action: Anchors and retracts the galea
	Nerve: Facial
Procerus	*Origin:* Fascia of the lower nasal bone; upper nasal cartilage
	Insertion: Skin between the eyebrows
	Action: Pulls skin between eyebrows downward; express anger
	Nerve: Cranial Nerve VII
Currugator supercilli	*Origin:* Supercilliary arches
	Insertion: Skin of forehead near the medial eyebrow
	Action: Wrinkle forehead, produce frowning, express suffering
	Nerve: Cranial Nerve VII
Orbicularis oculi	*Origin:* Orbital margin
	Insertion: Fascia between eyelids
	Action: Closes eyelids, produces squinting
	Nerve: Cranial Nerve VII
Nasalis	*Origin:* Maxilla
Includes dilator naris	*Insertion:* Nasal bone
	Action: Dilate nostrils, depress tip of the nose
	Nerve: Cranial Nerve VII
Levator labii superioris	*Origin:* Medial intra-orbital margin
	Insertion: Skin and muscle of the upper lip
	Action: Elevates the upper lip
	Nerve: Cranial Nerve VII

TABLE 6.36	**Muscles of the Body: Their Attachments, Actions, and Nerves (continued)**

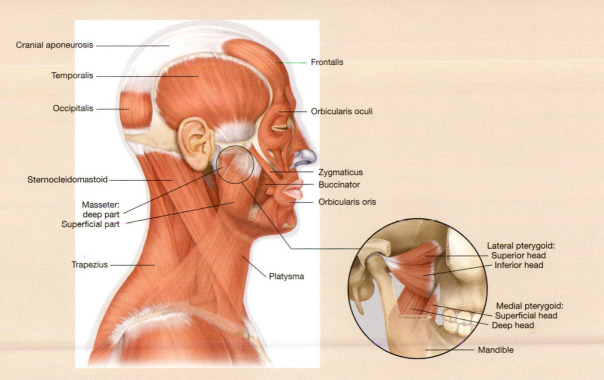

FIGURE 6.124

Head and face muscles.

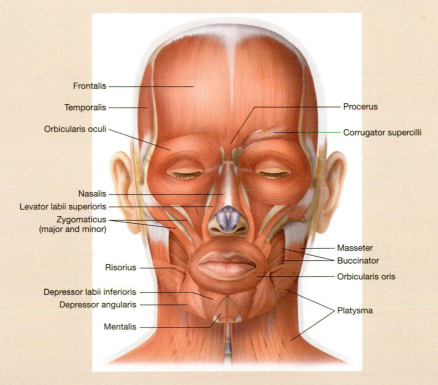

FIGURE 6.125

Muscles of facial expression.

TABLE 6.36   Muscles of the Body: Their Attachments, Actions, and Nerves (continued)

Zygomaticus *Subgroups* major, minor	*Origin:* Zygomatic arch *Insertion:* Corners of the mouth *Action:* Elevate the corners of the mouth, produce smiling *Nerve:* Cranial Nerve VII
Risorius	*Origin:* Fascia over parotid gland *Insertion:* Skin at corner of mouth *Action:* Pull back corners of mouth, assist in smiling *Nerve:* Cranial Nerve VII
Orbicularis oris	*Origin:* Maxilla, mandible, buccinator *Insertion:* Membranes and muscles of the lips *Action:* Close the lips, protrude and protract the lips, assists in eating, drinking, talking *Nerve:* Cranial Nerve VII
Depressor anguli oris	*Origin:* Tubercle of mandible *Insertion:* Lower side of mouth *Action:* Depress side of mouth, produce frowning *Nerve:* Cranial Nerve VII
Buccinator	*Origin:* Maxilla, mandible *Insertion:* Obicularis oris *Action:* Compress the cheeks, assists chewing *Nerve:* Cranial Nerve VII
Mentalis	*Origin:* Anterior mandible *Insertion:* Chin *Action:* Elevate chin, wrinkle chin, protrudes lower lip, produce pouting *Nerve:* Cranial Nerve VII
Platysma	*Origin:* Fascia covering upper pectoralis major *Insertion:* Edge of mandible, skin of lower face *Action:* Assists in depressing the mandible, tightens neck fascia *Nerve:* Cranial Nerve VII
Related Structure	
Galea aponeurotica	Network of cranial fascia that is connected to the hypodermis and slides over the periosteum of the cranium

Muscles of the Upper Extremities

- Found on the upper body, anterior and posterior
- Attach to shoulder girdle and arm bones
- Move the shoulders, arms, and hands

Upper Torso and Shoulder Muscles
(See Figure 6.126■)

Trapezius *Subsections* upper, middle, lower	*Origin:* External occipital protuberance, medial portion of superior nuchal line of occiput, nuchal ligament, spinous processes of C-7 to T-12 *Insertion:* Lateral third of clavicle, acromion, spine of scapula *Action:* Upper—Unilateral: laterally flex the head and neck, rotate the head and neck to the opposite side, elevate the scapula, upwardly rotate the scapula; Bilateral: extend the head and neck Middle—Adduct the scapula, stabilize the scapula Lower—Depress the scapula, upwardly rotate the scapula *Nerve:* Spinal accessory and cervical plexus

TABLE 6.36	Muscles of the Body: Their Attachments, Actions, and Nerves (continued)

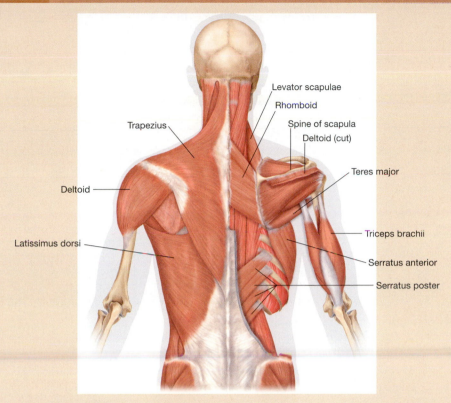

FIGURE 6.126

Upper back and shoulder muscles.

Deltoid *Subsections* anterior, posterior	*Origin:* Lateral third of clavicle, acromion, spine of scapula *Insertion:* Deltoid tuberosity *Action:* All—Abduct the shoulder Anterior—Flex the shoulder, medially rotate the shoulder, horizontally adduct the shoulder Posterior—Extend the shoulder, laterally rotate the shoulder, horizontally abduct the shoulder *Nerve:* Brachial plexus axillary
Latissimus dorsi	*Origin:* Spinous processes of T-7 to L-5; posterior suface of ribs 9–12, posterior iliac crest, posterior sacrum *Insertion:* Crest of lessor tubercle of humerus *Action:* Extend the shoulder, adduct the shoulder, medially rotate the shoulder *Nerve:* Brachial plexus
Teres major	*Origin:* Inferior third of posterior scapular border *Insertion:* Intertubercular groove of humerus *Action:* Extend the shoulder, adduct the shoulder, medially rotate the shoulder *Nerve:* Lower subscapular
Rhomboids *Subgroups* minor, major	*Origin:* Minor—Spinous processes of C-7 to T-1 Major—Spinous processes of T-2 to T-5 *Insertion:* Medial border of scapula *Action:* Adduct the scapula, elevate the scapula, downwardly rotate the scapula *Nerve:* Brachial plexus

TABLE 6.36 Muscles of the Body: Their Attachments, Actions, and Nerves (continued)

Levator scapula	*Origin:* Transverse processes of C-1 to C-4
	Insertion: Medial border and superior angle of scapula
	Action:
	Unilateral—Elevate the scapula, downwardly rotate the scapula, laterally flexes the head and neck, rotates the head and neck to the same side
	Bilateral—Extends the head and neck
	Nerve: Dorsal scapula nerve, cervical nerves
Serratus anterior	*Origin:* Surfaces of ribs 1–8
	Insertion: Anterior surface of medial border of scapula
	Action: Abduct the scapula, depress the scapula, hold scapula against rib cage; assist in forced inhalation
	Nerve: Brachial plexus
***Rotator cuff muscles* (supraspinatus, infraspinatus, teres minor, subscapularis)** (See Figure 6.127■)	
Supraspinatus	*Origin:* Supraspinatus fossa of scapula
	Insertion: Greater tubercle of humerus
	Action: Abduct the shoulder, stabilize the humerus head in glenoid cavity
	Nerve: Suprascapular
Infraspinatus	*Origin:* Infraspinous fossa of scapula
	Insertion: Greater tubercle of humerus
	Action: Laterally rotate the shoulder, adduct the shoulder, extend the shoulder, horizontally abduct the shoulder, stabilize the humerus head in glenoid cavity
	Nerve: Bracial plexus

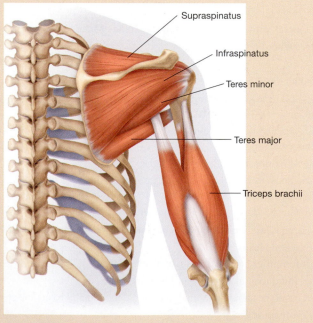 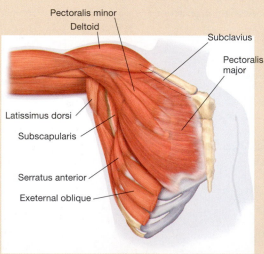

FIGURE 6.127
Rotator cuff muscles.

TABLE 6.36	Muscles of the Body: Their Attachments, Actions, and Nerves (continued)
Teres minor	*Origin:* Superior half of lateral border of scapula
	Insertion: Greater tubercle of humerus
	Action: Laterally rotates the shoulder, adducts the shoulder, extends the shoulder, horizontally abducts the shoulder, stabilizes the humerus head in glenoid cavity
	Nerve: Axillary
Subscapularis	*Origin:* Subscapular fossa of scapula
	Insertion: Lessor tubercle of humerus
	Action: Medially rotates the shoulder, stabilizes the humerus head in glenoid cavity
	Nerve: Subscapular
Chest Muscles (See Figure 6.127)	
Pectoralis major *Subsections* upper, lower	*Origin:* Medial half of clavicle, sternum, cartilage of ribs 1–6
	Insertion: Crest of greater tubercle of humerus
	Action:
	All—Adduct the shoulder, medially rotate the shoulder, assist in forced inhalation
	Upper—Flex the shoulder, horizontally adduct the shoulder
	Lower—Extends the shoulder
	Nerve: Brachial plexus
Pectoralis minor	*Origin:* Ribs 3–5
	Insertion: Coracoid process of scapula
	Action: Depress the scapula, abduct the scapula, tilt the scapula anteriorly, assist in forced inhalation
	Nerve: Brachial plexus
Subclavius	*Origin:* First rib and cartilage
	Insertion: Inferior clavicle
	Action: Elevates the clavicle, stabilizes the sternoclavicular joint
	Nerve: Cervical Nerves V and VI
Upper Arm Muscles (See Figure 6.128■)	
Biceps brachii *Subsections* short head, long head	*Origin:*
	Short head—coracoid process of scapula
	Long head—supraglenoid tubercle of scapula
	Insertion: Tuberosity of radius, aponeurosis of biceps brachii
	Action: Flex the elbow, supinate the forearm, flex the shoulder
	Nerve: Musculocutaneous
Triceps brachii *Subsections* long head, lateral head, medial head	*Origin:*
	Long head—Infraglenoid tubercle of scapula
	Lateral head—Posterior surface of proximal half of humerus
	Medial—posterior surface of distal half of humerus
	Insertion: Olecranon process of ulna
	Action:
	All heads—Extend the elbow
	Long head—Extend the shoulder, adduct the shoulder
	Nerve: Radial
Coracobrachialis	*Origin:* Coracoid process of scapula
	Insertion: Medial surface of mid-humerus
	Action: Flex the shoulder, adduct the shoulder
	Nerve: Musculocutaneous

TABLE 6.36 Muscles of the Body: Their Attachments, Actions, and Nerves (continued)

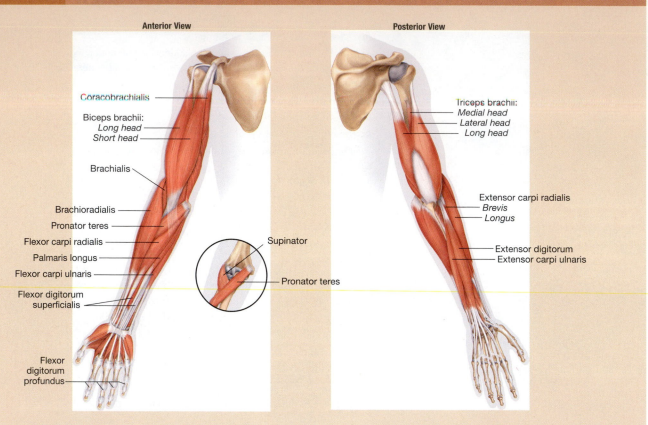

FIGURE 6.128

Upper arm muscles.

TABLE 6.36	**Muscles of the Body: Their Attachments, Actions, and Nerves (continued)**
Forearm Muscles (See Figure 6.128)	
Brachialis	*Origin:* Distal half of anterior humerus
	Insertion: Tuberosity and coronoid process of ulna
	Action: Flexes the elbow
	Nerve: Musculocutaneous
Brachioradialis	*Origin:* Lateral supracondylar ridge of humerus
	Insertion: Styloid process of radius
	Action: Flex the elbow, assist in pronation and supination of the forearm
	Nerve: Musculocutaneous and radial
Pronator teres	*Origin:* Medial epicondyle of humerus, common flexor tendon, coronoid process of ulna
	Insertion: middle and lateral surface of radius
	Action: Pronate the forearm, assist in elbow flexion
	Nerve: Median
Supinator	*Origin:* Lateral epicondyle of humerus, radial collateral ligament, annular ligament
	Insertion: Lateral surface of proximal shaft of radius
	Action: Supinates the forearm
	Nerve: Radial
Extensor muscle group (See Figure 6.128)	
Extensor carpi radialis *Subgroups* longus, brevis	*Origin:* Lateral supracondyle ridge of humerus
	Insertion:
	Longus—Base of second metacarpal
	Brevis—Base of third metacarpal
	Action: Extend the wrist, abduct the wrist, assists in elbow flexion
	Nerve: Radial
Extensor digitorum	*Origin:* Common extensor tendon from lateral epicondyle of humerus
	Insertion: Middle and distal phalanges of fingers 2–5
	Action: Extend fingers 2–5
	Nerve: Radial
Extensor carpi ulnaris	*Origin:* Common extensor tendon from lateral epicondyle of humerus
	Insertion: Base of fifth metacarpal
	Action: Extend the wrist, adduct the wrist
	Nerve: Radial
Flexor muscle group (See Figure 6.128)	
Flexor carpi radialis	*Origin:* Common flexor tendon from medial epicondyle of humerus
	Insertion: Base of second and third metacarpals
	Action: Flex the wrist, abduct the wrist, flex the elbow
	Nerve: Median
Palmaris longus	*Origin:* Common flexor tendon from medial epicondyle of humerus
	Insertion: Flexor retinaculum and palmar aponeurosis
	Action: Tense the palmar fascia, flex the wrist, flex the elbow
	Nerve: Median
Flexor carpi ulnaris	*Origin:* Common flexor tendon from medial epicondyle of humerus
	Insertion: Pisiform
	Action: Flex the wrist, adduct the wrist
	Nerve: Ulnar

TABLE 6.36	Muscles of the Body: Their Attachments, Actions, and Nerves (continued)
Flexor digitorum superficialis	*Origin:* Common flexor tendon from medial epicondyle of humerus, ulnar collateral ligament, coronoid process of radius
	Insertion: Middle phalanges of fingers 2–5
	Action: Flex fingers 2–5, flex the wrist
	Nerve: Ulnar
Flexor digitorum profundus	*Origin:* Anterior and medial surfaces of proximal ulna
	Insertion: Bases of distal phalanges of fingers 2–5
	Action: Flex fingers 2–5
	Nerve: Ulnar

Wrist and Hand Muscles
(See Figure 6.129■)

Thumb muscles

Opponens pollicis	*Origin:* Trapezium, transverse carpal ligament
	Insertion: Metacarpal 1
	Action: Flex the thumb, adduct the thumb
	Nerve: Median
Adductor pollicis	*Origin:* Capitate, metacarpals 2–3
	Insertion: Base of proximal phalange of thumb
	Action: Addicts the thumb, assists thumb flexion
	Nerve: Ulnar
Extensor policis *Subgroups* longus, brevis	*Origin:* Posterior surface of radius and ulna
	Insertion:
	Longus—Distal phalange of thumb
	Brevis—Proximal phalange of thumb
	Action: Extend the thumb
	Nerve: Radial
Flexor pollicis longus	*Origin:* Anterior surface of radius
	Insertion: Distal phalange of thumb
	Action: Flex the thumb
	Nerve: Median
Abductor pollicis longus	*Origin:* Posterior surface of radius and ulna
	Insertion: Base of first metacarpal
	Action: Abduct the thumb, extend the thumb
	Nerve: Radial

Thenar eminence: Five short muscles located at the base of the thumb on the palmar side

Hypothenar eminence: Three short muscles located on the ulnar side of the palm

Intrinsic muscles of the hand

Lumbricals	*Origin:* Sides of flexor digitorum profundus tendons
	Insertion: Extensor expansion
	Action: Extend the interphalangeal joints while flexing the metacarpophalangeal joint
	Nerve: Ulnar and median
Interossei	*Origin:* Metacarpals
	Insertion: Proximal phalanges
	Action: Abduct fingers
	Nerve: Ulnar

Related Structures

Palmar aponeurosis	Palmar fascia that connects the muscles of the palm

TABLE 6.36	**Muscles of the Body: Their Attachments, Actions, and Nerves (continued)**

Palmar View

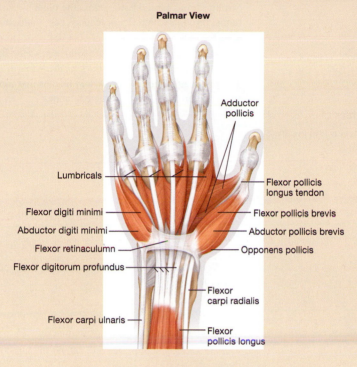

- Adductor pollicis
- Lumbricals
- Flexor pollicis longus tendon
- Flexor digiti minimi
- Flexor pollicis brevis
- Abductor digiti minimi
- Abductor pollicis brevis
- Flexor retinaculumn
- Opponens pollicis
- Flexor digitorum profundus
- Flexor carpi radialis
- Flexor carpi ulnaris
- Flexor pollicis longus

Dorsal View

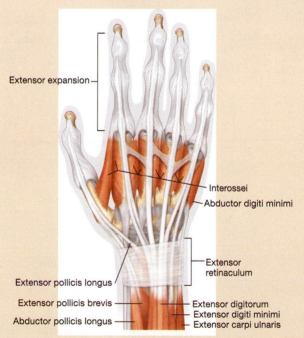

- Extensor expansion
- Interossei
- Abductor digiti minimi
- Extensor retinaculum
- Extensor pollicis longus
- Extensor pollicis brevis
- Extensor digitorum
- Abductor pollicis longus
- Extensor digiti minimi
- Extensor carpi ulnaris

FIGURE 6.129

Hand muscles. A. Palmar. B. Dorsal.

TABLE 6.36   Muscles of the Body: Their Attachments, Actions, and Nerves (continued)

Flexor retinaculum	Strong fibrous fascial band across the inner side of the wrist; forms the carpal tunnel through which flexor tendons run; continuous deep with palmar aponeurosis
Extensor retinaculum	Strong fibrous fascial band extending across the back of the wrist; consists of part of the deep fascia of the back of the forearm
Extensor expansion	The flattened tendons of extensor muscles that runs onto the back of the hand; spans the proximal and middle phalanges

Muscles of the Lower Extremities

- Found on the lower body, anterior and posterior
- Attach to scapula and leg bones
- Move the hip, thigh, lower leg, feet

Posterior Hip Muscles

(See Figure 6.130■)

Gluteus maximus	*Origin:* Coccyx, posterior sacrum, posterior iliac crest, sacrotuberous and sacroiliac ligaments
	Insertion: Gluteal tuberosity, iliotibial band
	Action: Extend the hip, laterally rotate the hip, abduct the hip, abduct the hip (lower fibers)
	Nerve: Gluteal
Gluteus medius	*Origin:* External ilium between anterior and posterior lines
	Insertion: Greater trochanter of femur
	Action: Abduct the hip, flex and extend the hip, medially and laterally rotate the hip
	Nerve: Gluteal
Gluteus minimus	*Origin:* External ilium between anterior and inferior lines
	Insertion: Greater trochanter of femur
	Action: Abduct the hip, medially rotate the hip, anteriorly rotate the pelvis
	Nerve: Gluteal

Deep Hip Lateral Rotators

(See Figure 6.131■)

Piriformis	*Origin:* Anterior sacrum
	Insertion: Greater trochanter of femur
	Action: Laterally rotate the hip, abduct the hip
	Nerve: Sciatic
Gemellus superior	*Origin:* Ischial spine
	Insertion: Greater trochanter of femur
	Action: Laterally rotate the hip
	Nerve: Sciatic nerve
Gemellus inferior	*Origin:* Superior ischial tuberosity
	Insertion: Greater trochanter of femur
	Action: Laterally rotate the hip
	Nerve: Sciatic nerve
Quadratus femoris	*Origin:* Lateral ischial tuberosity
	Insertion: Greater trochanter of femur
	Action: Laterally rotate the hip
	Nerve: Sciatic
Obterator internus	*Origin:* Obturator membrane, obturator margin
	Insertion: Greater trochanter of femur
	Action: Laterally rotate the hip
	Nerve: Sciatic

TABLE 6.36 **Muscles of the Body: Their Attachments, Actions, and Nerves (continued)**

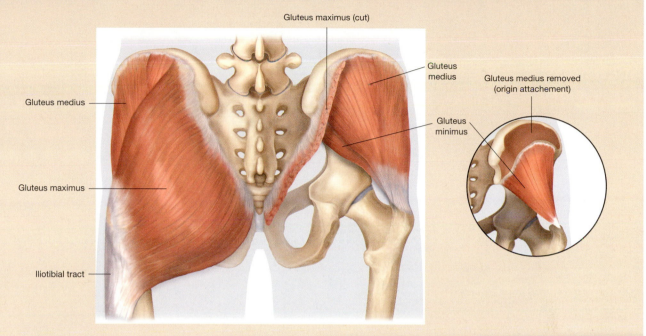

FIGURE 6.130

Posterior hip muscles. A. Posterior view of right buttock. B. Lateral posterior view of right buttock.

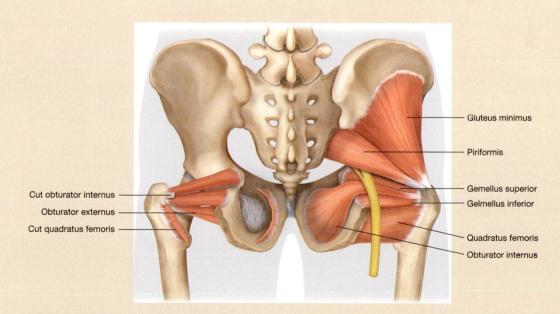

FIGURE 6.131

Deep hip rotator muscles.

TABLE 6.36	Muscles of the Body: Their Attachments, Actions, and Nerves (continued)
Obterator externus	*Origin:* Obturator membrane, pubic ramus, ischial ramus
	Insertion: Greater trochanter of femur
	Action: Laterally rotate the hip
	Nerve: Sciatic
Anterior Pelvic Muscles (See Figure 6.132■)	
Psoas major	*Origin:* Transverse processes of T-12 to L-5, vertebral bodies of T-12 to L-5, intervetebral disks of lumber region
	Insertion: Lesser trochanter of femur
	Action: Laterally rotates the hip, flexes the hip, flexes the spine, tilts the pelvis anteriorly
	Nerve: Lumbar plexus
Illiacus	*Origin:* Iliac fossa, anterior inferior iliac spine
	Insertion: Lesser trochanter of femur
	Action: Flex the hip, laterally rotate the hip, tilt the pelvis anteriorly
	Nerve: Femoral
Thigh Muscles *Quadriceps Femoris Group (Quads)* (See Figure 6.133■)	
Rectus femoris	*Origin:* Anterior inferior iliac spine
	Insertion: Tibial tuberosity
	Action: Extend the knee, flex the hip
	Nerve: Femoral
Vastus medialis	*Origin:* Medial linea aspera
	Insertion: Tibial tuberosity
	Action: Extend the knee
	Nerve:
Vastus lateralis	*Origin:* Lateral linea aspera, gluteal tuberosity
	Insertion: Tibial tuberosity
	Action: Extend the knee
	Nerve: Femoral
Vastus intermedius	*Origin:* Anterior and lateral shaft of femur
	Insertion: Tibial tuberosity
	Action: Extend the knee
	Nerve: Femoral

TABLE 6.36   **Muscles of the Body: Their Attachments, Actions, and Nerves (continued)**

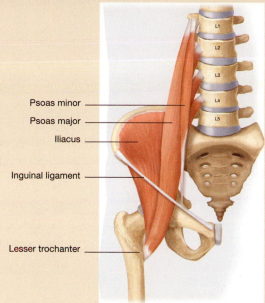

Psoas minor
Psoas major
Iliacus

Inguinal ligament

Lesser trochanter

L1
L2
L3
L4
L5

FIGURE 6.132

Anterior pelvic muscles.

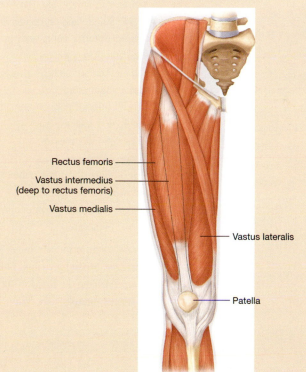

Rectus femoris
Vastus intermedius
(deep to rectus femoris)
Vastus medialis

Vastus lateralis

Patella

FIGURE 6.133

Anterior thigh muscles.

TABLE 6.36	Muscles of the Body: Their Attachments, Actions, and Nerves (continued)
Hamstrings group (See Figure 6.134■)	
Biceps femoris *Subsections* long head short head	*Origin:* Ischial tuberosity (long head), linea aspira (short head) *Insertion:* Head of fibula *Action:* Flex the knee, laterally rotate the leg and hip, extend the hip, tilt the pelvis posteriorly *Nerve:* Sciatic nerve
Semitendinosis	*Origin:* Ischial tuberosity *Insertion:* Medial proximal tibial shaft (pes anserinus) *Action:* Flex the knee, medially rotate the leg and hip, extend the hip, tilt the pelvis posteriorly *Nerve:* Tibial
Semimembranosis	*Origin:* Ischial tuberosity *Insertion:* Medial condyle of the tibia *Action:* Flex the knee, medially rotate the leg and hip, extend the hip, tilt the pelvis posteriorly *Nerve:* Tibial
Adductor group (See Figure 6.135■)	
Adductor magnus	*Origin:* Ischial tuberosity, inferior pubic ramus, ischial ramus *Insertion:* Linea aspera *Action:* Adduct the hip, flex the hip, extend the hip *Nerve:* Sciatic and obturator
Adductor longus	*Origin:* Anterior pubic body *Insertion:* Linea aspera *Action:* Adduct the hip *Nerve:* Obturator
Adductor brevis	*Origin:* Inferior pubic ramus *Insertion:* Linea aspera *Action:* Adduct the hip *Nerve:* Obturator
Pectineus	*Origin:* Superior pubic ramus *Insertion:* Linea aspera *Action:* Flex the hip, adduct the hip *Nerve:* Femoral
Gracilis	*Origin:* Interior pubic ramus *Insertion:* Medial proximal tibial shaft (pes anserinus) *Action:* Adduct the hip, flex the hip and knee, medially rotate the leg *Nerve:* Obturator

| **TABLE 6.36** | **Muscles of the Body: Their Attachments, Actions, and Nerves (continued)** |

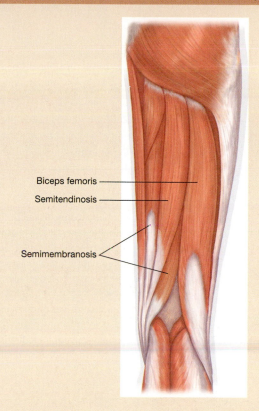

FIGURE 6.134

Posterior thigh muscles.

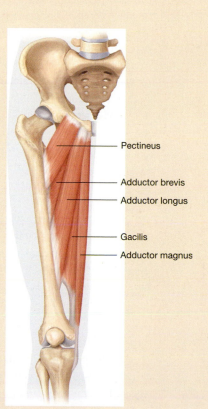

FIGURE 6.135

Adductor muscles.

TABLE 6.36	Muscles of the Body: Their Attachments, Actions, and Nerves (continued)
Lateral Thigh Muscles (See Figure 6.136■)	
Tensor fascia latae	*Origin:* Anterior iliac crest, anterior superior iliac spine
	Insertion: Iliotibial band
	Action: Abduct the hip, flex the hip, medially rotate the hip
	Nerve: Gluteal
Sartorius	*Origin:* Anterior superior iliac spine
	Insertion: Medial proximal tibial shaft
	Action: Flex the hip, laterally rotate the hip, abduct the hip, flex the knee, medially rotate the leg
	Nerve: Femoral
Related Structures	
Inguinal ligament	Band of connective tissue running from the anterior superior iliac spine (ASIS) to the pubic tubercle; forms the inguinal canal; continuous with the fascia lata of the thigh
Iliotibial band	Longitudinal fibrous reinforcement of the fascia lata that runs down the side of the thigh; serves as attachment site for gluteus maximus and tensor fascia lata muscles
Linea aspera	Longitudinal ridge of roughened surface on the mid-posterior femur that serves as the site of attachment for several muscles
Pes anserinus	Insertion of the conjoined tendons of the sartorius, gracillis, and semitendinosis on the front and inside surface of the proximal tibia (just below the knee)
Lower Leg Muscles *Extensors of the ankle (plantarflexors)* *Flexors of the toes* (See Figure 6.137■)	
Gastrocnemius	*Origin:* Posterior condyles of the femur
	Insertion: Calcaneus (Achilles' tendon)
	Action: Plantarflex the ankle, flex the knee
	Nerve: Tibial
Soleus	*Origin:* superior posterior tibia
	Insertion: Calcaneus (Achilles tendon)
	Action: Plantarflex the ankle
	Nerve: Tibial
Tibialis posterior	*Origin:* posterior tibia, posterior fibula, interosseous membrane
	Insertion: tarsals, bases of metatarsals 2–4
	Action: Invert the foot, plantarflex the ankle
	Nerve: Tibial
Plantaris	*Origin:* Lateral epicondyle of the femur
	Insertion: Calcaneus (Achilles' tendon)
	Action: Plantarflex the ankle, flex the knee
	Nerve: Tibial
Flexor digitorum longus	*Origin:* Posterior tibia
	Insertion: Distal phalanges 2–5 (plantar surface)
	Action: Flex toes 2–5, plantarflex the ankle, invert the foot
	Nerve: Tibial
Flexor hallicus longus	*Origin:* Mid-posterior tibia, interosseus membrane
	Insertion: Distal phlanx of the big toe
	Action: Flex toes 2–5, plantarflex the ankle, invert the foot, support the longitudinal arch
	Nerve: Tibial

TABLE 6.36 **Muscles of the Body: Their Attachments, Actions, and Nerves (continued)**

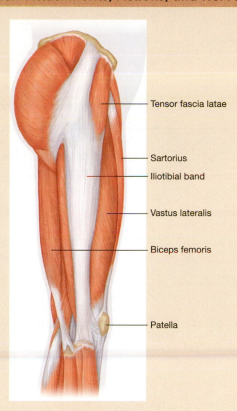

- Tensor fascia latae
- Sartorius
- Iliotibial band
- Vastus lateralis
- Biceps femoris
- Patella

FIGURE 6.136

Lateral view of thigh.

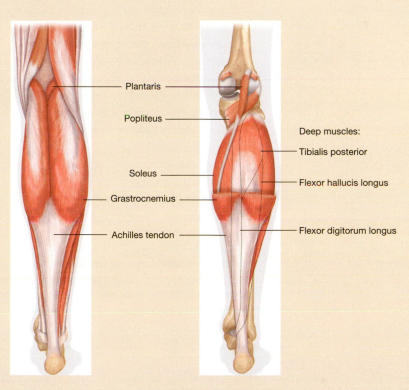

- Plantaris
- Popliteus
- Soleus
- Grastrocnemius
- Achilles tendon
- Deep muscles:
- Tibialis posterior
- Flexor hallucis longus
- Flexor digitorum longus

FIGURE 6.137

Posterior lower leg muscles.

TABLE 6.36   Muscles of the Body: Their Attachments, Actions, and Nerves (continued)

Flexor muscles of the ankle (Dorsiflexors)
Extenders of the toes
(See Figure 6.138■)

Tibialis anterior	*Origin:* Proximal lateral tibia
	Insertion: Metatarsal 1, cuneiform plantar surface
	Action: Dorsiflex the ankle, inverts the foot
	Nerve: Deep peroneal nerve
Extensor digitorum longus and brevis	*Origin:*
	Longus—Inferior head of fibula, proximal fibia shaft, lateral condyle of tibia, interosseus membrane
	Brevis—Calcaneus
	Insertion: Middle and distal phalanges of toes 2–5 (longus), tendons of longus to toes 2–4 (brevis)
	Action:
	Longus—Extend toes 2–5, dorsiflex ankle
	Brevis—Extend toes 1–4
	Nerve: Deep peroneal
Extensor hallucis longus	*Origin:* Anterior fibula, interosseous membrane
	Insertion: Distal phalanx of big toe
	Action: Extend the big toe, dorsiflex the ankle
	Nerve: Deep peroneal

Intrinsic Foot Muscles
(See Figure 6.139■)

Extensor digitorum brevis	*Origin:* Calcaneus (dorsal surface)
	Insertion: Toes 2–4 via extensor digitorum longus tendons
	Action: Extend toes 2–4
	Nerve: Peroneal
Flexor digitorum brevis	*Origin:* Calcaneus (plantar surface)
	Insertion: Middle phalanges of toes 2–4
	Action: Flexes toes 2–4
	Nerve: Plantar
Abductor hallicus	*Origin:* Calcaneus (plantar surface)
	Insertion: Proximal phalange of big toe
	Action: Abducts and flex the big toe
	Nerve: Plantar
Abductor digiti minimi	*Origin:* Calcaneus (plantar surface)
	Insertion: Proximal phalange of little toe
	Action: Abduct and flex the little toe
	Nerve: Plantar

Related Structures

Superior extensor retinaculum (transverse crural ligament)	Strong, broad connective tissue that binds the tendons that cross the superior ankle; continuous with the fascia of the leg
Plantar fascia	Thick connective tissue that runs from the calcaneus to the head of the metatarsals bones on the plantar side of the foot; supports the longitudinal arch

TABLE 6.36   **Muscles of the Body: Their Attachments, Actions, and Nerves (continued)**

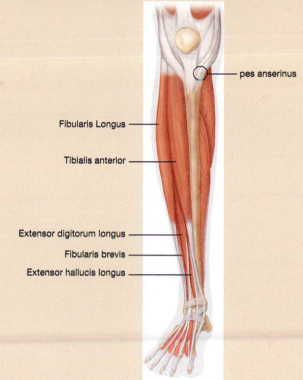

FIGURE 6.138
Anterior lower leg muscles.

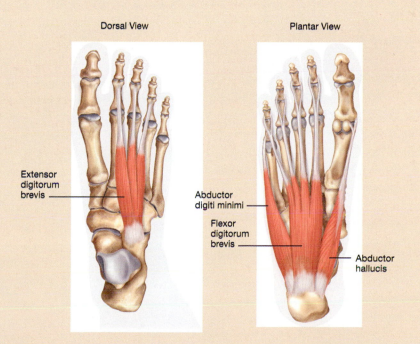

FIGURE 6.139
Intrinsic foot muscles. A. Dorsal view of right foot. B. and C. Plantar views of right foot.

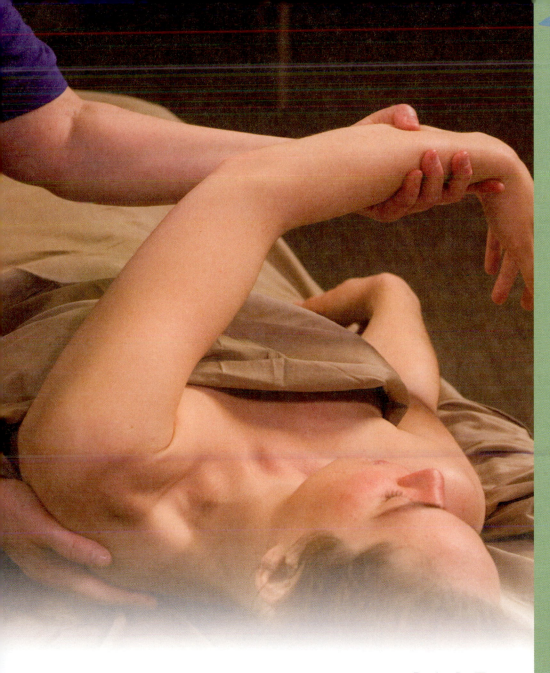

PART

2

Knowledge for Planning Massage Sessions

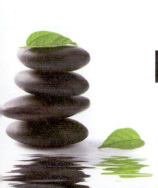

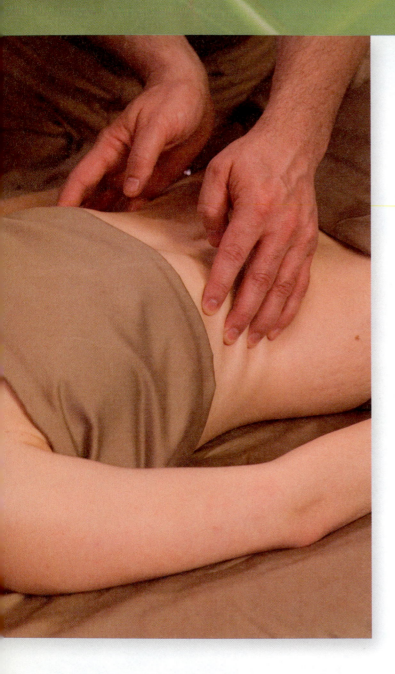

CHAPTER

7 Effects of Massage

 CHAPTER OUTLINE

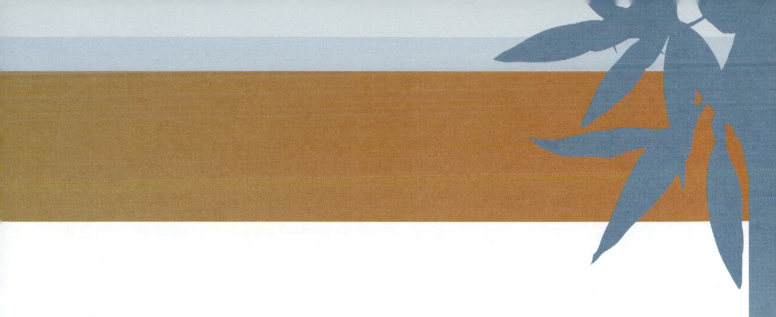

LEARNING OUTCOMES

After studying this chapter, you will have information to:

1. Discuss the effects of massage and its benefits for well-being.
2. Adopt a holistic view of the effects of massage.
3. Explain the meaning of evidence-based practice.
4. Locate and analyze research about the effects and applications of massage.
5. Explain the effects of massage at the tissue level.
6. Explain the effects of massage at the organ system level.
7. Explain the effects of massage at the whole organism level.
8. Describe the psychological effects of massage.
9. Discuss various mechanisms for the effects of massage.
10. Describe how different massage techniques are applied for different effects.

KEY TERMS

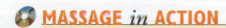

MASSAGE *in* ACTION

On your DVD, explore:
- Goal-Oriented 6-Step Planning

EFFECTS OF MASSAGE DEFINED

The term **effects of massage** refers to changes that occur in the body, mind, and emotions of the recipient as a result of soft tissue manipulation. These physiological and psychological changes can be beneficial or detrimental depending on the circumstances. They are benefits if they have a positive impact and lead toward healing and greater wellness. Stress reduction, improved tissue health, and increased feelings of well-being are examples of the general benefits of massage.

In referring to massage for the treatment of a medical condition, the term *indicated* is used. Massage is indicated if the effects contribute to healing the medical condition, alleviating symptoms, or making the recipient more comfortable. These benefits are the positive effects of clinical applications of massage and are discussed further in Chapter 8, Clinical Applications of Massage, on page 280.

In some cases, the effects of massage can be harmful. For example, increased blood and lymph circulation are healthy outcomes of massage most of the time. However, for someone with congestive heart failure or infection, increased fluid circulation would probably make matters worse. In these cases, massage is *contraindicated* and should not be applied. Contraindications for massage are covered in Chapter 9, Endangerment Sites, Contraindications, and Cautions, on page 294.

Time, Dose, and Effects

It is useful to make a distinction between the short- and long-term effects of massage. **Short-term effects** are changes that occur during a massage session. They may last for the time of the session and for a brief period afterward, perhaps a few hours or a day. Examples of short-term effects are decreased heart rate, muscle relaxation, and more positive mood.

Long-term effects are changes that start during a massage session and last for a longer period of time, such as a few days or weeks, or they may be more lasting changes that occur from massage received regularly over a period of time. For example, regular relaxation massage can lead to a decrease in a person's general state of stress and anxiety over time.

Some researchers believe that looking at single- and multiple-dose effects is also important. **Single-dose effects** refer to those changes that happen from one application of massage. **Multiple-dose effects** happen over time from repeated massage applications.

The idea of single-dose effects is similar to short-term effects, and the concept of multiple-dose effects is similar to long-term effects. However, it is possible for a single dose of massage to have a long-term effect (e.g., a massage session that relieves a tension headache), or each dose of multiple doses of massage may have only a short-term effect (e.g., regular lymphatic drainage for managing lymphedema).

How long the effects of massage last might also be affected by what happens to the recipient after the massage session. For example, the relaxation benefits of massage might wear off sooner if a person returns to a stressful environment, or they might be prolonged if he or she takes time to relax further by taking a restful walk or by soaking in a warm bath. It is important to understand the complexity of the situation when thinking about the effects of massage more critically.

Massage Techniques and Effects

Keep in mind that different massage techniques produce different effects. How techniques are applied may also influence the eventual outcomes. For example, tapotement has a stimulating effect if received for a short time and may have a sedating effect if received for a longer period of time. Effleurage applied slowly, rhythmically, and with light to moderate pressure usually has a relaxing effect, but applied briskly may feel invigorating.

When reading research about the effects of massage, it is important to understand what techniques or approaches were used in the study. The conclusion from the study can only be that a particular massage application had a certain effect. To speak of massage in general is not very useful for practical applications.

Practitioners who know how to apply massage techniques to obtain specific effects will be more successful in achieving session and treatment goals. Knowledge of the effects of the techniques they are using allows massage therapists to plan sessions to achieve therapeutic goals and avoid harming recipients. More information about Western massage techniques and how to apply them for specific effects is found in Part 3, Massage Guidelines and Applications, which begins on page 341.

Evidence for Effects

Information about the physiological and psychological effects of massage comes from several sources. Some beliefs about the effects of massage are passed down as tradition, and some come from personal observation and experience. Some massage outcomes statements are derived from an understanding of human anatomy and physiology, with deductions about what effects different massage applications might logically have. Other beliefs come from reports or anecdotes from massage recipients. Taken together, this knowledge constitutes the conventional wisdom about the effects of massage.

An increasing number of research studies are investigating the effects of massage to see if the conventional wisdom holds true scientifically. This is particularly important for massage therapists working in clinical settings where evidence-based therapies are preferred. Research may either confirm or cast doubts on effects that have been believed and accepted for some time. It can also refine our understanding of the effects of massage and the circumstance required to make certain effects happen.

Of course, one research project does not prove anything definitively, but if conducted well, adds to the collection of evidence. Evidence from scientific research accumulates over time as a body of knowledge is built up.

A *meta-analysis* of research looks at a number of studies on the same general topic to discover any consistent findings. Four meta-analyses of massage research have produced noteworthy evidence for the benefits of massage in certain cases. One meta-analysis showed tactile stimulation to be of benefit to the development of infants (Ottenbacher et al. 1987). Another confirmed the relaxation effects of back massage (Labyak and Metzger 1997). A third meta-analysis pointed toward massage therapy as a promising treatment for delayed-onset muscle soreness after exercise (Ernst 1998).

A more comprehensive meta-analysis looked at 37 well-designed research studies and nine variables. It found strong evidence that single massage applications can reduce state anxiety, blood pressure, and heart rate, and that multiple applications can reduce a client's experience of pain. The strongest evidence was found that massage therapy decreases state anxiety and depression (Moyer et al. 2004).

Not all theories about the effects of massage have been studied through research. When available, research that supports statements made about the effects of massage is cited in this chapter and also appears in Appendix H, References and Additional Resources, on page A-66. This is a sampling of relevant studies and is not meant to be an exhaustive review of literature. Students are encouraged to search in various databases (e.g., www.massagetherapyfoundation.org and www.miami.edu/touch-research) for further information and the most recent studies.

HOLISTIC VIEW OF EFFECTS

Some of the theories and research about the effects of massage and its benefits for health and well-being are reviewed in this chapter. The overall approach is based on the organization of standard human anatomy and physiology textbooks that first look at tissues, then organ systems, then whole organism interactions. Psychological effects are discussed at the whole organism level. The generally recognized effects of massage on the body and mind are summarized in Table 7.1■.

Equally important are theories about how these effects take place. What is it about manipulating the soft tissues of the body that causes the observed effects? Is it the mechanical action, physiological responses to touch, or something more complex? Theories about the mechanisms of massage are addressed throughout the chapter, as well as in a separate section on the topic.

Dividing the human organism into body, mind, and emotions can be useful for discussing the effects of massage at first. It is a product of Western thought and science to think of human beings as divided in this way. However, it should always be remembered that we live as whole persons, and that these effects interact with each other in complex ways. The interactions of different effects can produce an overall effect that is greater than the sum of its parts. A holistic view encompasses the whole person.

Massage as Body-Centered Therapy

Massage has been called a *body-centered therapy*. That is, it works primarily through touch and movement of the body. The center of attention in massage is the "body," which in bodywork theory includes both the physical and energetic body. This is in contrast to mind-centered therapies that rely on talk (e.g., psychotherapy) or listening (e.g., music therapy) or some other mind-centered approach.

This is not to say that verbal communication between massage practitioners and their clients is not important. Verbal communication can be very important for things such as giving directions and feedback, and expressing caring. However, the primary therapeutic benefits from massage are derived from touch and movement. In fact, some of the most important communication happens through skillful and caring touch.

An observer can see the massage therapist applying sliding, kneading, vibrating, and other manual techniques to the recipient's body. However, what the recipient experiences involves his or her whole being—body, mind, and spirit. For example, calming the nervous system, relaxing muscles, and providing pleasurable touch also influences the mental, emotional, and spiritual well-being of the recipient. These **body-mind effects** are discussed throughout this chapter.

Massage practitioners encounter the interconnectedness of human beings in many ways. For example, a practitioner may be focused on a physical aspect, such as relaxing hypertonic muscles. What the recipient experiences might also have an emotional component, such as painful memories of an accident that caused trauma to the area. Or massage therapists may witness the physical effects of stress in clients in the form of tension headaches. Awareness of how the mind, body, and emotions interact offers a more holistic view of what is happening during massage.

Indivisible Mind and Body

The mind and body function as a single unit, that is, in a holistic way. For example, emotions are felt in and expressed through the body. Love is felt deeply in the physical self, as

TABLE 7.1 Summary of the Effects of Massage

Body Level	Effects
Tissue Level	
	Enhance tissue repair and scar formation.
	Improve connective tissue health.
	Improve pliability of fascia.
	Release adhesions and separate tissues.
Organ System Level	
Integumentary system	Stimulate sensory receptors in skin.
	Increase superficial circulation.
	Remove dead skin.
	Add moisture with oil or lotion.
	Increase sebaceous gland secretions.
	Facilitate healthy scar formation.
Skeletal System	Promote smooth joint function.
	Promote optimal joint flexibility and range of motion.
	Promote proper skeletal alignment.
Muscular System	"Milk" metabolic wastes into venous and lymph flow.
	Elicit specific muscle relaxation.
	Promote general muscle relaxation.
	Enhance connective tissue health and pliability related to muscles and joints.
	Relieve myofascial trigger points.
	Release myofascial adhesions.
Nervous System	Stimulate parasympathetic nervous system (relaxation response).
	Reduce pain (e.g., neural-gating mechanism).
	Sharpen body awareness.
Endocrine System	Reduce stress and anxiety:
	• Increase dopamine level.
	• Lower cortisol level.
	• Lower norepinephrine/epinephrine level.
	Elevate mood:
	• Increase serotonin level.
Cardiovascular System	Increase general and local circulation.
	Enhance venous return.
	Reduce blood pressure and heart rate.
	Increase red blood cells in circulation.
Lymphatic System and Immunity	Increase lymph fluid movement.
	Improve immune function.
	• Reduce cortisol level
Respiratory System	Encourage diaphragmatic breathing.
	Relax muscles of respiration.
	Promote good structural alignment and rib cage expansion.
Digestive System	Improve digestion with relaxation.
	Facilitate bowel movement.
Urinary System	Enhance circulation to kidneys.
	Increase urinary production and bladder tension.
Reproductive System	Improve reproductive function with relaxation.
	Promote general breast health.
Organism Level	
Growth and Development	Promote growth and development in infants.

Body Level	Effects
Pain Reduction	Relieve muscle pain from tension and poor circulation.
	Deactivate myofascial trigger points.
	Activate neural-gating mechanism.
	Increase endorphins and enkephalins.
	Increase serotonin.
Stress Reduction	Trigger relaxation response:
	• Increase dopamine and serotonin levels.
Psychological Level	
	Increase mental clarity.
	Reduce anxiety.
	Facilitate emotional release.
	Promote feelings of general well-being.

*These effects do not occur during every massage session. The massage techniques used and the qualities of movement (e.g., rhythm, pacing, pressure, direction, duration) help determine which effects are likely to occur. The physical, mental, and emotional conditions of recipients and their openness to massage might also have impact on which effects occur.

is hate. Facial expressions are a window to our emotions. Mental and physical pain can be indistinguishable.

Physical manifestations of emotions include the blush of embarrassment, sweaty palms in nervousness, the clenched fist of anger, wide-eyed fear, and the quickened heartbeat of those in love. Some believe that body posture may be read for its emotional sources—for example, raised shoulders indicating fear, rounded shoulders carrying the weight of the world, or forward, hunched shoulders signifying self-protection and fear of being hurt.

The connectedness of mind and body can be traced to our beginnings as an embryo. In the third week of life, there are three layers of cells. The outer layer, or ectoderm, eventually develops into the skin, brain, and nervous system. Thus the physical structures that allow us to feel physical sensations are from the same source as those through which we experience emotions. It has been observed that "depending on how you look at it, the skin is the outer surface of the brain, or the brain is the deepest layer of the skin" (Juhan 1987, p. 35).

This connection between the skin and the nervous system has profound implications when studying the effects of massage on the mind and emotions. As massage therapists, when we touch the outermost part of the physical body, we are able to touch the innermost parts of our patients and clients.

Research on touch has borne out this connection. For example, babies deprived of touch fail to develop properly and suffer retarded bone growth, failure to gain weight, poor muscular coordination, immunological weakness, and general apathy. Massage, as a form of structured touch, has been used successfully to help premature infants gain weight and thrive.

RESEARCH LITERACY

While a detailed study of research is beyond the scope of this text, a few observations about research and massage will be useful here. **Research literacy** includes understanding the scientific method, locating and evaluating research articles, and gleaning practical information from research studies. It enables massage therapists to use research in planning effective massage sessions.

PRACTICAL APPLICATION

"Learning by doing" is particularly useful in a vocational program. In the case of massage, "learning by receiving" can be equally valuable. Receive two professional massages within a period of 2 weeks to see what beneficial effects it has on you.

1. What effects did you notice on your organ systems?
2. Did you experience any psychological effects?
3. Did the type of massage you received or the setting have particular effects?

Research is based on the **scientific method**, a systematic way of testing theories through gathering and analyzing relevant information to see if it supports the theory in question. It is based on observations about what actually happens, rather than taking the word of an authority or anecdotes from individuals.

Research studies start with a **hypothesis,** or an unproven theory about how something works or what will happen in a certain situation. For example, that massage will reduce the frequency and severity of chronic tension headaches might be the hypothesis of a study.

The measurement of results or *outcomes* after a particular massage application is an essential part of research. Measurement offers a concrete way of describing if and how something changed as a result of massage. In the earlier example, comparing the number of tension headaches before and after the massage application provides a useful measurement of the outcomes. Another measurement that might be used is the severity of the headaches, for example, on a scale of 1 (mild) to 10 (most severe). Comparing pre- and post-treatment measurements provides evidence that real change took place.

It is important to remember that research studies may have flaws that make their conclusions less valid. *External validity* is "the capacity of the findings to be generalized to a larger group than the one that participated in the study." *Internal validity* involves elements within the study design or execution that make it more or less credible (Menard 2009). Evaluation of research reports through careful reading allows you to judge their usefulness for clinical massage applications.

Levels of Evidence

There are different types of research studies that offer weaker or stronger evidence of cause and effect. For example, a *case study* might report that an individual client with chronic tension headaches had fewer headaches after massage therapy. This may be valuable information as far as it goes, but does not tell us if the results would be the same in others. A *case series* or number of similar cases would provide stronger evidence. A *randomized controlled trial,* comparing a number of clients who received a particular massage application with others who did not, would provide even stronger evidence. A *meta-analysis,* or systematic review of a number of different research studies looking at the same subject, provides an even more credible basis for evidence-based practice.

An example of how research has impacted a way of thinking in clinical massage therapy is the beliefs about massage for people with cancer. For many years massage therapists were taught that cancer was an absolute contraindication for massage. This was based on misunderstandings of cancer and the fear of doing harm with massage. An accumulation of research studies and experience has more recently shown this to be a false belief. Now massage is viewed as an effective complementary therapy in cancer treatment (Walton 2006).

Locating Research Studies

Locating research about clinical applications of massage has been made easier in recent years. Research study reports are listed in a number of online databases, and appear in various health professions publications. **Peer-reviewed journals** are credible sources of information about research studies. Peer-reviewed journals only publish research that meets certain standards and that has been evaluated by experts in the field. This is in contrast to reports by those with monetary interest in the outcomes of the research and anecdotal stories about massage often found in magazines.

The Massage Therapy Foundation funds research studies and maintains an online database of thousands of reports about the effects of massage and its clinical uses. The MTF also publishes a free, peer-reviewed online journal called the *International Journal of Therapeutic Massage & Bodywork: Research, Education, & Practice* (IJTMB) (http://journals .sfu.ca/ijtmb).

Two centers for the study of touch therapies have been established in North America. The Touch Research Institute (TRI) at the University of Miami School of Medicine and the Canadian Touch Research Center in Montreal conduct research on the use of massage in clinical settings. The National Library of Medicine search service, called PubMed, offers access to studies about massage reported in over 4,000 health-related journals. Websites for organiza-

REALITY CHECK

ALLISON: I don't plan on going into clinical massage therapy so research seems irrelevant to me. Did you ever read a research report once you graduated from school? Have you ever found it useful?

KELLY: When I graduated from school there wasn't much massage research to read. Now I find that some of the research being conducted is quite relevant to my practice and pretty interesting too. For instance, articles written in mainstream magazines about massage as a stress reducer and for relief from low back pain and tension headaches often cite recent research on the subject. Research on infant massage is often reported, too. Some of my clients have read about these benefits and come looking for that from me. I read the reports to see what massage application was used, what the study measured, and the results. Sometimes I pick up practical tips that I use in my massage sessions.

TABLE 7.2	Science as Conversation: Telling a Story*	
Sections of a Research Report	**The Conversation**	**Contents**
Abstract	"Here's why you should hear me out."	Quick overview of background, methods, results, and conclusion.
		Keywords (for database searching).
Introduction	"Here's what you need to know first."	Setting the plot: Why is this intriguing?
		Balanced relevant literature review.
		How is massage expected to help?
		Rationale for treatment and measurement choices.
Methods	"Here's what I decided to do."	Description of study subject(s).
		Description of massage application used, measurements, and other factors, such as session frequency and timing.
		Description of research design.
Results	"Here's what happened."	Case study—narrative summary of treatment and outcomes.
		Clinical trial—summary of outcome measurements.
		Organized display of results/findings.
Discussion	"Here's what I think it means, and where we go from here."	Connect results back to Introduction.
		Speculate on why the massage application worked or did not work as hypothesized.
		Comments on implications for practice.
		Ideas for future studies.
References	"Here are my sources of information."	Main sources of ideas and facts mentioned in the report.
		Citations of past research about the research topic.
		Establish confidence in approach to the study.

*Adapted with permission from a Massage Therapy Foundation presentation by Michael Hamm, LMP at the 2007 AMTA Convention in Cincinnati.

tions that support massage therapy research, or where relevant studies can be found, are listed under "Additional Resources" in Appendix H, References and Additional Resources, on page A-66.

Reading Research Reports

Reading and evaluating research reports require an understanding of their basic elements. Typical sections in research reports include the following: abstract, introduction, methods, results, discussion, and references. Research reports can be thought of as the researcher telling a story about what he or she did, how it turned out, and what it might mean. Table 7.2■ summarizes the part each section of a research report plays in telling the story.

It has been argued that the nature of massage as a holistic therapy makes it unsuited for scientific inquiry. For example, many practitioners distrust the formula approach to massage used in research to minimize variables in treatment. They understand the importance of varying the approach for the unique individual receiving the massage. Nevertheless, there are certain aspects of massage and its effects that can be measured objectively and provide valuable information to practitioners. Innovative research designs have also been proposed to address the unique considerations of holistic therapies such as massage.

PHYSIOLOGICAL EFFECTS— TISSUE LEVEL

Massage improves the overall health of cells and tissues of the body, primarily by increasing blood and lymph circulation. The "milking" action of petrissage techniques and the sliding movements of effleurage are very effective in moving body fluids to facilitate natural processes. Increased fluid circulation improves delivery of oxygen and nutrients to tissue cells and helps in removal of metabolic wastes and by-products of the inflammatory process (Yates 2004, p. 30). Two topics of special interest to massage therapists are tissue repair and the nature of connective tissue.

Tissue Repair

Healing from soft tissue injuries such as burns, bruises, sprains, and wounds has three physiological phases. The tissue repair process consists of *inflammation* to stabilize the injured area, *regeneration* to restore the tissue structure, and *remodeling* for healthy scar formation. Massage can play an important role in the tissue repair process. See Figure 7.1■ for a schematic drawing of the tissue repair process.

The initial reaction to injury, called inflammation, is designed to stabilize the situation and prepare damaged tissues for repair. Inflammation results in increased blood

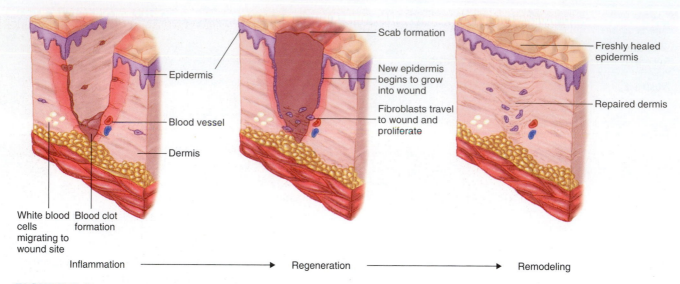

Scab formation

Epidermis

New epidermis begins to grow into wound

Blood vessel

Fibroblasts travel to wound and proliferate

Dermis

Freshly healed epidermis

Repaired dermis

White blood cells migrating to wound site

Blood clot formation

Inflammation → Regeneration → Remodeling

FIGURE 7.1

Three phases of the tissue/wound repair process.

flow to the area causing redness, warmth, swelling, pain, and decreased function. The lymphatic system plays an important role in the resolution of inflammation by removing fluid that creates swelling and surveying that fluid for harmful microorganisms. The length of the inflammatory phase will vary depending on the severity of the initial trauma and the strength of the individual's immune system.

Massage is contraindicated in the immediate location of an injury during the inflammatory phase, especially in the presence of infection. If there is no infection associated with an injury, lymphatic massage techniques may be used in some cases to reduce swelling in an area. Once the signs of inflammation subside, standard massage techniques can be applied safely around the injury site.

In the regeneration phase, the tissue structure is rebuilt and restored. New tissue replaces damaged tissue of the same type. This involves removing damaged cells, excess fluids, and other by-products of inflammation, as well as delivering the building blocks for new tissue formation. By improving general and local circulation, massage can facilitate this transportation process. The amount of pressure used at this phase of healing is limited to what the tissues can withstand without further damage.

Massage can also play a role in the remodeling phase of tissue repair by encouraging healthy scar formation. Deep transverse friction is used in rehabilitation to help form strong mobile scar tissue. Deep friction helps break interfiber adhesions by mechanically broadening the tissues. This in turn helps produce more parallel fiber arrangement and fewer transverse connections in the tissue that may inhibit movement (Cyriax and Cyriax 1993). Subcutaneous scar tissue may be loosened by careful and persistent friction; however, further research is needed to establish whether deeper scarring in connective tissue can be realigned once it is formed.

A less understood role for massage in tissue repair is related to its promotion of stress reduction. A study reported in *Lancet,* a British medical journal, showed that wounds healed more slowly in people suffering from chronic stress. Researchers found that the stressed group had lower levels of interleukin-1 beta, an immune system substance known to play a role in wound repair (Greene 1996, p. 16). To the extent that massage reduces stress, it may help wounds heal faster.

Connective Tissue

Connective tissue is the most pervasive tissue in the body. It fills internal spaces, provides structural support, and is a vehicle for fluid transportation and energy storage. Classifications of connective tissue include: fluid (e.g., blood and lymph); supporting (e.g., cartilage and bone); dense (e.g., tendons, ligaments, dermis), loose (e.g., fascia), and adipose tissue (i.e., fat). Figure 7.2■ shows common types and locations of connective tissue of interest to massage therapists. Some general connective tissue considerations and the nature of fascia are discussed briefly in the following section.

TENDONS, LIGAMENTS, FASCIA

The connective tissue in tendons, ligaments, and fascia has a property called *thixotropy,* which means that it becomes more fluid and pliable when it is mobile and firmer when it is immobile. Pressing, friction, stretching, and other movements of massage raise the temperature and the energy level of the tissue slightly and create a "greater degree of sol (fluidity) in organic systems that are already there but are behaving sluggishly" (Juhan 1987, pp. 69–70).

In addition to promoting healthy function, massage helps to prevent some connective tissue abnormalities and dysfunction. For example, massage techniques such as kneading and deep friction have been found to help prevent

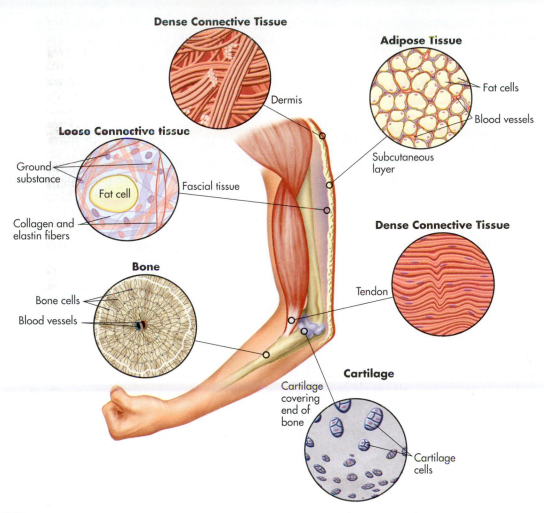

FIGURE 7.2

Types and locations of connective tissue.

the formation of abnormal collagenous connective tissue called *fibrosis* (Yates 2004, pp. 72–74).

Fascia is a type of connective tissue that surrounds all muscles, bones, and organs and helps to give them shape. Fascia literally holds the body together and can be thought of as continuous sheets of supportive tissue, which envelop the entire body and its parts. A theory of physical structure used by some bodyworkers views connective tissue, not bones, as the main support of the body.

In healthy bodies, fascial tissues are pliable and move freely. With chronic stress, chronic immobility, trauma, or disease, connective tissue may become thickened, rigid, or may stick to other tissues, forming adhesions. Adhesions result in restricted movement and impair the ability of the affected tissues to conduct exchanges of nutrients and cellular wastes. Massage can improve tissue function by helping to restore tissue pliability and eradicate adhesions.

Certain massage techniques remove adhesions formed when fascial tissues stick to each other or to other tissues. The simple mechanical action of some massage techniques separates tissues, for example, lifting, broadening, and applying a shearing force across the parallel organization of fibers. Kneading, skin rolling, deep transverse friction, broadening techniques, and myofascial techniques are examples of effective methods for separating and "unsticking" adhering tissues.

Chapter 18, Contemporary Massage and Bodywork, on page 520 provides more detailed information about myofascial techniques applied to improve the condition of fascial tissues. The discussion of increased joint mobility and flexibility in the "Muscular System" section of this chapter has further information on connective tissue and massage.

PHYSIOLOGICAL EFFECTS— ORGAN SYSTEM LEVEL

Massage has specific effects on the different organ systems of the body. In addition to keeping the organ tissues healthy and enhancing healing, massage can also improve the function of the system as a whole. And since organ systems interact in myriad ways, the effects of massage on any one system impacts others as well. Overlapping function is especially obvious in certain system pairings, such as muscular–skeletal, circulatory–lymphatic, nervous–endocrine, and respiratory–circulatory–muscular.

Integumentary System

The integumentary system includes the skin and its accessory structures such as hair, nails, and sebaceous and sweat glands. Sensory receptors in the skin detect touch, pressure, pain, and temperature and relay that information to the nervous system. There are three skin layers: the epidermis or outermost layer, dermis, and subcutaneous fascia. See Figure 6.9 on page 135. For further information about the integumentary system, see page 133 in Chapter 6, Anatomy & Physiology, Pathology, and Kinesiology.

The skin is the primary point of contact between the giver and receiver of massage. One of the major effects of pressure to the skin is stimulation of the sensory receptors found there. This stimulation may have beneficial effects such as general relaxation, pain reduction, and body awareness. Good body awareness enhances a person's sense of integrity and wholeness and is important for good mental and emotional health.

In order for the exocrine glands in the skin (sebaceous and sweat glands) to work properly, skin pores must be free from blockage. Pores may become blocked with substances such as dirt, makeup, dried oils, and sweat, or the accumulation of dead skin cells. Bathing with soap and water and hydrotherapy—such as whirlpool, steam room, and sauna—help open pores. Exfoliating, or removing dead skin cells by scraping or friction (e.g., with a loofa, brush, or coarse towel) is an old health and beauty practice. Read more about exfoliation on page 489 in Chapter 17, Spa Applications.

The friction of massage also increases superficial circulation and raises the temperature of skin. This promotes perspiration and increases sebaceous oil secretions. Oil and lotion applied to the skin during massage add moisture needed to prevent further drying or cracking. This is especially beneficial in dry climates, on aging skin, and with certain dry skin conditions.

Massage can facilitate the formation of healthy scar tissue on the skin surface following lacerations, surgery incisions, or burns. Applying cross-fiber and with-fiber friction techniques to scars during the remodeling or scar maturation phase helps form strong mobile scars, remove adhesions to underlying tissues, and reduce scar thickness. Skin lifting and rolling techniques stretch underlying fascia and remove superficial adhesions.

Skeletal System

The skeletal system includes the bones of the skeleton, associated cartilage, ligaments, and other stabilizing connective tissue structures. In addition to general tissue health promoted by good circulation, massage and related joint movements help maintain good joint function and range of motion. Movement of the joints stimulates production of synovial fluid that keeps joints moving smoothly. For further information about the skeletal system, see page 142 in Chapter 6, Anatomy & Physiology, Pathology, and Kinesiology. The skeletal system is illustrated in Figure 6.28 on page 143.

Optimal range of motion is achieved when the bones are in proper alignment and the tissues surrounding the joints are healthy, pliable, and relaxed. Joint flexibility (i.e., flexability) is enhanced with massage and stretching movements (Figure 7.3■). Flexibility is discussed in greater depth in the "Muscular System" section of this chapter.

Proper body alignment is necessary for optimal functioning of the skeletal system. Maintaining good posture is a function of the combined muscular, skeletal, and nervous systems and is discussed in more detail in the section that follows.

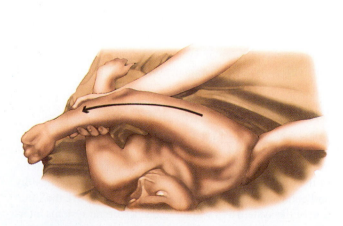

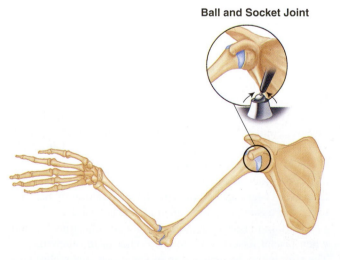

Ball and Socket Joint

FIGURE 7.3

Passive stretching enhances joint function.

Muscular System

The muscular system includes skeletal muscles, associated connective tissue (i.e., fascia and tendons), and motor and sensory neurons related to movement. Proprioceptors, important sensory neurons that monitor the movement and position of the body in space, are located in the skeletal muscles and associated connective tissue. For further information about the muscular system, see page 155 in Chapter 6. The muscular system is illustrated in Figure 6.49 on page 160–161.

The importance of muscular system health for overall well-being cannot be overestimated. It is through the musculature and the movement it produces that so many other health benefits derive, for example, good circulation, body heat, metabolism, kinesthetic awareness, and even emotional balance.

Problems in the musculature can cause severe pain and reduced quality of life. It is not surprising that massage therapy is valued so highly for its role in maintaining good health and function of the muscular system.

CELLULAR LEVEL ACTIVITY

Muscles maintain normal cellular level activity and balance through movement. Muscle contraction puts mechanical pressure on the veins and lymphatic vessels, thereby pushing fluids along and carrying away metabolic by-products. As the muscles relax, fresh blood flows into them, bringing nutrients to the area. This balancing action is disturbed through underactivity or overactivity.

Underactivity disturbs balance because the muscle contractions that provide the "milking" effect are less than needed for good fluid circulation. Waste products then accumulate in the muscle tissue, and the arrival of nutrients is slowed. When illness or injury results in muscular inactivity, massage techniques such as petrissage mimic the action of muscle contraction, thereby improving fluid circulation.

Overactivity (e.g., from strenuous exercise or work) also disturbs balance at the cellular level. Insufficient time between contractions decreases the inflow of nutritive products and oxygen to muscle tissues. In addition, metabolic waste products are formed faster than they can be eliminated. Muscle tension increases and muscles shorten due to reduced cellular nutrition. Muscle tension worsens the situation by further limiting fluid circulation.

Massage given immediately after strenuous activity reduces muscle stiffness and soreness. Massage has been found to reduce delayed-onset muscle soreness (DOMS) in some studies (Ernst 1998). A combination of effleurage (i.e., sliding) and petrissage (i.e., kneading or compression) flushes metabolic wastes, brings oxygen and nutrients to the area, and enhances tissue repair. These are important benefits of postevent, interevent, and recovery sports massage (Benjamin and Lamp 2005). For more information, see the discussion on increased blood circulation in the "Cardiovascular System" section of this chapter.

MUSCLE RELAXATION

Massage is often used to relax hypertonic or tense muscles. There are several ways that muscle relaxation may be effected. Reduction of general muscle tension may be due in part to stimulation of the parasympathetic nervous system via relaxation massage (Figure 7.4■). There may also be a conscious letting-go of muscle tension by the higher brain centers as the recipient assumes a passive state during a massage session.

General muscle relaxation may also be traced to increased sensory stimulation that accompanies the application of massage techniques. Yates (2004) reasons that massage causes a massive increase in the sensory input to the spinal cord, which results in readjustments in reflex pathways, which leads to spontaneous normalization of imbalances of tonic activity between individual muscles and muscle groups. Residual muscle tension left over from past activity or emotional stress is released as the system balances itself (p. 51). Thus, muscular relaxation results from the general application of a variety of basic massage techniques such as effleurage, petrissage, friction, tapotement, and vibration.

Manual techniques may be applied to relax specific muscles. For example, in a technique called *muscle approximation* the combined action of the muscular and nervous systems is utilized to reduce muscle tone. In this technique, the practitioner slowly and forcibly draws the attachments of the muscle closer together. This decreases stretch of the muscle spindles, which are composed of nerve filaments coiled around specialized muscle fibers. Muscle spindles cause contraction when muscles are suddenly elongated (i.e., stretch reflex). Approximation causes slack in the muscle and is held until the muscle spindles stop firing and the muscle fibers relax. Approximation is useful for treating muscle spasms.

Another muscle relaxation method called the *origin and insertion technique* is useful when direct work on the muscle belly is too painful. In the origin and insertion

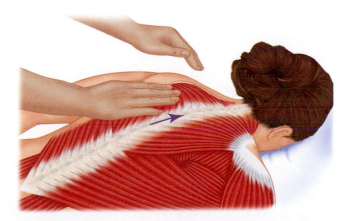

FIGURE 7.4

Massage reduces muscle tension and promotes relaxation.

technique, cross-fiber and with-fiber friction is performed on the attachments of the targeted muscle in small segments until the muscle fibers relax. Eventually, overall muscle tone is reduced. This works by stimulating sensory receptors called Golgi tendon organs, located in tendons near muscle attachments (see Figure 6.112 on page 219). When Golgi tendon organs fire, they inhibit contraction of the associated muscle (Rattray 1994). Since muscular relaxation is one of the fundamental effects of massage, there are many other manual techniques for promoting muscle relaxation discussed throughout the text.

INCREASED JOINT MOBILITY AND FLEXIBILITY

Flexibility refers to the degree of range of motion in a joint. It is a function of the combined muscular and skeletal systems with some nervous system involvement. Hypertonic muscles, scarring in muscle and connective tissues, myofascial adhesions, trigger points, and general connective tissue thickening and rigidity may all restrict movement at joints. Massage and passive joint movements can be used effectively to help maintain joint mobility and normal range of motion by addressing any abnormal conditions found in the soft tissues surrounding the joint.

In a study conducted by sport physical therapists and a massage therapist, massage was found to significantly increase range of motion in the hamstrings. The massage techniques used in the study were light and deep effleurage, stretching effleurage, petrissage (kneading), and friction (deep circular and deep transverse). Increased flexibility lasted for at least 7 days after the massage (Crosman, Chateauvert, and Weisburg 1985). Additional information on improving flexibility through joint movements may be found in Chapter 13, Western Massage Techniques, on page 398.

POSTURE

Proper body alignment or good posture is the combined function of the muscular, skeletal, and nervous systems. Poor posture usually results from a combination of factors such as ergonomically inadequate workstations or tools, injuries, or poor postural habits. Poor posture often leads to imbalances between muscle groups, hypertonic and shortened muscles, fascial adhesions, trigger points, and other problem conditions. Or vice versa: muscle imbalances or pathologies may result in poor body alignment.

Some forms of massage and bodywork specifically focus on helping clients improve their body alignment. After analyzing the client's posture and identifying the probable cause of misalignment, massage and related joint movements are applied with the goal of proper alignment. This might involve strategies such as relaxing and elongating muscles with massage, lengthening muscle groups with stretching, or removing fascial adhesions with myofascial techniques. Posture analysis is described in detail on page 324 in Chapter 10, Goal-Oriented Planning and Documentation.

Nervous and Endocrine Systems

The nervous and endocrine systems work together to coordinate organ system functions and respond to environmental stimuli. The nervous system controls relatively swift responses such as those related to movement, while the endocrine system regulates slower responses such as metabolic rate.

NERVOUS SYSTEM

Nervous system anatomy consists of the central nervous system (i.e., brain and spinal cord) and peripheral nervous system (i.e., sensory receptors and motor neurons). A division of the nervous system that regulates the activity of smooth muscle, cardiac muscle, and glands is called the autonomic nervous system, which plays an important role in relaxation massage. For further information about the nervous system, see page 163 in Chapter 6. The nervous system is illustrated in Figure 6.51 on page 164.

Some of the effects of massage related to the nervous system have already been discussed. For example, stimulation of sensory receptors in the skin enhances body awareness and plays an important role in muscle relaxation and pain reduction. The effects of massage on growth and development in infants are directly related to stimulation of the nervous system via the skin and through body movement (Field 2000; Ottenbacher et al. 1987).

Some massage and movement techniques use the nervous system to effect desired results. For example, some assisted stretching techniques deliberately activate proprioceptors in muscles to effect relaxation and elongation.

One of the most important effects of massage is its ability to elicit the relaxation response. This combined autonomic nervous system and endocrine system response is discussed in more detail in the "Physiological Effects—Organism Level" section of this chapter, because it involves many organ systems, as well as mental and emotional states.

ENDOCRINE SYSTEM

The endocrine system is composed of endocrine glands that secrete hormones that regulate important body processes such as cell growth and division, general metabolism, water loss, and blood calcium levels. For further information about the endocrine system, see page 170 in Chapter 6. The primary glands of the endocrine system are illustrated in Figure 6.60■ on page 171.

Endocrine system hormones related to massage include dopamine, cortisol, serotonin, norepinephrine, and epinephrine. The secretion of these hormones is regulated in conjunction with the central nervous system. Of particular interest for massage is the effect of the parasympathetic nervous system in increasing or reducing the release of these hormones. Massage can be understood as affecting the levels of these hormones via the relaxation response.

Levels of these five hormones have been used in research studies to measure the effects of massage on stress and anxiety levels. For example, massage has been linked to elevated levels of dopamine and lower levels of cortisol, which provides evidence of reduced stress. Elevated cortisol levels also inhibit the immune system, so massage is seen to reduce the negative effects of stress on immune function. Massage has also been linked to increased serotonin levels, which reduces pain and elevates mood. In addition, massage helps decrease levels of norepinephrine and epinephrine, as a result of turning off the fight-or-flight response (Field 2000; Rich 2002).

Cardiovascular System

Cardiovascular system anatomy includes the heart, blood vessels (i.e., arteries and veins), and blood, which is considered a fluid connective tissue. The cardiovascular system is essentially a fluid transportation system for nutrients, waste products, dissolved gases, hormones, and cells and molecules for body defense. For further information about the cardiovascular system, see page 175 in Chapter 6. An overview of the cardiovascular system is illustrated in Figure 6.65 on page 176.

The cardiovascular and lymphatic systems are transportation systems that rely specifically on the movement of fluids to carry out their functions. Good fluid circulation in these important body systems is a key to health at the cellular level.

The benefits of increased circulation include improved nutrient delivery and increased metabolic waste removal via the blood. It is also important for tissue repair, as building blocks for new tissues are brought to an area and damaged cells are removed. When pathogens enter the body, fluids deliver macrophages to attack the invaders and help prevent

disease. The team action of these two body systems is succinctly described by Yates (2004):

> Increases in blood and lymph circulation are the most widely recognized and frequently described of the physiological effects of massage therapy. Changes in blood and lymph circulation are appropriately discussed together because they have effects in common on the clearance of metabolic wastes, and the byproducts of tissue damage and inflammation, the absorption of excess of inflammatory exudate, and on the delivery of oxygen and nutrients to tissue cells. (p. 30)

BLOOD CIRCULATION

Massage increases both general and local blood circulation (Figure 7.5■). Several studies have shown that capillary vessel dilation and increased blood flow in an area occur with massage. Even light pressure was shown to have an effect (Wood and Becker 1981).

Superficial friction produces hyperemia or increased local circulation in the skin and underlying connective tissue. As a result the skin appears red and feels warm. This effect is the result of the release of the chemical *histamine* that causes dilation of capillaries in the area.

Deep effleurage and petrissage have specifically been shown to increase blood volume in an area. This increased flow is thought to last for some time after massage. For example, Bell (1964) reported that after a 10-minute massage of the calf, blood flow to the area doubled. This effect lasted 40 minutes. The benefits of increased circulation include improved nutrient delivery and increased metabolic waste removal via the blood.

FIGURE 7.5

Massage increases blood circulation.

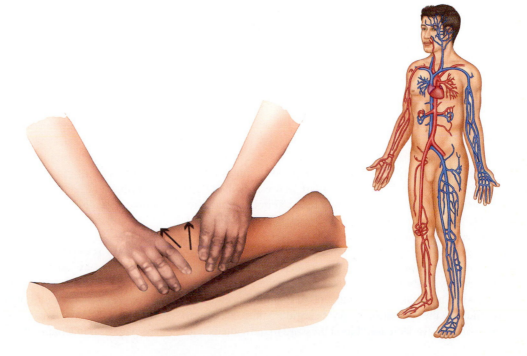

VENOUS RETURN

The mechanical action of deep effleurage enhances venous flow in the limbs. This technique physically pushes blood through venous circulation. The veins of the body are shown in Figure 6.70 on page 179.

The structure of veins dictates the direction of the application of deep stroking on the limbs. A dictum in classic Western massage states that deep stroking should always be "toward the heart," or moving distal (away from) to proximal (near the center).

Veins are low-pressure tubes. Movement of blood through them is aided by muscle contraction and by valves that prevent pooling due to the effects of gravity. Deep effleurage in the direction of the natural movement of blood enhances the flow. Conventional wisdom holds that applying massage in the opposite direction puts pressure on the valves and could possibly damage them.

Damage to valves results in a condition known as varicose veins (see Figure 6.78 on page 184). In varicose veins we find static, pooled blood. The constant pressure of pooled blood weakens the vein walls even further, causing a vicious cycle of pooling and weakening. Over time the veins become fragile. Under these conditions, massage might cause the vein to rupture, or release clots formed in the pools, into general circulation. Therefore, massage is locally contraindicated over superficial varicose veins and generally contraindicated for someone with a history of blood clots.

The mechanical action of kneading and other forms of petrissage also assist in venous return, much the same way muscle contraction does during exercise. Compression of the tissues increases local circulation and blood in the capillaries is moved along toward the larger veins.

Venostasis is a condition in which the normal flow of blood through a vein is slowed or halted. Lack of muscular activity can bring about venostasis, particularly in inactive or paralyzed limbs. Other causes for venostasis include varicose veins and pressure on the vessels from edema of the surrounding tissues. Massage given for this condition should first address the proximal aspects of an inactive limb before massage of the distal area. This ensures that the circulatory pathways are open enough to carry the venous flow from the distal area back toward the heart.

BLOOD PRESSURE

Researchers Barr and Taslitz (1970) found that blood pressure is temporarily decreased for about 40 minutes after a 1-hour massage session. The decrease in pressure is thought to result from a greater capacity for blood in the capillaries due to local vasodilation and greater permeability of capillary walls. The more blood in the capillaries, the less there is in other vessels to cause pressure on vessel walls. Reduction in both systolic and diastolic pressure was duplicated in research by Cady and Jones (1997).

Also, as mentioned earlier, one of the long-term effects of eliciting the relaxation response regularly and learning to control stress is decreased blood pressure in individuals with hypertension. This saves wear and tear on the circulatory system and improves circulation overall.

RED BLOOD CELLS

Massage increases the number of circulating red blood cells, thereby increasing the oxygen-carrying capacity of the blood. Red blood cells (RBC) stored in the liver and spleen are thought to be discharged during massage, as well as RBC in stagnant capillary beds returned to circulation (Mitchell 1894; Pemberton 1939).

Lymphatic System and Immunity

The lymphatic system is made up of a network of lymphatic vessels, a fluid called lymph, and organs (i.e., lymph nodes) that contain a large number of lymphocytes. The lymphatic system functions to return fluids from body tissues to the blood; transports hormones, nutrients, and waste products from tissues into general circulation; and defends the body from infection and disease via white blood cells or lymphocytes. For further information about the lymphatic system, see page 184 in Chapter 6. A schematic of the lymphatic system is illustrated in Figure 6.79 on page 185.

LYMPH FLUID MOVEMENT

Lymph is a viscous fluid that moves slowly through the lymphatic vessels. Lymphatic pressure is naturally lower, and lymph fluid movement slower, than venous blood flow.

The movement of lymph through the capillaries, ducts, and nodes of the lymphatic system depends on outside sources, such as the contraction of muscles, action of the diaphragm, and pressure generated by filtration of fluid from the capillaries. Lack of mobility due to a sedentary lifestyle, confinement to a bed or a wheelchair, pain, or paralysis seriously interferes with flow of lymph fluid.

It has been known for some time that massage techniques, especially effleurage and petrissage, mechanically assist general lymphatic flow (Drinker and Yoffey 1941; Elkins et al. 1953; Mortimer et al. 1990). In addition, special lymphatic facilitation techniques have been developed to maximize the effects of moving lymph through superficial capillaries (Figure 7.6■). Manual lymph drainage (MLD) techniques along with other therapies are used effectively in the treatment of a condition called *lymphedema* (Kelly 2002). Lymphatic facilitation techniques used to reduce swelling around musculo-skeletal injuries are described in Chapter 18, Contemporary Massage and Bodywork, on page 529.

IMMUNITY

Immunity is defined as "the resistance to injuries and disease caused by specific foreign chemical compounds and pathogens" (Martini and Bartholomew 1999, p. 269). It is a complex phenomenon in which the lymphatic system plays an important part. For further information about immunity, see page 186 in Chapter 6.

FIGURE 7.6

Lymphatic massage techniques improve the circulation of lymph fluid.

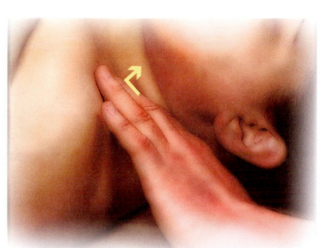
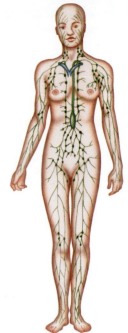

Massage affects immunity by enhancing the immune response, which is designed to destroy or inactivate pathogens, abnormal cells, and foreign molecules such as toxins. By improving lymphatic flow, as previously described, massage facilitates the transport of lymphocytes that participate in the immune response. This is a direct mechanical result of massage techniques such as effleurage and petrissage, both of which help move body fluids.

Massage also appears to improve immunity through a number of other mechanisms. Recent studies show massage to be associated with increased natural killer (NK) cells and increased CD4 cells, as well as decreased anxiety and cortisol levels. High cortisol levels inflict wear and tear on the body over time by inhibiting the production and release of white blood cells, blocking T and B cell function, and interfering with the production of interleukins, which are important for communication among white blood cells (Ironson et al. 1996; Zeitlin et al. 2000).

Respiratory System

The respiratory system includes the lungs and the passageways leading to the lungs (i.e., nose, nasal cavity and sinuses, trachea, bronchial tubes). It acts with the circulatory system to affect an exchange of gases between the body and the environment. The respiratory system relies on the diaphragm and other skeletal muscles to produce breathing. For further information about the respiratory system, see page 188 in Chapter 6. The organs of the respiratory system are illustrated in Figure 6-83 on page 189.

Massage enhances respiratory function by improving general blood circulation and encouraging relaxed diaphragmatic breathing. Massage can also address tension and shortening in skeletal muscles involved in respiration. To the extent that massage facilitates good posture, it helps achieve the structural alignment and rib cage expansion necessary for optimal vital capacity (i.e., the amount of air moved into or out of the lungs during a single respiratory cycle).

Digestive System

The digestive system consists of a muscular tube called the digestive tract (i.e., oral cavity, pharynx, esophagus, stomach, small intestine, large intestine, rectum, and anus) and accessory organs, including the salivary glands, gall bladder, liver, and pancreas. Functions of the digestive system include ingestion, mechanical processing, and chemical breakdown of food and drink, secretion of digestive enzymes, absorption of water and nutrients, and excretion of waste products. For further information about the digestive system, see page 195 in Chapter 6. The digestive system is illustrated in Figure 6.91 on page 195.

Massage enhances digestion through eliciting the relaxation response, in which digestive activity is increased. One of the negative effects of stress accumulated over a long period of time is disruption of the normal digestive processes, which can cause indigestion. Relaxation massage as part of a stress reduction program helps prevent digestive maladies.

Abdominal massage has been used for decades to facilitate bowel movement in people suffering from constipation. The direct mechanical effects of massage move the contents of the large intestine and initiate reflex effects that stimulate peristaltic movement (DeDomenico and Wood 1997). See Figure 7.7■. Abdominal techniques of infant

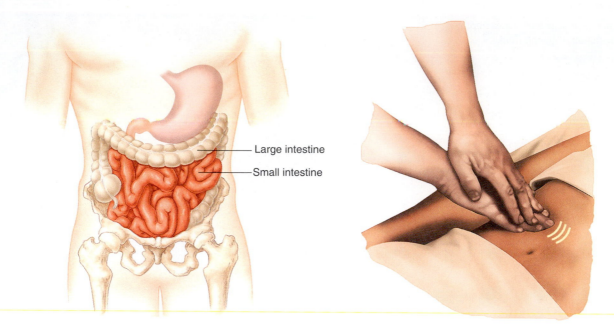

FIGURE 7.7

Abdominal massage facilitates bowel movement.

massage assist bowel and gas movement and help relieve distress. Abdominal massage for adults is described in Chapter 14, Full-Body Massage Sequence, on page 436, and for infants in Chapter 20, Special Populations and Adaptations, on page 593.

Urinary System

The structures of the urinary system include the kidneys, ureters, urinary bladder, and the urethra. The primary function of the urinary system is removal of waste products from the blood and their excretion out of the body. It also helps regulate blood volume and pressure, as well as blood composition. For further information about the urinary system, see page 201 in Chapter 6. The urinary system is illustrated in Figure 6.96 on page 201.

Because massage enhances function of the cardiovascular system, it indirectly affects the urinary system, which filters the blood. Better circulation to the kidneys leads to improved blood filtration overall. In addition, one of the results of activation of the parasympathetic nervous system via relaxation massage is increased urinary production and bladder tension. It is not uncommon to have to go to the bathroom after receiving a relaxing massage.

Reproductive System

The male and female reproductive organs are not appropriate targets for therapeutic massage. They do, however, benefit from improved general cardiovascular function, as do all body systems. There is evidence that chronic stress can impair sexual function, so to the extent that massage promotes relaxation, it could be said to benefit the reproductive function.

There are specialized approaches to massage for pregnant women. Postgraduate training in pregnancy massage is valuable for massage therapists in general practice or those working in places such as spas and salons. Some massage therapists are trained to work with midwives and health care practitioners during delivery. They often combine Western massage techniques with others such as shiatsu or, in some cases, folk-healing traditions. Chapter 20, Special Populations and Adaptations, describes pregnancy massage on page 588.

Women's breasts contain mammary glands and lymphatic vessels surrounded by pectoral fat pads and other connective tissues. A layer of loose connective tissue separates the mammary complex from underlying muscle. Breast massage is a specialized skill that helps promote well-breast health and is a complementary therapy for women undergoing treatment for breast cancer (Curties 1999). Breast massage requires informed consent from the client and may be beyond the legal scope of practice for some practitioners.

Occasionally in males, increased circulation to the groin area as a result of massage results in an erection. This does not necessarily indicate sexual arousal. With no sexual arousal, the erection will subside naturally. This is the situation in the vast majority of cases.

However, if there appears to be sexual arousal, it is advised to stop the session immediately, state your perception, and ask the client if your perception is correct. If you still believe that there is sexual arousal regardless of what the client says, or if you are uncomfortable, inform the client that the massage is over, and leave the massage room to allow the client to get dressed. The ethical issues with the client should be dealt with outside of the immediate massage environment. See the discussion about the intervention model on page 108 in Chapter 5, Ethics and the Therapeutic Relationship.

PHYSIOLOGICAL EFFECTS— ORGANISM LEVEL

The effects of massage at the organism level include phenomena that impact the person beyond the effects on any one or two organ systems. Important phenomena affected by massage include growth and development in infants, stress reduction, pain reduction, and certain psychological effects.

Growth and Development

Touch has been found to be essential for the proper growth and development of infants and children. Holding, cuddling, rocking, stroking, and other forms of touching are all necessary for infants to thrive. There is also evidence that adequate pleasurable tactile experience in early life can influence the development of personality traits such as calmness, gentleness, and nonaggressiveness (Brown 1984, pp. 41–120; Diego et al. 2002; Juhan 1987, pp. 43–55; Montageu 1978, pp. 76–157).

The importance of stimulation to the skin for proper growth and development cannot be overestimated. The skin develops from the same primitive cells as the brain and is a prime sensory organ. Stimulation of the tactile nerve endings in the skin provides information about the outside world and helps the brain organize its circuitry for proper development. This is also true for movement and information received through the kinesthetic sense. Thus "the use of touch and sensation to modify our experience of peripheral conditions exerts an active influence upon the organization of reflexes and body image deep within the central nervous system" (Juhan 1987, p. 40).

As infants learn about the world around them through touch and movement, they also learn about themselves and their own bodies. Juhan expresses this idea with these words: "by rubbing up against the world, I define myself to myself" (1987, p. 34).

Massage is an excellent way to provide systematic and regular touching to growing infants. See Figure 7.8■. The massage of infants has been practiced widely all over the world and has been increasing in use in the United States as more caregivers become aware of its benefits. Chapter 20, Special Populations and Adaptations, describes infant massage on page 000 in greater detail.

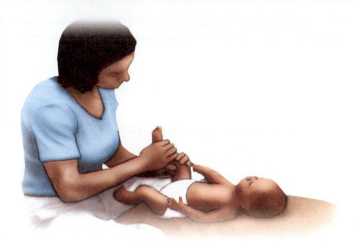

FIGURE 7.8

Massage promotes proper growth and development of infants.

Pain Reduction

Pain is an unpleasant sensation of discomfort, distress, or suffering caused by injury, disease, or emotional upset. It occurs in varying degrees of intensity from mild to severe. *Analgesia,* or pain reduction, is one of the benefits of massage that follows from its ability to elicit the relaxation response, reduce anxiety, relieve muscle tension, and improve circulation.

Some studies report massage to be effective in reducing chronic, long-term, and diffuse pain. Subjects reported reduced pain immediately after sessions, as well as in follow-up interviews (Hasson, Arnetz, Jelvis, and Edelstam 2004; Walach, Guthlin, and Konig 2003).

Massage may be used effectively to reduce pain caused by certain conditions. For example, muscle relaxation and improved local circulation can help relieve pain associated with tense muscles and the accompanying *ischemia* or lack of blood supply. Massage may also be used to help interrupt a pain–spasm–pain cycle induced by hypertonic or tense muscles. By relaxing the muscle and relieving the pain of the spasm, the cycle is broken and healing can take place. The use of specific techniques such as approximation, as described earlier, can be very effective for this purpose (Kresge 1983; Rattray 1994; Yates, 2004).

It is also thought that massage reduces pain by activating the neural-gating mechanism in the spinal cord through increase in sensory stimulation. The theory is that by activating fast, large nerve fibers that carry tactile information, transmission from slower, smaller pain-transmitting nerve fibers is blocked. The perception of pain may be reduced for minutes or hours through the additional sensory input created by massage techniques. Activation of the neural-gating mechanism has been suggested as an explanation for the temporary analgesia associated with deep friction massage in the treatment of injuries to tendons and ligaments (Yates 2004).

Research by de Bruijn (1984) noted that the high degree of analgesia resulting from deep transverse friction is preceded by painful irritation of the affected tissues. De Bruijn concluded that friction massage was a promising treatment for soft tissue injuries since the eventual pain-reduction effect allowed the patient to use the affected tissue for better healing.

Myofascial trigger points (TrPs) are known to cause pain at the site of the TrP, at satellite trigger points, and in muscles that lie within the reference zone of the TrP. Massage (e.g., ischemic compression and muscle stripping) and stretching are therapies often used in deactivating trigger points (Travell and Simons 1983, 1992). See Chapter 18, Contemporary Massage and Bodywork, on page 000 for further discussion of trigger point therapy.

There is also evidence that massage induces the release of neurochemicals called endorphins and enkephalins. These substances modulate pain-impulse transmission in the central nervous system and induce relaxation and feelings of general well-being. They are the body's natural painkillers. The mechanism involved is not clearly understood and may be a combination of psychological, as well as physical, reactions to massage (Yates 2004).

Stress Reduction

Soothing massage is commonly recognized as an effective relaxation technique. It is one of several stress-management methods known to trigger the relaxation response. Other popular methods include meditation, guided imagery, progressive relaxation, abdominal breathing, hatha yoga, and biofeedback.

Back massage is especially effective for stress management, and its application for relaxation is described in more detail in Chapter 14, Full-Body Massage Sequence, on page 421. Several studies have confirmed the benefits of back massage for reducing stress in hospitalized patients (Bauer and Dracup 1987; Fakouri and Jones 1987; Fraser and Kerr 1993). The value of back massage for stress reduction is directly related to its ability to activate the parasympathetic nervous system and elicit the physiological phenomenon called the *relaxation response.* Inducing the relaxation response counters the damaging effects of a chronic stress response by bringing balance to the body's systems.

Specific health benefits of the relaxation response cited by Robbins, Powers, and Burgess (1994, pp. 191–192) include:

- Decreased oxygen consumption and metabolic rate, and less strain on energy resources
- Increased intensity and frequency of alpha brain waves associated with deep relaxation
- Reduced blood lactates, blood substances associated with anxiety
- Reduced levels of cortisol, norepinephrine, and epinephrine
- Significantly decreased blood pressure in individuals with hypertension

- Reduced heart rate and slower respiration
- Decreased muscle tension
- Increased blood flow to internal organs
- Decreased anxiety, fear, and phobias, and increased positive mental health
- Improved quality of sleep

During the relaxation response, a person feels totally relaxed and is in a pleasant semi-awake state of consciousness.

Full-body massage consisting predominantly of effleurage and petrissage, with fewer specific techniques that cause discomfort, is very effective in eliciting the relaxation response. The qualities of such a session could be described as light, smooth, and flowing. The relaxing effects of this type of session may be enhanced with certain types of music, soft lighting, warm room temperatures, and minimal talking.

PSYCHOLOGICAL EFFECTS

The psychological effects of massage (i.e., on the mind and emotions) are less well understood than the physical effects, although they are related to the physical effects in many ways. The most well-studied mental and emotional effects of massage include increased mental clarity, reduced anxiety, and feelings of general well-being. A phenomenon called *emotional release,* which is an interesting interface of body, mind, and emotions, may also occur during massage.

Mental Clarity

Two studies performed at the Touch Research Institute in Miami suggest that massage helps improve mental clarity (i.e., sharpening cognitive skills like solving problems, remembering information, or paying focused attention). In one study, 15-minute massage sessions were given to hospital personnel over a 5-week period during their lunch breaks. People reported feeling more relaxed, in better moods, and more alert after receiving massage. Similarly, students who received massage during finals week reported being more relaxed and less anxious and said that they remembered information better after an 8-minute massage session (Field 2000).

In a job-stress study conducted in 1993, subjects received a 20-minute massage in a chair twice weekly for a month. They reported less fatigue and demonstrated greater clarity of thought, improved cognitive skills, and lower anxiety levels. See Figure 7.9■. EEG, alpha, beta, and theta waves were also altered in ways consistent with enhanced alertness (Field, Fox, Pickens, Ironsong, and Scafidi 1993).

Massage is used with athletes in pre-event situations to help spark the alertness necessary for competition. For pre-event readiness, sports massage sessions are 15–20 minutes in duration, have an upbeat tempo, and use techniques to increase circulation and joint mobility. Tapotement is frequently applied for stimulation.

In each of the cases mentioned, the massage sessions were relatively short—between 8 and 20 minutes. Increased mental alertness is most likely related to sensory stimulation

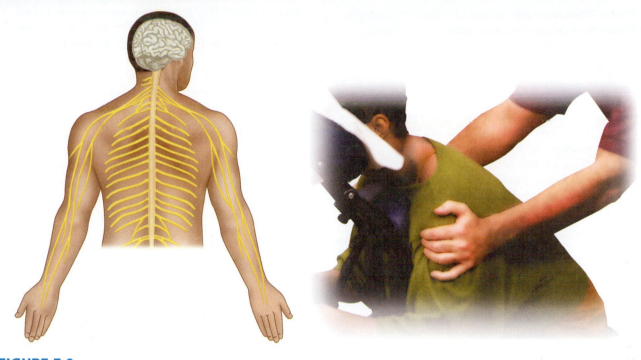

FIGURE 7.9

Short, upbeat massage sessions can improve mental alertness.

and enhanced circulation to the brain. Improved mental clarity may also be the result of a calmer mind and activation of the sympathetic nervous system.

Reduced Anxiety and Depression

A consistent finding of research on massage is that it reduces anxiety significantly. Interestingly, this is true for both the receiver and the giver. It is also true for the general public, as well as for those with chronic diseases and those hospitalized for different reasons. Anxiety is measured through subjective self-reporting instruments, as well as the more objective measure of cortisol levels in saliva and urine. Anxiety reduction would be an expected result of the relaxation response and action of the parasympathetic nervous system. It may also be related to the release of endorphins (Field 2000; Kaard and Tostinbo 1989; Moyer, Rounds and Hannum 2004; Rich 2002).

Character Armor and Emotional Release

Wilhelm Reich (1897–1957) introduced the concept of *character armor,* or muscular tension caused by suppression of emotions. For example, unexpressed anger often causes tension in the muscles of the back and arms that would have been used to strike out. Or unexpressed grief may result in shallow breathing and stiffening of muscles used in crying. In the process of relaxing the affected muscles, the suppressed emotions may be felt by the recipient. Massage practitioners sometimes encounter such armoring and should be prepared to help the patient or client understand the release of emotions that sometimes happens.

A phenomenon called *emotional release* sometimes occurs during a massage session. Unexpressed emotions that are held in the receiver's body may come to the surface in various forms, such as tearfulness, anger, fear, grief, or laughter and joy. Although emotional release is a phenomenon familiar to many massage practitioners, relatively little is known about the mechanisms involved. It is possible that during deep relaxation, a person's natural psychological defenses are lowered, allowing him or her to feel or express emotions held inside.

> Since the unconscious mind is actively involved in controlling experience and emotional flow, thereby maintaining the status quo, alteration of a person's body-mind patterns can threaten or loosen unconscious control of feelings and memories. If this control weakens, then what is stored or blocked in the unconscious can surface to consciousness and may be expressed emotionally in the form we know as emotional release. (Greene and Goodrich-Dunn 2004, p. 111)

Some forms of massage and bodywork specifically address the emotions, and practitioners are trained to deal with issues brought up during emotional release. Releasing unexpressed emotions can be an important step in a physical or psychological healing process.

Massage practitioners should be considerate of their clients during an emotional release and be good listeners, but at the same time be mindful of their own scope of practice. Clients should be referred to other health professionals as needed to resolve deep emotional problems.

Feelings of General Well-Being

Stated in positive terms, massage is shown to increase feelings of general well-being. This likely involves the same mechanisms as anxiety reduction, that is, relaxation response and release of endorphins. Tactile pleasure associated with relaxation massage and simple caring touch may also contribute to feelings of well-being.

It is interesting to note that prolonged exposure to pain and other stressors has been shown to deplete the stores of endorphins, leading to an increased perception of pain and despair. To the extent that massage helps to manage pain and stress, and to release endorphins, it may contribute to a more positive outlook.

Limbic System

The concept of the *limbic system* helps shed light on how the physical and emotional components of a person are related and how body memories are created (see Figure 17.24 on page 000). From a physiological perspective, the limbic system is defined as follows:

> The limbic (LIM-bik) system includes several groups of neurons and tracts of white matter along the border (*limbus* means border) between the cerebrum and diencephalon. This system is concerned with (1) the sense of smell and (2) long-term memory storage. One part of the limbic system, the hippocampus, plays a vital role in learning and storage of long-term memories . . . The limbic system also includes centers within the hypothalamus responsible for (1) emotional states, such as rage, fear, and sexual arousal, and, (2) the control of reflexes that can be consciously activated such as . . . movements associated with eating. (Martini and Bartholomew 1999, p. 173)

Memory researchers have been able to trace the flow of information from touch receptors in the skin through the spinal cord and brain stem into different parts of the brain. This activates the limbic system to experience emotions related to touch and to create memories or images of tactile experiences (Knaster 1996, pp. 123–124).

There is the possibility, therefore, that memories are activated, as well as created, by touch. This has a variety of important implications for practitioners. For example, if the recipient of massage has experienced caring touch primarily in a sexual context, the touch of the practitioner might bring up feelings and memories that would be confusing and inappropriate during a session. Or a recipient who has been physically or sexually abused may have difficulty accepting healing touch without hardening against it. Touch through massage is sometimes used to help in the healing and recovery process.

CASE FOR STUDY

Jim Learns about the Benefits of Massage

Jim is in his mid-30s. He works on a computer most of the day and likes to play sports on the weekends. He is in good physical condition but is feeling tired and sore lately. His job is stressing him out, too. A friend has suggested that Jim add massage to his wellness routine. Jim says he needs to learn more about the good things massage would do for him.

Question:

What information about the effects of massage might convince Jim to make a massage appointment?

Things to consider:

- What are Jim's major needs, given what you know about him?

- Which effects at the tissue or organ system level might he be interested in?
- Do any organism level or psychological effects seem relevant in this case?

Write a brief description of the effects of massage that might convince Jim that making an appointment would be to his benefit.

_____

_____

_____

TABLE 7.3	Mechanisms to Explain the Effects of Massage
Effects	**Mechanisms and Examples**
Mechanical effects	The result of physical forces such as compression, stretching, shearing, broadening, and vibration of tissues; occurs on the gross level of physical structure
	Examples: venous return, lymph flow, breaking adhesions
Physiological effects	Organic processes of the body on cellular, tissue, or organ system levels
	Examples: activation of parasympathetic nervous system; release of mood enhancing hormones
Reflex effects	The result of pressure or movement in one part of the body having an effect in another part; also effects mediated through the nervous system
	Examples: muscle relaxation, increased mental clarity, pain reduction, normalizing system function
Body–mind effects	The result of the interplay of body, mind, and emotions in health and disease processes
	Examples: relaxation response, anxiety reduction
Energetic effects	The result of balancing or improving the flow of energy within and around the body
	Examples: removing energy restrictions, dispersing pooled energy, strengthening deficient energy

MECHANISMS OF MASSAGE

Several mechanisms have been identified to explain how the effects of massage are produced. Some of these theories are recognized within the Western biomedical model, whereas others are on the cutting edge of alternative and body–mind studies. The mechanisms presented here include mechanical, physiological, reflex, body–mind, and energetic. Table 7.3■ outlines the mechanisms used to explain the effects of massage.

Some effects are produced by more than one mechanism. For example, changes in local blood circulation during and after massage are thought to occur through direct physical and mechanical effects on vessels; circulatory changes mediated by the local release of vasodilator chemicals (e.g., histamine); or circulatory changes elicited by reflex responses of the autonomic nervous system to tissue stimulation (Yates 2004).

Furthermore, a specific massage technique may produce a number of different effects. This is a further example of the holistic nature of human beings and the complexity of effects produced by something seemingly as simple as massage.

Mechanical Effects

Mechanical effects are the result of physical forces of massage, such as compression, stretching, shearing, broadening, and vibration of body tissues. These effects occur on the more gross level of physical structure. Examples of mechanical effects include enhanced venous return from deep effleurage; elongation of muscles by stretching; increased lymph flow from kneading and deep effleurage; and breaking tissue adhesions with deep transverse friction or myofascial massage.

Physiological Effects

Physiological effects refer to organic processes of the body. These effects involve biochemical processes at the cellular level, but may also occur at the tissue and organ system levels. Examples of physiological effects include the various results of the relaxation response produced by activating the parasympathetic nervous system; decrease in anxiety by facilitating the release of mood enhancing hormones; and proper development and growth in infants assisted by the tactile stimulation that occurs during massage.

CRITICAL THINKING

Think about the many effects of massage on human beings at the organ system and organism levels (refer to Table 7.1 on page 000). Analyze the primary mechanisms involved in creating these effects (refer to Table 7.3 above).

1. Are some effects elicited by more than one mechanism?
2. How are the mechanisms of different effects and massage techniques related?

3. Why is it important for massage therapists to understand the effects and mechanisms of massage?

Reflex Effects

Andrade and Clifford explain **reflex effects** as functional change mediated by the nervous system (2001, p. 12). Sensory receptors in the skin and proprioceptors in muscles are stimulated by massage and joint movements, thereby eliciting reflex effects. Some examples of reflex effects are muscle relaxation, enhanced mental clarity, and pain reduction.

A different type of reflex effect forms the theoretical basis for a type of bodywork called *reflexology*. In this largely unexplained phenomenon, pressing or massaging one part of the body (e.g., ears, hands, or feet) is believed to have a normalizing effect on an entirely different part of the body. It is not clear if the apparent effects occur through the nervous system or some other mechanism. Chapter 18, Contemporary Massage and Bodywork, explains more about foot reflexology on page 536.

Body–Mind Effects

Body–mind effects result from the interplay of body, mind, and emotions in health and disease. This concept has a long tradition in natural healing, in most indigenous cultures, and in healing traditions of China and India. Western medical science is beginning to confirm demonstrable links between our physical bodies and our mental and emotional states. The new science of psychoneuroimmunology (PNI) has grown out of these studies.

The body–mind connection can be seen clearly in the relaxation response, a physiological process involving the parasympathetic nervous system. The relaxation response is elicited by practices such as meditation, which quiets the mind, or by the tactile stimulation of massage. Other examples of body–mind effects of massage include reduction in anxiety and release of unexpressed emotions held in the body.

Energetic Effects

Massage and bodywork have been described as balancing and improving the flow of energy, thus providing **energetic effects.** What this energy is and how it relates to the body are yet to be determined in terms of Western science. How-ever, there are ancient traditions of massage and bodywork, primarily from China and India, based on concepts of energy flow. Therapeutic Touch is a form of energy work adopted by many nurses that addresses the energy field of the recipient. Other popular forms of energy bodywork include polarity therapy and Reiki (Claire 1995).

There are a variety of theories about how energy flows in and around the body, and many practitioners and receivers report "feeling" energy. Energy work is currently outside of the understanding and general acceptance of Western biomedicine, but it has persisted over time and is found to be useful by many people.

BENEFITS OF MASSAGE

When the effects of massage support general health and well-being or the ongoing healing process, there are benefits by definition. A general wellness or health massage aims to normalize body tissues and to optimize function. Everyone can benefit from the health-promoting effects of wellness massage.

The main intention in a general wellness massage is to elicit the relaxation response, promote muscular relaxation, and to enhance circulation of fluids, digestion, and elimination. The effects of general relaxation alone have an impact on many physiological and psychological aspects of health and well-being. Massage also provides healthy touch, which is a basic human need.

The effects of massage may be especially beneficial for people with special needs. These benefits are the natural effects of a wellness massage tailored for each unique individual. For example, athletes, pregnant women, infants, the elderly, the terminally ill, and clients with psychological problems or physical disabilities may find specific benefits derived from massage sessions planned to address their special needs. See Chapter 20, Special Populations and Adaptations, on page 000, for more information on how the benefits of massage can improve the quality of life—both physiologically and psychologically—for many people.

CHAPTER HIGHLIGHTS

- *Effects of massage* refer to changes that occur in the body, mind, and emotions of the recipient during a massage session.
  - Effects of massage can be beneficial or detrimental depending on the circumstances.
  - Effects are beneficial if they have a positive impact and lead toward healing and greater wellness.
  - Massage is *indicated* if its effects are likely to be beneficial to a person with a specific medical condition.
  - Massage is *contraindicated* if its effects are likely to be harmful to a person with a specific medical condition.
- Time and dose are important considerations when describing the effects of massage applications.
  - Short-term effects are changes that occur during a massage session and last for a few hours or a day afterward.
  - Long-term effects are changes that occur during a massage session and last for a longer period, such as a few days or weeks.

- ○ Single-dose effects occur after one massage application.
- ○ Multiple-dose effects occur over time from repeated massage applications.
- Different massage techniques and different methods of application can produce very different outcomes from massage.
- Information about the physiological and psychological effects of massage comes from several different sources.
  - ○ These sources include tradition, personal observation and experience, understanding of human anatomy and physiology, and anecdotes from recipients.
  - ○ Scientific research is conducted to examine theories about the effects of massage.
    - Meta-analyses look at a number of different studies on a specific topic to discover consistent findings.
- A holistic view of effects of massage looks at connections of body, mind, and emotions.
  - ○ In touching the outermost part of the physical body, we are able to touch the innermost parts of our clients.
  - ○ Massage is called a body-centered therapy, since it works primarily through touch and movement to create its effects.
- Research literacy includes understanding the scientific method, locating and evaluating research articles, and gleaning practical information from research studies.
- Scientific research is based on observations about what actually happens, rather than taking the word of an authority or anecdotes from individuals.
  - ○ Different types of research studies offer weaker or stronger evidence of cause and effect.
  - ○ Comparing pre- and post-treatment measurements provides evidence that real change took place.
  - ○ Research studies may have flaws that make their findings less valid.
- Research studies can be located in research databases found on the Internet.
- Peer-reviewed journals contain credible research reports that have been evaluated by experts in the field.
- Massage improves the overall health of cells and tissues of the body.
  - ○ Massage can assist in the tissue repair process, especially in the regeneration and remodeling phases, but is contraindicated in the inflammatory phase.
  - ○ Massage causes connective tissues to become more fluid and pliable, and prevents some connective tissue abnormalities and dysfunction.
- Massage improves the overall function of organ systems.
  - ○ *Integumentary system*—Oil applied during massage moisturizes the skin; massage stimulates

sensory receptors; friction techniques assist in healthy scar formation.
  - ○ *Skeletal system*—Massage promotes good joint mobility and flexibility and proper alignment.
  - ○ *Muscular system*—Massage can reduce muscle stiffness and soreness after strenuous activity and relax hypertonic or tense muscles; massage alleviates some of the negative effects of underactivity and overactivity of the muscular system.
  - ○ *Nervous and endocrine systems*—Massage works through the nervous system to increase body awareness, relax muscles, and reduce pain.
    - Massage helps trigger the release of stress, anxiety, and pain reducing hormones, and of mood enhancing hormones.
  - ○ *Cardiovascular system*—Massage improves the function of the cardiovascular and lymphatic systems by helping to move fluids through the systems.
    - Massage produces hyperemia locally, and increases blood volume in an area.
    - Mechanical action of deep effleurage enhances venous flow.
    - Massage can play a part in decreasing blood pressure and increasing the number of circulating red blood cells.
  - ○ *Lymphatic system*—Massage can assist in movement of lymph fluid through the lymphatic system and enhances immunity.
  - ○ *Respiratory system*—Massage enhances general circulation, relaxing muscles of respiration and encouraging deep diaphragmatic breathing.
  - ○ *Digestive system*—Relaxation massage improves digestive system function, and abdominal massage is used to treat constipation.
  - ○ *Reproductive system*—Although this system is not ordinarily a target for massage, massage can indirectly improve its function through improved circulation and general relaxation.
    - Massage can address the needs of pregnant women.
    - Breast massage is a specialty used for well-breast health and as complementary treatment for breast cancer.
    - Men can experience a nonsexual erection during massage due to increased circulation in the groin area.
- Massage can have a positive effect at the whole organism level.
  - ○ Massage enhances growth and development of infants.
  - ○ Massage has pain reduction effects and can elicit the relaxation response.
  - ○ Psychological effects of massage include increased mental clarity, reduced anxiety,

emotional release, and increased feelings of general well-being.

- Mechanisms through which the effects of massage are produced include mechanical, physiological, reflex, body–mind, and energetic.

- Everyone can benefit from the general health-promoting effects of massage.
- Special populations also benefit from massage planned to address their special needs.

EXAM REVIEW

Key Terms

Match the following key terms to their descriptions. For additional study, look up the key terms in the Interactive Glossary on page 000 and note other terms that compare or contrast with them.

_____ **1.** Body–mind effects
_____ **2.** Effects of massage
_____ **3.** Energetic effects
_____ **4.** Hypothesis
_____ **5.** Long-term effects
_____ **6.** Mechanical effects
_____ **7.** Multiple-dose effects
_____ **8.** Peer-reviewed journals
_____ **9.** Physiological effects
_____ **10.** Reflex effects
_____ **11.** Research literacy
_____ **12.** Scientific method
_____ **13.** Short-term effects
_____ **14.** Single-dose effects

a. Changes that start during a massage session and last for a longer period of time, such as a few days or weeks

b. Effects that happen over time from repeated massage applications

c. Publish research that meets certain standards and that has been evaluated by experts in the field

d. Functional changes mediated by the nervous system such as muscle relaxation, enhanced mental clarity, and pain reduction

e. Organic processes of the body that occur at the biochemical, cellular, tissue, and organ system levels

f. Changes that occur during a massage session and may last for the time of the session and for a brief period afterward

g. Understanding the scientific method, locating and evaluating research articles, and gleaning practical information from research studies

h. Systematic way of testing theories through gathering and analyzing relevant information to see if it supports the theory in question

i. Effects that result from the interplay of body, mind, and emotions in health and disease

j. Changes that happen from one application of massage

k. Balancing and improving the flow of energy

l. An unproven theory about how something works or what will happen in a certain situation

m. Changes that occur in the body, mind, and emotions of the recipient as a result of soft tissue manipulation

n. The result of physical forces of massage, such as compression, stretching, shearing, broadening, and vibration of body tissues

Memory Workout

To test your memory of the main concepts in this chapter, complete the following sentences by circling the most correct answer from the two choices provided.

1. Massage promotes the overall health of tissues, primarily through increased blood and (lymph) (waste) circulation.
2. Evidence from scientific research accumulates over time as a (body of knowledge) (case series) is built up.
3. A systematic review of a number of different research studies looking at the same subject is called a (case study) (meta-analysis).
4. The capacity of research findings to be generalized to a larger group than the one that participated in the study is called (external) (internal) validity.
5. A quick overview of background, methods, results, conclusion, and keywords in a research report is found in the (abstract) (discussion).
6. During the remodeling phase of tissue repair, deep friction massage helps in healthy (scab) (scar) formation.
7. Joint movement techniques stimulate production of (synovial fluid) (lymph fluid).
8. Muscles that are tense and in a state of partial contraction are said to be (hypotonic) (hypertonic).
9. The (fight or flight) (relaxation) response occurs with activation of the parasympathetic nervous system, which has effects on skeletal muscles as well as several other organ systems.
10. A condition in which normal blood flow in the veins is slowed or halted is called (venous return) (venostasis).
11. Resistance to injuries and disease caused by foreign substances is called (immunity) (approximation).
12. There is evidence that massage can produce the release of neurochemicals called (analgesia) (endorphins) that induce relaxation and feelings of well-being.
13. Effects of massage that are the result of physical forces such as compression, stretching, and vibration of body tissues are called (physiological) (mechanical) effects.
14. Character (development) (armor) is a concept used to explain muscular tension caused by suppressed emotions.

Test Prep

The following multiple-choice questions will help to prepare you for future school and professional exams.

1. Changes that occur over time from repeated massage applications are called:
   a. Short-term effects
   b. Single-dose effects
   c. Multiple-dose effects
   d. Indications
2. Understanding the scientific method, and locating and evaluating research articles are essential skills of:
   a. Research literacy
   b. Massage literacy
   c. Principle-based therapy
   d. Treatment planning
3. The type of research study that offers the strongest evidence of cause and effect is the:
   a. Case series
   b. Case study
   c. Randomized controlled trial
   d. Meta-analysis
4. Elements within the design or execution of a research study that make it more or less credible affect the study's:
   a. External validity
   b. Internal validity
   c. External reliability
   d. Statistical significance
5. "Here's what I decided to do" explained in some detail can be found in which section of a research report?
   a. Abstract
   b. Introduction
   c. Methods
   d. Discussion
6. The section of a research report that speculates on why the massage application worked or did not work as hypothesized is the:
   a. Introduction
   b. Methods
   c. Results
   d. Discussion
7. What is the primary mechanism of massage techniques that remove adhesions in fascial tissues?
   a. Reflex
   b. Body–mind
   c. Mechanical
   d. Energetic
8. Which of the following explains how massage promotes muscle relaxation?
   a. By evoking the relaxation response
   b. By providing an environment for recipients to consciously let go of tension
   c. By creating increased sensory input
   d. All of the above

9. Superficial friction produces an increase in local circulation in the skin and underlying connective tissue. This effect is called:
   a. Ischemia
   b. Hyperemia
   c. Hypertonicity
   d. Immunity

10. Which of the following massage techniques most effectively enhance venous circulation?
    a. Petrissage and deep effleurage
    b. Passive touch and direct pressure
    c. Deep and superficial friction
    d. Vibration and tapotement

11. A holistic view understands human beings as:
    a. Divided into body and mind
    b. Whole persons in body, mind, and spirit
    c. Separated into tissues and organ systems
    d. Body-centered beings with a mind

12. Which of the following statements about breast massage is *not* correct?
    a. Breast massage is a skill that requires specialized training.
    b. Breast massage is contraindicated for women undergoing treatment for breast cancer.
    c. Breast massage requires informed consent from the client.
    d. Breast massage may be beyond the legal scope of practice for some practitioners.

13. Massage techniques that promote better blood circulation are used to address a condition called:
    a. Ischemia
    b. Fibrosis
    c. Hyperemia
    d. Adhesion

14. Effects of massage that involve biochemical processes at the cellular, tissue, and organ system levels are called:
    a. Reflex effects
    b. Physiological effects
    c. Energetic effects
    d. Mechanical effects

15. What is the greatest benefit for infants of the tactile stimulation of regular massage?
    a. Better digestion
    b. Improved circulation
    c. Normal growth and development
    d. More relaxed muscles

Video Challenge

Watch the appropriate segment of the video on your DVD and then answer the following questions.

Effects of Massage

Goal-Oriented 6-Step Planning

1. How is knowledge of the effects of massage used in goal-oriented planning?

2. How might awareness of single-dose and multiple-dose effects influence a long-term plan for massage to treat a certain condition?

3. At what point in goal-oriented planning might you want to read research studies on the effects of massage?

Comprehension Exercises

The following short answer questions test your knowledge and understanding of chapter topics and provide practice in written communication skills. Explain in two to four complete sentences.

1. Explain how massage reduces pain using the neural-gating mechanism theory.

2. Explain the origin of the connection between skin, brain, and nervous system.

3. Name the parts of a research report and briefly describe the contents of each part.

For Greater Understanding

The following exercises are designed to take you from the realm of theory into the real world. They will help give you a deeper understanding of the subjects covered in this chapter. Action words are underlined to emphasize the variety of activities presented to address different learning styles and to encourage deeper thinking.

1. <u>Write</u> a brief personal health history for the past one or two years. Using the information in this chapter, <u>identify</u> any areas that might have benefited (or did benefit) from receiving massage. <u>Discuss</u> your conclusions with a study partner or group.

2. <u>Choose</u> one particular effect of massage to study in more depth. <u>Search</u> several sources for further information, including anatomy and physiology textbooks and research databases. <u>Discuss</u> your findings with a study partner or group.

3. <u>Choose</u> one research study to read, analyze, and evaluate. <u>Present</u> your findings and conclusions to a study partner or group.

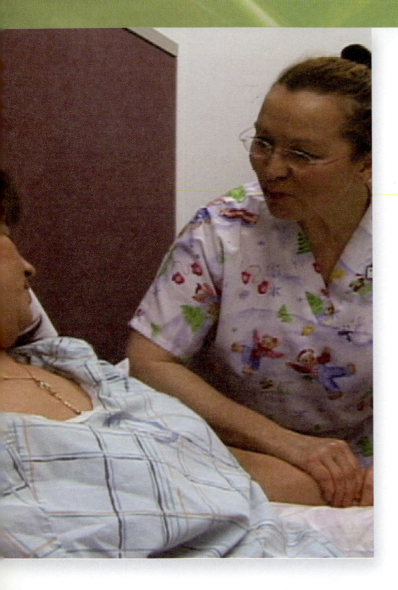

 CHAPTER OUTLINE

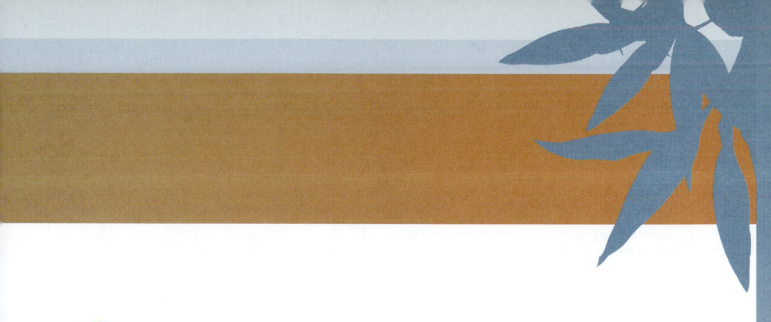

LEARNING OUTCOMES

After studying this chapter, you will have information to:

1. Define clinical massage therapy.
2. Explain the importance of evidence-based practice.
3. Explain the theory of client-centered massage.
4. Discuss different clinical approaches to massage.
5. Describe the benefits of massage in treatment of various pathologies.
6. Describe Therapeutic Touch and its healing potential.
7. Explain how massage is used to complement chiropractic care.

KEY TERMS

Client-centered massage *282*

Clinical massage therapy *282*

Direct therapeutic effects *283*

Evidence-based practice *282*

Indirect therapeutic effects *283*

Palliative care *283*

Principle-based therapy *282*

Recipe-based massage *282*

Therapeutic Touch *289*

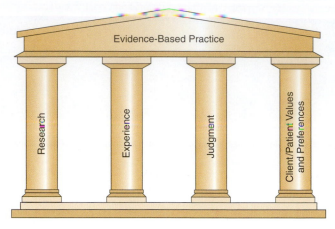

FIGURE 8.1

Four foundations of evidence-based practice.

MASSAGE *in* ACTION

On your DVD, explore:
- Documentation and SOAP Notes

CLINICAL MASSAGE THERAPY

Massage has been used to treat human ailments since ancient times and is currently being integrated into a number of medical settings as an effective therapy. The term **clinical massage therapy** describes applications of massage in the treatment of human pathologies.

Clinical massage therapy is not a technique or group of techniques. It includes Western massage, as well as specialized manual therapies that address specific tissues and organ systems. It also includes forms of energy bodywork and manual therapies from non-Western health care such as traditional Chinese medicine. Medical offices, hospitals, rehabilitation and sports medicine clinics, nursing homes, and medical spas are typical clinical settings. Some private massage practices specialize in clinical applications. Massage therapists working in clinical settings must understand the operating procedures there and develop the required skills, such as charting and note-taking.

Clinical applications require massage therapists to have greater knowledge of human pathology, how the body heals, and the effects of various medications. It is also important to know current standard and alternative treatments for pathologies being addressed, and to have an awareness of possible contraindications. Pathology textbooks written specifically for massage therapists are useful resources that contain information describing common ailments and their treatments, as well as contraindications and recommendations for massage therapy. Some of these books are listed in Appendix H, References and Additional Resources, on page A-67.

For clinical applications, it is essential to understand the effects that different massage techniques have and how to apply them for the greatest therapeutic benefit in each individual case. The growing interest in massage for treatment has led to an increased number of research studies about its efficacy. See page 257 in Chapter 7, Effects of Massage, for a discussion about research and its value to the practice of massage therapy.

EVIDENCE-BASED PRACTICE

In the emerging integrative health care scene, those therapies that are supported by scientific research are more likely to be used. This is called **evidence-based practice**, because research provides some verifiable objective evidence for the effectiveness of certain therapies. As stated in the Foreword to *Touch Therapy*:

One of the principal requirements of modern health care provision can be summed up by the term,

"evidence-based." It is no longer sufficient for any therapeutic approach to simply rely on a long history of use, or popularity, or widespread availability, to justify its continued acceptance (especially if insurance reimbursement is anticipated). (Field 2000, pp. vii)

Evidence from scientific studies can more clearly substantiate the benefits of massage in treating certain diseases, as well as identify contraindications. Applications of clinical massage therapy will become safer and more effective as the result of research.

The best evidence-based practice also takes into consideration the practitioner's experience and judgment, as well as the recipient's values and preferences. These factors taken together provide a more comprehensive view of what approach might be most effective for a particular individual. Figure 8.1■ shows the four foundations of evidence-based practice.

CLIENT-CENTERED MASSAGE

Knowledge gained from research is also essential to **client-centered massage**, which focuses on the client's unique situation, needs, and goals as the basis for treatment planning. This is in contrast to formula or **recipe-based massage**, in which every client receives exactly the same treatment (i.e., the same techniques applied in the same way) for a particular medical condition.

Client-centered massage is a form of **principle-based therapy** as described by Yates. The foundation of principle-based therapy is the creation of an overall treatment plan directed toward the achievement of specific treatment goals. Such a plan takes into consideration the pathology being treated, the condition of the individual, and most important, the therapeutic potential of different treatment methods. Principle-based therapy allows for variation:

Appropriate treatment techniques and modalities are selected, integrated, and adapted as necessary to

TABLE 8.1	Important Concepts in Clinical Massage Therapy
Concept	**Explanation**
Clinical massage therapy	Applications of massage in the treatment of human pathologies; sometimes referred to as medical massage therapy.
Evidence-based practice	Use of massage based on verifiable objective evidence such as scientific research.
Client-centered massage	Treatment planning based on the client's unique situation, needs, and goals; opposite of recipe-based massage.
Principle-based therapy	Treatment planning directed toward achievement of specific goals; takes into consideration the pathology, the client's condition, and the therapeutic potential of different treatment methods.
Recipe-based massage	Treatment based on predetermined formula or protocol for a specific pathology or condition; opposite of client-based massage.

achieve specific effects and are modified according to the changing physiological and psychological state of the patient as treatment proceeds. Treatment is therefore patient-centered rather than technique-centered. (Yates 1999, pp. 3–4)

Research can help sort out which massage techniques and approaches are most effective for clinical applications. However, research is most useful for adding to our understanding of the applications of massage, not as a means for developing recipes for treatment. There is room for consideration of research, experience, and the client in the client-centered practice of clinical massage therapy. A summary of important concepts in clinical massage therapy appears in Table 8.1■.

THERAPEUTIC APPROACHES

Approaches to clinical massage therapy and the research that supports its use are focused on its therapeutic outcomes. These approaches can be thought of as falling into three major categories: direct therapeutic effects, indirect therapeutic effects, and palliative care.

Direct therapeutic effects of clinical massage focus on the healing of a diagnosed medical condition, or easing of its symptoms. An example would be the use of deep transverse friction in treating repetitive strain injuries. Another is massage for healthy nervous system development and weight gain in preterm infants. Massage may be used to help manage chronic conditions such as asthma and autism. In these cases, massage may be the primary treatment approach, but is more often part of a multifaceted plan of care. This approach is frequently found in integrative and alternative health care settings.

Indirect therapeutic effects of clinical massage focus on enhancing the effectiveness of a primary treatment, or creating a more favorable environment for healing. For example, massage is used to help reduce anxiety, thereby improving the body's immune response. Massage may also help alleviate some of the negative effects of a primary treatment, for example, massage used to reduce nausea associated with some cancer treatments. In these cases, massage may be considered to be complementary health care.

In **palliative care**, massage is used to ease discomfort and to improve the quality of life for those with chronic medical conditions or terminal illness. Palliative care is provided for hospitalized or institutionalized patients. For example, massage has been suggested to help reduce the dehumanizing effects of nursing homes. It is also used in hospice care for a variety of outcomes, including positive physical, psychological, and social effects.

Although these categories are not mutually exclusive in all situations, they offer a way to sort out the intention behind clinical massage applications. They answer the question, What does massage contribute to the healing of this medical

CRITICAL THINKING

Locate a scientific research report about a clinical application of massage. Read, analyze, and evaluate the study reported. Read each section carefully to understand the researcher's approach to the study and the results. Refer to Table 7.2, Science as Conversation: Telling a Story on page 259.

1. What was the researcher trying to find out about massage? What was the hypothesis?

2. How did the researcher go about testing the hypothesis? What was the research method?

3. What did the research find out? What were the results?

4. What do the findings mean for clinical massage applications?

TABLE 8.2	Approaches to Clinical Massage Therapy
Approach	**Description**
Direct therapeutic effects	Focus on the healing of a diagnosed medical condition, or easing of its symptoms; alternative or integrated health care.
Indirect therapeutic effects	Focus on enhancing the effectiveness of a primary treatment, or creating a more favorable environment for healing; complementary health care.
Palliative care	Focus on easing discomfort and improving the quality of life for those with chronic medical conditions or terminal illness; often provided for hospitalized or institutionalized patients.

condition or to the well-being of this client/patient? A summary of these therapeutic approaches to clinical massage therapy can be found in Table 8.2■.

The remainder of this chapter discusses some of the uses of massage in medical settings and some of the promising research that has been done on its clinical applications. It is just a sampling of the growing amount of information available and points to areas where the study of the clinical applications of massage has been strong.

MUSCULOSKELETAL APPLICATIONS

Massage is routinely incorporated into the rehabilitation of musculoskeletal injuries by physical therapists, athletic trainers, and massage therapists (Figure 8.2■). It is also frequently used as a complement to chiropractic care.

Massage is particularly effective in relieving muscle tension, increasing flexibility and range of motion, promoting healthy connective tissue, and reducing muscular pain. These direct therapeutic effects on the muscular system were discussed in Chapter 7, Effects of Massage, on page 263.

Deep transverse friction has been especially effective in the treatment of repetitive strain injuries (RSI) such as tendinitis/tenosynovitis (i.e., inflammation of tendons and tendon sheaths) and bursitis (i.e., inflammation of the fluid sacs around joints). Deep friction techniques increase local circulation, help separate adhesions, and have an analgesic or pain-reducing effect (de Bruijin 1984; Hammer 1993).

Pain caused by hypertonic muscles can be relieved with massage. For example, chronic tension headaches caused by tense and shortened cervical muscles have been successfully treated using a combination of Western massage, myofascial release, and trigger point therapy (Puustjarvi, Airaksinen, and Pontinen 1990; Quinn, Chandler, and Moraska 2002). Massage has also been effective in treating subacute chronic low back pain (Preyde 2000; Cherkin et al. 2001). These findings are particularly encouraging because tension headaches and low back pain afflict so many people in the modern world.

Neuromuscular and myofascial massage are specialized techniques that relieve myofascial pain and dysfunction. Chapter 18, Contemporary Massage and Bodywork, discusses myofascial massage on page 520 and trigger point therapy on page 524 in more detail.

Fibromyalgia

Fibromyalgia syndrome (FMS) is a chronic condition characterized by widespread muscle pain and stiffness, and tenderness at specific body sites (see Figure 6.51 on page 162). The pain and fatigue associated with FMS can be debilitating. Other common symptoms of this syndrome are disturbed sleep, severe headaches, and osteoarthritis. Mental and emotional problems such as anxiety and depression often accompany FMS. Although there is no known cure for FMS, massage can address many of its symptoms. The general effects of massage that offer relief are reduction of stress and anxiety, more restful sleep, more positive outlook, improved

FIGURE 8.2

Massage is routinely incorporated into the rehabilitation of musculoskeletal injuries.

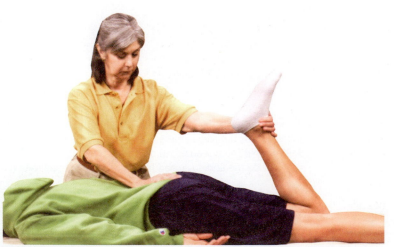

circulation, and relief for sore and stiff muscles (Sunshine et al. 1996; Field 2000).

CARDIOVASCULAR AND LYMPHATIC APPLICATIONS

Relaxation massage may be beneficial in treating some cardiovascular pathologies, such as hypertension (high blood pressure) and cardiac arrhythmia (Longworth 1982; Curtis 1994). It not only reduces heart rate and blood pressure, but also reduces anxiety, which helps give the patient a more positive outlook and improved feelings of well-being. These particular effects of massage are supported in a meta-analysis of massage research studies (Moyer, Rounds, and Hannum 2004).

A study by nurses Bauer and Dracup (1987) found that back massage consisting of effleurage had a positive effect on the perception of relaxation and comfort reported by patients with acute myocardial infarction. Although they could not confirm improvement in the pathology, the massage had no apparent detrimental effects.

In another study, patients hospitalized in a cardiovascular unit of a large medical center in New York City who received Therapeutic Touch had a significantly greater reduction in anxiety scores than those who received casual touch or no touch (Heidt 1981). A fuller discussion of Therapeutic Touch can be found later in this chapter.

Edema and Lymphedema

Edema, or excess interstitial fluid in the tissues, is not a disease, but rather a condition of fluid buildup or swelling. It may be caused by injury, tissue damage, inflammation, or poor circulation. The edema itself can cause pain from increased fluid pressure and the buildup of toxins in the tissues. Safe massage applications for edema require knowledge of the reason for the condition since some types of swelling are contraindications for massage. For example, circulatory massage is contraindicated in cases of heart failure, kidney disease, and liver congestion (Premkumar 1999; Werner 2005).

Traumatic edema occurs with minor muscular injuries such as strains and sprains. It is "localized swelling of tissue associated with soft tissue injury and the exertion of exercise." Lymphatic facilitation techniques can be used effectively for treatment of traumatic edema (Archer 2007). See page 529 in Chapter 18, Contemporary Massage and Bodywork, for more information about lymphatic facilitation techniques.

Lymphedema is a specific type of edema caused by lymphatic system defect or damage (see Figure 6.82 on page 188). Primary lymphedema results from congenital or hereditary defects. Secondary lymphedema occurs when nodes or vessels are damaged by trauma, surgery, infection, radiation, or chemotherapy (Kelly 2002). Manual lymphatic drainage (MLD) techniques have been developed as part of complete decongestive therapy to address lymphedema specifically.

The beneficial effects of manual lymph drainage for patients with chronic and postmastectomy lymphedema continues to be confirmed. Lymphatic massage in these cases is for management of the condition and must be received regularly for long-term benefit (Kurz et al. 1978; Zanolla, Monzeglio, Balzarini, and Martino 1984; Badger 1986; Bunce et al. 1994).

Immune Function

One of the basic positive effects of massage is improvement in immune function, as noted in Chapter 7, Effects of Massage, on page 266. One of the first major studies to link massage and improved immunity was conducted by the Touch Research Institute in 1996. In a group of HIV-positive men who received daily massage for a month, the majority had significant increase in the number and activity of natural killer (NK) cells. The men showed reduced anxiety and stress, lower cortisol levels, as well as increased serotonin levels during the month of massage.

Given that elevated stress hormones (catecholamines and cortisol) negatively affect immune function, the increase in NK cell activity probably derived from the decrease in these stress hormones following massage therapy (Field 2000, pp. 201–205).

To the extent that massage helps reduce stress and thus improves immune function, it can be considered an important disease prevention measure. Health problems caused by compromised immunity include frequent infections, autoimmune disorders, and possibly, cancer (Corwin 1996; Field 2000).

RESPIRATORY APPLICATIONS

Massage is used as a complementary therapy for people with respiratory conditions such as chronic bronchitis, emphysema, and asthma. The benefits of massage for these patients include anxiety reduction and relaxation that deepens breathing patterns, relaxation and lengthening of muscles tense from labored breathing, and reduced fatigue overall. Passive movement of the rib cage, as well as percussion on the back and chest, can help loosen mucus for more productive coughs.

Children with asthma have been the subjects of several recent research projects. In one study, children with asthma were found to have lower anxiety, improved attitude toward the asthma condition, and increased peak airflow after regular massage by their parents. Over a 1-month period, these children had fewer asthma attacks. The study suggested that daily massage may lead to improved airway tone, decreased airway irritability, and better control of asthma in children (Field 2000).

In another study, patients with asthma, bronchitis, and emphysema received a form of bodywork called Trager Psychophysical Integration®, which consists of gentle, painless, passive movements. Focus was on the neck, abdomen, and chest wall. After treatment, improvement was found in forced vital capacity, respiratory rate, and chest expansion. Patients reported general relaxation and decrease in anxiety and tension (Witt and MacKinnon 1986).

An increase in thoracic gas volume, peak flow, and forced vital capacity was found in four out of five chronic obstructive pulmonary disease (COPD) patients receiving a combination of massage and myofascial trigger point therapy. The trigger point techniques were specifically directed to improve the function of chronically hypertonic muscles involved in breathing (Beeken et al. 1998).

Note that the studies cited here used different massage therapy approaches to achieve their positive results. The overall objectives were to reduce stress, improve diaphragmatic breathing, and relax and lengthen the muscles of respiration. Studies help identify specific techniques that are effective for these goals.

BACK MASSAGE FOR HOSPITALIZED PATIENTS

The ability of massage to reduce anxiety, promote restful sleep, and manage pain accounts for much of its value as a complement to standard medical treatment in hospitals and nursing homes. Back massage in particular has been found useful in caring for patients hospitalized for a variety of conditions (Figure 8.3■). For example, back massage was found to be effective in promoting sleep in critically ill patients. It has been suggested as an alternative or adjunct to sleep medications in some cases (Culpepper-Richards 1998).

A randomized control study conducted in Veteran's Administration (VA) hospitals found back massage to be useful for patients who had just undergone major surgery.

Patients who received 20 minutes of effleurage on the back daily experienced short term decrease in pain intensity and unpleasantness. They also had a faster rate of decrease of pain intensity and unpleasantness over the first 4 postoperative days than the control group, which did not receive massage (Mitchinson et al. 2007).

Back massage was also found to be an effective, noninvasive technique for promoting relaxation and improving communication with elderly, institutionalized patients. The nurses who conducted the study noted the potential of massage for reducing the common dehumanizing effects of institutional care (Frazer and Kerr, 1993). Those results confirmed the results of a previous study of slow-stroke back rub for older adults by two nurses, Fakouri and Jones (1987).

MASSAGE FOR CANCER PATIENTS

Massage was once listed as a general contraindication for cancer patients. It is now recognized as a valuable complementary therapy. Cancer patients who receive massage are reporting relief from a number of physical, mental, and emotional discomforts related to the disease and its treatment (Walton 2006).

General benefits of massage especially important to cancer patients include reduced stress and anxiety, improved sleep, improved immune system function, pain relief, and the comfort of caring touch (Rhiner, Ferrell, Ferrell, and Grant 1993; Sims 1986; Weinrich and Weinrich 1990).

Cancer patients who undergo surgery may benefit from the effects of massage related to faster recovery from anesthesia, faster wound healing, separation of adhesions around incisions, healthy scar formation, and reduction of edema

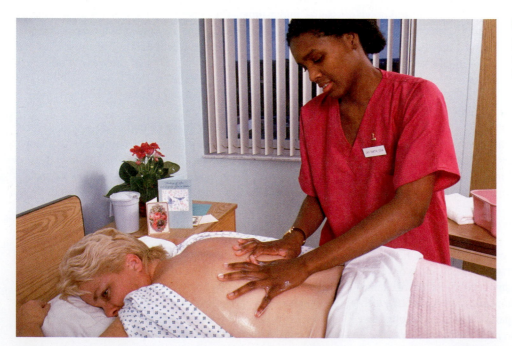

FIGURE 8.3

Massage is used as a complement to standard medical treatment in hospitals and nursing homes.

and lymphedema. Massage has also been linked to reduced pain and less need for pain medication. Hospitalized patients find relief from muscle soreness caused by prolonged bed rest. Improved circulation from massage helps prevent pressure and bed sores.

In one study, nurses examined the effects of therapeutic massage on hospitalized cancer patients. Primary techniques used were effleurage, petrissage, and trigger point therapy. They found that massage therapy significantly reduced the patients' perceived levels of pain and anxiety while enhancing their feelings of relaxation. Objective physiological measures (i.e., heart rate, respiratory rate, and blood pressure) tended to decrease, providing further indication of relaxation (Ferrell-Torry and Glick 1993).

Massage has also been found to reduce some of the negative side effects of radiation and chemotherapy, such as fatigue, nausea, diarrhea, loss of appetite, and insomnia (MacDonald 1995). However, the timing of massage in relation to treatment can be important; for example, the patient may be overtaxed and negative side effects worsened if massage is received too soon after a bout of chemotherapy.

The benefits of massage on the emotional level can be significant. Massage can help a cancer patient deal with depression and offer pleasant social interaction providing relief from isolation. It can help re-establish a positive body image and reclaim the body as an ally. It empowers patients to participate in their healing process and helps rebuild hope (Chamness 1996; Hernandez-Reif et al. 2004).

Breast massage is increasing in use as a clinical application for women who have experienced breast cancer. It is especially useful for postmastectomy patients, including for general wound healing, healthy scar formation, and treating lymphedema (Bunce et al. 1994; Curties 1999a, 1999b).

The concern about massage causing metastasis, or that massage may spread cancer, is still real in some cases. For example, massage should be avoided completely around the site of a tumor or where a tumor has recently been removed.

Massage practitioners should consult the patient's physician to assess the potential for harm from massage and to get advice on how to proceed safely (Walton 2006).

PEDIATRIC APPLICATIONS

Massage is being used increasingly in the care of hospitalized children, from infants to adolescents. Many of the uses of massage in pediatric care are similar to uses for adults (e.g., rehabilitation and anxiety reduction). A unique benefit for infants is the tactile stimulation provided by massage, which is essential for proper growth and development.

Much of the recent interest in massage for children has been generated by the work of Tiffany Field, PhD, who founded the Touch Research Institute (TRI) in 1991 at the University of Miami School of Medicine, Department of Pediatrics. The research being performed at TRI on a variety of pediatric conditions can be reviewed on their website (www.miami.edu/touch-research).

Preterm Infants

Building on research done in the 1970s, Field found that preterm infants who received tactile stimulation during their stays in transitional care nursery settings experienced greater weight gain, increased motor activity, more alertness, and improved performance on the Brazelton Neonatal Behavioral Assessment Scale. Tactile stimulation was applied by gentle stroking of the head and neck, across the shoulders, from upper back to the waist, from the thighs to the feet, and from the shoulders to the hands. Additional stimulation was provided by passive flexion/extension movements of the arms and legs (Field et al. 1986).

Subsequent research has shown that massage also benefits cocaine-exposed preterm infants. In addition to better weight gain, massaged infants showed significantly fewer postnatal complications and stress behaviors than the control infants did (Wheeden et al. 1993).

PRACTICAL APPLICATION

Investigate the uses of massage in the treatment of a particular pathology. Look at a variety of resources to locate information, for example, pathology textbooks, books about massage and/or the pathology, research reports, massage therapists with relevant experience, and other credible sources.

1. Is massage used for its direct therapeutic effects? Indirect effects? Palliative care?

2. What specific techniques are applied for the desired outcomes?
3. Are there contraindications or cautions to be aware of?
4. How would you defend the use of massage in the treatment of this pathology as evidence-based therapy?

Additional Pediatric Applications

A review of some of the research being done at TRI demonstrates the broad range of situations in which massage is found to be a useful treatment for children. Descriptions of the research for the results below, and for many other studies, can be found in the book *Touch Therapy* by Tiffany Field (2000) and on the TRI website (www.miami.edu/touch-research).

- *Asthmatic children.* Twenty-minute massages given to asthmatic children by their mothers for 1 month resulted in decreased anxiety levels and improved mood for both children and parents; the children's cortisol levels decreased; and they had fewer asthma attacks and were able to breathe better.

- *Autistic children.* After 1 month of massage therapy, the autistic children were less touch sensitive, less distracted by sounds, more attentive in class, related more to their teachers, and received better scores on the Autism Behavior Checklist and on the Early Social Communications Scales.

- *Diabetic children.* A pilot study showed that as a result of massage given to diabetic children by their parents, both children and parents showed lower anxiety and less depressed mood levels; the children's insulin and food regulation scores improved, and blood glucose levels decreased to the normal range.

- *Depressed adolescent mothers.* After 10 massage sessions over a 5-week period, depressed adolescent mothers reported lower anxiety; showed behavioral and stress hormone changes, including decreases in anxious behavior and in pulse and salivary cortisol levels; and a decrease in urine cortisol levels, suggesting lower stress levels.

- *Infants of depressed adolescent mothers.* Full-term infants born to depressed adolescent mothers were given 15 minutes of massage twice a week for 6 weeks. These infants gained more weight; showed greater improvement on emotionality, sociability, and soothability temperament dimensions, and on face-to-face interaction ratings; and had greater decreases in urinary stress catecholamines/hormones (norepinephrine, epinephrine, cortisol) than the control infants who were simply rocked.

- *Children with posttraumatic stress disorder.* Children traumatized by Hurricane Andrew were massaged at their schools twice a week for 1 month. The massaged children had less depression, lower anxiety levels, and lower cortisol (stress hormone) levels than children in the control group.

Although further research is needed to substantiate much of what has been found to date, massage appears to be a promising adjunct to treatment of children with a variety of disorders.

REALITY CHECK

ANTONIA

JERMAINE: I'm interested in working with clients in a substance abuse rehabilitation facility, but don't feel qualified right now. We learned a little in school, but not enough for me to feel confident. What can I do to gain the knowledge and skills needed for this career goal?

ANTONIA: Entry level training usually does not go very deeply into any of the wide variety of clinical applications of massage. For your career goal, I'd suggest a multifaceted approach. First look for articles on the subject in professional publications and in the index of books, and read them for background understanding. At the same time, search for relevant studies in massage research databases. Once you have this foundation, look for continuing education related to massage and substance abuse. Also try to interview a massage therapist working with this population. Locate a facility that fits your future employment goal and find out if they hire massage therapists and what qualifications they are looking for. A volunteer or internship position at a rehab facility might be a good place to get some experience and training. Or you might work with outpatient clients to begin learning about their characteristics and needs. Rather than learning additional massage techniques, it probably will be more important to learn how to apply techniques you already know to achieve the goals of this population, to keep proper boundaries, and to avoid some of the pitfalls of working in this setting. By reading, searching, interviewing, and getting some experience, you will eventually feel confident and ready to find the position you seek.

PSYCHOLOGICAL CLINICAL APPLICATIONS

Massage is sometimes used to address the psychological and emotional problems of patients receiving medical treatment. For example, several of the studies mentioned in this chapter found massage to be beneficial in the reduction of the anxiety of patients hospitalized for serious medical conditions.

Massage may also help in the treatment of patients with medical conditions significantly worsened by stress. For example, in a study by Joachim (1983), patients with chronic inflammatory bowel disease, ulcerative colitis, or Crohn's disease (ileitis) who received massage for relaxation had fewer episodes of pain and disability from the disease.

Massage may also help patients hospitalized for psychiatric reasons. In a study by Field et al. (1992), hospitalized depressed and adjustment-disorder children and adolescents who received massage were less depressed and anxious and had lower saliva cortisol levels (an indication of less depression) than patients who watched relaxation videotapes.

Psychotherapy patients not hospitalized may also benefit from the effects of massage related to stress and anxiety reduction, improved body awareness, and the ability to receive pleasurable nonsexual touch. For example, some massage therapists work with psychotherapists in the treatment of survivors of sexual and physical abuse. Massage has been found to be beneficial in helping these patients reconnect with their bodies, develop a more compassionate relationship with their physical being, and experience their bodies as a "source of groundedness and eventually of strength and even pleasure—good things instead of bad things" (Benjamin 1995, p. 28).

Reduction of depression and state anxiety were two of the effects of massage confirmed in a meta-analysis of massage research. A course of treatment for these conditions was seen to provide "benefits similar in magnitude to those of psychotherapy" (Moyer et al. 2004, p. 3).

THERAPEUTIC TOUCH

Therapeutic Touch is a form of manual therapy in which the energy field of the recipient is rebalanced, thus promoting health and healing. Although it does not fall directly into the category of soft tissue massage, it is performed by many massage practitioners and integrated into their work. It has found special acceptance by nurses, who find it effective in caring for patients.

Therapeutic Touch was developed by Dolores Krieger, PhD, RN, in the 1970s. She explains the technique as one of centering; then placing the hands in the recipient's energy field to detect a break in energy flow, pressure, or dysrhythmias; then rebalancing or repatterning the energy field by sweeping hand movements a few inches above the skin. She explains what happens as a profound relaxation response that has a positive effect on the immune system, which allows self-healing to reassert itself (Karpen 1995).

Kreiger explains that Therapeutic Touch has been found to have more effect on some conditions than others. For example, it seems to have a positive effect in working with fluid and electrolyte imbalances, dysfunctions of the autonomic nervous system, lymphatic and circulatory dysfunctions, and musculoskeletal problems. She further explains that:

Some collagen dysfunctions respond, such as rheumatoid arthritis, but lupus is resistant. Within the endocrine system, the thyroid, adrenals, and ovaries respond, but there is little success with the pituitary and variable success with the pancreas in treating diabetes. In psychiatric disorders, manic depressives and catatonics

---

CASE FOR STUDY

Marty Applies Massage for PTSD

Marty has a client who was diagnosed with posttraumatic stress disorder (PTSD). The client was referred for massage by her doctor, who thought that massage might be good to reduce stress and anxiety. Marty does not know much about PTSD but has an appointment with the client in a few days.

Question:

How can Marty find out about PTSD and massage in order to provide a safe environment for the client and apply massage most effectively?

Things to consider:

- Where can Marty go to find out about PTSD and its treatment?
- How can Marty find out if massage has been used successfully in the treatment of PTSD?

- What might the potential therapeutic outcomes be? The contraindications or cautions?
- What massage approaches or techniques are important to know for this clinical application?
- What are Marty's professional boundaries related to scope of practice in this situation?

Put yourself in Marty's shoes and prepare for this client with PTSD. From what you found out, what would be your general approach to the massage session? What cautions would you observe?

_____

_____

_____

respond, but there has been little success with schizophrenics. (Karpen 1995, pp. 142–146)

Therapeutic Touch was found to have potential in the treatment of tension headache pain (Keller and Bzdek, 1986). Therapeutic Touch has also been used successfully to help reduce the stress of hospitalized children (Kramer 1990). Research and articles about Therapeutic Touch can be found in nursing journals such as the *American Journal of Nursing* and *Nursing Research*. Further information about Therapeutic Touch research is available from Nurse Healers–Professional Associates (NH–PA), which was established in 1977 under the leadership of Dolores Kreiger (see Appendix A, 25 Forms of Therapeutic Massage and Bodywork, on page A-1). The NH–PA is a voluntary, nonprofit cooperative whose international exchange network facilitates the exchange of research findings, teaching strategies, and developments in the clinical practice of Therapeutic Touch (www.therapeutic-touch.org).

COMPLEMENT TO CHIROPRACTIC CARE

Chiropractic care is gaining recognition as an effective treatment for certain conditions, especially back pain. Massage is often given as a complement to chiropractic care to help prepare the body for chiropractic adjustments, to relieve tension and pain in muscles and related soft tissues, and to prevent future musculoskeletal misalignment.

The term *chiropractic adjustment* is used here to mean a technique in which bones and joints are manipulated to return the body to proper alignment. This often involves a forceful thrusting movement or manipulation. Such adjustments are performed on subluxations, a condition of misalignment in a joint, which often results in structural, nervous system, and chemical dysfunctions.

Local massage is sometimes used in preparation for an adjustment. Massage relieves muscle tension and warms up the soft tissues in the area, making joints more pliable and more easily adjusted. Massage may be given along with heat and ultrasound in this preparatory routine.

A general massage (30–60 minutes long) may also be good preparation for an adjustment. In addition to preparing the immediate area of concern, it helps induce general relaxation and accustoms the recipient to touch. The recipient may be more receptive to other hands-on treatment in such a relaxed state. Massage after an adjustment may help the muscles remain relaxed and prevent a tightening reaction to the treatment. Regular massage may help adjustments last longer by keeping muscles relaxed and lengthened.

Therapeutic massage may also be used to address some of the muscular problems that bring patients for adjustments. These include nerve constriction due to tight muscles, poor circulation, trigger points, damaged tissues, and the pain–spasm–pain cycle. Massage used with ice can help relieve muscles in spasm. Recent research shows massage to be an effective treatment for low back pain (Cherkin et al. 2001; Preyde 2000).

CHAPTER HIGHLIGHTS

- Clinical massage therapy refers to applications of massage for the treatment of pathologies.
- Client-centered massage puts the client's unique situation, needs, and goals as the focus of treatment planning.
  - This is in contrast to recipe-based massage, in which every client receives exactly the same treatment for a particular medical condition.
- Principle-based therapy takes into consideration the pathology being treated, the condition of the individual, and the therapeutic potential of different treatment methods.
- Approaches to clinical massage therapy are focused on its therapeutic outcomes.
  - Three major categories of approaches are direct therapeutic approaches, indirect therapeutic approaches, and palliative care.
- Massage has been found effective in relieving many musculoskeletal conditions, such as repetitive strain injuries, tension headaches, low back pain, and symptoms of fibromyalgia.

- Massage is used in treatment of cardiovascular and lymphatic disorders such as hypertension, edema, and lymphedema.
- Massage improves immune function, which is important in the treatment of many diseases.
- Massage is a useful complementary therapy for people with respiratory conditions, such as chronic bronchitis, emphysema, and asthma.
  - Several different massage therapy approaches have been studied for their effects on people suffering from COPD.
- Back massage has been used effectively with hospitalized patients to reduce anxiety and pain and to improve communication.
- Benefits of massage for cancer patients include reduced stress and anxiety, faster recovery from surgery, and reduction of the side effects from cancer treatment.
  - Emotional benefits for cancer patients include help in dealing with depression, re-establishing a positive body image, and rebuilding hope.

- Massage has been used successfully in pediatric care for children with asthma, autism, diabetes, depression, and posttraumatic stress disorder. It helps preterm infants gain weight and develop more normally.
- Massage is an effective complement to treatment of conditions worsened by stress. It relieves the anxiety and stress of psychiatric patients.
- Therapeutic Touch is a form of manual therapy that rebalances the energy field of the patient.
  - It has been found effective in treatment of fluid and electrolyte imbalances, dysfunction in the autonomic nervous system, and lymphatic and circulatory disorders.
  - Nurses have been particularly involved in the development of Therapeutic Touch and its use with patients.
- Massage is an effective complement to chiropractic care.
  - It helps prepare the body for adjustment and addresses some of the muscular problems of chiropractic patients.

EXAM REVIEW

Key Terms

To study the key terms listed at the beginning of this chapter, match the appropriate lettered meaning to each numbered key term listed below. For additional study, look up the key terms in the Interactive Glossary on page G-1 and note other terms that compare or contrast with them.

_____ **1.** Client-centered massage
_____ **2.** Clinical massage therapy
_____ **3.** Direct therapeutic effects
_____ **4.** Evidence-based practice
_____ **5.** Indirect therapeutic effects
_____ **6.** Palliative care
_____ **7.** Principle-based therapy
_____ **8.** Recipe-based massage
_____ **9.** Therapeutic Touch

a. Eases discomfort and improves the quality of life for those with chronic medical conditions or terminal illness
b. Enhance the effectiveness of a primary treatment, or create a more favorable environment for healing
c. Every client receives exactly the same treatment for a particular medical condition
d. The creation of an overall treatment plan directed toward the achievement of specific treatment goals
e. Focuses on the client's unique situation, needs, and goals as the basis for treatment planning
f. Form of manual therapy in which the energy field of the recipient is rebalanced, thus promoting health and healing
g. Focus on the healing of a diagnosed medical condition, or easing of its symptoms
h. Applications of massage in the treatment of human pathologies
i. Use of massage applications that are supported by scientific research

Memory Workout

To test your memory of the main concepts in this chapter, complete the following sentences by circling the most correct answer from the two choices provided.

1. The term (_clinical_) (_client-centered_) _massage therapy_ describes applications of massage in the treatment of human patholgies.
2. The growing interest in massage for (_rest and rejuvenation_) (_treatment of pathologies_) has led to an increased number of research studies about its efficacy.
3. Having verifiable (_objective_) (_anecdotal_) evidence for the effectiveness of therapies chosen for a treatment plan is the cornerstone of evidenced-based practice.
4. Massage that focuses on the client's unique situation, needs, and goals as the basis for treatment planning is called (_client-centered_) (_evidence-based_) massage.

5. Massage used to ease discomfort and to improve the quality of life for those with chronic medical conditions or terminal illness is referred to as (indirect) (palliative) care.

6. Research studies are most useful for adding to our understanding of the applications of massage, *not* as a means for developing (protocols) (principles) for treatment.

7. Two important effects of massage on the cardiovascular system are (reduced) (increased) heart rate and blood pressure.

8. The (Touch Research Institute) (Massage Therapy Foundation) at the University of Miami conducts and publishes many research studies on clinical massage applications.

9. A form of manual therapy sometimes used by nurses in clinical settings in which the energy field of the recipient is rebalanced is Therapeutic (Massage) (Touch).

10. One of the benefits of massage for cancer patients is reduction of the (therapeutic effects) (side effects) of cancer treatment.

Test Prep

The following multiple-choice questions will help to prepare you for future school and professional exams.

1. A complete description of evidence-based practice includes:
   a. Scientific research
   b. Scientific research and experience
   c. Scientific research and old traditions
   d. Scientific research, experience and judgment, and client values

2. Client-centered massage is the *opposite* of:
   a. Principle-based therapy
   b. Recipe-based massage
   c. Evidence-based practice
   d. Research-based massage

3. The use of deep transverse friction in treating repetitive strain injuries is an example of:
   a. Palliative care
   b. Indirect therapeutic effects
   c. Direct therapeutic effects
   d. Therapeutic Touch

4. Massage given to patients in hospices is an example of:
   a. Direct therapeutic effects
   b. Palliative care
   c. Acute care
   d. Intensive care

5. The effect of massage therapy for which there is the best evidence from scientific research is:
   a. Increased general circulation
   b. Relief from negative mood
   c. Reduction of trait anxiety
   d. General weight loss

6. In Therapeutic Touch, the energy field of the recipient is rebalanced or repatterned by sweeping hand movements performed:
   a. On the arms and legs
   b. A few inches above the skin
   c. Directly on the skin using light pressure
   d. On the back

7. A massage application found to be an effective, noninvasive technique for promoting relaxation and improving communication with elderly, institutionalized patients is:
   a. Abdominal massage
   b. Lymphatic drainage
   c. Deep transverse friction
   d. Back massage

8. Indirect therapeutic effects of massage:
   a. Create a favorable environment for healing
   b. Treat a pathology and ease its symptoms
   c. Address the comfort of the recipient
   d. Focus on cause and effect

9. In chiropractic care, a condition of misalignment in a joint, which often results in structural, nervous system, and chemical dysfunctions is called a(n):
   a. Mobilization
   b. Adjustment
   c. Subluxation
   d. Adhesion

10. The benefits of massage for patients with chronic inflammatory bowel disease, ulcerative colitis, and Crohn's disease are based on its ability to:
   a. Increase circulation
   b. Relieve stress
   c. Increase flexibility
   d. Increase body awareness

Video Challenge

Watch the appropriate segment of the video on your DVD and then answer the following questions.

Clinical Applications of Massage

Documentation and SOAP Notes

1. What do massage therapists in the video say about the usefulness of documentation for clinical massage applications?

2. How do SOAP notes as described in the video support evidence-based clinical massage therapy?

3. How are the Subjective and Objective sections of SOAP notes as described in the video used in client-centered massage?

Comprehension Exercises

The following short answer questions test your knowledge and understanding of chapter topics and provide practice in written communication skills. Explain in two to four complete sentences.

1. Describe the additional knowledge and skills needed for clinical massage therapy applications.

2. Explain the benefits of massage for hospitalized patients for which there is evidence from research studies.

For Greater Understanding

The following exercises are designed to take you from the realm of theory into the real world. They will help give you a deeper understanding of the subjects covered in this chapter. Action words are underlined to emphasize the variety of activities presented to address different learning styles, and to encourage deeper thinking.

1. Choose a specific pathology to study. Locate information about contraindications and cautions related to the pathology. Identify implications for giving massage to a person with the pathology studied. Discuss with a study partner or group.

2. Interview someone who is receiving massage as treatment for a particular pathology. Ask the individual to identify the benefits he or she feels from receiving massage. Compare this with conventional wisdom and available research.

3. Interview a massage practitioner who specializes in clinical applications or the director of a clinical massage setting. Ask the person about the types of pathologies seen in his or her practice and the benefits patients receive from massage. Report to a study partner or group.

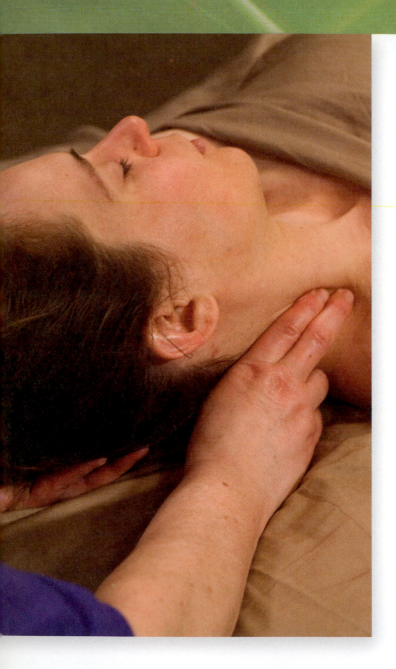

CHAPTER

9 Endangerment Sites, Contraindications, and Cautions

CHAPTER OUTLINE

Learning Outcomes

Key Terms

Do No Harm

Endangerment Sites

General Principles for Safety around Endangerment Sites

Contraindications

Principles for Contraindications and Cautions

Medications

Person-Centered Massage

Resources for the Practitioner

Chapter Highlights

Exam Review

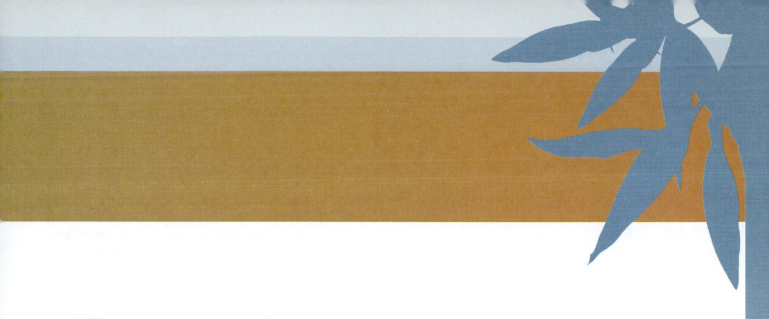

LEARNING OUTCOMES

After studying this chapter, you will have information to:

1. Locate endangerment sites on the body.
2. Apply massage safely around endangerment sites.
3. Recognize contraindications and cautions for massage.
4. Distinguish between general and regional contraindications for massage.
5. Adapt massage sessions for clients taking medications.
6. Demonstrate a person-centered approach to massage.
7. Locate information about endangerment sites and contraindications for massage in professional resources.

KEY TERMS

DO NO HARM

One of most basic principles of giving therapeutic massage is to **do no harm.** Guidelines for helping you make decisions about what to do and what to avoid to protect the health and safety of your clients are presented in this chapter. Topics addressed include endangerment sites, contraindications, cautions, medications, and resources for further information.

The variety of massage approaches used today complicates the issue somewhat. These forms vary from deep tissue structural massage of the physical body to light touch affecting the energy within and around the physical body. An endangerment site or a contraindication in one form of bodywork may be considered perfectly safe for a different form.

This chapter focuses on endangerment sites, contraindications, and cautions that are important when giving Western massage and forms that use similar techniques. This includes all techniques applied to the physical body that involve pressing, stroking, friction, kneading, tapping, and vibrating. Chapters devoted to other types of massage and bodywork address contraindications and cautions for that particular approach.

Knowledge of Western anatomy, physiology, and pathology is essential to ensure the safety of persons receiving massage and bodywork. It is particularly important to know the location of major nerves, blood vessels, glands, and visceral organs. Use Chapter 6, Anatomy & Physiology, Pathology, and Kinesiology, as a handy reference. Endangerment sites, contraindications, and cautions are discussed in this chapter in terms of Western biological science.

ENDANGERMENT SITES

Endangerment sites are areas of the body where delicate structures are less protected and, therefore, may be more easily damaged when receiving massage. Tissues and structures particularly vulnerable include blood vessels, nerves, lymph nodes, eyes, and all the internal organs. Caution is required when performing massage on or around endangerment sites. The following sections identify the location of endangerment sites and describe cautions when working in those areas. Figure 9.1■ shows the general location of endangerment sites on the anterior and posterior body.

Anterior Neck

The anterior neck is the triangular area on the front of the neck defined by the sternocleidomastoid (SCM) and includes the sternal notch, which is the depression found on the superior aspect of the sternum. Delicate structures located in the anterior neck triangle are the carotid artery, jugular vein, vagus nerve, larynx, and thyroid gland. Deep pressure on any of these structures can be harmful.

Pressure within the anterior triangle of the neck, including the depression formed by the sternal notch, should be avoided entirely in most forms of massage. Some advanced techniques address cervical muscles from the anterior neck, but they should be performed only by experienced therapists with special training. The gentle superficial stroking during lymphatic massage and noncontact forms of energy work are possible exceptions to the no-touch rule.

Great care should be taken when performing neck massage on older adults due to the likelihood of atherosclerosis and the potential for dislodging a thrombus that could lead to stroke. Too much pressure from massage could also cause further damage to blood vessels in the area. Moderate pressure on the posterior cervical muscles may be safe to apply with care.

Vertebral Column

The vertebral column protects the spinal cord of the central nervous system. The spinous processes of the cervical, thoracic, and lumbar vertebrae can be felt along the middle of the neck and back. Massage techniques that apply heavy pressure or that involve thrusting or percussion movements should not be performed directly over the spinous processes.

Thoracic Cage

The thoracic cage consists of the ribs and sternum. The thoracic cage is relatively flexible to allow for breathing. Ribs 1–10 attach to the sternum with cartilage, while ribs 11–12 do not attach and are called floating ribs. The inferior tip of the sternum, called the *xiphoid process,* is a slender piece of bone that can break under pressure and be driven into the liver, causing severe damage.

Avoid strong pressure or impact directly over the sternum, and especially on the xiphoid process. Heavy pressure over the rib cage should also be avoided, especially in older adults and those at risk for osteoporosis.

Shoulder and Axilla

Delicate circulatory and nerve structures are relatively exposed in the shoulder and axilla (i.e., armpit) area. These structures include the brachial artery, axillary artery and vein, cephalic vein, basilica vein, brachial plexus nerve complex, and axillary lymph nodes (Figure 9.2■). Deep specific pressure in this area should be approached with caution. Moderate broad pressure

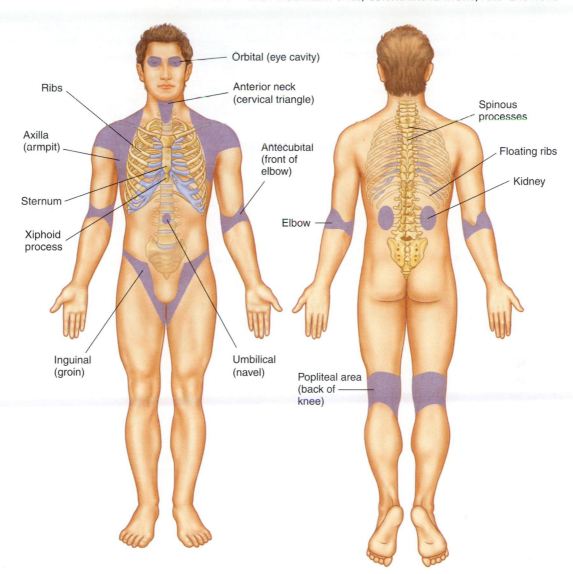

FIGURE 9.1

Endangerment sites—anterior and posterior views.

may be applied to the armpit, but deep specific pressure should be restricted to the surrounding musculature (e.g., pectoral and subscapularis muscles) and their attachments.

Elbow

Two places around the elbow or cubital area require caution. One is the space just medial to the olecranon process where the ulnar nerve is relatively exposed. This is the "funny bone" area that causes sharp pain when hit. Another sensitive place is the anterior fold of the elbow. This area is similar to the popliteal area found posterior to the knee. Vulnerable structures that pass through the elbow include the brachial vein and artery, median cubital vein, and median nerve. These structures are all close to the surface and unprotected by muscle. Moderate broad pressure may be applied to the area, but deep specific pressure should be restricted to the surround-

ing muscles and their attachments (e.g., forearm flexors and extensors).

Umbilicus

The umbilicus or "belly button" is a sensitive area superficial to the descending aorta and abdominal aorta. Avoid direct, heavy pressure to the umbilicus.

Kidney Area

The kidneys are located on either side of the spine, generally at the level between the third lumbar and twelfth thoracic vertebrae (see Figure 6.99 on page 204). They are positioned behind the parietal peritoneum and against the deep muscles of the back. Superficial or deep stroking and pressing techniques may be applied carefully to the muscles of the back located in the kidney area. However, only light pressure

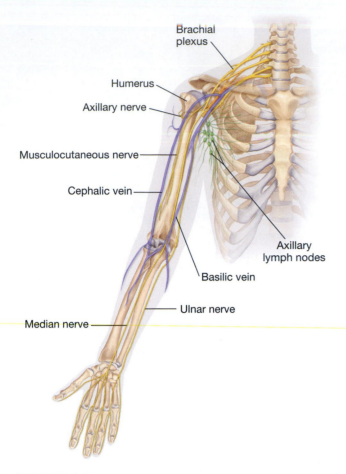

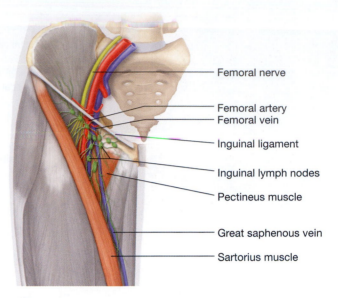

FIGURE 9.3

The inguinal area. Great care should be taken when applying deep pressure in this region.

FIGURE 9.2

The shoulder, axilla, and anticubital area. Deep pressure in this area should be approached with caution.

should be used when performing percussion techniques over this area.

Inguinal Area

The inguinal or groin area is located roughly where the thigh and the trunk meet on the anterior side of the body. The femoral nerve and major blood vessels to the lower extremities cross there (i.e., femoral artery, great saphenous and femoral veins). See Figure 9.3■. When the thigh is flexed, a depression is created in the area, exposing the more delicate structures. Great care should be taken when applying deep pressure into this area, for example, when addressing the iliopsoas muscle. This should be attempted by students only under supervision and by practitioners with adequate training.

Popliteal Area

The muscles of the posterior lower extremity cross the knee laterally and medially, leaving the center space relatively unprotected. This space is called the popliteal area. The

popliteal artery and vein and the tibial nerve are located there (Figure 9.4■). Broad flat hand strokes over this area may be safe, but avoid heavy specific pressure over the back of the knee joint. Follow the muscles around the popliteal area when massaging them.

Eyes

Take great care when working around the eyes. Be careful not to slip and hit the eyeball by accident. Only the very lightest pressure is used when stroking the eyelid.

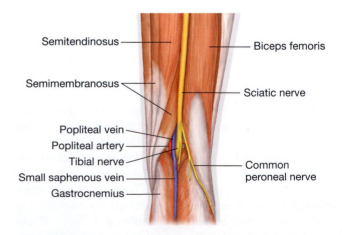

FIGURE 9.4

The popliteal area. Avoid heavy pressure over the back of the knee joint.

Major Veins in Extremities

Major veins in the extremities (see Figure 6.70 on page 179) are being included under endangerment sites because structural damage can occur to the valves within the veins if deep effleurage is applied improperly. Always apply deep flushing effleurage to the arms and legs from distal to proximal (i.e., toward the heart, and with the flow that opens the valves).

GENERAL PRINCIPLES FOR SAFETY AROUND ENDANGERMENT SITES

Here are some general principles to keep in mind to protect the receiver's body from structural damage during massage. Remember, your first responsibility is to do no harm.

1. Always adjust the pressure applied to match the part of the body, the condition of the tissues, and the recipient's comfort. Any part of the body can be damaged if too much pressure is used.
2. Avoid heavy pressure anyplace where nerves, blood vessels, or lymph vessels are close to the surface or are unprotected by muscle or bone.
3. Be careful around joints where delicate structures are less protected by skeletal muscle.
4. If you feel a pulse, it means that you are on a major artery. Move to a different place immediately.
5. If the receiver feels searing, burning, shooting, electrical sensations, "pins and needles," or numbness, you may be pressing on a nerve. Move to a different place immediately.
6. Any abnormal structure is a potential endangerment site. Get information about structural abnormalities, and proceed with caution when you are sure it is safe to do so.
7. Always work with awareness, and when in doubt, do not take a chance that might lead to injury.

CONTRAINDICATIONS

Contraindications are conditions or situations that make the receiving of massage inadvisable because of the harm it might do. In the treatment model, a contraindication is any symptom or condition that renders a particular medication, procedure, or treatment unwise given the circumstances. For **general contraindications,** avoid massage altogether. For regional or **local contraindications,** avoid only the specific area of the body affected.

Cautions are situations of potential danger that require thoughtful consideration and possible modifications of technique application. Cautions may or may not involve pathology.

Be alert to possible contraindications and cautions for every client. A **health history** taken during the initial visit provides information about previous conditions or health

REALITY CHECK

WENDY: The other day I was giving a massage and noticed that the client didn't have any toenails. It hadn't come up in the intake interview, and I was a little surprised. I didn't know what to say, but also didn't want to hurt her when massaging her feet. What can you do in a case like that?

ROB: Remember that many people have structural abnormalities that they have lived with for a long time and might forget to mention. If your demeanor is professional and you don't act embarrassed or overly concerned, it will put the client at ease in talking about the situation. Be matter of fact and say something like, "I notice that you don't have any toenails. Is there anything I need to know when massaging your feet? Are your toes tender?" This might be enough to get the person to talk to you about the situation. Then you can determine if any contraindications or cautions apply. The important thing is to acknowledge the situation, get the information you need to make good decisions, and document the condition on his or her health history after the session.

issues to be aware of. Chapter 10, Goal-Oriented Planning and Documentation, on page 319, discusses in greater detail the health history and intake interview, and Appendix G, Intake, Health History, and Note Forms, on page A-52, contains health history forms for general wellness massage, as well as treatment-oriented sessions. Check with regular clients at every session to see if their health status has changed in significant ways, especially if they are known to have conditions that are contraindications or for which special cautions apply.

Knowledge of normal anatomy and physiology, as well as the nature of common pathologies, is important for massage practitioners. Such knowledge may help prevent a well-meaning practitioner from causing harm. Those performing clinical applications need to be especially well versed in the pathologies that they are treating.

Be sure to fully understand the origin of any symptom of disease reported by a client. This information will help in the selection of appropriate techniques. It will also be useful in positioning clients to best support their health and comfort. If a client reports having a condition or disease that you are not familiar with, use your professional resources (as described in a later section of this chapter) to get more information before proceeding with the massage session.

Some general principles can be used to help determine whether receiving massage might be harmful. Some of the more common conditions and situations encountered in a massage practice are listed in the next section.

PRINCIPLES FOR CONTRAINDICATIONS AND CAUTIONS

1. **Severe Distress.** Do not perform massage when the recipient is experiencing severe distress.
   For example:
   - Feels physically ill or nauseated
   - Is in severe pain
   - Has a fever
   - Has been seriously injured recently

2. **Acute Inflammation.** Do not perform massage in the presence of acute inflammation. Signs of inflammation are redness, heat, swelling, and pain. Any diagnosed condition that ends in "itis" is either a general or local contraindication.
   For example:
   - **Appendicitis.** Massage will spread inflammation throughout abdomen; avoid massage entirely.
   - **Rheumatoid arthritis.** Avoid massage over acutely inflamed joints (local contraindication); use caution even when subacute; avoid traction of joints and spine.
   - **Phlebitis.** Inflammation of a vein; completely avoid site of disease, usually the legs.
   - **Locally inflamed tissues.** Signs are redness, heat, swelling, and pain; avoid the surrounding area; on limbs, only work proximal to the affected area.

3. **Loss of Structural Integrity.** Understand the physician's recommendations and the relevant anatomy and physiology in cases where there is a loss of integrity in an area.
   For example:
   - **Over recent surgery.** Only those specifically trained to work with scar tissue should attempt this work.
   - **Around burns.** Avoid any pressure over or around recent burns.
   - **Recent fractures.** With the client's permission, request information from his or her physician about the phase of healing of the fracture. See Figure 6.41 on page 153 for types of fractures. Acute or unset broken bones are contraindications for massage. Use

caution around plates and screws used to hold bones together. Avoid pressure to injured soft tissues. Lymphatic facilitation may be helpful to reduce related swelling.
   - **Artificial joint replacements.** Check recommended restrictions in range of motion in replaced joints. Comfortable positioning may also be affected by joint replacements in the knees or hips. Avoid positions that put pressure directly on joint replacements.

4. **Skin Conditions.** Do not touch areas of the skin where there is a pathological condition that is contagious or that may be worsened or spread by applying pressure or rubbing.
   For example:
   - **Acne vulgaris.** Avoid massage over acne lesions. Acne is a localized bacterial infection of the sebaceous glands in the face, neck, or upper back. Acne lesions include pimples, cysts, blackheads (open comedones), and whiteheads (closed comedomes). See Figure 6.12 on page 137.
   - **Rashes.** Avoid touching on or near contagious skin rashes. A rash is a general term for red spots on the skin. Inquire about the cause of the rash. Avoid massage altogether if the rash is caused by a systemic disease (e.g., Lyme disease, cellulitis, or lupus). Cellulitis is shown in Figure 6.15; and dermatitis is shown in Figure 6.16 on page 138.
   - **Boils.** Avoid touch on or near a boil. This is a localized staphylococcus infection of the skin.
   - **Athlete's foot.** Avoid touch on or near fungal infections such as athlete's foot.
   - **Ringworm.** Avoid touch on or near fungal infections such as ringworm (Figure 6.24 on page 141).
   - **Herpes simplex (e.g., cold sores).** Avoid massage altogether during an acute outbreak of herpes (Figure 6.18 on page 139). Avoid massage locally during the scabbing phase.
   - **Impetigo.** Avoid massage until lesions have completely healed. This is a highly contagious bacterial infection.
   - **Hives.** Avoid massage altogether in the acute phase of hives and locally in the subacute stage. Hives (urticaria) are areas of redness, itching, heat, and swelling that occur in reaction to an allergy or emotional distress (Figure 6.25 on page 141). Commons allergens that can result in hives are certain foods, pet dander, dust and mold, and certain materials such as latex.
   - **Skin cancer.** Cancerous skin lesions should be diagnosed by a doctor. If diagnosed as nonmalignant, a cancerous lesion is a local contraindication for massage. If it is diagnosed as metastasizing, massage may be generally contraindicated. The signs of malignant melanoma are discussed in detail on page 139 in Chapter 6, Anatomy and Physiology,

Pathology, and Kinesiology. See Figures 6.14, 6.19, and 6.23 for different types of skin cancers.

- *Allergies.* Clients with skin allergies may react negatively to certain oils or lotions used during massage. Check with recipient for substances to avoid, and be alert to skin reactions during the session.
- *Other skin disorders.* Some skin disorders such as benign moles (Figure 6.20 on page 140) and psoriasis (Figure 6.21 on page 140) are not contraindications for massage. See page 137 in Chapter 6 for further discussion of skin pathologies.

5. *Decreased Sensation.* Use extreme care in amount of pressure used when the client has decreased sensation, which may be caused by stroke, diabetes, spinal cord injury, or medication. Recipients cannot give accurate feedback regarding pressure and may also have abnormal vasomotor response to the massage.

6. *Increased Sensitivity to Touch.* Massage only to recipient's tolerance or comfort when there is increased sensitivity to touch. Clients who are ticklish or who have ticklish areas (e.g., feet) generally find light superficial stroking unpleasant and annoying. They may respond well to deeper, slower pressure, or to percussion techniques on the ticklish area.

7. *Cardiovascular Disorders.* For clients with cardiovascular system disorders, research the condition carefully, and with the client's permission, consult with his or her physician if the condition is advanced. Be aware of medications the client is taking and their potential as contraindications for massage.

For example:

- *High blood pressure.* If blood pressure is high, even with treatment, avoid massage approaches that increase general blood circulation.
- *Low blood pressure.* Someone with low blood pressure may be more susceptible to fainting after receiving massage either on a table or a massage chair. Orthostatic hypotension is a condition that causes light-headedness or fainting when changing from lying down or semireclining to standing up. Be sure that these clients get up slowly from a horizontal or semireclining position.
- *Cardiac arrhythmias or carotid bruit.* Avoid lateral and anterior neck.
- *Severe atherosclerosis.* Massage only with physician's permission and then only very superficially (Figure 6.72 on page 180).
- *Severe varicose veins.* Tissues can be easily damaged, and there may be a tendency to clotting; avoid massage of the area (Figure 6.78 on page 184).
- *Stroke.* Avoid circulatory massage, especially massage of neck. Blood thinners are usually prescribed after stroke, so use light pressure with all soft tissue manipulation.

8. *Spreading Disease by Circulation.* Do not perform circulatory massage when there is a pathological condition that might be spread through the lymph or cardiovascular systems.

For example:

- *Blood poisoning (lymphangitis).* Inflammation of the lymphatic vessels; appears as streaks of red on the skin.
- *Swollen glands (i.e., lymph nodes).* The immune system may be attempting to filter out bacteria or other pathogens, and draining them may cause an infection to spread.

9. *Bleeding and Bruising.* Do not perform massage near an area where there is bleeding or bruising.

For example:

- *Bruise.* Avoid pressure to immediate area in the acute stage, and use gentle pressure around the area after healing has begun. Bruises can be classified as hematoma (i.e., bleeding and pooling of blood between muscle sheaths) and ecchymosis (i.e., more superficial blood leakage).
- *Whiplash or other acute trauma.* Any situation in which there is tearing of tissue and where there may be bleeding into the tissue during the first 24–48 hours after the trauma; avoid massage in area, and if severe trauma avoid massage totally (see Principle #1 above).

10. *Edema.* Be sure of the cause of edema before proceeding with massage. Edema from inflammation due to bacterial or viral infection, pitted edema indicating tissue fragility, lymphatic obstruction due to parasites, and edema due to deep vein thrombosis are all contraindications for massage (Rattray and Ludwig 2000). In cases of general edema caused by cardiac, liver, or kidney disease, avoid massage altogether. Acute edema resulting from trauma may be treated with specialized lymphatic facilitation techniques.

11. *Compromised Immunity.* Take added sanitary precautions when working with clients who are ill or elderly. Be especially careful with personal and environmental hygiene when a client's immune function is depressed (e.g., after organ transplant when immune system is depressed with medication, with AIDS/HIV, or chronic fatigue syndrome).

12. *Osteoporosis.* Avoid deep pressure and vigorous joint movements with a client with diagnosed osteoporosis, someone whom you suspect to have the disease, or someone in a high-risk category. Osteoporosis is a disease in which bones become fragile, brittle, and fracture easily. The high-risk category includes small, sedentary postmenopausal women; frail older adults; or someone with hyperkyphosis or "dowager's hump." See Figure 6.42A on page 153.

13. *Cancer.* Massage may be contraindicated for a client with cancer in certain circumstances. Cancer is char-

acterized by uncontrollable growth in abnormal cells forming malignant tumors. Although cancer has been removed as a general category from the list of contraindications for massage, caution is still advised. With the client's permission, consult his or her health care provider before giving massage to a cancer patient. Patients undergoing treatment for cancer often find symptomatic relief from massage. Cautions related to wounds, burns, nausea, compromised immunity, and weakness may apply.

Massage therapists are advised to educate themselves about giving massage to people who have had or now have cancer. Physicians may not know or understand the different types of massage and their effects. They may also not be aware of current research about massage and cancer. See Chapter 8, Clinical Applications of Massage, on page 286, for further discussion of massage and cancer.

14. ***Personal Appliances.***   Avoid contact with personal appliances or aids that clients may be wearing. See Chapter 20, Special Populations and Adaptations, for a discussion of clients with medical appliances.

- ***Contact Lenses.***   If a client is wearing contact lenses, take special care when working around the eyes to avoid pressure on the lenses and to avoid dislodging or moving the lenses. Taking the contact lenses out during massage is preferable.
- ***Hearing Aid.***   If a client wears a hearing aid, be careful not to dislodge it while massaging around

the ears. If it is turned on, massage on the head or around the ears may make a lot of noise for the client and be annoying. Be sure that these clients can see you if you talk to them.

See Chapter 6, Anatomy & Physiology, Pathology, and Kinesiology, for more information about specific pathologies and their massage implications.

MEDICATIONS

Medications are used by an increasing number of people for a variety of ailments. This includes prescription drugs, as well as over-the-counter drugs. Some medications are for short-term use, for example, common cold medications and painkillers (analgesics) such as aspirin; and some are for long-term use, for example, heart medications or antidepressants. Massage practitioners need to be aware of what medications their clients are taking and understand the implications for massage therapy. Box 9.1 lists some of the most common considerations for massage and medications. It summarizes some important points to consider when working with clients taking medication. If in doubt, check with clients and their health care providers about potential for harm and how to avoid it.

A client's medications may affect the scheduling of massage sessions, the length of sessions, and techniques used and their application. They may also influence client

CASE FOR STUDY

Mindy Adapts Her Routine Massage

Mindy gave a health history interview to a new client. She discovered that the client has skin allergies, ticklish feet, varicose veins in her legs, and faints periodically. Several years ago the client broke her elbow in a fall and has a metal plate in her forearm. She has no major or chronic illnesses to report.

Question:

What precautions would Mindy take to ensure the health, safety, and comfort of her client during a massage therapy session?

Things to consider:

- Is anything the client mentioned a general contraindication for massage?

- Does any of the health information point to local contraindications?
- Are any cautions around certain body areas warranted?

Write a brief description of what Mindy can do to provide for the safety and comfort of this client during massage therapy.

_____

_____

_____

behavior. Types of medications that require caution include, but are not limited to, those that:

- Alter sensation (e.g., numbing, increase sensitivity)
- Affect the blood and circulation (e.g., prevent clotting, regulate blood sugar level)
- Compromise tissue integrity (e.g., corticosteroids)
- Alter mood (e.g., depressants, antidepressants)

Table 9.1■ presents a pharmacology overview, listing different classes of drugs, their functions, and generic and brand names. Additional information about common medications can be found in published pharmacology guides and on the Internet. Books that look specifically at medications and massage are also available. Be aware that new medications are continually being developed, and information about a particular drug's safety may change at any time.

Massage is generally contraindicated for persons under the influence of alcohol or recreational drugs. These drugs have the potential to alter sensation, affect mood, lessen the ability to give accurate feedback, and, in many cases, reduce good judgment. Giving massage therapy to a person "high" or in an altered state of consciousness is potentially dangerous for him or her and also for the massage practitioner.

PERSON-CENTERED MASSAGE

It is easy to lose sight of the person when there is pathology involved. From the wellness perspective, massage is best thought of as **person-centered** rather than pathology-centered. In other words, practitioners may give massage to people with pathologies, but the people are more than their pathologies. In fact, practitioners often find themselves working around pathologies.

This may be the case when a person has a condition for which deep or vigorous massage is contraindicated. A light massage may be appropriate to add an element of care, comfort, and stress reduction as a complement to standard medical care. For example, there would be few cases in which stroking the hand or head of a seriously ill person is contraindicated.

Most of the contraindications and cautions discussed in this chapter are based on common sense, given some knowledge of anatomy, physiology, and pathology. If the giver of massage is motivated by sincere concern, gentle in giving massage, and receptive and responsive to feedback from the recipient, the experience will most likely be a healthy one for both people. Even in the hands of a child, massage given with love and sensitivity can be supportive and helpful.

BOX 9.1   Guidelines for Massage and Medications

Scheduling of Sessions

- Massage **after** the client's scheduled dosage if the medication is needed for condition stability (i.e., to ensure maximum bioavailability of the medication). For example, with insulin-dependent diabetics, chronic pain clients, epileptic patients.
- Massage **before** or **shortly after** the client's scheduled dosage if medication decreases the client's perception of pain and his or her ability to give accurate feedback. For example, clients taking drugs such as nonsteroidal anti-inflammatories, narcotic analgesics, and central nervous system depressants.

Session Length

- **Shorten the session** if the medication significantly depletes the energy level of the client, causing abnormal fatigue. For example, clients taking hypertension medications, antianxiety drugs, and many antidepressants.
- **Shorten the session** if the medication significantly decreases the emotional stability of the client, causing him or her to feel emotionally volatile or easily overwhelmed. For example, clients taking corticosteroids (long term) or medications that have side effects that cause mood fluctuations, anxiety, or depression.

Selection of Massage Techniques

- **For drugs that alter clotting mechanisms** (e.g., anticoagulants, platelet inhibitors, and aspirin and other nonsteroidal anti-inflammatory drugs): Avoid high-pressure techniques such as muscle stripping, deep kneading, ischemic compression, and cross-fiber friction.
- **For drugs that alter protective responses** (e.g., centrally acting muscle relaxants, narcotic analgesics, antianxiety drugs): Avoid deep massage, tense–relax stretching, and any technique that requires accurate client feedback for safe application.
- **For drugs that compromise tissue integrity** (e.g., corticosteroids, long-term use or injected directly into joints or tissue): Avoid deep pressure techniques, heavy tapotement, forced stretching, skin rolling and wringing.
- **For drugs that mask pain responses** (e.g., anti-inflammatory drugs, analgesics): Rely less on client feedback and more on observation and palpation to determine appropriate pressure and technique applications.
- **For drugs that alter a client's cooperativeness or make him or her less communicative** (e.g., narcotic analgesics and antianxiety medications): Take time to ask questions as needed for accurate health histories and ongoing feedback during massage.

Information from Persad, Randall S., *Massage Therapy & Medications: General Treatment Principles* (Toronto, Canada: Curties-Overzet Publications, 2001).

TABLE 9.1 Pharmacology

Classification	Action	Generic and *Brand* Names
ACE inhibitor drugs	Cause vasodilation and decrease blood pressure	benazepril, *Lotensin* catopril, *Capoten*
Analgesics	Treat minor to moderate pain	salicylates, *Bayer Aspirin, Ecotrin* acetaminophen, *Tylenol* ibuprofen, *Aleve, Advil*
Androgen therapy	Replaces male hormones	testosterone cypionate, *Andronate, depAndro*
Anesthetics—topical	Applied to the skin to deaden pain	lidocaine, *Xylocaine* procaine, *Novocain*
Anesthetics	Produce a loss of consciousness or sensation	lidocaine, *Xylocaine* pentobarbital, *Nembutal* procaine, *Novocain*
Anorexiants	Treat obesity by suppressing appetite	phendimetrazine, *Adipost, Obezine* phentermine, *Zantryl, Adipex*
Antacids	Neutralize stomach acids	calcium carbonate, *Tums* aluminum hydroxide and magnesium hydroxide, *Maalox, Mylanta*
Antibiotic ointments	Kill bacteria causing skin infections	bacitracin, neomycin, Neosporin ointment
Antibiotics for the respiratory system	Kill bacteria causing infections	amoxicillin, *Amoxil* ciprofloxacin, *Cipro* ampicillin
Antibiotics for the urinary system	Treat bacterial infections of the urinary tract	ciprofloxacin, *Cipro* nitrfurantoin, *Macrobid*
Anticoagulants	Prevent blood clot formation by "thinning" the blood	heparin, *Heplock* warfarin sodium, *Coumadin, Warfarin*
Anticonvulsants	Prevent seizures by reducing the excitability of neurons	carbamazepine, *Tegretol* phenobarbital, *Nembutal*
Antidiarrheals	Control diarrhea	loperamide, *Imodium* diphenoxylate, *Lomotil* kaolin/pectin, *Kaopectate*
Antiemetics	Treat nausea, vomiting, and motion sickness	prochlorperazine, *Compazine* promethazine, *Phenergan*
Antifungals	Kill fungi infecting the skin	miconazole, *Monistat* clotrimazole, *Lotrimin*
Antihemorrhagics	Prevent or stop hemorrhaging	aminocaproic acid, *Amicar* vitamin K
Antihistamines	Block the effects of histamine released by the body during an allergic reaction	cetirizine, *Zyrtec* diphenhydramine, *Benadryl* fexofenadine, *Allegra* loratadine, *Claritan*
Antilipidemics	Reduce amount of cholesterol and lipids in the blood to treat hyperlipidemia	atorvastatin, *Lipitor* simvastin, *Zocor*
Antiparasitics	Kill lice or mites	lindane, *Kwell* permethrin, *Nix*
Antiplatelet agents	Prolong bleeding time by interfering with the action of platelets; used to prevent heart attacks and strokes	clopidogrel, *Plavix* ticlopidine, *Ticlid*

Classification	Action	Generic and *Brand* Names
Antiprostatic agents	Treat early stages of benign prostatic hypertrophy	finasteride, *Proscar* dutasteride, *Avodart*
Antipruritics	Reduce itching	diphenhydramine, *Benadryl* camphor/pramoxine/zinc, *Caladryl*
Antiseptics	Kill bacteria in cuts or wounds of the skin	isopropyl alcohol hydrogen peroxide
Antispasmodics	Prevent or reduce bladder muscle spasms	oxybutynin, *Ditropan* neostigmine, *Prostigmine*
Antithyroid agents	Block production of thyroid hormones in people with hypersecretion disorders	methimazole, *Tapazole* propylthiouracil
Antitussives	Relieve the urge to cough	hydrocodon, *Hycodan* dextromethorphan, *Vicks Formula 44*
Antivirals	Treat herpes simplex infection	valacyclovir, *Valtrex* famcyclovir, *Famvir* acyclovir, *Zovirax*
Beta-blockers	Lower the heart rate to treat hypertension and angina pectoris	metoprolol, *Lopressor* propranolol, *Inderal*
Bone reabsorption inhibitors	Reduce the reabsorption of bone in conditions such as osteoporosis	alendronate, *Fosamax* ibandronate, *Boniva*
Bronchodilators	Treat asthma by relaxing muscle spasms in bronchial tubes	albuterol, *Proventil, Ventolin* salmetrol, *Serevent* theophyllin, *Theo-Dur*
Calcium channel blockers	Cause the heart to beat less often and less forcefully to treat hypertension, angina pectoris, and congestive heart failure	diltiazem, *Cardizem* nifedipine, *Procardia*
Cardiotonics	Lower blood pressure by increasing urine production, which reduces blood volume	furosemide, *Lasix*
Corticosteroid creams	Anti-inflammatory creams applied topically	hydrocortisone, *Cortaid* triamcinolone, *Kenalog*
Corticosteroids	Anti-inflammatories used in conditions such as rheumatoid arthritis or other autoimmune diseases	prednisone methylprednisolone, *Medrol* dexamethasone, *Decadron*
Corticosteroids for the respiratory tract	Reduce inflammation and swelling	fluticasone, *Flonase* mometasone, *Nasonex* triamcinolone, *Azmacort*
Decongestants	Reduce congestion in the respiratory system	oxymetazoline, *Afrin, Dristan, Sinex* pseudoephedrine, *Drixoral, Sudafed*
Diuretics	Increase the volume of urine produced by the kidneys	furosemide, *Lasix* spironolactone, *Aldactone*
Dopaminergic drugs	Treat Parkinson's disease by replacing the dopamine that is lacking or increasing the strength of the dopamine that is present	levodopa L-dopa, *Laradopa* levodopa/carbidopa, *Sinemet*
Emetics	Induce vomiting	ipecac syrup
Expectorants	Improve the ability to cough up mucus from the respiratory tract	guaifenesin, *Robitussin, Mucinex*

(Continued)

TABLE 9.1 *(Continued)*

Classification	Action	Generic and *Brand* Names
Fertility drugs	Trigger ovulation	clomiphene, *Clomid* follitropin alfa, *Gonal-F*
H$_2$-receptor antagonists	Treat peptic ulcers and gastroesophageal reflux disease (GERD) by blocking H$_2$- receptors, which results in a low acid level in the stomach	ranitidine, *Zantac* cimetidine, *Tagament* famotidine, *Pepcid* esomeprazole, *Nexium*
Hematinics	Increases the amount of hemoglobin in the blood	epoetin alfa, *Procrit* darbepoetin alfa, *Aranesp*
Hormone replacement therapy (HRT)	Replaces estrogen in the postmenopausal woman	conjugated estrogens, *Cenestin, Premarin*
Human growth hormone therapy	Stimulates skeletal growth	somatropin, *Genotropin* somatrem, *Protropin*
Hypnotics	Promote sleep	secobarbital, *Seconal* temazepam, *Restoril*
Immunosuppressants	Prevent rejection of a transplanted organ by blocking certain actions of the immune system	mycophenolate mofetil, *CellCept* cyclosporine, *Neoral*
Insulin	Replaces insulin in type 1 diabetics or to treat type 2 diabetics	human insulin, *Humulin L*
Laxatives	Treat constipation by stimulating a bowel movement	senosides, *Senokot* psyllium, *Metamucil*
Mucolytics	Liquefy mucus so it is easier to cough up and clear from respiratory tract	N-acetyl-cysteine, *Mucomyst*
Narcotic analgesics	Used to treat severe pain; can be habit forming	morphine, *MS Contin* pxycodone, *OxyContin* meperidine, *Demerol*
Nonsteroidal anti-inflamatory drugs (NSAIDs)	Anti-inflammatory and mild pain relief for conditions such as arthritis	ibuprofen, *Advil, Motrin* naxoproxen, *Aleve, Naprosyn* salicylates, *Bayer Aspirin*
Oral contraceptive pills	Prevent conception by blocking ovulation	desogestrel/ethinyl estradiol, *Ortho-Cept* ethinyl estradiol/norgestrel, *Lo/Ovral*
Oral hypoglycemic agents	Cause a decrease in blood sugar	metformin, *Glucophage* glipizide, *Glucotrol*
Oxytocin	Begins or improves uterine contractions during labor and delivery	oxytocin, *Pitocin, Syntocinon*
Protease inhibitors	Stop viruses from reproducing by inhibiting the enzyme protease	indinavir, *Crixivan* saquinavir, *Fortovase*
Proton pump inhibitors	Block the stomach's ability to secrete acid	esomeprazole, *Nexium* omeprazole, *Prilosec*
Reverse transcriptase inhibitor drugs	Stop viruses from reproducing by inhibiting the enzyme reverse transcriptase	lamivudine, *Epivir* zidovudine, *Retrovir*
Sedatives	Produce a relaxing or calming effect	amobarbital, *Amytal* butabarbital, *Butisol*
Skeletal muscle relaxants	Relax skeletal muscles in order to reduce muscle spasms	cyclobenzaprine, *Flexeril* carisoprodol, *Soma*
Thrombolytics	Dissolve existing blood clots	clopidogrel, *Plavix* alteplase, *Activase* streptokinase, *Streptase*

Classification	Action	Generic and *Brand* Names
Thyroid replacement hormones	Replace thyroid hormones for people with hypothyroidism or who have had their thyroid glands surgically removed	levothyroxine, *Levo-T* liothyronine, *Cytomel*
Vasoconstrictors	Raise blood pressure by contracting smooth muscle in walls of blood vessels	metaraminol, *Aramine*
Vasodilators	Increase circulation to an ischemic area and reduces blood pressure by relaxing smooth muscle in artery walls	nitroglycerine, *Nitro-Dur* isoxsuprine, *Vasodilan*
Vasopressin	Controls diabetes insipidus and promotes reabsorption of water in the kidney tubules	desmopressin acetate, *Desmopressin* conivaptan, *Vaprisol*

RESOURCES FOR THE PRACTITIONER

Personal professional libraries should include some basic resources for information about conditions and pathologies commonly encountered in massage practices. This information can provide insights into possible contraindications and cautions, and implications for performing massage. See Chapter 6, Anatomy & Physiology, Pathology, and Kinesiology, for more information on specific pathologies as they relate to massage therapy. Pathologies may also be researched at a local library, a library at a school of medicine, and on the Internet.

A basic professional library for massage practitioners might include a good anatomy and physiology text, an atlas of human anatomy, a pathology text, a medical dictionary, and a pharmacology guide. Pathology books written especially for massage therapists are available and can be valu-able references that include special considerations for massage, including contraindications and cautions.

Practitioners working with special populations should have applicable references for basic information. There are books available on massage with specific populations (e.g., pregnant women, infants and children, older adults, cancer patients, and others). An up-to-date, general reference book for common medications and their effects and side effects would also be useful.

One of the best resources for information may be the recipient him- or herself. Recipients are often very knowledgeable about their own pathologies, especially if they have lived with a chronic condition for some time. The recipient's health care providers may also serve as valuable resources when there is any doubt as to the safety of an individual receiving massage.

PRACTICAL APPLICATION

Interview one of your practice clients using one of the health history forms that can be found in Appendix G (page A-52). Look over the information and identify contraindications and cautions relevant to this person receiving massage therapy.

1. Does he or she have a chronic illness or recent injury?
2. Are there structural anomalies?
3. Is the individual taking medications regularly or occasionally?

CRITICAL THINKING

Think about the contraindications and cautions identified in the Practical Application exercise for this chapter (page 307). Apply the Principles for Safety around Endangerment Sites and the Principles for Contraindications and Cautions to this case.

1. Are there specific techniques that you would avoid?
2. Are there certain areas of the body that require caution?
3. How might medications the client is taking affect your approach or choice of techniques?

CHAPTER HIGHLIGHTS

- One of the most basic principles of giving therapeutic massage is to do no harm.
- Awareness of endangerment sites, contraindications, and cautions ensure the health and safety of clients.
- Endangerment sites are areas of the body where delicate structures are less protected and therefore more easily damaged when receiving massage.
  - Endangerment sites include the anterior neck, vertebral column, thoracic cage, shoulder and axilla, elbow, umbilicus, kidney area, inguinal area, popliteal area, eyes, and the major veins in the extremities.
- General principles for performing massage related to endangerment sites include caution around delicate or abnormal anatomical structures, adjusting pressure to avoid damage, and always working with awareness.
- Contraindications are conditions that make receiving massage inadvisable because of the harm it might do.
  - For general contraindications, massage should be avoided altogether.
  - For local or regional contraindications, only the specific area of the body affected should be avoided.
- Cautions are areas of potential danger that require thoughtful consideration and possible modifications of technique application.

- Contraindications and cautions for massage include:
  - Severe distress, acute inflammation, skin problems, osteoporosis, decreased or increased sensation, compromised immunity.
  - Bleeding and bruising, some types of edema, cardiovascular disorders, diseases spread by circulation, loss of structural integrity.
  - Contact lenses and hearing aids.
- Medications including prescription and over-the-counter drugs that clients are taking must be considered.
  - Medications may affect the scheduling of massage sessions, the length of sessions, techniques used and their application, or the client's behavior.
  - Types of medications that require caution include those that alter sensation, affect the blood and circulation, compromise tissue integrity, or alter mood.
  - Persons under the influence of alcohol or recreational drugs should not receive massage because such substances alter sensation, affect mood, and reduce good judgment.
- From the wellness perspective, massage is person-centered, not pathology-centered.
- Personal professional libraries include books and other resources for information about contraindications and cautions for massage.

EXAM REVIEW

Key Terms

To study the key terms listed at the beginning of this chapter, match the appropriate lettered meaning to each numbered key term listed below. For additional study, look up the key terms in the Interactive Glossary on page G-1 and note other terms that compare or contrast with them.

_____ 1. Cautions
_____ 2. Contraindications
_____ 3. Do no harm
_____ 4. Endangerment site
_____ 5. General contraindications
_____ 6. Health history
_____ 7. Local contraindications
_____ 8. Person-centered

a. One of the most basic principles of giving therapeutic massage
b. For these, avoid only the specific area of the body affected
c. For these, avoid massage altogether
d. Provides information about previous medical conditions or health issues to be aware of
e. Focuses on the client rather than his or her pathologies
f. Situations of potential danger that require thoughtful consideration and possible modifications of technique application
g. Areas of the body where delicate structures are less protected and, therefore, may be more easily damaged when receiving massage
h. Conditions or situations that make the receiving of massage inadvisable because of the harm it might do

Memory Workout

To test your memory of the main concepts in this chapter, complete the following sentences by circling the most correct answer from the two choices provided.

1. Endangerment sites are areas of the body where delicate anatomical structures are (encased) (exposed) and, therefore, may be more easily damaged when receiving massage.
2. Always apply deep effleurage on the limbs from (distal to proximal) (medial to lateral) to avoid damage to the valves in the large veins.
3. Always adjust the amount of (pressure) (oil) you use to match the condition of the tissues being manipulated.
4. Avoid massage altogether for (general) (regional) contraindications.

5. A client health history should be taken to identify possible (preferences) (contraindications) for massage.
6. Acute inflammation is a general or local contraindication for massage, for example, almost any condition that ends in (osis) (itis).
7. Bruising is a (local) (mild) contraindication.
8. A client's compromised (immunity) (integrity) calls for extra care in personal and environmental hygiene.
9. If a medication significantly depletes a client's energy level, it may be advisable to (lengthen) (shorten) a massage session.
10. From a wellness perspective, massage is best thought of as (pathology-centered) (person-centered).

Test Prep

The following multiple-choice questions will help to prepare you for future school and professional exams.

1. Which region of the neck should be avoided during massage?
   a. Posterior
   b. Anterior triangle
   c. Lateral aspect
   d. Suboccipital

2. Forceful or heavy pressure techniques are generally contraindicated if a client has:
   a. Skin allergies
   b. Contact lenses
   c. Osteoporosis
   d. Low blood pressure

3. If you feel a pulse, it means that you are touching a(n):
   a. Nerve
   b. Artery
   c. Vein
   d. Lymph node

4. If the receiver feels a shooting or electrical sensation, you have probably hit a(n):
   a. Nerve
   b. Artery
   c. Tendon
   d. Ligament

5. For massage, skin acne is a:
   a. General contraindication
   b. Local contraindication
   c. Local indication
   d. Nonconsideration

6. Clients with diabetes usually have this condition in the feet:
   a. Warts
   b. Fallen arches
   c. Decreased sensation
   d. Increased sensation

7. If a client's medication decreases his or her sensitivity to pain, it is best to conduct the massage:
   a. Before the scheduled dosage
   b. After the scheduled dosage
   c. Not at all (contraindicated)
   d. Anytime

8. A primary concern related to long-term use of corticosteroids (e.g., for allergies or chronic inflammation) is that it tends to:
   a. Make a person less talkative
   b. Deplete energy
   c. Compromise tissue integrity
   d. Reduce blood clotting mechanisms

9. For a frail or seriously ill person, in addition to choosing less vigorous massage techniques, you might also:
   a. Make the session shorter
   b. Make the session longer
   c. Include a lot of joint movements
   d. Reduce the amount of lotion used

10. Which of the following precautions applies specifically to clients with low blood pressure?
    a. Avoid percussion techniques
    b. Get up slowly from a horizontal position
    c. Avoid massage of the feet
    d. Shorten the session

Video Challenge

Watch the appropriate segment of the video on your DVD and then answer the following questions.

Endangerment Sites, Contraindications, and Cautions

1. In what step of planning a massage session might a contraindication to massage be discovered?

2. How is knowledge of contraindications used in planning massage sessions?

Comprehension Exercises

The following short-answer questions test your knowledge and understanding of chapter topics and provide practice in written communication skills. Explain in two to four complete sentences.

1. Describe massage techniques that would be contraindicated and those that are safe to apply over the back of the knee or popliteal area.

2. Identify four types of medications that create conditions requiring caution for the application of massage techniques.

3. Explain why massage is contraindicated for a person under the influence of alcohol or recreational drugs.

For Greater Understanding

The following exercises are designed to take you from the realm of theory into the real world. They will help give you a deeper understanding of the subjects covered in this chapter. Action words are underlined to emphasize the variety of activities presented to address different learning styles and to encourage deeper thinking.

1. On yourself, or working with a study partner, explore the surface anatomy of the major endangerment sites. Carefully and safely feel the structure of the area and visualize the tissues and anatomical structures underneath the skin. Imagine how deep specific structures are to the surface and how exposed they are to pressure. Use an anatomy book or atlas as an aid to visualization.

2. Interview a massage practitioner who specializes in clinical applications or the director of a clinical massage setting. Ask the person about the types of pathologies he or she sees in his or her practice and the cautions taken in working with those clients. Report to a study partner or group.

3. Interview a person taking one or more medications. List the medications he or she takes and the related pathology for which the individual is being treated. Identify modifications you would make in a massage session with this person. Discuss your session plan with a study partner or group.

10 Goal-Oriented Planning and Documentation

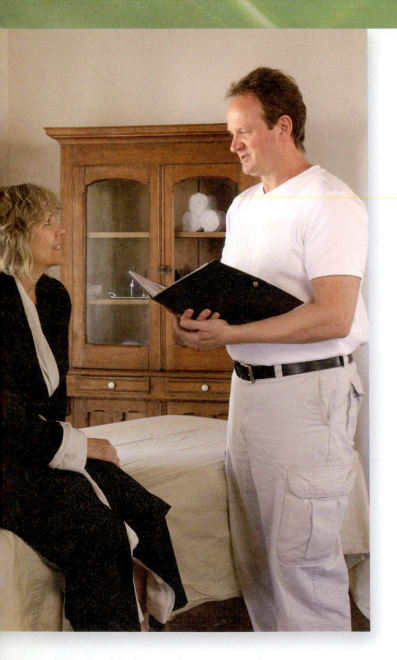

 CHAPTER OUTLINE

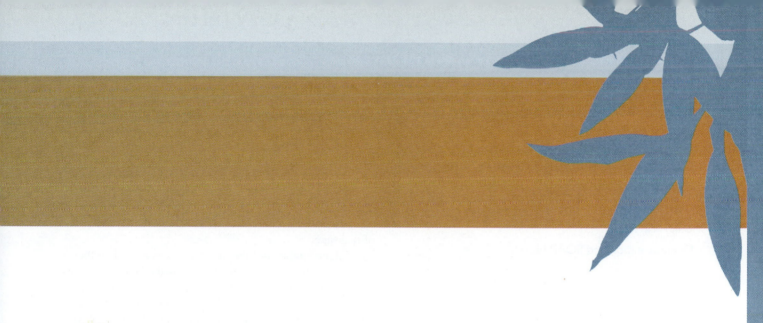

LEARNING OUTCOMES

After studying this chapter, you will have information to:

1. Use the six-step process for planning goal-oriented massage sessions.
2. Develop long-term, individual session, and treatment plans for meeting clients' goals.
3. Perform intake interviews to gather client information for planning.
4. Frame useful interview questions.
5. Use basic evaluation tools to collect objective information for planning.

6. Describe four types of SOAP notes.
7. Write SOAP notes clearly, concisely, and correctly.
8. Write simplified session notes.
9. Design a documentation system for a massage practice.
10. Identify legal and ethical issues related to documentation.

KEY TERMS

MASSAGE *in* ACTION

On your DVD, explore:

- Goal-Oriented, Six-Step Planning Process
- Observation: Posture, Biomechanics, and Gait
- Posture Analysis
- Biomechanical Analysis
- Gait Analysis
- Documentation and SOAP Notes

THE IMPORTANCE OF PLANNING

Every massage needs a plan. This is true whether you are giving a set massage routine to a healthy client, or designing a session to meet specific client goals. Session planning is the logical process of thinking through the massage. It includes collecting relevant information, assessing the situation and setting goals, choosing massage applications, performing the massage, and evaluating results.

The thoroughness of the session planning process varies with the situation. At a minimum, a short verbal or written intake to screen for contraindications may be sufficient before giving a standard massage routine. This is a common situation when offering sample massage at a health fair, postevent massage at a sports event, or signature massage to one-time clients at a destination spa. Planning in those cases is done quickly. Modifications to the routine are made during the session from client feedback. The *plan* in that case involves performing the standard massage and making changes necessary for the safety, comfort, and satisfaction of the client.

Goal-Oriented Planning

Goal-oriented planning focuses on meeting specific client needs, rather than giving a standardized massage routine. Planning to achieve client goals provides a focal point for organizing massage sessions and choosing appropriate techniques. It increases both practitioner and client awareness of positive results and improves satisfaction of regular clients. Goal-oriented planning is an intellectual process that provides a foundation for the artful and intuitive side of massage.

Clients come for massage for a reason. It is either to improve feelings of well-being, rejuvenate the mind/body, relax, reduce pain, improve mobility, alleviate symptoms of a disease, or some other specific desire. Goal-oriented planning can be applied to the entire Wellness Massage Pyramid (WMP). Figure 10.1■ shows the WMP and lists some of the many goals clients have related to massage therapy. The more aware you are of your clients' goals, the better you can serve them.

Clinical reasoning, the cognitive process used in goal-oriented planning, is essentially a problem-solving exercise. The client presents you with a problem to be solved (e.g., stress, muscle tension, pain), and you devise a plan using massage therapy to solve the problem. The goal-oriented planning process presented later uses a basic problem-solving approach.

In massage therapy, three variations of goal-oriented planning are long-range planning, individual session planning, and treatment planning. The steps in the process are the same, but are applied differently for the different circumstances.

STEPS IN GOAL-ORIENTED PLANNING

Goal-oriented planning involves six steps with a feedback loop for making adjustments. The general process is outlined in Box 10.1●.

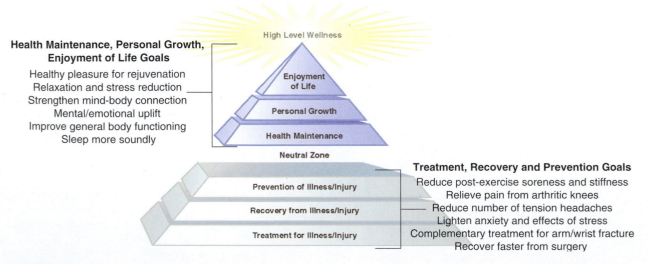

Health Maintenance, Personal Growth, Enjoyment of Life Goals

Healthy pleasure for rejuvenation
Relaxation and stress reduction
Strengthen mind-body connection
Mental/emotional uplift
Improve general body functioning
Sleep more soundly

High Level Wellness

Enjoyment of Life

Personal Growth

Health Maintenance

Neutral Zone

Prevention of Illness/Injury

Recovery from Illness/Injury

Treatment for Illness/Injury

Treatment, Recovery and Prevention Goals

Reduce post-exercise soreness and stiffness
Relieve pain from arthritic knees
Reduce number of tension headaches
Lighten anxiety and effects of stress
Complementary treatment for arm/wrist fracture
Recover faster from surgery

FIGURE 10.1

Sample client goals from the Wellness Massage Pyramid.

BOX 10.1	Six-Step Process for Goal-Oriented Planning

Step 1   Gather information from the client. Obtain subjective information from the client via written forms and verbal interviews.

Step 2   Collect information through observation and measurement. Compile objective information through practitioner observations, tests, and measurements.

Step 3   Assess the situation and set goals. Analyze the subjective and objective information obtained, make your conclusions, and determine client goals.

Step 4   Develop a plan to reach goals. Design a long-term program to achieve client goals. If it is an individual session, choose massage applications to achieve the day's goals.

Step 5   Implement your plan. Perform the massage therapy application

Step 6   Evaluate the results. Analyze the outcomes of a series of sessions, or of one specific session.

Adjust goals and/or plans based on new information and results.

Document the process in session notes (SOAP notes).

Planning is presented here as *steps,* which implies a linear process. In practice however, the thinking involved is not entirely linear. For example, subjective and objective information is gathered continuously as you listen to and observe your client before, during, and after a massage session. Information acquired during a massage from palpation or client feedback may signal a need to modify your session goals or massage application. Goal-oriented massage sessions are works in progress with adjustments as part of the process. Talking about the process as *steps* simply provides an orderly way to grasp the basic concepts and stay focused on the goals.

Taking time for goal-oriented planning is important. However, in most cases it does not need to be lengthy. For most wellness applications, a 5- to 10-minute interview in the initial massage session will suffice, followed by brief check-ins before subsequent sessions to review goals for the day. Treatment of injuries and the use of massage as complementary to medical treatment require more planning and discussion with the client. More time is taken for tests, measurements, and assessment in the initial and progress evaluation sessions for those clients. Many massage therapists schedule an extra 30 minutes for new client intake and interview.

LONG-TERM PLANNING

Long-term planning is typically part of an initial massage session. It is focused on gathering subjective and objective information to get a big picture of the situation, determining overall client goals, and planning out a series of massage sessions to reach those goals. The term *long term* is used here to mean more than one session, or the interval between an initial session and a progress session to check the extent to which goals have been reached. The interval might be anywhere from 1–8 weeks. The steps in long-term planning are summarized on page A-17 in Appendix E, Goal-Oriented Planning.

Step 1 Subjective information is gathered from the client intake form, health history form, and initial client interview.

Step 2 Objective information is collected from observing things such as the client's posture, movement, expression, and stress level. Tests are conducted and measurements are taken related to the client's stated goals, complaints, written referral, or prescription for massage. Tools for information gathering are described in more detail later in the chapter. Their purpose is to collect enough information to assess the situation and identify reachable goals.

Step 3 In Step 3 you assess the situation and establish long-term goals. Wellness goals that can be addressed with massage are identified, as well as problems for which massage is indicated. Also part of assessing the situation is identifying contraindications for massage and cautions to take into consideration later in planning. It may be determined at this point that the client should be referred for medical diagnosis before proceeding with massage.

For clients who receive regular massage as part of their general wellness plan, setting goals depends on what is happening in their lives at the time. They may go through a particularly stressful time, or participate in a seasonal activity like gardening or skiing. They may sustain injuries or get a new job with different physical requirements. Check in with regular clients on an ongoing basis for a continuous updating of long-term goals or goals for a particular session.

An important aspect of Step 3 is prioritizing goals with the client. This helps you determine what to focus on the most without losing sight of the bigger picture. It also brings the client into the process as he or she participates consciously in planning with you. Remember that it is the client's massage, and it is his or her goals that direct the sessions.

Step 4 With the results of Steps 1–3 in mind, an action plan is developed to achieve the client goals. For a long-term plan, this means suggesting the frequency and length of massage sessions. For example, to reduce chronic stress, the plan may be for the client to receive a 1-hour massage weekly at the end of the work week. Or during a competitive season, the plan may be for an athlete to get a weekly maintenance massage with an additional recovery massage the day after an event. Or to facilitate rehabilitation of soft tissue injury such as a sprain, a half-hour massage twice a week for 3 weeks may be the plan.

The action plan includes selecting a general approach, such as relaxation massage sessions, trigger point therapy, myofascial massage, passive joint movements, or some combination. Perhaps polarity therapy, or shiatsu/acupressure, lymphatic facilitation, or some other form of bodywork is called for. Massage therapists survey their repertory of techniques and methods to see which ones are most likely to effectively address client goals. Obviously, the larger your repertoire, the more choices you have. Also, the more knowledgeable you are about the effects of different

CASE FOR STUDY

Kate and Long-Term Planning

Kate has decided to add regular massage to her overall wellness lifestyle. She contacts a massage therapist recommended by a friend and schedules her first massage. She is not sure what to expect but believes that massage will be beneficial for her.

The massage therapist has Kate fill out intake and health history forms. Kate reports that she is taking medication for allergies, but otherwise has no major medical conditions. She broke her left arm a few years ago, but it has healed. She is also adjusting her diet for healthier eating and plans to exercise more.

The massage therapist observes that Kate has some limitation in motion in the upper extremities around the past fracture. She checks with Kate about her sensitivity to certain massage oils and lotions. They briefly discuss the potential health benefits of massage and Kate's expectations. They agree to focus on stress reduction and relief of tension in the left arm and shoulder for the next few sessions.

Kate plans to come for massage every other week. Before each session, the massage therapist checks on the effects the massage sessions are having. Additional goals are expected to be set as the client learns more about massage and expands her ideas about how it can help her achieve her wellness goals.

The massage therapist will apply Swedish massage techniques, adding trigger point therapy and stretching to the shoulders and arms, for the first few sessions. She writes intake information, observations, assessment, and the long-range plan in the session notes for the day. After 2 months, the massage therapist will evaluate progress toward the original goals and modify them as needed as the therapeutic relationship develops over time.

Questions for planning:

- What subjective information did Kate provide?
  _____

- What objective information was gathered by the massage therapist?
  _____

- What were the agreed upon goals for massage therapy?
  _____

- What was the resulting long-range plan?
  _____

---

techniques and approaches, the better able you will be to choose an approach to help clients reach their goals.

Home care is another important aspect of Step 4. Note that massage therapists do not *prescribe* activities for their clients, which is outside of their scope of practice. But they can suggest different additional activities to be done on the clients' own time at home that may help them achieve their goals more quickly or effectively. Common home-care activities include self-massage techniques, hot and cold applications, stretching, active exercises, and relaxation techniques.

Step 5 Implementing a long-term plan entails reviewing the plan with the client and making appointments. Being an educator is part of being a massage therapist as you teach your clients how to do their home-care activities.

Step 6 Long-term planning involves taking time to evaluate the results of a series of massage sessions and answering the question, "How well are the client's goals being met?" This is done in special progress sessions for well-defined goals, or on a less formal basis in presession interviews with the client, or with observations made during sessions.

The important point is to keep goals in mind and be aware of positive results toward those goals as time passes. You will thus gain from your experiences and become a better massage therapist than if you just give massage sessions without paying attention to the results. Your clients benefit from achieving their goals, and you benefit as you learn from your experiences.

Loop After the evaluation of results, the process loops to one or more of the steps described earlier as more information is gathered, and goals and plans are updated. Goal-oriented planning is less a linear process and more of a looping spiral.

Long-term plans are documented in notes that go into client files. These notes are essentially a recap of the steps in the planning process. Sections later in this chapter explain in detail what goes into the notes and how to write them.

A client who comes for massage to achieve a specific goal (e.g., to reduce tension headaches) may stop appointments once that goal is met. Many clients, however, benefit from regular massage to achieve high-level wellness or address a chronic health problem. Working with a client over time is a continuous process of assessing the situation and modifying your approach accordingly.

INDIVIDUAL SESSION PLANNING

Each individual massage session is a step toward achieving long-term client goals. Some basic questions to ask are, "Where are we today, and what can we do in this session to move closer to the long-term goals?" The goal-oriented planning process for individual massage sessions is summarized on page A-17 in Appendix E, Goal-Oriented Planning.

CRITICAL THINKING

Explore the truth of the statement: "Every massage needs a plan." Consider these questions:

1. What purpose does planning serve?
2. Can you give a massage without a plan?

3. How detailed does a plan for massage need to be?
4. When is a more detailed plan appropriate? When is an abbreviated plan a better choice?

Step 1 Before a client arrives, it is useful to do a quick review of previous session notes, and, in some cases, his or her intake and health history forms. Reacquaint yourself with the long-term goals and the results of the last session. From that point of orientation, you greet your client and perform a brief presession interview. In that interview, you ask the client about any changes in health status or medications and any progress or regression related to his or her goals since the last massage session.

Step 2 As you greet and interview your client, observe general posture, facial expression, voice quality, and other outward indicators of his or her state of being. Either before or during the session when the client is on the massage table, use brief tests and measurements to collect objective information (e.g., evaluating flexibility during a stretch, tissue quality while performing massage techniques, or ability to relax and let go of tension).

Step 3 Prior to beginning the massage, assess the current situation and prioritize the day's goals with the client. Determine any contraindications and cautions to be taken into consideration in this session. This may include long-standing conditions or temporary conditions, such as a recently acquired bruise or aspirin taken an hour before for a minor headache. Agree on goals for the session and briefly review your general plan for the day with the client.

Step 4 While assessing the situation in Step 3, begin formulating your plan for the day. This is a good example of the steps in the planning process as overlapping and blending, rather than being discrete sequential steps. The goals for the session will lead logically to an appropriate session organization and choice of techniques. While the client is undressing and getting onto the table, you can go over the plan in your mind, start your notes for the day, or prepare adjunct modalities such as hot packs.

Step 5 Begin the massage with the action plan in mind. For example, you begin at a certain place on the body using techniques chosen to achieve specific client goals. During the session, you might see reactions or results that either support the approach planned or signal a need to modify the plan. As you become aware of additional subjective and

objective information, you will modify the original action plan for best results.

Step 6 Evaluating progress during a massage session is an essential part of the implementation phase as explained in Step 5. A postsession evaluation is also important. When you are saying good-bye to the client, you can make general observations and conduct a brief postsession interview. Questions should be open-ended and designed to elicit information useful to evaluating the outcomes of the massage; for example, "How is your arm feeling now?" or "Are you feeling more relaxed?"

Each session is documented in notes that go into client files. The SOAP note format described later in this chapter is well suited for capturing the goal-oriented planning process. The notes from the last session become a point of departure for planning the next time the client comes for massage.

TREATMENT PLANNING

Treatment planning is a form of goal-oriented planning in which the goal is alleviation of symptoms, or facilitation of healing of a pathological condition. It is used for medical, clinical, and orthopedic massage applications, and the treatment and recovery levels of the Wellness Massage Pyramid. A treatment plan is sometimes called a *plan of care*. See Appendix E, Goal-Oriented Planning, on page A-18.

Treatment planning requires a greater knowledge of pathology and massage research, as well as more advanced assessment and manual skills than other massage applications. Massage therapists who treat structural problems learn advanced musculoskeletal anatomy, biomechanics, and kinesiology, the study of human movement.

The terms *clinical massage, medical massage,* and *orthopedic massage* are sometimes used to describe advanced specialties within the broader field of massage therapy that focus on treatment. These terms do not refer to a unique set of techniques, but rather to the application of massage in a treatment planning process (Lowe 2004; Rattray and Ludwig 2000).

CASE FOR STUDY

Steve and Individual-Session Planning

Steve signs up for a massage at the health club about once a month. He believes that regular massage helps him relax and relieves the aches and pains from his sports activities. Steve has been getting massage at the club for about 2 years. He sees whichever massage therapist is available at the time he wants to schedule the session.

While the massage therapist is waiting for Steve to arrive, he quickly reviews Steve's health history. He also looks at past session notes, especially from the last four massage sessions. He is looking for contraindications, past injuries, recent goals for sessions, and notes about results.

When Steve arrives, the massage therapist screens for changes in health status and current medications, and asks about Steve's specific goals for the session. Steve reports that his legs and feet are a little stiff, and that he has some bruises on his legs from a hiking trip the past weekend. Steve is looking for general relaxation, reduced stiffness, and overall rejuvenation.

The massage therapist plans a full-body basic maintenance sports massage session. He will spend a little extra time on the legs and feet, but will avoid deep pressure over bruised areas. The session will include effleurage and kneading techniques, trigger point therapy, and myofascial massage as needed. Joint mobilizing and stretching, especially in the lower extremities, will be done. Problems found through palpation and range-of-motion evaluation will be noted and addressed if there is time. The massage therapist writes observations, techniques applied, and results in the individual session notes.

Questions for planning:

● What subjective information did Steve provide?

_____

● What objective information was gathered by the massage therapist?

_____

● What were the agreed upon goals for massage therapy?

_____

● What was the resulting session plan

_____

One major difference between treatment planning and other types of goal-oriented planning is in Step 3, that is, assessment of the situation. In medical settings, assessment typically means identifying or diagnosing a pathological condition. Since massage therapists may not diagnose according to state laws, **assessment** is more about measuring function or loss of function (e.g., range of motion), or evaluating the condition of tissues (e.g., fibrosis and adhesions). It may be determining how massage can alleviate symptoms such as pain or facilitate healing. Clients often come to massage therapists seeking complementary care for a condition already medically diagnosed and under treatment by other health care professionals.

Yates (2004) sums up the critical competencies for developing treatment plans for medical conditions. First is the "ability to accurately *assess* the cause of the patient's presenting complaint in order to select and plan appropriate treatment." Second is the "capacity to *recognize* conditions for which some therapeutic approaches are contraindicated and to modify treatment accordingly." And third is "mastery of a sufficient variety of soft tissue techniques and other modalities to be able to safely and effectively *perform* the most appropriate form of treatment" (p. 13).

Another difference in treatment planning is the end point of treatment. Medical settings that take their lead from health insurance companies often define the point of discharge or end of treatment as reaching the neutral point. The neutral point is the point at which symptoms are relieved (e.g., pain),

normal function is restored, or sign of illness undetectable. However, in the wellness model, that is the jumping off point toward high-level wellness.

Collecting subjective and objective information from the client is the foundation of the goal-oriented planning process. These essential steps are explained in greater detail in the remainder of this chapter.

COLLECTING SUBJECTIVE INFORMATION

Intake is the process of gathering relevant information from a new client. This is considered to be subjective information. Intake forms are usually filled out by the client without direct help from the massage therapist. They contain general information about the client (e.g., name, address, phone, occupation); identification of the primary health care provider, and insurance company, if relevant; and the reason for the initial visit.

Intake forms also explain the nature and scope of the massage practice and fees and policies (e.g., fees, payment, and cancellation policy). Intake forms usually include a privacy statement explaining confidentiality policies and consent for care.

Give a copy of this form to the client to take home for reference and keep a signed copy for his or her client file. A basic intake form for massage therapy can be found in Appendix G, Intake, Health History, and Note Forms, on page A-52.

CASE FOR STUDY

Angela and Treatment Planning

Angela comes for massage complaining of frequent tension headaches. In the client intake interview, she reports having headaches at least 3 times a week. She mentions that her neck is stiff. The massage therapist notices that she has trouble turning her head from side to side. Angela takes aspirin, but that is becoming less effective. The headaches are more likely to occur in the afternoon after she works at her desk for a long period of time.

She has not been in an accident lately and has no other signs of contraindications for massage. Her doctor has ruled out any underlying medical conditions that might cause frequent headaches and prescribed moist heat and a pain reducer to alleviate the headache pain.

It appears to be a typical case of chronic tension headache with no contraindications for massage. After discussion, the massage therapist and Angela both agree that the goal for massage will be to reduce the intensity and frequency of the headaches. The plan is for Angela to come for massage twice a week for 2 weeks and perform home care of self-massage and stretching, as well as hot applications. She will also begin using a headset for the telephone and reposition her computer screen to achieve better neck alignment when working.

The general approach for massage sessions will be to focus on the shoulder, neck, and head muscles most often associated with tension headaches. General relaxation will be included for the beneficial effects of the relaxation response. Techniques will be drawn from Swedish massage, trigger point therapy, and myofascial massage.

The plan is to reassess the situation after 2 weeks to see if there are fewer or less severe headaches. Before and after each session, the massage therapist asks Angela to rate her headache pain on a scale from 1 to 10 (1 = no pain; 10 = severe pain). She also notes days when headaches occurred and how severe they were.

As her headaches subside, Angela reduces her sessions to once a week and then to twice a month. Regular massage and home care activities help keep shoulders and neck muscles relaxed and reduce the number of headaches and their intensity.

Questions for planning:

- What subjective information did Angela provide?

- What objective information was gathered by the massage therapist?

- What were the agreed upon goals for massage therapy?

- What was the resulting treatment plan?

Health/Medical History

A general health history is also filled out by the client as part of the intake process. The purpose of the health history is to learn more about the client's health and medical history, as well as to identify potential contraindications and cautions for massage. In treatment planning, information about medical conditions, diagnoses from health care providers, and treatment goals help massage therapists plan sessions specifically to address the condition for which massage is sought and indicated.

A sample health history form for general wellness applications, and a different form for more medically oriented situations, can be found in Appendix G, Intake, Health History, and Note Forms, on page A-55. The medically oriented form has more detail about past and current injuries, surgeries, diseases, and medications.

There are situations when intake forms and health histories are impractical or unnecessary, for example, for a short massage at a health fair, trade show, or sports event. In these cases, a minimum amount of information is necessary to provide a safe massage session. Some basic screening questions to ask are:

- Have you ever had massage before? (If no, provide more explanation and instructions.)

- Have you been ill recently?
- Do you have any skin conditions, injuries, or bruises I should avoid?
- Have you taken any medication today that affects your blood pressure or circulation?
- Have you taken any pain relievers today?
- If a woman: Are you pregnant?
- Is there any area that is especially tense that you'd like me to spend more time on?

The main purpose of these screening questions is to identify specific areas to focus on and contraindications or places to avoid massaging. A short consent statement and liability release form should also be signed before giving even a short massage. A sample intake list for massage events can be found in Appendix G, Intake, Health History, and Note Forms, on page A-59.

Intake Interview

After the client fills out the intake and health history forms, the massage therapist conducts a short intake interview. The purpose of the interview is to clarify items on the forms and fill in any gaps of information. For example, if a client says that he or she was in a car accident last week, you would want to ask further questions about medical treatment received, injuries sustained, or lingering aftereffects. This is also the opportunity to confirm the client's top priorities for massage and collect more specific information about problems the person may be having.

INTERVIEW SKILLS

Interview skills include a variety of methods for eliciting useful information from clients. These communication skills are important from the time you screen potential clients on the phone, to intake interviews with new clients, to taking health histories, and conducting pre- and postsession interviews.

Listening skills are essential to interviews, as are different methods for framing client answers. Some basic client interview methods are asking open-ended and multiple-choice questions, and using rating scales and body charts.

Open-Ended Questions   Open-ended questions steer clients to specific topics, but leave space for them to answer in their own words. Rather than dictating the form of response, the massage therapist listens to what the client has to say in answer to a simple question. Responses to open-ended questions often give clues for further questions. Examples of general open-ended questions used in presession interviews appear below.

- How are you feeling today?
- How has your shoulder been feeling since the last massage?
- How were your legs during the marathon last weekend?
- Has your stress level related to that work situation calmed down?
- Were you able to rearrange your workstation so you aren't straining your neck so much?
- What are your goals for the massage today?

Multiple-Choice Questions   Multiple-choice questions give clients a choice of descriptors, which helps them to be more specific and helps you to better assess the situation they are trying to describe. It gives them choices that they might not have thought of themselves, but that have meaning to you. Some useful descriptors for common complaints appear below.

- Is the sensation you feel numbness, tingling, or pain?
- Would you describe your pain as sharp, diffuse, dull, aching, or throbbing?
- Would you describe the pain as: mild, moderate, or severe?
- Would you describe movement at your shoulder as free, fluid, stiff, or restricted?
- Are your headaches seldom, occasional, frequent, or almost constant?

Rating Scales   Rating scales offer a rough measurement of things from the client's subjective view. Ratings use numbers to measure the degree or level of the client's experience of some factor related to their goals. Ratings give an indication of the client's experience of his or her condition and can be used to measure progress or regression from the client's perspective.

A scale from 1 to 10 is familiar to most clients, with 1 indicating the best scenario and 10 indicating the worst scenario for the item being rated. Below are examples of rating stress level, pain, and function.

- On a scale of 1 to 10—1 being pleasantly relaxed and 10 being totally stressed—how would you rate your level of stress today?
- On a scale of 1 to 10—1 being pain free and 10 being extreme pain—how would you rate how your back feels today?
- On a scale from 1 to 10—1 being easy and 10 being extremely limited—how would you rate your ability to walk up stairs today?

Body Charts   These forms show diagrams of the human figure (e.g., front, back, and side views) that are marked by the client to locate problem areas and indicate the nature of a complaint. They offer the client a visual and kinesthetic (as opposed to verbal) way to give subjective information. Body charts can be used in the initial interview, as well as before individual massage sessions.

Clients mark with a pen the exact spots of concern on an outline of a body. Symbols can be used to locate painful areas, recent injuries, or bruises. Symbols can also be used to indicate different feelings in the area, for example, tension, numbness, tingling, and pain.

A body chart marked by the client is similar to the body chart filled in as part of the massage therapist's written SOAP notes (see Figure 10.9 on page 332). Documentation should clearly indicate whether the client or the massage therapist is the source of information on the chart.

INTERVIEW GUIDELINES

In addition to framing relevant questions, conducting good interviews includes knowing how to create an openness to response, when to lead the questioning, what to avoid, and when to stop.

Clients feel more open to giving responses if they understand the reason for your questions. Explain why you are asking questions in the interview. For example, while setting up an appointment for a first-time client, say something like: "I'm going to ask you a few questions to see if massage therapy would help you reach your goals, and if so, to plan your first session." Before taking a health history explain: "I need a little more information about your health and any medications you are taking to plan the massage session."

Use body language that encourages answering. For example, look directly at the client and listen for the answer, rather than shuffling papers or looking around the room.

Give clients time to respond if you want thoughtful and accurate answers to questions. Do not rush the client's answers, and pause for 5–10 seconds before repeating the question or asking further questions. Remember that silence gives the client the space he or she needs to respond.

Some clients may need more direction, especially if you are relying on open-ended questions. Switch to multiple-choice questions, rating scales, or body charts for clients who have trouble expressing themselves verbally.

Ways to take more of a lead in questioning include asking for clarification of a statement, keeping clients on the topic if they are digressing, and helping them to get to the point. Ask clients to clarify conflicting statements. Ask for a final statement of agreement in important matters such as billing policies, informed consent, or goals of a massage session. For example, say, "Do we agree on those two primary goals for this session?"

Avoid creating an atmosphere in which clients feel like they're being interrogated, for example, by not smiling, or asking rapid-fire questions, or questioning their answers. Avoid being judgmental or dismissing their answers as unimportant. Do not deny their experiences.

Avoid questions not directly relevant to their massage therapy sessions. For example, it would be inappropriate to have a person coming to you for a relaxation massage go through an extensive medical history interview.

A good rule of thumb is to make interviews just long enough to get the essential information for planning a safe and effective massage session—no longer. Clients are coming for massage, which is a hands-on experience. Unnecessary questions take away from that valuable session time. A summary of interview guidelines is shown in Box 10.2●.

BOX 10.2	**Summary of Interview Guidelines**

When conducting client interviews, follow these guidelines:

1. Create an inviting and open atmosphere.
2. Explain to the client *why* you are asking questions.
3. Look directly at the client when asking a question.
4. Give clients time to think and speak.
5. Use affirmative listening for encouragement.
6. Use active listening to clarify what was said.
7. Lead back a client who is digressing.
8. Ask for clarification of conflicting statements.
9. Use open-ended questions to hear the client's own words.
10. Use multiple-choice, rating, or body charts to frame answers.
11. Ask only relevant questions.
12. Stop when you know enough.

Avoid:

1. Creating an atmosphere of interrogation
2. Asking rapid-fire questions
3. Speaking too fast
4. Being judgmental
5. Dismissing answers
6. Denying the client's experience
7. Posing unnecessary questions

COLLECTING OBJECTIVE INFORMATION

Objective methods of collecting information include the massage therapist's own observations, evaluations, and measurements. These methods do not rely on a client's subjective view, but come from the practitioner's objective or outside perspective.

The type of information collected varies according to the client's reason for seeking massage or to his or her initial complaint. Initial sessions and progress evaluation sessions will contain more evaluation than ongoing sessions. Methods for collecting objective information include making general observations about the client, palpation of the client's tissues, range-of-motion evaluation, posture analysis, biomechanics analysis, and gait analysis.

Be mindful that there is a difference between what you observe and your interpretation of those observations. For example, you might observe that a client is moving slowly and stiffly. It will take further investigation to assess why this might be the case. The cause might be any number of things, such as osteoarthritis, low mood, habitual movement pattern, a recent accident, or the marathon the individual ran the day before.

Be careful that you do not jump to conclusions or diagnose, that is, put the name of a pathology or medical condition to what you observe. Massage therapist are limited in their interpretations by their level of training. Beginning massage therapists have less knowledge to make interpretations than those with more training and experience. This means that you should sharpen your skills at observation, while understanding your limitations at interpretation of what you see.

General Observations

Observation is a basic tool for evaluation of the client's condition. Massage therapists use their senses to *observe* clients, that is, with their eyes, ears, noses, and hands. Some general observations and examples of descriptors are listed below.

- Skin: dry patches, blotches or red spots, acne, unusual marks or moles, rashes, bruises, wounds, scars
- Movement quality: slow, stiff, fluid, controlled, unstable, guarded
- Facial expression: smile, frown, nervous tick, furrowed brow, blank, serene
- Level of communication: nonstop talking, talkative, quiet, nonresponsive, silent
- Voice quality: loud, soft, weak, raspy, high pitched, low pitched
- Breathing: relaxed, diaphragmatic, chest breathing, labored, rapid, sighing, congested, wheezing, coughing
- Mental clarity: sharp, alert, fuzzy, vacant, distracted, forgetful, sleepy
- Emotional state: relaxed, agitated, nervous, angry, worried, anxious

For session notes, general descriptors are more useful if accompanied by specific or detailed descriptions of behaviors. For example, "The client seemed nervous and was tapping her pencil through the whole interview" is more informative than "The client seemed nervous." Another example, "The client's breathing was relaxed, from the diaphragm, and even" tells more than "The client seemed relaxed." Note that the simpler descriptions (e.g., nervous and relaxed) are actually interpretations of more specific behaviors that you observed.

Be as specific as you can in your notes. You may find out later that your interpretation of what you observed was incorrect. It is useful to be able to refer back to the original observation when reinterpreting or reviewing a situation. Although you observe many things about the client during the course of a massage, notes written about the session are limited to information used in planning and evaluating the current or future massage sessions. Session notes are discussed in more detail later in the chapter.

Palpation

Palpation is the act of sensing information about the client through touch. Palpation is about the *feel* of tissues and of movement at joints. Biel explains palpation as "an art and skill which involves 1) locating a structure, 2) becoming aware of its characteristics, and 3) assessing its quality or condition so you can determine how to treat it" (2001, p. 14). A fourth aspect of palpation is to detect changes in quality or condition of tissues as a result of massage.

Palpatory sensitivity can only be developed through hands-on practice, aided by describing in words what is felt. Chaitow states, "We need to unleash a torrent of descriptive words for what we feel when we palpate" and "to obtain a thesaurus and to look up as many words as possible to describe accurately the subtle variations in what is being palpated" (1997, p. 9). The physical skill of sensing qualities and the verbal skill of describing them accurately together make up palpatory literacy.

The first step in palpatory literacy for massage therapists is to be able to locate specific structures, that is, to feel where anatomical structures are located on the body. This is usually learned in anatomy class with a hands-on lab. Focus is on muscles, bones, joints, and related tissues and structures. This is useful knowledge for any type of massage therapy.

As palpation skills develop, you become more aware of differences in tissue temperature, texture, and firmness. You sense the ease of movement in healthy tissue and joints.

You are then able to detect abnormal tissue conditions. Descriptors for abnormal tissues include *spongy, hard, grainy, stringy, taut, taut bands, nodules, thick, congested, dehydrated,* and *adhering.* When assessing fascia, you feel for restrictions to movement or sticking. Abnormal joint movements may be described as *stiff, clicking, shortened, grinding,* or *bound.*

Some forms of massage therapy key into the body's rhythms that can be felt in the tissues. Body rhythms include circulatory rhythm or pulse, respiratory rhythm or breathing, and craniosacral rhythm in the circulation of cerebralspinal fluid. Practitioners of Chinese medicine read the subtle radial pulse and detect the health of each organ and flow of energy, or *chi,* in the body.

Some forms of energy bodywork rely on detection of the body's energy field and the flow of energy in and around the body. These include polarity therapy, reiki, and therapeutic touch.

Developing palpation skill takes time and attention. Biel offers three principles of palpation (2001, p. 18):

1. Move slowly. Haste only interferes with sensation.
2. Avoid using excessive pressure. Less is truly more.
3. Focus your awareness on what it is you are feeling. In other words, be present.

The more conscious hands-on time you log, the better your palpation skills will be. Palpation skills develop throughout your entire career as a massage therapist. Examples of useful terms to describe palpation findings are listed in Box 10.3•.

BOX 10.3   Descriptors for Documenting Palpation Findings

Words used to describe palpation findings are presented below in relative terms. Although most of these terms have inexact definitions, they are useful in describing general palpation findings.

Skin

hot / warm / cold
dry / damp / oily
hairless / hairy
smooth / rough
loose / taut
thin / thick
elastic / mobile
scarred

Soft Tissues (General)

spongy / firm
hard / tough / pliable / soft
dehydrated / puffy / swollen
congested
grainy / smooth

Muscles and Tendons

hypertonic / hypotonic
hard / firm / pliable
taut / taut bands / lax
knotty / smooth
ropey or ropelike
stringy
spasm / relaxed

BOX 10.3 *(Continued)*

Fascia

adhering / sticking / moving freely
restricted / unrestricted

Joint Movement

stiff / easy / free
clicking / hitches / glitches
crepetations
grinding / grating
stuck / bound / freely moving

Pulses

strong / weak
fast / slow
even / uneven
regular / irregular

Energy

stagnant / blocked / free flowing
pooled
fluid
excess / deficient

Range of Motion Evaluation

Objective information about the general condition and degree of flexibility at a specific joint can be obtained by a range of motion evaluation. This is done by active or passive movement of the joint through its range, while observing any restrictions or shortening and any discomfort experienced by the client. Normal range of motion at major joints is shown in Figure 6.110 on page 215.

For evaluating active range of motion (AROM) at a joint, first demonstrate the movement you want the client to perform. Ask him or her to move slowly and steadily. Observe the client's ease of movement and any limitations or weakness. The client may report pain or discomfort verbally or by facial expression. Compare movement on both sides of the body. Document any deviation from normal, pain-free movement in your session notes.

Three simple (AROM) tests for the shoulder are described by Hoppenfeld in *Physical Examination of the Spine and Extremities* (1976, p. 21). These are the Apley Scratch Test and two tests for internal rotation and adduction shown in Figure 10.2■. Tests like these are simple for clients to perform and offer quick, objective evaluations.

For evaluating passive range of motion (PROM) at a joint, have the client relax the muscles surrounding the joint while you move the joint through its range or apply a mild stretch. A passive stretch offers a good estimate of the degree of motion at a joint. For upper and lower extremities, compare the degree of flexibility on both the right and left sides. Note any restrictions in movement, differences in left and right sides, or discomfort experienced by the client. Document any positive findings, that is, any deviations from normal, pain-free movement at the joint.

You can also measure the range of motion quantitatively using an instrument called a goniometer, which is similar to a protractor used in geometry to measure angles (Figure 10.3■). There are specific protocols for measuring range of motion with this instrument that take some practice to master and are used primarily for medical applications.

Range of motion evaluation offers clues to potential muscle and tendon problems (AROM), or problems with ligaments and joint structures (PROM). Swelling, discoloration, or severe pain with passive joint movement signals

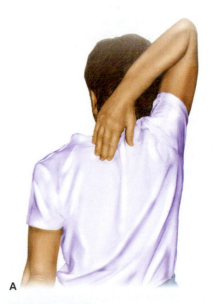
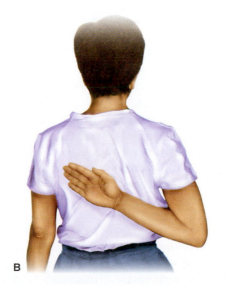
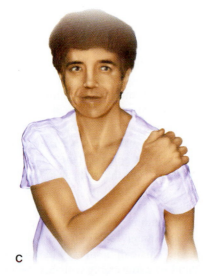

A   B   C

FIGURE 10.2

Active range of motion (AROM) tests for the shoulder. A. Apley Scratch Test. B. and C. Internal rotation and adduction tests.

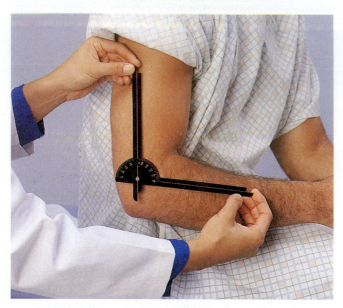

FIGURE 10.3

Using a goniometer to measure joint ROM.

that massage is contraindicated in the area. For any suspected joint injury, the client should see a health care provider for a diagnosis of his or her condition.

On the other hand, restricted range of motion may simply be a sign of tense, shortened muscles that can benefit from increased circulation in the area, muscle relaxation, and lengthening of muscles fibers. Joint movements are discussed in greater detail, along with examples of mobilizing techniques and stretches for the neck and upper and lower extremities, in Chapter 13, Western Massage Techniques, beginning on page 398.

Posture Analysis

Posture, or body alignment, can tell a lot about a client's physical and emotional state and reveals habitual patterns that can cause problems in the musculature. Standing, sitting, and sleeping posture are three basic points of reference for evaluating a client who complains about back, neck, and shoulder tension or pain. Evaluation of the body's structural alignment is called *posture analysis.*

Important guidelines for good posture include standing straight and tall while avoiding locking the knees. The weight of the body should be mostly over the balls of the feet, not back on the heels. The head should be in alignment on top of the neck and spine and the chin not pushed forward. To keep the head level, the chin can be tucked slightly. The arms hang naturally down at the sides of the body. The shoulders are relaxed.

Standing posture analysis can be as simple as asking a client to stand for a moment and observing his or her alignment. This can be done with the client clothed, shoes off, standing comfortably with feet slightly apart, and arms hanging at the sides. View the client from the front, back, and sides. Look for uneven height in shoulders or hips, leaning,

head and chin forward, stooping, head tilted to one side, twisting, one arm hanging lower than the other, and any other deviation from good body alignment. A vertical point of reference such as a door frame can be used to identify leaning or other asymmetry.

Wall grid charts are useful for formal postural analysis and essential for structurally focused massage therapists. Grid charts have both vertical and horizontal lines to measure more accurately any deviations from balanced posture. Photos taken of clients standing in front of grid charts are useful for the initial analysis, client education about posture, and evaluation of progress toward goals of improving posture. Body charts that show boney landmarks are useful for visual charting of posture deviations. See Figure 10.4■.

Sitting posture analysis is especially important for clients who work at desks or tables and complain of neck and shoulder tightness or pain. Some guidelines for good sitting posture are that the back is supported by the back of the chair, and the knees are aligned evenly with the hips, or slightly higher. Both feet are flat on the floor, or on a foot support. Slouching or sitting forward should be avoided, and the head should be aligned over the shoulders with the chin tucked slightly, as in good standing posture. If working at a desk, the arms should be flexed at a 75- to 90-degree angle, with shoulders squared and relaxed. Stretching breaks should be taken to avoid sitting in one position too long. Aligned sitting posture is shown in Figure 10.5■.

A client's sleeping posture may also cause problems. Subjective information about sleeping habits may reveal a source of muscular aggravation. Firm mattresses are generally better than soft ones for proper back support. Sleeping on the side or back offers better alignment than sleeping on the stomach, which can strain the neck and lower back. Pillows should help keep the natural curvature of the neck and not cause hyperextension or flexion. While the client is supine on the massage table, you can demonstrate using a neck roll for added support and the use of a pillow under the knees to relieve pressure on the lower back. You can also show proper use of pillows for good alignment while in the side-lying position.

Biomechanical Analysis

Biomechanics is the study of movement in living organisms. It takes into account principles of motion and the structure and function of the human body, especially the muscle and skeletal systems. Whereas posture analysis looks at the body at rest, biomechanics looks at the body in motion. It is a branch of kinesiology and an important aspect of sports medicine.

Biomechanical analysis of your own movements while performing massage is an important aspect of your training. It can help you avoid injuries from poor body mechanics and serve as a starting point for understanding your clients' body mechanics. Good body mechanics for massage therapists are described in greater detail in Chapter 12, Body Mechanics, Table Skills, and Application Guidelines, on page 362, and

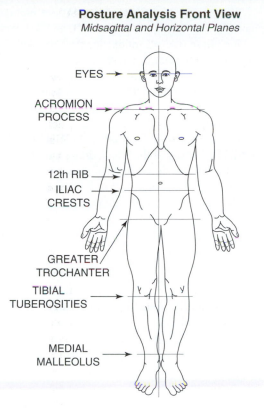

Posture Analysis Front View
Midsagittal and Horizontal Planes

EYES →

ACROMION PROCESS

12th RIB
ILIAC CRESTS

GREATER TROCHANTER

TIBIAL TUBEROSITIES →

MEDIAL MALLEOLUS →

Posture Analysis Side View
Coronal Planes

EAR →

HEAD OF HUMERUS →

0°
10°

GREATER TROCHANTER →

FEMORAL LATERAL CONDYLE →

LATERAL MALLEOLUS →

FIGURE 10.4

Body chart for standing posture assessment.

various aspects of self-care are discussed in Chapter 4, Physical Skills, Fitness, and Self-Care for the Massage Therapist, on page 82.

Knowledge of biomechanics is essential for massage therapists who work with athletes, dancers, musicians, artists, craftsmen, and others who use their bodies in their daily activities. Massage therapists who specialize in musculoskeletal complaints or structural bodywork should also be well versed in analyzing how the body moves, and how it applies and absorbs force.

Biomechanical analysis is the examination of common movements, such as lifting, and job-related movements, such as using a computer keyboard, and can help massage therapists identify points of stress and strain on their clients' bodies. This is especially helpful in providing objective information about clients with overuse injuries.

Biomechanical analysis not only points to specific structures affected by a movement (e.g., muscles, tendons, joints, ligaments), but also can suggest ways of correcting movement patterns that may be causing a client musculoskeletal problems.

Biomechanical analysis of lifting a heavy object with good alignment is shown in Figure 10.6■. Notice that the knees bend to reach the object, with the back bending as little as possible. In proper alignment, the leg muscles do the lifting, and not the lower back or arm muscles. Keep the weight of the object as close as possible to your center of gravity. Poor alignment when lifting puts strain on the lower back.

Advise your clients to carry heavy objects close to the body and switch arms frequently if carrying something in one hand, such as a suitcase. Balance equal weight on both sides if possible when carrying more than one object. When

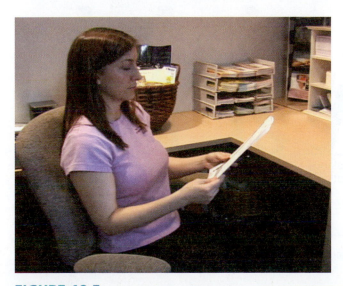

FIGURE 10.5

Good alignment for sitting posture.

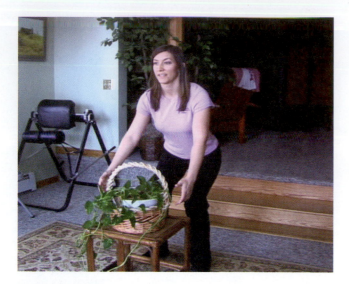

FIGURE 10.6

Good body mechanics for lifting heavy objects.

carrying a backpack, avoid leaning forward and rounding the shoulders. If unable to keep good alignment, consider using a pack or case with wheels.

Gait Analysis

Gait analysis looks at biomechanics while walking or running. Gait analysis starts when your client walks into the room, and you begin to observe his or her movement pattern. For further analysis, watch the client walk away from you and toward you. Figure 10.7■ shows the phases of walking.

The phases of walking for each foot include a stance phase (heel strike, flat foot, push off, and acceleration), and a swing phase (toe-off, midswing, and deceleration). While one foot is in the stance phase, the other foot is in the swing phase. Points to look for in walking are base width (2–4 inches from heel to heel), vertical movement of the center of gravity, knee flexion, lateral shifting, length of step, and pelvis rotation.

Deviations from normal include slow gait, limping, shuffling, twisting at the waist, dragging the feet, waddling (lateral movement), wide base, lurching. Compensations may also be made for arthritic or fused joints in the feet or legs. Some of the common causes of walking gait deviations are listed in Table 10.1■. More detailed analysis of gait is found in biomechanics, clinical massage, and orthopedic massage texts.

Orthopedic Tests

A number of orthopedic tests are available to assess pathology in musculoskeletal structures, movement and locomotor disorders, and sources of soft-tissue pain and dysfunction. Use of these tests is shared with other professionals, such as physical therapists, athletic trainers, and orthopedic doctors.

Orthopedic or clinical massage is an advanced specialty for massage therapists who focus on the use of massage to treat orthopedic conditions. Details about orthopedic massage and assessment skills are outside the scope of this foundations book, but can be found in other texts (see Appendix H, References and Additional Resources, on page A-63).

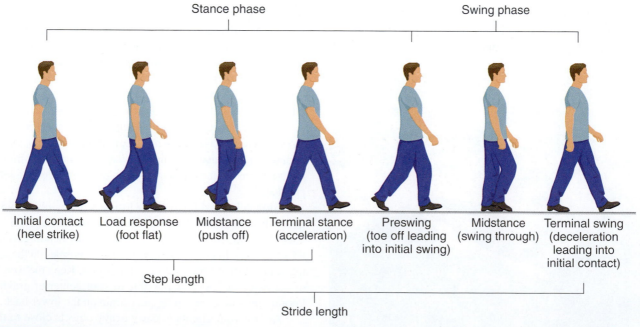

Stance phase   Swing phase

| Initial contact (heel strike) | Load response (foot flat) | Midstance (push off) | Terminal stance (acceleration) | Preswing (toe off leading into initial swing) | Midstance (swing through) | Terminal swing (deceleration leading into initial contact) |

Step length

Stride length

FIGURE 10.7

Phases of the normal walking gait.

TABLE 10.1	Common Causes of Walking Gait Deviations
Gait Deviation	**Common Causes**
Slow walk	Old age, neurological disorder, joint disease, or injury
Limping	Injury to foot or leg, short leg
Shuffling	Weak quadriceps, Parkinson's disease, neurological disorder
Twisting	Arms crossing midline during walk
Dragging	Tibialis anterior weakness (also called drop foot, toe scraping)
Waddling	Pain in lower back, hips, lower extremities
Wide base	Unsteadiness, dizziness, general weakness, vision problems
Lurching	Weakness in gluteal muscles

Massage therapists who apply these tests do so in the context of their scope of practice. They do not diagnose pathologies. The purpose of massage therapists using orthopedic tests is for observation of function, ruling out conditions and injuries that may be contraindications for massage, and for decisions about referrals to doctors for medical diagnosis.

IMPORTANCE OF DOCUMENTATION

Documentation is the process of writing massage session records for future reference. It is also called note-taking or charting. Session notes are kept on paper or in electronic form in client files.

Notes can be considered legal documents when used for insurance reporting, or may be subpoenaed as evidence in legal cases. Notes are official client health records. In clinical settings they are protected by **HIPAA privacy rules.** HIPAA stands for the Health Insurance Portability and Accountability Act, which was passed by the U. S. Congress in 1996 to protect the privacy of medical records. (Find more information about HIPAA on page 112 in Chapter 5, Ethics and the Therapeutic Relationship.)

Notes are also very practical. Notes assist the massage therapist in remembering what happened the last time a client came for massage and may show meaningful patterns over time. If two or more massage therapists share clients, they can review each other's notes while planning an upcoming session. Notes demonstrate the care taken to ensure a client's safety and well-being. Well-written SOAP notes also reflect a logical or clinical reasoning process by presenting information in an organized way and keeping the focus on goals for the massage sessions.

Documentation is not an extra chore or optional task. It is an important part of every massage session. Time can be set aside either between sessions or at the end of every day for completing client records.

Each massage practice or business creates its own system of keeping client notes. It is common for all regular clients to have personal files with an official record of their massage sessions. The systems of note-taking explained in this chapter contain the essential elements of documentation that can be adapted for your own or a specific employer's

PRACTICAL APPLICATION

Use the goal-oriented planning process to plan a 1-hour individual massage session with a practice client. Implement the plan. Afterward, write down your experience with each step. Ask yourself the following questions:

1. How long did it take to gather enough subjective and objective information to determine client goals for the session?

2. During the session, did you learn any information that caused you to modify the original plan?

3. Do you think that the approach and techniques you used helped achieve the goals for the session?

4. Did the practice client report results consistent with the goals you agreed on before the session?

REALITY CHECK

BARBARA

CHRISSY: How do you find the time to document massage sessions? I allow 30 minutes between sessions, and by the time one client leaves and the other arrives, I have no time.

BARBARA: There are some ways to make the time you need to document your massage sessions properly. For example, at the beginning of the day I pull all of the files for the clients I will see that day, and put them in a secure but accessible place. Then I write some notes about the previous client while the next client is getting undressed. Even if I can't complete the notes, I jot down some things I want to be sure to document later. Then I schedule in 30-40 minutes at the end of the day to finish my notes, return the files, and clean up the space. I've found that it takes less time to write notes now that I've had more practice, and I don't consider the day finished until the documentation is completed.

requirements. The goal-oriented SOAP note format and simplified formats for note-taking are presented in the remainder of the chapter.

SOAP NOTE OVERVIEW

SOAP notes have become a standard for charting massage sessions. *SOAP* refers to the format used to write the notes, and is an acronym for *subjective, objective, assessment,* and *plan.* The SOAP format helps sort information into meaningful categories and provides a standard outline for reports. SOAP notes are written in a kind of shorthand using standard abbreviations. SOAP notes capture the relevant information in a goal-oriented session plan. The SOAP format also serves as a guideline for planning sessions from the beginning. If you understand the planning process well, SOAP notes will be easier to write.

The SOAP format records the elements of logical and clinical reasoning. You start with subjective (S) and objective (O) information about the client, come to an **assessment** (A) of the situation (either the nature of a condition and/or goals for sessions), create a general plan (P) for achieving the goals

and a plan for each massage session. The initial session plan is followed in continuing sessions, and progress is evaluated regularly.

Even if you see a client for only one session, or have limited time for interviews, the session organizing and logical reasoning reflected in SOAP notes help you to aim the session at meeting client needs instead of giving exactly the same 1-hour massage routine to everyone. Even if the record forms or charts you use have only blank lines for recording session notes, you can use the SOAP format to better organize your thoughts about the client and the session.

Four types of notes are commonly reported on SOAP charts. These are intake notes, continuing session notes, progress notes, and discharge notes. The four types of notes reflect different stages in planning massage sessions. **Intake notes** are comprehensive and include the client's stated reason for massage or specific complaint, related subjective and objective information, agreed upon long-term goals, and a general plan. **Continuing session notes** are briefer and record the session-by-session history of a client's visits. **Progress notes** are for special sessions that re-evaluate a client's progress related to his or her long-term goals. Progress notes contain more assessment information than regular session notes and may identify new goals and plans. **Discharge notes** are a final summary of the client's progress and any comments about the course of treatment.

SOAP Note Format

Although originally designed for medical record keeping, the general format for SOAP notes can be adopted for nonmedical settings. The SOAP format is useful in settings such as health clubs, spas, and private offices. However, the detail required and abbreviations used in different settings may vary. Insurance companies may require that certain terms be used in SOAP notes to qualify for reimbursement.

Massage therapists working in the same office or with the same clients should use standard abbreviations so they can read each other's notes. The elements in notes are generally the same; however, a specific type of information may appear in different sections in different systems. Follow the format established and used in your current location.

Some massage therapists have adopted a variation called a *SOTAP note.* The *T* stands for *treatment,* and provides a separate section in the note for recording the massage and related techniques used in the session. In the SOAP format, the *T* description is often included in the *P* or *plan* section of the note.

SOAP Note Content

S stands for *subjective* and refers to subjective information reported by clients. It includes things like what clients say about their reasons for getting massage, how they feel overall, where they feel pain or tension, stresses in their lives, and recent accidents, illnesses, or other changes in health status. For continuing session notes, the *S* section summarizes complaints on the day of the session and any changes clients perceive from their last sessions to their current ones.

O stands for *objective* and refers to what the practitioner observes about the client. Objective information provides clues about the client's state of well-being. It includes observations (e.g., facial expression, general posture, or skin conditions); qualitative measurement from palpation of soft tissues or movement at joints; or results of standardized tests (quantitative measurement) for range of motion, muscle strength, posture, or specific muscle injuries.

A stands for assessment, and in medical charting, it is the practitioner's conclusions from the subjective and objective record. It is the assessment of the situation. For example, in an initial visit, a doctor may conclude that a patient has an arthritis flare up that is causing a swollen, painful knee. That is the diagnosis that goes into the *A* section of the note. Since diagnosis is *not* in the scope of practice of massage therapists, the *A* section can be used for other information.

A good use of the *A* section, from a wellness perspective, is to identify long-term goals for the client. Goals follow from an assessment of the client's needs (based on subjective and objective information), and ideally are agreed upon by the practitioner and client. This provides a basis from which to plan sessions that meet defined goals.

Examples of goals include reducing chronic muscle tension in the forearm, improving flexibility in the hip joint, or alleviating chronic stress or anxiety. Goals could be higher up the Wellness Massage Pyramid (see Figure 10.1 on page 314), for example, maintaining overall health, or body–mind–spirit rejuvenation. Another use suggested for the *A* section is to "summarize the patient's functional ability: limitations, previous ability, and current situation; and to set goals that, when accomplished, demonstrate functional progress" (Thompson 2005, p. 139).

For health care professionals whose scope of practice includes diagnosis of pathologies, the *A* section is fairly straightforward. *A* is used to record the diagnosis and prognosis of a medical condition as a prelude to writing a treatment plan. For wellness practitioners, the goals identified in the *A* section might fall anywhere within the full scope of the Wellness Massage Pyramid from treatment to health maintenance to life enjoyment.

P stands for plan and refers to the strategy for meeting the goals in the *A* section. It includes the plan as carried out for the current session, as well as long-term, general plans.

Additionally, *P* includes a description of the immediate massage application, including the length of the session, techniques used, and parts of the body massaged. Record specific work in more detail, such as when addressing neck and shoulder tension within the context of a general wellness massage.

In medical settings, *P* is the treatment plan for the diagnosed pathology. In massage therapy, the long-term plan might include the number and frequency of massage sessions to meet the goals; details about the massage and related therapies to be used; home care such as self-massage, relaxation exercises, or stretching; and a re-evaluation date.

For regular massage clients in nonmedical settings, the *A* and *P* sections can be revisited regularly to provide continuous focus on client needs and goal-oriented massage sessions. Although the goals of the regular sessions may change over time and may be special in any one session, meeting long-term client needs is the foundation of a successful practice. The more conscious you are of your clients' needs, the better you will be able to serve them. A summary of the SOAP note content appears in Table 10.2■.

WRITING SOAP NOTES

SOAP notes are written in shorthand using brief descriptions, abbreviations, and symbols. They tell a lot with few words, like text messaging on cell phones. With some practice, they can be written quickly using little space. However, they must be readable and able to be transcribed by others. Notes that cannot be read are not very useful. Common abbreviations and symbols used in SOAP notes are listed in Table 6.5, on page 126.

Notes do not contain complete sentences. They are typically strings of descriptions separated by commas and semicolons, or bulleted lists.

Notes contain anatomical terms for locations, adjectives, symptoms, measurements, and ratings. They might report quotes from the client such as "can't get to sleep at night," or "trouble turning my head when driving." Some examples of SOAP note entries are found in Figure 10.8■.

SOAP charts that include diagrams of the body are useful to manual therapists. They show front, back, and side views. Symbols can be used to locate problem areas visually, and indicate the general symptoms felt there, such as pain, numbness, inflammation, adhesions, or shortening. Elsewhere on the form there is space for the narrative SOAP notes. Figure 10.9■ is an example of a SOAP chart with body diagrams.

Entries are descriptions, *not* diagnoses, unless reporting a diagnosis made by a health care provider. In that case, the note would read something like, "client reported a diagnosis by his physician of arthritis in the R knee." A client's self-diagnosis should be reported as just that; for example, "client complained of arthritis in knees—not diagnosed by physician." The massage therapist's note might read, "R knee infl and P," meaning, "right knee inflamed and painful." This is a subtle but important point and must be observed to stay within the scope of practice of massage therapy.

If you or a client will be filling out health insurance claim forms for massage sessions, use terminology in your

TABLE 10.2   Summary of SOAP Note Content

SOAP Note Section		Content Possibilities
S	Subjective	Client's stated reason for massage
		Initial and subsequent complaints
		Health history information
		Report of medications taken
		Report of recent illness or injury
		Description of symptoms (e.g., pain, trouble sleeping)
		Report of functional limitations (e.g., walking, sitting)
		Qualitative description (e.g., tension, pain, numbness, stress)
		Quantitative rating (e.g., tension, pain, numbness, stress)
		Diagnosis from health care provider
O	Objective	Visual observations (e.g., posture, skin color, facial expression)
		Palpation (e.g., tissue quality, joint movement quality)
		Range-of-motion measurement
		Posture analysis
		Gait analysis
		Orthopedic tests of function
A	Assessment	Summary of conditions or limitations
		Identification of contraindications and cautions
		General goals for a series of massage sessions
		Goals for a specific massage session
P	Plan	General plan to achieve goals
		• Number of sessions and frequency of massage
		• Use of adjunct modalities (e.g., hot/cold packs)
		• Homework (e.g., stretching, relaxation exercises)
		Plan for specific massage session
		• Time spent on each body area
		• Techniques used
		• Adjunct modalities used
		• Results

Logical/clinical reasoning behind SOAP notes: *Subjective* information from the client and *objective* information gathered by the massage therapist are used in an *assessment* of the situation to set goals for the massage sessions, followed by the development of *plans* to achieve those goals.

notes that will be recognized by the insurance company, and learn current medical codes that apply. This is important because medical codes are used to process claims, and your records might be subpoenaed to support a client's insurance claim. Massage therapy covered may include hot and cold packs, massage, and manual therapy.

The medical codes change periodically, so if you do insurance billing, check with your state licensing or other appropriate agency for which codes are currently legally acceptable for massage therapy. Be aware that code numbers for physical and occupational therapy may be different from code numbers for massage therapy. Chapter 22, Private Practice and Finances, on page 640, discusses insurance issues as they pertain to massage therapy in more detail.

Guidelines for Writing SOAP Notes

The following guidelines summarize standard procedures for writing SOAP notes. They approach SOAP notes as legal documents and reflect some of the same standards used for legal contracts and accounting. With a little practice, these procedures can become second nature.

- Write legibly in blue or black ink.
- Write in concise, clear language using standard abbreviations and symbols; no need for complete sentences.
- Do not use so many symbols or abbreviations that the meaning of the note is lost; abbreviations make the most sense in context.

Intake SOAP Note – Example 1

S: CL 1° reason for M = stress ↓; 2° c/o is mild LBP with st in legs; Hx of LB ≈ 2 weeks ago; ↓ with use of CP and rest; CL walks and gardens for Ex; does mod lifting in job; previous M = 0.

O: CL walks slowly w/ st and mildly bent over; mm in LB felt ≡; flexibility in hams = poor; Mild ed in ST around knees; mm in shoulders and neck ≡ and short.

A: 1° LTG = stress ↓; 2° LTG = ↓ st in LB, legs, shoulders, neck.

P: GP = FBRM 1 X per wk w/ M for ↓ ≡ in mm in extremities and LB; HW of str in legs and back & gen relax Ex; CP if spasm in LB returns.

Continuing Session SOAP Note – Example 2

S: CL c/o ↑ stress at job from ↑ in workload; ↑ in # HA from ↑ ≡ in shoulders and neck; sev bruise on R lower arm; rpt ↑ mob in lower legs after str last M.

O: CL face looked ↑ tired; rubbed his neck; bruise on R lower arm ~ inch in diameter + dark color.

A: 1° goal = gen relax & ↓ ≡ in shoulders and neck; 2° = flex in hips and legs; bruise on R arm = local contra.

P: 1 hr M + NMT; 40 min on upper body + 20 min on hips & legs; DP to TrP in traps and neck mm + str; deep eff, pet & str to legs; used neck roll; enjoyed relax music; rpt feeling ↑ relax overall after M; HW: HP on shoulders and neck 2X day & str at night.

Continuing Session SOAP Note – Example 3

S: CL rpt feeling ↑ depression this wk; not heard from son in days; SD; yesterday in house all day & 0 visit w/ friends; skin dry; c/o cramp forearm mm.

O: Looked tired & sad; CL rated energy very L; skin dry; forearm mm ≡ on palp; held fist.

A: 1° goal ↑ feeling well-being & ↑ energy; 2° lube skin & ↓ forearm mm ≡.

P: 1 hr FBRM w/ mod pace & eff + gentle pet; 15 min M forearms and hands; music upbeat; oil & lotion to FB w/ more in dry areas; HW: relax Ex and str for forearms; CL ↑ talk and alter post Tx.

FIGURE 10.8

Examples of SOAP Note entries.

- Aim for spending only 5–10 minutes writing each SOAP note. Writing concise, useful, readable notes comes with practice.
- Start your note right after the last note entered so that it will always be in chronological order, and difficult for notes to be altered or added to.
- Date the note clearly at the beginning or in the space provided on the form.
- Print your name and initial or sign your note at the end.
- If you make a mistake, draw a single line through the mistake, and write "error" next to or above the area, and initial and date it. This makes it clear what was originally written and who altered the record and when. Never scribble over a note or use correction fluid over a mistake.

- Be objective, impersonal, and respectful in your notes.
- Stick to descriptions of symptoms and conditions (e.g., swollen, red, warm, painful), and do not make statements that could be mistaken for a medical diagnosis (e.g., tendinitis).
- Do not write anything that is personal, slanderous, or that you would not want the client to read. Clients have a legal and ethical right to see what is in their official records.
- Keep client records for at least 7 years, even if the client has stopped coming to you for massage. The records may be needed for legal or insurance purposes.
- Follow HIPAA Privacy Rules for storage and access to client records when applicable.

SOAP NOTE CHART
CONTINUING MASSAGE SESSION

Practitioner's Name _____   Date _____

Client's Name _____

S: Reason for massage, complaints, reports

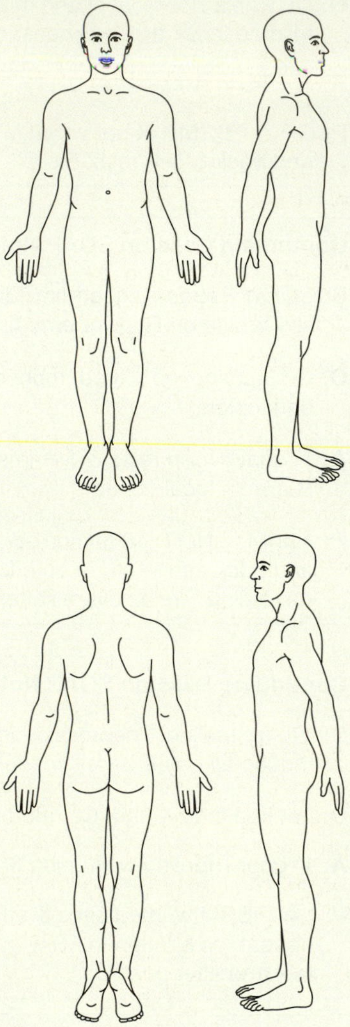

O: Observations, qualitative/quantitative measurements

A: Primary and secondary goals for the session;
contraindications

P: Duration of massage; areas addressed; techniques
used; results; suggested home care

Practitioner Signature _____   Date _____

Symbols:

Primary 1°	Secondary 2°	Change △	Increase ↑	Decrease ↓	Tension ≡
Adhesion **X**	Pain **P**	Numbness ∿	Inflammation ✱	TrP ⊗	

FIGURE 10.9

Example of SOAP chart with body diagram.

SIMPLIFIED DOCUMENTATION

There are circumstances in which documentation of a massage can be minimized, and postsession notes can be shortened or dispensed with altogether. However, at the very least, it is a good idea to keep a record of who received massage and to have clients sign a legal release form.

At venues such as health fairs, trade shows, sports events, and outreach events where people are receiving short, standard massage routines and will not be seen by the practitioner again, no postsession notes are necessary. An example of a form used at outreach events where massage recipients sign their names after reading a statement at the top is found in Appendix G, Intake, Health History, and Note Forms, on page A-59.

A simplified form can also be used for walk-in clients at a street venue, at a stand within a store or mall, or in public places such as airports. In those cases, adequate documentation might consist of a short intake form with a general statement about the massage to be given, a few questions asking for information about major contraindications, and the client's signature granting permission for the massage. This provides a record of who received massage and evidence that they knew what to expect. See Figure 10.10■. This type of form works well with one-time clients.

A simplified note system is adequate when a standard routine is given and then modified for a client's safety and/or preferences. It might also be appropriate at a spa or health club where clients come for massage periodically, but have no long-term goals in mind. Figure 10.11■ shows an example of a short note form with space for more than one date on a page for use with regular or periodic clients.

The short form contains some of the elements of a SOAP chart (e.g., subjective and objective information), but the *A* section is unnecessary, and a *C* section for general comments is added. The *P* section documents the length of the session, the routine performed (e.g., deluxe relaxation routine) and significant modifications made to address contraindications and cautions. If a client comes for a more goal-oriented massage, a regular SOAP chart can be used to document that session.

As with all documentation, it is recommended that even shortened and simplified records be kept for a period of 7 years. Legible and understandable entries are a must.

DESIGNING A SYSTEM OF DOCUMENTATION

Consider several factors when designing a note-taking system for your own practice. You may develop a few different forms for different circumstances. For example, if you have an office, do house calls, and work trade shows you may

want to use three different forms. Or if you have an office and offer routine massage as well as medical treatment, you may use two different forms.

As a general rule, use SOAP notes for goal-oriented or treatment sessions. A simplified form can be used for routine massage, or for one-time, walk-in clients. For a trade show or health fair, a signature list following a short statement might be adequate. See Appendix G, Intake, Health History, and Note Forms, on page A-52, for samples of different forms.

If you process claims for insurance reimbursement, be sure to document the services performed in claims. Design your note forms to include all the information required by the insurance companies you deal with.

Make a separate file for each regular client. File folders with fasteners are useful for keeping papers in order. In a file with two fasteners, general information (e.g., intake form, signed privacy and policy statement, health history, referral letter) can be kept on one side, and individual session notes on the other side.

Records for one-time clients can be kept in alphabetical order in a group file. If they become regular clients, you can make an individual file for them. Signature lists from events can have their own file in chronological order. The important thing is to have a system that allows you to locate records easily and one that works for your type of practice.

LEGAL AND ETHICAL ISSUES

Legal and ethical issues related to documentation and note-taking revolve around scope of practice, accuracy, honesty, confidentiality, and respect for the client. Since diagnosis is not in the scope of practice of massage therapists, no diagnoses by them should appear in session notes. References to others' diagnoses need to be clearly identified, for example, "condition as diagnosed by client's physician" or "client self-diagnosis." This is a legal as well as an ethical matter.

Write session notes to accurately reflect what happened in the session. Writing notes as soon as possible

PRACTICAL APPLICATION

Obtain a blank copy of the documentation form used in student clinic at your school. Examine the form to see how it is formatted and what information is requested for each massage session. Use the form to document practice sessions in preparation for your student clinic experience. Answering the following questions will help you with student clinic documentation.

1. What level of detail will be required at student clinic?
2. Is there a chart of standard abbreviations used in student clinic?
3. Does the clinic have specific guidelines related to completing documentation, for example, what information goes in each section and how each entry should be signed?

SHORT INTAKE and NOTE FORM

Client _____ Date _____

Address _____ Phone _____

Massage Therapist _____

Please answer the following questions to ensure a comfortable and safe massage session:

1. What is your primary goal for this massage?
   - ☐ Relaxation, stress reduction
   - ☐ Relieve muscle tension, specify area: _____
   - ☐ General health and wellbeing
   - ☐ Other, please specify _____

2. Have you had any illness, accidents, or injury recently? ☐ No ☐ Yes

   If so, please explain briefly _____

   _____

3. Are you experiencing any of the following today? Check all that apply.

   | ☐ pain or soreness | ☐ numbness or tingling | ☐ dizziness |
   | ☐ stiffness | ☐ swelling | ☐ nausea |

4. Do you have any allergies, especially to oils or lotions? ☐ No ☐ Yes

   If so, please explain briefly _____

   _____

5. For women – Are you pregnant? ☐ No ☐ Yes ☐ Maybe

6. Have you taken any medications today? ☐ No ☐ Yes

   If so, please list _____

I have answered the above questions to the best of my ability. I acknowledge that massage therapy does not include medical diagnosis and that I should see an appropriate health care provider to diagnose and treat medical problems. I give my consent for the massage session.

_____ Date _____
Signature

Plan:

Comments:

FIGURE 10.10

Examples of simplified note for one-time client.

---

after a session increases the likelihood of complete and accurate documentation. Record only those procedures that were performed in the session. Defrauding an insurance company is unlawful and unethical.

Keep session notes in a secure place such as a locked cabinet, and do not leave them lying around for others to see. Follow all HIPAA rules related to privacy of health records where applicable. Share the contents of clients' files only with their permission. See Chapter 5, Ethics and the

Therapeutic Relationship, on page 112, for more information about HIPAA confidentiality rules.

Write notes using respectful and professional language. Omit opinions and personal comments about clients that are unrelated to their massage session. Remember that clients have a right to look at their notes, and others may someday have access to the notes as well. Your notes are a reflection of your level of professionalism.

SHORT NOTE CHART

Client's Name _____

Date _____ Practitioner's Name _____

S: Comments, complaints, reports, recent illness or injury, medications

O: Visual observations, palpation

P: Length of session, routine given, significant modifications

C: General comments

MT Initials _____

Date _____ Practitioner's Name _____

S: Comments, complaints, reports, recent illness or injury, medications

O: Visual observations, palpation

P: Length of session, routine given, significant modifications

C: General comments

MT Initials _____

Date _____ Practitioner's Name/Initials _____

S: Comments, complaints, reports, recent illness or injury, medications

O: Visual observations, palpation

P: Length of session, routine given, significant modifications

C: General comments

MT Initials _____

FIGURE 10.11

Example of simplified non-medical setting.

CRITICAL THINKING

Obtain examples of three or four different note-taking forms used by massage therapists. Compare, contrast, and analyze the forms to determine which forms might be appropriate for different settings (e.g., spa, health club, clinic, private practice, outreach event). Redesign the forms to improve their appearance or usefulness. Consider the following:

1. Is the form complete? Is all important information included?
2. Is it easy to use? Is the format logical?
3. Is the form useful for the intended setting?
4. Does the spacing allow for writing entries?

CASE FOR STUDY

Jennifer and Simplified Documentation at the Salon

Jennifer, a massage therapist with a small practice within a community beauty salon, uses a simplified format for documentation of massage sessions given there. She has informed clients that the massage offered in the salon is primarily for relaxation and rejuvenation, and refers clients to other massage therapists for more clinical massage applications. The form she developed has three sections to document each massage session.

- The *H* section is for recording relevant health information including contraindications.
- The *MT* section is for a description of the massage therapy application for the day.
- The *C* section is for comments, including noteworthy events and results.

Jennifer can fit notes for four sessions with a client on one page and has learned to be concise in her documentation.

Session with Martha

Martha came in for her regular massage and in the brief presession interview reported that she had been to the doctor in the past week for a skin rash on her leg. The doctor thought it might be an allergic reaction and prescribed some oral medication and some anti-itch crème. Martha was stressed out from a family situation and was looking forward to relaxing. Jennifer gave her the relaxation massage as usual, but switched to a hypoallergenic lotion. She spent more time on the neck and shoulders, where Martha had reported tension, and avoided massage around the rash. Martha was a little more talkative than usual, and Jennifer tried to help her focus on her breathing and letting go of tension. She played special relaxation music for a calming atmosphere. Jennifer sensed that Martha was distracted, but did seem a little more relaxed at the end of the session. Martha thanked Jennifer and reported feeling less anxious.

Write notes for this session using Jennifer's system of documentation.

H _____

MT _____

C _____

Date _____ Time _____

CHAPTER HIGHLIGHTS

- Session planning is the logical process of thinking through the massage from beginning to end.
- Goal-oriented planning focuses on achieving specific client goals, as reflected in the Wellness Massage Pyramid.
- Clinical reasoning is the cognitive process used in goal-oriented planning and is essentially a problem-solving exercise.
- The six steps in goal-oriented planning are (1) collecting subjective information from the client; (2) collecting objective information through observation, tests, and measurements; (3) assessing the situation and setting client goals; (4) devising a plan to achieve client goals; (5) implementing the plan; and (6) evaluating the results. The plan is revised as needed based on the results obtained.
- Three basic variations of goal-oriented planning are long-range planning, individual session planning, and treatment planning.
  - Long-range planning is done in the initial session and in progress evaluation sessions.

- Individual session planning is done before each massage session.
  - Treatment planning is done when the goal is the alleviation of symptoms or facilitating healing of a pathological condition.
  - Each of the variations uses the six-step session planning process, modified for its specific application.
- Intake is the process of gathering relevant information from a new client.
- Intake involves the client filling out an intake form and a health history form and the therapist conducting a new client interview.
  - A health history provides information to identify contraindications and as background for planning sessions.
  - When providing routine massage at an outreach event, the intake process can be shortened to a few relevant questions and signing a consent form.
- Objective methods of collecting information include the massage therapist's own general observations, palpation, range-of-motion evaluation, posture analysis, biomechanical analysis, gait analysis, and orthopedic tests.
- Subjective and objective information gathered in Steps 1 and 2 of the session planning process is used in Step 3 to assess the situation and prioritize client goals.
- Documentation is the process of writing massage session records for future reference; also called note-taking or charting.
- Session notes are kept on paper or in electronic form in client files.
- Notes are legal documents, are used for insurance reporting, and may be subpoenaed as evidence in legal cases.
- Notes are official client health records and may be protected by HIPAA Privacy Rules.
  - Notes are also practical as an aid to memory and in planning sessions. Writing notes is an important part of completing a massage session.
- SOAP notes have become a standard for charting goal-oriented massage sessions.
- The SOAP format reflects a logical or clinical reasoning process.
  - Four types of SOAP notes are initial, continuing, progress, and discharge notes.
  - Massage therapists working in the same office should use standard abbreviations and symbols and follow the format required by their employer.
- SOAP is an acronym for subjective, objective, assessment, and plan.
  - The *S* or subjective section contains information provided by the client.

- The *O* or objective section contains observations, tests, and measurements made by the massage therapist.
- The *A* or assessment section identifies the goals for the massage session and any contraindications.
- The *P* or plan section lays out the steps planned to achieve identified goals.
- SOAP notes are written using brief descriptions, abbreviations, and symbols.
  - Notes are not complete sentences, but are strings of descriptions separated by commas or semicolons, or are bulleted lists.
  - Diagrams of the body are useful in writing notes.
  - Entries are descriptions and not diagnoses of conditions.
- SOAP notes are written legibly in clear, concise language in blue or black ink. They conform to standards for legal documents related to making and initialing changes, and are dated and initialed at the end.
  - Personal comments about clients should not be written.
  - Clients have the right to see their files.
  - Files are kept for at least 7 years.
- Simplified note formats may be used when routine massages are given, and with one-time, walk-in clients.
  - Documentation can include at a minimum a short intake form asking about contraindications, a description of the massage to be given, a date, and a signature from the client giving permission for the session.
- Massage therapists design systems of documentation and note-taking appropriate for the type of practice they have.
  - Therapists can design their own charting forms or use premade forms.
  - A separate file is created for each regular client.
- Legal and ethical issues related to documentation revolve around scope of practice, accuracy, honesty, confidentiality, and respect for clients.
- Client files should be kept secure and shared only with the client's permission.
  - The way you keep your files is a reflection of your level of professionalism.

EXAM REVIEW

Key Terms

To study the key terms listed at the beginning of this chapter, match the appropriate lettered meaning to each numbered key term listed below. For additional study, look up the key terms in the Interactive Glossary on page G-1 and note other terms that compare or contrast with them.

_____ 1. Assessment
_____ 2. Clinical reasoning
_____ 3. Continuing session notes
_____ 4. Discharge notes
_____ 5. Documentation
_____ 6. Goal-oriented planning
_____ 7. HIPAA privacy rules
_____ 8. Intake notes
_____ 9. Long-term planning
_____ 10. Progress notes
_____ 11. SOAP notes
_____ 12. Treatment planning

a. General process of planning massage sessions to meet client needs and goals
b. Notes related to the initial massage session with a client
c. Planning a series of massage sessions over time to reach specific goals
d. Step in goal-oriented planning in which the situation is analyzed and goals are prioritized
e. Common format used for documenting massage
f. Notes that evaluate achievement related to long-term goals
g. Record the session-by-session history of a client's visits
h. Process of planning massage sessions in which the goal is alleviation of symptoms or facilitation of healing of a pathological condition
i. Cognitive process used in goal-oriented planning
j. Protects the privacy of medical records
k. Process of writing massage session records for future reference; also called note-taking or charting
l. Final summary of the client's progress and any comments about the course of treatment

Memory Workout

To test your memory of the main concepts in this chapter, complete the following sentences by circling the most correct answer from the two choices provided.

1. Session planning is the (logical) (intuitive) process of thinking through a massage session.
2. Before (ending) (beginning) a massage session with a regular client, ask about any recent changes in his or her health status or medications.
3. The goal of treatment planning is the facilitation of healing of a (kinesiological) (pathological) condition.
4. The main purpose of a short intake interview before giving massage at outreach events is to identify possible (contraindications) (indications).
5. Rating scales offer a rough measurement of things from the client's (objective) (subjective) view.
6. Palpation is the act of sensing information about a client through (vision) (touch) and through the (look) (feel) of tissues.

7. In good standing posture, the head is in alignment over the shoulders, and the chin is slightly (tucked) (forward).
8. In proper lifting mechanics, power comes from the (shoulder) (leg) muscles.
9. Documentation is the process of writing detailed (records) (plans) of massage sessions for future reference.
10. The _O_ in SOAP notes stands for (other) (objective).
11. SOTAP is a variation of the SOAP note, and the _T_ stands for (theory) (treatment).
12. Body charts are good visual aids for collecting (objective) (subjective) information from clients.
13. Initial or sign your note at the (beginning) (end) of an entry.
14. Records for one-time clients can be kept in (alphabetical) (chronological) order in a group file.
15. Signature lists from events can have their own file in (alphabetical) (chronological) order.

Test Prep

The following multiple-choice questions will help to prepare you for future school and professional exams.

1. Which of the following is a method of collecting subjective information from clients?
   a. Range-of-motion evaluation
   b. Gait analysis
   c. Health history forms
   d. Palpation of tissues

2. Suggesting activities to be done outside of the massage session on the client's own time is correctly referred to as:
   a. A prescription
   b. Home care
   c. Contraindication
   d. An assignment

3. The goal-oriented planning process is best described as:
   a. Rigid and linear
   b. Logical but disorderly
   c. Linear and disorderly
   d. Looping spiral

4. Which of the following is *not* within the massage therapist's scope of practice?
   a. Measuring function or loss of function
   b. Assessing the condition of tissues
   c. Diagnosing a medical condition
   d. All of the above

5. At what point in a massage session does the massage therapist clarify the client's top goals for the massage?
   a. Presession interview
   b. Postsession interview
   c. Midpoint in the session
   d. When writing postsession notes

6. Which type of interview question steers clients to specific topics, but leaves space for them to answer in their own words?
   a. Open-ended question
   b. Multiple-choice question
   c. Rating scale
   d. Body chart

7. Which of the following tends to reduce the ability to feel or palpate the condition of tissues?
   a. Moving slowly
   b. Being focused and present
   c. Using heavy pressure
   d. Putting descriptive words to what your feel

8. In good sitting posture, the knees should be aligned with the hips or slightly:
   a. Lower
   b. Higher
   c. Turned in
   d. Turned out

9. The *S* section of a SOAP note contains:
   a. A transcription of the client's words from the intake interview
   b. A summary of subjective information from the client
   c. A summary of measurements taken during the intake interview
   d. A summary of the session plan

10. In the PSOAP variation of SOAP notes, the first *P* contains:
    a. Possible contraindications
    b. Plans developed in a prior session
    c. Permission to send records to the insurance company
    d. Prescription or diagnosis from a primary health care provider

11. In which section of SOAP notes for an individual massage session are the results of the day's massage typically recorded?
    a. S
    b. O
    c. A
    d. P

12. Once you have mastered writing SOAP notes, about how much time would you expect to spend after each massage session writing an entry?
    a. 1–2 minutes
    b. 5–10 minutes
    c. 25–30 minutes
    d. 45–50 minutes

13. Which of the following instructions for correcting a mistake made in SOAP notes is *not* acceptable?
    a. White-out or erase the mistake
    b. Put a single line through the mistake
    c. Write "error" above or next to the area
    d. Initial the correction

14. What is the recommended number of years that client records are kept?
    a. 1
    b. 3
    c. 5
    d. 7

15. The most acceptable place to store client records securely in a massage office is:
    a. In a locked file cabinet
    b. In a desk drawer
    c. In a box in the closet
    d. On a shelf behind the desk

Video Challenge

Watch the appropriate segment of the video on your DVD and then answer the following questions.

Goal-Oriented Planning and Documentation

Goal-Oriented Planning

1. Match the scenes in this video segment with the steps in the goal-oriented planning process. Which step does each scene illustrate?
2. Identify scenes in the video where massage therapists are collecting subjective data from clients. During which parts of massage sessions does subjective data collection occur?

Observation: Posture, Biomechanics, and Gait

3. For each scene in the video showing sitting posture, point out aspects of good alignment, as well as deviations that may result in muscle tension and pain.

4. Review scenes from the video explaining good standing alignment. What are important instructions for assessing a client's standing alignment?
5. List the different occupations illustrated in the video in the section on biomechanics. Identify potential musculoskeletal problems clients in these occupations might develop.

Documentation and SOAP Notes

6. List the many practical uses for session notes mentioned in the video.
7. Identify where the massage therapist gets the information contained in each section of the SOAP note as explained in the video.

Comprehension Exercises

The following short answer questions test your knowledge and understanding of chapter topics and provide practice in written communication skills. Explain in two to four complete sentences.

1. List the six steps in the goal-oriented planning process. Give an example of using the process for planning an individual massage session.

2. Describe good standing posture. List some anatomical markers for evaluating proper alignment when viewed from the front and from the side.
3. What is the difference between a *diagnosis* and a *description* of a complaint by a client? Which is within the scope of practice of massage therapists? Give an example.

For Greater Understanding

The following exercises are designed to take you from the realm of theory into the real world. They will help give you a deeper understanding of the subjects covered in this chapter. Action words are underlined to emphasize the variety of activities presented to address different learning styles and to encourage deeper thinking.

1. Interview a family member or friend after he or she has filled out a health history form. Lead the person in a discussion of the potential benefits of massage in helping to improve his or her overall wellness using the Wellness Massage Pyramid. Help the individual determine his or her top three goals for getting massage in the future.

2. Perform a posture, biomechanical, or gait analysis of a classmate's movements. Describe what you observe, and offer instructions for more balanced alignment or biomechanically sound movement.
3. Write a sample SOAP description in complete sentences without abbreviations or symbols. Give that description to a study partner and ask him or her to translate the longer descriptions using the SOAP shorthand format. Now give the abbreviated SOAP notes to a third study partner, and see if he or she can translate the note correctly back into longhand.

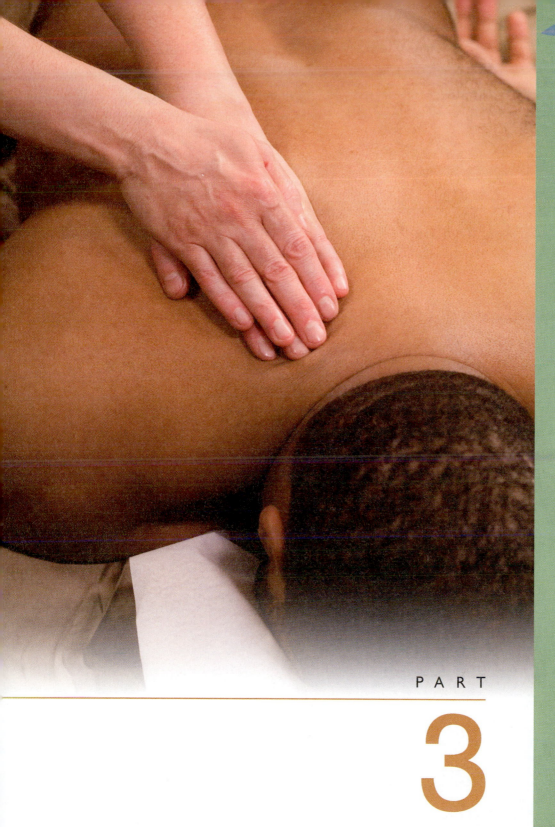

PART

3

Massage Guidelines and Applications

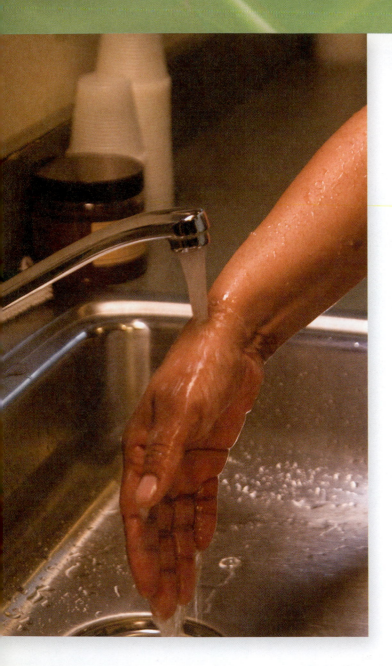

 CHAPTER OUTLINE

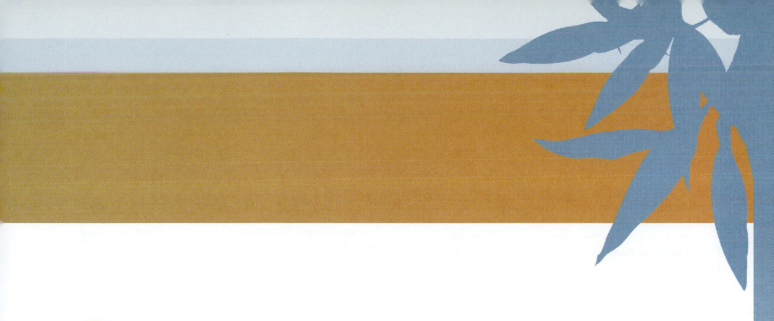

LEARNING OUTCOMES

After studying this chapter, you will have information to:

1. Practice good personal hygiene.
2. Wash hands thoroughly for massage therapy.
3. Evaluate massage tables and chairs in relation to practice needs.
4. Set up and care for massage tables and chairs properly.
5. Describe the variety of bolsters and pillows used in massage.
6. Describe the uses of sheets, blankets, and towels in massage.
7. Choose topical substances for their specific effects.
8. Keep equipment and supplies clean and sanitary.
9. Create a comfortable, sanitary, and safe environment for clients.
10. Follow infection control procedures to prevent the spread of serious diseases.

KEY TERMS

Bolsters *351*

Equipment *347*

Hygienic hand washing *344*

Massage chairs *349*

MRSA *356*

Personal hygiene *344*

Portable massage table *347*

Sanitation *344*

Topical substance *352*

Universal precautions *355*

MASSAGE *in* ACTION

On your DVD, explore:

• Hygienic Hand Washing

INTRODUCTION

Preparation for massage therapy includes consideration of hygiene, equipment, and environment. Hygiene is especially important when people are in close contact, such as when giving and receiving massage. Habits of personal and environmental hygiene are established from day one in massage training programs as you learn to keep yourself, your equipment, and your space clean.

Practicing massage therapy also requires knowledge of basic equipment and supplies. Massage tables and chairs provide the platform for massage applications and are essential tools of the profession. Additional basic tools are various accessories such as linens and bolsters and the oils and lotions typically used in Western massage.

Practicing massage techniques outside of school and experience in student clinic provide opportunities for learning to create a suitable environment for massage therapy. The goal is to provide for the comfort and safety of clients, as well as to organize a space conducive to relaxation and healing. Hygiene, equipment, and environment are interrelated aspects of preparation for massage and an essential foundation for hands-on applications.

PERSONAL HYGIENE AND HAND WASHING

Massage practitioners have a responsibility to follow good **hygiene** and **sanitation** practices that make the client comfortable and that prevent the spread of disease. While the original meaning of the words hygiene and sanitation referred generally to practices that promote good health, they are primarily used today to refer to cleanliness and removing disease-causing organisms. In this text, the word hygiene will be used in relation to personal cleanliness, while sanitation will be used when referring to cleaning equipment, supplies, and the massage space.

Personal Hygiene

The close physical contact inherent in massage therapy calls for excellent **personal hygiene.** Massage therapists must look neat and smell clean to inspire the confidence and trust of clients. This applies to clothes as well as to the body,

and especially to the hands. Professional appearance, grooming, and personal hygiene are discussed in greater detail in Chapter 3, Professional and Personal Development, on page 49.

In addition to looking clean and neat, avoid offensive odors. This includes odors from the body and clothes, including strong perfumes and colognes. Some practitioners bathe or change shirts during the day to stay fresh. After a spicy meal, or just a long day, consider using a breath freshener. Smokers should be particularly aware to eliminate odors on their clothes, hands, and breath.

The hands are the primary means for giving massage. The following hand-care guidelines for the practitioner help to make the massage a more pleasant experience for the recipient.

- Fingernails are clipped short and kept below the level of the fingertips. If you hold your hands up with the palms facing you, you should not be able to see the fingernails.
- Use lotion to keep the hands soft and moisturized. Smooth out rough spots and calluses that might feel scratchy to a receiver.
- Avoid wearing rings and bracelets. They can distract and possibly scratch the receiver.
- Wash hands thoroughly before and after each session, as described later in this chapter, to prevent the spread of disease. Remove odors from hands.
- Keep hands warm and dry before touching a client. They can be warmed beneath a heat lamp, by hot water, or by rubbing them together briskly. Dry wet hands thoroughly with a towel. Corn starch or powder may be used to keep hands dry.

Without good hygiene and sanitation, pathogens can be passed from practitioner to client or from client to client in various ways. One of the most basic personal hygiene measures for massage therapists is hand washing.

Hand Washing

The most effective method for preventing the transfer of pathogens during massage is **hygienic hand washing.** Massage practitioners wash their hands before and after each session. They may also wash during a session, for example, before touching the face after massaging the feet. A thorough hand-washing procedure includes nine steps, which are illustrated in Practice Sequence 11–1, Hygienic Hand Washing.

If washing with soap and water is not feasible, commercial hand sanitizers are an option. These gel-like substances typically contain ethyl alcohol to kill common pathogens. Choose a brand with a moisturizer included to prevent skin damage with frequent use. Be sure to follow directions.

PRACTICE SEQUENCE   11.1

Hygienic Hand Washing

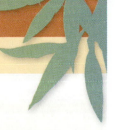

FIGURE 11.1 Adjust the water coming from the faucet so that the temperature is comfortable. Water too hot can damage your skin and is not necessary for cleaning. Water must be running to wash away pathogens.

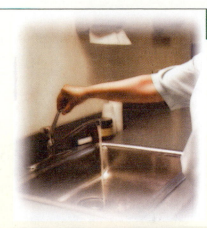

FIGURE 11.2 Wet the forearms and hands from elbow to fingertips. Keep the hands lower than the elbows. Water flows off the fingertips.

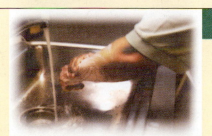

FIGURE 11.3 Scrub the nails with a nail brush to loosen oil and dirt. Clean the nail surface and under the nails.

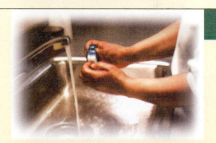

FIGURE 11.4 Create a soapy lather with the hands and spread the soap up to the elbows. Liquid soap is preferred. If using a bar of soap, be sure to rinse it after each use. Cover the entire skin surface, including the finger and thumb webs.

5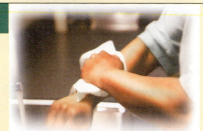

FIGURE 11.5 Rub for at least 15 seconds. Particles and pathogens become suspended in the soapy lather and are washed away.

6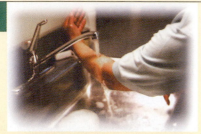

FIGURE 11.6 Rinse the soap off completely from fingertips to elbows. Water flows off the forearms near the elbows.

7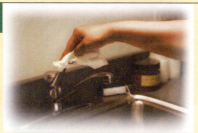

FIGURE 11.7 Dry hands and forearms thoroughly with clean paper towels to prevent chapping.

8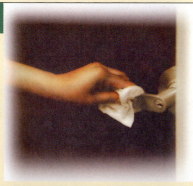

FIGURE 11.8 Use the same paper towels to turn off the faucet.

9

FIGURE 11.9 If before a massage, use the same paper towels to operate door handles and then discard in the massage room.

After you perform the Practice Sequence, evaluate how well you did by filling out Performance Evaluation Form 11–1, Hygienic Hand Washing. The form can be found in Appendix F, Performance Evaluation Forms, on page A-20 and on your DVD.

If you have cuts or scrapes on your hands or forearms, cover them when touching a client. Use either gloves or a finger cot if the exposure is just on one finger. Many people are allergic to latex, so if you have a skin reaction to it, use a nonlatex alternative. Also ask clients if they are allergic to latex, and use nonlatex alternatives if they are. If you have a skin abrasion on the forearm, avoid use of the forearm when applying techniques.

Other situations in which glove protection might be appropriate is when a client has a potentially contagious condition, or in the presence of blood or other body fluids. This may be necessary in some hospital and clinical settings and sometimes at sports events. Continuing to massage with gloves on assumes that there are no contraindications for massage present.

MASSAGE EQUIPMENT

Equipment refers to items that are relatively costly and that last for several years. Massage tables and massage chairs are the biggest equipment investments that beginning massage therapists make. Considering them as investments makes sense, since wise choices now will pay rich dividends in both the short and long terms. The aim is to select good quality massage tables and massage chairs to meet your needs in the foreseeable future.

You will begin learning about massage equipment as you set up, use, and take down massage tables and chairs in class. This presents a great opportunity to practice using and caring for equipment properly.

Massage Tables

Massage tables are specially designed for the needs of massage practitioners and may be stationary or portable. Massage tables are adjustable for height. Most have a removable, adjustable face cradle. Tables vary in length, width, and type of padding and covering. A typical portable massage table and adjustable face cradle are shown in Figure 11.10■.

The most appropriate table for a particular situation depends on the type of practice and the setting. For example, in settings where tables are rarely moved, stationary tables may be best for their stability. However, if the table will be carried from place to place, or set up and taken down frequently, then a **portable massage table** would be a better choice. A hinged table top is another option that allows easy positioning of clients in a semireclining position. This may be important when working with special populations or if specializing in a type of bodywork such as reflexology.

Table width, length, and height are also important considerations. Table widths vary from 27–32 inches or wider. Narrower tables are lighter weight, but may be less comfortable for larger clients. Wider tables are heavier to carry, but accommodate bigger people. If you are short, maintaining good body mechanics while reaching over a wider table may be a challenge.

Standard table length is 73 inches long, which fits people up to about 6 feet tall. Taller clients can be accommodated in various ways, including using special table extenders. A typical size massage table for Western/Swedish massage is 29–31 inches wide and 73 inches long.

Massage tables are adjustable for height. Massage therapists can then set up their tables at a height that allows for good body mechanics. Shorter massage therapists generally need lower tables, and taller people need higher tables. Proper table height might also vary depending on the size of the client, special client positioning (e.g., side-lying), or type of massage being given. Proper table height is the height that allows for massage applications without bending too much at the waist or neck. Massage tables typically have a height range of 8–10 inches, for example, a standard table is adjustable to 24–34 inches in height. Shorter massage therapists can get tables that start out lower (e.g., range of 18–26 inches); and taller massage therapists need tables that start out higher (e.g., range of 26–36 inches).

For sports massage, a narrower table is often preferred. Some shiatsu practitioners get up on the table for better

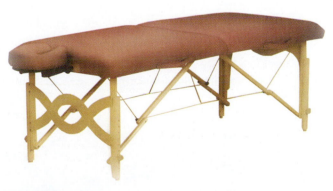

FIGURE 11.10

Adjustable massage table with face cradle.

leverage, and so a wider, stronger table is more desirable. There are special tables for pregnant clients, and tables with hinged tops that allow for a semireclining position.

A massage table is an important purchase for a student or recent graduate. To research a variety of tables, it is advisable to visit a massage supplies showroom, a trade show or convention, or check table manufacturers' websites. Avoid massage tables sold for personal, not professional, use. These lower-grade tables are not made to stand up to the use of a massage therapy practice. A good quality professional-grade massage table is a wise investment. A checklist of considerations for choosing a massage table is presented in Table 11.1■.

TABLE 11.1	Checklist for Choosing a Massage Table
1. Type of Massage or Bodywork	☐ Western/Swedish ☐ Deep tissue ☐ Sports massage ☐ Special populations ☐ Other _____
2. General Type of Table	☐ Portable ☐ Stationary ☐ Hinged table top for semireclining
3. Table Width	☐ Standard (29–31 inches) ☐ Narrow (28 inches or less) ☐ Wide (32 inches or more)
4. Table Length	☐ Standard (72–73 inches) ☐ Short (68–70 inches) ☐ Long (over 73 inches)
5. Table Height	☐ Standard (24–34 inches) ☐ Short (18–26 or 22–30 inches) ☐ Tall (26–36 inches)
6. Table Top Features	☐ Thick foam layer ☐ Thin foam layer ☐ Smooth vinyl cover ☐ Suede vinyl cover ☐ Other cover _____ ☐ Dark color ☐ Light color
7. Table Legs	☐ Wood ☐ Metal ☐ Height adjustment mechanism ☐ Leg stabilizing mechanism ☐ Special height needs
8. Weight of Table	☐ Light weight (25–28 lbs) ☐ Medium weight (29–34 lbs) ☐ Heavy weight (35+ lbs)
9. Table Strength*	☐ Strong enough for client ☐ Strong enough for client plus massage therapist *Standard maximum operating capacity: 300–600 lbs
10. Special Features Needed	☐ _____ ☐ _____ ☐ _____
11. Additional Factors	☐ Ease of set up and take down ☐ Ease of care and durability of table cover ☐ Cost

CRITICAL THINKING

Determine the ideal massage table for you at this time. Complete a features and cost comparison of massage table models from different companies. Pick one brand and model that seems best for you and your start-up practice after graduation.

1. Use the chart in Table 11.1 to identify important features of your ideal table.

2. Look at different massage tables in person or on company websites and pick out options for tables that have the features you want.

3. Determine the cost of your ideal table and think about how you will go about financing its purchase.

Massage Chairs

Massage chairs are specially designed to provide maximum comfort for people receiving massage in a seated position while fully clothed. Chairs typically have a seat, knee rests, armrest, chest cushion, and face cradle. A typical massage chair is shown in Figure 11.11■. This type of massage chair was introduced in the 1980s, and chairs are continually undergoing improvement in design.

Things to consider when choosing among different massage chair models are ease of set up, take down, and carrying from place to place. Massage chairs are designed to be used for on-site massage, that is, taken to a location such as a workplace, store, or community event. Look at the chair when it is folded up and try carrying it. Find out how much the massage chair weighs. Check to see if it has wheels. Set the chair up and then take it down a few times to see how easy or difficult it is.

Consider stability. Get onto the chair yourself to see how stable it feels. Is it easy to get onto and out of? Have someone else get on the chair while you apply a few massage techniques.

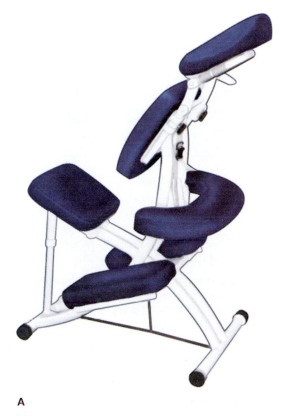

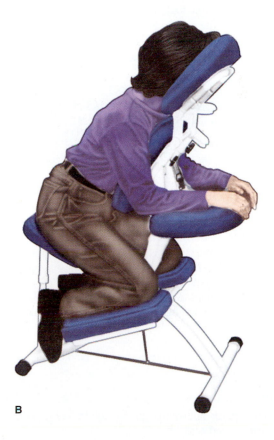

A   B

FIGURE 11.11

A. Adjustable massage chair. B. Recipient positioned in massage chair.

Does the chair move a lot or feel like it will tip over easily? A wider base helps prevent tipping from side-to-side, which is a client safety consideration.

Be aware of the range of clients the chair can accommodate. Chairs have a maximum weight allowance, for example, 300–600 pounds. How tall or short clients are can also make a difference. A typical chair can seat clients from 4 feet 6 inches to 6 feet 6 inches tall. Shorter or taller clients may have difficulty being positioned properly. Never place a client in a massage chair if you suspect the chair is not designed to handle his or her weight.

Look for adjustments in the face cradle, chest pad, armrest, and kneeler. Different massage chair models might also have special adjustments for client positioning variations. Some have seat and kneeler adjustments that allow clients to sit on the chair "backward" for different massage applications. Before purchasing a massage chair, investigate different models to find the features that you want.

Equipment Set Up and Care

Massage tables and chairs will remain in good condition longer with proper use and care. Follow the manufacturer's guidelines for basic care of equipment.

To set up a typical portable massage table, place it on the floor on its side with the handles up. Unlatch the closures and swing the table open to about 60 degrees. Remove the face cradle if it is stored inside. Then straighten out the legs and open the table completely. If there are two people, one stands at each end and they lift the table together, turning it onto its feet. One person can stand in the middle and pull the table onto its feet.

Once the table is set up, check to make sure the legs are straight and supporting cables or braces are in place properly.

The table can then be adjusted for height and the face cradle slid into place. Never sit on a portable massage table directly over the hinge in the middle. This weakens the table over time. Periodically check to make sure that nuts and bolts are tightened securely, since they can come loose from the movement of massage.

Massage chair designs differ greatly, and so there is no standard method of set up. Check the manufacturer's guidelines for instructions. Be sure that all attachments are in place properly. Get into the chair to check to make sure that it is stable. Tighten nuts and bolts as needed.

There are many choices of upholstery for massage tables. Some are softer and some harder. Some are suede-like and some smooth. Check the manufacturer's instructions for care of the upholstery on your equipment. Generally avoid cleaning with harsh chemicals that can dry out and damage the fabric. Depending on the type of massage or bodywork you practice, you may need to clean your table every day or week. Some recommend wiping the face cradle cushion after each client, even when a face cradle cover is used. Using a cloth or plastic barrier under the bottom drape can save wear and tear on upholstery.

Massage chairs should be wiped down after each client, especially the face cradle and armrests. Face cradle covers help keep sweat and makeup off the upholstery.

Alternatives to Tables and Chairs

Whenever possible, use equipment specially designed for massage. However, sometimes practitioners have to improvise in less than ideal situations. For example, massage is sometimes given to people in wheelchairs, to the bedridden elderly or ill, to workers at their desks, or even at poolside at

CASE FOR STUDY

Donna and Buying a Massage Chair

Donna has been given the opportunity to become an independent contractor providing on-site chair massage for the employees of a large corporation located close to her home-based massage therapy practice. However, Donna will need to purchase a massage chair before she can begin this new venture. She has discovered that there are many chairs available from which to choose and is concerned about finding the best quality chair within her budget.

Question:

What are the criteria Donna needs to bear in mind as she shops for a massage chair?

Things to consider:

- Is the chair sturdy but lightweight enough for her to set up and move around easily?

- Will the armrests hold up to the deep compression and friction techniques commonly used on the arms?
- Is the chair easy to adjust? What adjustments can be made?
- Are there any hinges or other metal components that could scratch or pinch the skin of either the therapist or client?
- Does the chair come with a warranty?

Investigate massage chairs by visiting manufacturers' showrooms or web sites or studying their catalogs. Has another massage therapist made a recommendation? Which chair would you choose if you were Donna? Why?

_____

_____

_____

a swim meet. In these circumstances, care should be taken to ensure the safety and comfort of the receiver while providing for good body mechanics for the practitioner.

SUPPLIES FOR MASSAGE

In addition to a massage table, some basic supplies are needed for massage therapy. Bolsters and pillows, draping materials, and topical substances such as oil and lotions are essential for most massage applications.

Bolsters and Pillows

Bolsters and pillows are used to position the client for comfort and safety. Body support may be provided in different positions as needed under the knees, neck, ankles, shoulders, and wrists (Figure 11.12■). Positioning clients correctly is addressed in Chapter 12, Body Mechanics, Table Skills, and Application Guidelines, on page 370.

Bolsters are long narrow pillows or cushions used to support or prop clients into position for massage. Massage bolsters are typically as wide as a standard table, and come in round, half-round, and quarter-round shapes. Small bolsters are useful for neck support. Soft wedges of various sizes and shapes are made for positioning different parts of the body. Some whole body support systems are available for pregnant and other special-needs clients.

Bolsters are usually covered with the same upholstery materials used on massage table tops. If a bolster touches a client's skin during massage, wash it afterward. Bolsters can also be covered or placed under the bottom drape for protection.

Standard bed pillows are sometimes useful for positioning clients, especially for those in the side-lying position. Be sure that pillows are washable. Pillows should be covered with liners and pillow cases, with cases changed after each client.

Sheets, Blankets, and Towels

Sheets are the most common draping material for Western massage (Figure 11.13■). The mechanics of draping with sheets are described on page 372 in Chapter 12, Body Mechanics, Table Skills, and Application Guidelines. Single bed sheets can be used on most massage tables, or sheets specially made for massage tables can be purchased. Sheets

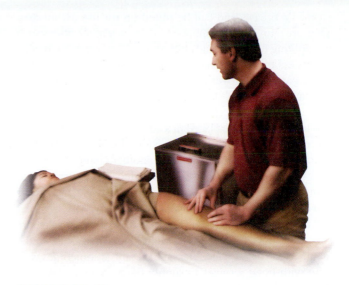

FIGURE 11.13

Sheets are the most commonly used draping material.

come in different fabrics with most made of cotton or cotton blends. Flannel sheets are sometimes used for warmth. Stock at least enough sets of sheets for the number of clients seen daily. Having extra sheets reduces the number of trips to the laundry.

Blankets are good to have when a client gets cold and can be placed over the top drape. Blankets sized for massage tables can be bought or made. Blankets that hang over the sides of the table too much are difficult to handle when draping and undraping arms and legs. Bulky and heavy blankets may feel uncomfortable to clients. Many find fleece and flannel blankets ideal for massage. In most circumstances, blankets that do not touch a client's skin may be used on other clients without washing first. In hospital or clinical settings, blankets would not be shared.

Having a variety of sizes of towels available is very practical (Figure 11.14■). Towels are serviceable for draping

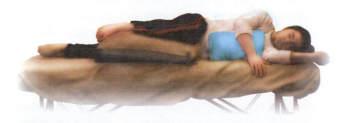

FIGURE 11.12

Bolsters and pillows are essential for most massage applications.

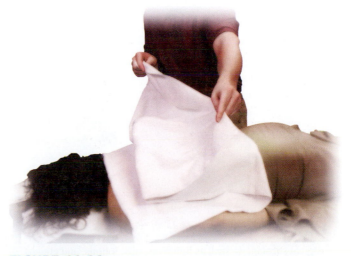

FIGURE 11.14

Towels have many uses during a massage therapy session.

women's breasts and can be rolled up for use as bolsters. They are employed for temperature therapy applications such as applying hot packs and cold packs. They are used to wipe off excess oil and lotion, and for cleaning up spills. A large towel can be laid over a top drape instead of a blanket for increased warmth.

Sheets must be changed after every client. Used sheets and towels should be placed in a covered or closed container, preferably away from the massage table. Never let a sheet or towel used on one client touch another client.

Wash sheets and towels as needed. An alternative to using a home washer and dryer is to take sheets and towels to a commercial self-service laundry. That way, you save wear and tear on your own machines and may be able to wash more sheets and towels in one load. Some businesses will do the laundry for you for a fee. Massage therapists sometimes contract with linen services to supply their sheets and towels. The service then takes care of laundering and delivers clean sheets as needed. This is a business decision that usually involves signing a contract so it should be entered into thoughtfully. Figure the time and cost of washing sheets and towels as part of the expense of your massage practice.

TOPICAL SUBSTANCES

Many forms of massage and bodywork use some kind of **topical substance** to enhance their effects or to minimize skin friction during the application of techniques. Topical substances are classified as liniments, oils, lotions, creams, or combinations of these (Figure 11.15■).

Uses of Different Topical Substances

Liniments have been used for centuries for sore and stiff muscles and for sprains and bruises. They are particularly popular with athletes. A liniment is a liquid or semiliquid preparation for rubbing on or applying to the skin for therapeutic purposes. Liniments are typically counterirritants

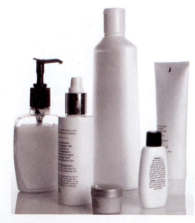

FIGURE 11.15

Topical substances, such as liniments, oils, lotions, and creams enhance the effects or minimize skin friction during the application of many massage techniques.

that produce a slight skin irritation to relieve symptoms of inflammation. They contain ingredients such as camphor, menthol, and turpentine. Herbal preparations might contain rosemary, wild marjoram, or cayenne pepper. Since they contain irritants, rubbing with them too vigorously may cause blistering. If liniments are used, they are usually rubbed onto the skin after massage of an area.

Oil serves as a lubricant to minimize uncomfortable skin friction during sliding and kneading techniques. Certain vegetable oils may also add moisture and nutrients to the skin. Commonly used vegetable oils include almond, olive, and grape seed. Mineral oils are sometimes used and generally wash out of sheets more easily than vegetable oils. Vegetable oils trapped in sheets can spoil and turn rancid, causing sheets to have an unpleasant odor. However, some consider vegetable oils healthier for both the giver and the receiver of massage.

Jojoba (pronounced ho-ho-ba) is an oil-like substance made from seeds of the jojoba plant found in the North American desert. Native Americans used jojoba for skin and hair care. Many massage practitioners use jojoba either by itself or in combination with lotions, because it is hypoallergenic, healthy for skin, and washes out of sheets easily.

Practitioners choose their oils based on a number of factors. These include properties such as the "feel" of the oil (e.g., thick or thin), inherent nutrients, and scent. Unscented oils are available. Massage oils should be of high quality and cold pressed. Oils developed specially for massage can be purchased from suppliers.

Lotions are semiliquid substances containing agents for moisturizing the skin or for therapeutic purposes such as reducing itching or local pain. Lotions are readily absorbed into the skin, unlike oils, which tend to stay on top of the skin longer. Lotions are good for situations in which lubrication is desired for a warm-up phase, but more friction is desired later in the session. Those who don't like the feel of oil on their skin may prefer lotions. Lotions also tend to be more water soluble than oils and are, therefore, more easily washed out of sheets.

Practitioners experiment with different topical substances and concoct combinations of substances to get the properties that best enhance their work. They frequently mix different oils or mix lotions and oils.

Some substances are more likely to cause allergic reactions. Also, some skin types are more easily irritated. Scent can be an important consideration. People going back to work after massage may desire an unscented substance. Men usually prefer different scents than women. Care should be taken in choosing a topical substance for each unique client or patient situation.

Sanitation and Topical Substances

A few simple practices can prevent cross-contamination from oils, lotions, and creams used in massage. First, wipe off bottles and jars after each session, and any topical substances spilled or dripped on surfaces in the massage room.

PRACTICAL APPLICATION

Experiment with various topical substances to become familiar with their different qualities and potential uses for massage therapy. Sample various liniments, oils, lotions, and creams. Use each one in a massage application and evaluate how it performs and how it compares to others.

1. What are the ingredients in each topical substance?
2. What are the advantages of each for different massage applications? Disadvantages?
3. Do you like some better than others? Why?

Use oil bottles with closeable spouts and keep them closed between uses. Pumps are available for dispensing lotion.

Do not dip your fingers into a jar to remove creams. Instead, take out what you intend to use with a little spatula and place it on a small plate or piece of paper. Wash the spatula after each use. Use the separated supply of cream for the massage, and discard any excess afterward. The original jar then remains uncontaminated. "Double dipping" can result in cross-contamination from one client to another.

Wash topical substances out of sheets and towels thoroughly. Some topical substance blends are formulated to be more easily washed out of sheets. Organic oils and lotions left in cloth can turn rancid over time, leaving a disagreeable odor. Once this happens, it is advisable to get rid of the sheets and buy new ones.

PHYSICAL ENVIRONMENT FOR MASSAGE

Regardless of the specific setting, there are certain environmental factors that will help maximize the benefits of massage. Important factors to consider include the configuration of the room, floor, wall, and window coverings, lighting and color, temperature and air quality, music or tranquil sounds, and dressing arrangements.

Room Set Up

The room in which massage is given must be large enough to accommodate the necessary furniture and equipment, plus the client and the massage therapist. At a minimum, a massage room contains a massage table and sitting stool on wheels, with adequate space for movement around the table. A step stool can help short or less mobile clients get onto the table. A nearby tabletop or countertop holds oils and lotions, small hand tools, hot packs, and other objects used during massage. A cabinet or closet is useful to store linens, lotions, and other supplies. Soiled linens are kept in a separate covered container. A chair and clothes rack for clients' belongings round out the furnishings in a well-equipped massage room.

Provide convenient dressing arrangements and a private space for clients to disrobe. If there is only one table in the room, then the practitioner may simply leave the room while the recipient is disrobing. A privacy screen or curtain can be used if needed. In situations where there is more than one table in the room, such as in a training room or clinic, gowns may be provided for clients to use when walking from the dressing area to the massage table. Robes are often provided for this purpose at spas.

It is considered a breach of professional boundaries for clients to be seen naked as they prepare for massage. Exceptions are in cases where the person receiving massage needs assistance undressing or dressing, such as with the elderly or disabled. Even in these cases, care should be taken to preserve the modesty of the recipient as much as possible.

Floors, Walls, and Windows

Floors in massage rooms should be able to be washed and disinfected regularly. Wood and tile floors are most easily washed, but can be cold for the client. Area rugs can add warmth, but look for those with rubber backing to avoid slipping when people walk on them. Carpet is the hardest floor covering to keep clean and is liable to stain if oil or lotion is spilled on it. Some local health ordinances may require a specific type of flooring for massage establishments.

Windows in a massage room allow for fresh air and natural sunlight. Be sure that curtains, shades, or blinds provide adequate privacy at all times.

Walls in a massage room may be decorated with artwork, and provide a place to hang certificates or anatomy charts. A small wall mirror is useful for clients to check their hair or makeup after massage. A typical massage room is shown in Figure 11.16■.

Keep a regular maintenance schedule for removing dust and dirt, and cleaning surfaces in massage rooms. Using some type of air cleaner can help keep dust to a minimum. Daily cleaning is a must, with more thorough cleaning on a weekly or monthly schedule.

Lighting and Color

Lighting is another important consideration. Soft and indirect lighting is more restful than harsh and direct lighting. Overhead lighting may shine in the receiver's eyes when he or

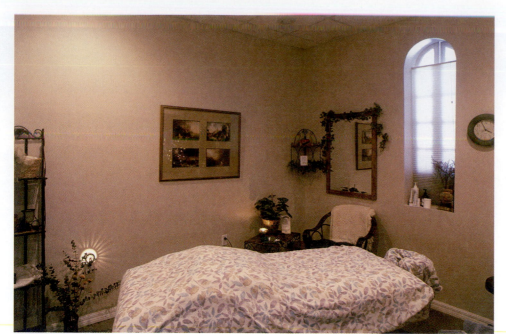

FIGURE 11.16

A typical massage room has adequate space for equipment and pleasant decorations.

she is supine on a table, as will the sun if doing massage in an outdoor setting such as at a spa or an athletic event. In places where overhead lighting cannot be controlled, you may provide the receiver with a light shield for the eyes when he or she is supine.

Temperature, Humidity, and Fresh Air

Keep the massage room temperature and humidity at a comfortable level. A good temperature is around 75 degrees Fahrenheit when the receiver is partially or fully unclothed under a drape. A comfortable humidity range is 45–50 percent. Lower humidity can cause drying of the skin and difficulty breathing, and damage equipment and furniture.

Clients often get cold during massage as they relax. Ways to help keep them warm include an electric mattress pad underneath the bottom sheet, a heat lamp overhead, or a blanket on top. Turning up the heat in the room is a less desirable solution, because the practitioner may then get overheated while working.

Well-ventilated rooms keep air quality fresh and pleasant. This may be a challenge in some places such as hospitals or beauty salons where strong odors are present. Eliminate allergens such as pollen and animal hair as much as possible. Electric air cleaners may be used, and in the summer, air conditioners can help keep air fresh. However, if using an air conditioner, be sure that the room does not get too cold for the client.

Music and Sound

Sound can help create a peaceful and healing environment or a stimulating one. Music elicits certain emotions and is often used to create a particular effect. In general, popular and vocal music should be avoided if the intent is to relax. Use of popular music may also confuse the profes-

sional relationship, since it is normally heard in social situations. Numerous CDs and tapes are available with music specifically designed for relaxation, some specifically for massage.

Sometimes it is desirable to have a background of more stimulating music, for example, when the receiver must go back to work immediately or for an athlete receiving massage just before an event. Music that is stimulating, while not stressful or frenetic, is appropriate in these situations. The receiver's taste in music should be taken into consideration and a variety of choices made available.

For some people, silence, or a fish tank bubbling in the background, is most restful. Fish tanks are known to have a relaxing effect on most people. There are also machines that produce "white noise" to mask annoying outside noises.

Safety

The safety of clients is the responsibility of massage therapists. Be aware of potential hazards in the massage environment and minimize them. Make sure that all equipment and furniture is stable and in good repair. Provide adequate lighting. Remove objects that clients might fall over or slip on. Make sure that wall hangings are secure, and that room dividers or screens will not fall over. Watch out for sharp edges on furniture, walls, doors, and other places that can cause harm. If something spills, wipe it up immediately to prevent falls.

There is a special responsibility with clients who are disabled or elderly. Help them onto and off of the massage table as necessary to prevent falls.

While "slip and fall" insurance protects you legally when accidents occur, you may be considered liable for injuries if you are deemed to have been negligent in your duty to provide a safe environment.

CASE FOR STUDY

Bobbie and Sanitation on the Road

Bobbie has a number of home-visit clients in her massage therapy practice. That means she must carry whatever she needs for massage to the client's home in her car. She has become more concerned recently about hygiene and sanitation, and wants to establish a more thorough cleaning and maintenance plan.

Question:

What might the elements of a thorough hygiene and sanitation plan look like for a home-visit massage practice?

Things to consider:

- What personal hygiene measures must be set up for a home visit?

- How might Bobbie plan for carrying clean linens? Removing used linens? Avoiding contamination of topical substances?
- What are some potential areas of difficulty for sanitation during a home visit session?
- What cleaning products might she need to have on hand and how might she carry them around?
- How might she best care for and sanitize her equipment?

Write a brief description of a hygiene and sanitation plan for Bobbie's home-visit massage practice.

_____

_____

_____

Maintenance Schedule

Overall cleanliness and neatness of the space where massage is given is essential. Not only does this provide a sanitary environment for the recipient, but also it helps create a calm, peaceful, and cheerful atmosphere. Neatly arrange oil bottles and wipe them clean. Stack and store clean linens. Place used sheets and towels in a closed container and keep them out of sight. Clean floors, vacuum carpets, and dust furniture regularly. Set time aside at the beginning and end of the day to care for the space. A checklist of daily maintenance tasks is provided in Box 11.1●.

There may be local health department regulations concerning sanitation in places where massage is provided. Requirements sometimes include washable floors, floors disinfected regularly, sheets and towels stored away, and other rules.

INFECTION CONTROL

The hygiene and sanitation measures discussed throughout this chapter help prevent infections from disease-causing organisms in the massage environment. This applies to the

massage school setting, as well as to a future massage practice. Infections can spread in school as students practice massage on one another, and also in student clinic. Infection control measures are important from the first day in massage school.

Two final topics related to infection control focus on less common situations, but important ones nonetheless because of their potential seriousness. These are universal precautions and MRSA.

Universal Precautions

The aim of **universal precautions,** sometimes called standard or sanitary precautions, is to prevent the transmission of serious communicable diseases. Among these are HIV, hepatitis B, and other blood- and fluid-borne pathogens. Although massage therapists are generally at low risk for coming into contact with blood and body fluids, it is prudent to know the standard precautions related to sanitation. Massage therapists who work in nursing homes, hospitals, hospice, or with the elderly or with athletes at competitive events have a special need to know about universal precautions.

Universal precautions apply to body fluids such as blood, semen and vaginal/cervical secretions, urine, feces, and vomit. They do not apply to nasal secretions, saliva, sweat, tears, and sputum, unless they contain visible blood. The risk of transmission of serious diseases from these latter substances is extremely low or negligible. Basic sanitary precautions are as follows:

1. Use protective barriers such as latex or nonlatex gloves to prevent contact with body fluids to which universal precautions apply. When removing gloves that have touched such fluids, hold them at the wrist and turn them inside out. This keeps the fluids from contact with the outside.

BOX 11.1	Massage Room Daily Maintenance Checklist

- ✔ Clean all furniture surfaces (e.g., tabletops, chairs).
- ✔ Wipe off oil and lotion bottles.
- ✔ Clean massage table upholstery.
- ✔ Stack and store clean linens.
- ✔ Remove dirty linens and store in closed container.
- ✔ Empty waste baskets.
- ✔ Clean or vacuum floors.

2. If your skin comes in contact with body fluids to which universal precautions apply, wash the area with a bleach solution of 1 part bleach to 10 parts water, or comparable disinfecting solution (Figure 11.17■).

3. If other surfaces, such as the massage table or chair, are exposed to contamination, immediately wash the surface with the bleach solution described. Wear protective gloves when washing the surface.

4. If sheets or towels come into contact with body fluids for which universal precautions apply, place them into a plastic bag separate from other laundry. Wear protective gloves. Wash the sheets or towels in a disinfecting solution.

MRSA

MRSA stands for methicillin-resistant staphylococcus aureus, which is a drug-resistant bacterial infection typically found on the skin but which can occur elsewhere in the body. MRSA (pronounced *mersa*) has become a serious problem in hospitals, schools, athletic facilities, and other places where people come in close contact or may share personal items such as towels and razors. If detected and treated early, MRSA is less difficult to control.

MSRA is a staph infection that is spread by direct contact with another person's infection or by contact with items that have touched an infection. MSRA appears as a bump or infection on the skin that is red, swollen, warm, painful, and with pus or other drainage. It is sometimes accompanied by a fever. If MRSA is suspected, cover the area and see a health care professional immediately. If you detect a suspicious bump or infection on a client, avoid touching the area and ask the client about the condition. Remember that fever is a general contraindication for massage. If you detect a suspicious skin condition while in school, tell a teacher or

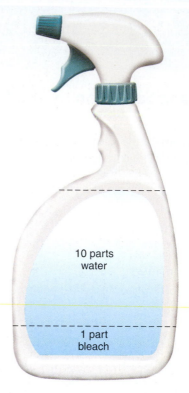

FIGURE 11.17

A good disinfecting solution you can make yourself consists of 1 part bleach to 10 parts water.

administrator immediately so that he or she can follow-up to prevent potential infection in the school.

For further information on infection control visit the U.S. Department of Health and Human Services, Centers for Disease Control and Prevention (CDC) website at www.cdc.gov.

CHAPTER HIGHLIGHTS

- A massage therapist's good personal hygiene helps the client feel comfortable with him or her and prevents the spread of disease.
- Massage practitioners wash their hands thoroughly (hygienic hand washing) before and after each session to prevent the spread of pathogens.
- When choosing a massage table, consider the type of massage or bodywork for which it will be used and the setting.
  - Evaluate the massage table for type (stationary or portable), height, width, length, padding, upholstery, weight, strength (operating capacity), and ease of set up and take down.
  - Special massage tables with hinged tops for semi-reclining positioning or other special features are available.
  - Choose a professional grade massage table, and check out table models at showrooms, trade shows or conventions, or look on table manufacturers' websites.
- Massage chairs are specially designed to provide maximum comfort while receiving massage in a seated position while fully clothed.
  - Massage chairs have a seat, knee rests, armrest, chest cushion, and face cradle.
  - When choosing a massage chair, consider its overall design, ease of set up and carrying, weight, stability, adjustments, and special features.
- Follow manufacturer's instructions for proper care of massage tables and chairs.
  - Clean upholstery regularly, but avoid using harsh chemicals.

- o Set up tables and chairs carefully to avoid damage to them.
  - o Do not sit directly in the center of a portable massage table over the hinge.
  - o Check nuts, bolts, and other hardware regularly and tighten or fix as needed.
- Sheets, blankets, and towels are supplies needed by massage therapists.
  - o Sheets are typically used for draping and should be easily washable.
  - o Blankets are used for added warmth.
  - o Various size towels are useful in massage therapy for draping, bolstering, wiping off oil, cleaning up spills, for hot and cold applications, and other uses.
- Many forms of massage and bodywork use some kind of topical substance (liniments, oils, lotions, creams, or combinations of these) to enhance their effects or to minimize skin friction during the application of techniques.
  - o Sanitation measures related to topical substances help prevent cross-contamination and the spread of disease.
  - o Wipe off bottles and jars after each session.
  - o Use oil bottles with closeable spouts and keep them closed between uses.
  - o Use pump jars for dispensing lotion.
  - o Do not dip your fingers into a jar to remove creams; instead, take out what you intend to use with a little spatula and place it on a small plate or piece of paper.
- Important factors to consider in creating the physical environment for massage include the configuration of the room, floor, wall, and window coverings, lighting and color, temperature and air quality, music or tranquil sounds, and dressing arrangements.
- Temperature, ventilation, lighting, and sound in a room can help set the tone for massage.

- Eliminate safety hazards in the massage environment such as slip and fall hazards.
- Set up a regular maintenance schedule for dusting, washing equipment, and cleaning floors and furniture in your massage room.
- Universal precautions are procedures for preventing contamination from certain body fluids that can carry serious diseases such as HIV and hepatitis B.
  - o Body fluids for which universal precautions apply include blood, semen, vaginal/cervical secretions, urine, feces, and vomit.
  - o Body fluids with extremely low or negligible potential for spreading serious disease include nasal secretions, saliva, sweat, tears, and sputum.
  - o Wear latex or nonlatex gloves in the presence of body fluids for which universal precautions apply.
  - o Wash contaminated surfaces with a bleach solution of 1 part bleach to 10 parts water, or comparable disinfectant.
  - o Isolate and dispose of contaminated items (gloves, sheets, towels) properly.
- MRSA stands for methicillin-resistant staphylococcus aureus, which is a drug-resistant bacterial infection typically found on the skin but which can occur elsewhere in the body.
  - o Signs of MRSA are a skin bump or infection that is red, warm, swollen, painful, with pus or other drainage, and may be accompanied by fever.
  - o MRSA is spread by direct contact with an infected area or contact with an item which has had direct contact with the infection.
  - o If MRSA is suspected, cover the area and have the client see a health care professional immediately.
- Good personal hygiene, environmental sanitation, and infection control are serious matters in the massage school environment to promote the health and safety of students, teachers, and clinic clients.

EXAM REVIEW

Key Terms

Match the following key terms to their descriptions. For additional study, look up the key terms in the Interactive Glossary on page G-1 and note other terms that compare or contrast with them.

_____ 1. Bolsters
_____ 2. Equipment
_____ 3. Hygienic hand washing
_____ 4. Massage chairs
_____ 5. MRSA
_____ 6. Personal hygiene
_____ 7. Portable massage table
_____ 8. Sanitation
_____ 9. Topical substance
_____ 10. Universal precautions

a. Drug-resistant bacterial infection typically found on the skin
b. Hinged table that can be carried from place to place and set up and taken down easily
c. Being clean and well groomed
d. Removing disease-causing organisms
e. Liniments, oils, lotions, and creams
f. Long narrow pillows or cushions used to support or prop clients
g. Procedures to prevent the transmission of serious communicable diseases
h. Most effective method for preventing the transfer of pathogens during massage
i. Designed to provide maximum comfort for people receiving massage in a seated position
j. Massage tables and massage chairs

Memory Workout

To test your memory of the main concepts in this chapter, complete the following sentences by circling the most correct answer from the two choices provided.

1. The words *hygiene* and *sanitation* refer to procedures that prevent the spread of (disease) (dust).
2. For hygienic hand washing, the water must be (hot) (running) to wash away pathogens.
3. If you have a cut or scrape on your finger, cover it with a (Band-Aid) (finger cot) before touching a client.
4. Keep fingernails clipped short (below) (above) the level of the fingertips.

5. It is a wise investment to buy a (professional) (personal) grade massage table.
6. Long narrow pillows used to support or prop clients into position for massage are called (cushions) (bolsters).
7. Used sheets and towels should be placed in a (plastic) (closed) container.
8. Since (lotions) (liniments) contain irritants, rubbing with them too vigorously may cause blistering.
9. Floors in massage room should be able to be washed and (sanitized) (refinished) regularly.
10. The aim of (universal) (therapeutic) precautions is to prevent the transmission of serious communicable diseases.

Test Prep

The following multiple-choice questions will help to prepare you for future school and professional exams.

1. Which of the following statements about hand washing before and after massage is *not* correct?
   a. Water must be running to wash away pathogens.
   b. Water should be as hot as possible to kill germs.
   c. Hands are rubbed for at least 15 seconds.
   d. Dry hands thoroughly to prevent chapping.
2. When rinsing off soap in hygienic hand washing, the arm is held at an angle so that water flows from:
   a. Wrist to fingers
   b. Elbow to fingers
   c. Fingers to wrist
   d. Fingers to elbow
3. A typical size massage table for Western/Swedish massage is:
   a. 30 inches wide and 73 inches long
   b. 28 inches wide and 80 inches long.
   c. 35 inches wide and 70 inches long
   d. 40 inches wide and 75 inches long
4. The width of the base of a massage chair helps determine its:
   a. Agility
   b. Adjustability
   c. Stability
   d. Portability

5. A topical substance that reduces friction during massage and that is readily absorbed into the skin is:
   a. Liniment
   b. Lotion
   c. Oil
   d. Corn starch
6. Camphor, menthol, rosemary, and cayenne pepper are ingredients commonly found in:
   a. Liniments
   b. Aromatherapy oils
   c. Infant massage lotions
   d. Natural cleaning solutions
7. Comfortable temperature and humidity for a massage room is about:
   a. 55 degrees Fahrenheit and 20% humidity
   b. 68 degrees Fahrenheit and 30% humidity
   c. 75 degrees Fahrenheit and 45% humidity
   d. 82 degrees Fahrenheit and 75% humidity
8. The ideal lighting for a massage room is:
   a. Overhead and direct.
   b. Soft and indirect
   c. Bright and direct
   d. Dark

9. Which of the following is *not* a good sanitary practice for handling topical substances?
   a. Using a pump to dispense lotion
   b. Wiping oil bottles clean after each massage
   c. Wiping up spills as soon as they happen
   d. Dipping your fingers into a jar to remove creams
10. Exposure to which of the following body fluids requires use of universal sanitary precautions?
    a. Tears
    b. Blood
    c. Sputum
    d. Sweat
11. The disinfecting solution used as a universal precaution is:
    a. 1 part bleach to 10 parts water
    b. 10 parts bleach to 1 part water
    c. 1 part bleach to 1 part water
    d. 100% bleach
12. MRSA is:
    a. A disinfectant cleaning solution
    b. A blood-borne disease-causing agent
    c. A drug-resistant staph infection
    d. A universal precaution procedure

Video Challenge

Watch the appropriate segment of the video on your DVD and then answer the following questions.

Equipment, Environment, and Hygiene
   Hygienic Hand Washing
1. How did the person in the video begin the hygienic hand washing procedure?

2. How would you describe the method of cleaning the fingernails shown in the video?
3. How did the person in the video turn off the water faucet?

Comprehension Exercises

The following short answer questions test your knowledge and understanding of chapter topics and provide practice in written communication skills. Explain in two to four complete sentences.

1. Describe the steps in hygienic hand washing. How is this different from ordinary hand washing?

2. Describe the important features of a portable massage table. What are the dimensions of a standard massage table for Western-style or Swedish massage.
3. Explain universal precautions. What body fluids are of concern? How would you handle sheets that were contaminated?

For Greater Understanding

The following exercises are designed to take you from the realm of theory into the real world. They will help give you a deeper understanding of the subjects covered in this chapter. Action words are underlined to emphasize the variety of activities presented to address different learning styles and to encourage deeper thinking.

1. Evaluate different models of massage chairs. Note special features of each and do a cost comparison of different models.

2. Take an inventory of your own massage therapy equipment and supplies. Note your method of storage and transport. Develop a maintenance plan for keeping them neater, cleaner, and more sanitary.
3. Visit a spa, health club, or other facility that offers massage therapy. Note the massage room set up, windows, walls, floors, lighting, sound, and air quality. Ask about hygiene and sanitary procedures. Evaluate your findings, and identify ways you might change that environment to make it more comfortable and safe for clients.

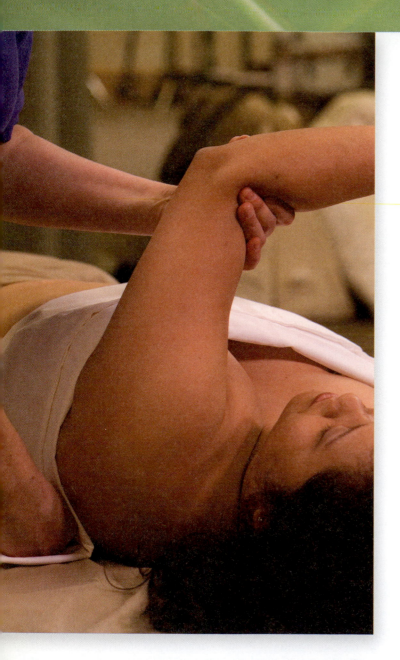

 CHAPTER OUTLINE

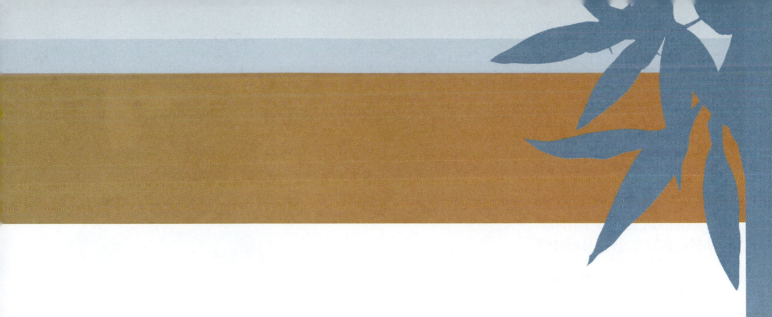

LEARNING OUTCOMES

After studying this chapter, you will have information to:

1. Practice good body mechanics and self-care.
2. Describe proper body mechanics for table massage.
3. Describe proper body mechanics for seated massage.
4. Use good hand mechanics for different massage applications.
5. Vary hand positions during massage to lessen strain.

6. Assist clients onto and off of the table as needed.
7. Position clients for safety, comfort, and accessibility.
8. Perform draping techniques skillfully.
9. Analyze massage application elements.

KEY TERMS

MASSAGE *in* ACTION

On your DVD, explore:

- Body Mechanics
- Positioning and Draping

PRINCIPLES OF HAND AND BODY MECHANICS

Practicing good body and hand mechanics is essential for well-being and your longevity as a massage therapist. **Body mechanics** refers to the overall alignment and use of the body while performing massage. Good body mechanics minimize shoulder, neck, and back problems, as well as injuries to the arms and hands. Good **hand mechanics** minimize strain on the fingers, thumb, and wrist.

A major concern for those performing massage on a regular basis is avoiding strain and overuse injuries. To prevent injuries, special attention must be paid to the care of the hands and wrists and to practicing good body mechanics.

PREVENTING INJURY AND OVERUSE

Avoiding undue strain and overuse injuries is accomplished in a number of ways. Being in good physical condition and using good hand and body mechanics are essential. See page 78 in Chapter 4, Physical Skills, Fitness, and Self-Care for the Massage Therapist, for information on physical fitness.

Common upper-body injuries for massage practitioners include repetitive strain injuries such as tendinitis, and nerve impingement syndromes such as carpal tunnel and thoracic outlet. In addition to strengthening and stretching exercises, self-massage and hydrotherapy can head off injuries due to the wear and tear of giving massage (Figure 12.1■).

The beginning of a massage session can also serve as a warm-up for the practitioner. It is like an athlete doing warm-ups before a competition. Begin the session slowly and gradually increase pressure and pace. This benefits both the giver and receiver, and eases both into the massage.

Using a variety of techniques in a session helps minimize repeated strain on a particular joint or body area. Some massage techniques are less strenuous than others, for example, light effleurage and passive touch. More strenuous techniques, such as compression and kneading, can be alternated with less stressful ones to provide a resting phase to a session. At the end of a session, the hands may feel hot or "charged" with energy. Running cold water over the wrists and hands after washing aids in recovery.

The number of massage sessions performed in 1 day and throughout the week is also important to take into consideration. The number that can be performed without leading to injury depends on several factors. These include the type of massage given, the practitioner's physical fitness, and the quality of his

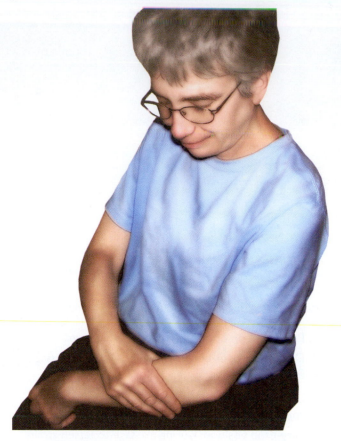

FIGURE 12.1

Self-massage of the forearm helps reduce the effects of stress on muscles used for massage.

or her body mechanics. Practitioners starting out in their careers must build strength and stamina to meet the physical stress on their bodies. A sudden increase in the number of sessions given per week can lead to strain, pain, and possible injury.

The following are guidelines for scheduling sessions per week. They project the number of massage sessions that can be given safely by most practitioners.

Schedule no more than:

- Five 1-hour sessions in 1 day, if you work 4 days per week
- Four 1-hour sessions in 1 day, if you work 5 days per week
- Twenty hours of massage per week total

In addition:

- Take 15- to 30-minute breaks between sessions.
- Take an additional 15- to 30-minute break after three consecutive 1-hour sessions.
- Do no more than four 1-hour sessions in 1 day if the type of massage is strenuous.

Hand and Wrist Care

The hands are the primary means for giving massage. Conditioning exercises for the hands, wrists, forearms, and shoulders can help prevent overuse injuries. These include both strengthening and stretching exercises. Simple strengthening exercises for the hands include squeezing a rubber ball and extending the fingers against resistance using a rubber band. Conditioning is especially important when learning massage and before embarking on a full-time practice.

HAND MECHANICS FOR DIFFERENT TECHNIQUES

Good hand mechanics emphasize joint alignment and efficient movement. Proper alignment reduces stress on hand and wrist joints, and efficient movement prevents muscle fatigue.

The thumb is especially vulnerable during high-pressure techniques such as direct pressure, trigger point therapy, and acupressure. A principle called **stacking the joints** can help protect the thumbs from damage. According to this principle, the bones of the thumb and wrist are lined up so that pressure passes in a straight line through the bones, as demonstrated in Figure 12.2A■. This avoids pressure applied at an angle to or across the joint, which causes strain on joint structures and tissues. Applying pressure with the thumb abducted is especially harmful (Figure 12.2B).

Other parts of the hand can be used to apply techniques, and to avoid strain on the thumb and fingers. A close look at the structure of the hand reveals a variety of points and flat surfaces that may be useful. For example, the point formed at the knuckle of the middle phalangeal joint of the middle finger can be used to apply direct pressure. The flat surface on the back of the fingers of a loose fist or of curled fingers can be used for broad sliding and friction tech-

niques. Hand position variations are demonstrated in Figure 12.3■

Keep the wrist in a **neutral position** (i.e., neither flexed nor extended) as much as possible when applying massage techniques (see Figure 12.4■). For compression techniques, avoid hyperextension of the wrist. To reinforce one hand with the other during compression techniques, place the top hand directly over the metacarpals of the bottom hand as demonstrated in Figure 12.5A■. Do not hold onto the bent wrist (Figure 12.5B), or hyperextend the wrists (12.5C).

The elbow and forearm can be very useful for applying heavier pressure to large muscles. For example, the forearm can be used to apply broad effleurage to the thighs or back muscles as demonstrated in Figure 12.6■.

BODY MECHANICS FOR TABLE MASSAGE

Good body mechanics help minimize shoulder and back problems. A key element is adjusting the table height to fit you properly. A table too high or too low can lead to poor body mechanics and put undue strain on your body. To determine the correct table height for you, stand facing the table with your hands at your sides as shown in Figure 12.7■. Adjust the legs so that your knuckles touch the tabletop. Notice your alignment when applying massage at this table height. Further adjust the table height up or down as needed to keep good alignment of the back and neck. For example, when working on large clients you can lower the table somewhat to avoid raising your shoulders when applying pressure downward.

To keep proper back alignment during a massage session, bend the knees to lower your body. Avoid bending the back excessively or dropping the head as depicted in

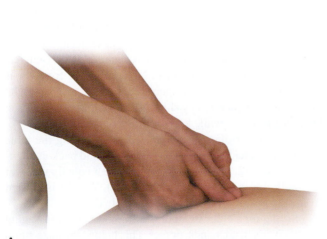

A

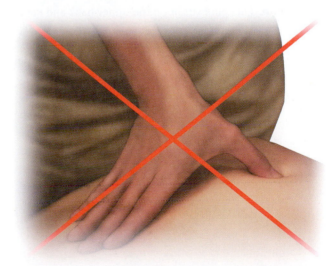

B

FIGURE 12.2

Stacking the joints. A. Correct thumb-wrist alignment for applying direct pressure. B. Incorrect position with thumb abducted will cause injury to the joints.

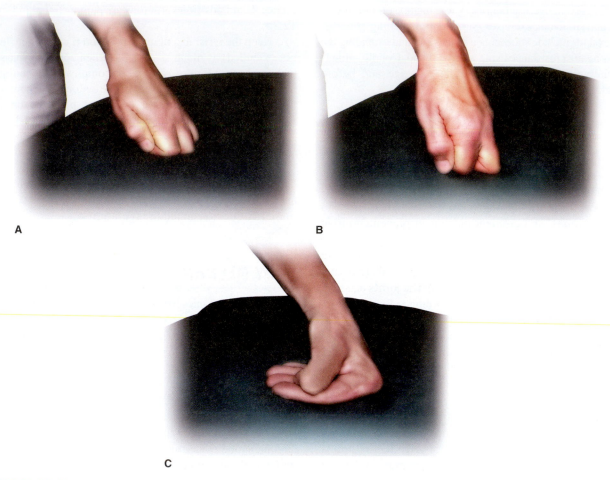

A B

C

FIGURE 12.3

Different hand positions and working surfaces for massage applications on large muscles. A. Flat surface between second and third finger joints. B. Point of second joint of the middle finger. C. Loose fist.

Figure 12.8■. This puts strain on the upper back and neck muscles.

Tai chi stances are effective for keeping good alignment when giving massage. They also position you to use body leverage to apply pressure. These stances emphasize

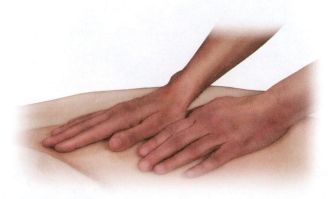

FIGURE 12.4

Wrist in neutral position while performing effleurage.

keeping the back in upright alignment while using the legs to generate power. Two stances especially useful for massage practitioners are the forward leaning or **bow and arrow stance,** and the side–side or **horse riding stance.**

The bow and arrow stance is used when facing the head or foot of the table as demonstrated in Figure 12.9A■. Both feet face the direction of movement. Notice that the front leg is bent more than the rear leg (Figure 12.9B). The torso is upright. Power can be generated by shifting the weight from the back leg to the front leg while keeping the back in alignment.

The horse riding stance is used when facing the table directly. Both feet face the table with head and back in alignment (Figure 12.10A■). The knees are bent equally to lower the body into position (Figure 12.10B). Weight is shifted from side to side as techniques are applied.

Sitting on a chair or stool is common when massaging the receiver's head, hands, or feet. This helps minimize strain on the body. Sit near the edge of the seat with the feet flat on the floor and upper body upright as shown in Figure 12.11■. Adjust the height of the chair to allow you to keep your wrists in a neutral position.

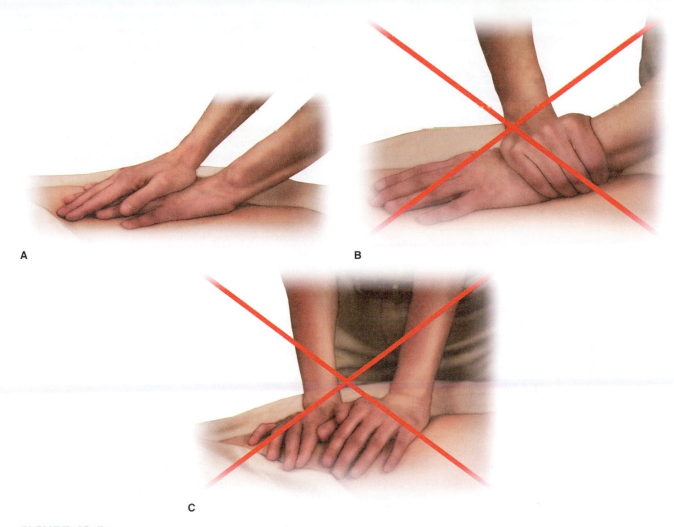

A

B

C

FIGURE 12.5

Correct wrist position while performing compression. A. Correct wrist position for compression techniques. B. Incorrect position with pressure directly on the wrist with the other hand will cause wrist injury. C. Incorrect position with wrist hyperextended will cause wrist injury.

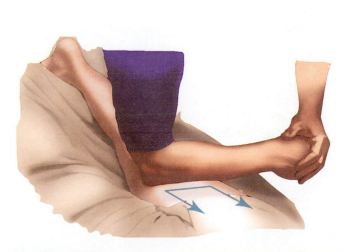

FIGURE 12.6

Use of forearm for performing effleurage on the hamstring muscles.

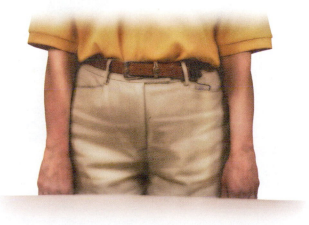

FIGURE 12.7

Determining a good table height. Stand facing the table with your hands at your sides. Adjust the table legs so that your knuckles touch the tabletop.

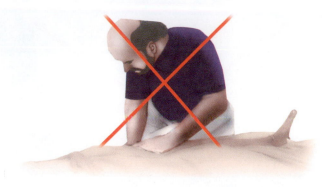

FIGURE 12.8

Incorrect body alignment with back bent and head forward.

BODY MECHANICS
FOR SEATED/CHAIR MASSAGE

The principles of good hand and body mechanics are the same whether the client is lying on a massage table or seated in a chair. Keeping the back upright and neck in good alignment are essential. Avoid hyperextending the wrists and applying pressure with the thumb abducted. Bend the knees, not the back, to lower the body.

With the client more or less vertical in the chair, you will experience some differences in body mechanics compared to working on a person who is horizontal on a table. You must be able to reach up to the head, as well as down to the hands. The bow and arrow stance and horse stance described in the preceding section are ideal for such changes

in level. Using a wider stance and bending the knees more lowers the body. Shortening the stance and straightening the legs raises the body. You can rise up on your toes for brief periods to gain more height. Avoid raising the shoulders when reaching upward.

Pressing into the recipient's back calls for more forward motion, rather than downward. Shift your weight forward, pushing from the rear leg to generate power. Joints are stacked from the shoulder through the elbow, wrist, and thumb when applying thumb pressure to the back, as shown in Figure 12.12■.

Applying pressure down onto the upper trapizius muscle can be done with the forearm. Lean your body weight into the forearm by sinking at the knees. The point of the elbow can be used with sensitivity to apply pressure to specific points. See Figure 12.13■.

Massage of the arms and hands requires lowering your body significantly. Options for keeping good alignment include sinking the knees farther in the bow and arrow stance, or kneeling on one or both knees (Figure 12.14■). If a chair or stool is accessible, massage of the arms and hands can be given from a sitting position.

With practice, keeping good body alignment becomes second nature. It may take a little experimentation at first to discover the most effective body mechanics for seated massage.

TABLE SKILLS

Table skills include a variety of actions required to position and drape a client properly on a massage table. The goals of table skills include the safety and comfort of the receiver and accessibility of different parts of the body for massage applications.

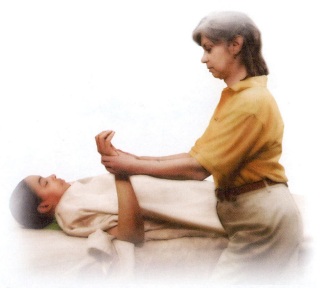

A

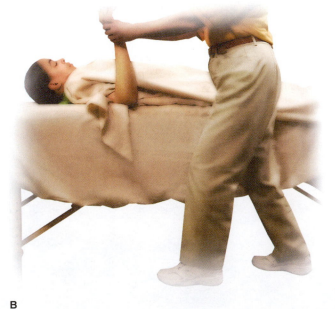

B

FIGURE 12.9

Good body mechanics when facing the head or foot of the table. A. Head and back in alignment. B. Legs and feet in forward leaning stance.

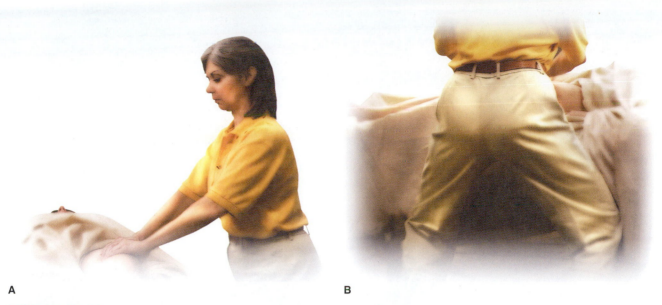

FIGURE 12.10

Good body mechanics when facing the table directly. A. Head and back in alignment. B. Legs and feet in horse riding stance.

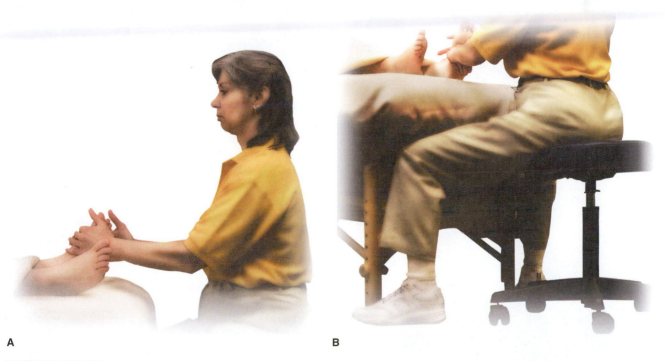

FIGURE 12.11

Good body mechanics for sitting on chair while performing massage. A. Sit with back and head in alignment. B. Sit near edge of chair with feet flat on floor.

Assistance Getting on and off the Table

Occasionally clients need assistance getting onto the massage table before the session, and off the table afterward. These include people with disabilities, the elderly, and pregnant women. Ask the client if he or she wants assistance, but take responsibility for helping anyone you believe needs assistance to be safe.

Keep a stepping stool available for use by clients. Make sure that it is stable and has a nonslip surface. If you are tall, and your table is set relatively high, shorter people may need a boost from a stepping stool to get onto the table safely. If you work in a place with a hydraulic table, you can set the table low for clients to get onto and raise it to the proper height for you before the session starts.

PRACTICAL APPLICATION

Experiment with different ways to apply effleurage or sliding techniques to various areas on a practice client. Focus on ease of application and avoiding strain on your body.

1. How do you maintain good overall body alignment when applying sliding techniques?

2. How do you apply effleurage to a long leg or arm without leaning forward too much?

3. What are different hand positions and surfaces you can use for different areas, for example, effleurage on the arm, shoulder, foot, neck, or face?

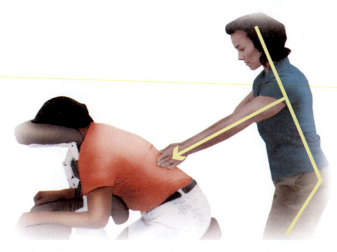

FIGURE 12.12

Good hand and body mechanics when applying thumb pressure to the back.

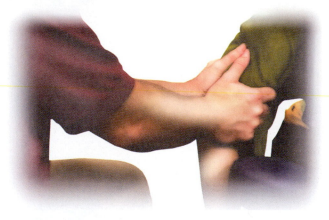

FIGURE 12.14

Kneeling on one knee to keep good alignment when massaging the arms and hands.

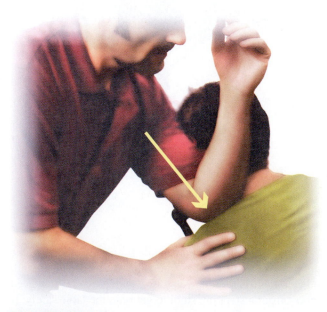

FIGURE 12.13

Use of the forearm to apply pressure to points on the upper trapezius muscle.

There are different degrees of assistance clients might need. In some cases, you might only need to stand close by to assist if necessary. Stand close enough to be able to react effectively if a client looses balance or cannot complete the movement he or she is attempting. In other cases, you might have to hold onto the client's arm, and/or put your arm around his or her shoulder while guiding the person onto or off the table.

For weak or frail individuals, a higher degree of assistance may be called for. In these cases, you can help clients to a sitting position on the side of the table, and then support their backs and heads as they lie down. They may also need help getting their legs up onto the table.

The reverse works well for getting off the table. Stand to the side of the table and put one arm around the client's shoulder, and the other under his or her knees (Figure 12.15■). As he or she attempts to sit up, offer as much assistance as necessary. Keep the drape covering the client during this process. Have him or her sit on the side of the table for a moment, especially if dizzy. Hold onto the client while he or she steps onto the stool and floor.

Maintain clients' modesty while you are helping them. In some cases, it might be too difficult for clients to take off all

CASE FOR STUDY

Nadia and Preventing Overuse Injuries

Nadia is finishing massage school in a few months and plans to begin a job at a spa when she graduates. She has recently begun to get pains in her hands and wrists, and has a lot of tension in her upper back after giving massage in class.

Question:

What can Nadia do to minimize the negative effects she is feeling from giving massage?

Things to consider:

- What aspects of body and hand mechanics might be causing her problems?

- What fitness exercises can she do to condition her body and especially her hands?
- How can she build up to a job doing massage full time?

What advice would you give Nadia as she prepares for her job at the spa?

_____

_____

_____

of their clothes for massage. They can be assisted onto the table fully clothed and then remove shoes and as much clothing as desired. Drape appropriately for modesty and warmth.

Assistance Turning Over

Clients may need assistance in turning from a supine to prone position or vice-versa. A skill called **tenting** keeps clients from getting rolled up in the drape. To create a tent, pin one side of the sheet against the table with your leg or hip. Then lift the sheet so that the client can turn over underneath the drape. Have him or her turn away from you. The client should be out of your sight and the sight of anyone else in the room, while turning over. See Figure 12.16■.

If clients have trouble turning over by themselves, you might consider using the semireclining, side-lying, or seated positions instead of supine and prone. This may be preferable for certain special populations such as the elderly and people with disabilities.

FIGURE 12.15

Assistance in getting off the massage table.

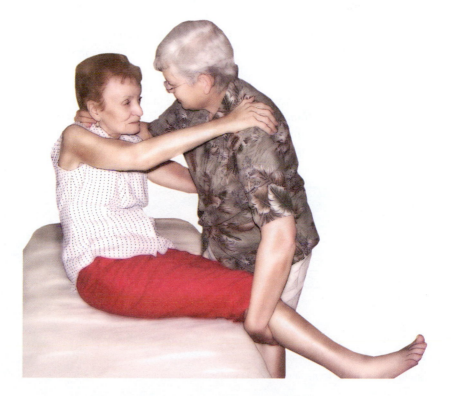

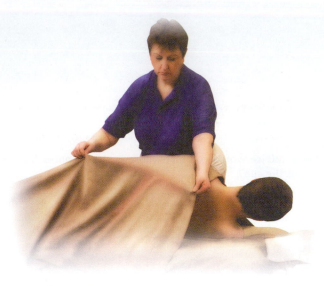

FIGURE 12.16

Creating a tent for turning from prone to supine or vice versa. Pin one side of the sheet against the table with the leg or hip, and lift the sheet so that the recipient can turn over underneath the sheet.

POSITIONING

Placing the receiver in a comfortable and safe position on the table, called **positioning,** is essential for effective application of massage. The recipient's position can also allow easier access to particular muscles or regions of the body.

The receiver should not have to exert muscular effort to stay in position or to hold draping in place. Various size bolsters, pillows, or rolled towels are used to support body areas and position receivers properly. See page 351 in Chapter 11, Hygiene, Equipment, and Environment, for more information about bolsters and pillows.

Supine

In the supine or face-up position, a bolster placed under the knees takes pressure off the lower back. A neck roll is sometimes used for support in the cervical area. This can be a small bolster or rolled up towel. See Figure 12.17■.

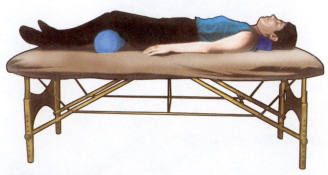

FIGURE 12.17

Supine position. Placement of bolsters under the knees and neck.

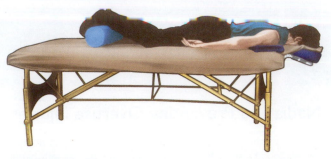

FIGURE 12.18

Prone position. Placement of bolsters under ankles and shoulders, head supported by face cradle.

If the table is wide enough, clients' arms can lie alongside of them on the table. If the table is narrow, clients can rest their hands on their abdomen. Attachable side-extenders are available to widen a table temporarily at the arms if needed. Sometimes clients' arms do not lie flat on the table due to their structure or muscular tightness. In those cases, small bolsters or rolled towels can be placed under the wrists or hands for support.

Prone

In the prone or facedown position, support is placed under the ankles to ease pressure on them. Small pillows may be placed under the shoulders for people with large chests. See Figure 12.18■. Positioning women with large breasts is discussed on page 601 in Chapter 20, Special Populations and Adaptations.

Face Cradle Adjustment

When a client is lying prone, using an adjustable face cradle provides the most options for positioning. Note that some face cradles are not adjustable and extend straight out from the table. This limits positioning and is less desirable for professional massage.

Most modern face-cradles have two adjustments. One adjustment elevates and lowers the entire face-cradle, and the other controls the angle. First adjust the face-cradle height so that the head is in proper alignment with the spine, and

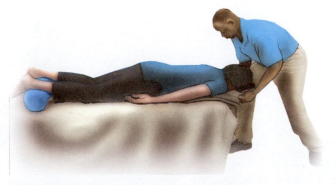

FIGURE 12.19

Face cradle adjustment for comfort of receiver.

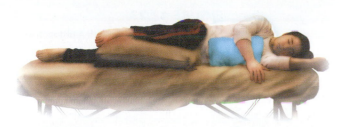

FIGURE 12.20

Side-lying position. Placement of bolsters under the superior leg, arm, and head.

then adjust the angle so that the face is tilted slightly downward. This opens the shoulder and neck region for better access. Always ask clients if the adjustment is comfortable for them. Practice adjusting the face cradle with different body types to learn to perform this essential table skill quickly and effectively. See Figure 12.19■.

Side-Lying and Semireclining

For the side-lying position, have the client straighten out his or her lower leg on the table and bend the upper leg at the hip and knee. Place one or two pillows under the upper leg for support. Ideally, from the knee down the upper leg ends up parallel to the table, which keeps the pelvis and spine in good alignment. Place another pillow under the upper arm. Some clients like to hug the pillow with both arms, while others prefer to place the lower arm on the table near the head. A pillow or bolster supports the head and keeps the neck in good alignment. The face cradle pad can be used for this purpose. See Figure 12.20■.

For the semireclining position, the client is sitting up at a 30–60 degree angle. A backrest is created either by adjusting a special hinged table or by propping the recipient up with a wedge-shaped bolster. A long round or quarter-round bolster is placed under the knees to prevent hyperextension. The arms lie alongside the body, or may be placed on the abdomen. A pillow is used under the head if needed for comfort. See Figure 12.21■.

Seated

Seated massage is given with the client positioned in a special massage chair or in a regular chair adapted for the

purpose. Special massage chairs offer the best options for receiving massage in the seated position and are described in detail on page 349 in Chapter 11, Hygiene, Equipment, and Environment.

Positioning in regular chairs is less than ideal but necessary in some cases. The use of regular household or folding chairs typically occurs in special circumstances. Examples are massage at a health fair, in offices at employee desks, with athletes at events, or at institutions such as senior centers.

If a massage chair is unavailable, choose a sturdy regular chair with a low back and comfortable seat. Clients should be able to place their feet flat on the floor. If the feet do not touch the floor, place a support under them so that the thighs are level. The rest of the positioning depends on the massage application.

One option for foot massage is to sit opposite the client and place his or her foot on your thigh. Place a towel on your leg to protect it from any lotion used. Change the protection for each client. For giving arm and hand massage, use an arm chair with a pillow over the chair arm for support. Place a protective covering over the pillow and change it for each client.

Head, neck, and shoulder massage can be given with the recipient in a regular chair with some consideration for bracing. Pressure applied against the posterior neck and back muscles tends to push the client forward. **Bracing** refers to offering a counter-resistance to prevent the movement of the body in the opposite direction. You can apply massage with one hand while bracing the client's head with the other hand to resist the push forward when massaging the neck (Figure 12.22■).

Better yet, have clients lean against a table or desk. They can place their forearms on the table and let their heads rest on them. For added comfort, they can place a pillow in

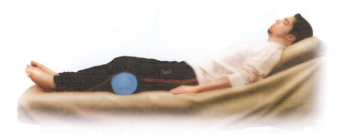

FIGURE 12.21

Semireclining position. Back supported and placement of bolster under the knees.

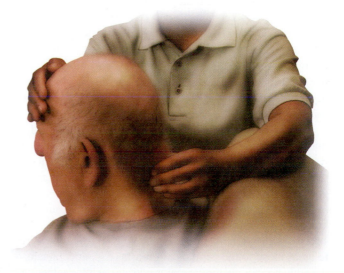

FIGURE 12.22

Bracing the head while applying pressure to the neck.

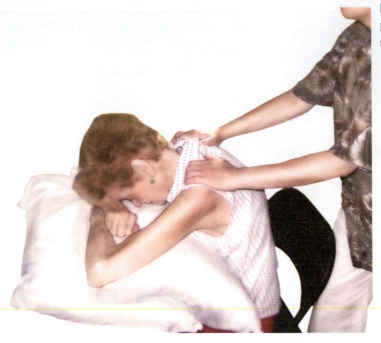

FIGURE 12.23

Leaning against a table with a pillow for support.

front of them and lean on that (Figure 12.23■). Some table top massage equipment provides a chest brace and face cradle for use with regular chairs at desks (Figure 12.24■). Remember the basic principles and use your creativity to provide stability, accessibility, and comfort for massage in regular chairs.

DRAPING

Covering the body during massage, or **draping,** serves to protect the receiver's privacy, maintains clear professional boundaries, and keeps the receiver warm. Skill in draping helps the client feel safe and allows for maximum relaxation. Choose draping material that is substantial enough to provide a sense of privacy and modesty. The use of thin sheets or small, narrow towels can leave the recipient feeling exposed, self-conscious, and uncomfortable.

When clients remove their clothing and are draped for massage, some general guidelines apply. The genitals and women's breasts should be draped at all times. Mutual consent or familiarity between practitioner and receiver are not good reasons to ignore this guideline. An exception might be during breast massage, but only after special training in breast massage for the practitioner and with informed consent from the client. Draping can be adjusted to allow access to areas close to the genitals or breasts (e.g., attachments to the adductors or pectoralis major muscle), while maintaining clear professional boundaries. This should be done only with informed consent.

Draping with a sheet provides maximum coverage. The part to be massaged is uncovered and then recovered during the session. Skillful tucking will enhance the security of the drape and prevent inadvertently exposing the receiver. Figure 12.25■ demonstrates undraping the arm prior to massage.

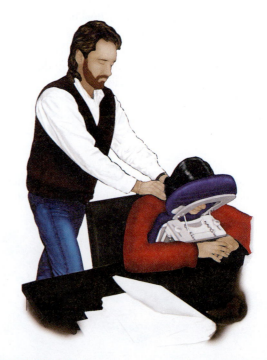

FIGURE 12.24

Portable tabletop equipment that provides support for recipients receiving massage.

CRITICAL THINKING

Think about the different positioning options for table massage. Analyze supine, prone, side-lying, and semireclining positions in terms of the client's alignment and the support needed.

1. In each position, what stresses are put on the joints when a client lies on a massage table without support?

2. What shape and size bolster gives the best support for each area of stress?

3. Why does each client's size and unique structure need to be taken into consideration? Give examples.

Preserve the client's modesty when undraping the leg. Lift the leg at the knee and then pull the drape underneath the thigh. Tuck the drape securely at the hip. The genitals, perineum, and gluteal cleft are covered at all times. Figure 12.26■ shows draping and undraping of the leg in a supine position, and Figure 12.27■ demonstrates undraping and securing the drape for the leg in a prone position.

Prior to massage of a woman's abdomen, the breasts are draped with a towel. This is done with informed consent. To begin, a towel is placed over the breasts on top of the sheet. Either you or the client can hold the towel in place as you pull the sheet down to the waist, exposing the abdomen. The towel remains covering the breasts. Tuck the sheet around the recipient's hips.

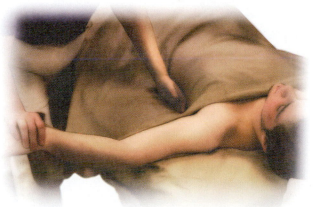

A

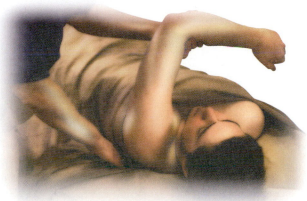

B

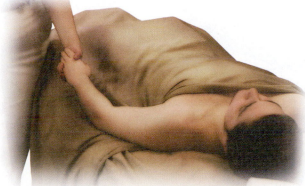

C

FIGURE 12.25

Draping for massage of arm. A. Hold arm to side and tuck drape at ribs. B. Lift arm across chest and tuck sheet underneath the shoulder. C. Place the arm on table ready for massage.

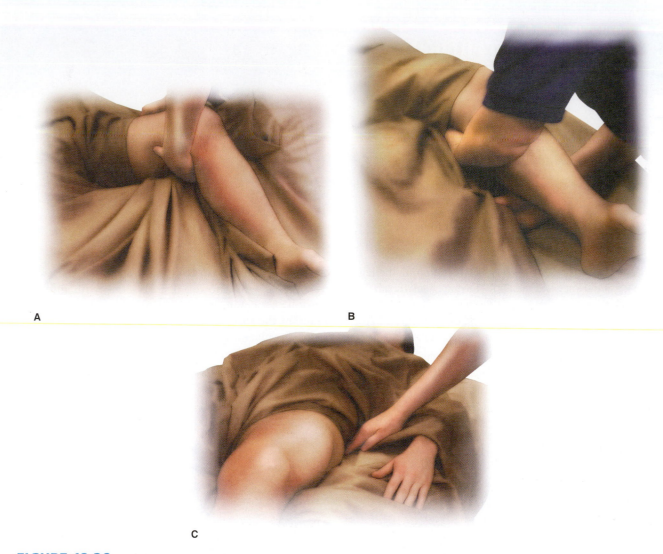

A

B

C

FIGURE 12.26

Draping for massage of leg in supine position. A. Lift the leg with one hand, and with the other hand pull the drape underneath the thigh. B. Pull the drape snugly around the thigh. C. Tuck top of drape under the hip.

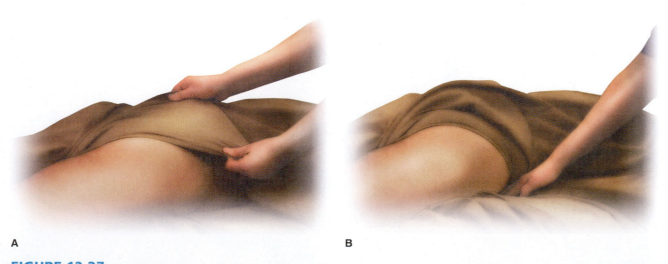

A

B

FIGURE 12.27

Draping for massage of leg in prone position. Pull the drape underneath the thigh. A. Uncover the buttocks muscles without exposing the gluteal cleft. B. Tuck the end of the drape under the hip.

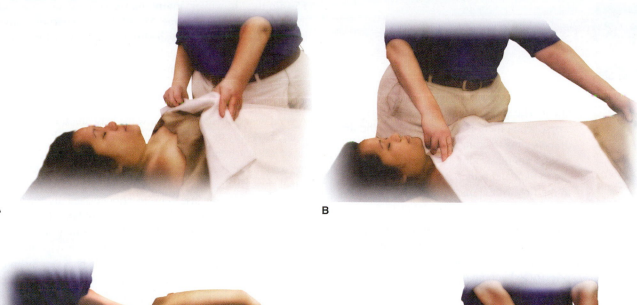

A

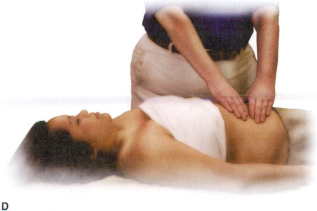

B

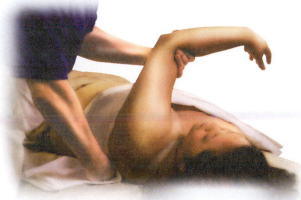

C

D

FIGURE 12.28

Draping for a woman's chest. A. Place a towel over the sheet on the upper chest. B. Hold the towel in place while you pull the sheet down to expose the abdomen. C. Tuck the towel securely at the sides. D. The towel remains in place while you massage the chest or abdomen.

Figure 12.28■ demonstrates proper draping for a woman's breasts.

Large towels may also be used for draping. The same general guidelines for modesty apply whatever type of drape is used.

In some situations, receivers do not remove their clothes and draping is unnecessary. For example, receivers usually remain clothed during pre- and postevent sports massage, chair massage, and some shiatsu and other energy-balancing sessions.

PRACTICAL APPLICATION

Practice draping for a recipient in different positions; for example, supine, prone, side-lying, and semireclining. Aim for skillful, secure, and effective draping.

1. Can you uncover and recover different parts of the body with ease?
2. Can you drape a woman properly for abdominal massage?
3. Do recipients feel that their modesty is preserved?

REALITY CHECK

LUTHER

LEE: I feel really awkward when I drape a client. The sheets seem bulky, and it is worse when there is also a blanket. And the drape seems to come loose a lot, especially when I am massaging the legs. I keep having to tuck and retuck, which is disruptive to the flow of the massage. What can I do to make draping easier?

LUTHER: Draping is an art in itself. It takes determination, practice, and the right draping materials to do the job smoothly. Make it a priority to become a draping expert early in your training, and good draping will come naturally after a while. First consider the size of your drape. If it is too large, it will hang over the sides of the table too much and will be difficult to handle. You can get sheets made specifically for massage tables or use standard twin-size sheets. Use light-weight blankets such as fleece to minimize bulk and consider cutting them to hang only about 8 inches over the sides and foot of the table. Don't rush through draping. Take time to tuck securely the first time. Through watching experienced massage therapists in person and on videos, you will see some of the draping tricks developed through the years. Practice and develop your own draping methods. Take pride in learning this skill as much as your massage techniques, and over time draping will not seem like such a chore.

MASSAGE APPLICATION GUIDELINES

There are a number of general performance elements to keep in mind when applying massage techniques. Important elements include the length of sessions, amount of lubricant to use, sequence of techniques and routines, specificity and direction, and pressure, rhythm, and pacing.

Length of Sessions

Session lengths vary depending on the goals of the massage and the setting in which it is given. For example, massage sessions for general health purposes typically last from 30–90 minutes. The most common length is 60 minutes. Seated massage given in the workplace may last from 15–20 minutes. Athletes may receive pre-event massage for 15 minutes, however, maintenance or recovery massage may last for 30–60 minutes. Massage that is part of a larger therapy session (e.g., physical therapy) may last for as little as 5–10 minutes. Guidelines for session lengths for different types of massage are suggested in later chapters.

Amount of Lubricant

A good general guideline is to use the least amount of lubricant needed to apply the massage techniques effectively. Too much oil or lotion prevents firm contact and causes slipping and sliding over the surface of the skin. Specific techniques applied to small areas, such as deep friction, use little or no lubricant. Too little lubricant can cause skin irritation, especially for people with fair or thin skin and those with a lot of body hair.

You may use more oil or lotion when warming an area with effleurage and petrissage techniques, and then wipe it off for more specific applications. Or you may finish an area by applying more lotion as a moisturizer if the recipient has dry skin.

The face is an area where little, if any, lubricant is usually needed. Also take care not to get oil or lotion in the client's hair when massaging the neck. Recipients can wear surgical or shower caps to keep lubricants out of their hair.

Lubricants absorb into the skin during massage, and the excess can be wiped off afterward. This avoids getting oily substances on the clothes. Some substances stain clothes, and certain scents may be difficult to wash out of fabrics. Rubbing the skin with a dry towel will remove most lotions and oils. Rubbing alcohol can be applied to the skin when more thorough cleaning is desired.

Sequence of Techniques and Routines

Different massage techniques are blended into sequences to create desired effects. Superficial warming techniques precede and follow deeper or more specific technique applications. Smooth transitions between techniques give a skillful feel to a session.

Routines are regular sequences of techniques performed in almost the same way every time. A routine may also include a standard sequence of body regions addressed during the session. For example, starting on the back with the recipient prone and ending on the head with the recipient supine. Practice Sequence 14–1 in Chapter 14, Full-Body Massage Sequence, on page 421, describes a full-body massage routine that can be used as a model for practice.

Experienced massage practitioners usually establish a routine way of approaching their massage sessions. They vary the routine depending on the needs and desires of the receiver. Routines are useful to establish a smooth pattern or flow for a session. They are also an effective way to learn new massage approaches. Several Practice Sequences or routines for different massage applications appear throughout the remaining chapters and can be viewed on your DVD.

Specificity and Direction

Many massage techniques are applied over large regions in sweeping movements. For example, the long, sliding strokes of effleurage are often used as a warming technique for large areas such as the back or the entire arm. And muscle groups are often kneaded and stretched, as opposed to individual muscles. This more general way of applying techniques is appropriate for effects such as warming an area, eliciting the relaxation response, relaxing muscle groups, or increasing general circulation. Transition and finishing techniques also usually cover larger areas.

There is greater specificity if techniques are focused on smaller areas or specific structures. For example, applying direct pressure with the thumb to a trigger point or deep transverse friction on a tendon are more specific applications. Working with specificity requires thorough knowledge of anatomical structures and good palpation skills.

The direction of technique application may be expressed in terms of general anatomical terminology (e.g., proximal, distal, medial, and lateral). An age-old dictum in massage is to apply deep effleurage to the limbs moving fluids from distal to proximal, or toward the heart. Lighter sliding movements using superficial pressure may be performed proximal to distal as when applying nerve strokes.

Direction also may be described in relation to a specific anatomical structure, for example, toward the muscle attachment. Or it could be said to be along the length of the muscle fibers as in stripping, or across the fibers as in cross-fiber friction. Massage approaches described in later chapters use the concepts of sequence, direction, and specificity to clarify their applications.

Pressure, Rhythm, and Pacing

Pressure, rhythm, and pacing describe different qualities of applying massage techniques. These qualities vary with the desired effect of the application of a single technique, a technique combination, or an entire session.

Pressure is related to the force used in applying techniques and to the degree of compaction of tissues that results.

The amount of pressure used in any one situation depends on the intended effect and on the tolerance or preference of the recipient. Generally speaking, when applying pressure to an area, it should start out light and then proceed to deeper pressure if desired. This allows tissues to warm up and become accustomed to the pressure. Tissues usually soften as pressure is applied gradually. Removing pressure slowly also allows tissues to adjust to the lightening of pressure over time. Pressure too light may cause tickling, while too deep too fast may elicit a tensing response. Either effect is undesirable during massage.

Rhythm refers to a recurring pattern of movement with a specific cadence, beat, or accent. The rhythm of massage may be described as smooth, regular, or in some cases, uneven. Rhythm is important for establishing the flow of a session. Working with specificity may slow or stop a regular rhythm, as when stopping to press a tender point. A smooth, flowing, regular rhythm tends to elicit the relaxation response. An uneven rhythm can be stimulating or sometimes distracting. A general rule is to avoid breaking contact with the skin once a session has begun, or breaking and resuming contact smoothly.

Playing music during massage sessions can help establish and keep a certain rhythm. Over time, massage practitioners tend to develop their own rhythm for working.

Pacing refers to the speed of the massage movements. Generally, a slower pace is more relaxing, while a faster pace is more stimulating. Relaxation massage tends to be slower, while pre-event sports massage is faster paced. Applying techniques too slowly and a lack of variation can actually seem boring to a recipient. Choose a pace that accomplishes the intended goals of the session.

The art of massage is the skillful blending of all of these performance elements. Massage practitioners apply techniques with these elements in mind to create healthy, satisfying experiences for their clients.

CHAPTER HIGHLIGHTS

- Good body mechanics minimize shoulder, neck, and back problems, as well as injuries to the arms and hands.
- Good hand mechanics minimize strain on the fingers, thumb, and wrist.
- Using a variety of techniques in a session helps minimize repeated strain on a particular joint or body area.
- Practitioners starting out on their careers must build strength and stamina to meet the physical stress on their bodies.
- Twenty hours of massage per week can be given safely by most practitioners; no more than 4–5 hours per day.
- Take 15- to 20-minute breaks between sessions, and at least a 30-minute break after three consecutive 1-hour sessions.
- Keep the hands and wrists in good alignment while applying massage techniques for minimal strain and injury; stack the joints of the thumb and wrist.
- Stack the joints so that the bones of the thumb and wrist line up and pressure passes in a straight line through the bones.
- Avoid pressure applied at an angle to or across the joint.
- Keep the wrist in a neutral position (i.e., neither flexed nor extended) as much as possible when applying massage techniques.
- To determine the correct table height for you, stand facing the table with your hands at your sides and adjust the legs so that your knuckles touch the tabletop.
- To keep proper back alignment during a massage session, bend the knees to lower your body, and avoid bending the back excessively or dropping the head.
- Use the bow and arrow stance when facing the head or foot of the table and the horse riding stance when facing the table directly.
  - Keep the back in upright alignment while using the legs to generate power.
- When sitting on a stool to give massage, sit on the edge of the seat with the feet flat on the floor.
- Body mechanics are adapted for applying massage with the client in a seated position.
  - With the recipient vertical, pressing into his or her back calls for more forward motion, rather than downward, which can be achieved by shifting your weight forward and pushing from the rear leg to generate power.
  - Massage of the arms and hands of a seated client requires lowering your body significantly to maintain good alignment.
- Positioning involves placing the receiver in a comfortable and safe position on the massage table; use bolsters, pillows, and rolled towels for positioning.
- Draping the body during massage serves to protect the receiver's modesty, provide clear professional boundaries, and keep the receiver warm; genitals and women's breasts are draped at all times.
- Massage sessions for general health purposes typically last from 30–90 minutes, with the most common length being 60 minutes.
- Use the least amount of lubricant needed to apply the massage techniques effectively and to prevent skin irritation.
- Massage routines are regular sequences of techniques performed in almost the same way every time.
- Superficial warming techniques precede and follow deep specific technique applications.
- The direction of technique application may be expressed in terms of general anatomical terminology (e.g., proximal, distal, medial, and lateral).
- Pressure, rhythm, and pacing describe different qualities of applying massage techniques.
  - Pressure is related to the force used in applying techniques and to the degree of compaction of tissues that results.
  - Rhythm refers to a recurring pattern of movement with a specific cadence, beat, or accent.
  - Pacing refers to the speed of the massage movements.
- The art of massage is the skillful blending of all application elements.
  - Application elements include the length of the session, the sequence of techniques, and the specificity and direction of applications.
  - The rhythm and pacing of massage sessions establish their flow.

EXAM REVIEW

Key Terms

Match the following key terms to their descriptions. For additional study, look up the key terms in the Interactive Glossary on page G-1 and note other terms that compare or contrast with them.

_____ 1. Body mechanics
_____ 2. Bow and arrow stance
_____ 3. Bracing
_____ 4. Draping
_____ 5. Hand mechanics
_____ 6. Horse riding stance
_____ 7. Neutral position
_____ 8. Positioning
_____ 9. Stacking the joints
_____ 10. Table skills
_____ 11. Tenting

a. Minimize strain on the fingers, thumb, and wrist
b. Neither flexed nor extended
c. Placing the receiver in a comfortable and safe position on the table
d. Overall alignment and use of the body while performing massage
e. Keeps clients from getting rolled up in the drape
f. Actions required to position and drape a client properly on a massage table
g. Avoids pressure applied at an angle to or across the joint
h. Forward-leaning stance used when facing the head or foot of the table
i. Tai chi side to side stance
j. Offering a counter-resistance to prevent the movement of the body in the opposite direction
k. Covering the body during massage

Memory Workout

To test your memory of the main concepts in this chapter, complete the following sentences by circling the most correct answer from the two choices provided.

1. The maximum number of massage hours per week that can be safely given by most massage therapists is (30) (20).
2. When joints are lined up so that pressure passes through them rather than across them, it is called (stacking) (extending) the joints.
3. When reinforcing one hand with the other during compression techniques, the top hand is placed over the (metacarpals) (wrist) of the other hand.
4. The wrist is kept in a (extended) (neutral) position as much as possible when applying massage techniques to prevent strain.
5. The (bow and arrow) (horse riding) stance is used when facing the massage table directly.
6. Actions required to position and drape a client properly on a massage table are called (table) (mechanical) skills.
7. Ask the client to turn over (away from) (toward) you when tenting to avoid getting wrapped up in the sheet.
8. Tilting the face cradle slightly (downward) (upward) opens the shoulder and neck region for better access.
9. A recurring pattern of movement with a specific cadence, beat, or accent is referred to as (pacing) (rhythm).
10. The (science) (art) of massage is the skillful blending of performance elements.

Test Prep

The following multiple-choice questions will help to prepare you for future school and professional exams.

1. Which of the following is *avoided* when applying direct pressure with the thumb?
   a. Stacking the joints
   b. Adduction
   c. Abduction
   d. Alignment with the wrist

2. In the bow and arrow stance, the body is lowered by:
   a. Widening the stance and bending the knees
   b. Narrowing the stance and straightening the knees
   c. Bending at the waist
   d. Bending the knees and the neck

3. Which of the following is the best option for lowering the body for massage applications to the forearms and hands of a person positioned in a massage chair?
   a. Kneeling on one or both knees
   b. Bending at the waist
   c. Taking an extra wide stance
   d. Bending forward and reaching down

4. Broad pressure to the upper trapezius muscle of a person positioned in a massage chair is best applied with your:
   a. Forearm
   b. Fingertips
   c. Palms
   d. Thumb

5. Where are bolsters typically placed to support a client in the supine position on a massage table?
   a. Neck and lower back
   b. Neck and knees
   c. Shoulders and feet
   d. Upper back and knees

6. When sitting on a stool to give massage, position yourself:
   a. Near the back with the ankles crossed
   b. Near the back with the feet flat on the floor
   c. Near the edge with the ankles crossed
   d. Near the edge with feet flat on the floor

7. When lying supine, if a client's arms do not lie flat on the table due to his or her structure or muscular tightness, support can be provided with a small bolster placed under the:
   a. Shoulder or upper arm
   b. Elbow
   c. Wrist or hand
   d. Fingertips

8. In the side-lying position, the upper leg is best supported so that it is:
   a. Perpendicular to the table
   b. Parallel to the table
   c. At a 45 degree angle to the table
   d. Touching the table

9. A good guideline for the use of lubricant for massage applications is:
   a. Use a lot of oil to provide maximum slide
   b. Use liberally for specific techniques such as deep friction
   c. Use no lubricant for people with a lot of body hair
   d. Use the least amount needed to apply techniques effectively

10. Pressure applied too deeply too fast during massage usually causes:
    a. Tension and pain
    b. Tickling
    c. Relaxation
    d. Sliding

Video Challenge

Watch the appropriate segment of the video on your DVD and then answer the following questions.

Body Mechanics, Table Skills, and Application Guidelines

Body Mechanics
1. What principles of good body mechanics did you see demonstrated in this video segment?

Positioning and Draping
2. How many bolsters were used, and where were they placed for the side-lying position?
3. How did the massage therapist's draping technique show a sense of respect for the client?

Comprehension Exercises

The following short answer questions test your knowledge and understanding of chapter topics and provide practice in written communication skills. Explain in two to four complete sentences.

1. Explain the principles of good hand mechanics for reducing stress on the thumb and wrist.

2. Describe the challenges to good practitioner body mechanics when applying massage techniques with the recipient in a vertical position.

3. Describe proper draping for abdominal massage for women.

For Greater Understanding

The following exercises are designed to take you from the realm of theory into the real world. They will help give you a deeper understanding of the subjects covered in this chapter. Action words are underlined to emphasize the variety of activities presented to address different learning styles and to encourage deeper thinking.

1. Make a video of yourself performing massage for about 10 minutes. Analyze your performance for good hand and wrist care, and general body mechanics. Get feedback from observers. Retape your performance, making corrections.

2. Observe someone giving a massage, and analyze the performance elements you see. Look at the technique sequence, direction, specificity, pressure, pacing, and rhythm. Explain how these elements put together in a specific application exemplify the art of massage.

3. Experiment with using different amounts of lubricant for a variety of massage applications. Notice how the skin in different areas of the body absorbs the oil or lotion, and what effect that has on different technique applications.

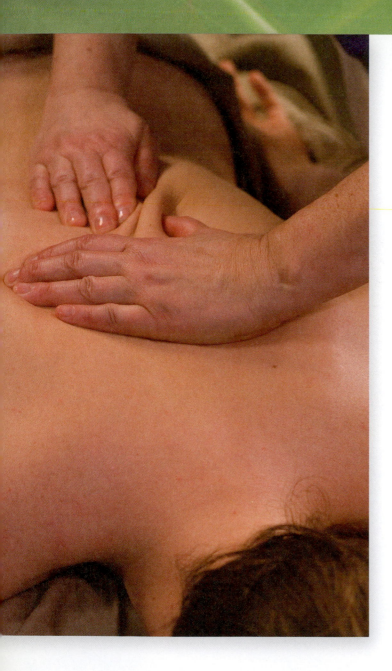

CHAPTER

13 Western Massage Techniques

 CHAPTER OUTLINE

Learning Outcomes

Key Terms

Western Massage Overview

Western Massage Techniques

Effleurage

Petrissage

Friction

Tapotement

Vibration

Touch without Movement

Overview of Joint Movements

Methods of Stretching

Safety

General Guidelines for Joint Movement Techniques

Regional Applications of Joint Movements

Chapter Highlights

Exam Review

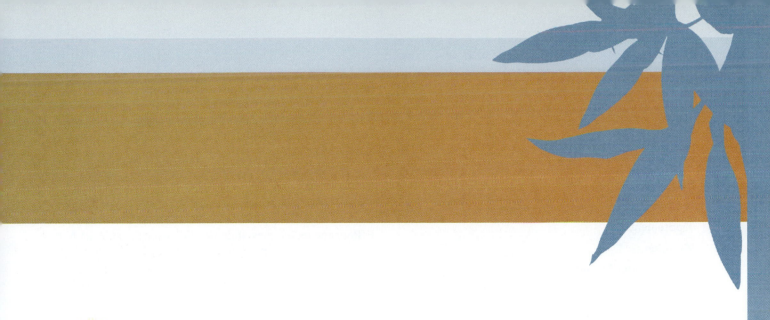

 ## LEARNING OUTCOMES

After studying this chapter, you will have information to:

1. Describe the seven Western massage technique categories.
2. Explain the effects of various massage techniques.
3. Apply massage technique variations for specific effects.
4. Use Western massage techniques effectively within a session.
5. Compare joint mobilizing techniques and stretching.

6. Describe four different stretching methods.
7. Explain the therapeutic benefits of joint movements.
8. Apply mobilizing techniques to different joints in the body.
9. Apply stretching techniques in different areas of the body.
10. Follow the general guidelines for applying joint movements.

 ## KEY TERMS

Assisted movements 397

Contract–relax–stretch
   (CRS) 399

Direct pressure 395

Effleurage 384

Friction 390

Mobilizing
   techniques 398

Petrissage 386

Resisted movements 397

Simple static stretch 399

Stretching 398

Tapotement 392

Touch without
   movement 395

Vibration 394

⊙ MASSAGE *in* ACTION

On your DVD, explore:

- Introduction
- Effleurage
- Petrissage
- Friction
- Tapotement
- Vibration
- Touch without Movement
- Joint Movements

WESTERN MASSAGE OVERVIEW

Western massage is the basis of most massage therapy performed in North America and Europe today. It is the most common form of massage found in spas, health clubs, and private practice. It is the foundation for therapeutic applications within the professions of massage therapy, physical therapy, athletic training, and nursing.

Today's Western massage began taking form in the nineteenth century in northern Europe. It is the legacy of people such as Ling (Swedish movements), Mezger (classic massage), Kellogg (massage in natural healing), McMillan (massage in physical therapy), and many others. Swedish massage is a form of Western massage popular for over 100 years. A more detailed view of the history of Western massage can be found in Chapter 2, The History of Massage as a Vocation, on page 28.

The effects, benefits, and indications for Western massage are understood in terms of Western concepts of anatomy and physiology and Western notions of health and disease. The techniques of Western massage are recognized as valuable for improving circulation of blood and lymph, relaxing muscles, improving joint mobility, inducing general relaxation, and promoting healthy skin. See Chapter 7, Effects of Massage, on page 252 and Chapter 8, Clinical Applications of Massage, on page 284 for a more thorough discussion of massage and Western science.

WESTERN MASSAGE TECHNIQUES

Western massage techniques fall into seven general categories: effleurage, petrissage, friction, tapotement, vibration, touch without movement, and joint movements. Within each category there are an endless number of variations. The techniques presented in this text represent only some of the many possibilities. The seven categories of Western massage are useful for thinking about how techniques are performed, their physiological effects, and common uses.

When practicing massage techniques and joint movements, always take into consideration endangerment sites, contraindications, and cautions, as described in Chapter 9, Endangerment Sites, Contraindications, and Cautions, on page 296. Use good hand and body mechanics, as presented in Chapter 12, Body Mechanics, Skills, and Application Guidelines, on page 362.

EFFLEURAGE

Effleurage techniques slide or glide over the skin with a smooth, continuous motion. Pressure may be light to moderate, as when applying oil or warming an area, or may be deep, as when facilitating venous return in heavily muscled areas. Experienced practitioners can perform effleurage in many different ways to suit the body area and to evoke specific effects.

Effleurage is perhaps the most versatile and frequently used Western massage technique. Effleurage is often used to begin a session, especially when oil or lotion is applied. It accustoms the receiver to the touch of the practitioner. It serves as a connecting or transition technique. Effleurage can provide a break from more specific techniques. It may also be applied to move gracefully from one area to another, to conclude work on an area, or to end the session.

While performing effleurage, a practitioner skilled in palpation can assess the general condition of the soft tissues and the firmness and shape of the musculature. Sensitive fingers may find areas of tension or holding. In some cases where there is pain, effleurage may be the only technique employed.

Effleurage can affect the recipient's body and mind in a variety of ways. The qualities of pressure, pacing, and rhythm may be varied for different effects. For example, when effleurage is performed with moderate pressure slowly and smoothly on the back, it may stimulate the parasympathetic nervous system and evoke the relaxation response. It enhances venous return in the limbs when performed with moderate to deep pressure moving distal to proximal. Deep effleurage may also provide a passive stretch to a muscle group.

Variations of Effleurage

Basic sliding effleurage is performed with the palms and fingers of the hands, thumbs, fists, or forearms. When using the palms and fingers, mold the hands to the surface of the body. This provides full contact, as shown in basic effleurage of the leg in Figure 13.1■. The thumbs may be used in small places such as between the metatarsals of the foot, as in Figure 13.2■. More pressure may be applied using the forearms or fists in broad places such as the back and hamstrings, as seen in Figure 13.3■.

Stripping is a type of basic sliding effleurage performed with deep pressure along the length of the muscle fibers, typically done with the thumb. See Figure 13.4■. It is commonly performed on the long muscles in the arms and legs, and on the cervical muscles. Stripping is specific to a particular muscle and usually follows the muscle to its site of attachment.

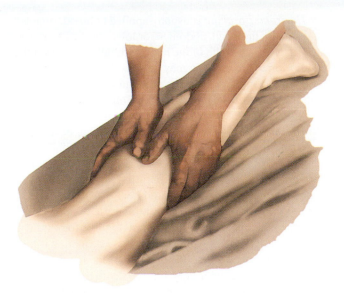

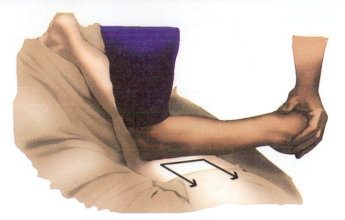

FIGURE 13.3

Basic sliding effleurage using the forearm applies broad, deep pressure to an area.

FIGURE 13.1

Basic sliding effleurage using the palms of the hands provides full contact with the leg.

If the muscle is wider than the thumb, stripping is performed in parallel lines to cover the entire muscle. Stripping separates and lengthens muscle fibers. It is a useful technique to apply after direct pressure to trigger points.

Shingles effleurage refers to alternate stroking, first one hand then the other in continuous motion, with the strokes overlaying each other like shingles on a roof. One hand always remains in contact with the receiver as the other hand

is lifted, which gives the feeling of unbroken contact. Shingles effleurage is commonly applied to the back with hands parallel to the spine and to the direction of movement as shown in Figure 13.5■. This is a good warming technique for the paraspinal muscles and is generally relaxing.

Bilateral tree stroking traces a pattern reminiscent of branches growing out from both sides of the trunk of a tree. It is usually performed on the back, starting with the hands on either side of the spine and moving laterally to and around the sides of the torso. This movement is repeated as you progress to cover the entire back. It may be performed standing at the head and progressing from the shoulders toward the hips, or moving from the hips to the shoulders. See Figure 13.6■.

Three-count stroking of the trapezius is applied in three movements, alternating hands with each movement. Count 1 begins at the origin of the lower trapezius and moves toward its insertion in the shoulder. Count 2 begins just as the first stroke concludes, moving from the origin of the middle trapezius toward its insertion. As soon as the first hand has completed its slide over the lower trapezius, it lifts and crosses over to the origin of the upper trapezius to begin

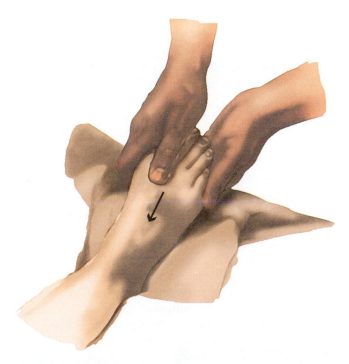

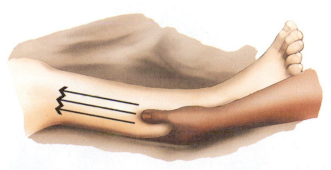

FIGURE 13.4

Stripping is performed with deep pressure along the length of a muscle to its attachment. Parallel strips are applied to cover the entire muscle width.

FIGURE 13.2

Basic sliding effleurage using the thumb gets into the small spaces between the metatarsals of the foot.

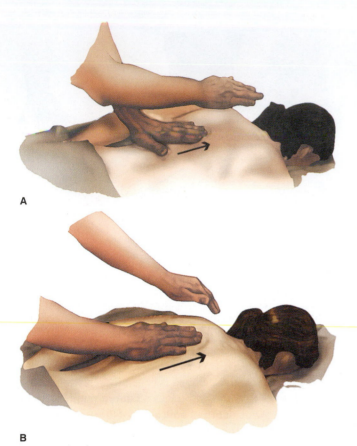

A

B

FIGURE 13.5

Shingles effleurage with hands parallel to the spine and to the direction of movement.

count 3. Count 3 moves laterally to the insertion to complete the sequence. Figure 13.7■ shows how the stroke is performed with the practitioner standing on the opposite side. The entire three-count sequence is repeated several times. The technique is timed so that the receiver feels unbroken contact.

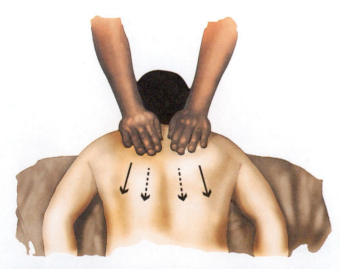

FIGURE 13.6

Bilateral tree stroking across the back.

Horizontal stroking is usually applied to broad, rounded areas such as the thigh, abdomen, or lower back. The movement is across the width of the body part, rather than over the length. Horizontal stroking may be considered a hybrid form of effleurage and petrissage because, in addition to sliding, there may be a lifting and pressing motion. Some call this technique *wringing,* as in wringing out a towel.

To perform horizontal stroking on the lower back, stand facing the side of the receiver near the waist. Place your hands lightly on the receiver's back, one hand on each side with the fingers of both hands pointing away from you, as shown in Figure 13.8■. Slide both hands toward the spine using firm pressure, and then continue the movement all the way to the other side. One hand will move forward and one hand backward, crossing at the spine. The motion is then reversed without changing the position of the hands.

Nerve strokes are a very light effleurage or brushing technique applied repeatedly in one direction. The fingertips gently brush the skin or the top of the drape. Nerve strokes are often used when finishing a section of the body or when ending a session. A few seconds of nerve strokes are usually enough to create a relaxing effect.

Knuckling effleurage is a variation in which the pressure is first applied with the back of the fingers in a loose fist, gradually turning the fist over as it slides over the skin, and finishing with the palm of the hand. Pressure starts lightly, becomes stronger, and then decreases again towards the end. See Figure 13.9■.

PETRISSAGE

Petrissage techniques lift, wring, or squeeze soft tissues in a kneading motion, or press or roll the tissues under or between the hands. Petrissage may be performed with one or two hands, depending on the size of the muscle or muscle group. There is minimal sliding over the skin as the tissues are lifted or pressed. The motions of petrissage serve to "milk" a muscle of accumulated metabolites (waste products), increase local circulation, and assist venous return. Petrissage may also help separate muscle fibers and evoke muscular relaxation.

Before performing petrissage, prepare and warm the area with effleurage. Use only a small amount of oil or lotion when warming up the area, since too much lubricant will make it difficult to grasp the tissues during petrissage. If you are working without lubricant, light compressions may be used to warm the area.

Take care to avoid pinching or bruising the tissues, and do not work too long in one area. Adjust the amount of pressure used to match the condition of the tissues, the recipient's preferences, and the area being massaged.

Variations of Petrissage

Basic two-handed kneading is performed by lifting, squeezing, and then releasing soft tissues with hands alternating in a rhythmical motion. In basic kneading, tissues are lifted with

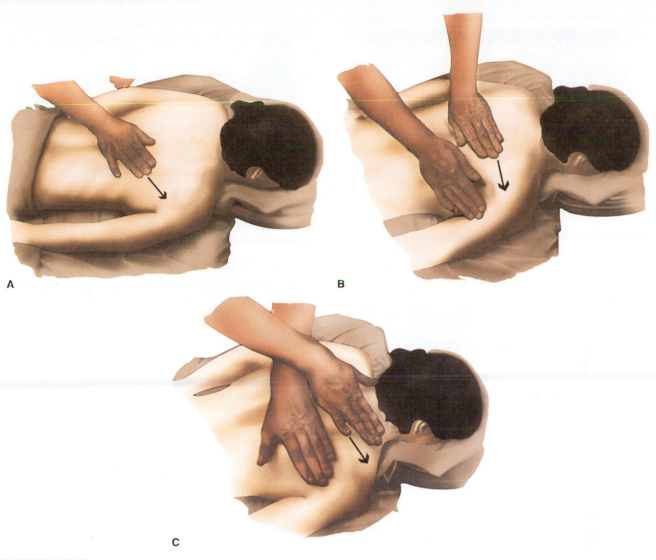

FIGURE 13.7

Three-count stroking of the trapezius. A. Count 1: lower trapezius. B. Count 2: middle trapezius. C. Count 3: upper trapezius.

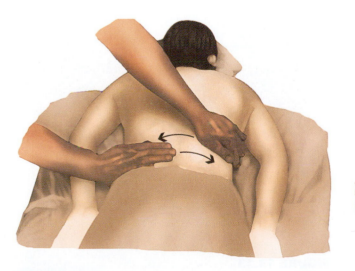

FIGURE 13.8

Horizontal stroking across the lower back.

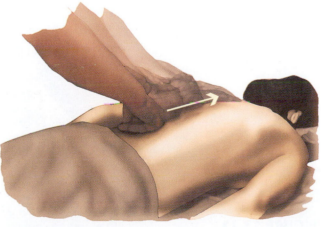

FIGURE 13.9

Knuckling effleurage (knuckle to palm) performed on the back.

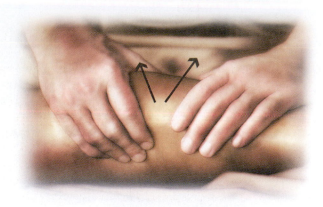

FIGURE 13.10

Basic two-handed kneading. Tissues are lifted with the whole hand in firm contact.

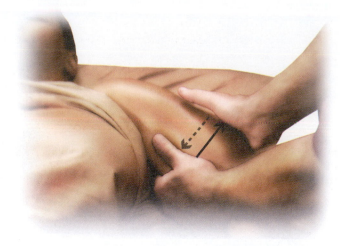

FIGURE 13.12

Alternating one-handed kneading. Alternate lifting and squeezing biceps and triceps in an even rhythm.

the whole hand in firm contact as shown in Figure 13.10■, rather than with just the fingertips. The movement is a lifting away from the underlying bone. Two-handed kneading works well on the larger muscles of the arms, shoulders, and legs.

One-handed kneading may be used on smaller areas, for example, on the arms. Place your hand around the part to be kneaded and pick up the muscle mass using your whole hand. The kneading movement may be described as circular—grasping the tissues on the up motion and relaxing the hand on the down motion without losing contact. As with two-handed kneading, use a slow and regular rhythm. Progression to a new position should follow three or four repetitions in the same place. In general, the movements should be performed distal to proximal on the limbs, and effleurage may be interspersed with petrissage or may follow it, to enhance venous return. The biceps is a good place to practice one-hand kneading, as shown in Figure 13.11■.

Alternating one-handed kneading may be used to work flexors and extensors at the same time. For example, on the upper arm, grasp the biceps with one hand and the triceps with the other hand. Alternate lifting and squeezing first the biceps and then the triceps using an even rhythm. See Figure 13.12■.

Circular two-handed petrissage is a skin lifting technique best performed on broad, flat areas such as the back. Warm the area first using deep effleurage. To practice this technique on the back, stand at the side of the recipient, and place your hands side by side on the skin. Fingers point in the same direction. The hands shape themselves to the contours of the back for firm contact. Move the hands in clockwise circles, timed so that when the hands pass each other, the soft tissues are picked up and pressed between the hands. Pick up tissues between the hands (not with the hands) as they pass each other, as shown in Figure 13.13■. After about

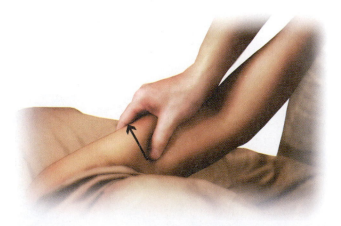

FIGURE 13.11

One-handed kneading. Tissues are lifted with the whole hand in firm contact.

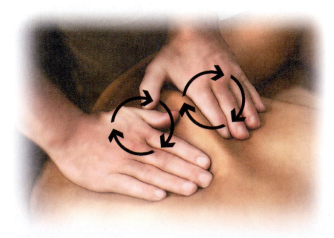

FIGURE 13.13

Circular two-handed petrissage. Tissues are picked up between the hands as they pass each other.

three repetitions of this technique in one place, slide the hands to the next area and repeat. A variation of circular petrissage can be performed on the forehead using the thumbs (see Figure 14.74 on page 441).

Alternating fingers-to-thumb petrissage is another lifting and pressing technique in which the soft tissues are pressed between the thumb of one hand and the first two fingers of the other hand. The hands alternate back and forth with an even rhythm. The fingers of one hand lift and move the tissues, pressing them against the opposite thumb. At the same time, the thumb is moving toward, and pressing the tissues against, the fingers of the opposite hand. Both skin and muscle tissue are affected. See Figure 13.14■. This same motion is repeated, alternating hands.

Skin lifting is a technique in which superficial tissues are picked up between the thumb and the first two fingers and gently pulled away from the deeper tissues. In *skin rolling*, the superficial tissues are pulled away, and then the thumbs push forward, lifting the tissues in a smooth, continuous rolling motion. Skin rolling stretches the underlying fascia and increases superficial circulation. Skin lifting and rolling are considered basic myofascial massage techniques (for more information about myofascial massage, see page 520 in Chapter 18, Contemporary Massage and Bodywork). These techniques are often performed on the back, but may be applied to almost any part of the body. Skin lifting is demonstrated in Figure 13.15■.

In *compression* techniques, tissues are pressed or rolled against underlying tissues and bone in rhythmic repetition. The effects are similar to other petrissage techniques as the tissues are compressed under the hands repeatedly. Figure 13.16■ shows compression using the palm of one hand, while the other hand provides additional force from above. Note that the heel of the top hand is placed so that it does not put pressure on the wrist of the bottom hand. Apply compressing force by leaning into the technique with your body weight. The force comes from

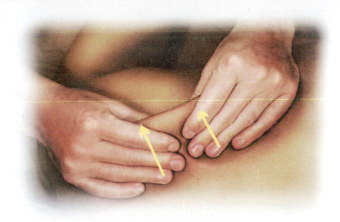

FIGURE 13.15

Skin lifting. Superficial tissues are picked up and gently pulled away from deeper tissues.

the legs through the torso and shoulders and into the arms and palms of the hands. Review the principles of good hand and body mechanics for compression in Chapter 12, Body Mechanics, Table Skills, and Application Guidelines, on page 363. A useful variation for massage of the buttocks is compression applied with a fist (see Figure 12.3C on page 364.

Rolling is a form of petrissage performed on the limbs. Grasp the limb lightly on opposite sides between the palms of the hands. Compress the muscles of the limb against each other as the hands press in and move back and forth. Rolling the limbs progresses from proximal to distal. In addition to compressing tissues, rolling causes movement in the shoulder or hip joint. The larger your hands are in proportion to the limb, the easier rolling is to perform. Rolling is an effective technique when the client's arm is hanging at the side, as in seated massage.

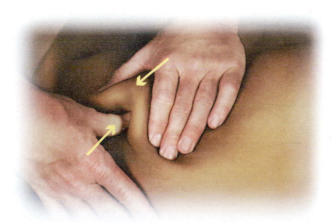

FIGURE 13.14

Fingers-to-thumb petrissage. The soft tissues are pressed between the thumb of one hand and the fingers of the other hand.

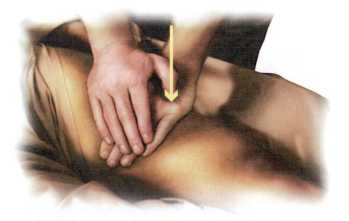

FIGURE 13.16

Compression using reinforced palm. The heel of the top hand is placed to avoid putting pressure on the wrist of the bottom hand.

FRICTION

Friction is performed by rubbing one surface over another repeatedly. For example, the hand is used to rub the skin for superficial warming, as in a traditional rubdown. The resistance to the motion provided by the surfaces creates heat and stimulates the skin.

Friction may also be created between the skin and deeper tissues. In deep friction, the practitioner's fingers do not move over the skin, but instead move the skin over the tissues underneath. Deep friction addresses one small area at a time and adds specificity to the massage by affecting specific structures, such as a particular section of a muscle or tendon. Cross-fiber, parallel, and circular friction are the basic forms of deep friction.

Variations of Friction

In *superficial warming friction,* the palm or some other part of the practitioner's hand is rubbed briskly over the skin. This generates heat and stimulates superficial circulation. Variations of warming friction use different parts of the hands to create the friction. Greater pressure may be applied to affect deeper tissues such as when using the knuckles (Figure 13.17■) and in *sawing,* also called *ulnar friction* (Figure 13.18■). Warming friction is best done "dry" or with little lubricant, since oil or lotion reduces the amount of resistance between the two surfaces and thus reduces the amount of friction. It can be applied over clothing, for example, during sports massage or seated massage.

Deep friction is used to create movement between the deeper tissues and helps keep them from adhering to one another. Tissues of the musculoskeletal system are designed for smooth and efficient movement and slide over each other without sticking. With lack of movement, stress, or trauma to an area, muscle fibers may stick together or tendons stick to tissues with which they come in contact. Deep friction can help keep tissues separated and functioning smoothly.

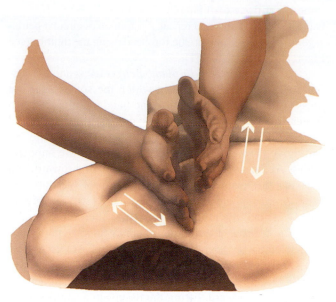

FIGURE 13.18

Warming friction created with a sawing motion (i.e., ulnar friction). The ulnar sides of the hands move back and forth on the skin to create friction in the area to be warmed.

Deep friction may also be used to create movement in tissues around joints such as the ankle and knee, reach into small spaces such as the suboccipital region, or be used in areas that lack muscle bulk such as on the head. Areas that don't lend themselves well to petrissage (e.g., at tendonous attachments) may be massaged with deep friction. See Figure 13.19■.

Deep friction may be performed in a cross-fiber, parallel, or circular motion. *Cross-fiber friction* refers to deep friction applied across the direction of the fibers, while *parallel friction* is applied in the same direction as the fibers. *Circular friction* is performed using circular movements, which move the underlying tissues in many directions. See Figure 6.48 on page 158 to review variations in muscle fiber directions. Figure 13.20■ shows cross-fiber friction being applied to the paraspinal muscles.

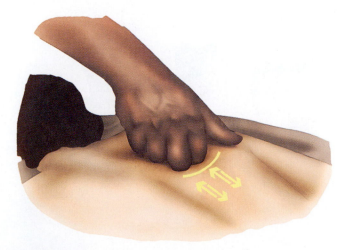

FIGURE 13.17

Warming friction using the knuckles. The first two knuckles move back and forth on the skin to create friction in the area to be warmed.

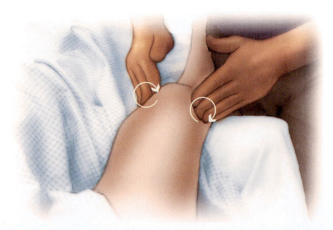

FIGURE 13.19

Circular friction around the knee with the fingertips.

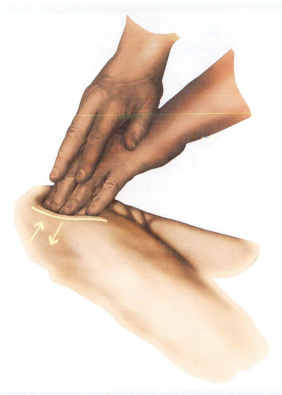

FIGURE 13.20

Cross-fiber friction to the paraspinal muscles. Friction is created by moving the more superficial muscle and connective tissues over the deeper tissues underneath.

Deep friction is performed with the tips of the fingers, the thumb, or the heel of the hand, depending on the size of the surface to be covered. For example, small tendons in places such as the wrist or around the ankle may be frictioned with the fingertips. In Figure 13.21■, circular friction is applied with the heel of the hand to free up the broad iliotibial band on the side of the leg.

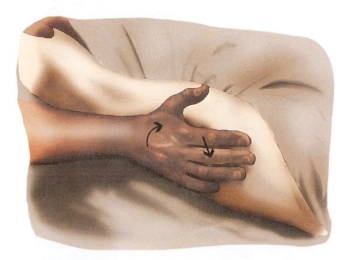

FIGURE 13.21

Circular friction to the broad iliotibial band. The heel of the hand is used to create friction between the skin and the underlying tendon, and between the tendon and underlying muscles.

Before deep friction is applied, warm the area thoroughly using effleurage and petrissage. The lubricant used in the warming-up phase may have to be wiped off before performing friction, to allow the hands to move the skin without sliding over it. Deep friction is a three-dimensional technique. Practitioners must be keenly aware of the depth at which they are working and the depth of the tissues they wish to affect. If the tissues are just beneath the skin, then lighter pressure may be effective. If the tissues are deep or under other tissues, then you must "work through" the more superficial tissues. It is helpful to visualize the tissues in cross-section and to develop palpation skills that will allow you to feel the layers of tissue. Care must be taken in applying deep pressure. Do not try to "muscle through" more superficial tissues, but instead soften them layer by layer. This process takes patience and sensitivity.

Friction Used in Rehabilitation

Deep transverse friction or *Cyriax friction* is a specific type of cross-fiber friction that is applied directly to the site of a lesion. It is used to facilitate healthy scar formation at an injury site. The mechanical action across tissues causes broadening and separation of fibers. Cyriax friction is "specifically intended to disrupt and break down existing and forming adhesions in muscles, tendons and ligaments using compression and motion" (Rattray and Ludwig 2000, p. 41). Deep transverse friction encourages a more parallel fiber arrangement of scar tissue and fewer cross-connections that limit movement. See Figure 13.22■.

Deep transverse friction is reserved for subacute and chronic musculoskeletal injuries, (e.g., repetitive strain injuries) and in the remodeling stage of tissue healing. It is contraindicated for acute injuries in the inflammatory and regeneration stages.

James Cyriax popularized the use of deep transverse friction in injury rehabilitation. He emphasized that the fingers and skin move together and that the amount of pressure used is less important than the friction created. The tissue must be held somewhat taut, and the friction must be over the exact site of the lesion. After warming the tissues thoroughly, friction is

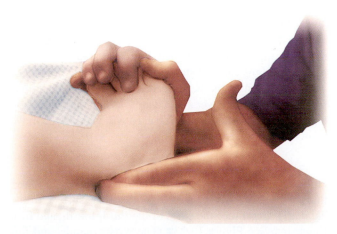

FIGURE 13.22

Deep transverse friction (i.e., Cyriax friction) on an ankle ligament.

applied for 1–5 minutes depending on the tolerance of the recipient and the tissue condition. (Cyriax and Cyriax 1993)

In addition to promoting healthy scar formation, circular and cross-fiber friction around an injury site can help keep normal tissues from adhering to the scarred area. Such adhering of tissues may cause chronic pain or inflammation. This is especially important where there is a large wound, such as after surgery.

TAPOTEMENT

Tapotement consists of a series of brisk percussive movements following each other in rapid, alternating fashion. Tapotement, also called *percussion,* has a stimulating effect and is pleasant to receive if performed skillfully. The most common forms of tapotement are hacking, rapping, cupping, clapping, slapping, tapping, and pincement.

The movement of tapotement is light, rapid, and rhythmic. The hands should "bounce off" the surface as they make contact, lightening the impact. The recipients should not feel like they are taking a beating, but should feel pleasantly stimulated.

The percussive sound itself can be pleasing and can add to the therapeutic effect. Different hand positions create different sounds, and different parts of the body sound different when struck. Quacking and squishes, described in the next section, are nontraditional forms of tapotement that make distinctive, interesting sounds.

Tapotement takes a certain rhythmic ability and much practice to master. The effort to learn it, though, is well worthwhile for the diversity it can bring to your work. Experiment with varying rhythms and hand positions for different effects.

Tapotement is often used in finishing either a section of the body, a side of the body, or the session itself. Because it can be stimulating if received for a short period of time, tapotement is useful in situations in which the receiver must be alert when leaving the session. For example, it may be used if the receiver must drive directly after a session or go back to work. Athletes benefit from tapotement before a competition. Some people simply like the tingling and alive feeling that tapotement can provide.

While performing tapotement, the amount of force used and the degree of stiffness of the hands depends on the area receiving the technique. Heavily muscular areas such as the back and thighs can withstand more force, while more delicate areas such as the head need a light touch. When performing tapotement over a broad area, as in ending a session on the back, the amount of force used will vary as you move from one section to another.

Variations of Tapotement

Hacking is performed with the hands facing each other, thumbs up. The striking surface is the ulnar surface of the hand and sometimes the sides of the third, fourth, and fifth fingertips. See Figure 13.23■. The wrists, hands, and fingers should be held loosely during the rapid percussion movement. Alternate hitting with the left and right hands.

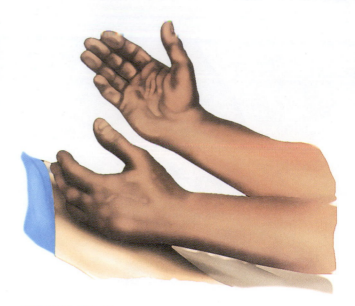

FIGURE 13.23

Hacking. Tapotement performed with the ulnar side of relaxed hands.

Performed correctly, the effect of hacking is one of pleasant stinging and stimulation.

A similar movement, called *rapping,* may be performed using lightly closed and loosely held fists. The fists may be held palms down as in rapping on a door as shown in Figure 13.24■. In side-rapping (sometimes called *beating*), the striking surface is the ulnar side of the fist. Keep the force of the blows light and "rebounding" in effect rather than jarring.

Cupping and *clapping* are applied with the same rhythmic, rapidly alternating force. For both techniques, cup the hand so that the thumb and fingers are slightly flexed and the palmar surface contracted. The thumb is held tightly

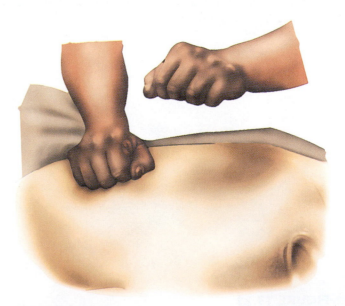

FIGURE 13.24

Rapping. Tapotement performed with the knuckles of a loosely closed fist, as if rapping lightly on a door.

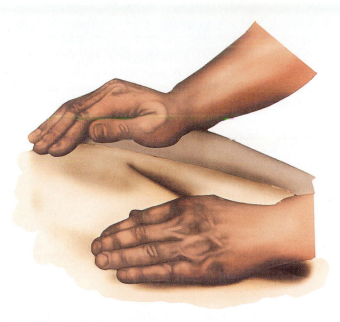

FIGURE 13.25

Cupping. Tapotement performed with the outside rim of a cupped hand.

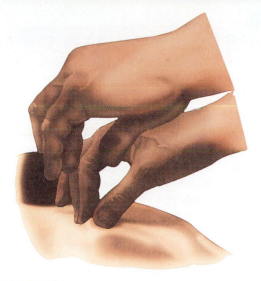

FIGURE 13.27

Pincement. Tapotement performed by gently picking up superficial tissues between the thumb and the first two fingers with a light rapid movement.

against the first finger. For cupping, strike the body surface with the outside rim of the cupped hand, keeping the palm contracted, as shown in Figure 13.25■. There will be a hollow sound. A slight vacuum is created with each blow, which some believe may loosen broad, flat areas of scar tissue or fascial adhesions. Cupping is also used for loosening congestion in the respiratory system.

Let the palm contact the body surface for *clapping*. This produces a less hollow sound and provides a broader contact surface. *Slapping* is performed with an open hand, the fingers held lightly together. Strike gently and briskly with the palmar surface of the fingers, rather than with the whole hand.

Tapping is done with the ends of the fingers. Sharp, light taps are applied with the padding of the fingers. See Figure 13.26■. *Pincement* is a rapid, gentle movement in which superficial tissues are picked up between the thumb and the first two fingers. It might be described as "plucking."

A rhythm is established alternating left and right hands. See Figure 13.27■.

Quacking is performed with the palms together and fingers loosely apart. The striking surface is the lateral edges of the tips of the fourth and fifth (little) fingers, as shown in Figure 13.28■. As the fingers hit the bony surface, they come together, making a quacking sound. This

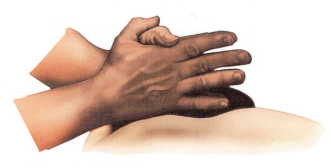

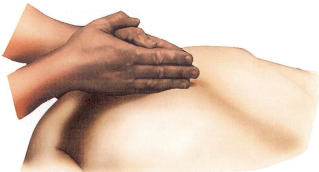

FIGURE 13.28

Quacking. Tapotement performed with the hands together and fingers loosely apart. Fingers come together as the little finger strikes, making a "quacking" sound.

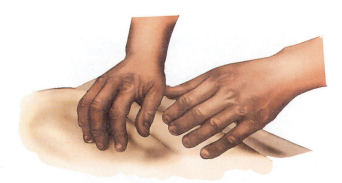

FIGURE 13.26

Tapping. Tapotement performed with the fingertips of a relaxed hand.

technique is sometimes called the *Thai chop* since it is also used in the traditional massage of Thailand.

Squishes are applied with the hands loosely folded, making an air pocket between the palms. The striking surface is the back of one of the hands. As the back of the hand hits, the palms push out the air between them, creating a "squishing" sound.

VIBRATION

Vibration may be described as an oscillating, quivering, or trembling motion, or movement back and forth or up and down performed quickly and repeatedly. The vibration may be fine and applied to a small area with the fingertips. Or it may be coarse and involve shaking a muscle belly back and forth.

Vibration over the abdomen is sometimes used to stimulate the organs of digestion and elimination. Coarse vibration, in the form of jostling, may be used to help a recipient become aware of holding tension, to bring greater circulation

to a muscle, and to help it relax. Fine vibration techniques impart an oscillating motion to the soft tissues and have a stimulating effect. They may also numb or relax specific muscles.

Electric vibrators may be used to impart fine vibration to tense muscles. The motion of vibration can be sustained for a longer period of time with a machine than if performed by hand. There are many types of handheld electric vibrators. Some impart a coarser vibration, others a finer oscillation. One type of vibrator straps to the back of the hand and causes vibration in the fingers. This allows the practitioner to stay in direct contact with the receiver and perform another technique such as light effleurage or friction. A standard handheld vibrator is shown in Figure 13.29■. A still finer vibration may be created by sound waves. There are devices that impart a lower frequency wave than ultrasound and are within the scope of practice of most practitioners.

Variations of Vibration

A *deep vibration* or trembling motion is imparted through the fingertips, but generated by the forearm. To practice deep vibration, place one hand on a muscle with the fingertips slightly apart. The trembling movement comes from the whole forearm, through the elbow, and the wrist and finger joints are kept in a fixed position. The elbow should be slightly flexed. This vibrating motion should be more in and out than side to side. The fingers remain in contact with the same spot during the vibration and are then lifted off the skin and placed on a new spot. Heavy pressure should be avoided. Deep vibration on the abdomen is shown in Figure 13.30■.

Light effleurage with vibration may be used for a soothing effect. While performing a light effleurage movement, add a slight vibration back and forth with the fingertips. Pressure can be so light that there is slight contact between the hand and the skin. It is a light, brushing movement. In cases of hypersensitive nerves, this technique has been credited with having a soothing effect.

Shaking is a coarse form of vibration that can assist muscular relaxation. For example, a muscle such as the biceps or gastrocnemius may be grasped with one hand and shaken

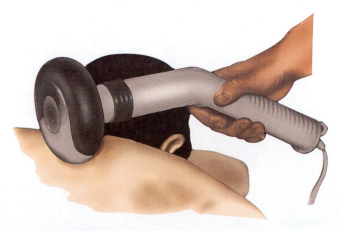

FIGURE 13.29

Fine vibration applied with a handheld electric vibrator.

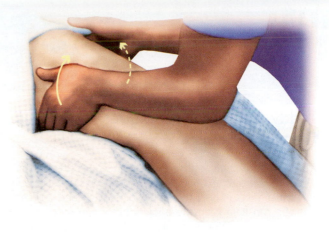

FIGURE 13.32

Jostling. A form of coarse vibration that includes mobilizing joints.

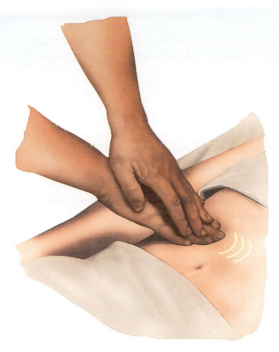

FIGURE 13.30

Deep vibration applied with fingertips to the abdomen.

gently back and forth. Figure 13.31■ shows shaking of the muscles of the leg.

In *jostling* the upper leg, two hands are used, one on each side of the leg. In this case, the muscle movement is back and forth from hand to hand, as shown in Figure 13.32■. It is helpful at times to jostle the entire limb gently to mobilize the surrounding joints and encourage relaxation and "letting go" of the whole area.

TOUCH WITHOUT MOVEMENT

Touch without movement is a unique massage technique category. It is defined by touch with the hands, but without any visible movement. Touch without movement is not casual or social touch, but is skilled touch with intention. Kellogg observes that this is not ordinary touch, but "touch applied with intelligence, with control, with a purpose; and simple as it is, is capable of producing decided physiological effects" (1895, p. 52).

Passive Touch

Passive touch is simply laying the fingers, one hand, or both hands lightly on the body. Passive touch may impart heat to an area, have a calming influence on the nervous system, or as some believe, help balance energy. Passive touch is often used to begin or end a session, or before the client turns over during a session. It is used effectively for its calming effects when applied to the feet or to the head, as shown in Figures 13.33■ and 13.34■.

Direct Pressure

Direct pressure, also called *direct static pressure,* may be applied with a thumb, finger, knuckle, or elbow. Tissues are compressed using light to heavy pressure. Once tissues are compressed, the technique is held for 5–30 seconds, depending on the intent. There is no movement after the initial compression.

Although this text categorizes direct pressure as touch without movement, it might also be considered *static friction,* or a form of compression. *Ischemic compression,* a form of direct pressure applied with enough force to cause blanching, causes vasodilation upon release of pressure, thus increasing local circulation. Ischemic compression is used to treat trigger points as described in Chapter 18, Contemporary Massage and Bodywork, on page 527.

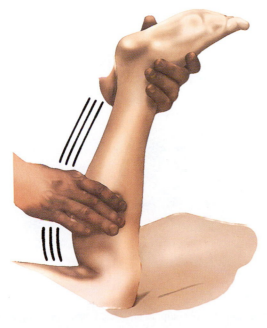

FIGURE 13.31

Shaking. A form of coarse vibration to a muscle or muscle group.

CASE FOR STUDY

Teddy Chooses Techniques to Address George's Goals

Teddy's client, George, wants a massage to reduce stress, enhance general circulation, and address occasional constipation. George has had stiffness in his arm and leg joints lately and wonders if massage can help keep those joints loose and moving freely. George also enjoys the mental alertness he feels after massage.

Question:

What massage techniques might Teddy incorporate into the massage session to meet George's goals?

Things to consider:

● Which technique variations directly address each of George's goals for his massage?

● When in the session might Teddy address each goal?
● Are some techniques more appropriate to apply at the beginning of the session? At the end? Somewhere in the middle?

Write a brief description of the techniques Teddy can include in George's massage session, and when they might be most effectively applied.

_____

_____

_____

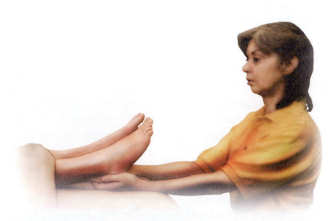

FIGURE 13.33

Passive touch by holding the head lightly.

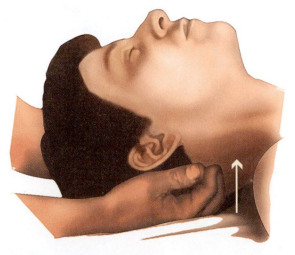

FIGURE 13.34

Passive touch by holding the feet lightly.

Apply pressure slowly and carefully to avoid bruising or damaging tissues. Direct pressure is often preceded by warming the area with effleurage or rhythmic compressions and followed with effleurage to "smooth out" the area or transition to another place. Figures 13.35■ and 13.36■ show two different uses for direct pressure.

Direct static pressure to various points on the body is known to relieve pain, diminish congestion, and help muscles relax. Theories about how it works have evolved over

FIGURE 13.35

Direct pressure to suboccipital muscles. Fingers press up into the cervical muscle attachments along the occipital ridge.

PRACTICAL APPLICATION

Verbally describe Western massage technique variations as you perform them. Explain to the recipient or to an observer what you are doing and why.

1. How are you moving your hands on the receiver's body?
2. How do you describe the manipulation of soft tissues?
3. What effects are you having as you apply different techniques?

CRITICAL THINKING

Think about the different categories of Western massage techniques. Compare the categories, noting their essential differences and any similarities.

1. What makes each technique category clearly different from the rest?

2. Does every technique variation fit neatly into only one of the categories?
3. Can you accurately categorize massage techniques that you observe in person or on a video of a massage session?

the years and include the concepts of zone therapy, motor points, stress points, reflex points, trigger points, and acupressure points. The intentions of practitioners using direct static pressure may differ, and the amount of pressure used, location of areas pressed, and duration of pressure may also vary. Use Performance Evaluation Form 13.1 in Appendix F, on page A-21, to rate your mastery of Western massage techniques.

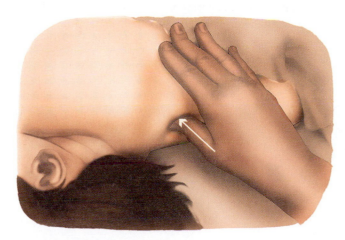

FIGURE 13.36

Ischemic compression (i.e., direct pressure) to a trigger point in the trapezius muscle.

OVERVIEW OF JOINT MOVEMENTS

Western massage traditionally includes joint movements, as well as soft tissue manipulation techniques. Joint movements are an integral part of Western massage sessions and are used along with soft tissue techniques for their therapeutic effects. Review joint movements beginning in Chapter 6, Anatomy & Physiology, Pathology, and Kinesiology.

Categories of Movements

Movements of the body can be categorized generally as either active or passive. *Active movements* are initiated and powered by the individual him- or herself. *Passive movements* refer to movements initiated and controlled by another person, while the recipient remains totally relaxed and receptive .

Movements can be further divided into free, assisted, and resisted. Free active movements are performed entirely by a person without assistance from anyone else. In **assisted movements,** a person initiates the movement, while another person helps him or her complete it. In **resisted movements,** a person initiates the movement, while a second person offers resistance, thereby challenging the muscles used. Resisted movements are sometimes used in rehabilitation to restore strength to a muscle. Assisted and resisted movements also can be used in conjunction with stretching techniques.

TABLE 13.1	Comparison of Joint Mobilizing and Stretching Techniques	
	Joint Mobilizing Techniques	Stretching Techniques
Definition	Nonspecific passive movements of joints within their normal range of motion	Joint movements applied to the limit of the normal range in a specific direction
Qualities	Free, smooth, loose	Slow, sustained, controlled (static stretching)
Effects	Warms associated soft tissues; stimulates proprioceptors; elicits muscle relaxation; stimulates production of synovial fluid	Elongates targeted muscles and associated connective tissue; elicits muscle relaxation
Benefits	Freer movement of joints; increases kinesthetic awareness; decreases muscle tension	Greater flexibility; decreases muscle tension and stiffness
Example	Passive shoulder roll (Figure 13.41 on page 402)	Horizontal stretch (Figure 13.43 on page 403)

Joint Movement Techniques

In massage therapy, joint movements are used for a variety of therapeutic goals. Joint movement techniques can be categorized as joint mobilizing and stretching techniques. A comparison of the two types of joint movement techniques is made in Table 13.1■.

A third category, joint manipulations or adjustments (sometimes called chiropractic adjustments), is important to know about, but is outside of the scope of massage therapy. By joint manipulations and adjustments, we mean techniques that take a joint beyond its normal range of motion. They are direct attempts to realign a misaligned joint, or free a frozen joint, usually using a thrusting movement. They should be performed only by those trained to do so within their legal scope of practice. "Cracking" necks and backs and "popping" toes are potentially dangerous and are not within the scope of standard Western massage.

Mobilizing techniques or free joint movements used in massage therapy are nonspecific passive movements applied within the normal range of motion. Joint mobilizing techniques are applied with a smooth, free, and loose quality.

These free joint movements warm the surrounding soft tissues and elicit muscle relaxation. They stimulate proprioceptors in the surrounding area, which develops kinesthetic awareness. These techniques free up motion at the joints involved and stimulate the production of synovial fluid. Recipients can learn to let go of tension and unconscious holding patterns during passive joint movements.

Some contemporary systems of bodywork, such as Trager Psychophysical Integration®, use joint mobilizing techniques to affect the nervous system. Mobilizing techniques that are free and easy help re-educate muscles and integrate function.

Stretching is a type of joint movement applied to the limit of a joint's normal range in a specific direction. Stretching elongates the muscles and connective tissues that cross the joint. It is used to increase flexibility at the joint and for muscle relaxation. Stretching techniques typically target a specific muscle or muscle group. Different methods of stretching are discussed later in the chapter.

Joint movements add a kinetic dimension to massage sessions and provide diversity of technique. They are useful for increasing flexibility and improving posture and body alignment. Athletes find joint movements particularly beneficial for improving performance, preventing injuries, and rehabilitating injuries.

The next section focuses on joint movement techniques that fall under the categories of nonspecific joint mobilizing and stretching. These movements can be incorporated into a general massage session or used for achieving specific therapeutic goals.

PRACTICAL APPLICATION

Visualize the anatomical structure of the joints as you practice mobilizing and stretching techniques. Compare the picture in your mind and in your textbooks to what you palpate with your hands.

1. How is the movement of the joint related to its bony structure and to associated muscles and other soft tissues?

2. What limitations does the structure place on the movement of the joint?

3. Does this particular joint show deviation from what is considered normal? How do you modify your technique to account for such deviations?

METHODS OF STRETCHING

Four basic methods of stretching are the (1) simple static stretch, (2) contract–relax–stretch (CRS), (3) CRS using reciprocal inhibition, and (4) active assisted stretch. With practice, these methods of stretching can easily be integrated into a massage session.

A **simple static stretch** is a type of passive stretch characterized by slow, sustained, and even application. Sudden, forceful, or bouncing movements are avoided when applying static stretches.

To apply a simple static stretch, move the body part to be stretched into position and hold at the limit of range of motion. The limit is determined by feeling for the point of resistance from the tissues involved. The receiver is passive during the entire stretch. Use feedback from the recipient for safety. The recipient should feel the stretch, but not feel pain. Hold for 10–15 seconds, and then try to increase the stretch. The muscles will often relax after a short time, allowing further stretch (30 seconds overall).

Stretches can be facilitated with techniques that utilize muscle physiology. Review information on muscle spindles and Golgi tendon organs in Chapter 6, Anatomy & Physiology, Pathology, and Kinesiology on page 218. See Figure 6.111 (page 218) and Figure 6.112 (page 219). In **contract–relax–stretch (CRS)** techniques, the practitioner gets into position to apply the stretch, but first asks the client to contract the muscle to be stretched against a resistance (resisted movement). Immediately following the targeted muscle's relaxation, the stretch is applied.

When CRS incorporating *reciprocal inhibition* is used, the practitioner gets into position to apply the stretch, but first asks the client to contract the target muscle's antagonist against a resistance. The target muscle relaxes as its antagonist contracts. Immediately following the antagonist's relaxation, the stretch is applied.

Applying the stretch during the recipient's exhalation can enhance the stretch. The body is more relaxed during exhalation than during inhalation, and holding the breath causes tension in the musculature and restricts movement. So it is better to stretch a muscle on the exhalation. Once you and the recipient are in position to apply a stretch, ask him or her to "take a deep breath and then let it out slowly." During the exhalation, apply the stretch.

For an *active assisted stretch,* the practitioner gets into position to apply the stretch and then directs the recipient to actively move the body part in the desired direction. The practitioner then assists the stretch, providing additional force in the direction of the movement. Have the recipient breathe normally during the active stretch; however, move more deeply into the stretch on an exhale.

The four methods of stretching are summarized in Table 13.2.

SAFETY

Being familiar with the bony structure and soft tissues around joints is essential for the safe and effective application of joint movements. Anatomical structures determine the type and degree of movement possible at the joint. Review of musculoskeletal anatomy and kinesiology related to joints is useful before attempting to perform joint movement techniques. For a review of skeletal and muscular anatomy and kinesiology, see Chapter 6, beginning on page 120.

TABLE 13.2 Methods of Static Stretching

Method	Description	Example Using Quadriceps Stretch (see Figure 13.58 on page 408)
Simple static stretch	• Position targeted muscle • Apply static stretch • Recipient is passive	Relax the entire leg during the stretch
Contract–relax–stretch (CRS)	• Position targeted muscle • Contract targeted muscle against resistance • Relax targeted muscle • Apply static stretch	Resistance to quadriceps contraction applied before the stretch
CRS using reciprocal inhibition	• Position targeted muscle • Contract antagonist against resistance • Relax antagonist • Apply static stretch	Resistance to hamstrings contraction applied before the stretch
Active assisted stretch	• Position targeted muscle • Client actively performs the stretch • Practitioner assists by applying additional force in the desired direction	Assistance for the stretch is applied by the practitioner

CRITICAL THINKING

Think about the variations on static stretching that utilize the principles of contract–relax–stretch and reciprocal inhibition. Evaluate each stretch you apply to determine if one of these variations might enhance the effect. Determine how to best make the application.

1. Can you name the primary muscle targeted with the stretch and its antagonist?
2. Can you apply adequate resistance to the muscle you want the recipient to contract?
3. Can you give clear instructions to the recipient to perform the technique correctly?

Normal range of motion refers to the degree of movement typically found at a particular joint (see Figure 6.110 on page 215). Normal range of motion is a point of comparison for assessing the degree of flexibility of a joint in a specific person and how it might vary from the norm. Knowing the limitations of movement at each joint also decreases the likelihood of inadvertently damaging a joint or the surrounding tissues and increases safety for the recipient.

Palpation skills are important for learning how joints move. Practitioners can learn much about the condition of the joint and surrounding tissues from the kinesthetic feel of its movement. Sensations such as "drag" and "end feel" offer clues to restrictions to normal range of motion, areas of tightness, patterns of holding, and the limits of stretches. *Drag* refers to resistance felt as the soft tissues around a joint are stretched, and *end feel* refers to resistance as the limit of the stretch is approached. Clicking or grinding in a joint may signal misalignment or some abnormality or pathology such as osteoarthritis.

Cautions and Contraindications

Caution is advised in cases of abnormal joint conditions. Joint abnormalities may be congenital or may be the result of accidents, injuries, or diseases. Range of motion at an abnormal joint may be limited, or the joint may be hypermobile and unstable. Remember that massage and joint movements are contraindicated when acute inflammation is present.

Past trauma to a joint can cause unusual conditions in the area. These include shortening or loss of muscle tissue, scarring in connective tissues, or abnormal joint structure. Recent soft tissue injuries around a joint can leave swelling and inflammation that affect the joint itself.

After a fracture, care is warranted when moving joints in the vicinity. Even if the break is a distance from a joint, muscles that cross the joint may be affected. Hardware, such as metal pins and plates, may have been used to treat a fracture and may still be attached, thus limiting movement. Joint replacements are also becoming more common, and movement around artificial joints may be restricted. Hip and knee replacements are especially common in older adults.

Diseases that affect joints directly can cause pain, swelling, periods of inflammation, and loss of mobility. Osteoarthritis, also called degenerative joint disease, is caused by wear and tear of the joint structures. Bursitis, or inflammation of the fluid sacks in synovial joints, results in pain and limited mobility. Osteoporosis, or loss of bone tissue, leaves bones thin, brittle, and prone to injury (see Figure 6.43 on page 154). These and other joint pathologies have implications for applications of joint movements and massage. Table 6.14, Common Pathologies of the Skeletal System, on page 152 lists skeletal and joint pathologies and their massage implications.

Take the time to learn about joint conditions presented by clients and note them in their health history files. Additional information can be obtained from a recipient's medical records or from the recipient's physician. Make the effort to learn more about unfamiliar conditions by consulting anatomical and medical references. Greater knowledge helps to ensure a safe application of joint movements.

GENERAL GUIDELINES FOR JOINT MOVEMENT TECHNIQUES

The following is a summary of the general guidelines for performing joint mobilizing and stretching techniques:

- Check for contraindications before applying joint movements.
- Adapt techniques for structural abnormalities.
- Stay within the normal range of motion of the joint.
- Stay within the comfort range of the recipient.
- Warm surrounding soft tissues before stretching.
- Apply joint mobilizing techniques with smooth, free, loose quality.
- Apply stretching techniques with slow, sustained, even motion.
- Apply a stretch as the recipient exhales.
- Use contract–relax and reciprocal inhibition to enhance a stretch.
- Use client feedback to determine the limit of a stretch.

REGIONAL APPLICATIONS OF JOINT MOVEMENTS

The following sections discuss applications of joint movements to the neck, shoulder girdle, elbow, wrist, hand, chest, hip, knee, ankle, and foot. See Figure 6.109 to review joint movements and Box 6.1 on page 214 in Chapter 6 to review the terminology of joint movements.

Neck

Structure and Movement The *neck* is a general term for the region between the head and the trunk. It includes the seven cervical vertebrae and the surrounding soft tissues.

The musculature in the neck region is complex, with deeper, smaller muscles entirely within the neck, and larger and more superficial muscles attaching superior and inferior. Movements at the neck include flexion, extension, lateral flexion, and rotation.

Mobilizing Techniques Mobilizing techniques for the neck are performed when the recipient is lying supine. The mobilizing movement occurs between the cervical vertebrae and in the suboccipital region. All the following examples may be performed with the practitioner seated at the head of the recipient. It is useful to have an adjustable stool or chair on wheels so that you can get in good position, for both leverage and good body mechanics.

Simple mobilizing movements of the neck may be performed by lifting the head slightly off the table and moving the neck into lateral flexion, rotation, forward flexion, or hyperextension. Be sure to have a firm grip on the head. You may have to remind the recipient to relax, since it takes great trust to let someone hold and move your head. You may also assure the individual that you will not "crack" his or her neck, and that such manipulations are not part of this type of joint movement. Keep the movements small at first and gradually increase the range of motion as the recipient allows.

Finger push-ups may be used to produce gentle movement between the cervical vertebrae. First warm up the neck muscles with effleurage and circular friction along each side. Straighten the neck so that the recipient is facing up. Simply place the fingers at the base of the neck on either side, palms up, and push up with the fingers, applying direct pressure. Move your hands about an inch at a time along the neck, pressing up at each spot as you move along. You will feel movement between the vertebrae and notice movement at the head. Variations of finger push-ups include alternating pressing from side to side.

A *wave movement* may be created in the neck by simply applying deep effleurage on both sides at the same time, moving from the base to the suboccipital region. You exaggerate the natural curve of the neck by pressing up as you slide along. The neck will return to its normal curve as you finish the movement (see Figure 14.68 on page 439). At the end of the movement, give a gentle pull on the occiput to straighten any hyperextension remaining from the movement.

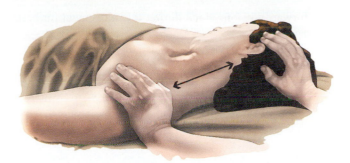

FIGURE 13.37

Stretch of trapezius and cervical muscles with neck in lateral flexion.

Stretches Massage and simple mobilizing techniques are used to warm up the neck thoroughly before applying stretches. The following stretches may be performed when the recipient is lying supine on a table.

A stretch in *lateral flexion* helps lengthen the muscles on the sides of the neck. Place the head in position to one side at a point where you feel the tissues just starting to stretch. The head placement, either face up or turned to the side, will determine which muscles are stretched most. Place one hand on the shoulder and the other on the side of the head. You can create a gentle stretch of tissues by pushing the head and shoulders in opposite directions, as shown in Figure 13.37■. Guide the recipient to exhale as you apply the stretch. Repeat on the other side.

Range of *rotation* may be enhanced with a simple stretch. Position the head face up so that the neck is straight. Then rotate the head to one side, keeping the neck vertically aligned. Gently push the head into greater rotation, stretching the neck muscles. Repeat on the other side.

Position the head face up to stretch the neck in *forward flexion*. Lift the head with one hand, and with the other hand, reach under the head and across to the tip of the shoulder. The head rests on the forearm. Reach under that arm with the free hand and place it on the other shoulder. The head should be cradled safely at the place where the forearms cross, as shown in Figure 13.38■. Slowly stretch the neck

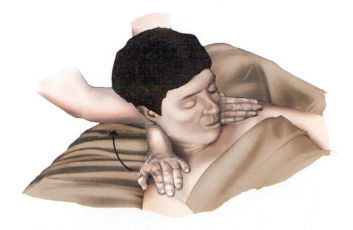

FIGURE 13.38

Cross-arm stretch of cervical muscles with neck in forward flexion.

into forward flexion. Stand during this movement for best leverage.

The *cross-arm stretch* may also be performed with the head rotated. This will stretch neck muscles at a different angle. After forward flexion, return to the starting position and turn the head to one side. Repeat the forward flexion to each side with the head in rotation. For safety, be sure that the stretch is pain free.

Shoulder

Structure and Movement The shoulder is the most mobile area of the body. It includes the glenohumeral, acromio-clavicular, and scapulocostal joints. Movements possible in the shoulder include the upper arm movements of flexion, extension, abduction, adduction, rotation, and horizontal flexion. Movements of the scapulae themselves include elevation, depression, upward and downward rotation and tilt, and retraction and protraction. The entire shoulder is structured to accomplish circumduction.

Mobilizing Techniques Mobilizing movements of the shoulder girdle can be performed with the recipient in supine, prone, side-lying, or seated position. Mobilizing the joints of the shoulder may be accomplished indirectly by movement of the arm or by movement of the scapula.

To mobilize the shoulder girdle with the recipient in the supine position, take hold of the hand and lift and wag the arm as shown in Figure 13.39■. While *wagging* the arm, there will also be movement at the wrist and elbow. *Shaking* is performed by creating a slight traction of the arm toward the feet, holding onto the hand and leaning back, as shown in Figure 13.40■. Loosely shake the arm up and down. Movement will be felt at the wrist, elbow, and shoulder.

The *passive shoulder roll* may be used for mobilizing the shoulder. Hold onto the upper arm with one hand with the other hand at the tip of the shoulder. Simply move the shoulder through the full range of motion possible in the supine position. The quality of movement should be smooth, free, and loose. Figure 13.41■ shows the passive shoulder roll with the recipient supine. This same technique is effective in the prone, side-lying, and seated positions.

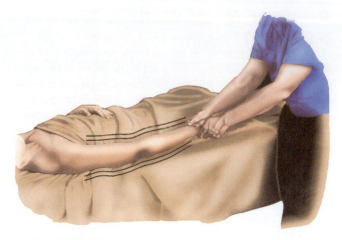

FIGURE 13.40

Shaking: an arm and shoulder mobilizing technique.

With the recipient prone, *scapula mobilizing* may be accomplished using pressure applied at the top of the shoulder. Position the recipient's arm on the table with elbow bent and hand near the waist. Then place your hand on top of the shoulder near the tip and pressing lightly toward the feet. The scapula will move and lift if the attached muscles are relaxed, as shown in Figure 13.42■. Don't force the movement, but encourage relaxation by gentle motions and reminding the recipient to let go of tension in the area. Once the medial border lifts, you may apply effleurage to massage the muscles that attach there.

Stretches Use massage and mobilizing techniques to warm up the shoulder girdle before stretching. Shoulder girdle stretches are effective in the supine, prone, and side-lying positions. The muscles of the shoulder girdle are stretched primarily with movements of the upper arm.

In the supine position, a stretch in *horizontal flexion* may be performed by moving the arm over the chest. This

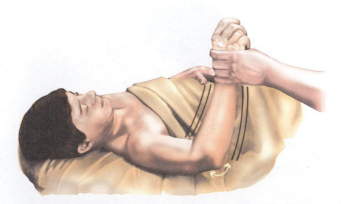

FIGURE 13.39

Wagging: an arm and shoulder mobilizing technique.

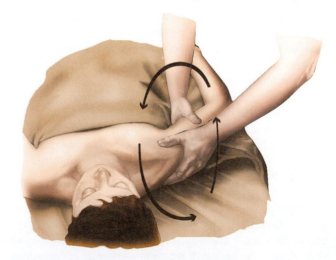

FIGURE 13.41

Passive shoulder roll: mobilizing technique for the shoulder with recipient in supine position.

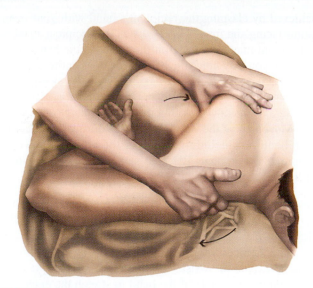

FIGURE 13.42

Scapula mobilizing technique: move and lift the scapula by pulling back at the shoulder.

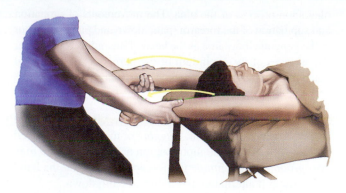

FIGURE 13.44

Overhead stretch for the shoulder muscles. Lean back to create the stretch using your body weight.

elongates the muscles that attach to the medial border of the scapula, including the rhomboids, as well as the posterior shoulder muscles. Hold onto the recipient's lower arm near the wrist with one hand, while the other hand reaches under to the medial border of the scapula. Stretch the arm over the chest, and enhance the stretch by gently pulling back on the scapula at the same time. See Figure 13.43■.

A very pleasant stretch may be applied with the recipient's arms extended overhead. This *overhead stretch* may be performed one arm at a time or both arms at the same time. For a two-arm stretch, simply place the arms overhead, grasping the forearm near the wrist. Lean back to create the stretch at the shoulder, as shown in Figure 13.44■. This technique stretches all of the muscles of the shoulder girdle, including the latissimus dorsi and pectoral muscles.

A similar stretch may be applied with the recipient seated in a massage chair. Grasp the forearm with both hands and move the arm overhead to a position in line with the

angle of the body. You should be facing in the same direction as the recipient. Lift the arm upward and give it a gentle shake, as shown in Figure 13.45■.

Elbow

Structure and Movement The elbow joint is formed by the junction of the distal end of the humerus and the proximal ends of the radius and the ulna. Movements of the humeroulnar hinge joint are limited to flexion and extension. The bony structure of the joint further limits the range of motion in extension. What we think of as the point of the elbow is the

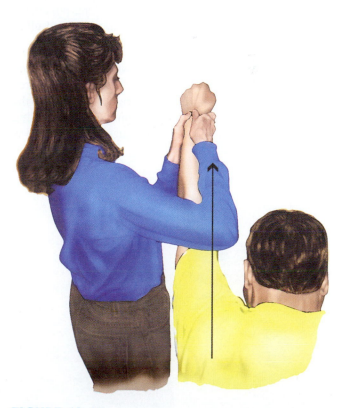

FIGURE 13.45

Overhead stretch of the shoulder muscles. Recipient in a massage chair.

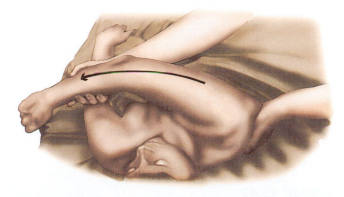

FIGURE 13.43

Stretching the shoulder muscles with arm in horizontal flexion.

olecranon process of the ulna. The movements of pronation and supination of the forearm (palm down and palm up) occur in the general elbow area as the head of the radius rotates over the surfaces of the capitulum of the humerus and the radial notch of the ulna. At the same time, the distal ends of the radius and ulna glide over one another.

Mobilizing Techniques   Movements at the elbow are limited by the structure of the joint. *Wagging* of the arm as described previously offers some mobilization at the elbow. You may also *pronate and supinate* the forearm by holding the hand and turning it alternately palm up and palm down.

To perform a simple mobilizing technique at the elbow called *circling the forearm,* bend the arm at the elbow so that it is perpendicular to the table. Hold the arm just below the wrist. Trace a circle with the hand creating movement at the elbow, as shown in Figure 13.46■.

Stretches   Stretches of muscles that cross the elbow are accomplished largely by stretching the whole arm as in the *overhead stretch* of the shoulder described earlier. If the biceps muscles are shortened, the stretch is created by simply straightening out the arm at the elbow.

Wrist

Structure and Movement   The wrist joint is formed by the union of the slightly concave surface of the proximal row of carpal bones with the distal end of the radius and the midcarpal joint. What people commonly call the "wrist bone" is actually the distal end of the ulna. Movements possible at this juncture include flexion, extension, radial and ulnar deviation (side-to-side movement), and circumduction.

Mobilizing Techniques   Mobilizing the wrist is best performed with the recipient supine. The soft tissues in the wrist area may be warmed up with small effleurage movements with the thumbs prior to mobilizing and stretching. A useful starting position for basic mobilizing techniques and stretching is achieved by clasping the recipient's hand with your own, palms facing and fingers interwoven. The recipient's elbow is bent and may be resting on the table. In the hand-clasp position, you may move the hand through its entire range of motion at the wrist including flexion, extension, side-to-side in radial and ulnar deviation, and circumduction. Keep the passive movement well within the possible range of motion.

Movement at the wrist also occurs during less specific mobilizations, including wagging the arm, as shown in Figure 13.39 on page 402, and supination and pronation of the forearm.

Stretches   *Flexion* and *hyperextension* are the major stretches performed at the wrist. Figure 13.47■ shows stretching the flexors of the forearm by extending the wrist to the limit of its range. Press down gently on the palm side of the fingers to hyperextend the wrist. Now flex the wrist by pressing down on the back side of the hand to stretch the extensors of the forearm, as shown in Figure 13.48■. During these stretches, be careful to approach the limit of motion slowly.

Hand

Structure and Movement   Joints within the hand and distal to the wrist include the metacarpophalangeal juncture (i.e., knuckles) and the small joints between phalanges. Movements of the fingers include flexion, extension, abduction, and adduction. The hand as a whole is capable of holding and grasping objects.

Mobilizing Techniques   Perform mobilizing techniques of the hand joints very carefully, matching the force used to the size and strength of the hand you are working with. Warm the muscles in the recipient's hands with effleurage

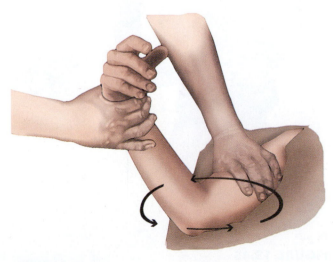

FIGURE 13.46

Circling the forearm to create movement at the elbow.

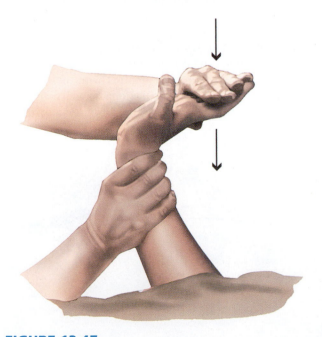

FIGURE 13.47

Stretching the flexor muscles of the forearm by hyperextending the wrist.

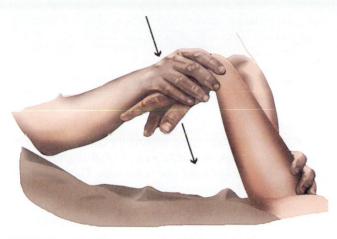

FIGURE 13.48

Stretching the extensor muscles of the forearm by flexing the wrist.

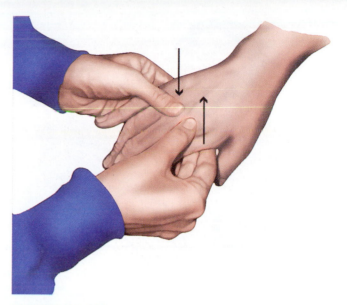

FIGURE 13.50

Scissoring motion to create movement between the metacarpals of the hand.

and light frictions before performing mobilizing techniques and stretches.

Mobilizing the knuckles, one at a time, may be achieved making *figure-8s*. Hold the recipient's hand with one of your hands, his or her fingers pointing toward you, palm down. With your other hand, grasp the fifth (little) finger firmly near the knuckle and move in a small figure-8 pattern two or three times, mobilizing the joint. See Figure 13.49■. Repeat for each knuckle joint.

You can mobilize the soft tissues between the metacarpals with a *scissoring* motion. With the recipient's palm down, take hold of the knuckles of the fifth and fourth fingers as shown in Figure 13.50■. Simply move one knuckle up and the other down at the same time, alternating in a scissoring motion. Repeat along all of the knuckles.

Stretches   There are a few simple stretches for the joints of the hand. Perform them slowly and with care. The fingers can be *extended* at the knuckles. Interlace your fingers with the recipient's, palm to palm, placing the tips of your fingers just below the recipient's knuckles. Gently press between the back of the hand, bending the recipient's fingers into extension.

Taking the whole hand into *hyperextension* can stretch all of the flexor muscles within the hand and the wrist flexors in the forearm. Hold the forearm with one hand, and with the other hand, press back on the phalanges, causing hyperextension at the knuckles and at the wrist. Gently stretch the tissues of the hand and the forearm. See Figure 13.47.

Chest

Structure and Movement   The *chest* is a common term for the area on the front and sides of the upper body generally defined by the ribs, sternum, and clavicle. Several slightly moveable joints are located in the general chest area, including those linking the ribs to the sternum, the clavicle to the sternum, and the clavicle to the acromion process of the scapula. Several muscles involved in shoulder movement attach to the chest.

The chest is the part of the thorax accessible when lying supine. The entire thorax, including the chest, expands and contracts with the inhalation and exhalation of breathing.

Mobilizing Techniques   The rib cage may be mobilized by *gentle rocking* from the side. Stand facing the side of the table in line with the rib cage. Put one hand on top of the other and place them on the rib cage, as shown in Figure 13.51■. Gently rock the rib cage by repeatedly pushing and then letting up the pressure in a rhythmic manner. Move around on the rib cage to mobilize different areas. You will feel the elastic quality of the rib cage as it springs back after you push.

If you can reach far enough with your arms, you can cause movement in the chest from both sides. Face the rib

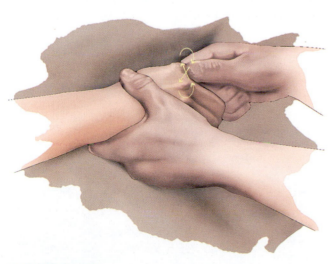

FIGURE 13.49

Figure-8s at the knuckles of the hand.

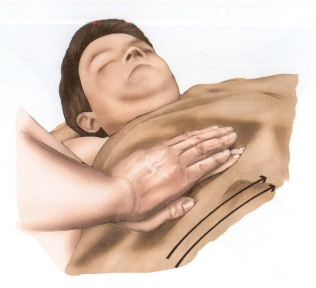

FIGURE 13.51

Placement of hands for mobilizing the rib cage from one side.

cage from the side of the table, reach over with one hand to the far side of the chest, fingers pointing down toward the table. Place the other hand on the near side, fingers pointing up. See Figure 13.52■. Gently rock the rib cage by alternately pulling with the far hand and pushing with the near hand. Establish a smooth rhythm to encourage relaxation of the surrounding musculature.

Stretches There are no highly movable joints on the chest itself. However, the pectoral muscles of the shoulder girdle attach there. Use the *overhead stretch* of the arms, as shown in Figure 13.44, to lengthen the pectorals.

Hip

Structure and Movement The hip area includes the hip joint and related muscles. The hip joint is a typical ball-and-socket joint. The muscles that move the hip joint are located primarily on the thigh and the buttocks. Movements possible at the hip joint include flexion, extension, abduction, adduction, diagonal abduction and adduction, outward and inward rotation, and circumduction.

Mobilizing Techniques Most hip movements are performed with the recipient in the supine position. Mobilizing techniques are an excellent way to affect the deeper muscles that move the hip.

With the recipient supine, remove the bolster from under the knees. The legs should be straight and slightly apart. Stand facing the thigh at the side of the table. Gently *rock the leg* into rotation by placing the hands palms down on the top of the thigh and pressing down and away. See Figure 13.53■. The leg will usually rotate back, especially if the gluteals are tight. Repeat with a rhythmic rocking motion.

To achieve *passive movement through full range of motion* of the hip, bend the leg, placing the foot in one hand and using the other hand for support at the knee. See Figure 13.54■. Let the knee trace a circle as the hip flexes, adducts diagonally, extends, abducts diagonally, and goes round again in circumduction. The movement should be smooth and loose.

Stretches The muscles that move the hip can be stretched in many directions. The following are a few simple useful stretches for the hip joint.

A stretch for the gluteals may be applied with the hip in flexion by pressing the knee toward the chest in the supine position (*knee to chest flexion*). See Figure 13.55■. The hamstrings may be stretched with the leg straight and in flexion (*straight leg flexion*), as shown in Figure 13.56■. To enhance the stretch and involve all of the gluteal and leg muscles, dorsiflex the foot while you bring the leg into flexion as close to perpendicular as possible.

Diagonal adduction of the thigh while lying supine will also stretch the gluteals. Bring the knee toward the chest, and then let it cross the body diagonally, as shown in Figure 13.57■. The recipient's shoulders remain flat on the table, while the spine rotates and the hip muscles stretch. This is also a good stretch for the lower back.

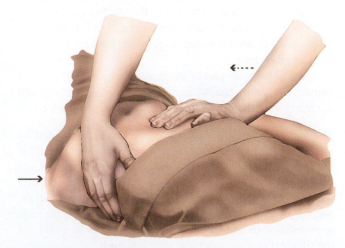

FIGURE 13.52

Placement of hands for mobilizing the rib cage from both sides.

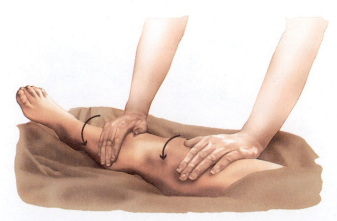

FIGURE 13.53

Rocking the leg to create rotation in the hip joint.

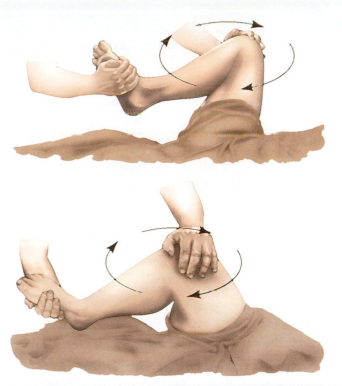

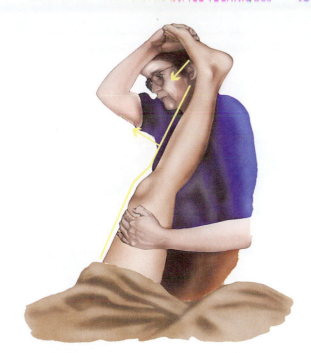

FIGURE 13.56

Stretching the hamstrings with straight leg flexion.

FIGURE 13.54

Moving the hip through its full range of motion.

Knee

Structure and Movement The knee is a hinge joint formed by the articulation of the distal end of the femur with the proximal end of the tibia. A large sesamoid bone embedded in the connective tissues that cross the joint forms the knee cap or patella. The major movements of the knee joint are flexion and extension. Some minor inward and outward rotation of the tibia is possible when the knee is flexed in a non-weight-bearing situation.

Mobilizing Techniques The knee joint is best mobilized with the recipient in the prone position. A simple mobilization at the knee involves tossing the lower leg back and forth from

hand to hand. This *leg toss* technique helps the recipient learn to relax and let go of tension in the legs. After the leg toss, you may perform a different knee mobilization by *circling the lower leg*. Place one hand on the thigh to steady it and grasp the lower leg near the ankle with the other hand. Make small circles with the lower leg. Stay well within the small range of this circular motion.

Stretches A few of the stretches for the hip joint, performed with a straight leg, also stretch muscles that cross the knee. See Figure 13.56. An additional stretch (*heel to buttocks*) for the knee extensors can be created with the recipient in the prone position by bringing the heel of the foot toward the buttocks. See Figure 13.58■. Table 13.2, on page 399, describes four different methods of applying this stretch.

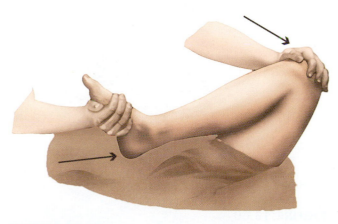

FIGURE 13.55

Stretching the gluteals by bringing knee to chest.

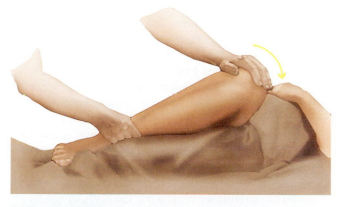

FIGURE 13.57

Stretching the muscles of the hip and lower back with diagonal adduction of the bent leg.

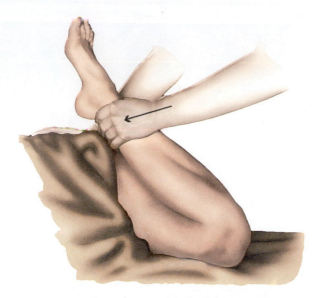

FIGURE 13.58

Stretching the quadriceps by bringing the heel of the foot toward the buttocks.

Ankle

Structure and Movement   The ankle is a hinge joint formed by the junction of the talus with the malleoli of the tibia and fibula. The structure is bound together with many ligaments for stability. The tendons of the muscles of the lower leg that attach to the foot all pass over the ankle. They are bound neatly at the ankle by a band of connective tissue called the retinaculum. Movements possible at the ankle include dorsiflexion (flexion), plantar flexion (extension), pronation (eversion and abduction), and supination (inversion and adduction).

Mobilizing Techniques   When the recipient is prone, the ankle may be accessed by lifting the lower leg so that the foot comes off the table. For mobilizing with *dorsiflexion,* stand at the feet facing the end of the table. Lift one leg and place both hands on the foot, thumbs on the bottom of the foot. Lean into the foot with the thumbs in the arch, moving the foot into dorsiflexion, as shown in Figure 13.59■. Repeat the mobilization several times in a rhythmic manner, changing the location of the thumbs to affect different spots on the feet.

   With the lower leg lifted so that it is perpendicular to the table, the ankle can be put through a *full range of motion through passive movement.* Grasp the bottom of the foot from above and move the ankle through dorsiflexion, pronation, plantar flexion, and supination in a circular movement. This is also an excellent position from which to apply simple dorsiflexion and plantar flexion.

   With the recipient supine, the ankle can be put through *side-to-side mobilizing* by placing the heels of the hands on the foot just under the malleoli of the tibia and fibula (ankle bones) and alternately pressing one side and then the other. The movement is rapid, and causes the heel of

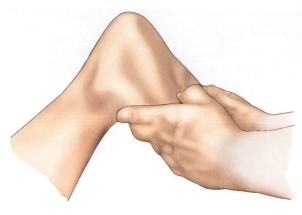

FIGURE 13.59

Dorsiflexion of the foot with direct pressure to bottom of foot with the thumbs.

the foot to move from side to side at the articulation of the talus and malleoli of the tibia and fibula. (See Figure 14.36 on page 430.)

Stretches   Stretches at the ankle are primarily performed in *dorsiflexion* and *plantar flexion* and may easily be done with the recipient prone or supine. Stretches may be applied from any of the positions mentioned for mobilizations. Simply move the foot into dorsiflexion or plantar flexion and take it to the limit of range of motion. Figure 13.60■ shows the ankle and foot stretching in plantar flexion. This movement helps elongate the foot flexors located on the front of the lower leg and may be felt across the top of the foot.

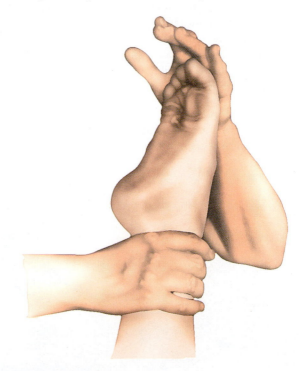

FIGURE 13.60

Stretching the flexors of the foot in plantarflexion, recipient prone. Lower leg perpendicular to the table.

Foot

Structure and Movement The foot may be described as an elastic arched structure made up of 26 bones and designed for support and propulsion. There is a longitudinal and a transverse arch. The intertarsal joints allow for slight gliding movements, and the joints of the toes allow for flexion and extension.

Mobilizing Techniques Mobilizing techniques for the feet are similar to those for the hands. They are best performed with the recipient supine. The soft tissues in the feet may be warmed up with small sliding effleurage movements with the thumbs or fingers and compressions with the fist on the bottom of the foot.

Hold the foot steady with one hand and with your other hand, grasp the fifth (little) toe firmly near the knuckle and move in a small *figure-8* pattern two or three times, mobilizing the joint. Repeat for each knuckle joint. You can mobilize the tissues between the metatarsals with a *scissoring* motion. Take hold of the knuckles of the fifth and fourth toes. Simply move one knuckle up and the other down at the same time, alternating in a scissoring motion. Repeat for all of the metatarsals.

Sometimes the toes curl under due to shortening of the toe flexors that are located on the bottom of the feet. The toes can be mobilized into extension using *effleurage* along the underside of the toes. This is usually performed with the thumbs. Do not "pop" or forcefully pull on the toes straightening them out, which is uncomfortable to most recipients and can be dangerous.

Stretches There are a few stretches for the intrinsic tissues of the foot itself. As described earlier, you can plantar flex the foot from either the prone or supine positions, stretching the tissues on the top of the foot, including the extensor muscles. The toes alone may easily be stretched back at the ball of the foot or pressed forward for a stretch (*hyperextension*). The

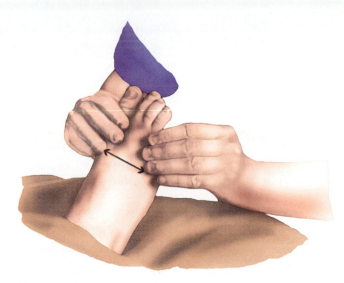

FIGURE 13.61

Creating space between metatarsals by pulling sides of foot away from each other.

foot may be spread stretching the spaces between the metatarsals and the muscles that run across them. Simply grasp both sides of the foot and pull in opposite directions, *widening the foot at the metatarsals* and stretching related tissues, as shown in Figure 13.61■.

Since the foot is a small part of the body with many joints, it can be massaged thoroughly rather quickly combining soft tissue techniques with mobilizations and stretches. Joint movements help recipients regain a sense of their feet as having moving parts and help sharpen their kinesthetic sense. This is important, especially for those who live in cultures where shoes are worn all day.

Table 13.3■ provides a quick, at-a-glance overview of joint movement techniques. Use Performance Evaluation Form 13.2 in Appendix F, on page A-24, to rate your mastery of joint movement techniques.

TABLE 13.3	At-a-Glance Joint Movement Techniques	
Region	**Mobilizing Techniques**	**Stretches**
Neck	Finger push-ups	Cross-arm stretch
	Meltdown	Forward flexion
	Simple mobilizing movements	Lateral flexion
	Wavelike movement	Rotation
Shoulder	Passive shoulder roll	Horizontal flexion
	Scapula mobilizing (prone)	Overhead stretch
	Shaking	
	Wagging	
Elbow	Circling the forearm	Overhead stretch
	Pronation and supination	
	Wagging	

(Continued)

TABLE 13.3 (Continued)

Region	Mobilizing Techniques	Stretches
Wrist	Passive movement through full range of motion Waving	Hyperextension Flexion
Hand	Figure-8s Passive movements of all joints Scissoring	Flexion Hyperextension of fingers and wrist
Chest	Gentle rocking of rib cage	Overhead stretch
Hip	Passive movement through full range of motion Rhythmic rocking of straight leg	Diagonal adduction with flexed knee Knee to chest flexion Straight leg flexion Straight leg hyperextension— prone and side-lying
Knee	Circling the lower leg Leg toss Wagging	Heel to buttocks
Ankle	Dorsiflexing foot with thumb pressure Passive movement through full range of motion Side-to-side mobilizing	Dorsiflexion Plantar flexion
Foot	Figure-8s of toes Scissoring metatarsals Straightening toes with effleurage	Fingers interlocked between toes Foot widening at metatarsals Hyperextension of toes

CASE FOR STUDY

Shirley Applies Joint Movements to Improve Roger's Walk

Shirley has a client named Roger who complains of stiffness in his legs and feet. Roger sits for long periods of time at work, and when he stands up has a hard time moving smoothly. He can barely touch his toes anymore with his legs straight and has tripped a few times from not picking up his toes high enough as he walks. Other people have commented that he seems to be limping a little.

Question:

How can Shirley incorporate joint movements into Roger's massage sessions to help improve his walking?

Things to consider:

- Does Roger have any recent injuries to his lower limbs or other contraindications for joint movements?
- Does Roger have good flexibility in his legs at the ankles, knees, and hips?
- Are there specific leg muscles that seem tight or shortened?

Write a brief description of which joint mobilizations and stretches to include in Roger's next massage session. Assume that there are no contraindications.

_____

_____

_____

CHAPTER HIGHLIGHTS

- Western massage is the most common form of massage found in Europe and North America and is used for a variety of wellness and therapeutic applications.
- Western massage is understood in terms of Western science and Western beliefs about health and disease.
- Western massage techniques fall into seven broad categories: effleurage, petrissage, friction, tapotement, vibration, touch without movement, and joint movements.
- Effleurage techniques slide or glide over the skin with a smooth, continuous motion.
  - Effleurage is used to begin a session, apply lubricant, accustom the receiver to touch, connect, or transition from one body region to another, assess the condition of tissues, and conclude work on an area.
  - The pressure, rhythm, and pace of effleurage are varied for different effects.
- Petrissage techniques lift, wring, or squeeze soft tissues in a kneading motion, or press or roll the tissues under or between the hands.
  - Petrissage is used to increase local circulation, "milk" tissues of accumulated waste products, assist venous return, separate muscle fibers, and evoke muscular relaxation.
- Friction is performed by rubbing one surface over another repeatedly.
  - Superficial friction is used for warming tissues and is performed by rubbing the palms briskly over the skin.
  - Deep friction is used to separate tissues, break adhesions, form healthy scar tissue, or to create movement in less-muscled areas, such as around joints and over the head; types: cross-fiber, parallel, or circular.
  - Cyriax friction is a form of deep transverse friction used in injury rehabilitation.
- Tapotement consists of a series of brisk percussive movements following each other in rapid, alternating fashion.
  - Tapotement is used for stimulation and as a finishing technique.
- Vibration is an oscillating, quivering, or trembling motion, or movement back and forth or up and down performed quickly and repeatedly.
  - Deep vibration is applied with the fingertips or with an electric vibrator.
  - Coarse vibration is applied with the whole hand over a larger area and includes light effleurage with vibration, shaking, and jostling.
- Touch without movement is defined by touch with the hands, but without any visible movement.
  - Touch without movement is used to impart heat, have a calming effect, or balance energy.
  - Variations include passive touch and holding.
  - Direct pressure (e.g., ischemic compression) is applied to specific points for a number of effects.
- Joint movement techniques are traditionally part of Western massage.
  - Joint movements within the scope of massage therapy are nonspecific joint mobilizing and stretching techniques.
  - Joint manipulations or adjustments that involve thrusting movements are not within the scope of massage therapy.
- Movements of the body may be generally categorized as active and passive.
  - Active movements are initiated and powered by the person him- or herself.
  - During passive movements, the recipient remains totally relaxed and receptive while the practitioner initiates and controls the movement.
- Movements may be free, assisted, or resisted.
- Joint mobilizing techniques are nonspecific passive movements performed within the normal range of joint motion.
  - Qualities are smooth, free, and loose.
  - They warm surrounding tissues, elicit muscle relaxation, stimulate proprioceptors, free up motion, and stimulate production of synovial fluid.
- Stretching is a type of joint movement that is performed to the limit of the range of motion in a specific direction
  - Stretching elongates muscles and connective tissue and elicits muscle relaxation.
- Four basic stretching methods are used in massage therapy.
  - A simple, static stretch is a slow, smooth, and even stretch application, holding the end point for up to 30 seconds.
  - Contract–relax–stretch (CRS) involves contracting the targeted muscle before a stretch.
  - CRS with reciprocal inhibition involves contracting the antagonist of the targeted muscle before a stretch.
  - Active assisted stretch involves the recipient initiating the stretch and the practitioner assisting by applying additional force in the desired direction.
- Practical knowledge of the structure and the movement possible at each joint is essential to ensure the safety of the recipient during joint movements.
- Joint movements add a kinetic dimension to a massage session and provide diversity of technique.

EXAM REVIEW

Key Terms

Match the following key terms to their descriptions. For additional study, look up the key terms in the Interactive Glossary on page G-1 and note other terms that compare or contrast with them.

_____ 1. Assisted movements
_____ 2. Contract–relax–stretch (CRS)
_____ 3. Direct pressure
_____ 4. Effleurage
_____ 5. Friction
_____ 6. Mobilizing techniques
_____ 7. Petrissage
_____ 8. Resisted movements
_____ 9. Simple static stretch
_____ 10. Stretching
_____ 11. Tapotement
_____ 12. Touch without movement
_____ 13. Vibration

a. Nonspecific passive movements applied within the normal range of motion
b. Technique in which a person initiates the movement, while a second person offers resistance, thereby challenging the muscles used
c. Technique that lifts, wrings, or squeezes soft tissues in a kneading motion, or presses the tissues under or between the hands
d. A person initiates the movement, while another person helps him or her complete it
e. Series of brisk percussive movements following each other in rapid, alternating fashion
f. Technique used to increase flexibility at the joint and for muscle relaxation
g. Touch with the hands, but without any visible movement
h. An oscillating, quivering, or trembling motion, or movement back and forth or up and down performed quickly and repeatedly
i. Tissues are compressed using light to heavy pressure and applied with a thumb, finger, knuckle, or elbow
j. Technique performed by rubbing one surface over another repeatedly
k. First the client contracts the muscle to be stretched against a resistance (resisted movement); immediately following the targeted muscle's relaxation, the stretch is applied
l. Type of passive stretch characterized by slow, sustained, and even application
m. Technique that slides or glides over the skin with a smooth, continuous motion

Memory Workout

To test your memory of the main concepts in this chapter, complete the following sentences by circling the most correct answer from the two choices provided.

1. Classic Western massage includes (five) (seven) technique categories.
2. (Effleurage) (Friction) techniques slide over the skin with a smooth, continuous motion.
3. (Pacing) (Pressure) used during petrissage should avoid bruising the tissues.
4. (Superficial) (Subcutaneous) friction generates heat on the skin by brisk rubbing over the skin surface and is done best with little or no lubricant.
5. (Cyriax) (Deep) friction is applied in parallel fiber, cross fiber, or circular movements.
6. Tapotement consists of a series of brisk (percussive) (sliding) movements following each other in light, rapid, rhythmic, alternating fashion.
7. Variations of tapotement are achieved by altering (hand position) (force used).

8. Deep vibration or trembling motion is imparted by the fingertips, but generated by (forearm) (shoulder).
9. A variation of shaking with movement back and forth from hand to hand, usually of a limb, that causes movement in related joints is called (jostling) (wagging).
10. In (resisted) (assisted) movements, the client initiates the movement, while the practitioner helps complete it.
11. Joint manipulations intended to realign misaligned joints by sudden thrusting movements (are) (are not) within the scope of massage therapy.
12. Stay within the (extended) (normal) range of motion of the joint when performing joint movement techniques.

13. Joint mobilizing techniques can be characterized as (smooth, loose) (controlled, precise).
14. When using reciprocal inhibition to enhance a stretch, the (agonist) (antagonist) of the targeted muscle is contracted prior to the stretch.
15. Use client (feedback) (height) to determine the limits of a stretch.
16. Joint abnormalities may be (congenital) (constitutional) or may be the result of accidents, injuries, or diseases.

Test Prep

The following multiple-choice questions will help to prepare you for future school and professional exams.

1. The variation of effleurage that is applied with deep pressure along the length of the muscle fibers, often with the thumb, is:
   a. Basic sliding effleurage
   b. Stripping
   c. Shingles effleurage
   d. Bilateral tree stroking
2. Horizontal stroking applied to broad, rounded areas such as the thigh and lower back can be considered a hybrid form of:
   a. Basic stroking and vibration
   b. Petrissage and friction
   c. Vibration and tapotement
   d. Effleurage and petrissage
3. If your intention were to increase superficial circulation *and* remove fascial adhesions in the skin on the recipient's back, your best choice of technique would be:
   a. Basic effleurage
   b. Skin rolling
   c. Tapping
   d. Deep vibration
4. The form of tapotement that makes a hollow sound, creates a slight vacuum when applied, and is used on the back and chest for treating respiratory congestion is:
   a. Hacking
   b. Pincement
   c. Rapping
   d. Cupping
5. For ending a session with a calming technique that is also thought to help balance energy in the body, your best choice of the following techniques would be:
   a. Passive touch
   b. Ischemic compression
   c. Fine vibration
   d. Quacking
6. The best technique for moving soft tissues around boney joints such as the knee, ankle, and wrist is:
   a. Nerve strokes
   b. Knuckling
   c. Fingertip friction
   d. Passive touch

7. A form of compression that is sometimes referred to as *static friction* is:
   a. Deep friction
   b. Direct pressure
   c. Pincement
   d. One-handed kneading
8. In deep transverse or Cyriax friction:
   a. Fingers slide over the skin to stretch deeper tissues.
   b. Fingers and skin move together over deeper tissues.
   c. Friction on the skin increases superficial circulation.
   d. Fingertips move in circular motion around a tender spot.
9. How is full, firm contact best achieved when applying effleurage techniques with the hands?
   a. Hands mold to the surface of the body.
   b. Hands are held stiffly and only the palms touch the body.
   c. Hands are relaxed and only fingertips touch the body.
   d. Fingers are spread and rake the skin.
10. Before applying deep massage techniques, tissues in the area should be thoroughly:
    a. Cooled off
    b. Warmed up
    c. Frictioned
    d. Lubricated
11. Movements performed entirely by a person without assistance from anyone else are called:
    a. Passive resisted
    b. Free active
    c. Active assisted
    d. Free resisted
12. Which of the following joint movements is not within the scope of massage therapy?
    a. Figure-8s of the toes
    b. Extension of the arm overhead
    c. Thrusting on the back
    d. Flexion of the ankle
13. A simple, static stretch is a type of stretch characterized by:
    a. Slow, sustained, and even application
    b. Sudden, forceful movements
    c. Forceful bouncing
    d. Slow, even bouncing

14. A contraindication for joint movement techniques is:
    a. Muscle soreness
    b. Muscle shortening
    c. Acute inflammation
    d. Osteoarthritis
15. Time the stretch to the client's:
    a. Holding his or her breath
    b. Inhale
    c. Exhale
    d. Diaphragmatic breath
16. For the contract–relax–stretch technique, the client contracts the:
    a. Target muscle just before the stretch
    b. Target muscle right after the stretch
    c. Antagonist to the target muscle just before the stretch
    d. Antagonist to the target muscle right after the stretch

17. Which is the best indication that a stretch is at its safe limit?
    a. When the practitioner feels a little resistance in the tissues
    b. When the skin in the area turns color
    c. When the practitioner hears a snap
    d. When the client tells the practitioner the limit has been reached
18. Care around hypermobile joints is advised because they may be prone to:
    a. Dislocation
    b. Adhesions
    c. Swelling
    d. Hyperextension

Video Challenge

Watch the appropriate segment of the video on your DVD and then answer the following questions.

Western Massage Techniques

Petrissage
1. Notice that various types of petrissage are demonstrated on different parts of the body. Why were specific body areas chosen for these petrissage demonstrations?

Tapotement
2. Notice that variations of the technique make different sounds. Can you describe the different sounds made by these tapotement variations?

Effleurage, Petrissage, and Friction
3. What do you notice about the color of the receiver's skin in the area of the technique application? Why does this change in color occur?

Joint Movements
4. What are the three guidelines mentioned in the video for joint mobilizations?
5. Describe the technique shown in the video for mobilizing the shoulder with the client in the supine position.
6. What are the four guidelines mentioned in the video for stretching techniques?

Comprehension Exercises

The following short-answer questions test your knowledge and understanding of chapter topics and provide practice in written communication skills. Explain in two to four complete sentences.

1. Describe superficial and deep friction. Why are both of these techniques considered friction? How are they different?

2. Describe the use of lubricant when applying Western massage techniques. How does the optimal amount of lubricant differ among different techniques? Give an example.
3. Explain how the principle of reciprocal inhibition can enhance a simple static stretch.

For Greater Understanding

The following exercises are designed to take you from the realm of theory into the real world. They will help give you a deeper understanding of the subjects covered in this chapter. Action words are underlined to emphasize the variety of activities presented to address different learning styles and to encourage deeper thinking.

1. After developing skill in the techniques illustrated in the book, underline{experiment} with your own technique variations. underline{Explain} to a practice partner why you think your variation would be effective.
2. underline{Watch} a video of a full-body Western massage (or portion of a session), underline{identify} the techniques and how they are used in the session (e.g., warming, transition, ending), and note their different effects (e.g., circulatory, muscle relaxation, general relaxation). You may substitute a live massage session for the video.
3. In a group of three, one person underline{talks} another through performing a particular stretch on a receiver lying on the massage table. He or she underline{describes} step-by-step how the technique is performed. Include static, contract–relax–stretch, CRS with reciprocal inhibition, and active assisted stretching.

14 Full-Body Western Massage

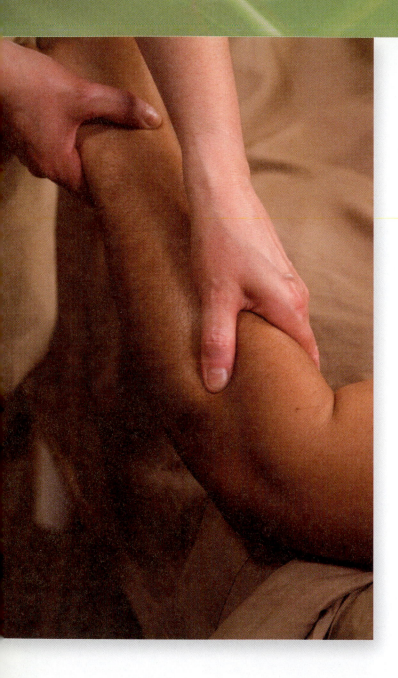

 CHAPTER OUTLINE

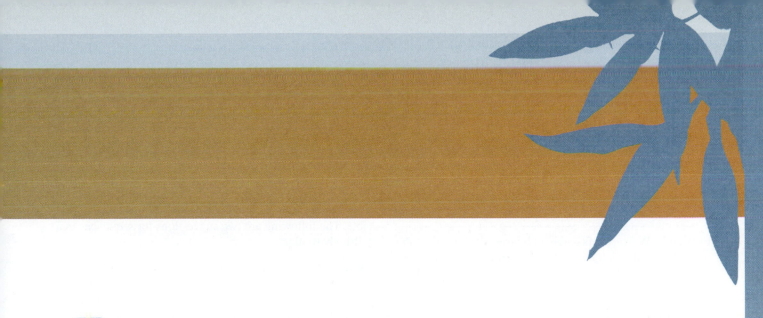

 LEARNING OUTCOMES

After studying this chapter, you will have information to:

1. Describe a full-body Western massage.
2. Organize a massage session from body region to body region.
3. Apply techniques in appropriate order within each body region.
4. Choose opening, warm-up, transition, and finishing techniques appropriately.
5. Apply the principles of continuity, rhythm, pacing, specificity, and pressure.
6. Perform a 1-hour full-body Western massage for health promotion.

 KEY TERMS

Continuity *420*
Finishing techniques *419*
Flow *420*
Full-body Western massage *418*

Opening technique *418*
Pacing *420*
Pressure *420*
Rhythm *420*

Specificity *420*
Transition techniques *419*
Warming technique *418*

OVERVIEW

Full-body Western massage addresses all regions of the body. It usually includes techniques from all seven of the basic Western massage technique categories. Oil, lotion, or other lubricant is typically used to enhance sliding over the skin and to prevent chafing. Full-body massage sessions last from 30–90 minutes, with the 60-minute format being the most common.

Performed from a wellness perspective, these sessions focus on general health and well-being, as well as meeting the specific therapeutic needs of the recipient. The goals for health promotion include improving circulation, relaxing the muscles, improving joint mobility, inducing the relaxation response, promoting healthy skin, and creating a general sense of well-being.

GUIDELINES FOR FULL-BODY MASSAGE

Although each practitioner combines and blends various massage techniques in different ways, there are some general guidelines for giving a full-body massage. These guidelines address draping, sequence of body parts, order of techniques, continuity, rhythm, pacing, specificity, and pressure. Table 14.1■ summarizes the guidelines for performing full-body massage.

Draping

Draping is done with a sheet or large towel, and body parts are skillfully uncovered and recovered as needed. Genitals are covered at all times. Women's breasts are always covered, except when breast massage is performed by a practitioner with special training and then only with informed consent of the recipient. Breast massage is not yet common in the United States and, therefore, will not be included in the general full-body routine described in this chapter.

Sequence of Body Regions

In a full-body session, the practitioner massages each region of the body (e.g., back, arms, and legs) in a particular sequence. The sequence usually includes supine and prone positions, and has a starting point, direction (e.g., clockwise), and an ending point. This establishes a routine way of working.

Recipients lie prone or supine for the first part of the massage, and then turn over for the second part. Whether they start prone or supine is a matter of preference for the practitioner and the recipient. Sometimes the side-lying or semireclining positions are used, for example, with special populations.

There are no hard and fast rules for sequence, but it should facilitate a smooth flow from one region of the body to the next. Some advocate moving clockwise around the table. The following are two suggestions for sequences in a full-body routine.

- If a session starts with the recipient in the prone position, a commonly used sequence of body sections would be the back, buttocks, and legs. The neck and feet are sometimes addressed prone, but are more easily accessed supine. Then turn over to the supine position with a sequence moving from legs and feet, shoulders, arms and hands, chest and abdomen, neck, and ending with the head and face.
- If the session starts with the recipient in the supine position, a commonly used sequence of body sections would be head and face, neck and shoulders, arms and hands, chest and abdomen, legs and feet. Then turn over to the prone position with a sequence moving from buttocks to legs and ending on the back.

The advantages of starting in the prone position include that it may feel safer to a recipient new to massage, and back massage triggers the relaxation response sooner. It also allows those who need to be more alert at the end of the session to finish face-up. An advantage of starting in the supine position is that the practitioner can massage the head, face, and neck right away, which may be appreciated by recipients who do a lot of desk or computer work.

Order of Techniques

The general order of techniques for each region of the body is similar. Once a part is undraped, opening and warming techniques are applied. These are followed by a combination of techniques for general health promotion, as well as techniques for specific therapeutic effects. Finishing and transition techniques complete work on the region.

The most common **opening technique** and **warming technique** for each area to be massaged is effleurage. It is used to apply oil or lotion, to warm the area, and to facilitate circulation. It is applied first using lighter and then deeper pressure. Effleurage on the limbs should always be performed moving distal to proximal, unless the pressure used is very light. Compressions may also serve as an opening or warming technique.

The opening is followed by a combination of techniques to improve circulation, relax muscles, improve joint

TABLE 14.1	Summary of the Elements of a Full-Body Western Massage Routine
Goals	General health promotion
	Improved circulation, relaxed muscles, improved joint mobility, relaxation response, healthy skin, sense of well-being
	Therapeutic needs (e.g., reduce muscle stiffness and soreness, relieve trigger points, injury recovery)
Length of Time	30–90 minutes (typically 60 minutes)
Draping	Full sheet or large towel
	Body regions uncovered for massage and then recovered
	Genitals and women's breasts covered at all times
Sequence of Body Regions	Starting prone:
Starting point	Start on back
Direction (e.g., clockwise)	Buttocks, legs
Ending point	*Turn to supine*
	Legs/feet, arms/shoulders, chest, abdomen
	End with neck, head, and face
	Starting supine:
	Start on head and face
	Neck, arms/shoulders, chest, abdomen, legs/feet
	Turn to prone
	Legs, buttocks
	End with back
Order of Techniques on a Specific Body Region	Opening technique (e.g., effleurage to apply oil or compressions)
	Warming techniques (e.g., effleurage or compressions)
	Combination of techniques
	For general health (e.g., effleurage, petrissage, superficial warming friction, joint movements)
	Specific therapeutic goals (e.g., deep friction, vibration, direct pressure)
	Transition techniques (e.g., effleurage, tapotement, compression)
	Finishing techniques (e.g., effleurage, tapotement, compression)
Continuity	Sense of continuous touch throughout the session
	Avoid abrupt removal of touch
Flow	Orderly sequence and smooth transitions
	Skillful draping
Rhythm	Smooth and even rhythm
Pacing	Moderate speed
Specificity	For attention to specific muscle or small area
	Shorter length session = less specificity in full-body massage
Pressure	Medium to light pressure, heavier pressure by request
	Vary according to part of body massaged and condition of tissues
	Feedback from recipient at the beginning of the session, and after moving to a different area

mobility, and other health promotion goals. Technique combinations at this stage usually include effleurage, petrissage, warming friction, and joint movements. Deep friction, vibration, and direct pressure are applied as appropriate for more specific applications. Finish massage of the area with effleurage, tapotement, and/or compression.

Transition techniques serve to provide continuity and flow from one section to another. For example, when moving from massage of the upper leg to the lower leg, a few effleurage strokes to the entire leg help tie the regions together kinesthetically for the recipient.

When ending work on a specific part of the body, the prone or supine side, or the entire session, some thought should be given to finishing techniques. **Finishing techniques** may be used to reconnect parts of the body that have been worked on more specifically or to further sedate or stimulate the recipient. Effleurage, tapotement, and compression are typical finishing techniques that can create a sense of wholeness, connectedness, and completeness. Light effleurage, sometimes called nerve strokes, is more soothing, while tapotement is more stimulating. Passive touch in the form of simple holding at the head or feet is calming and is sometimes used to end a session.

Continuity and Flow

A skillful full-body massage has a sense of continuity and flow. **Continuity** is achieved by creating a sense of continuous contact throughout the session from the initial touch to the finishing touches. Establishment or removal of touch is never abrupt. This does not mean that you may never take your hands off a recipient during a session, but that doing so is kept to a minimum and is done as imperceptibly as possible.

A sense of **flow** is achieved through an orderly sequence and smooth transitions from one part of the body to the next. Skill in draping, including uncovering and recovering, can add to the sense of smooth transitions.

Rhythm, Pacing, Specificity, Pressure

The **rhythm** of a classic full-body massage session may be described as smooth and even, and the **pacing** as moderate

in speed. Trying to perform a full-body session in half an hour will necessitate a faster pace with less attention to detail. A session focusing on general relaxation will be slower paced and usually minimize or eliminate such stimulating techniques as tapotement. **Specificity** is required for attention to a specific muscle or small area. If the recipient requests more attention to certain parts of the body, such as the back and neck, then those areas would receive more time and specific techniques, while the rest of the body would receive less specific massage. The amount of **pressure** used for full-body massage varies from medium to light, although some clients may like heavy pressure. Vary the pressure used according to the part of the body massaged. For example, use lighter pressure on the face and medium to heavy pressure on more muscular areas. Ask for feedback about pressure near the beginning of the session to get a sense of the client's preference and after moving to a new region.

FULL-BODY WESTERN MASSAGE PRACTICE SEQUENCE

There is no one best way to perform a full-body Western massage. Practitioners usually develop their own styles and routine ways of performing a massage session. Routines generally involve a regular starting point and opening techniques, a specific sequence of body regions, a certain order of techniques in each body region, and a regular way of ending the session. These routines typically change with further training and experience, and are modified to meet the needs of the recipient on the table. Today's eclectic practitioners may use a full-body Western routine as a starting point and then integrate contemporary techniques as appropriate to accomplish the therapeutic goals of the session.

Some spas and salons offer what they call a *signature massage,* which is a massage routine that is given uniformly by all massage therapists in the establishment. This provides some standardization, and customers know what to expect. Establishments train their employees to perform their signature massages.

The following Practice Sequence is an example of a 1-hour full-body routine that may be used to practice the basic Western massage techniques on different parts of the body. By having a routine as a framework, the learner is free to focus on specific skills, including good body mechanics, draping, specific techniques, smooth transitions, continuity, rhythm, and pacing.

It is impossible to describe every single movement of a routine in writing. Use the Practice Sequence offered here as a framework, but feel free to add variations of techniques as you become more attuned to the work. Experiment with what feels right to you. To lengthen the routine, you may repeat techniques or insert additional techniques as appropriate.

REALITY CHECK

ESTEBAN

JENNIFER: I think I'm using too much pressure in my full-body massage. I can feel my practice clients tensing up, and sometimes they tell me to "lighten up." I don't realize I'm hurting them until they say something to me. I'm just really strong. How can I learn to develop a better sense of the pressure I'm using?

ESTEBAN: Varying pressure according to the situation is part of the art of massage. Work with a practice partner to learn to vary the pressure you are applying. It doesn't matter how strong you are, you can learn to control how much pressure you use. And remember that individual preferences regarding pressure vary a lot. Some people have lower tolerance for pressure for reasons that are not always apparent. That's why it's good to start with what you think is medium pressure (less than your heaviest pressure), and ask for feedback. You can go lighter or heavier from there. Also look for nonverbal signs earlier. Be prepared to go as light or heavy as clients want within reasonable limits.

PRACTICE SEQUENCE

14.1
I-hour massage

Full-Body Western Massage

Preliminary Instructions

• Before leaving the recipient alone to undress in private, request that he or she be covered with the drape and lying face down on the table when you return. Show the recipient how the face cradle works.
• Before the session starts, adjust the position of the face cradle and place a bolster under the ankles.

Recipient prone
Region: Back (15 minutes)

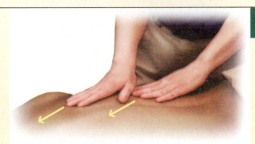

FIGURE 14.1 Uncover the back down to the waist. Stand at the head to apply lubricant to the back using long effleurage strokes. Cover the entire back and sides using light to moderate pressure.

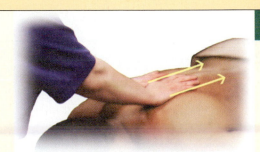

FIGURE 14.2 Without losing contact, move to the recipient's right side. Stand at the hip and face the head. Apply shingles effleurage along the right side of the spine with fingers pointing toward the head. Use moderate to deep pressure. Repeat 3–4 times.

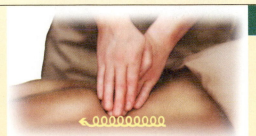

FIGURE 14.3 Apply deep circular friction with the fingertips to the erector muscles on the right side, moving from the sacrum to the neck. To apply deeper pressure, use both hands, placing one hand on top of the other. Circle away from the spine. Repeat twice.

4

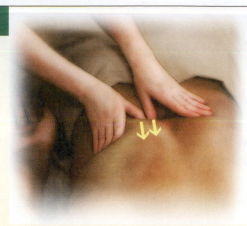

FIGURE 14.4 Apply deep effleurage with the thumbs between the iliac crest and the last three ribs. Keep the thumbs in proper alignment. Repeat this technique in two or three strips, moving out laterally from the spine. Alternative (not shown): Warming friction using the knuckles may be substituted as easier on the hands. Less lubricant is used so that friction can be created.

5

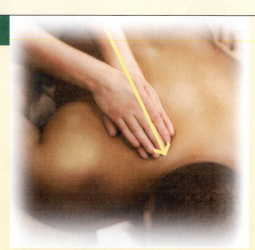

FIGURE 14.5 Reconnect the lower back with the shoulder with a few deep effleurage strokes. Then place one hand over the other to apply greater pressure for a circular movement around the shoulder. Repeat 3–4 times.

6

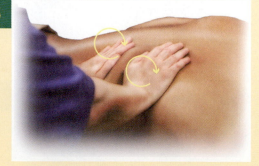

FIGURE 14.6 Starting at the waist, apply circular two-handed petrissage over the entire right side. Keep hands flat with full contact on the back surface. Both hands move clockwise. Lift superficial soft tissues as hands pass each other.
Alternative (not shown): Use skin rolling if the skin does not lift easily and appears to be adhering to soft tissues underneath. It can be applied to the entire back or in specific areas of adhering.

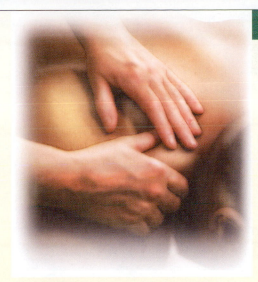

7

FIGURE 14.7 Knead the upper trapezius with one or two hands. Lift, squeeze, and release the soft tissues in a rhythmical motion.

Apply kneading across the shoulder and up the neck. Get feedback from client about the amount of pressure you are using.

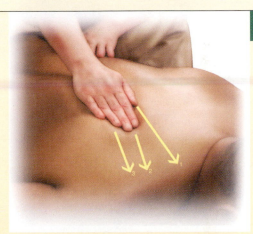

8

FIGURE 14.8 Walk around the head of the table to the left side and reach across to perform three-count stroking to the right shoulder (trapezius). Cover the lower, middle, and upper trapezius. Keep flat, firm contact that conforms to the body contour. Repeat 3–4 times.

Note: Perform from same side if it is too difficult to reach across the table.

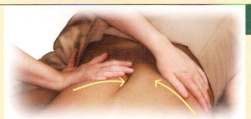

9

FIGURE 14.9 Reconnect the lower and upper back with horizontal stroking from lower back to shoulders. Keep flat, firm contact that conforms to the body contour. Repeat twice.

Repeat Steps 2–9 on the left side.

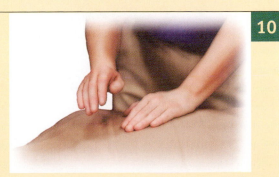

10

FIGURE 14.10 When both sides of the back have been massaged, redrape the back. With light to moderate force, use rapping or some other form of tapotement as a finishing technique for the entire back.

Region: Lower Limbs and Buttocks (10 minutes)

11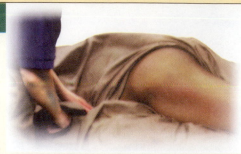

FIGURE 14.11 Undrape the left leg up to the waist, being careful not to expose the gluteal cleft. Tuck the drape securely under the hip and at the waist. When massaging the legs and buttocks, your hands should never touch or come unreasonably close to the genital area.

12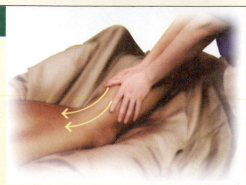

FIGURE 14.12 Stand at the side of the table facing the head. Apply lubricant with effleurage from ankle to hip following the curves of the leg and using moderate pressure. Contact the sides and posterior surfaces. The inside hand will slide onto the back of the leg about half way up the thigh and follow the outside hand around the buttocks and hip. Hands return together to the ankle with a light sliding motion.

13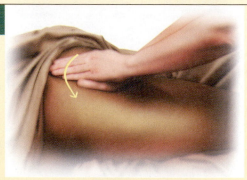

FIGURE 14.13 Apply deep circular effleurage to the buttocks muscles as a warming technique. Place one hand on top of the other for reinforcement. Follow the contour of the area moving medial to lateral and around the hip.

14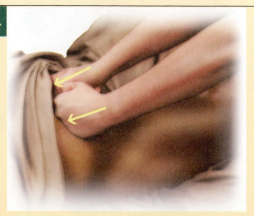

FIGURE 14.14 Apply compressions over the entire buttocks region with the fist using moderate to heavy pressure. Include the attachments along the iliac crest. Finish with circular effleurage, using either the hand-over-hand position or the fist. Transition with 2–3 long effleurage strokes to the entire leg.

FIGURE 14.15 Apply effleurage to hamstring muscles with fists from just above the popliteal fossa to the superior attachments of the hamstring muscles. Alternative: Use the forearm to apply the effleurage for more pressure.

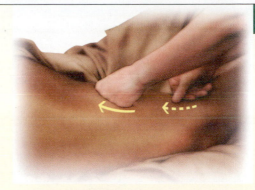

FIGURE 14.16 Continuing with one fist, perform effleurage along the iliotibial band and the tensor fascia lata muscle moving from the hip to the knee. This broad band of fascia and muscle can accept moderate to deep pressure.

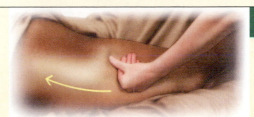

FIGURE 14.17 Place one hand on the medial and one on the lateral thigh to begin horizontal stroking. Slide hands up and around the thigh, exchanging positions with a smooth sliding and lifting motion. Apply from the knee to just below the attachments of the adductors. Be mindful of professional boundaries when touching the inside of the leg.

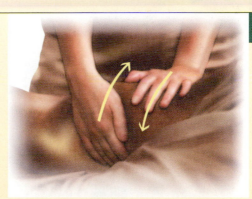

FIGURE 14.18 Two-handed kneading on the upper leg. Apply kneading to medial, posterior, and lateral muscles of the thigh.

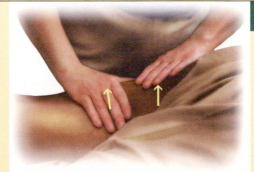

19

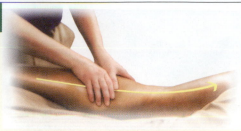

FIGURE 14.19 Basic effleurage distal to proximal as a transition technique. Apply first to the upper thigh and then to the entire leg.

20

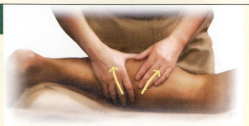

FIGURE 14.20 Two-handed kneading to lower leg muscles. Knead the belly of the calf muscles using two hands alternating in an even rhythm.

21

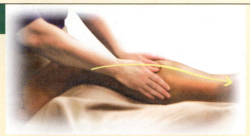

FIGURE 14.21 Basic sliding effleurage to the lower leg. Apply from heel of foot to knee. Conform hands to contour of leg for full contact.

22

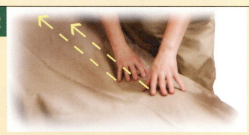

FIGURE 14.22 Finishing techniques to entire leg. Start with basic effleurage from ankle to hip. Redrape the leg. Finish with a few nerve strokes from the buttocks to the ankle.

Repeat Steps 11–22 on the right side. Afterward, continue with Step 23.

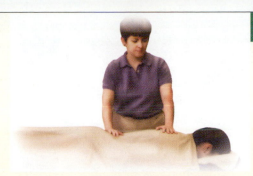

FIGURE 14.23 Finishing techniques for the back of the body. With the recipient fully draped, gently rock the body from side to side, from back to hips to legs for about 5 seconds. Perform 2–3 light effleurage stokes from shoulders to feet over the drape as a connecting maneuver, and to signal the end of the massage on the back side of the body.

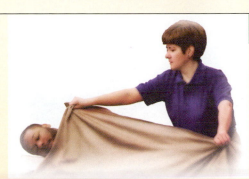

FIGURE 14.24 Turning over technique: Use tenting to assist the recipient turning to supine position. Anchor the drape with your leg against the side of the table and hold the other side of the drape up slightly. Have the recipient roll away from you to prevent him or her from getting wrapped up in the sheet. Lower the drape.

Note: The recipient should have been out of your sight as he or she turned over under the tent. If there is more than one session going on in the room, be sure that you do not expose the recipient to others.

Recipient supine
Region: Lower limbs (10 minutes)

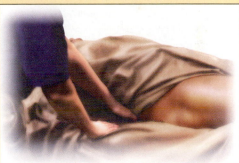

FIGURE 14.25 Undrape the right leg. Tuck the drape securely under the thigh.

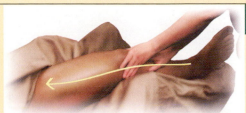

FIGURE 14.26 Apply lubricant to the entire right limb using basic sliding effleurage. Apply moderate pressure distal to proximal, and slide back with light touch. Hands conform to the contour of the leg for maximal contact. Lighten pressure over knee. Cover anterior, medial, and lateral aspects of the limb.

27

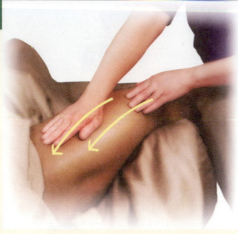

FIGURE 14.27 Apply deep effleurage to the thigh from knee to superior thigh. Cover anterior, medial, and lateral aspects of the thigh. Use flat hands or loose fists to apply pressure.

28

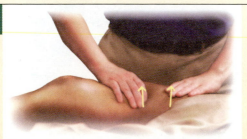

FIGURE 14.28 Apply two-handed kneading to quadriceps, adductor, and abductor muscles of the thigh.

29

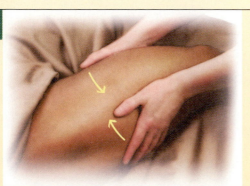

FIGURE 14.29 Jostle the thigh, tossing from side to side, hand to hand. Causes loose, free movement in the hip and knee joints.

30

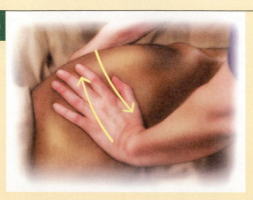

FIGURE 14.30 Place one hand on the medial and one on the lateral thigh to begin horizontal stroking. Slide hands up and around the thigh, exchanging positions with a smooth sliding and lifting motion.   Apply from the knee to the superior thigh. Be mindful of professional boundaries when touching the inside of the leg.

FIGURE 14.31 Effleurage to transition to lower leg—distal to proximal. Apply effleurage with moderate pressure to thigh first, and then to entire limb from ankle to thigh. Follow with effleurage from ankle to knee.

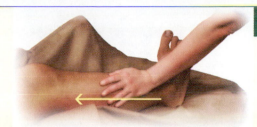

FIGURE 14.32 Apply circular friction around the knee with the heels of the hands moving the skin over soft tissues underneath. Stay to sides of the kneecap.

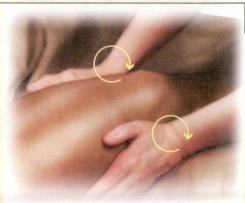

FIGURE 14.33 Use thumbs to apply stripping effleurage to the muscle just lateral to the shin bone (tibialis anterior). Apply from ankle to the attachments near the lateral condyle of the tibia. Complete 2–4 strips, depending on the size of the muscle.

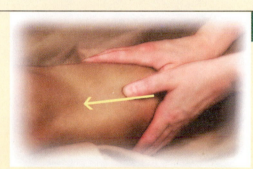

FIGURE 14.34 Direct thumb pressure along the tibialis anterior. Start at proximal end, moving about 1 inch at a time to distal end. Keep thumb and wrist in good alignment. Use moderate to heavy pressure. Transition with effleurage over lower limb.

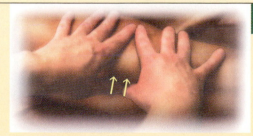

35

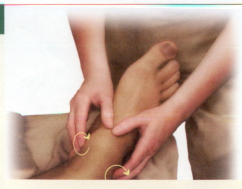

FIGURE 14.35 Circular friction around the ankle with the fingertips. Applying pressure with the fingertips, move the skin around the ankle over underlying soft tissues. Follow the contour of the ankle bones.

36

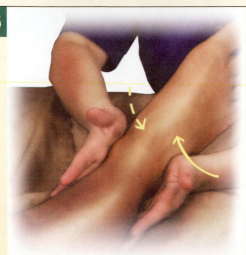

FIGURE 14.36 Mobilize the ankle using the heels of the hands. Place the heels of the hands just under the ankle bones. Shift the hands back and forth causing movement side to side in the ankle. Action is free and loose.

37

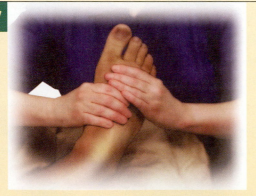

FIGURE 14.37 Squeeze the foot lightly from heel to toes. Fingers of hands on top with thumbs around the sides and underneath. Apply slight pressure to the sides to spread the metatarsals.

FIGURE 14.38 Effleurage between the metatarsals using the thumb or fingers. Slide between the metatarsals one-by-one from the toes to the ankle.

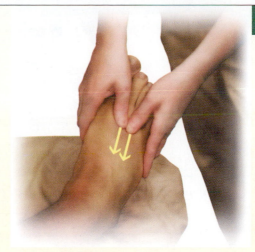

38

FIGURE 14.39 Slide along the bottom of the foot with the fist. Apply from the ball of the foot to the heel. Use moderate to deep pressure. Other hand supports the foot from the dorsal side.

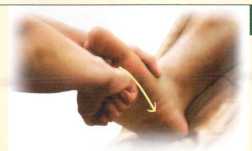

39

FIGURE 14.40 Slapping tapotement on the bottom of the foot. Slap lightly 4–5 times.

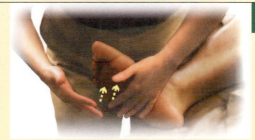

40

FIGURE 14.41 Effleurage to the entire limb with moderate pressure, followed by nerve strokes as a finishing technique. Apply effleurage distal to proximal, and then redrape the leg. Apply nerve strokes proximal to distal over the drape to finish.

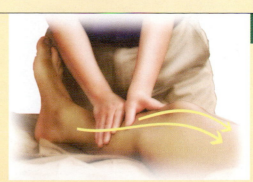

41

Repeat Steps 25–41 on the left leg. Afterward, continue with Step 42.

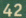

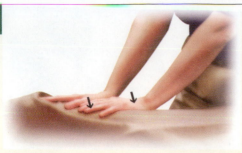

FIGURE 14.42 Transition from the lower to the upper limbs with compression over the drape. Apply compression with palms over the leg and then up the arm to the shoulder as a connecting and transition technique.

Region: Arms, Shoulders, Chest (10 minutes)

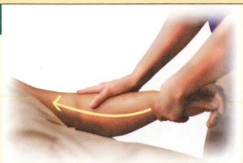

FIGURE 14.43 Uncover the left arm and shoulder. Apply oil or lotion to the arm with effleurage from hand to shoulder, including the deltoid muscle.

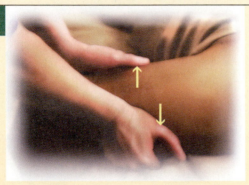

FIGURE 14.44 Alternating one-hand kneading to the upper arm. Squeeze the biceps side, then the triceps side, alternating in a rhythmical motion. Cover the entire upper arm from the shoulder to the elbow.

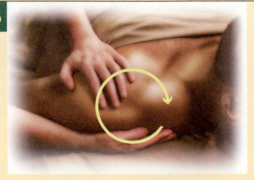

FIGURE 14.45 Passive shoulder roll. Place one hand on the anterior and the other on the posterior shoulder. Circle the shoulder clockwise, then counterclockwise twice in each direction.

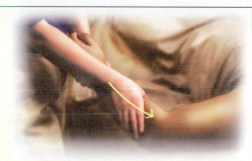

FIGURE 14.46 Effleurage to transition to forearm—distal to proximal. Apply effleurage with moderate pressure to upper arm first, and then to entire arm from wrist to shoulder. Follow with deep effleurage from wrist to elbow.

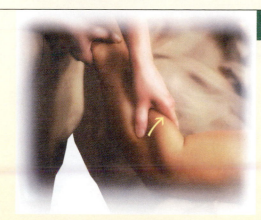

FIGURE 14.47 One hand kneads the forearm muscles, while the other hand stabilizes the arm at the wrist.

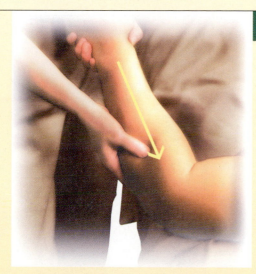

FIGURE 14.48 Apply stripping effleurage with the thumb to the flexor and extensor muscles of the forearm. Apply from the wrist to their attachments near the elbow.

49

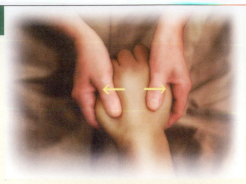

FIGURE 14.49 Warm wrist and hand. Palm down, hold the hand on the little finger and thumb sides, then gently squeeze the hand while broadening the palm and separating the metacarpals. Apply effleurage with the thumbs to back of the wrist, and then between metacarpals. Turn the palm up to apply effleurage to the palm of the hand.

50

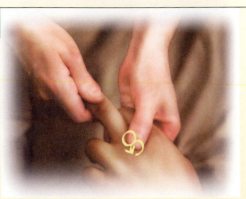

FIGURE 14.50 Mobilize the joints in the hand. Follow with figure-8s at the knuckles and scissoring the metacarpals.

51

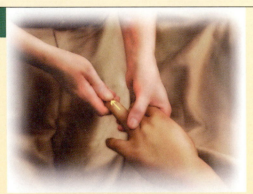

FIGURE 14.51 Lightly squeeze along each finger applying pressure first near the knuckle and then moving along the finger to the tip.

52

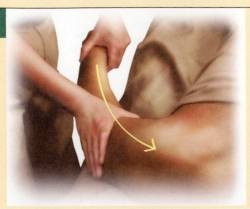

FIGURE 14.52 Effleurage to entire arm to reconnect and transition to the chest. Apply effleurage with moderate pressure from hand to shoulder 2–3 times.

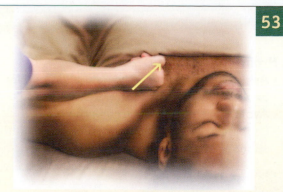

FIGURE 14.53 Effleurage to pectoral muscles using fist. Lift the arm, holding just below the wrist. Apply effleurage over the pectoral muscles with a loose fist, moving lateral to medial and stopping at the breast tissue.

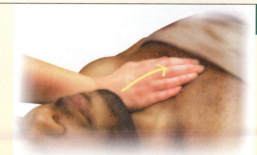

FIGURE 14.54 Effleurage over sternum. Apply with the palm of the hand between breast tissue. Omit this technique if a woman recipient has large breasts or if she might feel it is an invasion of her personal boundaries. Ask permission if in doubt.

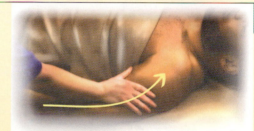

FIGURE 14.55 Effleurage to the entire area with moderate pressure as a finishing technique. Apply effleurage distal to proximal, and then redrape the arm and shoulder.

Repeat Steps 43–55 on the right arm. Afterward, continue with Step 56.

Region: Abdomen (5 minutes)

Preliminary Considerations:
• Ask permission to massage the abdomen if the recipient is new to massage or new to you.
• Explain to women that the breasts will be draped.
• Avoid if recipient has eaten in the last hour.
• People experiencing constipation or gas in the bowels may be sensitive to pressure. Get feedback about their comfort.

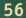

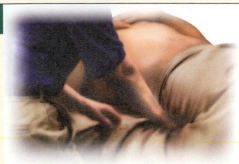

FIGURE 14.56 Drape recipient for abdominal massage. Tuck drape along sides for secure anchoring. Do not expose the pubic area. (Cover women's breasts before pulling the sheet to the iliac crest exposing the abdomen.)

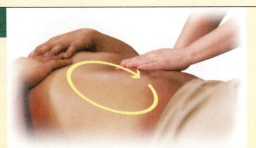

FIGURE 14.57 Circular clockwise pattern. Gently lay a hand on the abdomen to establish contact. Apply effleurage with one hand while the other rests on top. Move in a large circle along the bottom of the ribs and around the outline of the pelvis. Check with the recipient to make sure the pressure is comfortable.

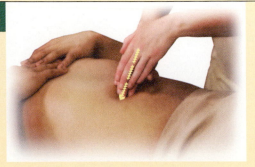

FIGURE 14.58 Vibration to the abdomen with the fingertips. Apply vibration from spot to spot in a clockwise pattern. Stop if the recipient reports feeling pain.

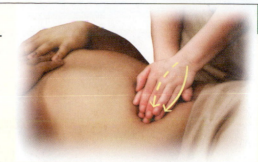

FIGURE 14.59 Petrissage with a flat hand. Apply compression across the abdomen in a wavelike motion. Push in first with the heel of the hand and then roll onto the fingertips, repeating the wave with rhythmic movement.

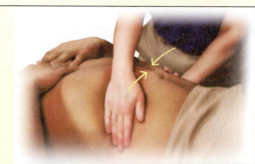

FIGURE 14.60 Horizontal stroking of the abdomen. Place a hand on either side of the waist, fingers pointing away from you. Slide and lift the hands to the other side simultaneously. Hands cross in the middle. Repeat 3–4 times.

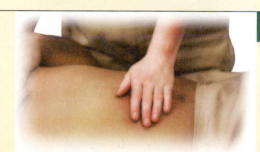

FIGURE 14.61 Passive touch in center of abdomen as finishing technique. Place a hand gently in the center of the abdomen and rest there for a moment. Remove your hand and recover the recipient to the shoulders with the larger drape. (If the recipient is a woman, the breast drape may remain in place for warmth or may be removed at this time.)

Region: Neck and Shoulders (5 minutes)

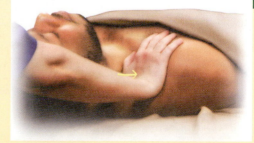

FIGURE 14.62 Mobilize shoulders with "cat paw" technique. Place a hand on each shoulder to establish contact. Mobilize the shoulders by alternating pushing one side and then the other with a slow rhythmical motion. Perform from a sitting position or a low horse stance at the head of the table.

63

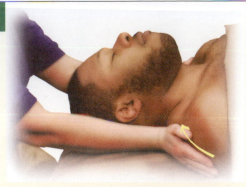

FIGURE 14.63 Apply oil or lotion with effleurage to both sides of the neck. With recipient face-up, apply oil or lotion with both hands (one on each side of the neck) sliding along the upper trapezius from the shoulder tips to the occipital ridge.

Note: Steps 64–67 are all applied to one side of the neck at a time before proceeding with Step 68.

64

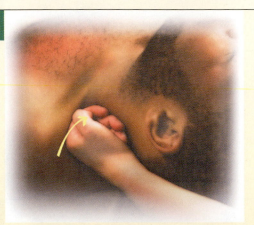

FIGURE 14.64 Effleurage with loose fist to left side of neck. Turn the head slightly to the right side, exposing the left side of the neck. Perform effleurage with the fist on the upper trapezius from the occipital ridge to the shoulder. Creates a mild stretch in the upper trapezius.

65

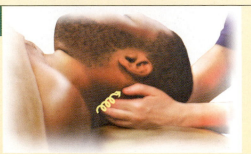

FIGURE 14.65 Apply circular friction to the left side of the neck along cervical muscles with the fingertips of your left hand. Start at the base of the neck moving up along the cervical muscles to the suboccipital region. Use moderate pressure to warm the deeper muscles.

66

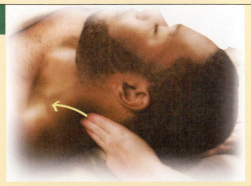

FIGURE 14.66 Stripping effleurage along cervical muscles. Using the fingertips or a knuckle to apply deep effleurage to the posterior cervical muscles from the suboccipital region to the base of the neck. Feel the stretching and broadening of the cervical muscles.

FIGURE 14.67 Effleurage as a finishing and transition technique. Finish the left side with effleurage moving back and forth from the tip of the shoulder to the suboccipital region. Use palm of hand or fist. Return the head to face upward.

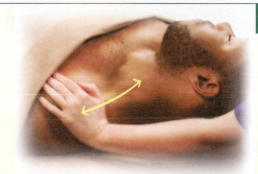

Repeat Steps 64–67 on the right side. Afterward, continue with Step 68.

FIGURE 14.68 Wavelike neck mobilization. Place the hands palms up at the base of the neck, one on either side of the spine, with fingertips pressing up on the cervical muscles. Draw the fingers toward the occiput, maintaining pressure upward. The cervical vertebrae will rise and fall as the fingers pass underneath. If the muscles are relaxed, this will create a wavelike motion in the neck.

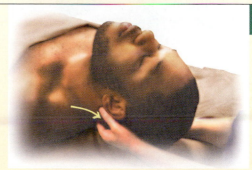

FIGURE 14.69 Finish with effleurage and passive touch. Apply effleurage to both sides simultaneously, starting at the tips of the shoulders and drawing the hands toward the base of the neck and up to the occipital ridge. Repeat twice.

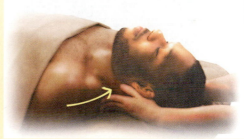

FIGURE 14.70 Cradle the head briefly in both hands to end this section.

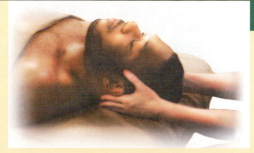

Region: Face and Head (5 minutes).

Preliminary Considerations:
• Ask permission to massage the face, especially if the recipient is wearing makeup.
• Do not use oil on the face and use lotion only if the skin is dry.

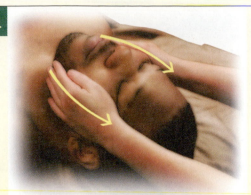

FIGURE 14.71 Apply effleurage to face with palms. Place the hands gently on the face with fingertips at the jaw. Draw the hands toward the temples using the full palm-side of the hands. Repeat 2–3 times.

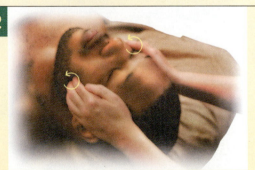

FIGURE 14.72 Circular friction to jaw muscles and temples. Apply circular friction with the fingertips over the masseter and then the temporalis muscles.

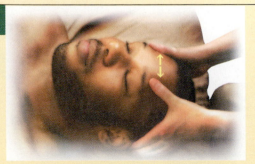

FIGURE 14.73 Effleurage to forehead. Use the thumbs to stroke the muscles of the forehead, applying effleurage medial to lateral. Repeat 2–3 times.

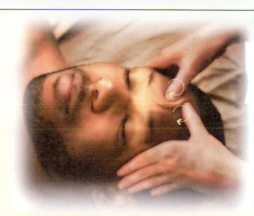

FIGURE 14.74 Circular petrissage to forehead. Use the thumbs moving in counterclockwise circles. The movement is timed so that the tissues are lifted and pressed as the thumbs move past one another.

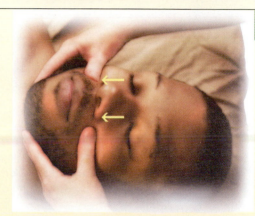

FIGURE 14.75 Stroke alongside the nose and under the cheekbones. Use the thumbs to slide down the sides of the nose, ending in the indentation at the inferior end. Continue under the cheekbones, moving bilaterally. Repeat twice.

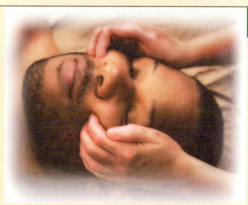

FIGURE 14.76 Press up under the cheekbones. Use light to moderate pressure to press into the soft tissues up against the underside of the cheekbones.

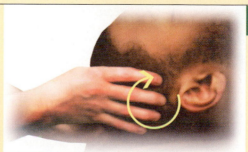

FIGURE 14.77 Loosen the scalp by applying circular friction to the sides, back, and top of head (over entire hair area). The fingers and scalp move together over a spot before moving to the next spot. Do not slide over the skin or hair.

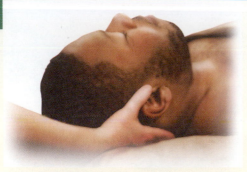

FIGURE 14.78 Cradle the head briefly in both hands to end this section. Hold for a few seconds until you can feel the recipient completely relax.

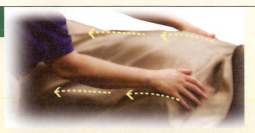

FIGURE 14.79 Finish the entire session with brushing over front of the body. Apply brushing movements with fingertips from head and shoulder areas to toes. Sweep along the sides in the genital area. Hold feet gently and tell the recipient that the session has ended.

 After you perform the Practice Sequence, evaluate how well you did by filling out Performance Evaluation Form 14–1, Full-Body Western Massage. The form can be found in Appendix F, Performance Evaluation Forms, on page A-28 and on your DVD.

PRACTICAL APPLICATION

Use the Practice Sequence presented in this chapter to develop skill in combining techniques for a full-body Western massage session. With practice, you will be able to complete a full-body session in 60 minutes.

1. Can you complete the routine for each separate region in the time allotted?
2. Are your transitions smooth?
3. Can you maintain awareness of the recipient's comfort and safety while practicing?

CRITICAL THINKING

Think about the sequence of techniques used in the Practice Sequence and the flow of the entire session. Analyze one region closely and describe how you might alter or add to it to make it more effective.

1. How might you transition from one technique to the next to create better continuity or flow?
2. How might you create more specificity?
3. How much can you add and still stay within the time allotted in the 60-minute session?

CHAPTER HIGHLIGHTS

- A typical full-body Western massage lasts 60 minutes, and includes massage of the back, legs, abdomen, chest, arms, neck, and head.
- Wellness massage sessions focus on general health and well-being, as well as meeting the therapeutic needs of the recipient.
- Practitioners develop their own styles and routine ways of performing a massage session.
- The recipient is typically unclothed and draped with a sheet for modesty.
- The seven basic Western massage techniques are blended into a sequence to create a routine.
- The sequence usually includes both supine and prone positions, and has a starting point, a direction (e.g., clockwise), and an ending point.
- Oil or lotion is used to enhance movement over the skin and to prevent chafing.
- The order of techniques for each part of the body includes opening and warming techniques such as effleurage or compressions, followed by technique combinations for general health and specific therapeutic effects.
- Massage of a particular area is concluded with finishing techniques to reconnect, smooth out, and gradually lighten touch.

- ○ Finishing techniques typically include light effleurage, tapotement, or passive touch, such as holding.
- A full-body massage has a sense of continuity and flow.
  - ○ Touch is established at the beginning of a session and maintained continuously throughout, with minimal interruption.
  - ○ A sense of flow is achieved through an orderly sequence and smooth transitions from one part of the body to the next.
- The rhythm of a full-body massage is smooth and even, and the pacing is moderate in speed.
- Specificity is required when giving attention to small areas or applying techniques for specific therapeutic purposes.
- Pressure varies according to the part of body receiving massage, and the preference of the client; usually medium to light, but heavier upon request.
- Eclectic practitioners may use full-body Western massage as a starting point, and then integrate other massage forms as appropriate to meet the client's needs.

EXAM REVIEW

Key Terms

Match the following key terms to their descriptions. For additional study, look up the key terms in the Interactive Glossary on page G-1 and note other terms that compare or contrast with them.

_____ 1. Continuity
_____ 2. Finishing techniques
_____ 3. Flow
_____ 4. Full-body Western massage
_____ 5. Opening technique
_____ 6. Pacing
_____ 7. Pressure
_____ 8. Rhythm
_____ 9. Specificity
_____ 10. Transition techniques
_____ 11. Warming technique

a. Type of massage developed in Europe and North America
b. Attention to a specific muscle or small area
c. The speed of a massage session
d. Techniques that provide a sense of continuity when moving from one section of the body to another
e. Element of full-body massage described as smooth and even
f. Sense of continuous touch throughout a massage session
g. Sense of fluid movement or smoothness in a massage session
h. Technique used to prepare and warm tissues for massage
i. Techniques to create a sense of wholeness and completion
j. Technique used to begin a massage
k. Force used in applying massage

Memory Workout

To test your memory of the main concepts in this chapter, complete the following sentences by circling the most correct answer from the two choices provided.

1. A typical full-body massage lasts for (60) (120) minutes.
2. Practitioners blend massage techniques into logical sequences or (routines) (treatments).
3. Recipients are usually draped with a (towel) (sheet).
4. The (genitals) (buttocks) should always be covered.
5. A massage (sequence) (technique) has a beginning, a middle, and an end point.
6. Advantages of starting prone are that it often feels (safer) (lighter) to those new to massage.
7. Massage of each region of the body begins with (warming) (transition) techniques.
8. Establishment or removal of touch should never be (made) (abrupt).
9. The (shorter) (longer) the session, the less specificity is possible on any one region.
10. Routines are (lengthened) (modified) to meet the needs of the recipient on the table.

Test Prep

The following multiple-choice questions will help to prepare you for future school and professional exams.

1. Which of the following is an appropriate goal for a full-body Western massage?
   a. Improve circulation
   b. General relaxation
   c. Reduce muscle soreness
   d. Any of the above
2. When is it considered ethical to uncover a client completely during a massage?
   a. Only if he or she requests it
   b. Only if it is hot in the room
   c. Only if the drape interferes with technique application
   d. Never
3. Which of the following is the most versatile transition technique?
   a. Effleurage
   b. Petrissage
   c. Friction
   d. Vibration
4. Which of the following statements about the continuity of touch during a full-body massage session is *most* correct?
   a. Once a session has begun, never remove your hands from the body until the session is finished.
   b. Re-establish touch quickly if you remove your hands from the body during a session.
   c. Establishment or removal of touch during a session should not be abrupt.
   d. Continuity of touch during a session is not important to its flow.
5. Which of the following would be the *least* appropriate place to begin a full-body Western massage session?
   a. Face and head
   b. Back
   c. Abdomen
   d. Feet
6. Which of the following is the best choice for a finishing technique for a massage session if the recipient needs to be alert and ready to go back to work afterward?
   a. Nerve strokes over the drape from head to feet
   b. Holding the feet with passive touch
   c. Light tapotement from shoulders to feet
   d. Holding the head with passive touch
7. A massage session focusing on general relaxation would be:
   a. Faster paced with stimulating techniques
   b. Slower paced and avoiding stimulating techniques
   c. Medium paced with deep specific techniques
   d. Slower paced with deep specific techniques
8. When draping for abdominal massage to a woman:
   a. Simply pull the large drape down to the waist and tuck securely
   b. Use a separate drape to cover the breasts, then pull the large drape down to the waist and tuck securely
   c. Always apply abdominal massage through the drape
   d. Any of the above
9. Experienced massage therapists usually develop:
   a. A routine way of approaching their massage sessions
   b. A specific set routine that they use for all clients
   c. Their own unique approaches to massage sessions
   d. A routine for women and a different routine for men
10. If a portion of a massage session is focused on a particular anatomical structure or a small area, it is referred to as working with:
    a. Continuity
    b. Flow
    c. Specificity
    d. Generality

Video Challenge

Watch the appropriate segment of the video on your DVD and then answer the following questions.

Full-Body Western Massage

1. In the full body session demonstrated in the video, in what order are the body regions massaged?

2. How are transitions made from one region to another in the full body session?
3. What is the intent of each massage technique used in the full body session? Analyze the applications in one or more body regions.

Comprehension Exercises

The following short answer questions test your knowledge and understanding of chapter topics and provide practice in written communication skills. Explain in two to four complete sentences.

1. What is the purpose of applying finishing techniques at the end of full-body Western massage session? Give two examples of different ways to end a massage session.

2. Discuss the decision to begin a massage session with the recipient prone or supine. What are the factors to consider? What are the advantages of each starting position?
3. Explain the concept of *specificity*. Describe a massage application that shows specificity in a session.

For Greater Understanding

The following exercises are designed to take you from the realm of theory into the real world. They will help give you a deeper understanding of the subjects covered in this chapter. Action words are underlined to emphasize the variety of activities presented to address different learning styles and to encourage deeper thinking.

1. Receive two professional massages from the same person. Compare and contrast the two experiences. Did you notice a routine way of working, favorite techniques, and other similarities? Were there differ-

ences in the two sessions? If yes, what were they, and why do you think there were differences?
2. Receive a 60-minute full-body massage and, at a later time, a 30-minute full-body massage from the same practitioner. Analyze how the practitioner shortened the second session. How did the two experiences compare?
3. Watch a video of a full-body Western massage routine. Analyze the elements of the routine with particular attention to the techniques chosen and the continuity and flow. Discuss with a study partner or group.

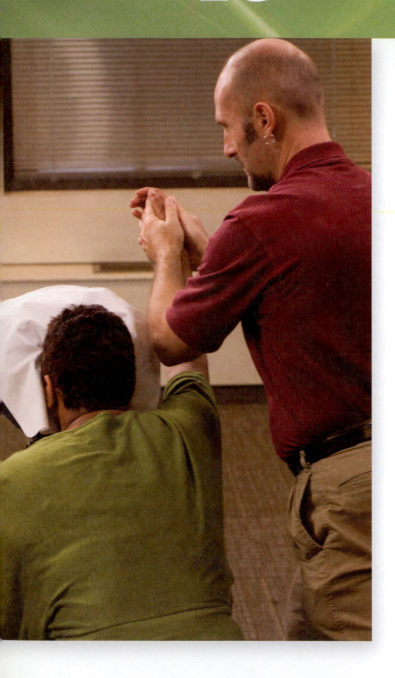

15 Seated Massage

CHAPTER OUTLINE

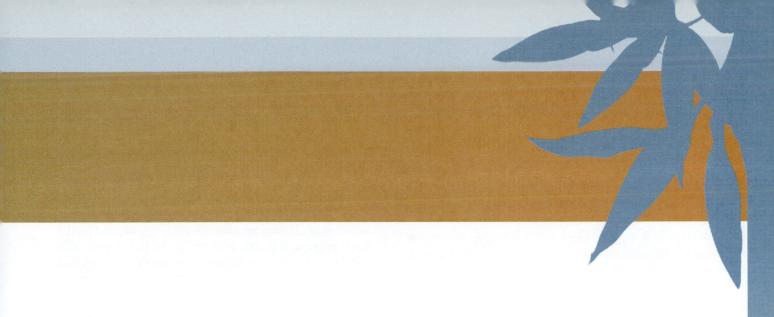

LEARNING OUTCOMES

After studying this chapter, you will have the information to:

1. Trace the history of seated massage.

2. Explain the benefits of seated massage.

3. Define on-site massage.

4. Practice good body mechanics for seated massage.

5. Screen for contraindications and cautions.

6. Position clients comfortably on massage chairs.

7. Perform a seated massage Practice Sequence.

8. Plan for seated massage given at events and on-site.

KEY TERMS

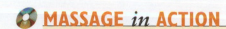

MASSAGE *in* ACTION

On your DVD, explore:
- Seated Massage

SEATED MASSAGE OVERVIEW

Massage is sometimes given with the recipient sitting on a special massage chair or on a regular chair adapted for the purpose. This is referred to as **seated massage** or *chair massage*. Being skilled in seated massage offers massage therapists more options for positioning clients and for giving massage in public venues such as community heath fairs and workplaces. The massage techniques are the same for seated massage and table massage; however, there are some special considerations for client positioning and body mechanics. Seated massage is not new in the history of massage, but has regained popularity recently with the development of the portable massage chair in the 1980s.

Brief History

Throughout the centuries, massage has been given wherever it was convenient to do so, including with recipients seated on the ground, on stools, chairs, and tables. Some examples are a servant giving a foot massage to a lady sitting on a stool after a bath, a village healer treating a headache by rubbing the head of a man sitting on a tree stump, an athletic masseur rubbing the leg's of an athlete sitting on a training table, and a physiotherapist in an army hospital massaging a soldier's arm while he is sitting on a chair. The body part to be massaged was easily accessed with the recipient sitting on some surface.

It was not until the early 1900s that full-body massage with the recipient lying on a padded table gained popularity. Swedish massage in particular became so popular during the twentieth century that for most people, the word *massage* conjured up a picture of someone lying on a table underneath a sheet.

That changed in the 1980s with the invention of a chair designed specifically for positioning a client for massage. The first modern **massage chair** was developed in the 1980s by David Palmer of San Francisco. The original idea of the massage chair was to make receiving massage readily available to the general public. The chair can be transported easily, allows recipients to receive massage sitting up and with their clothes on, and can be used in public areas. Massage techniques that do not need oil for their application are generally used for seated massage. A typical modern massage chair is shown in Figure 11.11A on page 349.

The first massage chairs were promoted as the foundation for **on-site massage.** On-site massage means that the massage practitioner goes to where the potential clients are, therefore making massage more accessible. One of the first large corporations to provide on-site massage for its employees was Apple Computer Corporation in 1985 (Palmer 1995). Massage chairs are now familiar sights in a number of public places, such as in stores and day spas, at trade shows and conventions, at shopping malls and airports, and even on the street and in parks.

The availability of the massage chair has sparked renewed interest in the potential for giving massage to seated clients. In addition to massage for relaxation and rejuvenation, clinical massage applications are being adapted for the seated position. It is also used for special populations such as athletes, the elderly, and people with disabilities. Offering seated massage can provide additional income for a massage therapist, promote an office-based massage practice, or constitute a full-time massage therapy practice.

BENEFITS OF SEATED MASSAGE

The benefits of seated massage are largely the same as for table massage. It promotes general relaxation, improved circulation, muscle relaxation, and mental clarity. Having a massage chair available in a massage office can be useful as an alternative or as an adjunct to table massage. Some clients may prefer massage in a chair, but more often a massage chair is used to give better positioning for certain therapetic applications, for example, the shoulder, arm, or back.

Outside of the massage therapy office, seated massage has the added benefit of being more convenient for those with less discretionary time, and the massage therapist and chair can travel easily to where potential clients are located. Some benefits are related to the specific venues where seated massage takes place.

Public Places and Events

Seated massage at airports and train stations provides a respite from the stresses of traveling. It relieves muscle tension from sitting in uncomfortable positions and gets the circulation going after long periods of sitting. It also presents a pleasurable pastime for those waiting for the next leg of their journeys. Because travelers do not have to get undressed for massage, and the time is relatively short, seated massage can be squeezed in between flights or trains.

Seated massage in malls and stores is a walk-by opportunity. Shoppers not planning or scheduling a massage ahead of time have the chance to stop for a brief session. It may motivate people new to massage to give it a try. Such a public venue may seem safe and too convenient to pass up. Seated massage gives shoppers a chance to get off their feet and be rejuvenated for the rest of the day's activities.

Seated massage at trade shows can be an attraction that brings attendees to a specific booth. It serves as a break from walking exhibition halls and sitting in meetings and lectures.

Besides its physical benefits, massage can help attendees stay alert for long days of meetings and networking.

Health fairs, fund-raising runs and walks, and other community events are also prime venues for seated massage. They are places to expose potential clients to massage in general and to the massage therapists in their communities. Recipients reap the overall health benefits of massage at a convenient time and place.

In the Workplace

Massage is increasingly popular in **workplace wellness programs.** These employer-sponsored programs make services and activities available to employees to improve their overall health and well-being. Seated massage, in particular, is popular with businesses exploring ways to reduce employee stress on the job and to minimize job-related injuries.

Many tasks performed by workers in the past are now done by sophisticated machines run by computers. However, many workers still sit at workstations for long periods of time performing repetitive tasks such as using computer keyboards, sorting objects, or assembling parts. Tradesmen, craftsmen, artists, and musicians repeat certain movements over and over, stressing their bodies. These repetitive movements can lead to debilitating musculoskeletal problems.

Repetitive strain injuries (RSIs) are common in a number of occupations. RSIs may involve tendinitis (inflammation of tendons), bursitis (inflammation of fluid sacs around a joint), ganglion cysts (a mass formed over a tendon), or nerve impingement (Table 6.17 on page 162 describes some of these types of pathologies and their massage implications). Symptoms of RSI include aching, tenderness, swelling, tingling, numbness, weakness, loss of flexibility, and spasms in the muscles affected. RSI can result in chronic pain, loss of mobility, and, eventually, disability. Massage is effective for preventing and treating various forms of RSI.

Tension headaches are also common at work. They have a variety of causes, including poor posture, lack of movement, mental tension, and poor nutrition. Headaches are more common toward the end of the day with the accumulation of stresses. Massage that addresses tension and trigger points in the shoulders and neck can be very effective in treating tension headaches. See Figure 18.8 on page 526 for trigger points related to tension headaches.

The stress level of employees is a major wellness factor in the workplace. Meeting deadlines, working long hours, and relationships with coworkers are just some of the stressful aspects of work life. The dizzying pace of modern times, at work and in everyday life, also adds to the stress of employees. A high level of chronic stress is known to have a negative effect on health. It compromises the immune system and reduces the ability to concentrate. In the workplace, massage can be an oasis of relaxation in an otherwise stressful environment.

Massage also has been found to increase mental clarity and alertness. Studies show that workers who received seated massage got more work done and made fewer mistakes (Field et al. 1993; Massage 1996). Practitioners can adapt massage sessions to address the needs of workers, and the use of massage chairs makes offering this service in the workplace convenient.

A recent study on work-site acupressure massage (WSAM) found that the group receiving the specific massage protocol enjoyed significant health benefits. The massage was a 20-minute session received twice weekly for a period of 8 weeks. The recipients were fully clothed. Techniques included Western massage, acupressure, and reflexology. Results showed that people receiving massage had a significant decrease in anxiety, an increase in emotional control, a decrease in perceived sleep disturbances, decreased blood pressure, improved cognition, and a decrease in perception of muscle tightness (Hodge, Boehmer, and Klein 2002). Training is available for massage practitioners desiring to specialize in chair massage. Visit the website for the TouchPro Institute (www.touchpro.org) for more information about chair massage and scheduled seminars and workshops.

Popularity of Seated Massage

Seated massage is popular for a number of different reasons. It takes less time than table massage and eliminates having to undress. It has immediate positive effects, since recipients usually feel better right away. It may alleviate some of the physical aches and pains developed from sitting, standing, or walking for long periods of time. In contrast to other wellness practices, massage requires no practice and little effort on the part of the recipient. It complements other health practices such as exercise and stress-reduction programs.

Seated massage in the workplace helps increase good feelings about the employer and promotes loyalty. It boosts productivity and can be taken advantage of by most workers.

BODY AND HAND MECHANICS

Body and hand mechanics for giving seated massage are based on the same principles as for table massage, but are adapted for a client in a more vertical position than horizontal. In summary, keep your spine and head in good alignment, shoulders down, joints stacked, and wrists in a neutral position. Apply pressure forward or downward by leaning into the technique with your body weight rather than just pushing with the arms. Use a bow-and-arrow stance for most techniques, and lower the body by bending the knees. Kneel if necessary to reach the arms and hands to keep your back and neck in alignment. For more detailed information on hand and body mechanics for seated massage, see page 366 in Chapter 12, Body Mechanics, Table Skills, and Application Guidelines.

REALITY CHECK

RANDY: I'm having a hard time adapting my massage techniques to work with someone clothed sitting upright. And my back and my thumbs hurt after I do seated massage for a while. How can I get more skilled at this?

ANTONIA: Seated massage does take some getting used to at first. You have to be really aware of maintaining good body and hand mechanics until they become more natural. Seated massage requires a lot more bending of the knees, and wider stances. Many people incorporate techniques from Eastern bodywork forms such as acupressure that do not use oil or lotion. Learn the practice sequence presented in class, and then experiment with variations of techniques such as compression, kneading, and direct pressure.

SCREENING FOR SEATED MASSAGE

Before giving seated massage, screen for contraindications and cautions. When massaging repeat clients, for example at a regular workplace appointment, you may be familiar with recipients and their health histories. However, at events and places such as airports and trade shows, you may be seeing clients on a one-time basis. A brief **screening interview** will reveal important information. At a minimum, ask the recipient:

1. Have you ever had a massage before? In a massage chair?
2. Have you had any illness or injuries recently?
3. Are you taking any medication?
4. If a woman: Are you pregnant?
5. Do you wear contact lenses?
6. Are there any areas you want me to avoid when giving the massage?
7. Do you have low blood pressure or are you prone to fainting?

The answer to the first question lets you know how much instruction to offer the recipient during the session. Questions 2 and 3 may reveal general and regional contraindications or cautions for massage. See page 300 in Chapter 9, Endangerment Sites, Contraindications, and Cautions, to review contraindications.

If a woman is pregnant (question 4), ask follow-up questions to screen further for contraindications relevant to pregnancy. Some authorities consider pregnancy to be a general contraindication for seated massage, while others advise appropriate cautions. Techniques applied to the back that result in heavy pressure against the abdomen should be avoided. See page 588 in Chapter 20, Special Populations and Adaptations, for more information on contraindications for massage during pregnancy.

If the recipient wears contact lenses (question 5), be sure that the face cradle does not press against the eyes or will not displace the contact lenses. Question 6 offers the recipient the opportunity to set personal boundaries. It may also lead to further information about regional contraindications. The last question (7) is important because massage may temporarily lower blood pressure further. When lying on a massage table, this usually does not present a problem. But when sitting up, a drop in blood pressure can result in light-headedness, dizziness, or fainting. If any of these symptoms occur during the seated massage, help the recipient off the chair and have him or her lie on the ground. Elevating the legs helps bring blood pressure back to normal.

POSITIONING FOR SEATED MASSAGE

Positioning clients for seated massage takes into consideration the type of chair available, the parts of the body to be massaged, and the types of techniques to be applied. Review page 371 in Chapter 12, Body Mechanics, Table Skills, and Application Guidelines, for a description of positioning recipients in regular chairs when a massage chair is unavailable. A portable tabletop device designed to offer support for the chest and head when the recipient is seated at a desk or table is shown in Figure 12.24 on page 372.

Positioning in specially designed massage chairs simulates lying prone on a massage table in many ways. Of course, a big difference is that clients are in a more **vertical position** supported on their buttocks, lower legs, and chest instead of lying facedown on a horizontal surface. Done properly, positioning in a massage chair can be very comfortable and relaxing.

There are several models of massage chairs, and each has its own features for positioning a client comfortably. Standard **massage chair adjustments** include the height of the chest pad and the angle of the face cradle. Other adjustments may include the height and/or angle of the seat, the kneeling pads, and the armrest. Examine the model available to you for its adjustment features.

Note that different massage chair models have limits on body types and weights that they can accommodate safely and comfortably. For example, the maximum weight a chair can typically hold is about 300 pounds. People less than 4 feet tall or more than 6 feet tall, or with a large girth, may have trouble fitting into a particular massage chair properly. Be familiar with your chair's limitations. See Case for Study, Donna and Buying a Massage Chair, on page 350 in Chapter 11, Hygiene, Equipment, and Environment, for a list of criteria to consider if you are buying a massage chair.

To position a client for massage, first have him or her sit down and kneel on the pads provided. Check the angle of the kneeling pads and seat and the overall fit of the client in the chair. The client should be able sit comfortably in this basic position. If kneeling is uncomfortable or painful, have the client put his or her feet flat on the floor instead. The seat may have to be adjusted to be more horizontal in this case.

Next adjust the height of the chest pad and ask the client to lean forward. Special chest pads are available to position large breasted women comfortably. Some chairs have an additional chest pad angle adjustment. Then raise or lower the face cradle and tilt it down, so that the client's neck is flexed slightly. If the face cradle is too low, the neck will be shortened with an exaggerated curve. If it is too high, the top of the face cradle pad will not rest on the forehead, or the chin will be tilted up out of good alignment.

Last, adjust the angle of the arm rest. Ask for feedback about the overall comfort of this position. Make further adjustments as needed. Proper positioning for seated massage is shown in Figure 11.11B on page 349.

Some chairs can be adjusted to allow clients to sit facing out with their backs against the chest pad. This allows access to the front of the body for some massage applications. With this feature, anterior leg and foot massage may be added to a seated massage session.

SEATED MASSAGE SESSIONS

Seated massage sessions commonly focus on the upper body. Areas addressed include the neck and shoulders, head and scalp, upper and lower back, forearms, wrists, and hands. Techniques that are effective without the use of oil are used. The most common are petrissage (i.e., kneading and compression), friction, direct pressure, tapotement, light stroking, and joint movements. Forms of energy balancing such as polarity therapy may be incorporated into a session. Shiatsu and other forms of Asian bodywork are particularly adaptable for seated massage, because they are given without lubricant and include techniques such as thumb and finger pressure, compressions, and percussion.

Before beginning sessions, ask recipients to remove large pieces of jewelry, ties, jackets, and sweaters, eyeglasses, and other obstacles to massage. Ask permission to work on the face if the recipient is wearing makeup. Also get the recipient's consent to massage the scalp, which can disturb the hair.

The following Practice Sequence for seated massage is designed for general relaxation and for treating common areas of muscular tension. Techniques can be added to address the needs of each specific recipient.

PRACTICAL APPLICATION

Practice positioning different people in a massage chair. Make adjustments for different body types, shapes, and sizes.

1. What adjustments are possible on the massage chair you are using? How does the chair work mechanically?

2. In what order are the adjustments made? What do you look for to determine proper positioning in the massage chair?

3. What role does the recipient play in positioning?

4. Practice a few massage techniques to see if the recipient is positioned well to receive them.

PRACTICE SEQUENCE 15.1

Seated Massage 20 minutes

Preliminary Instructions

• Screen for contraindications and cautions.
• Ask recipient to remove jewelry, bulky clothing, eyeglasses, etc.
• Give instructions for getting onto the massage chair.
• Adjust chest pad, face cradle, and other areas as needed.

1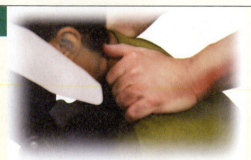

FIGURE 15.1 Stand behind the recipient. Lay your hands on the shoulders to establish contact. Squeeze the shoulders (upper trapezius and deltoid muscles) several times. Gradually increase the force of the squeezes.

2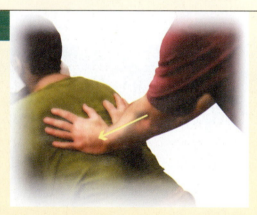

FIGURE 15.2 Press the back muscles, using the palms or loose fists to apply compression. Do not hyperextend your wrists. Press along the sides as well as along the spine, but not over the spine.

3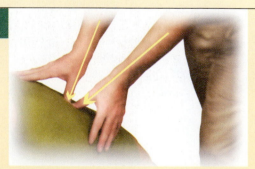

FIGURE 15.3 Apply thumb pressure to points along the spine bilaterally from superior or inferior. Space points about every 2 inches. Keep joints stacked. Shift weight to apply pressure.

FIGURE 15.4 Apply direct pressure to points along the shoulders. Stand to one side and use your forearm to apply broad pressure to one shoulder. Move from medial to lateral. Repeat with your elbow, pressing points about every 2 inches. Only press into muscle. Repeat on other side.

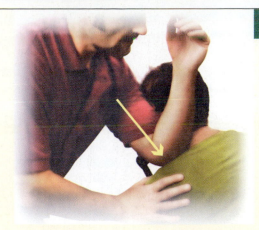

FIGURE 15.5 Standing behind the recipient, squeeze the shoulders and down the upper arms. Squeeze muscles bilaterally across the shoulders and down the upper arms. Use for finishing and transition to arms.

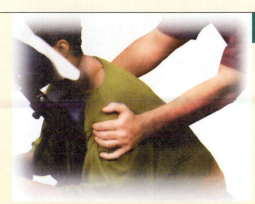

FIGURE 15.6 Shift to one side. Let the recipient's arm hang down. Knead upper and lower arm muscles from armpit to wrist. Afterward position the arm back on the armrest.

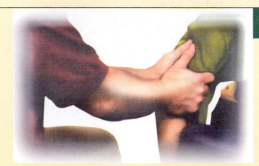

7

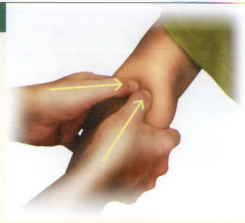

FIGURE 15.7 Apply thumb pressure to forearm muscles, particularly the extensors muscles. Apply circular friction to tender spots. Finish with squeezes from elbow to wrist.

8

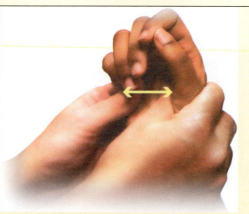

FIGURE 15.8 Squeeze hands and fingers. Compress and broaden the hand. Squeeze along each finger.

9

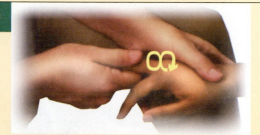

FIGURE 15.9 Move joints in hands. Apply scissoring to metacarpals and figure-8s to fingers.

10

FIGURE 15.10 Stretch arm overhead. Stand to the side facing the same direction as the recipient. Hold onto the hand and stretch the arm upward in line with the recipient's body angle. Lean into the stretch. Replace the arm onto armrest. Brush off to finish before moving to the other arm.

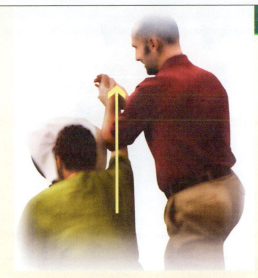

Repeat Steps 6–10 on the other arm.

11

FIGURE 15.11 Knead neck muscles. Use one hand to knead muscles on both sides of the neck.

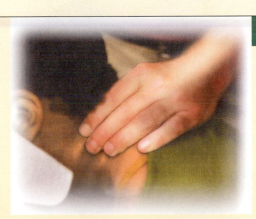

12

FIGURE 15.12 Press into points along the neck with your thumb, one side at a time. Apply circular friction to tender spots. Move from the base of the neck up to and across the suboccipital region.

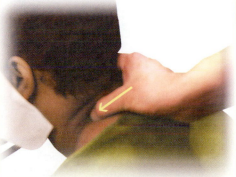

13

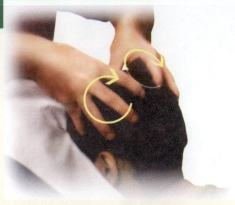

FIGURE 15.13 Apply circular friction with both hands to mobilize the scalp.

14

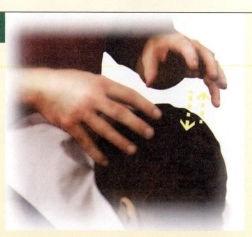

FIGURE 15.14 Tap the head. Apply light fingertip tapotement to the head: top, sides, and back.

15

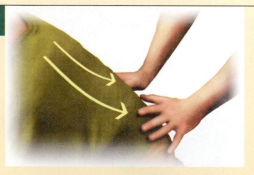

FIGURE 15.15 Brush off the back. Apply several long brushing strokes from head to hips to finish the session.

Assist the recipient as needed to get up and out of the chair.

After you perform the Practice Sequence, evaluate how well you did by filling out Performance Evaluation Form 15–1, Seated Massage. The form can be found in Appendix F, Performance Evaluation Forms, on page A-29 and on your DVD.

CASE FOR STUDY

Ramón Addresses Forearm Strain

Ramón gives seated massage to workers twice a month at a small office. One of his clients, Maria, works part time as a hair stylist in addition to working at a computer for hours at the office. She is starting to experience pain in her forearms and hands from the repeated stress in her upper body. She has asked Ramón to focus on those areas during her regular seated massage.

Question:

What can Ramón do to address Maria's complaints?

Things to consider:

- What musculoskeletal structures are likely involved?
- Can Ramón consider using massage techniques that require lotion in this case?

- How would the arm be positioned most effectively for applying techniques?
- What can Ramón do to maintain good body mechanics and reduce stress on his own body?

Outline a 20-minute seated massage sequence to address Maria's complaints. Be specific about massage techniques and timing. List home care suggestions (stretches, self-massage, cold applications).

_____

_____

_____

PREPARING FOR DIFFERENT VENUES

Giving seated massage in different venues involves some preparation, especially for places away from your regular office. Equipment and supplies need to be gathered and transported to the site. Space must be set up, and a method for scheduling and screening clients determined. Products for sanitizing equipment must be available, as well as a way of washing your hands between clients.

Supplies needed for seated massage events include disposable face cradle covers, something to wipe the chair after each client, hand sanitizer, and a garbage bag for used supplies. Dispose of used face cradle covers, and put on a fresh one after each massage. Antibacterial or antimicrobial disposable wipes can be used to sanitize the face support, armrests, chest pad, and leg rests of the massage chair after each session. A hand sanitizer is essential when working on-site because washroom facilities may not be available or convenient to use.

Additional supplies include a clipboard, pen, and intake/release forms for keeping records of clients seen. Other useful items include a small table to set things on and a little tray or dish for holding clients' jewelry or eye glasses. Depending on the setting, you may want to bring a device to play appropriate music.

The space for seated massage can be flexible. If at the workplace, it may be at the recipient's workstation, or in an empty office or cubicle or in a conference or workroom. It may be in a booth at a tradeshow or the lobby of a health club. It may be under a tent at a street fair or in a space at the back of a store. The only requirement is enough space for the practitioner to move around and keep good body mechanics. An ideal space would be quiet and somewhat removed from the hectic activity of the surrounding environment.

Time is also a factor. Seated massage sessions typically last from 15–20 minutes. A minimum 10-minute break between sessions allows for necessary transition from one client to the next. During this time, equipment is sanitized, and the face cradle cover is changed. The incoming client can be screened and given instructions.

Be sure to take regular breaks to avoid undue stress and strain. Scheduling sessions on the half-hour provides for a short break between clients. Take at least a 30-minute break after four sessions. Do no more than 5 hours of seated massage in 1 day.

With adequate preparation, taking seated massage on-the-road can run smoothly. It can be a rewarding addition to a general massage practice or may provide a specialty for a full-time seated massage business.

CRITICAL THINKING

Think about the various places where seated massage is offered other than the workplace, for example, at street fairs, in airports, at trade shows, and in shopping malls. Analyze how seated massage might be adapted to meet the needs of people in four different venues.

1. What physical and mental stresses do people in each venue face?

2. What goals for a seated massage might be appropriate to meeting their needs?
3. How might a session be adapted for the circumstances?
4. What equipment and supplies would you need to take to each venue?

CHAPTER HIGHLIGHTS

- Giving massage to a client sitting on a special massage chair or regular chair is referred to as seated massage or chair massage.
- Throughout history, massage has been given in the seated position whenever it was convenient to do so.
- The invention of the modern massage chair in the 1980s sparked an interest in seated massage that continues today.
- The benefits of seated massage are largely the same as for table massage, with the addition of convenience and accessibility.
- Massage in the workplace is useful to minimize job-related injuries and health problems, such as repetitive strain injuries, tension headaches, and high stress levels.
  - Seated massage increases mental clarity and worker productivity.
- Basic principles of good body and hand mechanics apply to seated massage.
  - Body mechanics are adapted for applying massage with the client in a vertical position.
- Seated massage clients are screened for contraindications and cautions.
  - Important questions include information on previous massage experience, recent injuries or illnesses,

medications being taken, pregnancy, contact lenses, areas to avoid, and low blood pressure.
- Positioning a client properly on a massage chair requires adjustments in the chair seat, kneeling pads, arm pad, chest pad, and face cradle.
- Massage techniques that do not require oil are used for seated massage, for example, compression and kneading (petrissage), friction, tapotement, and other forms of bodywork such as shiatsu, and polarity therapy.
- Areas of focus for seated massage include neck and shoulders, head and scalp, upper and lower back, forearms, wrists and hands.
- Clients remove jewelry, jackets and sweaters, ties, eyeglasses, and other potential obstacles to massage. Ask permission to massage the face or scalp.
- Giving seated massage in different venues involves preparation of equipment, supplies, and the space; scheduling and screening; sanitizing and hygiene.
- At events, scheduling clients on the half hour allows time for a short break between sessions and time to sanitize equipment.
  - Take a 30-minute break after four sessions, and do no more than 5 hours of massage in 1 day.

EXAM REVIEW

Key Terms

To study the key terms listed at the beginning of this chapter, match the appropriate lettered meaning to each numbered key term listed below. For additional study, look up the key terms in the Interactive Glossary on page G-1 and note other terms that compare or contrast with them.

_____ **1.** Massage chair
_____ **2.** Massage chair adjustments
_____ **3.** On-site massage
_____ **4.** Repetitive strain injuries (RSIs)
_____ **5.** Screening interview
_____ **6.** Seated massage
_____ **7.** Vertical position
_____ **8.** Workplace wellness programs

a. The massage practitioner goes to where the potential clients are
b. Questions to ask prospective clients for massage that can reveal important information regarding health conditions and possible contraindications for massage
c. Massage given with the recipient sitting on a special massage chair or on a regular chair adapted for the purpose
d. Can be transported easily and allows recipients to receive massage sitting up and with their clothes on
e. Massage clients are supported on their buttocks, lower legs, and chest instead of lying facedown on a horizontal surface.
f. Services and activities for employees sponsored by employers to improve people's overall health and well-being
g. Can include the height of the chest pad, the angle of the face cradle, the height and/or angle of the seat, the kneeling pads, and the armrest
h. Debilitating musculoskeletal problems resulting from repeated overwork or overload

Memory Workout

To test your memory of the main concepts in this chapter, complete the following sentences by circling the most correct answer from the two choices provided.

1. The first modern massage chair was developed in the (1950s) (1980s) by (David Palmer) (Janet Travell).
2. When the massage therapist goes to where the clients are located, for example, at their workplace, it is often referred to as (on-site) (chair) massage.
3. One of the main attractions of seated massage is that it is (convenient) (relaxing) for clients.
4. Seated massage has been found to increase mental (relaxation) (alertness) that can only enhance worker productivity.
5. For office workers, tension headaches are more common toward the (middle) (end) of the day.
6. Body and hand mechanics for seated massage take into consideration the (reclining) (vertical) position of the client on the chair.
7. People with low blood pressure may be prone to (fainting) (shaking).
8. Pressing into the back of someone in a massage chair calls for more (forward) (upward) motion, rather than downward.
9. To position a client on a massage chair, tilt the face cradle slightly (downward) (upward).
10. Ask for the client's (assistance) (permission) to massage the face or scalp.

Test Prep

The following multiple-choice questions will help to prepare you for future school and professional exams.

1. One of the first large corporations to provide on-site massage for its employees in 1985 was:
   a. Boeing Aircraft
   b. Apple Computer Corporation
   c. Hartford Insurance
   d. Coca-Cola Corporation
2. For seated massage techniques, pressure is most often applied by:
   a. Pushing with the arms
   b. Bending from the waist
   c. Lifting your shoulders
   d. Leaning with your body weight
3. Pressing into the back of a seated client is best done from a:
   a. Bow-and-arrow stance
   b. Horse stance
   c. Kneeling stance
   d. Sitting position
4. If a client receiving seated massage suddenly feels faint or dizzy, the best action is to:
   a. Call 911
   b. Have the person stand up immediately
   c. Have the person lie on the ground with his or her feet elevated
   d. Switch to tapotement to increase his or her alertness
5. If a person with knee pain wants to receive massage in a massage chair, a good alternative for positioning is to:
   a. Raise the chest pad to take pressure off of the knees
   b. Raise the seat to take pressure off of the knees
   c. Have him place his feet flat on the floor instead of on the knee pads
   d. Adjust the angle of the knee pads to be more horizontal
6. If a pregnant woman in her third trimester signs up for seated massage at a health fair and she is otherwise healthy, the best action is to:
   a. Adjust the massage chair to fit her current shape and size and give the usual massage
   b. Let her get into the massage chair but avoid pressing hard on her back
   c. Ask her to sit in regular chair and give her a head, neck, and shoulders massage
   d. Politely refuse to give her massage because of contraindications
7. Seated massage sessions in the workplace or at community events typically last:
   a. 5 minutes
   b. 15 to 20 minutes
   c. 30 to 40 minutes
   d. 60 minutes
8. In the bow-and-arrow stance, the body is lowered by:
   a. Widening the stance and bending the knees
   b. Narrowing the stance and straightening the knees
   c. Bending at the waist
   d. Widening the stance and bending at the waist
9. A thoroughly sanitized face cradle for each seated massage client is best achieved by:
   a. Changing the disposable face cradle cover for each client
   b. Washing the face cradle after the last client
   c. Both washing the face cradle and using a clean cover for each client
   d. Sanitizing after every third client
10. As a self-care measure, take regular breaks when providing seated massage at events. A good rule of thumb is to take at least a:
    a. 30-minute break after each session
    b. 30-minute break after every four sessions
    c. 15-minute break after 2 hours of massage
    d. 30-minute break after 4 hours of massage

Video Challenge

Watch the appropriate segment of the video on your DVD and then answer the following questions.

Seated Massage

1. What type of massage techniques were used most often in the seated massage demonstration in the video?
2. For which technique applications were shifting the body weight most obvious?
3. How did the practitioner in the video keep good body mechanics when massaging the arms and hands?

Comprehension Exercises

The following short answer questions test your knowledge and understanding of chapter topics and provide practice in written communication skills. Explain in two to four complete sentences.

1. Describe equipment, space, and time requirements for seated massage in the workplace.

2. Give four reasons for the popularity of seated massage in workplace wellness programs.
3. What screening questions are asked prior to seated massage? How do you use the information from the client's answers?

For Greater Understanding

The following exercises are designed to take you from the realm of theory into the real world. They will help give you a deeper understanding of the subjects covered in this chapter. Action words are underlined to emphasize the variety of activities presented to address different learning styles and to encourage deeper thinking.

1. Receive a seated massage offered in a public place such as a shopping mall, airport, or street fair. Describe your experience: How did the practitioner prepare you for the session? Did he or she adjust the chair? What techniques were used? How long did it last? How did you feel afterward?

2. Interview people who receive massage at their workplaces. Ask them to describe the seated massage sessions. What benefits do they experience personally?
3. Compare the features of several different massage chairs available for purchase. How many adjustments can be made? How stable and sturdy is each chair? How easy is each to transport and store? Prepare a written cost and features comparison.

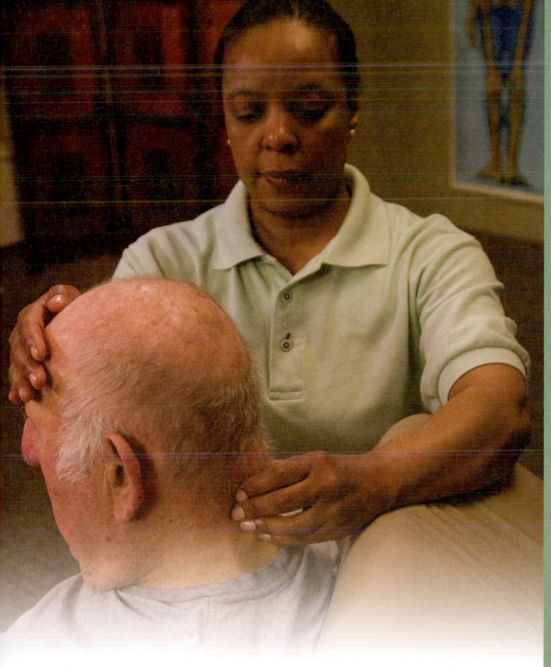

PART

4

Adjunct Therapies and Special Applications

16 Hydrotherapy and Temperature Therapies

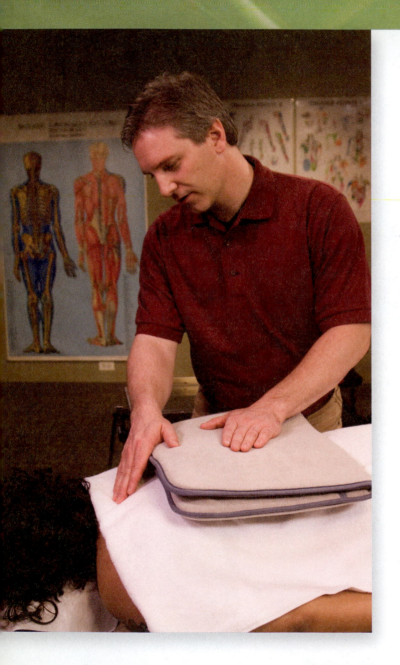

 CHAPTER OUTLINE

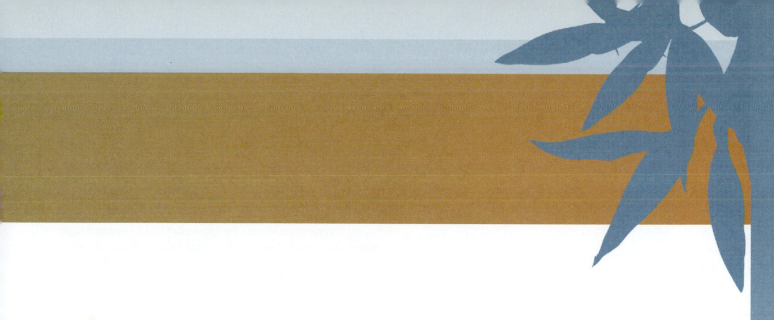

LEARNING OUTCOMES

After studying this chapter, you will have information to:

1. Discuss the history of hydrotherapy.
2. Describe the healing properties of water.
3. Describe hydrotherapy facilities found in spas and health clubs.
4. Compare degree ranges for different temperature therapy modalities.
5. Recognize contraindications for hydrotherapy and temperature therapy.
6. Use hydrotherapy facilities effectively and safely.
7. Apply thermotherapy and cryotherapy effectively and safely.
8. Use hot packs within the scope of massage therapy.
9. Use cold packs within the scope of massage therapy.
10. Apply ice massage for therapeutic benefit.

KEY TERMS

Cold packs 475
Cryotherapy 467
Hydrotherapy 466
Hot pack 471

Ice massage 475
Sauna 469
Steam rooms 469
Temperature therapy 466

Thermotherapy 467
Whirlpool bath 468

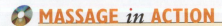

MASSAGE *in* **ACTION**

On your DVD, explore:

- Hot Application on Upper Back
- Cold Application for Knee
- Ice Massage for Elbow

INTRODUCTION

Hydrotherapy is the use of water in health and healing practices. The trio of water, massage, and exercise is a natural combination found all over the globe in bathhouses, spas, and health clubs. The word *spa* is an acronym for the Latin *salus per aquam* meaning "health from water." A more general term for therapeutic applications of hot and cold, whether or not water is involved, is **temperature therapy.**

This chapter explores some of the more common hydrotherapy methods and hot and cold applications within the scope of massage therapy. For more in-depth information on the use of physical agents overall and within the context of rehabilitation, refer to specialty textbooks listed for this chapter in Appendix H, References and Additional Resources, on page A-71.

HISTORY OF HYDROTHERAPY

The use of water for bathing, relaxation, and recreation is universal. From time immemorial, humans have enjoyed mineral and hot springs for their soothing and cleansing effects. Native Americans are said to have frequented natural springs for their healing properties. Later, in places such as Saratoga Springs, New York; Hot Springs, Arkansas; and Calistoga, California, resorts were built where the hot and cold mineral waters were taken internally as well as used for bathing. At spas today, hot and bubbling mineral waters are collected in pools for bathers seeking relaxation and healing.

Archaeologists studying the ancient Maya and Aztec civilizations have found the ruins of sweat baths throughout Central America. The oldest of the sweat baths date from about 1350 BCE. These structures, called *temezcalli,* are described in the first written history of Mexico by Friar Diego Duran in 1567. Most were small buildings with low ceilings and small entranceways, and held about 10 people. Steam was created by pouring water over hot rocks. Herbs were used with the steam for their healing effects. Sweating was thought to purify the body and cure illnesses. Mayan sweat baths are the antecedents of today's *temescal* or sweat houses still found in Central America

In North America, the sweat lodge ceremony is one of the most important traditional practices of Native Americans. In the past, sweat lodges were circular domed structures constructed from animal skins stretched over frames made of tree branches, but today sweat lodges take many forms. In this ritual for spiritual cleansing, stones are heated in a central fire pit and added in increments to increase the heat in the lodge. Water is added to the stones to increase steam, and herbs (sage, copal, lavender) are placed on the stones for therapeutic purposes. Native American spiritual objects and rituals are typically part of the traditional sweat lodge ceremony.

The sauna was developed centuries ago in Finland. The sauna is typically a wood-lined room or shed heated to a high temperature by hot rocks. Water is poured on the rocks periodically to add some moisture to the room. After sitting and sweating in these superheated rooms, hardy Finns would jump into cold rivers and snow banks to cool off. It is a practice that many believe builds stamina, energy, and strength.

Today's spa and health club facilities such as whirlpool baths, showers, and steam rooms can be traced in Western civilization directly to the ancient Greek gymnasia and Roman baths. Turkish baths, based on the Roman prototype, became popular in Europe and the United States in the latter nineteenth century. Baths were also popular in ancient Asia, particularly India, China, Korea, and Japan. Massage and bodywork was and still is an integral part of the bathhouse experience.

The Water Cure

The healing effects of water applications were known in ancient Greece. The famous Greek physician Hippocrates (c. 460 BCE) used compresses, sponging, bathing, and drinking water in his treatments.

Water therapies of various kinds were among the natural healing methods that blossomed in the 1800s. Vincent Priessnitz, a farmer in the Austro-Hungarian Empire, was well known for the methods of water therapy he developed from 1829 to 1849. Priessnitz created an entire system of baths, compresses, and other hot and cold applications to treat various diseases.

Sebastian Kneipp, born in 1821 in Bavaria, is perhaps the most famous water cure practitioner of his era. Kneipp was a priest who built on Priessnitz's water-based therapies and his own knowledge of herbal remedies, becoming the foremost authority on the subject. His book, *My Water Cure,* first written in 1889, was translated into many languages through the years. People flocked to him from all over Europe to be cured of a variety of ailments.

European spas, which cater to people seeking healing as well as relaxation, adopted the methods of Priessnitz and Kneipp. An example of a Kneipp treatment given at the Biltz Sanitarium in Weisbaden, Germany, in 1898 is shown in Figure 16.1■. The great spas at Baden-Baden and Weisbaden in Germany, Montecatini Terme in Italy, and Evian-les-Bains in France, as well as many smaller hydrotherapy establishments, carry on the tradition of the water cure.

The idea of the natural healing resort was imported to the United States in places such as J. Harvey Kellogg's Battle Creek Sanitarium in Michigan. Kellogg wrote *Home Hand-*

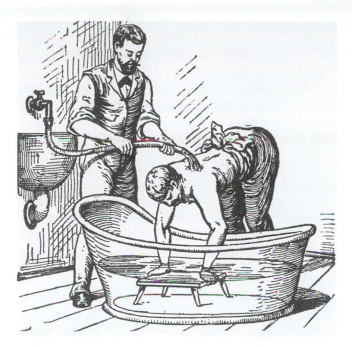

FIGURE 16.1

Kneipp treatment: Upper affusion with hose at the Biltz Sanitarium in Weisbaden, Germany, 1898.

book of *Domestic Hygiene and Rational Medicine* in 1880, which covered hydrotherapy, electrotherapy, and Swedish remedial gymnastics. His book *Rational Hydrotherapy*, written in1900, described 200 water treatments.

Hydrotherapy versus Hydropathy

Sir John Floyer, a physician in Lichfield, England, wrote a treatise in 1702 titled *The History of Cold Bathing to the Ancient and Modern*. Later that century, Dr. Currie of Liverpool, England, wrote *Medical Reports on the Effects of Water, Both Warm and Cold, as a Remedy in Fevers and Other Diseases* (1797). The use of water as a therapeutic agent was being recognized within the developing field of biomedicine by the eighteenth century.

Almost a century later in Vienna, Winternitz (1835–1917) experimented with various forms of external water applications to treat a variety of diseases. He used the shower, spray, alternating hot and cold baths, along with manipulations and massage. He varied the temperature of the water and the force with which it was applied for his results (Graham 1923).

Mineral water hospitals were opened in England starting with Bath in 1738, Harrogate in 1824, Droitwich in 1836, and Buxton in 1858. Physicians controlled the larger spas, but had competition from lay natural healers whom they considered quacks. The medical-versus-lay healer split widened, although each side adopted methods of the other.

By the 1890s, the use of water as a therapeutic agent had two main branches and two terms to describe it. At places such as Nauheim, Germany, and Bath and Malvern in England, where the medical influence was strong, the term used was *hydrotherapy*, a rational system of baths, exercises, and electricity. The term *hydropathy* was reserved for "barefoot back-to-nature cults masterminded by lay philosophers" practiced at continental mountain resorts (Barclay 1994, p. 3).

Methods of natural healing and those of modern biomedicine were diverging into separate paths by the turn of the nineteenth century. Biomedicine opted largely for treatments with drugs and surgery. The old hydrotherapy became the province of naturopaths and other natural healers. Hydrotherapy retained its association with massage and movement therapies.

Members of the Chartered Society of Trained Masseuses (later Physiotherapy) in England treated injured servicemen during World War I (1914–1918) with hydrotherapy, massage, and related therapies (Barclay 1994). This idea was imported to the United States at about the same time, and the profession of physical therapy as we know it here was born. Physical therapists continue to research the therapeutic uses of water and temperature as a science.

HEALING PROPERTIES OF WATER

Water is relaxing to look at in rivers, lakes, and ponds, and to listen to by the seashore, at a waterfall, or in a desktop water fountain. Flowing water feels pleasurable on the skin.

Taken internally and experienced externally, water is the basis of many natural healing methods. The therapeutic use of water taken internally is outside of the scope of massage therapy, aside from encouraging clients to drink water to stay hydrated.

External applications of water in various forms and immersion in water, however, have an association with massage that goes back to ancient times. Hydrotherapy and temperature therapy may be roughly divided into *thermo, neutro,* and *cryo*. **Thermotherapy** involves methods above normal body temperature. Neutrotherapy uses methods at about body temperature. **Cryotherapy** involves methods below body temperature. Table 16.1■ outlines the sensations associated with these temperature ranges.

Methods within the scope of massage therapy include types of hydrotherapy used for health promotion, such as those found in health clubs and spas. It also includes therapeutic uses of hot and cold applications in the forms of hot and cold packs, and ice. The general temperature ranges for these methods are listed in Table 16.2■.

Healing properties of water are related to its use in cleansing the body, and its ability to raise and lower the core body temperature or the temperature of specific body tissues. Water can assume different forms—liquid, steam, and ice—each with its own contribution to healing. Water pressure from a shower, hose, or water jets is also used for a type of massage of the soft tissues.

TABLE 16.1	Temperature Sensations for Thermo-, Neutro-, and Cryo-Hydrotherapy

Descriptions are based on perception of temperature on the skin. These perceptions are subjective and vary from person to person.

Type	Description	Fahrenheit	Celsius*
Thermo	Very hot	111° to 120°	44° to 49°
	Hot	101° to 110°	38° to 43°
	Warm	94° to 100°	34° to 38°
Neutro	Neutral	90° to 93°	32° to 34°
Cryo	Tepid	80° to 92°	27° to 33°
	Cool	70° to 79°	21° to 26°
	Cold	55° to 69°	13° to 21°
	Very cold	31° to 54°	1° to 12°
	Freezing	32° and below	0° and below

*Temperature conversion Fahrenheit (°F) to Celsius (°C):
°F = °C × 9/5 + 32.

Source: Adapted from Miller, E. (1996). *Day Spa Techniques.* Albany, NY: Milady Publishers; Belanger, A. (2002). *Evidenced-Based Guide to Therapeutic Physical Agents.* Philadelphia: Lippincott Williams & Wilkins.

HYDROTHERAPY FACILITIES

Typical spa and health club settings offer whirlpool baths, showers, steam rooms, and/or saunas in addition to massage services. Hot tubs and Esalen massage have been part of the California scene since the 1970s. Massage practitioners should know something about these facilities to be able to give clients guidance and to suggest their safe and effective use in relation to massage.

The benefits of warm to hot forms of hydrotherapy include raising the body temperature, producing sweating, cleansing skin pores, increasing superficial circulation, muscular relaxation, and general relaxation. These are best used before receiving massage.

The benefits of cool to cold forms of hydrotherapy include lowering body temperature, closing skin pores, decreasing superficial circulation, and general invigoration or stimulation. The cold shower is the most common form of cryo-hydrotherapy in the spa setting. Cold showers, or a contrasting hot to cold shower, are best taken after massage. See Table 16.3■ for major effects of hot and cold hydrotherapy.

A **whirlpool bath** consists of a water-filled tub that has air or water jets causing movement or churning of the water. Private whirlpool bathtubs are deep enough so that a person can lie down. In the spa, health club, or bathhouse, whirlpools are usually communal baths, in which people sit on benches and are immersed with just their shoulders and heads above water. Whirlpool baths within the context of physiotherapy may be smaller to accommodate an arm or a leg and are made of stainless steel.

TABLE 16.2	Degree Ranges for Hydrotherapy and Temperature Therapy Methods from Cold to Hot Applications

Method	Temperature Range
Ice	23° to 32°F (25° to 0°C)
Cold pack	33° to 50°F (1° to 10°C)
Cold water	50° to 80°F (10° to 27°C)
Bath—cool/cold	70° to 80°F (21° to 27°C)
Whirlpool bath—warm	95° to 104°F (35° to 40°C)
Whirlpool bath—hot	105° to 110° (41° to 43°C)
Steam room*	105° to 130° (41° to 54°C)
Sauna**	160° to 180° (71° to 82°C)
Hot pack—wet	165° 2 170°F (74° to 77°C)

*Wet heat with 100% humidity
**Dry heat with 6–8% humidity

Source: Adapted from Miller, E. (1996). *Day Spa Techniques.* Albany, NY: Milady Publishers; Belanger, A. (2002). *Evidenced-Based Guide to Therapeutic Physical Agents.* Philadelphia: Lippincott Williams & Wilkins.

TABLE 16.3	General Effects of Hydrotherapy Comparing Thermo-Hydrotherapy and Cryo-Hydrotherapy

Hydrotherapy refers here to methods that are applied to the whole body, e.g., whirlpool, shower, steam room, and sauna.

Thermo-hydrotherapy	Cryo-Hydrotherapy
• Increase core body temperature	• Decrease core body temperature
• Increase pulse rate	• Decrease pulse rate
• Decrease blood pressure	• Increase blood pressure
• Increase respiratory rate	• Decrease respiratory rate
• Decrease muscle tone	• Increase muscle tone
• Induce sweating	• Induce shivering
• Relaxing/sedative effect	• Invigorating/stimulating effect
	• Reduce inflammation
	• Decrease pain

Note: The actual effects of specific hydrotherapy methods depend on the health of the client, the actual temperature of the water or room, and the length of time a person is exposed to the heat or cold.

Source: Adapted from Table 14.4, Body Systemic Effects Generally Associated with Cryo-, Thermo-, and Neutro-hydrotherapy, in Belanger, A. (2002). *Evidenced-Based Guide to Therapeutic Physical Agents.* Philadelphia: Lippincott Williams & Wilkins.

The temperature of the water in a whirlpool bath is generally hot, but may vary considerably depending on the purpose of the bath and the health of the patron. The recommended water temperature for relaxation ranges from about 95° to 105°.

The healing effects of the whirlpool bath stem from the water heat and the pressure of the water coming out of the jets and hitting the body. The churning of the water helps sustain the heat of the water on the skin and stimulates the touch receptors of the skin.

A hot tub is a barrel-shaped tub made with wood slats and a rubber or plastic liner. Hot tubs have water heaters and may have whirlpool jets. The guidelines for whirlpool baths apply also to hot tubs.

Showers are created by water streaming out of showerheads mounted on the wall. Showers may have no added pressure, that is, falling like rain, or may have added pressure or pulsing pressure. Showers may be hot or cold. Hot showers have a similar effect as whirlpool baths, that is, relaxation and increased superficial circulation.

Cold showers are stimulating and help reduce general body heat. They may be taken as a cool down after thermo-hydrotherapy or exercise. Variations of the showers found in spas include the Swiss shower in which showerheads surround the bather at different levels from head to toe. The Vichy shower is given with the patron lying down on a table with water showering down from about 4 feet above (see Figure 17.3 on page 487). The Vichy shower can be varied with pulsating water, with alternating hot and cold water, or with a salt or shampoo scrub. An attendant controls the water pressure and temperature from a panel.

Steam rooms are typically spaces tiled from floor to ceiling with benches for sitting. Steam comes out from jets in the walls and fills the space with wet heat from 105° to 130°F (41° to 54°C) with 100 percent humidity. Patrons in the steam room inhale the steam, which helps clear sinuses and relieve respiratory congestion. Steam also raises the body temperature and causes sweating. It is a relaxing, cleansing experience.

A variation of the stream room is the steam cabinet. The patron sits on a stool in an enclosed box with his or her head sticking out. Steam is pumped into the box, raising core body temperature and causing sweating. Since the head is out of the box, the steam is not inhaled. A cold shower following a steam room or steam cabinet experience can help wash off sweat and bring body temperature down to normal.

When raising the core body temperature is contraindicated or undesirable, facial steam may be beneficial. Facial steam devices focus steam to the face and are used in skin care, as well as to improve respiration.

Taking a **sauna** involves sitting in a room with dry heat from 160° to 180°F (71° to 82°C) with 6 to 8 percent humidity. The sauna is typically a wood-lined room heated without steam, and the air is very dry. Patrons sit on wooden benches.

BOX 16.1   Contraindications for Thermo-Hydrotherapy

These contraindications apply to hydrotherapy methods that raise the core body temperature. In some cases, using water with lower temperature and/or limiting the time in the hot water or steam may make their use safer.

Contraindications

- High or low blood pressure
- Heart or circulatory problems
- Pregnancy
- Systemic diseases such as hepatitis
- Seizures
- Multiple sclerosis
- Infection or inflammatory condition
- Vascular problems associated with phlebitis, varicose veins, diabetes
- Skin rashes
- Allergies to water additives
- Contagious conditions
- Some cancers and cancer treatments

Certain medications may make hydrotherapy unsafe for a client. These include drugs that:

- Alter how blood vessels react to hot and cold
- Change skin sensitivity to hot and cold
- Alter the body's temperature control or cooling mechanism

Source: Adapted from Miller, E. (1996). *Day Spa Techniques*. Albany, NY: Milady Publishers; Persad, R. S. (2001). *Massage Therapy and Medications*. Toronto: Curties-Overzet Publications; Belanger, A. (2002). *Evidenced-Based Guide to Therapeutic Physical Agents*. Philadelphia: Lippincott Williams & Wilkins.

Occasionally, water may be poured over hot rocks to produce steam, adding some moisture to the air. A cold shower or a plunge into a swimming pool or lake (or snowbank) after sitting in a sauna is stimulating, closes the skin pores, and helps reduce body temperature.

Contraindications for thermo-hydrotherapy are listed in Box 16.1●. The most serious contraindications are related to heart, circulatory, and other systemic diseases. People with skin rashes should also avoid the increase in superficial circulation that results from immersing in hot water. Of course, people using public facilities should be careful not to spread contagious disease of any kind.

Although it is possible to overdo cryo-hydrotherapy causing adverse reactions, it is more common for people to stay too long in the heat of the thermo-hydrotherapy baths and rooms. First-time bathers should only stay 5–15 minutes in hot water, while healthy, experienced bathers may stay up to 30 minutes. People who are weak or over 60 years old should limit their exposure to hot baths and steam to 5–15 minutes (Miller 1996).

See Box 16.1 on page 469.

BOX 16.2   Guidelines for Safe Use of Thermo-Hydrotherapy Facilities: Whirlpool, Shower, Steam Room, and Sauna

Check to make sure that no contraindications are present before using thermo-facilities. See Box 16.1 on page 469.

1. Wait for at least 1 hour after eating before using thermo-facilities.
2. Avoid alcohol before or during use of thermo-facilities.
3. Wear sandals or shoes with nonslip bottoms to avoid slipping and falling.
4. Check temperature of the water or room (steam and sauna) for therapeutic range (see Table 16.2 on page 468) and for individual tolerance.
5. Limit use according to experience in thermo-facilities and factors such as general health and age. In general, for those less experienced, less healthy, weaker, or over age 60, limit use to 15 minutes; otherwise 15–30 minutes is appropriate.
6. Drink plenty of water during and after thermo-hydrotherapy to replace loss through sweating.
7. Always have someone to call for help if needed.
8. Monitor how you feel, and if weak, dizzy, or nauseous get out of the water or room. Lie or sit down in a cooler place, and replace fluids by sipping a cool drink of water.
9. If reaction to heat is severe or lasts a long time, consider seeking medical evaluation.

Note: Use of thermo-hydrotherapy facilities *before massage* is beneficial for initiating general relaxation, muscle relaxation, and increased superficial circulation and connective tissue pliability. Use of the thermo-hydrotherapy facilities *after massage* may continue the benefits described. Be sure to drink water to replenish fluids, and wash off oil and lotion thoroughly before entering thermo-facilities. Lubricants can contaminate water and leave slippery films on benches and floors.

If a client reports feeling lightheaded or dizzy, is nauseous, or develops a headache, he or she probably stayed immersed too long in hot water or steam. Take measures to reduce the body temperature gradually, such as sitting or lying in a neutral temperature environment and sipping tepid to cool water. If symptoms persist or get worse, consider medical evaluation. Guidelines for safe use of thermo-hydrotherapy facilities are summarized in Box 16.2•.

The most commonly used methods of temperature therapy within the scope of massage therapy are hot packs, ice, cold packs, and ice massage. The focus of the following section is on local applications of temperature therapy.

HOT APPLICATIONS

Heat applied locally to muscles and related soft tissues not only feels good, but also helps muscles relax, increases local circulation, and makes connective tissues more pliable. Sore, stiff muscles benefit from the increased circulation and heat.

Raising tissue temperature to between 104° and 113°F (40°–45°C) increases cell metabolism and blood flow for various therapeutic results. Lower temperatures have little therapeutic effect, and higher temperatures will damage cells (Belanger 2002).

Although heat is applied locally, use of hot packs can raise core body temperature. In that case, contraindications for thermo-hydrotherapy also apply. See Box 16.1 on page 469. Local contraindications for the use of hot packs include burns, wounds, swelling, inflammation, and skin conditions (e.g., rashes) that could be made worse by heat. Check the area visually and/or by palpation for evidence of contraindications before deciding to use hot packs.

CRITICAL THINKING

Experiment with three different heat sources or hot packs for thermotherapy applications. Compare their ease of application, safety considerations, and overall effectiveness.

1. What materials is each heat source or hot pack made from?

2. How do you get the application to the desired temperature? Is additional equipment required?

3. What are the most cost-effective methods for different therapeutic goals?

Hot Packs and Massage

The application of **hot packs** prior to massage can help begin muscle relaxation, enhance circulation locally, and prepare the area for deeper massage techniques. After massage of an area, hot packs can enhance muscle relaxation and prolong increased local circulation.

Heat sources include moist hot packs or dry hot packs or pads. Moist hot packs are more penetrating. A rubber hot water bottle is an inexpensive yet effective heat source. Some newer types of hot packs heated in microwave ovens can be good heat sources and are generally easy to use. They can be applied over warm, damp cloths to create moist heat.

Typical moist hot packs come in various sizes and shapes, and are heated in hot water. Hydrocollator units are metal containers with electrical heating elements used to keep the water within a constant range: 158°–168°F (51°–54°C). Hot packs are suspended in the hot water to a therapeutic temperature and then applied to the client.

Always check how the hot pack feels on your own skin (e.g., at the wrist) prior to applying it to a client. Packs that have been sitting in the hydrocollator for a long time (i.e., over 60 minutes) will be hotter than packs that are rotated in and out often, or that have been heating for only a few minutes.

Take care not to burn the client's skin. This is accomplished by placing towels between the hot pack and the skin. Ask the client for feedback every 5–7 minutes about how the pack feels (i.e., if it feels too hot). A visual and tactile check is also a good idea. Clients taking medications that reduce skin sensation, or alter the reaction of blood vessels to heat, or reduce their body heat control mechanisms, are not good candidates for hot packs. See Box 16.3 for guidelines for the use of moist hot packs with massage. Practice Sequence 16-1 shows a hot application on the upper back.

REALITY CHECK

KELLY

TAMIKA: I'd like to use heat applications for clients, especially in the winter, but it takes so many towels. I end up having to do a lot of extra laundry. Do you have any suggestions for alternatives?

KELLY: Hot packs heated in hydrocollators are very wet, so you have to use several towels to protect the client's skin from burning. This type of wet heat is best in clinical situations. But if your goal is to provide warmth, comfort, and some muscle relaxation, other heat sources that can be applied over the drape may be adequate. This type of hot pack is generally filled with therapeutic beads, gel, aromatic herbs, or rice and is typically heated in a microwave oven, so is more convenient for nonclinical settings. Some hot pack fillings also generate some moisture when heated, but not so much that towels are needed.

BOX 16.3 Summary of Guidelines for Safe Use of Moist Hot Packs before and during Massage

1. Be clear about your goals for using hot packs in association with massage.
2. Check to make sure that no contraindications are present and that the client is not taking medications that reduce sensation or alter circulation.
3. Get informed consent from the client to apply hot packs.
4. Instruct the client on the need for feedback about how the hot pack feels to him or her, especially if it feels too hot.
5. Check the hot pack to make sure it is the correct temperature. Touch it to your own skin (e.g., wrist) to judge if it is hot enough or too hot, and how many layers of towels to use.
6. Apply layers of towels between the client's skin and the hot pack to help avoid burns. Use more layers for more sensitive skin and for clients over 60 years old.
7. Apply a towel over the hot pack to help keep heat from escaping.
8. Ask for feedback from the client every 5 to 7 minutes or more if needed. Heat of tissues increases the longer the hot pack is applied.
9. Add additional towels beneath the hot pack if the client complains of too much heat.
10. Remove hot pack immediately if you judge potential for damage to skin or if client is having negative reaction to heat (e.g., dizziness, nausea).
11. Maximum time for hot pack use on a local area is about 20 minutes.

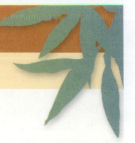

PRACTICE SEQUENCE 16.1

Hot Application on Upper Back

15 minutes
Recipient prone

Preliminary Instructions

• Prepare heat source ahead of time.
• Check for contraindications for heat applications.
• Get informed consent for the hot application.
• Get frequent feedback about heat intensity from recipient.

1

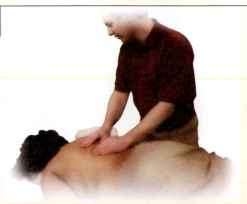

FIGURE 16.2 Prepare upper back for hot application. Undrape upper back. Check tissues visually and through palpation.

2

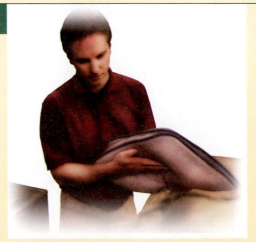

FIGURE 16.3 Check heat source for temperature. Evaluate the amount of heat given off from the source using your own sense of touch. Use your judgment on how thick a heat barrier to start with.

FIGURE 16.4 Place sheet or towel over area to be heated. Use sufficient heat barrier for the heat source used. Use at least one depth of towel under moist heat source.

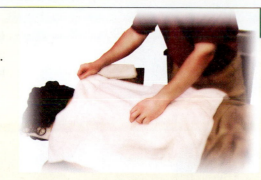

3

FIGURE 16.5 Apply the heat source and ask for immediate feedback on the heat intensity felt by the recipient. Heat should not cause pain, but feel soothing. Add or subtract heat barriers as needed to protect the skin.

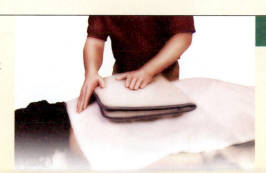

4

FIGURE 16.6 Instruct recipient on giving you feedback immediately if heat becomes too intense. Remind the person that the effects of heat can build over time.

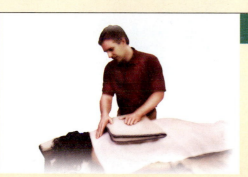

5

FIGURE 16.7 Cover heat source to slow cooling by placing a towel over it.

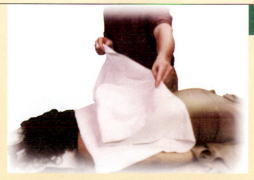

6

7

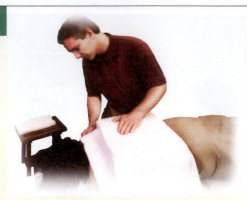

FIGURE 16.8 Get feedback every 5–7 minutes about heat intensity. Add or subtract heat barriers to maintain therapeutic effect. Massage other areas while heat is on upper back.

8

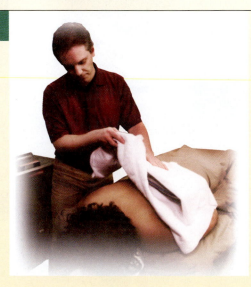

FIGURE 16.9 Remove the heat source and check the skin for redness. Massage the area and notice muscle relaxation that has occurred.

After you perform this practice sequence, evaluate how well you did by filling out Performance Evaluation Form 16–1, Hot Application on Upper Back. The form can be found in Appendix F, Performance Evaluation Forms, on page A-30 and also on your DVD.

COLD APPLICATIONS

Cryotherapy, which is cold applied locally to muscles and related soft tissues, causes vasoconstriction and decreased local circulation. There is also decrease in cell metabolism, nerve conduction velocity, pain, muscle spindle activity, and spasm in the cold area. After about 20 to 30 minutes of continuous application, cold-induced vasodilation is thought to occur. This may lead to increased circulation, but it is doubtful that circulation rises to a baseline of what it was before the cold was applied. Cold applied locally can also act eventually to lower core body temperature.

Cold applications after trauma or injury can decrease secondary cell and tissue damage. Cold helps prevent the worsening of a soft tissue injury by causing vasoconstriction. This limits internal and external bleeding. It also reduces acute inflammation and swelling.

First aid for a strain or sprain, or a blow to soft tissues, includes immediate application of cold, preferably ice cold. This limits hemorrhaging, swelling, and secondary cell hypoxia or damage. If a limb is involved, the RICES first aid principle applies (i.e., rest, ice, compression, elevation, and stabilization).

Cryotherapy is used most often with massage in settings where clients are likely to have soft tissue injury or pain. These include sports medicine and rehabilitation settings and chiropractic offices. However, any client may have had a recent injury or have muscle spasms, so knowledge of the use of cold applications can be useful. Contraindications to local cold applications include circulatory insufficiency, such as with Raynaud's disease and diabetes, allergic reaction to cold, cold sensitivity, and low core body temperature or chilling. Clients with multiple sclerosis or asthma may not react well to cold. Take special care with clients taking medications that reduce skin sensation, alter the reaction of blood vessels to heat and cold, or reduce their body temperature control mechanisms. See Box 16.4● for a summary of contraindications for cryo-hydrotherapy and cold applications.

The person receiving the cold application will normally feel the following stages: (1) a sensation of cold, (2) tingling or itching, (3) pain, aching, or burning, and (4) numbing or analgesia. It is good to inform the client about what he or she will feel, since some of the sensations can be uncomfortable. Be careful not to apply very cold applications for too long (1-hour maximum) to avoid tissue damage and frostbite. Guidelines for cold applications are summarized in Box 16.5●.

Cold Packs and Massage

Cold packs of various kinds are commercially available. They are usually made of materials that hold cold over a period of time and stay pliable even when near freezing. They have coverings for comfortable contact with skin.

Ice packs are made with ice cubes or crushed ice inside plastic bags that can be sealed. A disadvantage of ice is that it melts over time, and plastic bags can leak water. Ice,

---

| BOX 16.5 | **Summary of Guidelines for Safe Use of Cold and Ice Packs before and during Massage** |

1. Be clear about your goals for using cold applications in association with massage.
2. Check to make sure that no contraindications are present and that the client is not taking medications that reduce sensation or alter circulation.
3. Get informed consent from the client to apply cold packs.
4. Instruct the client on the need for feedback about how the cold application feels to him or her.
5. Inform the client of the stages of sensation to expect with cold applications, i.e., (1) cold sensation, (2) tingling or itching, (3) aching or burning, and (4) numbness or analgesia.
6. Apply the cold or ice pack directly to the desired area.
7. Take care when applying a cold-gel pack directly to the skin under a compression bandage, since it may cause frostbite over time.
8. Use the RICES principle if the injury is to a limb: rest, ice, compression, elevation, stabilization.
9. Ask for feedback on the cold application every 5 to 7 minutes.
10. Remove the cold pack immediately if it causes an adverse reaction (e.g., skin rash, chilling).
11. Maximum time for continuous cold application is 1 hour; 15 minutes is usually sufficient in the context of a massage session.

| BOX 16.4 | **Contraindications for Cryo-Hydrotherapy and Cold Applications** |

These contraindications and cautions apply to cryo-hydrotherapy methods that lower the core body temperature.

Contraindications

- Circulatory insufficiency or vasospastic disorders (e.g., Raynaud's disease, diabetes)
- Cardiac disorder
- Allergy to cold
- Cold hypersensitivity or chilling
- Multiple sclerosis
- Asthma
- Rheumatoid arthritis
- Osteoarthritis
- Some cancers and cancer treatments
- Infection
- Depression
- Pregnancy

Certain medications may make hydrotherapy unsafe for a client. These include drugs that:

- Alter how blood vessels react to hot and cold
- Change skin sensitivity to hot and cold
- Alter the body's temperature control or cooling mechanisms

Source: Adapted from Knight, K. L. (1995). *Cryotherapy in Sports Injury Management.* Champaign, IL: Human Kinetics; Belanger, A. (2002). *Evidenced-Based Guide to Therapeutic Physical Agents.* Philadelphia: Lippincott Williams & Wilkins; Persad, R .S. (2001). *Massage Therapy and Medications.* Toronto: Curties-Overzet Publications.

---

water below 32°F (0°C), is also hard to the touch and may be less comfortable over injuries. However, ice is readily available and generally stays cold longer than cold packs. Ice can be replaced in bags as needed to hold a freezing temperature.

Cold packs are used as adjuncts to massage to reduce muscle spasm or muscle pain, or if a client has swelling from a recent injury such as a sprained ankle. Cold may be applied to reduce spasm and pain so that the area can be massaged. It can also be used instead of massage if massage would further aggravate the injury or spasm. Cold or ice may be applied to a specific area during massage of other parts of the body. Practice Sequence 16-2 illustrates a cold application for the knee.

Ice Massage

Ice massage involves rubbing ice directly on the skin using an ice cube or ice cup. Ice cups are made by filling paper cups with water and putting them in the freezer to harden. The paper is peeled back to expose the ice with some paper left on for holding the cup.

Ice massage is performed in a circular motion over a small area for about 5–10 minutes, until the area becomes numb. Ice massage may be used to numb an area before performing deep transverse friction such as in a case of tendinitis. It allows the therapist to work deep enough without causing severe pain. Ice is also used after this treatment to continue to numb the area. Ice massage for the elbow is demonstrated in Practice Sequence 16-3.

PRACTICE SEQUENCE   16.2

Cold Application for Knee

15 minutes
Recipient supine

Preliminary Instructions

• Use a cold source that will conform to the shape of the knee.
• Check for contraindications for the cold application.
• Get informed consent for the cold application.
• Get frequent feedback about cold intensity from recipient.

1

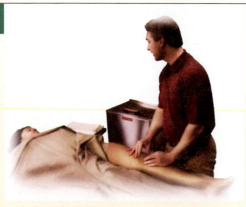

FIGURE 16.10 Prepare knee for cold application. Undrape the leg. Check tissues visually and through palpation and notice any swelling

2

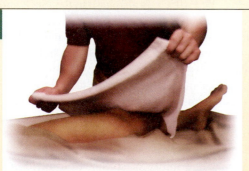

FIGURE 16.11 Place a towel or sheet over knee area. Use a thin barrier to protect skin from cold source.

3

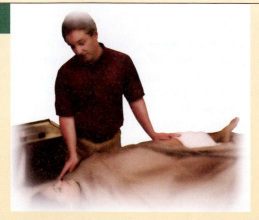

FIGURE 16.12 Instruct recipient on stages of feeling cold. Tell the recipient to let you know right away if cold becomes too intense.

FIGURE 16.13 Apply the cold source and ask for immediate feedback. Conform the cold source to the shape of the knee covering the knee cap and lateral areas.

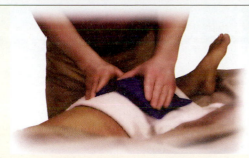

4

FIGURE 16.14 Cover and secure the cold source in place. Wrap the cold source using a towel or elastic bandage to keep it in place. Let the cold source remain in place for about 12 minutes.

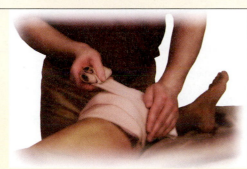

5

FIGURE 16.15 Get feedback every 5–7 minutes about cold intensity. Massage other areas while cold source is on the knee.

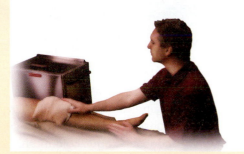

6

FIGURE 16.16 Remove cold source and check the knee for changes. Notice skin color and changes in swelling around the knee.

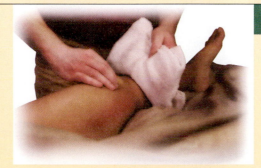

7

 After you perform this practice sequence, evaluate how well you did by filling out Performance Evaluation Form 16–2, Cold Application for Knee. The form can be found in Appendix F, Performance Evaluation Forms, on page A-31 and also on your DVD.

CASE FOR STUDY

Rod and Temperature Therapy Home Care

Rod is a client in his fifties who exercises regularly. He is usually stiff and tight in his shoulders when he comes for massage. His massage therapist thinks that temperature therapy applied between massage sessions can benefit Rod.

Question:

What temperature therapy methods might Rod's massage therapist suggest for home care?

Things to consider:

- Would thermotherapy or cryotherapy be most effective to reduce stiffness and tightness?

- What questions would help identify contraindications?
- What temperature therapy methods would be readily available to Rod at home?
- What safety considerations should the massage therapist caution Rob about?

Your Recommendation to Rod for Home Care:

_____

_____

_____

PRACTICE SEQUENCE   16.3

Ice Massage for Elbow

10 minutes
Recipient supine

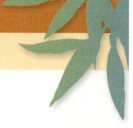

Preliminary Instructions
- Prepare ice in paper cups ahead of time.
- Check for contraindications for ice massage in the elbow area.
- Get informed consent for the ice massage.
- Get frequent feedback about cold intensity from recipient.

1

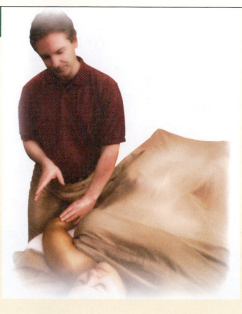

FIGURE 16.17 Position the forearm for ice massage of the tendons around the elbow. Rest the forearm comfortably on a towel. Palm is down. Instruct recipient on stages of feeling cold, and to let you know right away if the cold becomes too intense.

FIGURE 16.18 Massage extensor muscles and apply transverse friction over tendons. Knead and press into forearm muscles just distal to the elbow to locate tense muscles and tender points. Apply transverse friction to tendons in the area for about 1 minute.

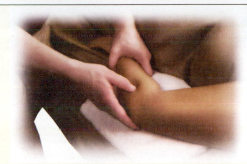

2

FIGURE 16.19 Circular movement of ice over lateral area just distal to the elbow. Use medium pressure to apply ice massage to the skin over the extensor tendons. Move ice in circular motion the entire time. Continue ice massage for 10 minutes.

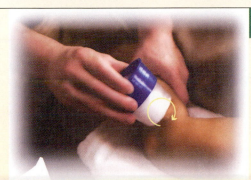

3

FIGURE 16.20 Apply superficial friction with the towel to warm and dry the area.

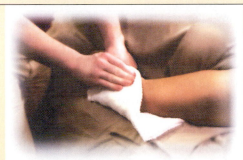

4

 After you perform this practice sequence, evaluate how well you did by filling out Performance Evaluation Form 16–3, Ice Massage for Elbow. The form can be found in Appendix F, Performance Evaluation Forms, on page A-32 and also on your DVD.

PRACTICAL APPLICATION

Perform the ice massage practice sequence on a practice client. Interview him or her to find a site that may benefit from the application and to identify any contraindications.

1. Did the practice client feel the four stages of sensation for cold applications?
2. How long did it take to cause numbness?
3. What changes did you notice in tissues receiving the ice massage?

CHAPTER HIGHLIGHTS

- Hydrotherapy is the use of water in health and healing practices.
- Temperature therapy is the application of hot or cold for therapeutic effects.
- The history of hydrotherapy can be traced to ancient times in all parts of the globe.
  - Native American traditions include the use of sweat baths and the sweat lodge ceremony.
  - Western traditions of hydrotherapy include the work of Priessnitz, Kneipp, Winternitz, Kellogg, and the Chartered Society of Trained Masseuses in England.
- Temperature therapy can be roughly divided into thermotherapy, neutrotherapy, and cryotherapy based on the temperature of the application.
  - Thermotherapy involves heat applications higher than normal body temperature.
  - Neutrotherapy involves applications at about normal body temperature.
  - Cryotherapy involves cold applications lower than normal body temperature.
- Water is used in temperature therapy in the form of liquid, steam, or ice.
- Water pressure from shower, hose, or water jets can serve as a type of massage of the soft tissues.
- Hot forms of hydrotherapy include whirlpool baths, showers, steam rooms, and sauna.
  - Effects of hot hydrotherapy include raising the body temperature, producing sweating, cleansing skin pores, increasing superficial circulation, and general relaxation.
  - Hot hydrotherapies are best used before a massage session.
  - Guidelines should be observed for safe use of these therapies
- Heat applied locally to muscles and related soft tissues feels good, helps muscles relax, increases local circulation, and makes tissues more pliable.
  - Moist hot packs are typically used for thermotherapy.
  - Measures to avoid burning the client's skin include using towels as a safety barrier and limiting the time the hot pack is applied.
- Cold applications or cryotherapy causes vasoconstriction and decreased local circulation, cell metabolism, nerve conduction, and reduced pain and spasm.
  - Cold applications are used in first aid for trauma and injury.
  - Cryotherapy methods include cold and ice packs, and ice massage.
- Contraindications and safety guidelines for all forms of hydrotherapy and thermal therapies should be observed to avoid harm to the client.

EXAM REVIEW

Key Terms

To study the key terms listed at the beginning of this chapter, match the appropriate lettered meaning to each numbered key term listed below. For additional study, look up the key terms in the Interactive Glossary on page G-1 and note other terms that compare or contrast with them.

_____ 1. Cold packs
_____ 2. Cryotherapy
_____ 3. Hydrotherapy
_____ 4. Hot pack
_____ 5. Ice massage
_____ 6. Sauna
_____ 7. Steam rooms
_____ 8. Temperature therapy
_____ 9. Thermotherapy
_____ 10. Whirlpool bath

a. Application prior to massage can help begin muscle relaxation, enhance circulation locally
b. Facility that clears sinuses, relieves respiratory congestion, raises body temperature and causes sweating
c. Wood-lined room with dry heat and low humidity
d. Involves applications above normal body temperature
e. Involves applications below body temperature
f. Therapeutic applications of hot and cold
g. Healing effects stem from the water heat and the pressure of the water coming out of the jets and hitting the body
h. Made of materials that hold cold over a period of time and stay pliable even when near freezing
i. Used to numb an area, allowing the therapist to work deep enough without causing severe pain
j. The use of water in health and healing practices

Memory Workout

To test your memory of the main concepts in this chapter, complete the following sentences by circling the most correct answer from the two choices provided.

1. Hydrotherapy is the use of (heat) (water) in health and healing practices.
2. Therapeutic use of hot and cold applications is called (temperature) (physical) therapy.
3. Sebastian (Kneipp) (Kellogg) from Bavaria further developed therapeutic use of water adding his knowledge of herbs (c. 1880).
4. Therapeutic use of water taken (internally) (externally) is outside the scope of massage therapy except for encouraging clients to drink plenty of clean pure water.
5. The (Vichy) (whirlpool) bath consists of a water tub with water jets that cause water movement or churning.
6. To prevent burns, towels are placed between the hot pack and the (top drape) (client's skin).
7. Increasing the temperature of tissues, increases cell (division) (metabolism) and blood flow locally.
8. Cold applied locally causes (decreased) (increased) local circulation.
9. Cold applied to tissues after trauma (decreases) (increases) secondary cell or tissue damage.
10. Get (written consent) (informed consent) from clients before giving hot or cold applications along with a massage session.

Test Prep

The following multiple-choice questions will help to prepare you for future school and professional exams.

1. Temperature therapy that is below the body's normal temperature is called:
   a. Thermotherapy
   b. Neutrotherapy
   c. Cryotherapy
   d. Vichy therapy
2. The humidity in a steam room is typically:
   a. 10%
   b. 40%
   c. 60%
   d. 100%
3. A sauna provides:
   a. Dry heat
   b. Wet heat
   c. Cold plunge
   d. Steam heat
4. It is best to replenish fluids during and after using a steam room or sauna by:
   a. Drinking plenty of water
   b. Drinking an alcoholic beverage
   c. Draping a wet towel over your head
   d. Soaking your feet in a tub of water
5. The temperature sensation for an application at 31° degrees Fahrenheit (1° C) is:
   a. Tepid
   b. Warm
   c. Neutral
   d. Very cold

6. Exercise caution when giving hot or cold applications to clients taking medications that:
   a. Reduce sensation
   b. Alter circulation
   c. Affect temperature regulation
   d. All of the above
7. Which of the following is *not* an effect of thermo-hydrotherapy?
   a. Increased pulse rate
   b. Increased core body temperature
   c. Increased muscle tone
   d. Sweating
8. For a person with high blood pressure, using a steam room is:
   a. Highly beneficial
   b. Contraindicated
   c. Therapeutic
   d. Advised
9. First aid for an ankle sprain would include a:
   a. Hot moist pack
   b. Hot dry pack
   c. Cold pack
   d. Hot whirlpool treatment
10. The third stage of sensation during an ice application is:
   a. Burning or aching
   b. Tingling or itching
   c. Cold
   d. Numbness

Video Challenge

Watch the appropriate segment of the video on your DVD and then answer the following questions.

Hydrotherapy and Temperature Therapies

Hot Application on Upper Back

1. In the video demonstration of a hot application, what precautions did the massage therapist take to avoid burning the client?

Cold Application for Knee

2. How did the massage therapist in the video secure the cold pack to the recipient's knee? Why?

Ice Massage for Elbow

3. In the ice massage demonstration on the video, why did the massage therapist keep the ice moving in a circle?

Comprehension Exercises

The following short answer questions test your knowledge and understanding of chapter topics and provide practice in written communication skills. Explain in two to four complete sentences.

1. Explain how to use thermo-hydrotherapy facilities in relation to a massage session.

2. Describe how you would ensure the comfort and safety of your client during hot and cold applications.
3. Describe the application of ice massage.

For Greater Understanding

The following exercises are designed to take you from the realm of theory into the real world. They will help give you a deeper understanding of the subjects covered in this chapter. Action words are underlined to emphasize the variety of activities presented to address different learning styles and to encourage deeper thinking.

1. Visit a spa or health club with hydrotherapy facilities. Observe how other people use the facilities. Was there anything you thought they needed instruction about, for example, contraindications or how best to enjoy the experience? Were there any signs or people to instruct patrons on how to use the facilities?

2. Immerse your foot or hand into a bucket of ice water. Notice the phases of sensation you experience. Say them out loud to a study partner as you experience them. (Variation: Apply a cold pack instead.)

3. Visit a training room with a certified athletic trainer. Observe how the trainer uses hydrotherapy and thermal therapy in treatment of athletes. Report your observations to a study partner or group.

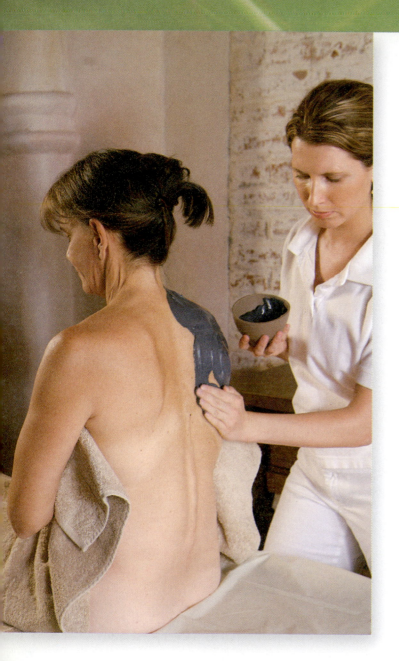

CHAPTER OUTLINE

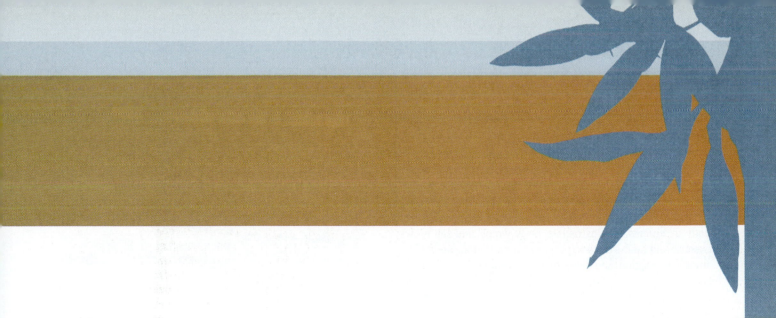

 LEARNING OUTCOMES

After studying this chapter, you will have information to:

1. Describe equipment and supplies needed for spa applications.

2. Explain the sanitation practices necessary for a spa practice.

3. Help clients choose spa treatments for themselves.

4. Describe exfoliation and its benefits.

5. Explain full body and quick prep dry brushing.

6. Describe how to perform scrubs.

7. Explain chemical, enzyme, and dissolving exfoliations.

8. Describe how to perform body wraps.

9. List the features of 10 foundational essential oils.

10. Explain how aromatherapy can be used in a massage practice.

11. Describe stone massage.

 KEY TERMS

Aromatherapy *504*

Clays *496*

Dry brushing *490*

Body polishes *491*

Body wraps *496*

Carrier oil *505*

Chemical, enzyme, or dissolving exfoliation *490*

Emollient *491*

Essential oils *504*

Exfoliation *489*

Infusion *503*

Limbic system *505*

Manual exfoliation *490*

Muds *496*

Peat *496*

Scrubs *491*

Stone massage *510*

OVERVIEW

Spa applications are typically offered within spa establishments but can also be used by massage practitioners in private practice. Spa venues range from hair salons and day spas to destination spas offering multiple-day stays and every amenity imaginable, including strategies for major lifestyle changes. Depending on the type of spa, the services can include bodywork such as massage therapy, shiatsu, and Thai massage; body treatments such as facials, body wraps, and salt glows; exercise and fitness classes; programs for nutrition, weight loss, smoking cessation, and detoxification; spiritual renewal classes such as yoga, meditation, and labyrinth walking; and cosmetic treatments for skin rejuvenation, liposuction, and plastic surgery. Many massage therapists augment their offerings with spa applications but do not consider their practices to be spas.

Note that the terms *application, service,* and *treatment* are used interchangeably in the spa setting. Although in most health settings, the word *treatment* is reserved for approaches to healing a medical condition, the spa setting has traditionally used the term to describe spa services, for example, a seaweed body wrap treatment. This stems from their history as natural healing establishments over a century ago. See page 7 in Chapter 1, The Massage Therapy Profession, for more information on personal care settings, types of spas, and typical spa services. Also see page 28 in Chapter 2, The History of Massage as a Vocation, for a historical look at personal care and natural healing venues.

There are many different spa applications and, because innovation is the hallmark of the spa industry, more are being developed all the time. Individual spas can differ greatly in what services they offer and in the equipment and supplies available. Spa staff members are expected to become familiar with and proficient at using what the spa has, and each spa provides its staff with proper training.

This chapter illustrates methods and techniques commonly provided by massage therapists in spa and private practice settings. The focus is on the spa applications of exfoliation, body wraps, aromatherapy, and stone massage.

EQUIPMENT AND SUPPLIES

There are certain pieces of equipment and categories of supplies practitioners are likely to encounter at any spa establishment, and from which massage therapists with their own practices can choose when offering spa services.

Equipment

Equipment encompasses everything from brushes used in exfoliations to Vichy showers. The following are some examples of the equipment practitioners may use while working in a spa.

- *Hot towel cabi.* This piece of equipment stores rolled moist towels at a temperature of about 175° F. Many have a built-in UV sanitizer that keeps the towels hygienic until they can be used. See Figure 17.1■.

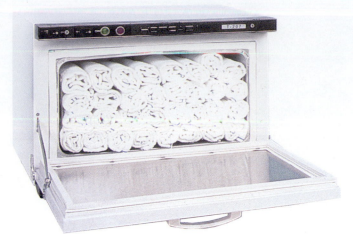

FIGURE 17.1

Hot towel cabi.

Courtesy of YCC Products, Inc.

- *Wet table.* This type of table has a drain in it. Clients lie on the table for treatments involving substances that need to be rinsed off, such as muds and seaweed. Rather than have the client go to a separate shower facility, the practitioner rinses the client using a Vichy shower or other water source while the client is on the table.
- *Wet room.* This is a specially constructed room for the use of water in treatments and may contain equipment such as wet tables, Vichy showers or other handheld showers (to remove spa substance residue from clients' bodies), whirlpool tubs, or other specialty showers or hoses. The room is usually tiled on the walls and floor, and also has drains in the floor. Figure 17.2■ shows a wet table in a wet room.
- *Vichy shower.* This shower has multiple nozzles that hang above the client. The practitioner controls the temperature, pressure, and amount of water used to rinse off the client. See Figure 17.3■.
- *Small equipment.* These include bowls used for treatment substances, spatulas, eye pillows, stones for hot and cold stone treatments, music CDs, and table warmer pads.

Supplies

Everything from substances used during treatments to footwear given to clients to wear in the spa are considered to be supplies. While there are broad categories of supplies, it is important for practitioners to remember that most spas have their own lines of signature treatments and products, and it is important for spa employees to become knowledgeable about them.

- *Linens.* These include sheets used during treatments, face-rest covers, blankets, towels, washcloths, plastic sheeting using during certain treatments (like wraps), robes, or staff uniforms (these may be laundered on-site

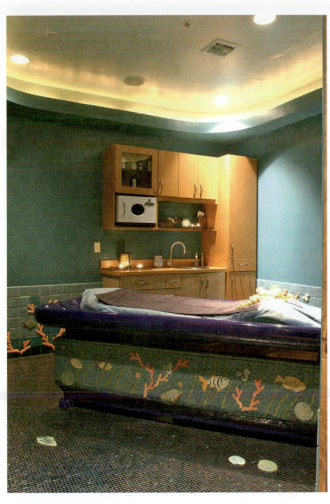

FIGURE 17.2

Wet table in a wet room.

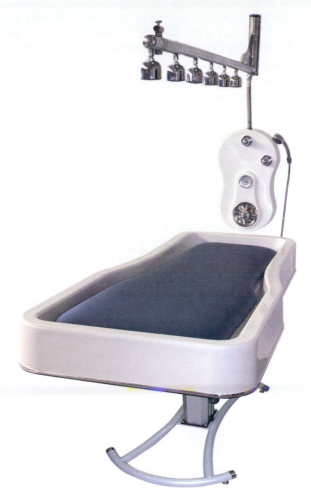

FIGURE 17.3

Athlegen Neptune Wet Table and Vichy Shower.

Courtesy of Athlegen Consolidated Enterprises

or practitioners may be expected to launder their own). Practitioners will be instructed in what the spa's protocols for handling the linen are, such as where clean ones are kept, and how to dispose of used linens.

- *Substances.* These are applied to the client's body or used as aromatherapy during the various treatments and include muds, seaweed, peat, creams, gels, exfoliation substances (salt, sugar, ground coffee, etc.), essential oils, and herbs (for herbal infusions). Practitioners will be instructed in the safe use, handling, storage, and disposal methods of each substance used within the spa.
- *Disposables.* Supplies needed during the performance of treatments, including disposable undergarments for clients, disposable spatulas to mix substances, and so forth. Disposable gloves should be available for staff use when there is contact with body fluids in a procedure.
- *Toiletries.* These are offered for client cleanliness and convenience. For spas that offer showers for client

use, they can include body washes, bath scrubbies and shower footwear, deodorant, shampoo, hair conditioner, hair spray, hair gel, combs, cotton swabs, and cotton balls. It may be the responsibility of practitioners to make sure these items are readily available for client use, or it may be a duty of other spa staff.

- *Cleaning supplies.* These are necessary for hygiene and sanitation, and include rubbing alcohol, bleach, and other sanitizers and disinfectants.

PURCHASING SUPPLIES

Most supplies can be purchased at local stores, beauty supply stores, natural foods stores (for herbs, some muds, and seaweed), and on the Internet. When considering what to buy, it is important for practitioners to consider that the supplies and equipment need to be able to stand up to a lot of treatments. Something may seem like a bargain but turn out not to be if it has to be replaced often. For example, towels that are inexpensive initially may end up being quite expensive in the long run if they are so thin that they wear out after just five or six uses. Thicker, plusher towels that cost more at first are more cost effective because they can last for 25 to 30 treatments. For more information on equipment and supplies, visit the websites listed under Chapter 17 in Appendix H, References and Additional Resources, on page A-72.

Sanitation

As discussed in Chapter 11, Hygiene, Equipment, and Environment, practitioners need to be aware of the risk of transferring pathogens from one client to another. Aside from the human factor, pathogens can also be found on supplies and equipment, as well as in any of the substances used in spa treatments. This is important to note since many pathogens grow in dark, warm, damp places, which makes spa treatment settings especially vulnerable to mold growth and disease transmission.

In addition to following personal health and hygiene practices, practitioners should know that it is important that everything is cleaned between clients, including linens, equipment, floors, tables, countertops, and so on. There are many good antibacterial sprays and disinfectants on the market; research them to find the ones that work best for you.

HELPING CLIENTS CHOOSE SPA TREATMENTS

Receiving spa treatments may be a totally new experience for the client, who may be feeling excited and apprehensive at the same time. It is the responsibility of practitioners to be knowledgeable about all the services they perform, to be able to answer clients' questions as completely as possible, and to give in-depth explanations of treatments, including:

- Benefits, indications, contraindications
- How the treatment is performed
- What results the client can expect
- How the client can expect to feel after the treatment

Some spa treatments involve a certain amount of nudity for the client. For example, a client may have mud from a mud wrap rinsed off with a Vichy shower and is either totally nude or covered only minimally for this process. Other treatments may involve minimal coverage of the breasts, genitals, and buttocks throughout the treatment. While practitioners are used to this, it may be unexpected or embarrassing for a new client. Clients need to be tactfully informed about their possible levels of nudity during treatments and given the opportunity to refuse a treatment if there is anything with which they are not comfortable. Clients may also choose to receive treatments that usually involve minimal coverage but request more conservative draping. It is up to the practitioner to modify draping as necessary to make the client feel at ease. See page 372 in Chapter 12, Body Mechanics, Table Skills, and Application Guidelines, for more information about draping.

Practitioner's Role

There are so many spa treatments available it is sometimes difficult for a client to choose which one to try. Sometimes the treatment a client really wants to experience is not one he or she should receive, or perhaps there is a treatment the client does not know about that would suit his or her needs perfectly. Practitioners need to know how to elicit information from clients so they can recommend the best spa applications for them.

There are times when clients want treatments that would not be the best for them. For example, a woman may have spent the morning sunbathing and arrives for an afternoon spa treatment, an exfoliation, with a sunburn. The scheduled treatment is not possible because it would be painful and damaging to the skin. It is up to the practitioner to explain this clearly and tactfully to the client. Most clients will accept the expertise of the practitioner and allow themselves to be directed to another treatment more appropriate under the circumstances or to reschedule the appointment. If clients insist on receiving treatments that are not in their best interests or could even be harmful to them, the practitioner who is employed in a spa should consult the spa supervisor for support in managing the situation. The practitioner can use conflict resolution skills if this occurs.

Health and Medical Considerations

The following questions need to be answered by the client on an intake form to get a picture of his or her health and medical history. This also will provide a good framework for designing the treatment session. Review the completed form and follow up by asking the client for clarification as needed.

- *Do you have any medical conditions?* This can include chronic and acute conditions. For example, uncontrolled hypertension and vascular disorders are contraindicated for herbal and mud wraps; pregnancy is a contraindication for certain spa applications and the use of some essential oils.
- *What prescription or over-the-counter medications do you take?* If a client is taking an analgesic (pain reliever), it could interfere with the ability to give accurate feedback about temperature and pressure; a hot stone treatment would therefore be contraindicated. Also, some essential oils inhibit the actions of certain medications.
- *Do you have any allergies?* Clients can be allergic to any and all spa treatment substances, including muds, peat, clays, ginger, essential oils, and sea products, including sea salt and sea mud. It is best if the client notes any allergies on an intake form so there is written documentation. People can develop allergies throughout their lives, so every time a client arrives for a treatment, the practitioner should check for any updates.

A common allergy is to shellfish. Clients who are allergic to shellfish and/or iodine should *never* receive treatments with sea products such as sea salt, seaweed, and sea mud. Clients may not realize that an allergy to shellfish and/or iodine also means allergies to sea products so it is important for the practitioner to discuss this with clients. Another common allergy is to nuts. Clients with nut allergies should not receive treatments with nut-based oils or exfoliants.

Clients may not be aware of allergies they have, so before any treatment is performed, apply the substance to a small area on the client's skin, usually the forearm, to see if there is an allergic reaction.

Allergic reactions run a wide gamut. They can be as simple as a few localized hives and itching all the way up to a full-blown anaphylactic reaction, which interferes with the client's ability to breathe.

If a client has an allergic reaction, the most important thing the practitioner should do is to stay calm and stop the treatment immediately. The substance should be removed and the client thoroughly rinsed off. If the client's condition worsens, for example, numerous hives, impaired breathing, and/or widespread inflammation, emergency care, such as calling 911, should be initiated immediately.

- *Do you have any areas of inflammation, rashes, or other skin conditions?* Skin disorders may cause certain treatments to be contraindicated, such as exfoliations. On the other hand, there are treatments that can be soothing for some skin conditions, such as a mud wrap.

- *How often do you get sick? How fast do you recover?* If robust and not prone to illness, and provided there are no other contraindicated conditions, the client can receive just about any treatment. If, however, the client is in fragile health, then treatments using hot and cold such as stone massage would need to use less extreme temperatures or are contraindicated all together. Sedating treatments may be more beneficial; invigorating treatments could possibly deplete the client further.

- *What is your temperature tolerance?* Clients who have a low tolerance to hot temperatures may not be the best candidates for hot stone treatments, or would need the temperatures lowered. Likewise, clients who have low tolerance to cold temperatures may not be the best candidates for receiving cold stone therapy, or would need the temperatures raised.

Other Considerations

There are a few other things to consider when helping a client choose spa treatments. These are related to the client's level of spa experience, goals for the visit, and plans afterwards.

- *Have you had a spa treatment before?* If there is no prior experience, then the client may need detailed explanations of all treatments. For example, the client may ask for a wrap, but after the practitioner explains that minimal draping is involved, the client may opt for a stone massage instead.

If the client has had spa treatments before, the practitioner should ask the client what the results were and whether the client liked it. Perhaps the client is looking to repeat a great experience or to try something new. If the client did not have good results or did not like the treatments, a different treatment should be suggested.

Practitioners should also let clients know that some spa treatment products have particular odors to them. Muds and peat have an earthy aroma; seaweed smells like the ocean. Practitioners can let clients smell the substances and, if the odor is displeasing, they can choose other treatments.

- *What are your desired goals for the treatment?* Does the client want softer, smoother skin? An exfoliation treatment followed by a seaweed wrap could be suggested. Does the client have a specific area of discomfort, such as wanting some muscle tension relief in the back? A hot stone massage on the area might be the best treatment. If the client has some sinus congestion, an inhalation treatment with eucalyptus essential oil could be performed.

- *What will you be doing after the treatment session?* Is it acceptable for the client to feel sedated afterward, or does the client need to be energized? This can determine what treatments to suggest. For example, if an important presentation is planned for later on in the day, then perhaps a relaxing body wrap that makes the client feel sleepy is not the best choice; a salt glow with peppermint essential oil may be better.

EXFOLIATION

Exfoliation is the peeling and sloughing off of dead skin cells from the surface of the body. An overabundance of dead skin cells can cause skin pores to clog with natural body oils, dirt, and debris, which can lead to dryness and flakiness, and the formation of pustules. Removal of the dead cells brightens skin color and clarity by encouraging the body to produce new skin cells. It also unclogs the follicles and pores, improves skin texture by making it smoother, and allows moisturizers, lotions, serums, and other preparations to better hydrate and nourish the skin. Exfoliation leaves the skin invigorated and increases vasodilation of skin blood vessels so that blood is brought to the surface of the body. It also energizes superficial lymphatic flow and stimulates nerve endings.

A full body exfoliation is a powerful therapy in and of itself that can have a positive impact on the entire body. The removal of dead skin cells, the vasodilation of skin blood vessels, and the stimulation of nerve endings make it an invigorating treatment. Exfoliation can also be a prelude to another treatment, such as a mud or herbal wrap. It not only prepares the skin for the wrap, but also it gives clients the benefit of receiving more than one treatment, enhancing their spa experience.

Contraindications for exfoliations include:

- Skin irritations
- Rashes
- Sunburn
- Allergy to substances being used
- Contagious skin condition
- Athlete's foot—only the feet would be contraindicated; the rest of the body could be exfoliated
- Recent tattoo
- Area shaved 24 hours prior to treatment

Methods of Exfoliation

The term *exfoliant* encompasses both the substances and the tools used to remove dead skin cells. There are two main methods of exfoliation. The physical process of applying friction with abrasives is called **manual exfoliation.** Manual exfoliants include tools such as dry brushes, mitts, loofahs, and abrasive cloths, and natural substances such as salt, sugar, cornmeal, and ground coffee beans that are abrasive. These substances are typically mixed with water, oils, or creams before being rubbed over the surface of the skin.

The other method is **chemical, enzyme, or dissolving exfoliation.** This consists of chemicals or enzymes that work by dissolving dead skin cells, but do not overstimulate the skin the way manual abrasives can. After application, the enzymes are washed or rubbed off. Natural substances such as yogurt, milk, and papaya contain acids and enzymes that act as natural exfoliants. There are also many different commercial preparations, and the manufacturer's instructions need to be followed carefully when they are used.

Manual Exfoliation

Manual exfoliation can be done using many different tools and substances, depending on the level of abrasion needed.

DRY BRUSHING

Exfoliation using brushes or fiber tools is known as **dry brushing** or *body brushing.* Other manual exfoliation tools that can be used for dry brushing include loofahs, nylon mitts, sisal mitts (sisal is a coarse fiber), ayate cloths (a woven fiber that is less coarse than sisal), and other abrasive cloths depending on the level of abrasion desired. See Figure 17.4■ for examples of manual exfoliation tools. Dry brushing can be performed from mild to moderate to vigorous.

A full-body dry brushing takes about 30 minutes and can be offered as an individual treatment or in conjunction with other therapies. For example, body brushing can be done before a body wrap. When the dead skin cells are removed, the substances used in body wraps, such as mud or cream, can have a much better effect on the skin. An abbreviated version is called quick prep dry brushing. It addresses the entire body and usually only takes a total of 10 minutes—5 minutes with the client prone and 5 minutes with the client supine.

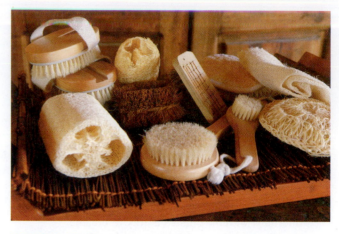

FIGURE 17.4

Examples of manual exfoliation tools: lower left—loofah; top and center—various brushes; top right—ayate cloth; bottom right—sisal mitt.

Dry brushing and all manual exfoliation methods help to stimulate the flow of lymph. Dry brushing strokes applied to the extremities, face, neck, upper chest, abdomen, and back are done lightly to stimulate the flow of lymph in superficial lymphatic vessels. See page 184 in Chapter 6, Anatomy & Physiology, Pathology, and Kinesiology, for more information about the lymphatic system and review the section on lymphatic facilitation on page 529 in Chapter 18, Contemporary Massage and Bodywork. The strokes performed in dry brushing and other manual exfoliation techniques travel along the pathway of lymph flow:

- In the extremities, the strokes are performed toward the client's heart.
- Strokes on the face, neck, and upper chest are performed downward.
- Abdominal strokes are performed in a clockwise direction, then up each side to the center of the abdomen.
- Back strokes are performed downward from the neck and shoulders to the mid-back, then from the lumbar area up to the mid-back.

When using the body brush or exfoliation tool, the most efficient stroke is a brisk half-moon stroke, using a flick of the wrist. These brisk movements remove the maximum amount of dead skin cells with each stroke (see Figure 17.5■).

For clients who have mild edema not due to medical conditions, such as from standing for long periods of time, dry brushing may be useful. Practitioners, however, should never go beyond their scope of practice. There are specific courses of study in lymphatic drainage, including certification courses, that give practitioners the skills and tools needed to address more serious medical conditions such as lymphedema.

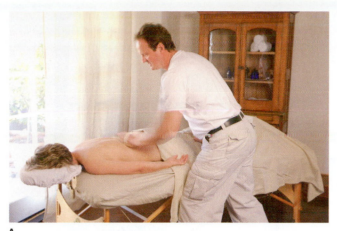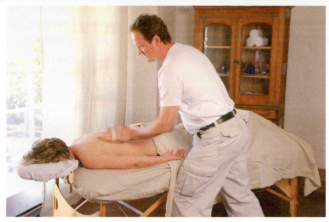

A   B

FIGURE 17.5

A brisk half-moon stroke is the most efficient stroke to use with the body brush or exfoliation tool because it removes the maximum amount of dead skin cells with each stroke.

SCRUBS AND BODY POLISHES

Other manual exfoliation methods are **scrubs** or *frictions using salts, sugar, or coarser organic substances.* These tend to be brisk treatments that leave the client energized. The exfoliant substance is mixed with a fluid such as water, oil, cream, milk, yogurt, vinegar, water, or a body wash. Essential oils can be added to the mixture to enhance the treatment with fragrance. Since these treatments both remove the top layers of the skin and cause vasodilation of skin blood vessels, the person is left with brighter skin characterized as a "glow." Because of this, scrubs using salt and sugar are often referred to as *salt glows* and *sugar glows.*

Unlike salt, sugar has moisturizing properties; like salt, it leaves the skin soft and smooth. The salt or sugar is usually mixed with a few drops of oil and a little water, to make it the consistency of snow. The amount of water needed to make the mixture is minimal enough that it does not dissolve the salt and sugar crystals. The salt or sugar can be mixed completely with oil for the exfoliation but this makes for a messier treatment. The oil is difficult to remove from the client's body and to launder from the sheets.

Salts and sugars are particularly useful because, in addition to being abrasive, they contain glycolic acid that dissolves away dead skin cells so they can be considered chemical or enzymatic exfoliants as well. Additionally, salt is an excellent substance to use in spa and hydrotherapy treatments because it can:

- Act as a natural antibacterial agent.
- Draw impurities out of the skin.
- Ease certain skin disorders such as eczema and psoriasis.

There are several major types of salts used in spa treatments. Sea salt is often used, and the salts harvested from the Dead Sea, which is located between the West Bank of Israel and Jordan, are popular. The magnesium and potassium in Dead Sea salts have cleansing, detoxification, and restorative properties, especially for the skin and muscles.

Desert mineral salts are gathered from deserts that are the remnants of prehistoric oceans. The most common desert mineral salt is borax. Borax, or sodium borate, is a complex mineral, mined near Death Valley, California, as well as in Tibet and Italy. It is naturally fine-grained so is ideal for use in body polishes. Redmond salt is another type of desert mineral salt. It gets its name from the part of the world in which it was initially discovered, Redmond, Utah. Redmond salt contains over 50 trace minerals, which gives it a slight pink color.

Epsom salt is named for the mineral-rich waters of Epsom, England. The therapeutic agent in Epsom's water is magnesium sulfate, a mineral salt. Epsom salt can be used for exfoliation; soothing, stress-reducing soaks; reducing inflammation; and calming muscle aches and pains.

Unrefined salt is always the best choice to use in spa treatments because it has no additives nor has it undergone chemical processing. Dead Sea salt, sea salt, and natural mineral salts come in different size grains. A fine- or medium-grain salt is best for a salt glow exfoliation or body polish.

Body polishes are a gentler form of exfoliation using softer granules such as those found in fine blue cornmeal or finely ground natural substances like crushed almonds or grape seed meal. A skin **emollient** such as oil, lotion, or cream can be used as part of the mixture. A skin emollient is a substance that makes the skin soft and supple. For coarser grains, the emollient should be thicker; for smaller grains, the emollient can be thinner.

Many different substances can be used for scrubs and body polishes. Just about anything that occurs in granular form, or that can be ground into granules, can be used as long as it is natural. When using natural substances, it is best to grind them to a desired consistency and make them into a paste or slurry using water, oil, cream, milk, yogurt, vinegar, a body wash, or any other liquid of choice.

Additionally, practitioners can explore the use of materials found in their geographic areas. For example, grape seeds, wine, and grape-seed oil are used for scrubs at spa and bodywork practices in the Napa Valley wine country of California. The Spa at the Hotel Hershey in Hershey, Pennsylvania, offers a chocolate sugar scrub. Substances used in scrubs and body polishes include:

- Coffee grounds
- Cornmeal—blue, white, yellow
- Crushed pearls
- Ground nuts—almonds, peanuts, hazel nuts, etc.
- Pulverized pumice (crushed volcanic rock)
- Salt—sea salt, Epsom salt, Dead Sea salt, desert mineral salt
- Seeds—grape, poppy, flax, sunflower, sesame
- Sugar—table sugar, raw sugar, brown sugar
- Oatmeal
- Barley

Figure 17.6■ shows some substances used in scrubs and body polishes.

There are several factors to consider when helping clients choose which exfoliation substances would work best for them. For delicate or sensitive skin, milder abrasives such as those used in body polishes would be appropriate. Clients with dry skin may benefit from the hydrating aspects of a sugar scrub. Salt scrubs may be useful for a client with oily skin. Pumice tends to be more abrasive than many other exfoliation substances, making it an excellent scrub for the feet.

An exfoliation can be very invigorating, so practitioners need to keep communicating with the client about pressure of application. Sometimes deeper pressure and more time are needed to exfoliate the soles of the feet, palms of the hands, elbows, and knees.

Natural exfoliation substances leave residue on the body; therefore, it may be best to use them in locations where there is access to a shower. Some spas will have wet tables or Vichy showers available for rinsing clients thoroughly. This will involve a level of client nudity and, as discussed earlier in the chapter, it is very important that practitioners explain clearly to clients how the procedure is performed and what the client can expect.

If the exfoliation is being done in a dry room with no access to a shower, the exfoliation substance can be removed using the dry room substance removal technique as described in Box 17.1●.

Preparing for a Scrub Application

Gather the supplies needed for the scrub application before the client arrives. Essential supplies and equipment are shown in Figure 17.7■ and include:

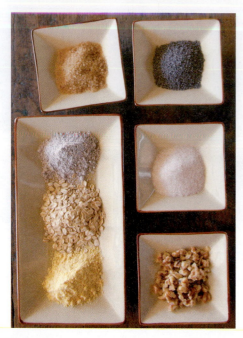

FIGURE 17.6

Common substances for scrubs and/or body polishes: top left—flax seeds; top right—poppy seeds; middle left (top to bottom)—blue cornmeal, oatmeal, yellow cornmeal; middle right—sea salt; bottom right—grape seeds.

- Small, nonmetal bowl for exfoliation substance—nonmetal because the substance may react chemically with metal, changing the substance's properties.
- Natural exfoliating substance (one-quarter to one-half cup). If performing a salt glow, use 50 percent fine salt and 50 percent medium grain salt (sea salt, Epsom salt, Dead Sea salt, desert mineral salt). If performing a sugar glow, use table, brown, or raw sugar.
- Essential oil(s). If using an essential oil, a couple of drops of a carrier oil will also be needed. For more information on essential oils, see the Aromatherapy section in this chapter on page 504.
- Liquid to make a paste or slurry (water, milk, yogurt, oil, etc.).
- Three cloth sheets (one fitted and two flat) or two sheets (one fitted and one flat) and one large towel, approximately 30″ × 60″, can also be used. The client's drape can be a flat sheet or a large towel.

BOX 17.1	Dry Room Substance Removal Technique

1. Place a warm, moist towel on the exfoliated area of the body for a few seconds, patting it down firmly.
2. Remove the substance with one firm, smooth stroke, taking care not to scrub or wipe with the towel.
3. A new warm, moist towel is used for each area of the body from which the exfoliation substance needs to be removed.

PRACTICAL APPLICATION

Make and try out your own natural exfoliants for scrubs. Compare cost of supplies, ease of application, and overall effectiveness.

1. Which substances and liquids go together the best?

2. What considerations (such as allergies) do you need to keep in mind when using these exfoliants on clients?
3. How could you pair scrubs with other treatments to make them more effective and appealing to clients?

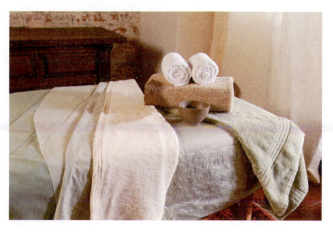

FIGURE 17.7

Equipment and supplies needed for manual exfoliation using natural substances.

- One large towel, approximately 30″ × 60″, to be used for draping the chest area when applying the scrub to the client's abdomen.
- If there is no access to a shower, a basin of warm water and three or four towels, approximately 18″ × 30″, are needed for substance removal. A towel cabi or electric cooking pot such as a Crock Pot™ filled with moist towels can also be used. More towels may be necessary for large clients or for those with a lot of body hair.

After the supplies are gathered, prepare the work space in this manner:

- Place three sheets, or two sheets and one large towel, lengthwise on top of the table.
- Put the exfoliation substance, liquid, and small bowl within easy reach.
- If working in a dry room and using an electric pot or cabi, turn on the warmer to heat the towels for substance removal at the end of the treatment. Moisten the towels and put them in the electric pot or cabi. If using a basin of warm water to heat and moisten the

towels, place the basin in a convenient spot so it can be filled with warm water during the treatment.

Performing a Scrub Application

To begin, the client gets on the table in supine position underneath the top sheet or large towel. He or she will be lying on top of two sheets. Throughout the application, be sure to ask the client for feedback about the amount of pressure you are using and adjust as necessary.

1. Blend the natural exfoliating substance with the fluid in the bowl until it resembles a slurry. Just enough fluid is added to make the salt or sugar the consistency of snow; if desired, an essential oil (mixed well with a couple of drops of carrier oil) can be added to the mixture.
2. Undrape one of the client's legs. Pour some water into your hands and, starting at the right foot, apply it up the client's leg.
3. Rub a small amount of the exfoliation mixture between your hands and apply to the top surface of the client's foot using small circular strokes to thoroughly exfoliate it.
4. Continue using small circular strokes up the ankle and anterior right leg, taking more exfoliation mixture as needed (Figure 17.8■). Redrape the leg, and repeat on the left leg.
5. Move to one side of the client's upper body and undrape the arm. Use small, circular strokes to thoroughly exfoliate the client's hand and arm, up to the shoulder. Redrape and repeat on the other arm.
6. Standing at the head of the table, accordion the large chest draping towel vertically over the client's chest area and grasp the top of the large, horizontal towel on top of the client. As you unfold the vertical towel (Figure 17.9A), fold down the horizontal towel until the client's chest is draped by the vertical towel and the abdomen is undraped (Figure 17.9B■).
7. Using smaller movements and a lighter touch, stroke in a clockwise direction on the abdominal area. Finish

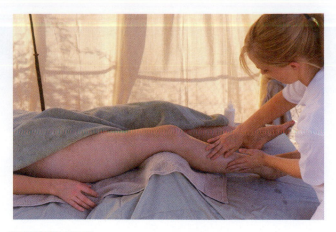

FIGURE 17.8

Use small circular strokes up the ankle and leg.

this area by exfoliating each of the client's sides and coming back to the center of the abdomen. Pull the towel up over the client's abdomen and draping towel on the client's chest area, then gently pull the chest draping towel out from under the sheet.

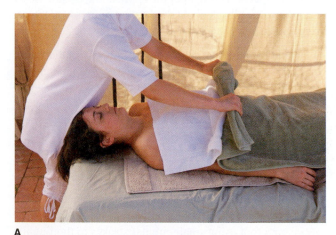

A

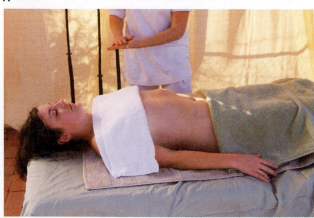

B

FIGURE 17.9

Undrape the abdomen.

8. Move to the head of the table to exfoliate the client's upper chest area. Use smaller movements and a lighter touch, working downward from the collarbone. If the client's face is to be included, a light touch is also used. With small gentle strokes, exfoliate from the chin to forehead.

9. Before the client turns over to prone position, remove the exfoliation substance (it can be left on and removed all at once at the end of the treatment, if preferred). If using a wet table or Vichy shower, rinse the client thoroughly. If working in a dry room, use the dry room substance removal technique described earlier in Box 17.1.

10. Help the client turn over. Undrape the left leg and exfoliate the bottom of the foot using small circular strokes, then continue using small circular strokes up the posterior leg, including the gluteal area, taking care to use less pressure on the back of the knee. Redrape and repeat on the right leg.

11. Move to the head of the table and undrape the client's back. Using small, circular strokes, apply the exfoliating substance to the client's neck and back (Figure 17.10■), moving around to the side of the table to include the lateral sides of the back. The exfoliation process is now complete.

12. If using a wet table or Vichy shower, rinse the client thoroughly. If there is a separate shower facility, help the client off the table, draping the top sheet or large towel around him or her for modesty. Guide the client to the shower and then back to the treatment table after rinsing off. While the client is in the shower, remove the top sheet on the massage table, uncovering the fresh, fitted sheet underneath.

13. If the exfoliation is being done in a dry room with no access to a shower, use the dry room removal tech-

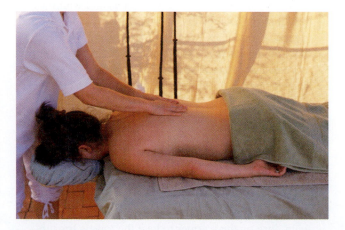

FIGURE 17.10

Using small, circular strokes, exfoliate the client's neck and back.

nique as described in Box 17.1, then remove the sheet the client is lying on using the dry room sheet removal technique described in Box 17.2● and shown in Figure 17.11■.

14. Whichever method is used to remove the exfoliation substance, and once the client is lying on a clean sheet, apply a moisturizing oil or lotion to the body.

Chemical Exfoliation

Another type of exfoliation uses chemical, enzyme, or dissolving exfoliants. Enzymes and alphahydroxy acids (AHA) or betahydroxy acids (BHAS) are found in commercial products. They are also found in nature as:

- Citric acid in citrus fruits
- Malic acid in apples
- Tartaric acid in grapes
- Lactic acid in dairy products like milk, cream, and yogurt
- Glycolic acid in sugar and sugar cane

When these acids are applied to the skin, they loosen the keratin that holds skin cells together, allowing the cells to be easily sloughed off. Papaya (papain) and pineapple (bromelain) also contain enzymes that are effective exfoliants. Because they are nonacid enzymes, they are considered the safest for sensitive skin, unless there is an allergy to papaya or pineapple.

A chemical exfoliation can be very gentle on the skin or very aggressive, as in a medical facial peel. It is recommended that a reputable esthetician be consulted regarding the use of any over-the-counter chemical, enzyme, or dissolving exfoliation products. It is very likely that spas will carry chemical, enzyme, or dissolving exfoliation products. Spa staff members who are expected to use these on clients will receive training on how to apply them properly.

A full-body chemical, enzyme, or dissolving exfoliation treatment can be done in much the same way as a scrub application with a few modifications:

- Approximately one-half cup of the exfoliation substance is needed and no additional liquid should be needed.
- Preparation is the same with the addition of a large towel placed horizontally at the head of the table
- The application is similar, with the exfoliation substance being applied either by hand or by painting it on the client's body with a brush. Once the exfoliation substance has been applied to both the front and back of the client, instead of being immediately removed, the practitioner wraps the two top sheets around the client securely, then wraps the towel around the client over the sheets (Figure 17.12■). The client stays wrapped for about 20 minutes, after which the exfoliation substance is either rinsed off or removed using the dry room substance removal technique described in Box 17.1.

<table>
<tr><td>**BOX 17.2**   **Dry Room Sheet Removal Technique**</td></tr>
</table>

1. Have the client lift his or her head slightly, then reach across the client's body, grasp the sheet on both sides, and gently pull down.
2. With the client's head back down on the table, have him or her lift the shoulders, then lay the shoulders down, then lift the hips and lay the hips down as you continue pulling the sheet toward the foot of the table.

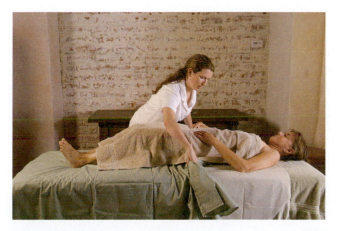

FIGURE 17.11

Removing the sheet from underneath the client.

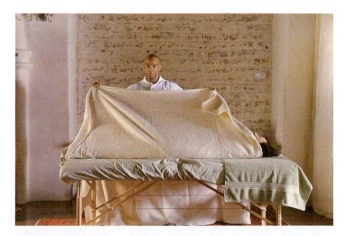

FIGURE 17.12

Wrap the two top sheets around the client securely.

- Once the exfoliation is complete, another treatment can be performed, such as a massage or body wrap.

BODY WRAPS

A popular spa treatment is the **body wrap.** Its primary purpose is to detoxify the body by stimulating blood and lymph circulation. Body wraps can be used in conjunction with many different substances. Muds, peats, and seaweed are commonly used materials, as well as sheets soaked in an herbal infusion (herbal wraps). After the substance is applied, the body is wrapped in sheets, blankets, and/or a plastic covering.

New wraps are being continually developed. For example, avocado, aloe, and chocolate wraps are currently popular. Spas and individual therapists can offer regional specialties, such as a prickly pear gel wrap in the southwest. As more and more organic substances are discovered to have healing properties, innovations in body wrap materials are inevitable. Treatments also can be packaged together, such as a desert mineral salt scrub applied before a desert herbal wrap, a sea salt glow coupled with a seaweed body wrap, or a coffee scrub preceding a chocolate wrap.

It is important to begin with an exfoliation. Removing the dead skin cells enables the substance being used to work more efficiently. This can be done with any exfoliation treatment, although the quick-prep dry-brushing technique is usually a standard exfoliation that can be done before any body wrap. The full-body dry brushing can be performed if clients desire a longer treatment.

There are many ways to perform wraps. Generally, each spa has its own body wrap protocols and trains their practitioners accordingly. What is presented in this chapter may or may not be consistent with how individual spas perform their wraps. However, by practicing the procedures in this chapter, practitioners, whether they work in a spa, clinic, or private practice, will acquire foundational skills, become comfortable handling supplies and equipment, and become able to discuss body wrap options with clients in a knowledgeable manner.

The body wrap treatment itself typically takes 35–40 minutes. The time can be extended to 60–90 minutes when supplemented with other bodywork treatments, such as full-body dry brushing, massage therapy, shiatsu, acupressure, or reflexology. Some body wraps use creams and gels, such as aloe vera, cocoa butter, or shea butter to smooth and hydrate the skin. An ideal way to conclude the wrap is to perform a short gliding massage so the body wrap substance is evenly distributed and absorbed.

Contraindications for body wraps include:

- Heart conditions
- Untreated hypertension
- Allergy to iodine or shellfish (seaweed wraps)
- Inflammation
- Vascular disease, including varicose veins
- Numbness/loss of sensation in area; neuropathy

- Flare-up stages of autoimmune disorders such as lupus, rheumatoid arthritis, and multiple sclerosis (the heat from a wrap would be painful and debilitating)
- Skin conditions made worse by heat; burns
- Intolerance to heat
- Broken or irritated skin
- High body temperature (fever)
- Claustrophobia
- Pregnancy

Muds and Clays

Sometimes the terms *mud* and *clay* are used interchangeably because they can resemble each other. However, they have different constituents and different properties, and need to be considered separately.

Muds are differentiated based on the soils and marine sediments from which they are derived. Inorganic muds contain mostly minerals that result from lake and river sedimentation and have very little organic material. Volcanic muds can be found near hot mineral springs. Organic muds are formed from algae, plant, and animal matter that have mixed with lime, clay, and sand in the soil. The colors of the muds depend on the amounts of various minerals in them. For instance, muds that are red contain a high amount of iron.

One of several properties of muds that can make them therapeutic is their mineral content. The minerals help with deep skin cleansing and aid in the removal of waste products by their drawing action, which also can stimulate local blood and lymphatic flow. When applied, mud forms a covering that acts as an insulator on the body, trapping heat and keeping it from radiating away and keeping water from evaporating from the body. Thus muds are excellent warming and hydrating treatments. The trapped heat also serves to increase local blood circulation.

Overall, muds are used therapeutically to help relieve pain in muscles and joints, and pain from tendinitis, muscle strain, joint injuries such as sprains, noninflammatory stages of arthritis and bursitis, and to soothe certain skin conditions.

The therapeutic effects of both marine-based and soil-based **clays** lie in their mineral content and ability to suspend easily in an emulsion with water or other liquid. Clays draw impurities from the body, aiding deep skin cleansing and the removal of waste products. Because clays are porous and hold water molecules they hold heat especially well, making them excellent for heat applications.

Muds and clays are categorized based on their region of origin and composition. New ones are continually being discovered, and new treatments are developed that are location specific. Table 17.1 ■ shows representative examples of muds and clays from the United States and around the world.

Peat

For the past 200 years, peat has been used therapeutically in baths and packs. **Peat** is an organic soil that contains minerals, organic material, water, and trapped air. It is formed by

TABLE 17.1	Examples of Muds and Clays from the United States and Around the World	
Mud/Clay	Location	Comments
Calistoga mud	Calistoga, CA	Volcanic mud and hot springs known for their healing properties; Native Americans first made use of the mud baths and later the Spaniards; today, many spas are located in the area
Natural red clay	Glen Ivy Hot Springs, Corona, CA	Clay known for healing and purifying; Native Americans designated the area as sacred; later the Spaniards took advantage of the healing benefits; today a spa on the site offers treatments from local mud
Dead Sea mud	Dead Sea, Israel	Mineral-rich, highly saline mud that draws impurities and retains heat; used for a wide range of skin disorders such as psoriasis and eczema; especially beneficial for muscle pain and stiffness, arthritis, and other joint pain
Rotorua thermal mud	New Zealand	Volcanic mud; silky in texture and rich in minerals and trace elements; QE Health (formerly known as the Queen Elizabeth Hospital) in Rotorua uses the mud as part of its standard care in the treatment of arthritis and other joint conditions
Muds and clays	Australia	Muds and clays found near mineral-rich, natural springs; harvested from undeveloped areas so are essentially free from chemical pollutants; sun dried after being harvested; used for over 60,000 years by Aboriginal tribes for healing, sacred and ceremonial purposes; only recently available outside Aboriginal culture
Rasul (Rhassoul)	Morocco	Lava clay mined in the Atlas Mountains of Eastern Morocco; used alone or in a combination mud and steam treatment originating in the Middle East

Sources: Calistoga Spas, "The Mud Baths" (2008); Glen Ivy Hot Springs Spa, "Hot Springs Spa, History" (2008); Minton, M., "Mud: Dig It!" (2008); Williams, A., *Spa Bodywork, A Guide for Massage Therapists* (2007).

the decomposition of layers of plants, mainly mosses, and animal matter under bodies of water. The properties of the different peats depend on the local flora and fauna that made up the layers. Most peats used in spa therapies are a combination of moss and sedge, a marshland plant. Peats are mostly cultivated in Ireland, Austria, Germany, the Czech Republic, and other Eastern European countries.

The substances in peat that contribute to its therapeutic effectiveness are organic acids and minerals. The acids contribute to peat's ability to draw and absorb toxins from the body. Physically, peat contains micropores that allow it to take in water like a sponge. Like muds and clays, peat can form a covering that acts an insulator on the body. It keeps heat from radiating away from the body and keeps water from evaporating from the body. Thus, peats are excellent warming and hydrating treatments. The heat also increases local blood and lymph circulation.

Peats are used to help relieve aching muscles and joints, and pain from muscle injuries, noninflammatory stages of arthritis, and to soothe skin disorders.

Moor Mud

Moor mud is a type of peat that is also known as *black mud,* because of its appearance. It is the mineral-rich sedimentation that is deposited at the bottom of lakes and rivers fed by both hot springs and cool springs. The hot springs contribute volcanic ash to the mixture of plant material settling to the bottom of the water. The lakes from which moor mud is taken maintain a temperature around 86° F, but the combination of hot and cool water creates a great deal of circulation in the lake. This enhances the decomposition of organic mate-

rial; layers and layers build up over time. The Neydharting Moor is in a glacial valley that was once a lake, and the moor has been developing for over 20,000 to 30,000 years. Neydharting moor mud is an organic mud and is known for being pure and nutrient-rich.

Moor mud has a very low pH, usually around 3.54. The application of moor mud can assist in the regeneration of the acid mantel of the skin, which protects the body from harmful bacteria. High grade moor muds come from Austria, Germany, Hungary, and the Czech Republic. In North America, Canadian moor mud is known for its mineral rich qualities (Figure 17.13■).

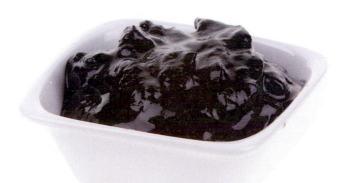

FIGURE 17.13

Hungarian Moor Mud can assist in the regeneration of the acid mantel of the skin, which protects the body from harmful bacteria.

Courtesy of Universal Companies, Inc.

Seaweed and Sea Mud

Seaweed and sea mud are organic materials that have more than 60 salts, vitamins, and other trace elements essential to the body. Seaweed and sea mud have the same therapeutic benefits to the body as other muds. In addition, they are also antibacterial agents; the minerals and salts in these sea products kill certain bacteria.

The term *seaweed* has become an umbrella term for any marine plant or algae. However, seaweed is not technically a true plant. While it does have chlorophyll, which allows it to produce oxygen like plants do, it does not have true roots, stems, or leaves. It is actually *algae.* Often, the terms algae and seaweed are used interchangeably. Algae are groups of aquatic organisms that perform photosynthesis. They are found in almost every habitat in the world. Species of algae can be anything from single-celled and microscopic, such as plankton, to multicellular and huge, such as a brown seaweed that has fronds (leaves) 200 feet long. There are many different types of seaweed, and some are harvested from beaches where they have washed up, some are harvested from the water close to shore, and some are harvested from the deep oceans.

The three major categories of seaweed are based on their colors: green, brown, and red. *Green seaweeds* are found near shores in shallow waters. One of the most common green seaweeds used in spa treatments is sea lettuce (*Ulva lactuca),* which is used to relieve inflammation and muscle soreness.

Brown seaweeds have a brown pigment that masks the green of the chlorophyll. There are two major groups of brown seaweeds used in spa treatments, the *Laminaria* species (kelp) and the *Fucus* species (wracks). Brown seaweeds are used in spa treatments and hydrotherapy treatments for detoxification, revitalization (through increased local blood and lymph circulation), slimming, and skin tightening.

The *red seaweeds* are mostly delicate and fernlike. One red seaweed, *Chondrus crispus,* actually grows in more shallow waters, especially around the British Isles. Because it is harvested extensively in Ireland, it is called Irish moss. Another name for it is carrageen (or carrageen moss). Irish moss is used in spa and hydrotherapy treatments for detoxification, revitalization (through increased local blood and lymph circulation), slimming, skin tightening, and moisturizing.

There are other algae that are not seaweed; some of these are also used in spa therapy treatments. These include spirulina, a type of blue-green algae, and white algae, which is actually a lichen. Lichens are a combination of a fungus and an organism, usually a type of green algae, which produces food for the lichen from sunlight. Spirulina and white algae treatments are used in spa treatments for detoxification, revitalization (through increased local blood and lymph circulation), slimming, skin tightening, and moisturizing.

Sea mud is collected from beaches at low tide and mixed with seawater. Like all sea products, it is used for its analgesic, warming, and sedative properties, as well as for detoxification. Sea mud can be used by itself or mixed with clays.

Preparing for a Body Wrap Application

Gather the supplies needed for the body wrap application before the client arrives or while he or she is undressing. Essential supplies and equipment are shown in Figure 17.14■ and include:

- Exfoliation tools or ingredients for a scrub.
- Mud, seaweed or peat; or powders of any of these mixed with water; or gels or cream of any of these (one-quarter to one-half cup).
- Small, nonmetal bowl—nonmetal because mud and peat react chemically with metal and their properties will change. Likewise, mud and peat should not be stored in metal containers.
- Three cloth sheets (one fitted and two flat).
- Insulating sheet (rubber, plastic, Mylar, etc.).
- Wool blanket.
- One extra large towel, approximately 35″ × 65″.
- Two large towels, approximately 30″ × 60″.
- Textured washcloth or bath scrubby the client can use to remove the mud or peat if there is access to a shower.
- If there is no access to a shower, a basin of warm water and three to four towels, approximately 18″ × 30″, for substance removal are needed. A towel cabi or electric pot filled with moist towels can also be used. More towels may be necessary for large clients or for those with a lot of body hair.
- Washcloth.
- Small bowl.
- Cool water.

After the supplies are gathered, prepare the work space in this manner:

- Layer the table in the following order, as shown in Figure 17.15■:
  ○ Fitted sheet to protect table
  ○ One large towel placed horizontally across the head of the table

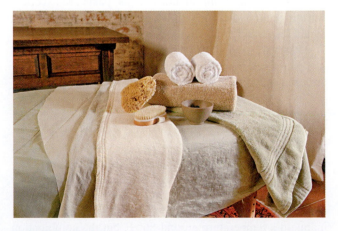

FIGURE 17.14

Equipment and supplies for a mud or peat body wrap.

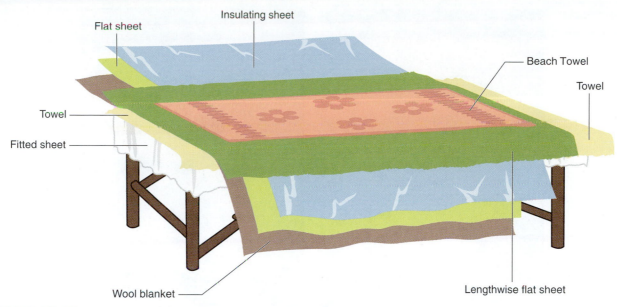

Flat sheet

Insulating sheet

Beach Towel

Towel

Towel

Fitted sheet

Wool blanket

Lengthwise flat sheet

FIGURE 17.15

Layers of sheets and towels on the table.

- ○ Wool blanket placed horizontally across the table, on top of the towel, leaving enough room for the head to rest on the towel
  - ○ One large towel placed horizontally across the end of the table, on top of the wool blanket
  - ○ Flat sheet placed horizontally on top of the wool blanket
  - ○ Insulating sheet placed horizontally on top of the cloth sheet
  - ○ One flat sheet placed lengthwise on top of the insulating sheet
  - ○ Extra large towel placed lengthwise on top of the flat sheet
- Place the body wrap substance (mud, peat, seaweed) in the small bowl; position the bowl within easy reach.
- If working in a dry room and using an electric pot or cabi, turn it on to warm the smaller towels for substance removal at the end of the treatment. Moisten the towels and put them in the electric pot or cabi. If using the basin of warm water and towels, place the basin in a convenient place so it can be filled it with warm water during the treatment.
- Fill the small bowl with cool water and place the washcloth in it. Position it within easy reach.
- Leave the room while the client gets on the table under the extra large towel, lying prone.
- It is important to stay near the client while he or she is wrapped. Some clients may become claustrophobic or overheated and need to have the wrappings removed as soon as they start feeling uncomfortable.

Performing a Body Wrap Application

1. Perform a pre–body wrap exfoliation starting with the client prone and ending with the client supine.
2. Remove the sheet immediately under the client. Use the dry room sheet removal technique described earlier. Set the sheet aside. Make sure that the client's shoulders are slightly below the top of the insulating sheet.
3. Help the client sit up and quickly apply the body wrap substance to the back with long, smooth strokes, covering the area thoroughly (Figure 17.16■). Help the client lie back down.
4. Move to the client's left leg and ask him or her to flex the knee while draping carefully and securely. To stabilize the client's leg, gently sit on the foot (Figure 17.17A■). Apply the substance to the posterior leg with one smooth stroke (Figure 17.17B). Grasp the client's ankle and lay the leg flat.
5. Apply the substance to the client's left anterior leg with long, smooth strokes. Cover the left leg with the insulating sheet to prevent chilling (Figure 17.18■). Move to the client's right leg and apply the substance to the posterior and anterior leg in the same manner as for the left leg. Cover the right leg with the insulating sheet to prevent chilling.
6. Move to the client's abdomen and drape one of the large towels across the client's chest area and have the client hold it firmly. Pull the bottom draping towel inferiorly until the client's abdomen is undraped. Apply the substance to the abdomen in a clockwise motion (Figure 17.19■).
7. Move to the client's left arm and apply the substance to the posterior and anterior arm with long, smooth

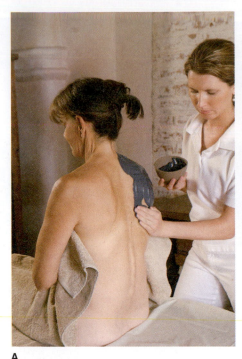
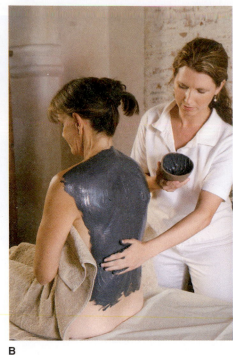

A   B

FIGURE 17.16

Apply the body wrap substance to the back with long, smooth strokes, covering the area thoroughly.

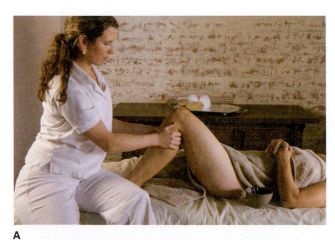
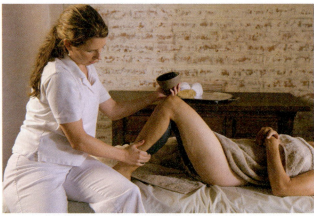

A   B

FIGURE 17.17

A. To stabilize the client's leg, gently sit on her foot. B. Apply the substance to the client's posterior leg with one smooth stroke.

strokes (Figure 17.20■ A). Cover the left arm and abdomen with the insulating sheet to prevent chilling (Figure 17.20 B). Move to the client's right arm and apply the substance the same as for the left arm. Cover the right arm with the insulating sheet to prevent chill.

8. Move to the head of the table and apply the substance to the client's upper chest (Figure 17.21■).

9. Wrap the client securely with each of the layers on the table, one at a time, except for the bottom sheet (Figure 17.22■).

10. Use the towel at the head of the table to wrap around the client's neck securely.

11. Make sure the client is comfortable using bolsters, pillows, or other props as needed. An extra blanket can be added for more warmth. The client should remain wrapped for 25–30 minutes. During this time a scalp and facial massage can be given or the client's feet can be unwrapped for a foot massage. Another option is to sit quietly at the head or foot of the table. Place a cool, moist washcloth on the client's face or forehead if needed.

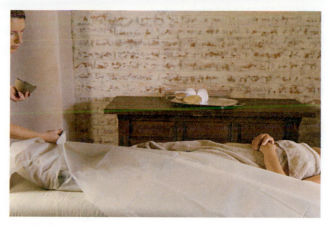

FIGURE 17.18

Cover the client's leg with the insulating sheet to prevent chilling.

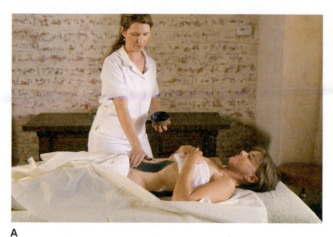

A

B

FIGURE 17.19

Apply the substance to the abdomen in a clockwise motion.

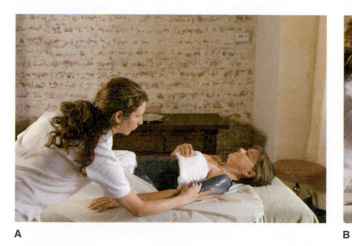

A

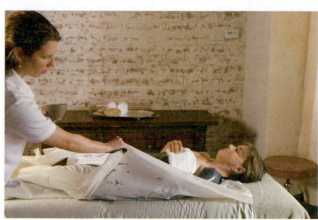

B

FIGURE 17.20

A. Apply the substance to the arm with long, smooth strokes. B. Cover the arm and abdomen with the insulating sheet to prevent chilling.

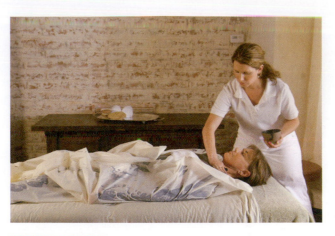

FIGURE 17.21

Apply the substance to the client's upper chest.

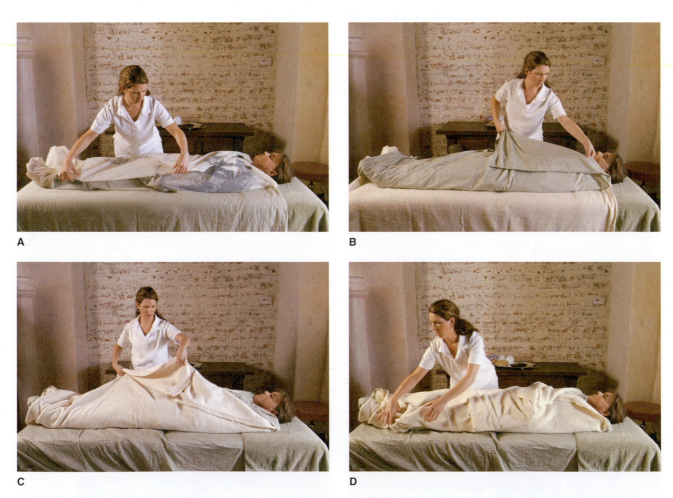

A

B

C

D

FIGURE 17.22

Wrap the client securely on the table with each of the layers, one at a time, except for the bottom sheet.

12. When the time is up, unwrap each of the layers until the client is covered by just the plastic sheet and the towels with which he or she was initially draped (Figure 17.23■ A and B). Place a large towel lengthwise over the client. Gently pull the plastic sheet out from underneath the towel (Figure 17.23 C).

13. Help the client sit up with legs hanging off the side of the table. Use a warm, moist towel to remove residue from the client's back.

14. If using a wet table or Vichy shower, rinse the client thoroughly to remove residue. If there is a separate shower facility, help the client off the table, offering a bathrobe

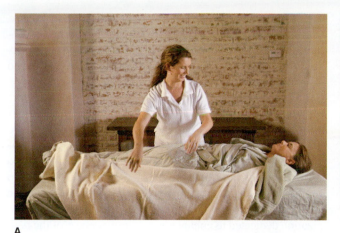

A

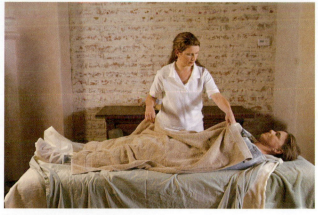

B

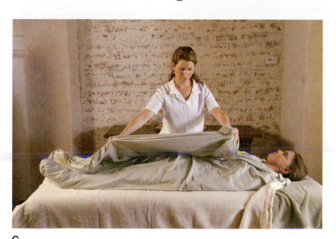

C

FIGURE 17.23

A. Unwrap each of the layers until the client is covered by just the plastic sheet and the towels with which the client was initially draped. B. Place a large towel lengthwise over the client. C. Gently pull the plastic sheet out from underneath the towel.

or draping a large towel for modesty. Give the client the textured washcloth or bath scrubby and guide him or her to the shower and then back to the massage table after rinsing off. If working in a dry room, use the dry room substance removal technique described earlier in Box 17.1 on page 492. Once the residue has been removed thoroughly from the skin, help the client off the table.

Herbal Wraps

The herbal wrap is probably the most popular and best known herbal spa treatment. It is a full-body moist heat treatment, using multiple towels or muslin sheets soaked in an herbal infusion. The herbal wrap treatment can easily be incorporated into a 60-minute treatment; the wrap itself typically takes 20–30 minutes. It can be an individual treatment, or it can be preceded by an exfoliation and followed by a complementary therapy.

HERBS

Herbs are invaluable additions to spa treatments in the form of infusions for wraps, inhalations, and aromatherapy applications. You may discover useful plants that are indigenous to your geographic area. For example, in the southwest, poultices can be made from prickly pear pads (after the needles are

removed, of course). In the northeast, chickweed can be used for body wraps. Hayflower grows abundantly in Germany, and spas there have long incorporated it into treatments. Hayflower treatments are now becoming popular in the United States. Table 17.2■ shows the effects of common herbs and plants.

Organic and natural food stores are good places to find a variety of high-quality herbs; there are also many Internet sources. Herbs can be purchased either fresh or dried. If fresh plants are desired, only purchase as much as will be used for specific treatments to ensure they do not spoil before the next use. Plants can also be dried by gathering them in small bundles, tying them together with string, and hanging them upside down. Hanging them this way makes it easier to pull leaves off stems.

When the herbs are fully dried, they can be stored in glass jars with tight lids. Even dried plants do not last more than a couple of months before they lose their potency. If a continual supply of high quality, fresh plants is desired, planting an herb garden may be the solution.

HERBAL INFUSIONS

Infusions are one of the easiest methods to prepare herbs for use in spa treatments. An **infusion** involves immersing the leaves, flowers, or berries of a fragrant plant in boiling water.

TABLE 17.2	Effects of Common Herbs in Spa Treatments	
Stress Relief and Relaxation	**Energizing and Balancing**	**Detoxification**
Lavender	Chamomile	Juniper
Chamomile	Clary sage	Ginger
Clary Sage	Rosemary	Grapefruit zest
Jasmine	Geranium	Eucalyptus
Marjoram	Lemongrass	Clove
Linden flowers	Orange zest	Lemon balm
Hops	Ylang ylang	Hayflower
Valerian		Oatstraw
Passionflower		Fennel
		Nettle

Sources: Ody, P., *Essential Guide to Natural Home Remedies* (2002); Ody, P., *The Medicinal Herbal* (1993).

The mixture is then left to stand for 15–30 minutes, or longer for a stronger infusion. The infusion water can then be used in simple inhalations and facial saunas (discussed in the Aromatherapy section in this chapter) and herbal wraps.

AROMATHERAPY

Aromatherapy is the therapeutic use of the preparation of fragrant essential oils extracted from plants. According to the National Association for Holistic Therapy, "Aromatherapy can be defined as the art and science of utilizing naturally extracted aromatic essences from plants to balance, harmonize and promote the health of the body, mind and spirit" (NAHA 2005a). Aromatherapy has many effects on the body and it is because of this that aromatherapy can be used in many different ways.

There are so many different ways scents can be used in the spa and bodywork profession, as well as in everyday life, that aromatherapy in popular culture has come to mean anything that is scented in a pleasant way. Air fresheners, candles, and even flower-scented detergents are now called aromatherapy. Scented spray mists to freshen the face or feet, dishes of aromatic beads placed in the treatment room, and lavender-scented lubricants are all examples of what may be considered aromatherapy in the spa and bodywork realm.

One particular type of substance, however, requires more research and education. These are essential oils, and their effects can be so powerful that, in order to truly understand how they should be used, it is recommended that practitioners who are interested in becoming aromatherapists attend formal courses in aromatherapy. The National Association for Holistic Aromatherapy (www.naha.org) is a valuable source of information. This is an educational, nonprofit organization dedicated to enhancing public awareness of the benefits of true aromatherapy.

This section discusses basic aromatherapy concepts for practitioners who are beginners in the use of essential oils. Information on common essential oils is presented, such as characteristics, uses, and cautions, along with methods of incorporating essential oils into the spa and bodywork setting and treatments.

It is important to note that practitioners should never go beyond their scope of practice. Check with local and/or state regulations regarding the use of essential oils in the spa setting or a massage therapy practice. Some areas require that anyone who applies essential oils topically to another person be professionally licensed, such as for massage therapy, energy work, cosmetology, and other practices. Check with all pertinent regulatory bodies to be sure of compliance with laws governing the application of essential oils.

Essential Oils

Essential oils are the volatile oils that aromatic plants, trees, and grasses produce. The term *volatile* means able to vaporize easily at low temperatures. It is the volatility of essential oils that causes their scents to spread so rapidly. These oils can be obtained from any part of the plant. Usually they are distilled from the flowers, roots, rinds of fruits, stalks, sap or resin, nuts, or bark of plants. For example, sandalwood is gathered from the heart of the tree, but only after the tree is at least 40 years old. Eucalyptus is obtained from the leaves of the

CRITICAL THINKING

Of the different types of substances that can be used in a body wrap treatment, such as muds, peats, seaweed, and herbal infusions, which one would you want to experience? Compare the benefits, contraindications, equipment, supplies and procedures of each.

1. Do you have a specific condition that would benefit from this body wrap?
2. What do you think you would like about this body wrap?
3. What do you think you would not like about it?
4. How would you expect to feel after the treatment?

eucalyptus tree. Neroli, rose, jasmine, and lavender come from the plants' flowers. Various species of frankincense trees grow wild throughout western India, northeastern Africa, and southern Saudi Arabia. The oil is distilled from the gum resin that oozes from incisions made in the bark of the trees. Myrrh comes from a shrub that grows in Ethiopia, Sudan, and Somalia. The shrubs exude a resin that hardens into reddish brown tear-shaped drops—this is myrrh.

How Essential Oils Work

About 200 different essential oils have been extracted from plants for use in aromatherapy, and are employed for many different purposes:

- Antiseptics against viruses, bacteria, and fungi
- Analgesics
- Acts on the central nervous system to reduce anxiety and insomnia or to be stimulating and energizing
- Acts on the endocrine system and metabolism
- Stimulates the immune system

Essential oil preparations that are taken internally may stimulate the immune system and function as antibiotics. Since these are pharmacological uses of essential oils, recommending internal use of essential oils is beyond the scope of practice of massage therapists and bodyworkers and is not discussed in this text.

Other essential oils that are applied to the skin activate thermal (heat) receptors and kill dermal microbes and fungi. They can also be absorbed through the skin from baths, massage treatments, and compresses. Essential oils are readily absorbed through the skin due to their lipid-solubility and the small size of the aromatic molecules. The molecules enter the bloodstream quickly and easily cross the blood-brain barrier to have an effect on the brain. The natural oiliness of the skin also enhances the up-take of essential oils.

Essential oils used for their aromas stimulate a specific part of the brain called the **limbic system.** The limbic system (Figure 17.24■) is located within the higher brain, or cerebrum. It is sometimes referred to as the *emotional brain* because it has a major role in a variety of emotions—pleasure, affection, passivity, fear, sorrow, sexual feelings, and anger. It is also involved in memory and *olfaction,* which is the term for the sense of smell. This is why our sense of smell evokes memories much more strongly than any of our other senses. *Olfaction bulbs,* components of the limbic system, are formed of nervous tissue, which play a role in the brain's interpretation and differentiation of all the diverse aromas we are able to detect.

The limbic system is closely associated with the part of the brain called the hypothalamus that controls many physiological functions and plays a major role in the regulation of homeostasis. It is responsible for, among other things, controlling the autonomic nervous system and regulating emotional and behavioral patterns.

From the olfactory bulbs, the impulses travel along the olfactory tract. The olfactory tract extends into parts of the brain that identify odors, so a person can put a name to them, and to parts of the brain that distinguish different odors so a person can sort them out. This tract extends into the part of the brain where conscious awareness of smell begins, as well as into the limbic system and hypothalamus. It is this connection to the limbic system and hypothalamus that accounts for emotional and memory-based responses to aromas.

PRECAUTIONS FOR WORKING WITH ESSENTIAL OILS

Essential oils are highly concentrated and volatile, and they need to be handled with care. There are only two essential oils that can be applied directly to the skin—lavender and tea tree. All other essential oils must be diluted in **carrier oil,** also called *base oil,* before applying to the body. These are typically plant-based oils used to dilute essential oils for use on the skin, as in massage. They can also serve to moisturize the skin and keep essential oils on the skin longer. The carrier oil can be any high-quality vegetable oil such as:

- Sweet almond
- Apricot

FIGURE 17.24

The limbic system is located within the higher brain, or cerebrum.

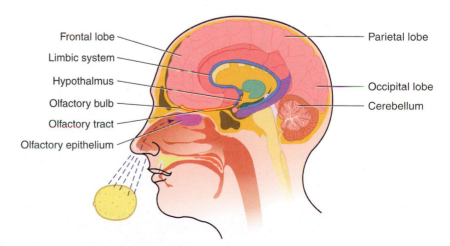

Frontal lobe

Limbic system

Hypothalmus

Olfactory bulb

Olfactory tract

Olfactory epithelium

Parietal lobe

Occipital lobe

Cerebellum

- Grapeseed
- Olive
- Coconut
- Sunflower
- Jojoba
- Sesame
- Canola
- Sunflower
- Safflower
- Peanut

See Table 17.3■ for a list of dilutions of common essential oils within a carrier oil.

Additional precautions to keep in mind when working with essential oils:

- A skin test should always be done on clients and on practitioners themselves before any essential oil is used, even if the essential oil has been used before. As stated previously, people can develop allergies throughout their lives, even to substances to which they have not previously been allergic.
- Essential oils are *never* used near the eyes.
- Pregnancy can be a contraindication, especially during the first trimester. A qualified aromatherapist can be consulted for information about essential oils that work well and those that are contraindicated. Some safe essential oils for use during pregnancy are rose, neroli, lavender, ylang-ylang, chamomile, sandalwood, spearmint, frankincense, and the citruses. A 1 percent dilution of essential oil to carrier oil should be used on pregnant clients, or one drop added to bath water. When in doubt, do not use essential oils.
- Use essential oils cautiously with clients who are fragile, including babies, small children, the aged, and those who have serious health problems such as asthma, epilepsy, or heart disease. No more than a 1 percent dilution of essential oil to carrier oil, or one drop added to bath water, should be used for these clients. When in doubt, do not use essential oils.
- Caution should be used with essential oils that can result in photosensitivity. For example, bergamot contains a natural chemical called bergaptene that causes the skin to become very sensitive to ultraviolet light. If bergamot is applied and the skin is exposed to sunlight, or light from sun lamps or tanning beds, the reaction can be anywhere from mild (just reddening of

REALITY CHECK

BARBARA

JACKIE: My client forgot to mention that she had an allergy to nuts, and she is having an allergic reaction to the KuKui nut oil I am using. What should I do?

BARBARA: Stay calm and stop the treatment. Immediately remove all of the oil and rinse the skin. If the reaction is mild and has stopped, ask your client if she would like to continue with the treatment. If so, be sure to check the ingredients on the new lubricant you use. And remember to add the information about her allergy to her health history file and document the incident in session notes.

the skin) to severe (acute lesions and brown spots). Mild reactions usually resolve within a day or so. However, severe reactions can take weeks to resolve, with the accompanying brown spots taking months or years to completely disappear. Removing the bergaptene does not hinder the benefits of the essential oil, so it is recommended that bergaptene-free bergamot be used whenever possible.

- If a client is taking homeopathic remedies, consult a qualified aromatherapist before using essential oils on him or her. Essential oils may counteract the action of the homeopathic remedy.

PURCHASING AND CARE OF ESSENTIAL OILS

It is best to buy only pure, organic, good quality essential oils. "Organic" means that the plant material was grown without the use of pesticides, herbicides, or fungicides made from synthetic chemicals or petrochemicals.

Avoid synthetic fragrance oils. They have no therapeutic value. Labels on bottles may say "organic," "pure," and "natural," but the oil may, in fact, be synthetic. If the label says "fragrant oil," "perfume oil," or "aromatherapy oil," it is an indication that the oils are not pure oils and have been mixed with other substances. For example, the oil may have been diluted with vegetable oils. A good way to test for this is to place a couple of drops of the essential oil on a piece of paper. If an oily stain is left behind when the essential oil evaporates, it was most likely diluted with vegetable oil.

True essential oils will have the botanical name, not just the common name, on the label. The label will also state that it is a "pure essential oil" or "100% essential oil." If the label is not clear about this information, do not buy it.

Price can also be an indication. Pure, organic oils cost more than synthetic oils or blends. Some are quite expensive. While orange, lemon, and lime may be reasonably

TABLE 17.3	Dilutions of Essential Oils in Carrier Oil	
Dilution	Drops of Essential Oil per Ounce of Carrier Oil
1%	5–6
2%	10–12
3%	15–18

priced, jasmine, neroli, and rose are very costly. The bottle itself can be a guide. The best quality oils will always be in dark glass bottles to protect them from sunlight. A product line of aromatherapy oils in clear glass bottles that are all the same price are most likely synthetic fragrance oils.

Essential oils are best stored tightly sealed in amber, brown, or blue glass bottles. Oxygen, sunlight, and heat can damage oils, causing them to lose their therapeutic properties. The average shelf life for most essential oils is 2 years, although the citrus oils have a somewhat shorter life expectancy. Unused oils that have reached the end of their shelf life should be discarded. Interestingly, the heavy, woodsy resin-type oils can last much longer (up to 6 years), and are said to actually improve with age.

Classification by Notes

Essential oils have been classified by the French perfume industry according to their *notes,* or scent characteristics, and by the rate at which they evaporate. There are top notes (T), middle notes (M), and base (B) notes. Some oils are a combination of top and middle (T/M), or middle and base (M/B) notes.

Top notes have light, fresh, and uplifting qualities. They typically have antiviral properties. Since they evaporate quickly, their scents are usually not long lasting. *Middle notes* comprise the bulk of the essential oils. They have warm, soft fragrances that unfold gradually. Also known as the heart notes, they are the balancing and harmonizing scents. *Base*

notes are intense, heavy, long-lasting fragrances that evaporate slowly. They are rich and relaxing, and usually are the most expensive essential oils. See Table 17.4■ for more information on essential oils and notes.

Ten Foundational Essential Oils

With almost 200 essential oils to choose from, practitioners may not know where to start when beginning their work with aromatherapy. Some practitioners may want to learn as much as they can as fast as they can, while others may want to find a few they can use regularly and in many different ways.

Table 17.5■ lists and describes 10 essential oils that have many different uses. Purchasing these would provide a good "starter set" of essential oils without investing a large amount of money. As practitioners become more comfortable working with essential oils, they may discover that they want more oils in their collection. Or they may discover that just having these is enough for the treatments they perform.

The information in Table 17.5 provides an introduction to essential oils and does not contain in-depth descriptions. The information is not intended to treat, cure, prevent, or diagnose any disease, disorder, or health condition.

BLENDING ESSENTIAL OILS

Used individually, essential oils can have powerful effects. Sometimes, though, blending different essential oils together creates a more optimal outcome. The main thing to keep in

TABLE 17.4 Essential Oils and Notes			
Note	Top Notes (T)	Middle Notes (M)	Base Notes (B)
Characteristics	Light and airy	Harmonizing	Deep
	Evaporates quickly	Soothing, soft undertones	Intense
	Penetrating or sharp scent	Scent unfolds gradually	Powerful
	Fresh smell		Long lasting
			Warm and sensuous
Examples	Peppermint (T/M)	Chamomile	Rose absolute
	Orange	Cypress	Patchouli
	Lemon	Marjoram	Vetiver
	Lime	Lavender	Jasmine
	Tangerine	Geranium	Myrrh
	Grapefruit	Dill	Frankincense
	Melissa	Celery	Sandalwood
	Lemongrass	Coriander	Benzoin
	Mandarin	Black pepper	Spikenard
	Eucalyptus (T/M)	Juniper	Cedarwood
	Basil	Thyme	
		Rose (M/B)	
		Neroli (M/B)	
		Rosemary	
		Pine	

Source: Pure Essential, Inc., "Esssential Oils and Perfume Notes" (2007).

TABLE 17.5   Ten Foundational Essential Oils

Essential Oil	Characteristics	Uses	Cautions
Bergamot (T) *Citrus bergamia*	Relaxing, refreshing, uplifting, cooling; the flavor of Earl Grey tea; can be a good substitute for rose oil.	Reduces allergies, acne, psoriasis and gas; relieves anxiety; alleviates depression	Avoid exposing skin to sunlight after using this oil until after bathing or showering to remove the oil
Peppermint (T) *Mentha piperta*	Stimulating, refreshing, cooling, restorative; uplifts the mind and body; one of the most useful essential oils	Relaxes the muscles of the digestive system and stimulates bile flow; relieves gas, colic, and indigestion; refreshes tired head and feet; inhale briefly from bottle or apply one drop on a tissue and inhale to revive during travel; blend with rosemary and juniper to makes a stimulating morning bath.	Can cause a burning sensation and irritate skin if too much is used or it is not diluted properly; can neutralize homeopathic medicines
Eucalyptus (T) *Eucalyptus globulus*	Energizing and stimulating; cleanses and purifies	Helps relieve respiratory congestion, colds, fevers, and pain; kills airborne bacteria	Do not use on pregnant clients, by pregnant therapists, or by people who have epilepsy; can neutralize homeopathic medicines.
Tea Tree (T) *Melaleuca alternifolia, M. linariifolia, M. uncintata*	Powerful antiseptic, antifungal, and antiviral agent	Reduces acne, cold sores, warts, and burns; cleansing agent for the skin; can be used as a vapor to kill airborne germs; helps combat foot odor and athlete's foot	May be used full strength as a first aid application; do a patch test first on extremely sensitive skin; limit usage to problem area if using undiluted
Geranium (M/T) *Pelargonium graveolen*	Uplifting and calming	Soothes certain skin conditions; helps relieve PMS, cramps, menstrual and menopausal issues, tension, anxiety, and depression; is an immunostimulant, can be used as an aromatic insect repellant.	Do not use if pregnant or on pregnant clients; do not use on persons with a history of estrogen-dependent cancer
Lavender (M/T) *Lavendula augustifolia, L. officinalis, L. vera*	Most versatile and valuable essential oil; helpful in many ways for the mind and body; safe to use on children; blends easily with many other oils	Helps heal wounds, cuts, burns; relieves headaches; acts as a local anesthetic to relieve pain from sunburn, asthma, and throat infections; relieves irritability and sleeplessness; is an immunostimulant; can be used as an aromatic insect repellant.	Avoid high doses during pregnancy; can cause uterine contractions
Chamomile (Roman Chamomile) (M) *Chamaemelum nobile (formerly known as Anthemis noblis)*	Relaxing; safe to use on children	Relieves pain; increases mental clarity; decreases anxiety, nervous tension, depression, anger, and irritability; soothes sunburn, earaches, toothaches, and headaches	Can neutralize homeopathic medicines
Cypress (M) *Cupressus sempervirens*	Distilled from the twigs, needles, and cones of the cypress tree; has a spicy, smoky, pungent pinelike scent	Antispasmodic; warming; diuretic; helps relieve edema, asthma, hot flashes; assists in balancing hormonal levels; helps relieve pain from varicose veins and hemorrhoids; decreases the appearance of thread veins; supports weight reduction	Do not use if pregnant or on pregnant clients; do not use on persons with a history of estrogen-dependent cancer
Marjoram (M) *Origanum Marjorana, Majorana hortensis*	Calming, relaxing, and sedating	Relieves pain, insomnia, headaches, constipation, and colds; increases circulation; helps regulate menstrual cycle; helps relieve anxiety; makes an excellent after-sports rub because of its pain-relieving ability	Do not use if pregnant or on pregnant clients; do not use on persons with a history of estrogen-dependent cancer
Rosemary (M) *Rosemarinus officinalis, R. coronarium*	Revives, warms, stimulates, and restores	Refreshes tired muscles and feet; increases mental concentration; perfect in pre– and post–sports rubs to maintain suppleness; helps combat water retention; combats fatigue; clears a stuffy atmosphere	Do not use by or on people who are pregnant, by or on people who have epilepsy, or by people who have untreated high blood pressure; can neutralize homeopathic medicines

Sources: Buckle, J., *Clinical Aromatherapy, Essential Oils in Practice* (2007); Price, S. and Price. L., *Aromatherapy for Health Professionals,* 3rd ed. (2007); Rose, J., *375 Essential Oils and Hydrosols* (1999); Shutes, J. and Weaver, C., *Aromatherapy for Bodyworkers* (2008); Tisserand, R. B., *The Art of Aromatherapy* (1985); Worwood, V. A., *The Fragrant Heavens* (1999).

mind when considering which essential oils to blend together is the intention behind the blend. For example, if the goal is the creation of pleasant and relaxing ambiance for the treatment area, any essential oils that are soothing can be blended and placed in a diffuser. On the other hand, if a client has muscle pain, other essential oils can be chosen specifically for their muscle tightness relieving properties, and a muscle relief blend can be created.

The French perfume industry considers a well-rounded blend to contain top, middle, and base notes. Top notes can be up to 20 percent of the blend, middle notes are approximately 50–80 percent of the blend, while the deep base notes can be up to 5 percent of the blend. Using this as a guideline, the majority of the blend should contain middle note essential oils because they tend to harmonize with other oils the best. Because top note oils are lighter and more quickly detected by the nose, they are used in a lesser amount. Base note oils are intense and longer lasting, so they are usually used in the least amount.

For example, if a 2 percent well-rounded blend is desired, that means that 10–12 drops of essential oil will be added to 1 ounce of carrier oil, according to Table 17.3. Of those 10–12 drops, 2 can be a top note oil, 5–8 drops can be a middle note oil, and 1–3 drops can be a base note oil.

However, all three notes do not always have to be used in a blend; it all depends on the individual properties of the essential oils, what they will be used for, and the blender's preference of oils and the desired final scent.

Using Essential Oils in a Spa or Massage Therapy Practice

There are numerous ways to use essential oils for aromatherapy purposes. These include diffusers, aromastones, scented candles, scented massage oils and lotions, simple inhalation treatments, and scubs.

- *Diffusers.* Aromatherapy diffusers come in many sizes, shapes, and styles. The basic diffuser is a ceramic pot with a small bowl to hold water and essential oils (4–6 drops), heated by a small candle (Figure 17.25■). The warmth of the candle releases the properties in the essential oils. Another type of

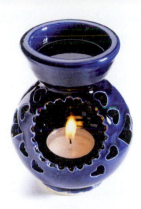

FIGURE 17.25

Aromatherapy diffuser. The warmth of the candle releases the properties in the essential oils.

aromatherapy diffuser uses the warmth of hot water indirectly. A plate is placed over a pot filled with hot water, and 4–6 drops of essential oil are placed on the plate. As the plate warms, the essential oil evaporates and diffuses into the air. There are also electric diffusers, some with fans, some made of glass. These diffusers disinfect and scent the atmosphere by releasing droplets of essential oil as a cool mist.

- *Aromastones.* Aromastones are made of porcelain or ceramic and plug into electrical outlets. Essential oil is poured directly onto the heated porcelain or ceramic surface; no water is needed.
- *Scented Candles.* Candles come in all different sizes and shapes and scents. They can be made of paraffin, soy wax, or beeswax. High-quality candles that burn cleanly and are scented with pure essential oils are the best to use.
- *Scented Massage Oils, Lotions, and Cream.* To prepare one application, dilute 10–12 drops of essential oil with 1 ounce of an unscented carrier oil, lotion, or cream. If preparing a 4–8 ounce bottle of oil or lotion, or a 4–8 ounce jar of cream, the addition of a few drops of jojoba oil, vitamin E oil, or wheat germ oil will act as a preservative.

CRITICAL THINKING

Experiment with using aromatherapy therapy three different ways. Compare the therapeutic benefits and safety precautions of each essential oil.

1. What essential oils blend well together?

2. How would you make aromatherapy massage oils, lotions and creams that are soothing, invigorating, or "sports blends" effective for working on tight muscles?

3. How cost effective is it to incorporate aromatherapy into a massage practice?

- *Simple Inhalation Treatments.* Simple inhalation treatments using essential oils are excellent for relieving head congestion and sinus infections. Pour 1 quart of boiling water into a large bowl. Add 5–8 drops of the desired essential oil and stir. Cover head with a towel and lean over water. Keep eyes closed and breathe deeply through the nose for 5–15 minutes, depending on your level of comfort. Rinse face with cool water and gently blot skin dry. Essential oils can also be used in steam cabinets; just add 5–8 drops to the water.
- *Scrubs.* The scrubs discussed previously in this chapter can be enhanced by adding 2–3 drops of desired essential oil to the manual exfoliation mixture.

STONE MASSAGE

Stone massage involves the use of hot or cold stones for therapeutic purposes. Basically, a stone is a collection of minerals with a very dense structure. The main type of stone used in hot stone therapy is basalt, because its chemical structure makes it ideal for retaining heat (Figure 17.26■). Round, smooth basalt stones are heated and then placed on or tucked around the client, and used in the palms of the practitioner's hands to massage the body. Marble, jade, and sardonyx are often used for cold stone therapy, because their chemical structures retain coolness (Figure 17.27■). Chilled stones are applied after deep focus work or during deep tissue and trigger point therapy. The beneficial effects of stone massage and its contraindications are shown in Table 17.6■.

There are currently many different types of hot and cold stone therapy options. Treatments can range from simple

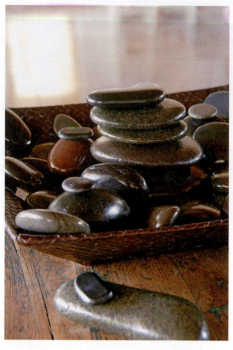

FIGURE 17.26

The main type of stone used in hot stone therapy is basalt.

treatments using a few stones to elaborate setups using multiple sets of stones. The stones are adaptable to a variety of modalities. There are custom sets especially for estheticians, reflexologists, practitioners of Asian bodywork, physical therapists, chiropractors, sports massage therapists, and spa practitioners.

Because of the heat involved in stone massage treatments, it is highly recommended that practitioners learn how to use

TABLE 17.6	Stone Massage: Beneficial Effects, Therapeutic Uses, and Contraindications		
Beneficial Effects of Hot Stone Massage	**Beneficial Effects of Cold Stone Massage**	**Therapeutic Uses of Both Hot and Cold Stone Massage**	**Contraindications for Stone Massage**
• Increases blood flow to soft tissues • Relaxes tight muscles • Makes connective tissue more pliable • Warms the joints so that they move more easily • Creates an overall sense of relaxation	• Decreases inflammation and swelling (cold acts as a vasoconstrictor) • Enhances tissue repair after deep tissue work • Slows down nerve or pain impulses • Provides analgesic effects	• Injuries both acute and chronic • Muscle spasms • Osteoarthritis, tendinitis, and bursitis (cold for acute stages; heat for non-inflammatory stages) • Sprains, strains (cold for acute stages; heat for non-inflammatory stages) • Headache • Stress	• Heart conditions • Hypertension • Fever • Vascular disease in area stones would be applied • Numbness or loss of sensation in area stones would be applied • Broken or irritated skin • Inflammation (contraindication for heat) • Pregnancy • Physical frailty • Intolerance to heat • Intolerance to cold

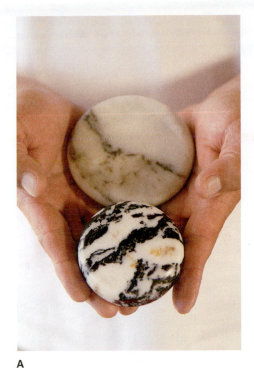

A

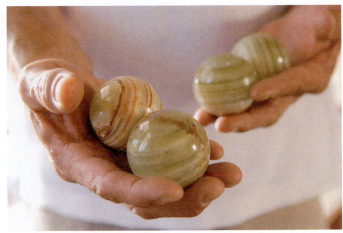

B

FIGURE 17.27

Marble (A) and sardonyx (B) are used often for cold stone therapy.

them from experienced and credentialed instructors. The risk of practitioners injuring clients and themselves due to lack of proper supervised instruction is otherwise too great.

Preparing for Stone Massage

For a hot stone application, the basalt stones need to be heated in water that is 130°–140° F for 45–60 minutes. They retain the heat for a relatively long time, but the body draws heat from the stones so newly heated stones need to be continually reapplied during a treatment.

If the stones are used at 120° F or below, they tend to lose heat rapidly and are not as beneficial. However, 110°–120° F is a good temperature to use on people who are frail or have a low tolerance to heat. When the treatment is being learned, it is best to begin at the lower temperatures.

Cold stones are able to draw a great deal of heat away from the body. Chilling time for stones is about 15 minutes using ice or an hour using a freezer. Their temperature should be at or just above freezing (32° F) in order to be effective.

Both hot and cold stones can be used in the same treatment to achieve different effects. The weight of the stones also provides benefits during treatments, because the weight helps heat to penetrate the body or, if cold stones are being used, to draw heat from the body more readily.

Oil is the lubricant of choice for stone massage; lotions and creams do not provide enough glide. Because of its thickness, jojoba oil is recommended. A generous amount of oil is needed to perform stone massage because of the heat of the stones and their weight.

Performing Hot Stone Massage

1. Remove stones from hot water and dry off.
2. With the client prone and draped with an extra large towel, approximately 35″ × 65″, place a large, flat stone under the abdomen (protected by a towel), another on the towel over the sacrum, others up the client's back, and into each of the client's palms (Figure 17.28■). Let the heat penetrate into the body for a period of time.

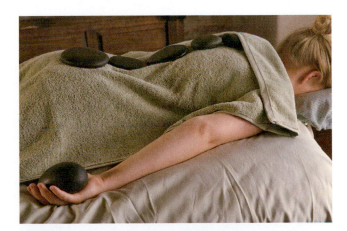

FIGURE 17.28

Hot stones placed on the sacrum, up the back, and into each of the palms.

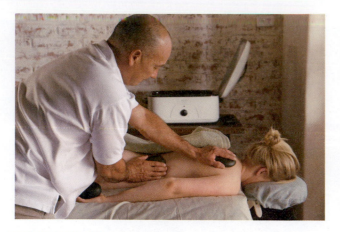

FIGURE 17.29

Placing hot stones on the back.

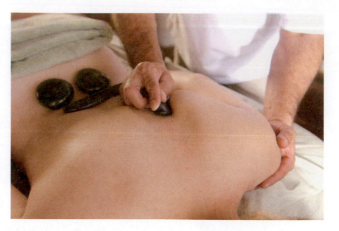

FIGURE 17.31

Using hot stones for specific applications under the scapula.

3. Choose a pair of stones to use for massage and uncover the area to be massaged.

4. After massaging oil on the client's body, apply the stones with firm pressure and long, gliding strokes, making several passes. Keep the stones on muscle tissue and avoid the bony areas. Strokes on the extremities should always be performed toward the shoulder.

5. When the stones start to lose their heat, return them to the heating unit and use another pair.

6. Hot stones can be used on the client's back (Figure 17.29■), posterior arms, posterior legs and gluteals (Figure 17.30■), feet, and posterior neck.

7. Specific work can also be performed with stones (Figure 17.31■).

8. When finished with the client's posterior side, help the client turn over, making sure he or she stays draped, as described on page 369 in Chapter 12, Body Mechanics, Table Skills, and Application Guidelines.

9. With the client supine, place the hot hand stones in the client's hands and the toe stones between the client's toes. Cold stones can also be placed along the client's

torso and on the forehead. A hot stone can be placed under the client's neck (Figure 17.32■).

10. Hot stones can be used to massage the client's anterior arms, hands, anterior legs, upper chest, neck (Figure 17.33■) and face (Figure 17.34■).

11. Finish by removing the stones placed on the client's body and then performing some long, gliding strokes to close the treatment.

When to Use Cold Stones

Chilled stones can be used in place of heated stones anywhere in a stone massage application. They can be used in combination with heated stones, tucked under the abdomen,

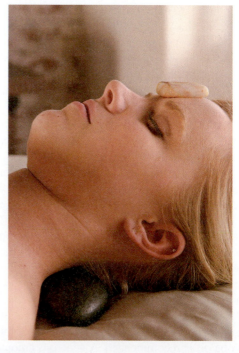

FIGURE 17.32

A hot stone placed under the client's neck.

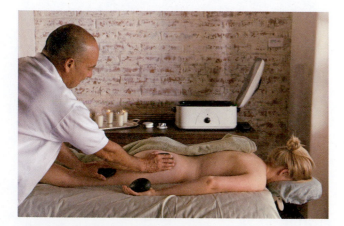

FIGURE 17.30

Hot stones on the gluteals and posterior leg.

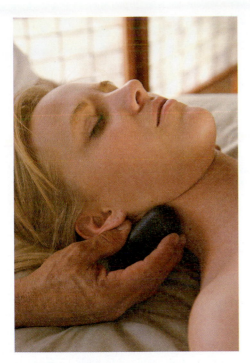

FIGURE 17.33

Using a hot stone to massage the neck.

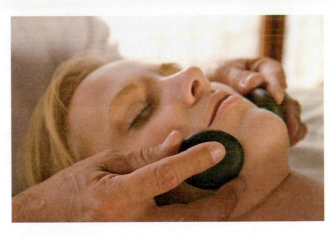

FIGURE 17.34

Using hot stones to massage the face.

or placed along either side of the spine when the client is supine. But they are primarily used following hot stones on a focus area. They are extremely effective when used to chill an area either before or after specific work. The cold stones draw heat from the body so they are effective where there is inflammation or to ease the discomfort of sunburn.

As a consideration to the client, it is important to verbally announce cold stones before you apply to them to the client's body. Ask the client to take a deep breath as the stone is applied, and to let the breath out immediately after the stone is applied. Having the client focus on the breath is a way to draw attention away from the chill of the stone, and breathing deeply helps the client release muscle tension caused by the application of the cold stone. The application of chilled stones is done slowly and gradually, giving the client time to adjust to the change in temperature. Cold stones are applied with firm pressure, held in place momentarily, and then moved slowly around the area until it is thoroughly chilled.

CASE FOR STUDY

Carolina and Her First Spa Application

Carolina has been "burning the candle at both ends." She is working on her master's degree while struggling to keep up with increased demands in her job as a school administrator. She hasn't been eating as well as she normally does and feels depleted. She receives massage sporadically from Jaime. During their last massage, Jaime mentioned that he has learned some spa applications and shared some of their benefits with her. Carolina has decided to take some time for herself and try one of Jaime's spa treatments.

Question:

Which spa treatments would help her feel rejuvenated?

Things to consider:

- What questions should Jaime ask Carolina to determine which application would be most beneficial?
- What are the benefits and indications of these applications?
- What are the equipment and supplies needed for these applications?
- How are these applications performed?

Which application do you think Jaime should recommend to Carolina?

_____

_____

_____

_____

CHAPTER HIGHLIGHTS

- Spa applications are treatments that are used within spa establishments but can also be used by massage therapists in private practice.
- The applications that form the foundation of most spa menus are exfoliation, body wraps, aromatherapy, and stone massage.
- Spa equipment and supplies include hot towel cabi, wet table, Vichy shower, wet room, linens, substances, toiletries, cleaning supplies, and disposable gloves
- Follow sanitation guidelines for spa application equipment and supplies because spa treatment settings are especially vulnerable to mold growth and disease transmission.
- Spa treatments need to be explained to clients in depth and include:
  - Benefits, indications, and contraindications
  - How the treatment is performed
  - What results the client can expect
  - How the client can expect to feel after the treatment
  - Levels of nudity involved for certain treatments
- A health and medical history of the client is important to obtain before beginning any treatments.
- Eliciting information from clients about their likes and dislikes and previous spa treatment experiences is important, so that practitioners can recommend the best spa application for them.
- Contraindications and safety guidelines for all forms of spa applications should be observed to avoid harm to the client.
- Exfoliation is the peeling and sloughing off of dead skin cells from the surface of the body. Benefits include brightening the skin, encouraging the production of new skin cells, making the skin smoother, allowing other preparations to hydrate and nourish the skin, and stimulating superficial blood and lymph flow.
  - Manual exfoliation is the physical process of applying friction with abrasives. It includes dry body brushing, scrubs (frictions), and body polishes.

- Chemical, enzyme, or dissolving exfoliations use chemicals or enzymes that work by dissolving dead skin cells.
- Body wraps can be used in conjunction with many different substances. Muds, peats, and seaweed are all commonly used materials, as well as sheets soaked in an herbal infusion (herbal wraps).
  - Muds help with deep skin cleansing and aid in the removal of waste products, stimulate local blood and lymphatic flow, and are excellent warming and hydrating treatments.
  - Peats draw and absorb toxins from the body, are warming and hydrating, and increase local blood and lymph circulation.
  - Seaweed and sea mud firm the skin, help eliminate toxins, stimulate blood circulation, and are moisturizing.
  - Herbs and plants used in herbal wraps can be for stress-relief and relaxation, energizing and balancing, or detoxification.
- Aromatherapy is the therapeutic use of fragrant essential oils extracted from plants.
- Follow all precaution guidelines when working with essential oils.
- Buy only pure, organic, good quality essential oils.
- Essential oils can be used in spa applications and massage practices in diffusers, lightbulb rings, aromastones, scented candles, scented oils, lotions and creams, and scrubs.
- Stone massage involves the use of hot and cold stones during a treatment.
- Heat from warmed basalt stones applied to the body increases blood flow to soft tissues, relaxes tight muscles, and makes connective tissue more pliable.
- Cold from chilled marble, jade, or sardonyx stones is very effective in decreasing inflammation and swelling. Cold also slows down nerve impulses, including pain impulses, which makes it an ideal analgesic.

EXAM REVIEW

Key Terms

Match the following key terms to their descriptions. For additional study, look up the key terms in the Interactive Glossary on page G-1 and note other terms that compare or contrast with them.

_____ 1. Aromatherapy
_____ 2. Dry brushing
_____ 3. Body polishes
_____ 4. Body wraps
_____ 5. Carrier oil
_____ 6. Chemical, enzyme, or dissolving exfoliation
_____ 7. Emollient
_____ 8. Essential oils
_____ 9. Exfoliation
_____ 10. Clays
_____ 11. Infusion
_____ 12. Limbic system
_____ 13. Manual exfoliation
_____ 14. Muds
_____ 15. Peat
_____ 16. Scrubs
_____ 17. Stone massage

a. Substance that makes the skin soft and supple
b. Organic soil that contains minerals, organic material, water, and trapped air
c. Created by immersing the leaves, flowers, or berries of a fragrant plant in boiling water
d. Therapeutic use of fragrant essential oils extracted from plants
e. Physical process of applying friction with abrasives
f. Derived from different soils and marine sediments
g. Gentler form of exfoliation using finely ground natural substances such as crushed almonds or grape seed meal
h. Located within the cerebrum, it plays a major role in memory and the sense of smell
i. Exfoliation method using salts, sugar, or coarser organic substances
j. Exfoliation using brushes or fiber tools
k. Peeling and sloughing off of dead skin cells from the surface of the body
l. Exfoliation using substances that loosen the keratin that holds skin cells together, allowing the cells to be easily sloughed off
m. The use of hot or cold stones for therapeutic purposes
n. Treatment used for detoxification in which a substance is applied and the body is wrapped in sheets, blankets, and/or a plastic covering
o. Volatile oils that aromatic plants, trees, and grasses produce
p. Aid deep skin cleansing by drawing impurities from the body
q. Plant-based oil used to dilute essential oils for use on the skin

Memory Workout

To test your memory of the main concepts in this chapter, complete the following sentences by circling the most correct answer from the two choices provided.

1. A (Vichy) (hot cabi) shower has multiple nozzles that hang above the client.
2. It is the responsibility of practitioners to be knowledgeable about all (exercises) (applications) they provide.
3. Contraindications for certain spa applications include allergies to the common foods (shellfish) (wheat) and nuts.
4. To help clients choose spa treatments, practitioners should ask what their desired (goals) (expenses) are for the treatment.
5. The physical process of applying friction with coarse substances or textures is called (body polish) (manual exfoliation).
6. Exfoliation using brushes or fiber tools is known as (dry) (coarse) brushing or (manual) (body) brushing.
7. For a scrub, the salt or sugar is usually mixed with just enough water to make it the consistency of (oatmeal) (snow).
8. Body polishes would be best used on clients who have (sensitive) (pale) skin.
9. Muds are categorized based on their region of origin and (density) (composition).
10. The substances in peat that contribute to its therapeutic effectiveness are organic acids and (minerals) (marine sediments).
11. After applying the body wrap substance to each extremity, it is important to cover the extremity with the insulating sheet to prevent (smearing) (chilling).
12. Seaweed and other sea products are organic materials that have more than (60) (25) salts, vitamins, and other trace elements essential to the body.
13. Two herbs that can be used for a detoxifying herbal wrap are (lemon balm) (sage) and (ginger) (anise).
14. Jasmine, lavender, and chamomile are all herbs that can be used for (pain) (stress) relief.
15. Harmonizing and soothing are terms used to describe essential oils that are (low) (middle) notes.
16. An essential oil that should not be used on clients with epilepsy is (eucalyptus) (lavender).
17. The main type of stone used in hot stone therapy is (marble) (basalt).
18. For clients who are frail or have a low tolerance to heat, stones should be heated to a temperature of (110°–120° F) (130°–140° F).

Test Prep

The following multiple-choice questions will help to prepare you for future school and professional exams.

1. Which of the following is one of the ways practitioners can help clients choose appropriate spa and hydrotherapy treatments?
   a. Respect client privacy by avoiding questions about medical history
   b. Give the treatment the client asks for, even if there are contraindications
   c. Offer the client discounts on treatments that would be ineffective for the client
   d. Determine whether the client has any skin rashes or allergies
2. If a client wants a body wrap but dislikes the smell of seaweed, the practitioner could:
   a. Offer the client a different treatment
   b. Explain the benefits of a seaweed treatment
   c. Refuse to do the treatment
   d. Reschedule the client for another time
3. If a client is uncomfortable with minimal draping during a treatment, the practitioner can:
   a. Reassure the client that everyone feels that way
   b. Explain that that is what the treatment requires
   c. Refuse to do the treatment
   d. Adjust coverings until the client is comfortable
4. In addition to being an exfoliant, salt is a natural:
   a. Moisturizer
   b. Detoxifer
   c. Emollient
   d. Vasodilator
5. On which of the following should dry brushing strokes be applied lightly?
   a. Abdomen
   b. Back
   c. Feet
   d. Neck
6. When making an exfoliant with natural substances, which of the following fluids can be combined with an abrasive?
   a. Milk
   b. Oil
   c. Water
   d. Any of the above
7. A therapeutic property of mud is that it is:
   a. Dehydrating to the skin
   b. Cooling to the body
   c. An effective vasoconstrictor
   d. Warming to the body

8. Which of the following describes a correct way to layer the table to prepare for a body wrap?
   a. Wool blanket, insulating sheet, cotton sheet, extra large towel
   b. Cotton sheet, wool blanket, insulating sheet, cotton sheet
   c. Insulating sheet, cotton sheet, wool blanket, extra large towel
   d. Cotton sheet, wool blanket, cotton sheet, insulating sheet

9. In a body wrap treatment, the typical length of time a client remains wrapped is:
   a. 10–15 minutes
   b. 25–30 minutes
   c. 30–45 minutes
   d. 45–60 minutes

10. Which of the following is used in spa treatments to relieve inflammation and muscle soreness?
    a. Spirulina
    b. Red seaweed
    c. Green seaweed
    d. White algae

11. What is the *minimum* amount of time herbs should be allowed to steep while making an infusion?
    a. 5 minutes
    b. 15 minutes
    c. 20 minutes
    d. 25 minutes

12. Essential oils are used for the purposes of:
    a. Increasing pain sensations
    b. Increasing anxiety and insomnia
    c. Stimulating the immune system
    d. Stimulating bacterial growth

13. Which of the following oils would be safe to use on a pregnant client?
    a. Cypress
    b. Bergamot
    c. Geranium
    d. Eucalyptus

14. Which of the following is a contraindication for hot stone therapy?
    a. Pregnancy
    b. Low back pain
    c. Chest congestion
    d. Headache

15. Which of the following can be used for cold stone therapy?
    a. Marble
    b. Basalt
    c. Sardonyx
    d. a and c

Comprehension Exercises

The following short answer questions test your knowledge and understanding of chapter topics and provide practice in written communication skills. Explain in two to four complete sentences.

1. Explain how practitioners can communicate with clients in order to provide them with the best spa application possible.

2. Describe how aromatherapy can be incorporated into a massage practice.

3. Identify the beneficial effects of hot stone therapy and cold stone therapy.

For Greater Understanding

The following exercises are designed to take you from the realm of theory into the real world. They will help give you a deeper understanding of the subjects covered in this chapter. Action words are underlined to emphasize the variety of activities presented to address different learning styles and to encourage deeper thinking.

1. Visit a spa or massage practice that provides spa applications. Observe how the staff and practitioners communicate with you about such matters as choosing a treatment, contraindications, draping practices, or how best to enjoy the spa experience. What did they communicate especially well? What could they have communicated better? Report to your study partner or group about your experience, and explain how you would improve client communications.

2. Create a regional aromatherapy or body scrub treatment utilizing an herb, plant, or other substance found in your geographic area. Consider the equipment and supplies you will need, as well as the amount of time needed to perform the applications.

3. Design your own spa treatment menu based on the treatments you have developed. Think about which treatments can be successfully paired with others to offer distinctive, personalized spa experiences to clients. Discuss your spa menu with your study partner or group.

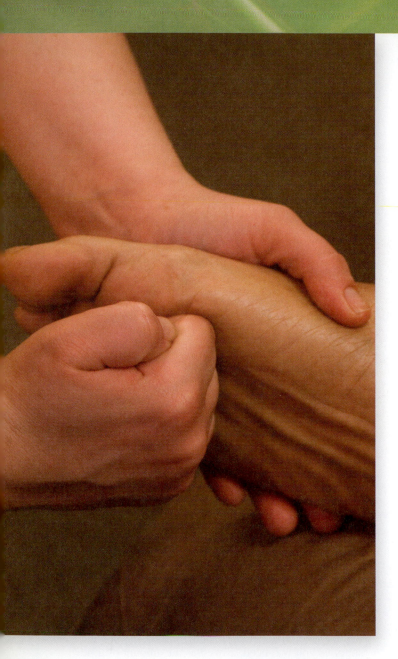

CHAPTER OUTLINE

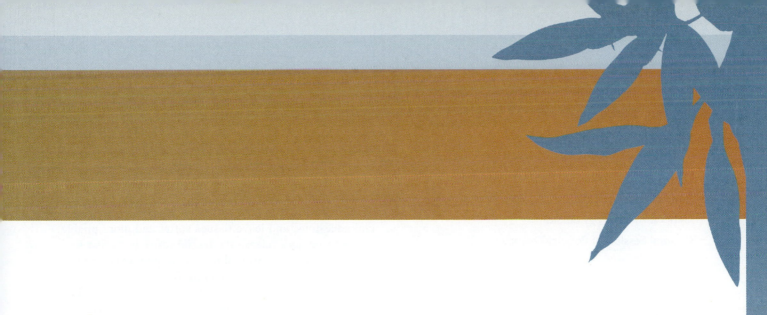

LEARNING OUTCOMES

After studying this chapter, you will have information to:

1. Explain the theories behind contemporary massage and bodywork applications.
2. Define key terms related to forms of modern bodywork.
3. Discuss the history of modern bodywork approaches.
4. Describe basic myofascial massage techniques.
5. Describe trigger point deactivation techniques.
6. Explain lymphatic facilitation techniques and applications.
7. Describe reflexology techniques and applications.
8. Describe polarity therapy techniques.
9. Compare and contrast different forms of contemporary massage and bodywork.
10. Perform basic techniques from different forms of contemporary massage and bodywork.

KEY TERMS

MASSAGE *in* ACTION

On your DVD, explore:

- Myofascial Massage of the Back
- Trigger Point Therapy for Tension Headaches
- Lymphatic Facilitation for the Head and Neck
- Lymphatic Facilitation for the Lower Extremity
- General Reflexology Session
- General Session of Polarity Therapy

INTRODUCTION

Classic Western massage is defined by a wide variety of techniques and a broad range of applications. Over the past century, more focused forms of manual therapy have been developed to affect specific body tissues and systems and to address specific therapeutic goals. Examples are myofascial massage to address the health of myofascial tissues, trigger point therapy to remove a common source of muscular pain and dysfunction, and lymphatic facilitation to reduce edema from a variety of causes.

At the same time, knowledge about human anatomy, physiology, and psychology has evolved, opening the possibility of explaining more clearly why certain techniques have therapeutic results. Today, scientific studies are examining alternative therapies, such as reflexology, to see if their apparent therapeutic effects can be verified and explained according to modern science.

In addition, Western audiences have become more open to ideas about energy or a life force affecting human health and disease. Forms of manual therapy from different parts of the world, which include some notion of energy, have been introduced into Western countries. For example, Chapter 19, Eastern Bodywork, on page 552 describes bodywork systems from China, India, and Thailand that strive to balance or affect energy flow to promote health. Polarity therapy, a form of energy bodywork derived from ancient sources, is presented later in this chapter.

Contemporary massage and bodywork is a term that describes the broad range of unique systems, approaches, and techniques of manual therapy in use today. Individual massage therapists may learn a particular system in depth as a specialization. More commonly, they integrate some of the basic techniques and applications into a more eclectic approach to massage therapy. This expands the massage therapist's tool box to address a client's goals.

The forms of contemporary massage and bodywork described in this chapter are some of the most accepted and useful approaches of interest to practitioners of manual therapy today. Their underpinning theory and basic techniques enrich the practice of massage therapy and expand its therapeutic potential.

MYOFASCIAL MASSAGE

Myofascial massage addresses the body's fascial anatomy, that is, the fibrous connective tissue that holds the body together and gives it shape. The general intent of myofascial massage is to release restrictions in superficial fascia, in deep fascia surrounding muscles, and in fascia related to overall body alignment.

Myofascial techniques stretch fascial sheets, break fascial adhesions, and leave tissues softer and more pliable. These techniques release the fascial restrictions that limit mobility and cause postural distortion, poor cellular nutrition, pain, and a variety of other dysfunctions.

Myofascial techniques were pioneered by Ida Rolf (1896–1979), who developed an approach to bodywork known today as Rolfing. Rolf's work spawned a number of subsequent systems known variously as myofascial release, myofascial unwinding, myofascial manipulation, and myofascial massage. The first International Fascia Research Congress was held at Harvard Medical School in 2007.

Fascia and Fascial Anatomy

Fascia is loose, irregular connective tissue found throughout the body. Fascia surrounds every muscle, nerve, blood vessel, and organ. It holds structures together giving them their characteristic shapes, offers support, and connects the body as a whole. It can be thought of as winding through the body in a continuous sheet. Fascia is also discussed in Chapter 6, Anatomy & Physiology, Pathology, and Kinesiology, on page 128.

A metaphor often used to describe fascia is a knitted sweater. Because all of the threads of yarn in a sweater are connected, a pull in one section may cause distortion in a spot distant from the original pull. Likewise, a restriction in fascia in one place can cause distortion in another area. Restrictions in fascia surrounding muscles can limit their ability to stretch and lengthen.

Fascial tissue is composed of three primary elements: ground substance, collagen, and elastin. Ground substance is a gel-like mucopolysaccharide, the same fluid that forms interstitial fluid. Collagen fibers are long, straight proteins that are strong yet flexible. Elastic fibers are wavy, branched proteins that return to their original shape when stretched. Sheets of fascia are formed by hydrogen bonds between collagen fibers. The multidirectional nature and low density of typical fascia is depicted in Figure 18.1■.

Fascia has a greater amount of ground substance than other types of connective tissue. It is the immediate environment of every cell in the body and forms the interstitial spaces. It has important functions in support, protection, separation, cellular respiration, elimination, metabolism, fluid flow, and immune system function. Any restriction or dysfunction in fascia can lead to a variety of problems, including poor exchange of cellular nutrients and wastes, pain, and loss of mobility.

Fascia displays an intriguing property called **thixotropy**, that is, it can change from a more solid to a more fluid consis-

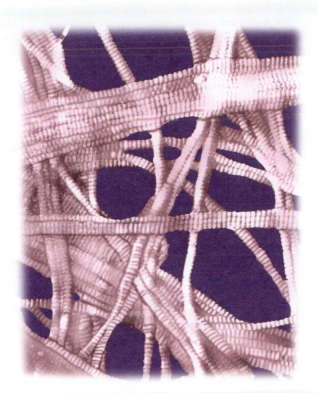

FIGURE 18.1

Multi-directional nature and low density of typical fascia.

Guidelines for Myofascial Applications

Myofascial massage applications involve identifying and releasing myofascial restrictions. Guidelines for these applications follow from the nature of fascial tissue and fascial structures. A summary of guidelines for myofascial massage appears in Box 18.1●.

Myofascial restrictions are located in two primary ways, that is, by observation and palpation. Visual analysis of a client's posture can reveal areas of fascial shortening and distortion in fascial anatomy. Restrictions may also be detected through palpation of soft tissues, or feeling where tissues seem "stuck together" and resist lengthening. Knowledge of fascial structures points to likely areas for restrictions.

Choose myofascial techniques suitable for the area and for the depth of the application. Some techniques address more superficial fascia, while others penetrate to deeper fascia.

Use no lubricant, or very little, on the skin. You must be able to feel subtle restrictions in the movement of soft tissues and the letting go that occurs as fascia elongates, becomes more pliable, and fascial sheets get unstuck. These subtleties are lost if the hands are sliding over the skin. Myofascial techniques also require traction on the skin as tissues are slowly and gently pushed, pulled, and stretched.

tency as a result of movement, stretching, and increase in temperature. Myofascial release techniques, and the method of their application, are based on these characteristics of fascia.

DEPTHS OF FASCIA

Fascia is distinguished as lying at different depths in the body. The most superficial is *subcutaneous fascia*, which forms a continuous layer of connective tissue over the entire body between the skin and the deep fascia. *Deep fascia* is an intricate series of dense connective sheets and bands that hold the muscles and other structures in place throughout the body. *Subserous fascia* lies between the deep fascia and the serous membranes lining the body cavities. Myofascial massage focuses mainly on subcutaneous and deep fascia related to the musculature.

FASCIAL STRUCTURES

Fascial anatomy includes identifiable fascial structures that shape and connect the body. For example, there are the *retinaculae* or straps at the wrist and ankle, which secure the tendons that cross there, like bungee cords keeping computer cables in place. There are also seven bands that give characteristic shape to the human torso. These bands run horizontally at the level of the pubic area, the lower abdomen (inguinal), the abdomen (umbilical), the chest just below the nipples, the collar bone, the chin, and the eyes. And there are fascial sheaths surrounding and linking muscles and muscle groups, for example, the large muscles of the back of the body as shown in Figure 18.2■.

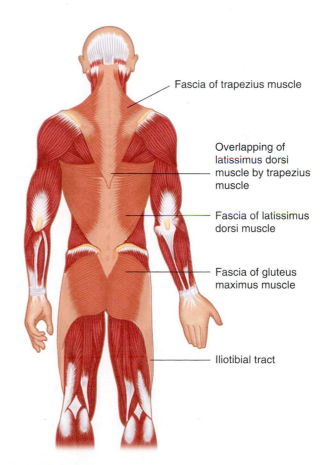

Fascia of trapezius muscle

Overlapping of latissimus dorsi muscle by trapezius muscle

Fascia of latissimus dorsi muscle

Fascia of gluteus maximus muscle

Iliotibial tract

FIGURE 18.2

Fascial sheaths surrounding and linking the muscles of the back of the body.

BOX 18.1 Guidelines for Myofascial Massage

1. Use observation of posture, palpation skills, and knowledge of fascial anatomy to identify areas of fascial restriction.
2. Choose myofascial massage techniques suitable for the area and for the depth at which you are working.
3. Use no or very little lubricant so that you can feel fascial restrictions and apply techniques without sliding over the skin.
4. Make gentle contact and enter tissues slowly until a point or area of resistance is felt.
5. Shift tissues horizontally once you are at the depth you wish to affect.
   - Avoid compressing tissues into bone.
6. Hold a stretch of fascial tissues until they release, usually in 2–5 minutes.
   - Maintain a continuous stretch.
   - Release feels like "melting," softening, or "giving" in tissues.
7. Flow with the tissues. Let the direction of the stretch be determined by which way the tissues seem to want to release.
8. Exit tissues with as much care and awareness as when you entered into them.
9. Let fascial tissues rest and integrate after a stretch.

Note: This list of myofascial massage guidelines summarizes instructions from many sources cited in this chapter.

Myofascial techniques are characteristically gentle, slow, and sustained. Movements are very subtle. The stretch of tissues is typically held from 2–5 minutes. The elastin stretches first. The collagen barriers and bonds take longer to release, and respond later to sustained gentle pressure. When they release, a melting, elongation, or sinking into tissues is felt.

For superficial applications involving skin lifting, make gentle contact, pick up the skin, and slowly pull it away from underlying tissues (see Figure 18.3A). Feel for areas of resistance to the lifting action. Hold the tension until a subtle stretch or giving way is felt.

For deep myofascial applications, make gentle contact and enter the soft tissues slowly until a point or area of resistance is felt. Once you are at the depth you wish to effect, shift the tissues horizontally (see Figure 18.5A). Avoid compressing tissues into bone. After a time, a melting or letting go will be felt in the tissues. There will be subtle movement and lengthening.

For some applications, it makes sense to flow with the restrictions and releases, letting the tissues lead the direction. This occurs in myofascial unwinding, which addresses fascia from a more three-dimensional view. Unwinding restores structural integrity and proper alignment of tissues, and promotes improved tissue health and organ function.

Exit tissues slowly with care and awareness. Let fascial tissues rest after stretching them. Avoid overworking tissues in one area.

Myofascial applications can be integrated into a full-body massage as needed, or may be used as the primary approach in a session. For treatment of specific problems, myofascial release techniques are sometimes combined with other soft tissue approaches such as trigger point therapy, as well as exercise, nutrition, relaxation, and psychotherapy.

CONTRAINDICATIONS

Myofascial massage is contraindicated locally if the tissues are damaged in some way, for example, if there is bruising, a wound, a burn, a fracture, local infection, or edema due to trauma. Arthritis with inflammation and gout are contraindications for fascial manipulation in the immediate area. General contraindications for myofascial massage include cellulitis, fever, systemic infection, lymphedema, advanced osteoporosis, and advanced diabetes. Avoid fascial applications if a client is taking medication that decreases sensitivity to pain, that reduces the ability of the blood to clot (i.e., anticoagulants), or compromises tissue integrity (e.g., steroids). See Table 9.1 on page 304 for information about classes of drugs and their actions.

Myofascial Techniques

The myofascial techniques presented in this chapter address subcutaneous fascia and deep fascia related to the muscula-

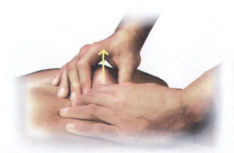
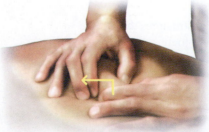
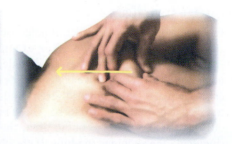

A   B   C

FIGURE 18.3

Skin lifting techniques. A. Basic skin lifting. B. Lifting with directional shift. C. Skin rolling.

ture. Their intent is to make fascial tissues more pliable and to release adhesions that cause restrictions to free movement. This is accomplished by stretching, pulling, and pushing movements that separate tissues mechanically. In addition, the practitioner's hand or arm imparts heat, which, together with the stretch, produces a softer consistency in fascial tissues (an example of thixotropy), breaks adhesions, and frees restrictions.

The quality of application of myofascial techniques is essential to their success. That includes slow sustained stretching of myofascial membranes in a direction that releases their adherence to each other. Little if any lubricant is used to prevent the hands from sliding superficially over the skin.

Myofascial technique categories include skin lifting, fascial stretching, and fascial mobilizations. There are many variations within each category. The techniques presented here are useful for learning the basics of myofascial applications and can be readily integrated into a massage session.

SKIN LIFTING TECHNIQUES

Skin lifting techniques free restrictions in subcutaneous fascia. They release adhering tissues and increase local superficial circulation. The skin is gently picked up with the fingers and slowly pulled away from underlying tissues. Maintain the pull until tissues are more pliable and shift direction more easily. This usually takes 2–3 minutes for problem areas. Do not overwork an area by staying too long at one time, or by repeated applications in one session.

Skin lifting techniques include basic lifting, lifting with directional shift, and skin rolling (Figure 18.3■). In basic skin lifting, the tissues are picked up vertically only. While sustaining the vertical lift, you may also gently pull or push in more horizontal directions feeling for restrictions. For skin rolling, lift the skin vertically and then crawl your fingers along the skin pushing up from behind with the thumbs. This creates a rolling wave of tissue that moves across the surface.

FASCIAL STRETCHING TECHNIQUES

Fascial stretching techniques elongate fascial tissues in broad areas. They can be applied at different depths. For all fascial stretches, hold the tension steadily for 2–5 minutes until you feel the tissue give way or elongate, and avoid sliding over the skin. This category includes dual and single direction stretches and anchored stretches (Figure 18.4■).

The cross-hand stretch is a dual direction stretch for subcutaneous fascia. Place crossed hands parallel to and adjacent to the spine, with one hand in the thoracic region and the other in the lumbar region. Engage the tissue, and slowly apply horizontal pressure to spread the tissue between the hands.

To make the cross-hand stretch a single direction stretch, anchor the skin with one hand, while the other hand pushes horizontally in the opposite direction. Hold and wait for an elongation of tissues. For a smaller area, use a thumb to anchor the skin in place, while the fingers of the other hand pull and stretch the fascia in the opposite direction.

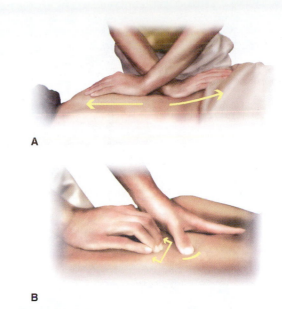

A

B

FIGURE 18.4

Fascial stretching techniques. A. Cross-hand dual direction stretch. B. Pin and stretch with the thumb and fingers.

FASCIAL MOBILIZATIONS

Fascial mobilizations are used to apply a shearing force across the surface of fascial sheets to release bonding between the sheets. The general direction of this stretch is horizontal to the adhering tissues. Fascial mobilizations are entered into slowly to the depth desired followed by a horizontal stretch. The stretch is held steadily for 2–5 minutes until a release is felt. Fascial mobilizations can be applied with the palms, forearm, or fingertips (Figure 18.5■).

A reinforced palm can be used to apply pressure to a broad area such as the lower back (Figure 18.5A). Press into the tissue with the palm until you engage the surface of the muscular layer, and then sift the tissues horizontally toward the pelvis. Hold until a release is felt.

Fascial mobilization over the round surface of the thigh is applied with a flat hand (Figure 18.5B). In this broad plane shift, the entire hand makes contact with the skin surface; however, the heel is used to engage tissues and shift the fascia around the leg toward the table. The recipient is in side-lying position for this technique.

The forearm can also be used for fascial mobilization on both flat (Figure 18.5C) and rounded surfaces. Note in the example of fascial mobilization around the shoulder (Figure 18.5D) that the proximal third of the forearm is used to engage the tissues and the upper arm is held away from the body. Avoid applying pressure with the point of the elbow.

The fingertips can be used for deeper pressure in smaller areas. Pressure is applied vertically into tissues (Figure 18.5E) until the desired depth is attained, and then tissues are shifted more horizontally. Sensitive fingers can feel in which direction the fascial sheets seem to be adhering (point of resistance) or in which direction the tissues seem to want to release (point of

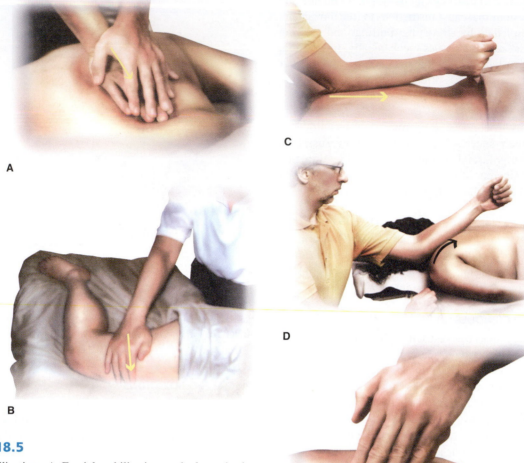

FIGURE 18.5

Fascial Mobilizations. A. Fascial mobilization on the lower back using the palm. B. Broad plane shift around the thigh using the heel of the hand. C. Fascial mobilization on the flat upper back using the forearm. D. Fascial mobilization around the top of the shoulder using the forearm. E. Fascial mobilization using the fingertips.

least resistance). With experience, you will develop a kinesthetic feel for which way to go to best unwind the fascial sheets.

Be sure to let the tissues rest after myofascial massage applications (Figure 18.6■). This allows the tissues to integrate the changes that have occurred. See video of Myofascial Massage of the Back on the accompanying DVD.

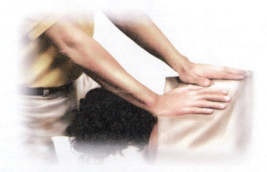

FIGURE 18.6

Allow tissues to rest after myofascial applications.

TRIGGER POINT THERAPY

Trigger point therapy involves the identification and deactivation of painful fibrous nodules called trigger points that occur in muscle and connective tissue. **Trigger points (TrPs)** are felt in muscles as taut bands of tissue that elicit pain if pressed and that refer pain to other areas in predictable patterns. They cause pain, weakness, and loss of flexibility. Manual techniques such as direct pressure to TrPs are effective in deactivating the points and relieving the accompanying pain and dysfunction. Trigger point therapy can be easily integrated into massage sessions as needed.

Trigger point therapy was popularized in the United States by Janet Travell (1901–1997) who developed a treatment for myofascial pain syndrome caused by trigger points. Travell was appointed White House physician to Presidents Kennedy and Johnson in the 1960s. She, along with coauthor David Simons, wrote the definitive work on the subject, *Myofascial Pain and Dynsfunction: The Trigger Point Manual*, Vols. 1 & 2 (1992, 1999).

TrPs and Reference Zones

Trigger points feel like small tense spots or taut bands of tissue in a muscle or tendon. They are tender to the touch, and active TrPs radiate pain when pressed. A microscopic view of the muscle would reveal tiny contraction knots along the muscle fibers. This accounts for the nodular and taut feel of TrPs.

Trigger points are categorized as:

- Latent or active
- Primary or secondary
- Satellite
- Associated

Latent TrPs are painful only when pressed. *Active* TrPs are always tender, prevent full lengthening of the muscle, weaken the muscle, and refer pain with direct compression. *Primary* TrPs are activated by acute or chronic overload of a muscle, while *secondary* TrPs become active in reaction to a primary TrP. *Satellite* TrPs are in the zone of reference of a primary TrP. Secondary and satellite TrPs are also called

TABLE 18.1	Varieties of Trigger Points
Type of TrP	Characteristics
Latent TrP	Painful only when pressed
Active TrP	Always tender, weakens and shortens the muscle, refers pain
Primary TrP	Activated by acute or chronic muscle overload
Associated TrP	Activated by primary TrP (also called secondary TrP)
	Activated by being in reference zone of primary TrP (also called satellite TrP)

associated TrPs. Table 18.1■ summarizes the varieties of trigger points.

Trigger points can occur anywhere in muscles or tendons, but some TrP locations are more common. These are at typical points of stress in the body such as the shoulders, neck, buttocks, and legs (Figure 18.7■).

FIGURE 18.7

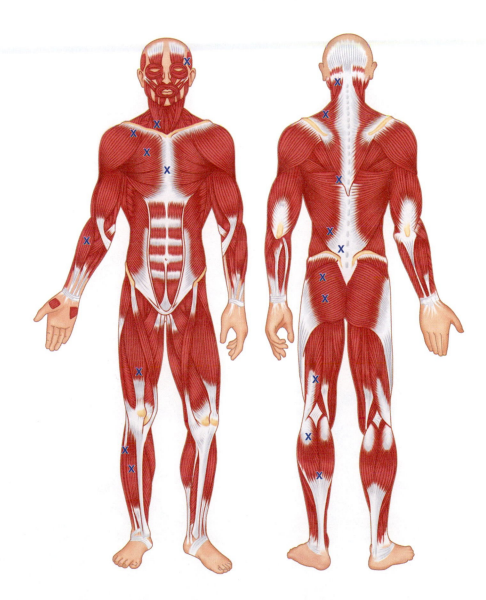

Common trigger point locations.

REFERENCE ZONES

Trigger points radiate pain in predictable patterns. The area of the body affected by a particular TrP is called its **reference zone**. For example, TrPs in the shoulders and neck refer pain to the head, which is experienced as a tension headache (Figure 18.8■). A TrP reference zone might be some distance from the TrP itself. For example, TrPs in the suboccipital muscles refer pain to an area on the side of the head above the ear.

TrPs elicit pain when pressed, but active points may be tender and painful without pressure. The referred pain of TrPs has been described as dull, aching, and deep. TrPs can cause minor discomfort to severe debilitating pain. The muscle involved is typically stiff, weak, and restricted in its range of motion. It may feel tense and ropelike, and stretching the muscle increases the pain. While trigger point charts are useful for confirming common TrP locations and referral patterns, you may find points and patterns unique to an individual client.

Other sensory, motor, or autonomic phenomena may be "triggered" by active TrPs. These include spasm, vasoconstriction, coldness, sweating, pilomotor response (goose bumps), vasodilation, and increased gland secretion.

ORIGINS OF TrPs

Trigger points can be activated by direct stimuli such as acute overload or overwork of a muscle, chilling, or trauma. Indirect stimuli that may activate TrPs include arthritis, emotional stress, certain visceral diseases, and other TrPs.

People who perform repetitive tasks are prone to TrPs, for example, athletes, musicians, artists, and physical laborers. Poor posture can also stress muscles and cause TrPs especially when sitting at a desk or in a car for long periods of time. Forward head posture, which places the upper body in a round-shoulder, slumped forward position, produces TrPs in the pectoral and posterior cervical muscles. Something as simple as habitually carrying a heavy backpack with straps that press into the shoulder muscles can cause the muscle overload that leads to trigger points.

TrP Deactivation Techniques

A variety of manual techniques are used to deactivate trigger points. The most common manual technique used by massage therapists is direct pressure on the TrP using the thumb, the fingers, or a simple hand tool (Figure 18.9■). Deep effleurage (stripping) along the muscle fibers affected by the TrP and deep transverse friction at the TrP site can also be effective.

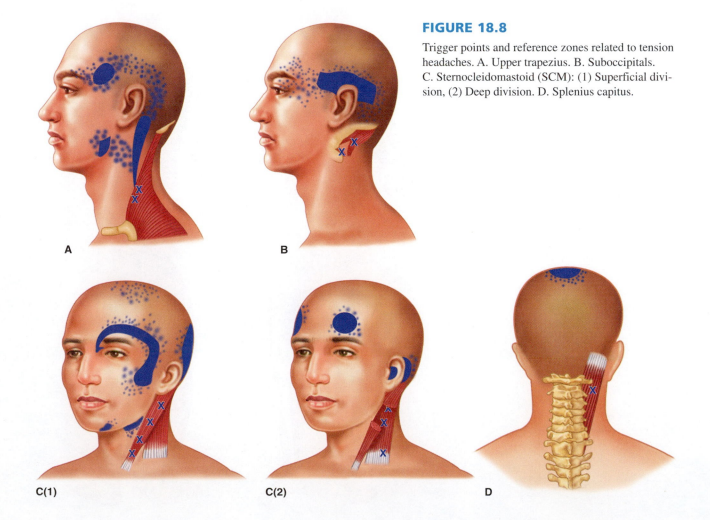

FIGURE 18.8

Trigger points and reference zones related to tension headaches. A. Upper trapezius. B. Suboccipitals. C. Sternocleidomastoid (SCM): (1) Superficial division, (2) Deep division. D. Splenius capitus.

A

B

C(1)

C(2)

D

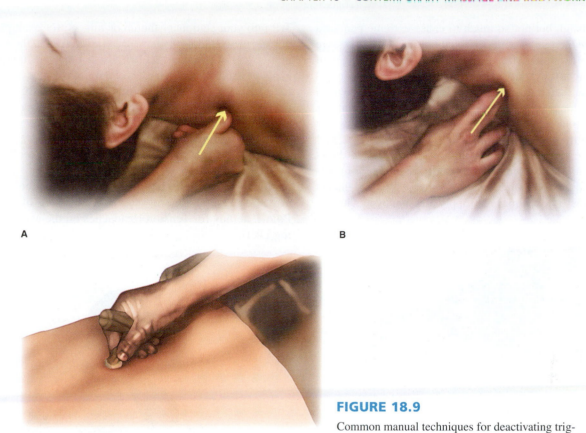

FIGURE 18.9

Common manual techniques for deactivating trigger points. A. Thumb. B. Fingers. C. Hand tool.

These soft tissue applications are typically followed by a stretch of the affected muscle. This is especially important to complete the TrP deactivation and return the affected muscle to a normal state.

LOCATING TrPS

Suspect myofascial trigger points when clients complain of muscle tension causing pain or when you find localized muscle soreness and shortening. Clients might also describe one of the common pain patterns of TrPs. The more knowledgeable you are about TrPs and their predicable referral patterns, the more easily you will be able to locate specific points.

Massage therapists often discover latent TrPs during a massage session. Affected muscles are painful and often feel ropelike. The taut bands at exact TrP locations can be palpated. Clients can give feedback about pain referred to other areas of the body when a TrP is pressed.

Clients may point to the exact location of active TrPs. He or she might say, "It hurts when I press here," or may rub the muscle in which the TrP is located. You can also have clients mark painful spots on a body chart during an intake interview.

It is helpful to know the origin of a client's TrPs. Was the client in an accident? Did he fall down, or get hit with something? Does she perform a repetitive motion in her job or recreation activity? Does he or she have poor posture, or sit or stand for long periods of time? A person must stop or modify whatever it was that caused the TrP to prevent it from coming back.

CONTRAINDICATIONS AND CAUTIONS

Trigger point therapy is contraindicated for undiagnosed conditions that cause severe pain or that are related to recent accidents or trauma. It is locally contraindicated over bruises, wounds, and other instances of soft tissue damage. Caution is advised for clients taking medication that prevents blood from clotting or that compromises tissue integrity.

DIRECT PRESSURE TECHNIQUES

Direct pressure techniques involve compressing tissues directly over the taut band of the TrP. This is sometimes called ischemic compression because the compressed tissues become temporarily white from lack of blood, followed by increased local circulation to the spot when pressure is released.

Direct pressure to the TrP site is thought to push apart the small contractile units in muscles called sarcomeres, thus releasing the tiny contraction. When this happens a softening or relaxation of the taut band can be felt.

Direct pressure is applied after warming surrounding tissues with effleurage and petrissage techniques. The amount of pressure necessary to deactivate a TrP is enough to engage the taut band, but not so much to cause extreme pain or a protective tightening of the affected muscle. Apply pressure into a TrP by slowly sinking into the point and holding until a softening is felt. Increase pressure gradually as tension and pain at the site seem to decrease. Release pressure when the TrP is no longer tender. Do not overwork a TrP site in one session. Hold points for 30–90 seconds total. Follow with a stretch of the affected muscles.

There are a variety of techniques for applying direct pressure to trigger points. When using the thumb or fingers to apply direct pressure, keep the joints in good alignment (Figure 18.10■). You may also apply pressure by moving the TrP into your stationary thumb or fingers, for example, by turning the head into fingers placed over TrPs in the suboccipital region (Figure 18.11■). Use a pincer technique to apply pressure when both sides of a muscle can be accessed, for example, for TrPs in the sternocleidomastoid (SCM) muscle (Figure 18.12■). The tip of your elbow is effective for applying pressure to TrPs in the upper trapezius when the client is seated in a massage chair (Figure 18.13■).

Whenever possible, follow direct pressure techniques with muscle stripping over the site. It often provides additional relief. End TrP applications with a stretch of the affected muscle (Figure 18.14■). See video of Trigger Point Therapy for Tension Headaches on the accompanying DVD.

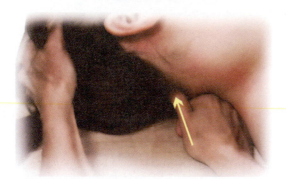

FIGURE 18.10

Thumb and wrist in alignment when applying direct pressure.

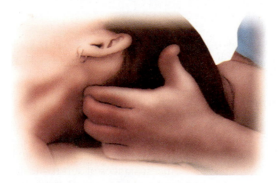

FIGURE 18.11

Turn the head into stationary fingers to apply pressure to TrPs in the suboccipital muscles.

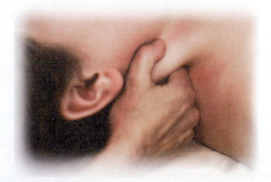

FIGURE 18.12

Pincer technique for TrPs in the sternocleidomastoid muscle.

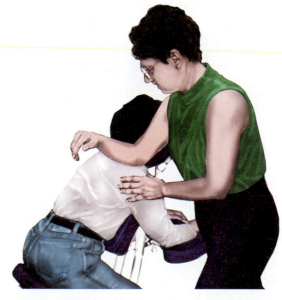

FIGURE 18.13

Tip of the elbow used to apply pressure to TrPs in the upper trapezius muscle when the client is seated in a massage chair.

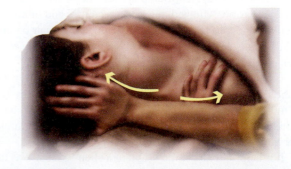

FIGURE 18.14

Follow TrP deactivation techniques with stretching of the affected muscles.

PRACTICAL APPLICATION

Perform a massage practice session for the head, neck, and shoulders. After warming the area with Western massage techniques, search for trigger points commonly associated with tension headache (Figure 18.8). Apply appropriate TrP deactivation techniques.

1. Before the session, did the recipient complain of tension in the neck and shoulders or of having a headache?
2. Could you locate trigger points through palpation?
3. What role did the recipient play in providing feedback? Was it useful?

LYMPHATIC FACILITATION

Lymphatic facilitation (LF) is a light and gentle massage technique used to facilitate the removal of excess fluid that collects in tissues for a variety of reasons, including traumatic injury, inflammation, and allergies. Certain pathologies that cause fluid accumulation or edema are contraindications for LF and are discussed further in another section of this chapter.

Fluid accumulation can cause irritation, pressure, and pain, as well as limited movement due to swelling around affected joints, reduced nutrient delivery to the surrounding area, and restrictions in fascial tissues. LF techniques facilitate transportation of fluids through interstitial spaces, into the lymph capillaries, around the lymph system, and back into general circulation.

Current approaches to lymphatic massage trace their histories to Emil and Astrid Vodder, Danish physiotherapists, who developed Manual Lymphatic Drainage (MLD) in the 1930s. MLD was designed as a precise protocol for the treatment of lymphedema and is part of complete decongestive therapy (CDT), that is, skin care, MLD, compression bandaging, exercise, and patient self-care. Drs. John and Judith Casley-Smith of Australia subsequently developed complex decongestive therapy for lymphedema that uses a simplified manual technique in place of the MLD protocol. The lymphatic facilitation techniques described in this chapter are a further evolution of lymphatic massage designed initially for treating common musculoskeletal injuries.

Lymphatic System

Knowledge of the structure and function of the lymphatic system is essential for understanding lymphatic facilitation applications. The techniques themselves, and the order in which they are applied, are based on the unique character of this complex body system. It will be helpful for you to review basic lymphatic system anatomy in preparation for the following discussion which focuses on information related to LF applications. See page 184 in Chapter 6 for more information about lymphatic system anatomy, physiology, and pathology.

Lymphatic system components include a network of lymph vessels, lymph fluid, lymph nodes, the cisterna chyli, and the spleen and thymus. An overview of lymphatic system structures appears in Figure 18.15■. Note that the flow of lymph fluid in the system is in an asymmetrical pattern. Lymph fluid from the legs, lower abdomen, and left side of the body flows to the thoracic duct (left lymphatic duct) and into the left subclavian vein. Lymph from the right side of the body above the diaphragm flows to the right lymphatic duct and into the right subclavian vein. Lymphatic facilitation applications direct flow toward the appropriate lymphatic duct.

Lymphatic system functions include the production and distribution of lymphocytes and the transport of fluid, hormones, waste products, and cellular debris back to the cardiovascular system from the tissues. Normally, about 10 percent of interstitial fluid is returned to the cardiovascular system via the lymphatic system.

If the blood and lymph capillaries in an area become blocked or damaged, fluid will build up in the tissues, resulting in edema. This typically happens with traumatic injury and common musculoskeletal injuries such as strains and sprains. The lymphatic system has the ability to increase its capacity up to 50 percent for a short period of time to help remove excess fluid in an area. The skillful application of lymphatic facilitation increases fluid absorption and flow, thus re-establishing homeostatic fluid balance in tissues.

LYMPH

Lymph is the colorless fluid in the lymph vessels that contains water, protein molecules, cellular components, and fatty acids that need to be transported back into blood circulation. Before it enters the lymph system, this fluid resides in and moves through the intercellular spaces as interstitial fluid.

Molecules, proteins, and cellular wastes too large to enter blood capillaries are returned to general circulation via the lymph capillaries. Without the lymph system, this material would accumulate in the tissues, causing inflammation, irritation, and pain.

INTERSTITIAL MATRIX

Matrix is a more accurate description of what is often called the interstitial space. The word space implies a vacant open area between cells. However, this space is more structured than usually depicted. The matrix is created by collagen fibers that form "scaffolding" within which fluids such as water and plasma flow (Figure 18.16■). This matrix is

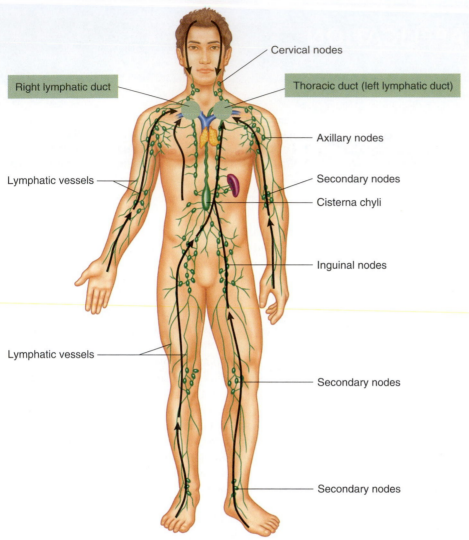

FIGURE 18.15

Overview of the lymphatic system.

Cervical nodes

Right lymphatic duct

Thoracic duct (left lymphatic duct)

Axillary nodes

Lymphatic vessels

Secondary nodes

Cisterna chyli

Inguinal nodes

Lymphatic vessels

Secondary nodes

Secondary nodes

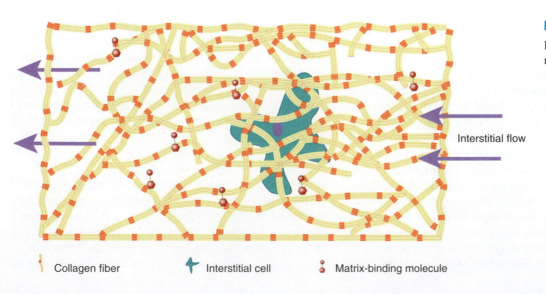

FIGURE 18.16

Interstitial space or matrix.

Interstitial flow

Collagen fiber   Interstitial cell   Matrix-binding molecule

referred to as a *prelymphatic channel* in many manual lymph drainage texts.

The optimal delivery of nutrients and removal of waste products requires that the interstitial matrix be free of debris and restrictions. Lymphatic facilitation applications help maintain the health of this matrix by moving interstitial fluid through the system. And if lymphatic vessels are damaged in a certain area, LF techniques can move interstitial fluid through the matrix into a different watershed (drainage area) to facilitate its eventual removal via the blood and lymph capillaries.

LYMPHATIC SYSTEM VESSELS AND STRUCTURES

The lymphatic system is composed of hollow vessels that carry lymph from peripheral tissues back to venous circulation (Figure 18.17■). The smallest vessels dead end in the interstitial spaces and are known as lymph capillaries or **initial/terminal lymph vessels**. These initial/terminal (I/T) vessels flow into progressively larger vessels called collector vessels and then into transport vessels. The lymphatic vessels finally empty into two large collecting ducts in the chest.

I/T Vessels I/T vessels are the entry point for excess fluid, proteins, and various waste products. They are the smallest lymph vessels, with walls that are only one cell thick (Figure 18.18■). It is at this point in the system that LF techniques have their greatest effect. About 40 percent of all I/T vessels are found in the skin.

The cell junctions in I/T vessels must open for interstitial fluid to enter. This is accomplished by tiny anchoring filaments attached to the cell wall on one end and the surrounding connective tissue on the other end. An increase in interstitial fluid, as well as gentle skin traction, can pull on the anchoring filaments and open the flaps. Too much pressure (e.g., as used in most massage techniques) closes the flaps and slows or stops the flow of fluid into the I/T ves-

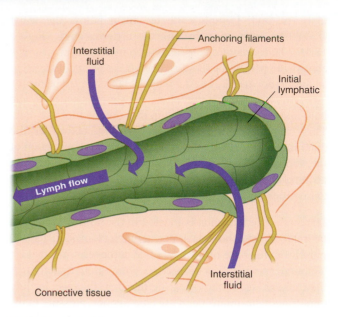

FIGURE 18.18

Schematic drawing of initial/terminal (I/T) lymph vessels.

sels. That is why LF techniques use only enough pressure to create traction and movement in the superficial skin layers.

Collector Vessels Collector vessels gather lymph from I/T vessels, and take it to the transport vessels or lymphangia. Collector vessel walls are one or two cells thick and do not contain valves. They extend from I/T vessels in the interstitial spaces to the deeper transport vessels.

Transport Vessels Transport vessels or lymphangia are segmented, with each segment approximately 2–10cm in length. Each segment is referred to as a *lymphangion* and has a valve at each end. Once lymph enters the transport vessels, manual techniques cannot change its direction, but can increase transport capacity and flow.

Transport vessels have an outer, middle, and inner layer of tissues similar to veins. The middle layer contains smooth muscle. As the vessels fill with fluid, the pressure on the walls stimulates the muscle to contract (i.e., stretch reflex). This sets off a peristaltic wave that moves fluid through the system toward the lymphatic ducts.

The lymphangia contraction rate is estimated to be 4–10 times per minute at rest. That rate can increase up to 40 times a minute as a result of skeletal muscle contraction, increased heart rate, diaphragmatic breathing, and increased fluid moving through the system. Because LF techniques bring more fluid into I/T vessels, a substantial increase in the rate of lymphangia contraction may follow as the amount of fluid in the system increases overall.

If transport vessels in an area become damaged or blocked, an emergency pathway called the *anastomosis* is used to clear fluid from the area (Figure 18.17). This system of tiny vessels links one lymphangion to another providing an alternate route for lymph flow. This is especially important in areas of trauma and injury.

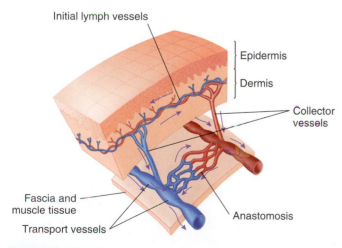

FIGURE 18.17

Lymphatic system vessels and the flow of lymph.

Cisterna Chyli Lymph collected from below the waist watershed must pass through the cisterna chyli (Figure 18.15). This structure is located deep in the abdomen and is considered part of the thoracic duct. It has been compared to an upside-down turkey baster with the bulb situated below the tube. To clear the cisterna chyli, we simply "squeeze" the bulb and the lymph is pushed up through the thoracic duct. This can be accomplished through the action of the diaphragm in deep breathing and through the contraction of the abdominal muscles such as when doing sit-ups. The cisterna chyli is important for LF applications in the lower extremities.

Terminus The terminus is located in the hollow space just lateral to the attachments of the sternocleidomastoid (SCM) muscles at the base of the neck. It is at the terminus that LF techniques are applied to increase lymph flow directly into the thoracic ducts, thus clearing the area. Increase in fluid uptake at the terminus decreases the internal pressure in the lymphatic system as a whole, relative to the pressure in I/T vessels. Because of this pressure differential, more fluid enters I/T vessels until the pressure is equalized. It has been suggested that this alone can increase the lymph uptake at I/T vessels by up to 30 percent and last for several hours after the LF session.

Lymph Nodes Lymph nodes are spongy structures located throughout the lymphatic system. They contain chambers through which lymph must pass, and, therefore, tend to slow transport. The function of lymph nodes is to filter lymph and house cells of the immune system. Clusters of lymph nodes are found in the popliteal, inguinal, axilla, and neck areas (Figure 18.15).

General Drainage Patterns

Superficial drainage patterns in different areas of the body are divided into areas called *watersheds*. Lymph traveling in the lymphangia moves within its watershed toward the concentration of lymph nodes or *catchments* nearby. The direction of lymph flow in major watersheds and the major catchments are shown in Figure 18.19■. LF techniques direct lymph fluid toward the nearest proximal catchments.

FIGURE 18.19

Superficial drainage pathways or watersheds. Circles indicate clusters of lymph nodes or catchments.

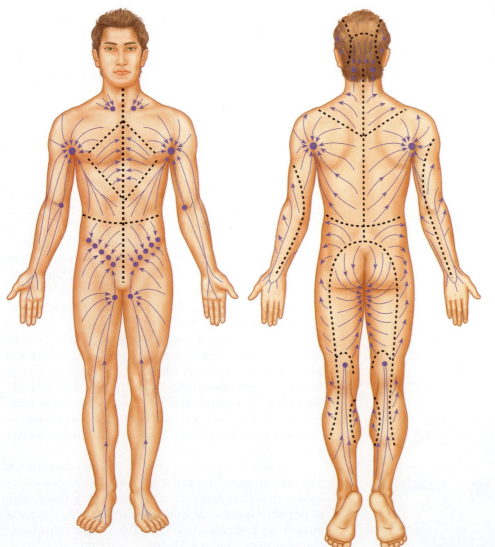

Contraindications for LF

There are few absolute contraindications for LF. One of these is lymphedema, for which complete decongestive therapy has been developed. CDT encompasses manual lymph drainage techniques in combination with other therapies.

Other contraindications for LF include infection, blood clots, phlebitis, pitting edema, and major heart problems such as congestive heart failure. Any conditions that can be worsened by increased fluid circulation warrant caution for LF applications. This includes kidney disease, asthma, thyroid conditions, and menstruation in women.

It was believed in the past that massage, and specifically manual lymphatic drainage, would cause cancer to spread to other parts of the body. At this point, there is no evidence to support this belief. When working with a cancer patient, the massage therapist is advised to discuss the merits and cautions related to massage for a particular patient with his or her physician.

LF may be appropriate at different stages of a cancer patient's treatment; for example, postsurgery to enhance removal of secondary edema, promote fewer adhesions, and support the healing cycle. It may also be beneficial postradiation treatment for the same reasons. If the lymph system has been compromised during treatment and lymphedema results, it is important to refer the patient to a CDT specialist and not use LF alone for treatment. Consultation with a cancer patient's physician is advised before providing lymphatic massage of any kind.

LF Strokes and Guidelines

LF techniques are designed to increase absorption of fluid at I/T vessels, move fluid through the interstitial matrix, increase the rate of lymphangia contraction, and generally improve the flow of lymph within lymphatic vessels. LF can also direct the direction of lymph flow in superficial tissues.

L STROKE, LONG STROKE

The two basic LF strokes are the L stroke and the long stroke. The L stroke is applied by stretching the skin in an L-shaped pattern. The fingertips, finger pads, thumb pads, flat fingers, or full hand is used for applying the L stroke. One of the stretch directions must be in the desired direction of lymph flow. See Figure 18.20■ in the following Practice Sequence. Stretch the skin within its willingness to move without increasing pressure into the tissues. The L stroke ends with a release of the tissue so that it snaps back into position. This is repeated 10–15 times.

The long stroke resembles effleurage, but the skin is stretched as the hands slide toward the nearest catchment.

The long stroke is applied with the palm and fingers of the open hands. Pressure is light, and the stretch is maintained over the full length of the stroke. The distance covered is usually no farther that the closest proximal joint in the extremities or catchment area in the torso. See Figure 18.24■ in the following Practice Sequence. Hands are released quickly at the end so that the skin snaps back before repeating the long stoke 10–15 times.

GUIDELINES

LF is effective if strokes are applied with the correct attributes. These attributes are light, slow, repeated and rhythmic, and stretch/snap back. Strokes are applied in a certain order and direction, that is, proximal before distal, and in the direction of lymph flow. To begin every LF session, the left and right thoracic ducts are cleared first.

Light Pressure Use only 4–5 grams of pressure. This is about as much pressure as you would use to move your eyelid over your eye. Using more pressure would close I/T vessel flaps and prevent fluid from entering the capillaries.

Slow Pace Apply strokes at a relatively slow steady pace. Lymph flow cannot be forced. About 2 liters of lymph fluid flows through the thoracic duct in 24 hours.

Repeated and Rhythmic Strokes are repeated in the same place 10–15 times in an even rhythm to set up a pressure wave of fluid entering the I/T vessels.

Stretch/Snap Back Skin is stretched superficially and then released quickly so that it snaps back into place. This alternately opens and closes the I/T vessels flaps to help set up the pressure wave of fluid.

Direction and Order of Application LF strokes are directed toward the nearest proximal catchment area. Proximal areas are cleared before more distal areas to create space into which lymph can flow.

Clear Left and Right Thoracic Ducts At the beginning of every LF application, the left and right thoracic ducts are cleared with strokes on the sides of the neck and at the terminus. For applications below the diaphragm, the cisterna chyli is also cleared.

LF Practice Sequence for the Lower Extremity

Practice Sequence 18-1, Lymphatic Facilitation for the Lower Extremity, demonstrates the basic strokes and guidelines described previously. Steps 1–3 begin the process of lymphatic drainage in the entire body.

PRACTICE SEQUENCE 18.1

Lymphatic Facilitation for the Lower Extremity

30 minutes
Recipient supine

Preliminary Instructions
• Drape appropriately for access to the leg.
• Screen for contraindication and cautions.
• Determine cause and nature of trauma or indications for LF.
• Stand at the side of the table facing the head.

1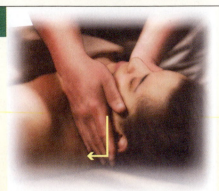

FIGURE 18.20 Apply L-strokes to both sides of the neck with flat fingers. Hands are placed just under the ears with fingers pointing towards the table. The stretch is toward the back of the neck and then toward the shoulders. Release and let the skin snap back. Repeat 10–15 times.

2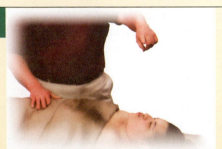

FIGURE 18.21 Apply L-strokes to the terminus. Place your index and middle fingers on the left and right terminus. The stretch is toward the clavicle and then toward the midline. Release and let the skin snap back. Repeat 10–15 times.

3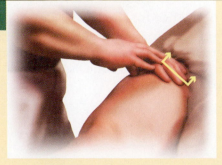

FIGURE 18.22 Clear the cisterna chyli by having the recipient breathe out forcefully. Have the recipient take a deep breath and then exhale forcefully as if blowing out a candle about 2 feet away. Repeat 5–6 times.

4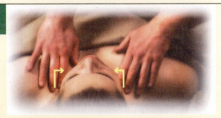

FIGURE 18.23 Clear the inguinal catchment area. Place one hand across the thigh inferior and parallel to the inguinal ligament, little finger side towards the torso, and place the other hand on top. Gently press straight down toward the table using medium pressure, and then stretch the skin toward the abdomen. Release and let the tissue snap back. Repeat 10–15 times.

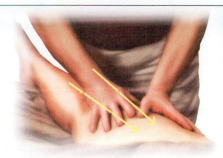

FIGURE 18.24 Apply long strokes to the thigh. Place the full flat of the hand on the thigh just superior to the knee. Stretch the skin toward the inguinal nodes, and then continue sliding toward the inguinal area while maintaining the stretch. Release and let the skin snap back. Repeat 10–15 times.

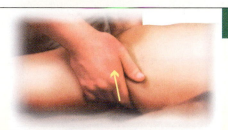

FIGURE 18.25 Clear the popliteal catchment area. Face the head of the table, and place both hands under the recipient's knee with palms up and fingers interlaced. Lift up into the popliteal space until the knee begins to bend. Maintain this upward pressure as you stretch the skin toward the torso. Release quickly and let the skin snap back. Repeat 10–15 times.

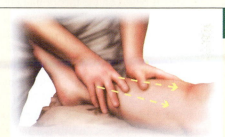

FIGURE 18.26 Apply long strokes to the lower leg, anterior and posterior. Begin with long strokes to the anterior lower leg from ankle to knee. Repeat 10–15 times. Then bend the knee to access the posterior leg, and apply 10–15 long strokes (not shown). Let the skin snap back after each stroke.

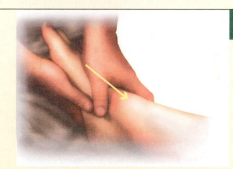

FIGURE 18.27 Apply short strokes to the foot. Place the flat of the hand over the dorsal foot, thumb on medial side. The other hand stabilizes the foot from the plantar side. Stretch the skin toward the knee and release. Repeat 10–15 times.

Note: Modify this protocol to meet the needs of each client. If the pathology being addressed is located at the knee, then the practitioner need only clear down to the knee and not below. This will prevent additional fluid from being pushed into an area of existing edema or inflammation and allow the most effective clearing of the area of pathology.

 After you perform the Practice Sequence, evaluate how well you did by filling out Performance Evaluation Form 18-1, Lymphatic Facilitation for the Lower Extremity. The form can be found in Appendix F, Performance Evaluation Forms on page A-33 and on your DVD.

See video of Lymphatic Facilitation for the Head and Neck on the accompanying DVD.

CRITICAL THINKING

Think about the structure of the lymphatic system and the guidelines for lymphatic facilitation applications. Analyze the LF application for the lower extremities presented in this chapter.

1. Why did the application begin with techniques not applied directly to the leg? What were they and what was their purpose?

2. In what order were different areas on the leg addressed? Why?

3. Which specific manual techniques were used at each step of the application? Why was each chosen for that step?

REFLEXOLOGY

Foot reflexology is based on the theory that pressure applied to specific spots on the feet (called **reflexes**) produces positive changes in corresponding parts of the body. For example, pressing just under the tips of the toes at the sinus reflex affects the sinuses. There are reflex areas on the feet that correspond to all systems and structures of the body. Maps of the feet identify reflex locations (Figure 18.28■).

Pressure applied to reflexes is thought to marshal the body's innate healing forces and to normalize body functions. Different reflexology techniques apply pressure in ways that cause the desired reflex action.

Reflexology has ancient roots in many parts of the world, including Asia and the Americas. Evidence of its ancient origins is found in foot maps that appeared in India about five thousand years ago. Modern Western reflexology developed along its own path with European writings on zone therapy in the late 1500s. In 1771 German physiologist Johann Unzer coined the term *reflex* to explain motor reactions to applied pressure. American reflexology can be traced to the early 1900s and the book *Zone Therapy* by Dr. William Fitzgerald of Hartford, Connecticut. Dr. Joseph Shelby Riley built on Fitzgerald's ideas and made the first detailed diagrams of reflex points on the feet. A physiotherapist named Eunice Ingham (1889–1974), who worked for Riley, combined zone therapy with compression massage of the feet. The special techniques for applying pressure to the feet that Ingham developed became the basis for modern reflexology. Ingham has often been called the "Mother of Modern Foot Reflexology." Mildred Carter (1912–2005), a student of Ingham, expanded the theory of reflexology by locating reflex areas throughout the body and focusing on reflexes in the hands and feet.

Reflexology Theory

A number of theories have been proposed to explain the therapeutic effects of reflexology. Physiological theories focus on body systems such as the nervous, circulatory, and lymphatic systems. Energetic theories relate reflexology to bioelectrical energy and the meridians of traditional Chinese medicine.

The theory of zone therapy has been a foundation of American reflexology. In zone therapy, the body is divided lengthwise into 10 imaginary longitudinal zones with five zones on each side of the body, and end points on the head, hands, and feet (Figure 18.29■). The belief is that pressure applied anywhere in a zone affects all of the anatomical structures and organs in that zone. Reflexology charts are derived from zone therapy, and show which structures and organs are located in each zone and are affected by pressure to specific spots on the feet and hands.

Eunice Ingham took zone therapy and combined it with compression massage of the feet. She believed that the techniques of reflexology dissolved crystalline deposits in the feet that interfered with nerve and blood supplies to the organs in the corresponding zones. Today this concept has expanded to include all types of congestion that might inhibit the optimal functioning of body systems. Possible inhibiting factors include buildup of cellular debris, excess fluid, toxins, and by-products of inflammation.

Over the years, other theories have evolved to explain reflexology. Nerve theory proposes that reflexology techniques stimulate the thousands of nerve endings in the feet. This stimulation results in normalization of body systems. Others believe that reflexology acts to keep energy flowing freely, similar to acupoints in traditional Chinese medicine. According to these theories, pressure on the feet maintains harmony and balance in life energy or Qi.

More recently, research studies have been conducted to investigate the effectiveness of reflexology for improving health and for treatment of a variety of ailments. For example, a two-year study funded by the National Institutes of Health (NIH) found that reflexology produced a significant reduction in pain and anxiety in cancer patients. The Research Analysis Document published by the International Council of Reflexologists summarizes more than three hundred studies from around the world. Citations are also found on various research databases, including that of the Massage Therapy Foundation (www.massagetherapyfoundation.org).

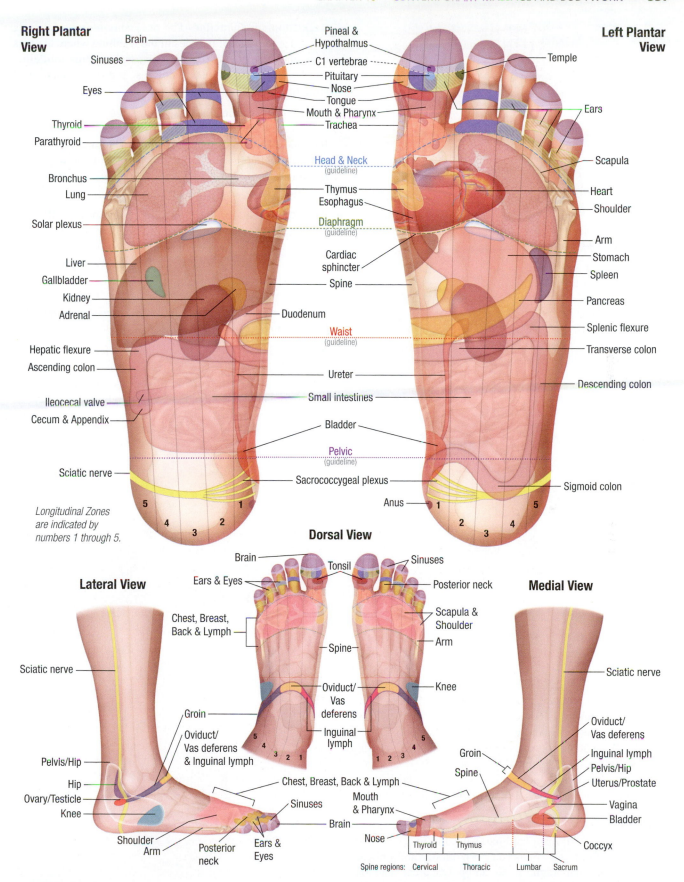

Right Plantar View

Brain
Sinuses
Eyes
Thyroid
Parathyroid
Bronchus
Lung
Solar plexus
Liver
Gallbladder
Kidney
Adrenal
Hepatic flexure
Ascending colon
Ileocecal valve
Cecum & Appendix
Sciatic nerve

Longitudinal Zones are indicated by numbers 1 through 5.

Pineal & Hypothalmus
C1 vertebrae
Pituitary
Nose
Tongue
Mouth & Pharynx
Trachea
Head & Neck (guideline)
Thymus
Esophagus
Diaphragm (guideline)
Cardiac sphincter
Spine
Duodenum
Waist (guideline)
Ureter
Small intestines
Bladder
Pelvic (guideline)
Sacrococcygeal plexus
Anus

Left Plantar View

Temple
Ears
Scapula
Heart
Shoulder
Arm
Stomach
Spleen
Pancreas
Splenic flexure
Transverse colon
Descending colon
Sigmoid colon

Dorsal View

Brain
Tonsil
Ears & Eyes
Chest, Breast, Back & Lymph
Spine
Oviduct/ Vas deferens
Groin
Oviduct/ Vas deferens & Inguinal lymph
Inguinal lymph
Sinuses
Posterior neck
Scapula & Shoulder
Arm
Knee

Lateral View

Sciatic nerve
Pelvis/Hip
Hip
Ovary/Testicle
Knee
Shoulder Arm
Posterior neck
Ears & Eyes
Sinuses
Brain
Nose

Chest, Breast, Back & Lymph
Mouth & Pharynx

Medial View

Sciatic nerve
Oviduct/ Vas deferens
Inguinal lymph
Pelvis/Hip
Uterus/Prostate
Vagina
Bladder
Coccyx
Groin
Spine

Thyroid
Thymus
Spine regions: Cervical   Thoracic   Lumbar   Sacrum

FIGURE 18.28

Foot reflexology chart showing the location of reflexes with corresponding anatomical structures and organs.

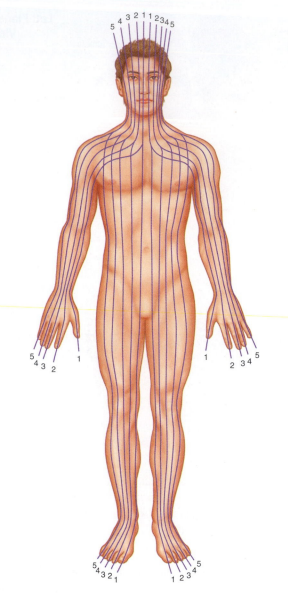

FIGURE 18.29

Ten longitudinal zones of zone therapy.

Zones and Guidelines

As previously mentioned, reflexology charts are based on zone therapy and show which reflexes on the feet to press to affect anatomical structures and organs in the corresponding zones. When looking at the bottoms of the feet with a person sitting or lying supine, the 10 longitudinal zones can be imagined as bordered by 10 vertical lines running from toes to heel, five on each foot. The vertical lines lie approximately along each toe.

GUIDELINES

Guidelines are additional landmarks used to locate reflexes on the feet. Four guidelines run horizontally and indicate neck/shoulder, diaphragm, waist, and pelvic areas. The longitudinal tendon guideline is parallel to the zones. Together the zones and guidelines form a grid that map the feet. Guidelines are shown in Figure 18.30■.

Neck/Shoulder Guideline The neck/shoulder guideline is located at the base of the toes in the webbing where the toes meet the ball of the foot. Reflexes along this guideline address neck and shoulder muscles, and other anatomical structures in the area.

Diaphragm Guideline The diaphragm guideline runs along the base of the metatarsal heads from medial to lateral foot. It divides the body into the chest and abdominal cavities. It is also the diaphragm reflex that is stimulated to release tension in the thoracic region to improve breathing and digestion and relieve stress and anxiety.

Waist Guideline The waist guideline runs horizontally from the tuberosity of the fifth metatarsal on the lateral foot (often felt as a bulge) to the medial side. This guideline bisects the abdominal cavity into upper and lower. The upper region contains the liver, gallbladder, kidneys, adrenal glands, stomach, pancreas, duodenum, and spleen. The lower region contains the small intestine, large intestine, appendix, kidneys, ureters, and bladder.

Pelvic Guideline The pelvic guideline is found on the heel, typically where the tougher heel tissue changes into the softer arch. It identifies the location of the pelvic girdle, reproductive organs, and colon. It also forms a bridge between the lateral and medial pelvis, whose reflex areas are located on the lateral and medial ankle.

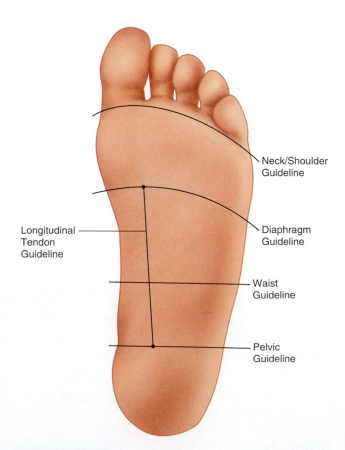

FIGURE 18.30

Guidelines.

Longitudinal Guideline The longitudinal guideline is located in zone 1 between the diaphragm and pelvic guidelines. It helps to accurately locate the adrenal glands, kidneys, ureters, and bladder.

Reflexology Techniques

Pressure is applied to reflexes using techniques specifically designed for reflexology. These include thumbwalking, fingerwalking, rolling, hook-and-backup, and press-and-flex. Direct pressure and deep friction are also used to stimulate reflex points. Reflexes can be simulated by joint movements in the ankles and feet.

For many reflexology techniques, one hand stabilizes the foot, while the other hand applies the pressure. The hand applying the techniques is called the *working hand*. The hand providing the brace or backstop is called the *stabilizing hand*.

Thumbwalking Thumbwalking is used to apply pressure rapidly along lines on the feet. To practice thumbwalking, place your thumb at the heel of the foot on the medial side, and "walk" your thumb along the spinal reflex, that is, up the side of the foot to the toes. See Figure 18.34■ in the following Reflexology Practice Sequence. Stabilize the foot with one hand, while the working hand performs the technique. Bend your thumb at the first joint, press into the tissues, then straighten the thumb and move to the next spot. Repeat this action as the thumb walks along in a line. Apply pressure with the top center of the thumb, or the top edge of the thumb just to the side of the nail. The movement is rhythmical and steady, much like the action of a sewing machine needle as it travels over a piece of cloth.

Fingerwalking Fingerwalking is a similar technique applied to larger areas, such as the flat medial ankle area of the pelvic reflex. See the placement of the fingers on the pelvic reflex (refer to Figure 18.39A■). The finger joints bend and straighten as the fingertips "walk" over the area. *Rolling* is an alternative to walking. In rolling, the thumb or finger is held in place on a reflex, and the body part rotated into the point to apply pressure. See Figure 18.39 A & B in the following Reflexology Practice Sequence.

Dorsal Fulling Dorsal fulling is applied to the lymphatic reflex on the top of the foot. The skin is stretched toward the toes using light pressure, and then released so that it snaps back into place. Eight fingers are placed on top with the thumbs stabilizing the foot from the bottom. See Figure 18.36■ in the following Reflexology Practice Sequence. The stretch is applied first near the toes (chest/back reflex), and then repeated moving row by row to the ankle (groin reflex). Dorsal fulling affects the entire back, as well as the muscular, nervous, lymphatic, and respiratory systems.

Hook-and-Backup The hook-and-backup technique is used to apply deep pressure to a specific area or reflex. Locate the reflex you wish to press, and place your thumb directly on the spot. Bend the first joint to apply pressure, and then pull the thumb to the side across the spot to deepen the pressure. This technique is useful to apply deep pressure to small reflexes such as the gallbladder reflex. See Figure 18.38■ in the following Reflexology Practice Sequence.

Press-and-Flex In the press-and-flex technique, pressure is applied by flexing a joint so that reflex point is pressed deeper into the thumb or finger. This is demonstrated in Figure 18.40■ in the following Reflexology Practice Sequence. Pressure can be applied to reflexes on the toes with simple squeezing between the thumb and index finger. See Figure 18.41■ in the following Reflexology Practice Sequence.

Contraindications

Because reflexology affects anatomical structures and organs indirectly, it is relatively safe to use with most clients. In fact, it can be an effective complementary therapy, since the intent is to activate the innate healing force through a reflex mechanism.

Before beginning foot reflexology sessions, check the condition of the feet for local contraindications. These include fractures, bruises, burns, skin lesions, cysts, damaged veins, warts, and contagious infections such as athlete's foot. Use caution around arthritic joints, bunions, heel spurs, Morton's neuroma, and tarsal tunnel syndrome. Do not apply reflexology to feet with acutely inflamed joints or excessive swelling.

Ask the origin of any prominent scars and the history of injuries or surgery in the area. Be cautious around prior fractures, especially if metal pins, plates, or other medical hardware are present.

Use lighter pressure for reflexology techniques if the recipient has decreased sensitivity in the feet, for example, those with diabetes or multiple sclerosis. If the client is weak for some reason, consider shortening the session to about 10 minutes per foot. Some general contraindications for massage apply, for example, fever, nausea, severe distress, blood clots, and acute inflammation.

Reflexology Sessions

Foot reflexology sessions commonly last from 30–60 minutes. Time is divided equally between the two feet. Sessions usually begin with a general foot massage to warm the tissues and joints, followed by systematic application of pressure to various reflexes.

The recipient is positioned supine or semireclining on a massage table. A bolster may be placed under the knees to relieve pressure on the knee joints. Recliner chairs that tilt back and elevate the legs may also be used for reflexology. Recipients remain clothed, but a drape over the legs may be used for warmth. The feet are at a level that allows the practitioner to maintain good body mechanics. The practitioner is typically seated with the head, neck, and back in proper alignment (Figure 18.31).

SENSATIONS DURING AND AFTER REFLEXOLOGY SESSIONS

Recipients of reflexology report a wide variety of sensations during and after sessions. These include relaxation, tenderness, ticklishness, electrical or energy bursts, emotions, deep rest, and rejuvenation.

A completely healthy person would experience no discomfort or pain during a reflexology session.

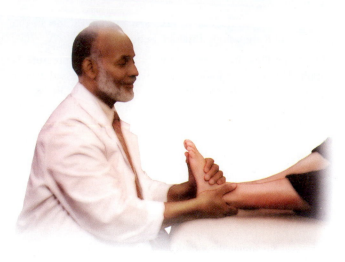

FIGURE 18.31

Client and practitioner positioning for foot reflexology.

The feet may be tender because of fluid buildup (swollen feet), foot injuries, or other common foot problems such as bunions and corns. Ill-fitting shoes can cause chronic foot pain. Some clients have low pain tolerance.

Tenderness or pain when pressing a specific reflex may indicate an imbalance or congestion in the corresponding area. It may signal overall tension, stress, and fatigue. Medications, drugs, or poor nutrition may cause toxicity in the body reflected in tenderness in the feet. In reflexology, pressure is repeatedly applied to tender reflexes until the discomfort declines or dissipates, and the body re-establishes balance.

Reflexology Practice Sequence for General Well-Being

The following reflexology Practice Sequence addresses the entire body, and provides opportunity to practice a variety of reflexology techniques.

PRACTICE SEQUENCE 18.2

General Reflexology Session

30 minutes
Recipient semireclining in chair or on table

Preliminary Considerations
- Before beginning, conduct a verbal screening for contraindications for massage (e.g., fever or extreme nausea).
- Ask about any structural problems with the feet and any contagious foot conditions such as athlete's foot.
- Do not perform reflexology on a foot if it might cause structural damage or spread contagious skin conditions.
- Place a bolster under recipient's knees and raise the legs so that you can keep your spine in good alignment while applying techniques.
- Sit at the feet of the recipient.
- You may wear latex (or nonlatex substitute) for protection in certain cases.
- If a foot soak is used prior to the reflexology session, towel dry the feet thoroughly and sprinkle with corn starch or nontalc foot powder. Reflexology techniques require that pressure be applied without gliding or slipping over the skin.

1

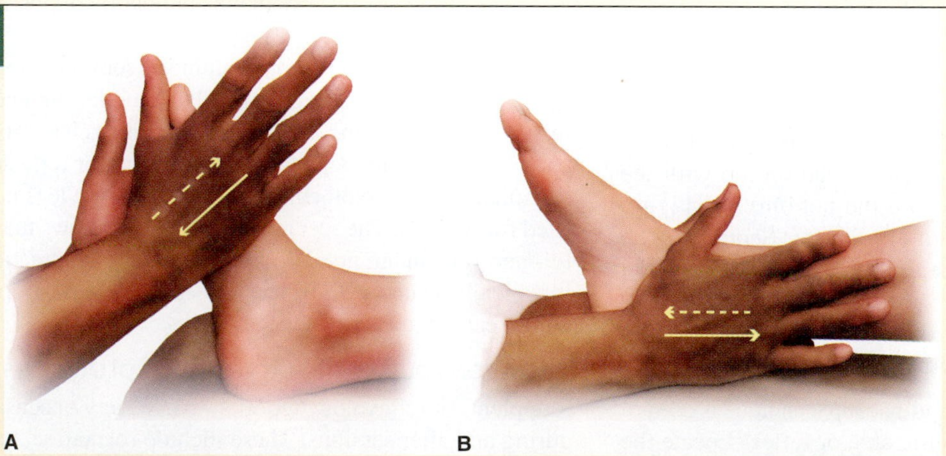

A   B

FIGURE 18.32 Warm up the foot soft tissues and joints of the feet with (A) massage techniques, and (B) joint movements.

FIGURE 18.33 Spinal twist. Use two hands to apply three quick rhythmical twists at the pelvic, waist, and diaphragm guidelines. This releases tension in the lumbar and thoracic spine.

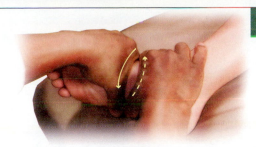

2

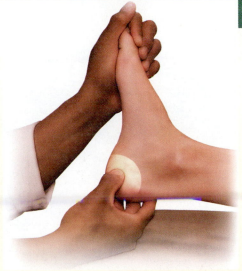

3

FIGURE 18.34 Thumbwalk the spinal reflex on the medial side of the foot, from the sacrum reflex at the heel to the cervical reflex at the top of the big toe. Move up and down the spinal reflex several times to affect the entire central nervous system.

FIGURE 18.35 Direct thumb pressure across the base of the big toe along the neck and occipital ridge reflex. This eases neck tension and improves blood supply to the head.

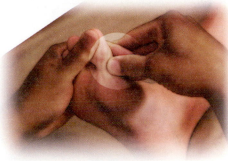

4

FIGURE 18.36 Dorsal fulling with ankle rotation. Stretch the skin in rows over the top of the foot, and then move the ankle through its full range. This affects the entire back and the internal organs.

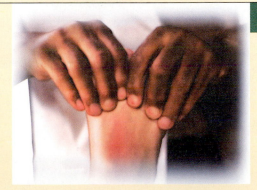

5

6

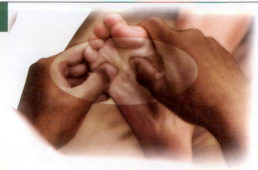

FIGURE 18.37 Direct thumb pressure over the entire foot bottom to affect chest and abdominal reflexes. Use both thumbs to apply pressure simultaneously. Place the thumbs on the reflexes. Start with your elbows out to the sides and then push them down as the thumbs sink into the foot bottom.

7

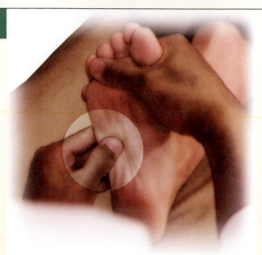

FIGURE 18.38 Hook and backup applied to the gallbladder reflex.

8

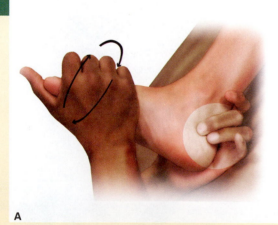
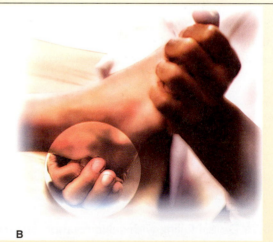

A   B

FIGURE 18.39 Roll the foot into the fingers placed over (A) the pelvis/hip reflex on the medial ankle, and (B) the genital reflexes on lateral ankle.

cheeks flush, blood pressure drops, salivation increases, heart rate slows, eyes may tear, and the stomach grumbles. These are objective signs of the relaxation response of the parasympathetic nervous system.

Some of these physiological changes can be explained with a closer examination of polarity therapy techniques. For example, in one technique a very light oscillating pressure is applied over the pressure sensitive baroreceptors in the carotid arteries on the sides of the neck. It is probable that this is sufficient to activate the neurological reflex that slows heart rate and lowers blood pressure.

Polarity techniques that involve rocking motions of the limbs and torso stimulate mechanoreceptors in joints. It appears that when these receptors are stimulated, a reflex response is activated that lowers muscle tone, increases circulation, and results in endorphin release.

The rhythmic quality of other polarity techniques can induce a light hypnotic state. This brings calming and peace of mind. Sometimes this state of quiet awareness allows people to see their problems from a broader perspective, or allows hidden feelings to surface. Polarity therapy can be a valuable adjunct to psychotherapy.

Many polarity techniques are as easily set within the framework of modern science as they are within Ayurvedic and energy theories. It is as if the basic principle that Stone sought transcends all ideas, ancient or modern, and is instead embodied in the actual experience of the hands-on work, rather than in the particular theories used to explain it. Energy is simply an abstract metaphor, one way of looking at the results obtained through polarity therapy. Neurological reflex is another abstract metaphor, a way of explaining a mechanism we cannot see, except in its effects.

Principles of Polarity Therapy

Polarity therapy is based on concepts of energy, love, removing obstructions, and understanding. These concepts guide the application of the gentle polarity techniques.

Energy Polarity therapy practitioners develop an awareness of feeling energy in their hands. These sensations can be picked up and amplified with practice. For example, rub your hands together to wake up the nerve endings, and bring your awareness to your palms. Then hold your palms about six inches apart, and focus your awareness on how they feel. Experiment with moving your palms closer and farther apart. Note changes in the feeling and a sense of the palms plugging into each other energetically.

Love Another important polarity therapy concept is *love*. Love in this sense is not a sentimental attachment or affection. It can be thought of as caring for someone else with no agenda or objective in mind, not even that of healing or helping. It is an attitude of surrender or openness. It is getting out of the way and letting the body's tendency to wholeness and healing take place.

One way to explore this quality of love is a simple front-to-back polarity technique. Have the recipient sit up straight but relaxed. Stand on the person's left side, and place your left hand over his or her heart and the right hand on the upper back between the shoulder blades (Figure 18.43■). Move your hands around slowly until you feel a sense of the palms "plugging in" to each other, as if they are connected by a flow of energy. Simply hold your hands in place and feel the connection. Note any reaction in the recipient. After a few minutes, slowly withdraw your hands.

Removing Obstructions Another principle of polarity is **removing obstructions** to the free flow of energy. An energy obstruction can be seen in the body where there is holding, tension, or misalignment. An alert polarity practitioner begins assessing clients visually as soon as they arrive. Obstructions can be further detected through palpation.

To develop skill in locating energy obstructions, practice the *tummy rock* technique. Have the recipient lie supine with the hands at his or her sides. Stand at the right side and place your right hand lightly on his or her abdomen below the navel (Figure 18.44■). Become aware of his or her breathing pattern, skin temperature, and muscular tension. Make certain that your own hand and arm muscles are completely relaxed, and that your breathing is calm. Increase the pressure slightly, and introduce a wavelike movement by pressing first with the heel and then the fingers of your hand, repeating the motion gently. Place your hand on the person's forehead, and feel for a sensation of plugging in. Gently rock the abdomen while keeping the hand on the forehead still. Note any tingling in your own hands, and watch for subtle changes in the recipient such as deeper breathing or muscle relaxation. These are signs of removing obstructions.

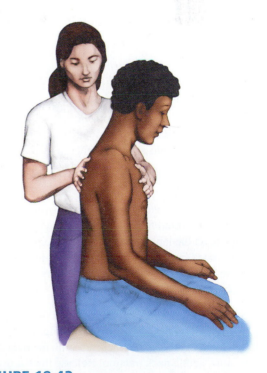

FIGURE 18.43

Feeling the palms "plugging into each other."

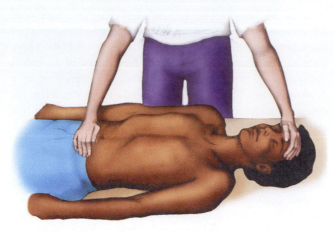

FIGURE 18.44

Tummy rock to release energy blocks in the torso and head.

Understanding The fourth principle is understanding, a concept that invites the practitioner to be open to the recipient's experience and to the effects of polarity therapy. Each recipient will react to polarity therapy differently, and understanding calls for knowledge of the broader picture of what might be happening physiologically and psychologically in a session.

Polarity is a gentle art. Nothing is ever forced. The recipient is experiencing the effects of past actions and present decisions. The giver is not there to rescue the receiver, but to plant seeds of letting go and trusting, and to be an accepting observer. This attitude protects the practitioner from taking on the recipient's ailments in a misguided attempt to heal. A commonsense approach emphasizes a caring attitude, acceptance, and trust that whatever happens is from a clearing of obstructions and is for the best.

Polarity Therapy Techniques

Polarity therapy techniques are gentle holding, rocking, and probing movements. They come from a variety of sources, including Stone's studies of healing practices from around the world. The following are samples of polarity techniques that can be easily integrated into a massage therapy session when energy obstructions are suspected or used as transition and finishing techniques.

The Cradle Position your hands palms up, and overlap the last three fingers of each hand to form a cradle (Figure 18.45■). Rest your hands on the table, supporting the recipient's head in your palms. Index fingers lie beside the sternocleidomastoid (SCM) muscle. Hold 1–2 minutes, or until a current of energy is felt strongly.

The Neck Stretch Rest the receiver's head on your right palm, and take a firm hold on the base of the skull (Figure 18.46■). Rest your left hand lightly on the forehead. With the right hand only, apply slow, gentle neck traction. Release the traction as the receiver exhales, and increase it on the inhale. Repeat this traction-release movement 5–10 times.

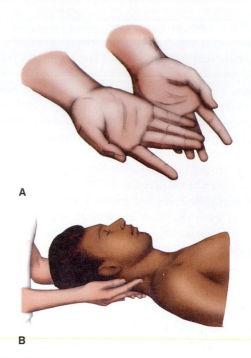

A

B

FIGURE 18.45

The cradle. A. Hand position. B. The cradle supporting the recipient's head.

The Leg Pull Grasp both feet behind the heels, and gently pull the legs straight toward you several inches above the table (Figure 18.47■). Slowly rest the legs back on the table and place your hands over the feet for a few moments before proceeding.

Thumb Web–Forearm Stimulation Walk to the recipient's right side. With your left hand (thumb and index finger) squeeze the webbing of the recipient's thumb (Figure 18.48■). With your right hand, press your thumb into a point about 1 inch below the recipient's elbow crease and a half-inch from the medial side of the arm. Stimulate the two points alternately in a rhythmic movement 10 times. Repeat on the left side.

Pelvic Rock From the right side, place your right hand over the recipient's left hip bone and your left hand on the right shoulder (Figure 18.49■). Stabilize the shoulder and gently rock the torso with the right hand. Gradually increase the rocking movement

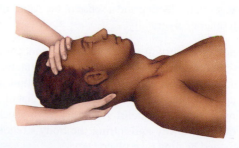

FIGURE 18.46

Neck stretch.

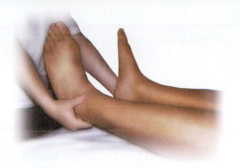

FIGURE 18.47

Leg pull.

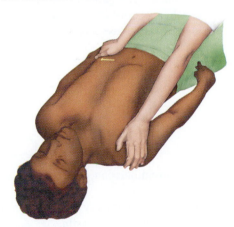

FIGURE 18.48

Thumb web-forearm stimulation.

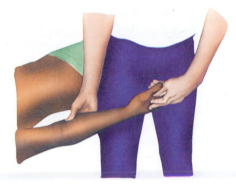

FIGURE 18.49

Pelvic rock.

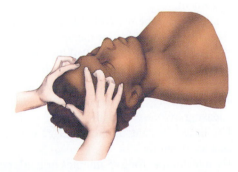

FIGURE 18.50

Cranial polarization.

for 20 seconds and then gradually decrease the movement. Hold for a moment before proceeding to the left side.

Cranial Polarization Place both thumbs lightly on the anterior fontanel and both index fingers touching the "third eye" on the forehead (Figure 18.50■). The remaining fingers are spread out touching the forehead lightly. Relax your hands and arms, and breathe calmly. Hold this position for 1 minute or until a gentle pulsation is felt.

Brush Off to Finish Have the recipient sit on the edge of the table with his or her hands on the thighs. Stand behind the recipient and place your hands on the shoulders. With a sweeping movement, brush your hands across the spine, then down to the sacrum, and out to the hips (Figure 18.51A■).

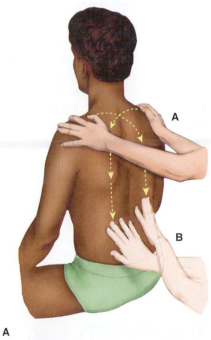

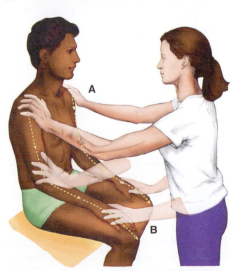

FIGURE 18.51

Brushing off to finish. A. The back. B. The front.

Repeat three times. Stand in front of the recipient and place your hands on the shoulders. With a sweeping movement, brush down the arms to the knees and down the legs (Figure 18.51B). Repeat three times. See video of a General Session of Polarity Therapy on the accompanying DVD.

SOME FINAL THOUGHTS

Each of the therapies presented in this chapter can stand alone as a specialization beyond entry-level training in massage therapy. The theory and practice of any one form could be the entire focus of a massage therapist's career. Such expertise adds greatly to the therapeutic possibilities of massage and bodywork.

More commonly, and of equal value, are the knowledge, basic techniques, and applications that different forms of contemporary massage and bodywork bring to the field as a whole. The specialized knowledge that underpins different forms of bodywork expands our understanding of humanity, health, and healing. Basic techniques and applications can be integrated in massage sessions to help achieve client goals. Eclectic massage therapists develop a large tool box of approaches over the years. And even basic knowledge of different forms of contemporary massage and bodywork enhances the work of a well-rounded practitioner.

ESTEBAN

REALITY CHECK

NADIA: My hands hurt after practicing trigger point therapy and reflexology—especially my thumbs. Is this normal, and I just have to get used to it? Is there anything I can do about it?

ESTEBAN: There could be a few things going on to cause your hands to hurt. Maybe you're pressing too hard or using poor hand mechanics. Be sure that your wrist and thumb joints are in good alignment when you apply pressure. Then see how little pressure you can use and still get good results. You need to apply adequate pressure, but people often press harder than they need to be effective. Harder doesn't mean better. And when your hands hurt after practicing massage, soak them in ice water for about ten minutes to reduce swelling and inflammation. You can also try doing more to condition your hands. Getting the strength for doing massage develops over time. Get a hand strengthening device and use it daily to build up the strength you need.

CHAPTER HIGHLIGHTS

- Contemporary massage and bodywork is a term that describes the broad range of unique systems, approaches, and techniques of manual therapy in use today.
  - Over the past century, forms of manual therapy have been developed to affect specific body tissues and systems, and to address specific therapeutic goals.
- Myofascial massage addresses the body's fascial anatomy.
  - The general intent is to release restrictions in superficial fascia, in deep fascia surrounding muscles, and in fascia related to overall body alignment.
  - Myofascial techniques stretch fascial sheets, break fascial adhesions, and leave tissues softer and more pliable.
  - Myofascial techniques were pioneered by Ida Rolf (1896–1979), who developed an approach to bodywork known today as Rolfing.

- Fascia is loose, irregular connective tissue found throughout the body.
  - Composed of three primary elements: ground substance, collagen, and elastin.
  - Lies at three depths: superficial, deep surrounding muscles, continuous sheet related to overall body alignment.
  - Can change to be more pliable as a result of movement, stretching, or increase in temperature; this is due to a property called thixotropy.
  - Fascial structures include retinaculae, body straps, and fascia related to the musculature.
- Myofascial massage applications involve identifying and releasing myofascial restrictions.
  - Use little lubricant; applications are gentle, slow, sustained, subtle.
  - Hold technique for 2–5 minutes or until melting is felt.
  - Exit tissues slowly, and let them rest.

- Basic myofascial techniques include skin lifting, fascial stretching, and fascial mobilizations.
- Trigger point therapy involves the identification and deactivation of painful fibrous nodules called trigger points that occur in muscle and connective tissue.
- Trigger points are felt as taut bands of tissue that elicit pain if pressed and that refer pain to other areas in predictable patterns called reference zones.
- Trigger point therapy was popularized in the United States by Janet Travell (1901–1997), who developed a treatment for myofascial pain syndrome caused by trigger points.
- Trigger points are categorized as latent or active, primary or secondary, satellite, or associated.
  - Latent TrPs hurt only when pressed.
  - Active TrPs are always tender, prevent full lengthening of the muscle, weaken the muscle, and refer pain with direct compression.
- The referred pain of TrPs has been described as dull, aching, and deep.
  - The muscle involved is typically stiff, weak, and restricted in its range of motion; and may feel tense and ropelike.
- Origins of TrPs include direct stimuli such as acute overload or overwork of a muscle, chilling, trauma, or indirect stimuli such as arthritis, emotional stress, certain visceral diseases, and other TrPs.
- Techniques for applying direct pressure to trigger points to deactivate them include direct pressure with the thumb, fingers, or elbow, squeezing, and use of a hand tool.
- Lymphatic facilitation (LF) is a light and gentle massage technique used to facilitate the removal of excess fluid that collects in tissues for a variety of reasons, including traumatic injury, inflammation, and allergies.
- Current approaches to lymphatic massage trace their histories to Emil and Astrid Vodder, Danish physiotherapists, who developed Manual Lymphatic Drainage (MLD) in the 1930s.
- LF techniques are based on lymphatic system anatomy, including lymph flow patterns, lymph vessels and structures, watersheds, and catchments.
  - LF techniques mainly affect I/T vessels or lymph capillaries; about 40 percent of all I/T vessels are found in the skin.
- LF strokes include the L stroke and the long stroke.
- Guidelines for LF applications are light pressure; slow, rhythmic, repeated movements; stretch/snap back; correct direction and order of application.
  - To begin, clear left and right thoracic ducts at the terminus.
  - Order: clear proximal before distal, and proceed in the direction of lymph flow.
- Foot reflexology is based on the theory that pressure applied to specific spots on the feet (called reflexes) produces positive changes in corresponding parts of the body.
- Eunice Ingham (1889–1974) is called the "Mother of Modern Foot Reflexology."
- Foot reflexology charts map the location of important reflexes on the feet.
  - Based on zone therapy; the body is divided into 10 longitudinal zones with endpoints in the head, hands, and feet.
  - Guidelines help locate reflexes: neck/shoulder, diaphragm, waist, pelvic, and longitudinal guidelines.
- Reflexes are stimulated using direct pressure and joint movements.
  - Techniques include thumbwalking, fingerwalking, rolling, dorsal fulling, hook-and-backup, and stretch-and-flex.
- Tenderness on pressure to reflexes may indicate an imbalance in the corresponding part of the body.
- Polarity therapy techniques involve simple touching and gentle movements designed to release obstructions to the free flow of energy in the body.
- Polarity therapy was developed in the early 1900s by Randolph Stone (1890–1981), an eclectic natural healer who studied Ayurvedic medicine from India.
- Principles of polarity therapy include energy, love, removing obstructions, and understanding.
- Polarity therapy techniques include the tummy rock, the cradle, neck stretch, leg pull, thumb web–forearm stimulations, pelvic rock, and cranial polarization.
- Forms of contemporary massage and bodywork can be a specialization beyond entry-level training, or their basic knowledge and techniques can be integrated into massage therapy sessions.

EXAM REVIEW

Key Terms

Match the following key terms to their descriptions. For additional study, look up the key terms in the Interactive Glossary on page G-1 and note other terms that compare or contrast with them.

_____ **1.** Contemporary massage and bodywork
_____ **2.** Fascia
_____ **3.** Foot reflexology
_____ **4.** Initial/terminal lymph vessels
_____ **5.** Lymphatic facilitation (LF)
_____ **6.** Myofascial massage
_____ **7.** Polarity therapy
_____ **8.** Reflexes
_____ **9.** Removing obstructions
_____ **10.** Trigger points (TrPs)
_____ **11.** Trigger point therapy
_____ **12.** Reference zone

a. Locate with zones and guidelines
b. Anchoring filaments open flaps
c. Broad range of manual therapy today
d. Compression massage and zone therapy
e. Reduce traumatic edema
f. Free adhesions and restrictions in fascia
g. Remove obstructions to energy flow
h. Taut band of tissue
i. Ground substance, collagen, elastin
j. Principle of polarity therapy
k. Area of the body affected by a particular TrP
l. Deactivation of painful fibrous nodules that occur in muscle and connective tissue

Memory Workout

To test your memory of the main concepts in this chapter, complete the following sentences by circling the most correct answer from the two choices provided.

1. Fascia has a property called (mobilization) (thixotropy) that means it can become more pliable with movement, heat, and stretching.
2. Fascia is loose, irregular (connective) (muscle) tissue found throughout the body.
3. Muscles in the immediate area of a trigger point often feel (stringy) (ropelike).
4. Direct pressure to soft tissues that causes blanching is called (deep) (ischemic) compression.
5. A concentration of lymph nodes in a specific drainage area is called a (watershed) (catchment).
6. A more accurate description of interstitial space is (matrix) (anastomosis).
7. According to zone therapy, the body is divided into 10 (longitudinal) (diagonal) zones.
8. The guideline located near the heel of the foot is the (pelvic) (waist) guideline.
9. Observable changes during polarity therapy include signs of deep (hypnosis) (relaxation).
10. In polarity therapy, the principle of (love) (removing obstructions) refers to responding to the recipient's needs without attachment to the results.

Test Prep

The following multiple-choice questions will help to prepare you for future school and professional exams.

1. The primary mechanism of myofascial techniques is:
   a. Physiological
   b. Reflexive
   c. Mechanical
   d. Energetic
2. When myofascial restrictions release, it feels to the massage therapist like:
   a. Hardening and shortening
   b. Gathering and contracting
   c. Melting and shortening
   d. Melting and lengthening
3. Trigger points that are painful only when pressed are categorized as:
   a. Associated
   b. Latent
   c. Active
   d. Satellite
4. Direct pressure to a trigger point is typically sustained for:
   a. 10 seconds
   b. 10–20 seconds
   c. 30–90 seconds
   d. 3 minutes

5. The repeated and rhythmic application of LF strokes creates a:
   a. Pressure wave inside the interstitial space
   b. Pressure wave inside the lymphatic vessels
   c. Blockage at I/T vessels
   d. Blockage at the thoracic ducts
6. When applying long strokes, the skin is stretched in the direction of the:
   a. Nearest distal catchment
   b. Nearest proximal catchment
   c. Farthest distal catchment
   d. Deepest transport vessels
7. On which foot is the corresponding reflex area for the kidneys?
   a. Left foot only
   b. Right foot only
   c. Outside ankles
   d. Bottoms of both feet

8. According to zone therapy theory, pressure applied anywhere in a particular zone affects the:
   a. Entire zone
   b. Adjacent zone
   c. Entire body
   d. Corresponding area of the brain
9. The original theory of polarity therapy was heavily influenced by:
   a. European folk remedies
   b. Ayurvedic medicine from India
   c. Western medicine from Europe
   d. Mayan healing practices from Central America
10. If the recipient feels pain during the neck stretch technique of polarity therapy, it means that:
    a. The technique may be contraindicated
    b. Energy is flowing freely
    c. You should pull harder
    d. You should pull on the exhale instead of the inhale

Video Challenge

Watch the appropriate segment of the video on your DVD and then answer the following questions.

Contemporary Massage and Bodywork

Myofascial Massage
1. How would you describe the elements of the myofascial massage applications demonstrated in the video, for example, pace, depth, direction, quality of touch?

Trigger Point Therapy
2. What principles of good body and hand mechanics are in evidence in the trigger point therapy demonstration in the video?

Reflexology
3. During the thumb- and fingerwalking techniques, what is the practitioner's other hand doing to assist in the applications?

Comprehension Exercises

The following short answer questions test your knowledge and understanding of chapter topics and provide practice in written communication skills. Explain in two to four complete sentences.

1. Contrast myofascial mobilization with the pin-and-stretch technique. How is each applied? How do they affect myofascial tissues differently?
2. Explain the cause of trigger points in the musculature. Give two common examples of how they might develop.
3. Describe the intent of lymphatic facilitation techniques. In what ways do they improve lymph flow?
4. Describe the mechanics of the thumbwalking technique of foot reflexology. What is it used for? Where would it be best applied?
5. Describe the observable physiological changes that might occur in a polarity therapy session as energy blockages are cleared.

For Greater Understanding

The following exercises are designed to take you from the realm of theory into the real world. They will help give you a deeper understanding of the subjects covered in this chapter. Action words are underlined to emphasize the variety of activities presented to address different learning styles and to encourage deeper thinking.

1. Receive or observe a myofascial massage *or* trigger point therapy session performed by someone with advanced training in the technique. What verbal interaction took place? Which specific technique variations were used? How did the recipient respond?
2. Search a research database for studies related to one of the contemporary massage and bodywork approaches presented in this chapter. List five of the most recent studies, and summarize their findings.
3. Visit the website of a professional specialty association for one of the contemporary massage and bodywork approaches presented in this chapter. Be sure that the website address ends in ".org." Locate information about the association's mission, whether it offers professional certification, and if so, the educational and other requirements.

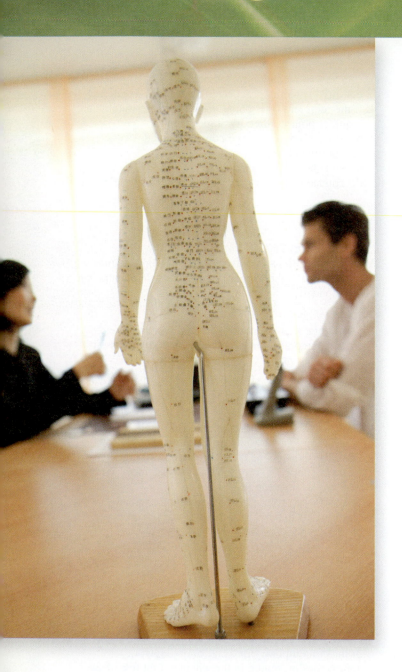

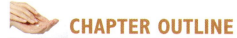 **CHAPTER OUTLINE**

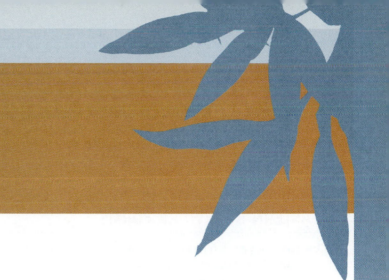

 ## LEARNING OUTCOMES

After studying this chapter, you will have information to:

1. Describe forms of bodywork from China, India, and Thailand.
2. Explain key concepts of traditional Chinese medicine.
3. Demonstrate basic acupressure techniques.
4. Describe qi gong exercises.
5. Explain key concepts of Ayurvedic philosophy.

6. Describe Ayurvedic massage.
7. Describe yoga postures.
8. Explain the theory underlying Thai massage.
9. Describe a Thai massage session.

 ## KEY TERMS

MASSAGE *in* ACTION

On your DVD, explore:

- AMI for the Back
- Qi Gong Twenty Form Routine

EASTERN BODYWORK FORMS

Eastern bodywork refers to traditional forms of manual therapy from the continent of Asia. The term distinguishes these forms from Western massage as developed in Europe and America in the past few centuries.

Three forms of Eastern bodywork that are particularly popular in Western countries are Asian bodywork therapies from China and Japan, Ayurvedic massage from India, and Thai bodywork from Thailand. Although some of the manual techniques in these approaches have similarities to Western massage techniques, their applications and the underlying theory are dramatically different. This chapter provides a survey of these popular Eastern bodywork forms to familiarize massage therapists with some of their basic concepts and techniques. For sources of additional information, refer to the References and Additional Resources listed in Appendix H on page A-74.

Eastern bodywork forms developed within cultures with roots that go back thousands of years in time. They predate modern science and are embedded in whole systems of medicine. These systems are based on certain beliefs about the nature of the universe, of human beings, and of health and healing. There are differences as well as some striking similarities in these beliefs.

One overarching similarity is the holistic view of human beings as body, mind, and spirit. Unlike the relatively recent interest of Western medicine in the concept, a holistic perspective is nothing new to these ancient systems of medicine. Another similarity of the Eastern forms is their consideration of human beings as essentially part of nature and as influenced by their relationships to the natural world. They also incorporate some notion of energy or life force that flows in, around, and through the physical body.

Ancient systems of medicine used herbs, temperature therapy, physical exercise, and manual therapy as mainstays of treatment. In these systems manual therapies and related exercises are used to balance life energy and remove obstructions to its free flow.

As we explore Eastern forms of massage and bodywork that are so different from Western approaches, keep an open mind and heart. Understand that they come from worldviews different from Western thinking and have endured for centuries. You do not have to accept the ideas presented in this chapter as "true" in the sense of scientifically proven facts. They are ways of thinking about health and disease that grew out of a particular culture long ago and that continue to evolve. These theories have spawned practices and treatments that are accepted today as valuable and effective approaches to health and healing.

Truly understanding these systems takes years of study and practice. This introduction provides a broad overview. In studying these forms, we enlarge our understanding of the world.

TRADITIONAL CHINESE MEDICINE OVERVIEW

Traditional Chinese medicine (TCM) is thought to have originated in the barren lands north of the Yellow River in China. Long ago, the inhabitants of this area used herbs, acupuncture, *anmo* (manual or bodywork methods), and other methods to heal various ailments. Over the centuries, these folk healing practices became formalized into a system of medicine unique to China. Later these practices spread to Korea and Japan.

The earliest known text on Chinese medicine is the *Huang Di Nei Jing,* or the *Yellow Emperor's Classic of Internal Medicine.* It is traditionally ascribed to the legendary Yellow Emperor, Huang Di, who is thought to have lived around 2500 BCE. The concepts of Yin and Yang, Qi or energy, Five Elements, energy channels, and acupoints were developed over time to form the foundation of traditional Chinese medicine. An ancient drawing of energy channels is shown in Figure 19.1■. The aim of TCM is to restore and maintain natural balance and harmony in the body, mind, and spirit.

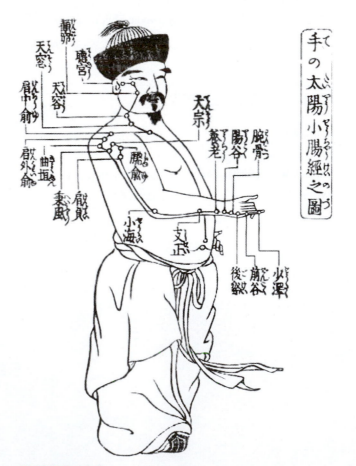

FIGURE 19.1

Ancient drawing of energy channels and acupoints.

Yin and Yang

The concepts of **Yin and Yang** are used to illustrate the relatedness and interconnectedness of all. The Ying/Yang symbol has been described as two comets chasing each other (Figure 19.2■). It reminds one of the movement and constant change of the universe, which is a fundamental idea in TCM. Yin and Yang are always considered in relationship to each other.

Yin is represented by the dark side of the Yin/Yang symbol. The Chinese character for Yin depicts the shady side of a hill. Yin is the dark, deep, dense aspect of the universe. It is characterized as feminine, interior, still, substantial, cool, and contracting in contrast to Yang.

Yang is represented by the light side of the Yin/Yang symbol. The Chinese character for Yang depicts the sunny side of a hill. Yang is the light, energetic, and spacious or heavenly aspect of the universe. Yang is characterized as masculine, exterior, moving, insubstantial, warm, and expanding in contrast to Yin.

Notice that there is a dot of Yang in the Yin side of the symbol, and a dot of Yin in the Yang side. This symbolizes that nothing is pure Yin or Yang, but that these aspects are continually morphing and changing in relationship to each other.

FIVE PRINCIPLES OF YIN/YANG

Five principles explain the relationship of Yin and Yang. The principle of *interdependence* reminds us that these are relative concepts that cannot exist in isolation. The principle of *mutual/supporting relationship* points out that Yin and Yang must be in constant dynamic balance. The principle of *opposition* means that Yin and Yang control and restrict each other. *Intertransformation* explains that Yin and Yang are not static, but are constantly transforming into each other. Lastly, Yin and Yang are *infinitely divisible* and can exist in small or large amounts in everything.

THE BODY IN TERMS OF YIN/YANG

In TCM, the human body is considered in terms of Yin and Yang. Yang corresponds to the back, head, exterior, and lateral/posterior aspects of the limbs. Yang organs, which are hollow, transform, digest, and excrete impure products of food and fluids. Yin corresponds to the front, interior, medial/interior aspects of the limbs. Yin organs, which are solid, store the pure essences extracted from food by the Yang organs. Each of the energy channels described later in this chapter is also designated as Yin or Yang.

Qi

Qi (pronounced *chee*) refers to the energy of the universe. In a larger sense, everything in the universe is Qi, sometimes referred to as Big Qi. When Big Qi condenses, it becomes material, and when it disperses, it becomes nonmaterial.

The Chinese character for Qi depicts rice cooking in a pot with steam escaping. Qi is the rice and the steam, the material and the energy. Qi condensed becomes material, forming rocks, trees, raindrops, birds, and human beings. Qi dispersed becomes energy, sunshine, starlight, and the movement of the wind. This is similar to the idea of quantum physics, in which matter and energy are seen as interchangeable, merely vibrating at different frequencies.

In a more narrow sense, Qi is the *life force* or *life energy* that flows through the body and makes people alive. This energy is extracted from the food we eat and the air we breathe. This useable Qi circulates through the body in a network of energy channels bringing life and health.

Qi's functions in the body are summarized as transforming, transporting, holding, protecting, and warming. Disease is the result of disharmony or disruption of these functions.

BALANCING QI

TCM focuses on harmonizing and balancing Qi, and enhancing its flow throughout the body. If Qi is deficient, you tonify or strengthen it. If it is in excess in some place, you disperse it. If it is stagnant, you move it. If it is sinking, you uplift it. If it is rebellious, you rectify or calm it. Bodywork based in TCM uses manual techniques to tonify, disperse, move, uplift, and rectify Qi as needed to create harmony and balance.

Another goal of TCM is to harmonize the ease and flow of Qi along with the other fundamental substances: Shen or *Spirit,* Jing or *Essense,* Xue or *Blood,* and Jin/Ye or *Fluids.* Qi, Spirit, and Essence are known as the "Three Treasures" in Chinese medicine, and harmony among them is considered essential for good health.

The Five Elements

In TCM, the **Five Elements** or *Five Elemental Energies* are Wood, Fire, Earth, Metal, and Water. The Five Elements are a way of thinking about nature, human beings, and relationships among all natural phenomena. They are used in a metaphorical sense, and do not refer to the chemical elements found in Western science.

The Five Elements are used in TCM to explore the causes of imbalances that lead to poor health and disease. They have relationships to Yin and Yang, energy channels, and other TCM concepts. Table 19.1■ lays out some of these important relationships.

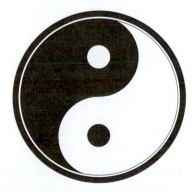

FIGURE 19.2

Yin/Yang in traditional Asian medicine.

TABLE 19.1 Attributes of Major Energy Channels According to Traditional Chinese Medicine

Energy Channel	Symbol	Yin/ Yang	Element	Acupoints*	Flow	Body Clock	Connects With
Lung	Lu	Yin	Metal	11 × 2	Chest to hand	3 A.M.–5 A.M.	LI
Large Intestine	LI	Yang	Metal	20 × 2	Hand to head	5 A.M.–7 A.M.	Lu
Stomach	St	Yang	Earth	45 × 2	Head to foot	7 A.M.–9 A.M.	Sp
Spleen	Sp	Yin	Earth	21 × 2	Foot to chest	9 A.M.–11 A.M.	St
Heart	Ht	Yin	Fire	9 × 2	Chest to hand	11 A.M.–1 P.M.	SI
Small Intestine	SI	Yang	Fire	19 × 2	Hand to head	1 P.M.–3 P.M.	Ht
Bladder	Bl	Yang	Water	67 × 2	Head to foot	3 P.M.–5 P.M.	Ki
Kidney	Ki	Yin	Water	27 × 2	Foot to chest	5 P.M.–7 P.M.	Bl
Pericardium	Pc	Yin	Fire	9 × 2	Chest to hand	7 P.M.–9 P.M.	TW
Triple Warmer	TW	Yang	Fire	23 × 2	Hand to head	9 P.M.–11 P.M.	Pc
Gallbladder	GB	Yang	Wood	44 × 2	Head to foot	11 P.M.–1 A.M.	Lv
Liver	Lv	Yin	Wood	14 × 2	Foot to chest	1 A.M.–3 A.M.	GB
Conception Vessel	CV	Yin		24 midline front		Anytime	6 Yin Primary Channels
Governing Vessel	GV	Yang		28 midline back		Anytime	6 Yang Primary Channels

* (x 2 = bilateral).

Wood Wood is a Yang element. Wood energy is expanding. The Wood element is evident in spring when seeds germinate and young plants push out of the ground. It is seen at sunrise, heard in shouting, and felt in anger. Wood is associated with green, wind, sour taste, and sight. Balanced Wood energy results in benevolence, discernment, and patience. Unbalanced Wood energy can lead to being argumentative, timid, rigid, or unable to make decisions.

Fire Fire is the most Yang element. Fire energy is fusing. The Fire element provides heat and light, and is evident in summer. It affects our ability to feel warm both physically and emotionally. The Fire element is associated with laughter, joy, sweat, and bitter taste. Fire affects a person's capacity for love, passion, self-realization, and confidence. Unbalanced Fire energy may appear as being guarded, vulnerable, controlling, or apathetic.

Earth Earth is a Yin element felt in late summer when the weather is humid and damp. Earth energy is moderating. It is felt in the change of seasons and has a transformative quality. Earth energy allows for being rooted, secure, and centered to flow with changes. Earth is heard in singing, tasted in sweet, and smelled in fragrant. Balanced Earth energy is displayed in integrity, altruism, and adaptability. Individuals with unbalanced Earth energy tend to be selfish, martyrs, self-sufficient or needy, stubborn, or wishy-washy.

Metal Metal is a Yin element felt most in autumn and associated with letting go. Metal energy is condensing. It is felt at dusk, in grief, and heard in crying. Metal has a pungent taste and rank smell. It is related to a sense of smell, dryness, and mucus. Individuals with balanced Metal energy

appear inspired, receptive, and discriminating. Unbalanced Metal energy can appear as vanity, anguish, zealotry, or despondency.

Water Water is the most Yin element and the most yielding. Water energy is conserving. The Water element is felt in the cold, dark, quiet winter, and at night. It is related to body fluids such as blood, sweat, tears, saliva, and urine. Water is associated with hearing, fear, the sound of groaning, rotten smell, and salty taste. Body parts influenced by Water energy are the bones, ears, kidneys, and bladder. Balanced Water energy manifests as wisdom, concentration, and contemplation. Imbalance in Water energy may appear as extreme recklessness, scattered attention, profound conservativeness, or physical or emotional isolation.

SHENG AND KO CYCLES

Relationships among the Five Elements are described in the Sheng and Ko cycles. In these cycles, each of the Five Elements is seen as supporting another and also as being controlled by another in a predictable pattern. These relationships are summarized in Figure 19.3■.

Sheng Cycle The Sheng cycle is also called the creation, generating, or promoting cycle. In the Sheng cycle, each Element supports the next. For example, Wood feeds Fire, which creates ash residue, which becomes Earth. Deep within the Earth, metals are developed that are then found in trace amounts in the Water that springs out from the ground. The waters nourish the trees or Wood and the cycle continues.

Ko Cycle The Ko cycle is also called the controlling or acting cycle. Each Element controls another and is also controlled by another Element. Metal, such as an ax, will control wood.

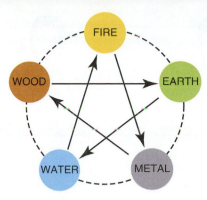

FIGURE 19.3
Sheng and Ko cycles.

Wood controls Earth, such as the trees covering the ground or the roots of trees holding the earth to prevent erosion. Earth can dam or channel Water. Water will control or extinguish Fire. Fire will melt the metal blade of the ax. The Ko cycle balances the Sheng cycle to avoid unrestrained growth.

Certain Elements, if especially strong, can either nourish or control another Element. If especially weak, it will fail to nourish or can be easily overcome. The balanced cyclic relationship of the Elements maintaining one another is considered to foster the healthiest life. The therapies of TCM, including bodywork and exercises like qi gong, aim to restore natural balance and equilibrium among the Five Elements.

Energy Channels

Qi travels through the body in a network of **energy channels** or meridians. Every part of the body is enlivened, nourished, and warmed by Qi flowing through this network. There are 12 primary energy channels, 8 extraordinary vessels, and various other channels. Two extraordinary vessels are especially important, the Conception Vessel (CV) and the Governing Vessel (GV). The paths of the 12 primary channels and the CV and GV vessels are traced in Figure 19.4■.

Each energy channel is named for a body organ it affects and is considered either Yin or Yang. Each is associated with one of the Five Elements. There are a number of acupoints or spots on the channel where Qi is more easily accessed. Each channel flows in a certain direction and connects and communicates with other channels. Important attributes of the 12 primary channels and 2 extraordinary vessels are summarized in Table 19.1

CHINESE BODY CLOCK

The channels flow through the body according to a natural, rhythmic cycle called the **Chinese body clock.** The day is divided roughly into 2-hour periods, and during that 2 hours, a certain primary channel is most active. During the next 2-hour period a different channel is most active—and so on throughout the day. For example, the Stomach channel is most active from 7 A.M.–9 A.M., followed by the Spleen channel from 9 A.M.–11 A.M., and the Heart channel from 11 A.M.–1 P.M. The channels cycle through their peak periods in a consistent pattern every day (see Table 19.1).

TCM practitioners use the knowledge of the location of channels, and the flow of Qi within them, to diagnose energy imbalances and to plan treatment. Also taken into consideration are the correspondences to Yin/Yang, the Five Elements, and location of acupoints.

Acupoints

Acupoints are places in the body where Qi collects and where it can be accessed and influenced. There are 365 classic acupoints located along the primary energy channels. In the ancient practice of acupuncture, acupoints are stimulated by inserting needles. Acupoints can also be stimulated by applying pressure, as in the manual therapies of acupressure and shiatsu.

Acupoints are designated by the name of the energy channel on which they are found and by a number, indicating their place in the sequence of points on that channel. For example, GB-20 is located on the Gall Bladder energy channel, and is the twentieth acupoint from the beginning of that channel. Each acupoint can also be located in reference to anatomical structures in the area. GB-20 is located in the suboccipital area in a recess between the sternocleidomastoid and trapezius muscles. Each acupoint also has a Chinese name. GB-20 is also known as *Fengchi* or Wind Pond. Refer to Figure 19.4 for the location of acupoints along the primary channels.

Acupoints are useful in the diagnosis and treatment of energy imbalances. Certain acupoints have been associated with treating specific ailments. Pressing GB-20 has been found to be effective for treating tension headaches, stiff neck or shoulders, dizziness, vertigo, and insomnia. Table 19.2■ lists some useful acupoints for common ailments.

However, it is important to remember that in TCM acupoints are not used as "pills" that treat disease. So pressing a point will not automatically cure an ailment or remove symptoms. Acupoints are treated as part of a broad approach that aims for harmony and balance in Yin/Yang, the Five Elements, and Qi. Acupoints are selected specifically to support a person's movement into greater balance.

KYO AND JITSU

Shiatsu, an Asian bodywork form from Japan, uses the concepts of Kyo and Jitsu to indicate acupoints (called *tsubos* in Japanese) and surrounding tissues with an imbalance of Ki (same as Qi). Kyo is energy deficiency and is felt in the tissues as a soft, hollow spot with no tone. Jitsu is energy excess and is felt in the tissues as hardness, resistance, or sensitivity. Areas of kyo and jitsu are treated differently with manual techniques.

When a kyo or deficient point is found, the practitioner presses into the spot and holds it for 7–10 seconds. The intention is to tonify or strengthen the area.

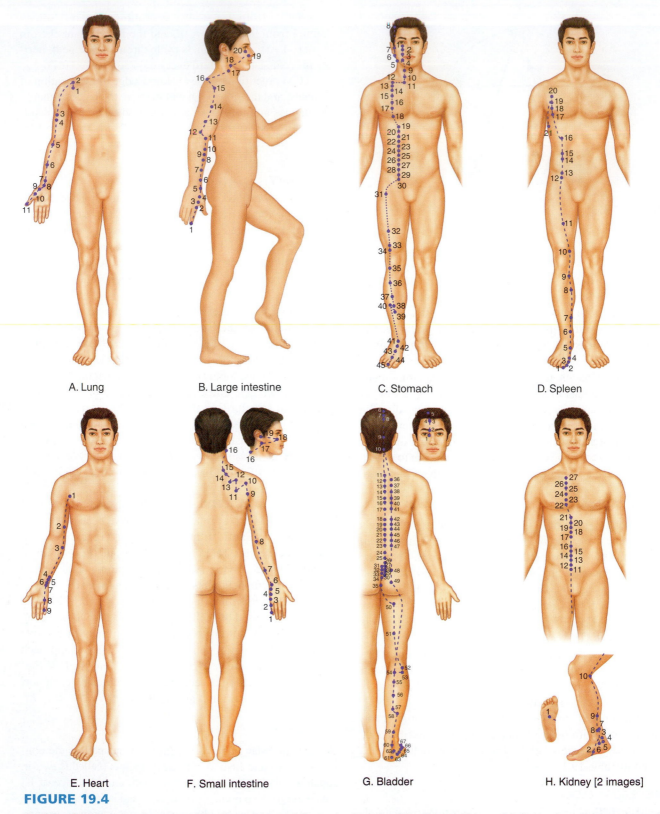

A. Lung

B. Large intestine

C. Stomach

D. Spleen

E. Heart

F. Small intestine

G. Bladder

H. Kidney [2 images]

FIGURE 19.4

Twelve primary energy channels and the Conception and Governing Vessels of Traditional Chinese Medicine. Acupoints are denoted by numbers along the energy channels.

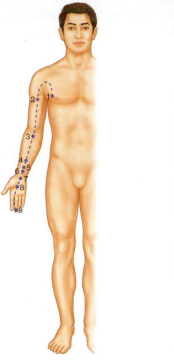

I. Pericardium

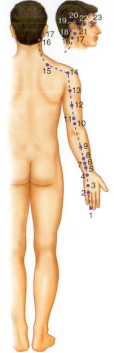

J. Triple warmer

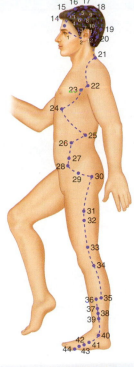

K. Gallbladder

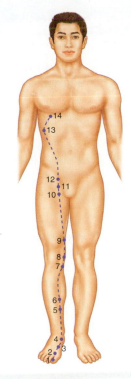

L. Liver

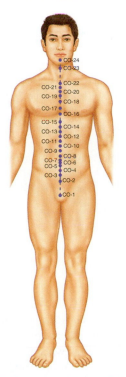

M. Conception Vessel (CV)

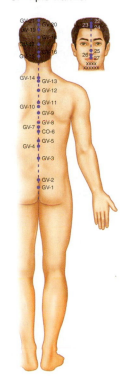

N. Governing Vessel (GV)

FIGURE 19.4

Continued

When an area of jitsu or excess is found, the spot is pressed for 3–5 seconds and then released. This is repeated about 10 times or until a change is felt. The intention is to disperse the excess energy and sedate the area.

Assessment and Treatment in TCM

A TCM practitioner uses various methods of assessment to locate energy imbalances and disharmony in Yin/Yang and the Five Elements. This is very different from diagnosis in Western medicine, which looks at organic disease processes.

The traditional pillars assessment are looking, touching, smelling, listening, and asking. For example, the TCM clinician observes a person's physical appearance, general demeanor, and movement. He or she looks at the condition of the hair and skin, and listens to the quality of the voice. The tongue is fully assessed, including its shape, color, and coating. Energy pulses on each hand are felt. This is different from the cardiovascular pulse. Clients are asked about their physical and emotional state. From this information, an assessment of imbalances is made.

In some forms of shiatsu, a *hara* diagnosis is conducted by feeling the abdominal area (roughly the area below the ribs and the sternum to just above the pubic bone). Diagnostic areas for each of the 12 primary meridians are found in this region. The practitioner palpates the abdomen to detect

TABLE 19.2   Useful Acupoints

Acupoint	Name	General Location	Indications
Lu-1	Central Treasury	Lateral chest, between ribs 1–2	Lung congestion, asthma
Lu-7	Broken Sequence	Lateral interior forearm, proximal to thumb	Common cold, asthma, stiff neck, dry throat and eyes, worry and sadness
LI-4	Tiger's Mouth	Dorsal side of thumb web	Frontal headache, toothache, hay fever symptoms, excessive sweating (contraindicated during pregnancy)
LI-11	Crooked Pond	Distal humerus on lateral side just above elbow crease	Sore throat, skin eruptions, hypertension, elbow pain
LI-15	Shoulder Bone	Depression in center of deltoid muscle when arm is raised	Shoulder pain and dysfunction
LI-20	Welcome Fragrance	Groove at lateral edge of nostril	Nasal congestion, nosebleed, sneezing, facial paralysis, facial tics
St-36	3 Mile Point	Just below lateral knee	Stomach pain, indigestion, vomiting, diarrhea, knee/wrist pan, postpartum dizziness, energy deficiency
St-40	Bountiful Bulge	Lower leg midway between knee and ankle and lateral to tibial crest	Upper respiratory congestion, asthma, heavy feeling, mental disturbance
Sp-6	Yin Intersection	Just above medial ankle bone on posterior edge of tibia	Abdominal pain, menstrual disorders, medial knee pain, diarrhea, sexual dysfunction, urination problems (contraindicated during pregnancy)
SI-3	Back Stream	Ulnar side of hand, just proximal to the fifth metacarpal head (little finger side)	Stiff neck, shoulders or back, occipital headache, weak spine, convulsions, lacking courage
Bl-10	Celestial Pillar	Suboccipital region lateral to cervical spine at hair line	Tension headache
Bl-40	Entrusting Middle	Back of knee in center at crease	Lower back pain, hip problems, abdominal pain, vomiting, diarrhea, burning urination
Bl-60	Kunlun Mountain	Depression between lateral ankle and Achilles tendon	Occipital headache, chronic stiff neck, shoulders or back, heel pain (contraindicated during pregnancy)
Pc-6	Inner Gate	Inner forearm above wrist crease	Nausea, vomiting, hiccups, chest pain, insomnia, agitation, nervousness
TW-5	Outer Gate	Back of forearm just above wrist	Fever and chills, headache, ear problems, red/swollen eyes, pain in ribs
GB-20	Wind Pond	Suboccipital region	Tension headache, stiff neck or shoulders, dizziness, vertigo, and insomnia
GB-21	Shoulder Well	Highest point on the shoulder	Tension headache, stiff shoulder (contraindicated during pregnancy)
GB-30	Jumping Round	Hip	Sciatica, lumbar pain, frustration
GB-34	Sunny Side of Mountain	Depression anterior and inferior to head of fibula	Numbness, weakness or pain in lower extremities, bitter taste in mouth, frequent sighing or irritability

meridians that are out of balance or show signs of kyo or jitsu. He or she then applies pressure to acupoints along those energy meridians to correct imbalances found.

TREATMENT OF ENERGY IMBALANCES

Treatment of energy imbalances in TCM can take several forms. Acupuncture with thin needles inserted at acupoints is perhaps the most recognizable treatment. Different Asian bodywork therapies (ABT) are also familiar in the West. These include tuina and acupressure from China, and amma and shiatsu from Japan. Tuina and amma are more massage-like, while acupressure and shiatsu rely on direct pressure to acupoints.

Other common TCM treatments are Chinese herbs, *moxibustion* (burning mugwort), and *guasha* (scraping the skin). Moxibustion warms the vessels when there are symptoms of cold, and guasha moves Qi and Blood when there is stagnation. Qi gong, a form of active exercise, is also used to stimulate and balance Qi. Qi gong is performed for prevention, as well as treatment of energy imbalances, and is discussed further in a later section of this chapter.

Acupuncture is a licensed profession in many states. Asian bodywork practitioners may also need state licenses. This differs from state to state. TCM practitioners are certified through the National Certification Commission for Acupuncture and Oriental Medicine (NCCAOM).

ACUPRESSURE MASSAGE INTEGRATION

Massage therapists can integrate principles and techniques of acupressure with standard Western massage to address both the physical and energetic wellness of their clients. **Acupressure massage integration (AMI)** utilizes the massage therapist's knowledge of Western anatomy, energy pathways, and location of key acupoints. In an AMI session, both Western massage techniques and ABT finger pressure techniques are applied systematically for their wellness effects.

The intent of AMI is to balance the body's vital energy (Qi) overall, release tension, and improve circulation. Acupressure techniques can tonify areas of Qi deficiency and disperse excess Qi that is pooling in one place. Stimulating specific acupoints restores Qi, strengthens weaknesses, relieves common ailments, and prevents health problems.

Acupressure massage integration combines some of the theory and techniques of Chinese massage with Western massage techniques. It uses Western massage style manipulations to balance the free flow of Qi in the body.

Basic AMI Approach

The basic approach in acupressure massage integration is to apply massage techniques region by region along major energy pathways, feeling for signs of deficiency (kyo) or excess (jitsu), and pressing important acupoints. When areas needing attention are found, appropriate techniques are performed to restore energy balance and flow.

When integrating acupressure and massage, practitioners are aware of both the physical condition of the musculature and signs of energy balance or imbalance. Manual techniques are applied to the body's soft tissues along classic energy pathways and to key acupoints.

Practitioners aim for certain effects when applying techniques. Keeping your intention in mind during AMI guides the energy as needed. Your intention may be to increase energy flow generally in energy channels, to stimulate key acupoints, or to address specific areas of energy deficiency or excess. It is an important principle that energy follows intention.

AMI uses a combination of classic Western massage and Asian bodywork techniques. Effleurage or sliding techniques are used to spread oil or lotion. When applying effleurage, especially over energy pathways, palpate for areas of deficiency (kyo) or excess (jitsu). Petrissage or lifting and pressing techniques influence energy flow in broad areas. Cross-tissue and circular fiber applied with the fingertips or knuckles addresses smaller areas with more specificity.

The thumb or elbow is used to apply pressure to key acupoints. When areas of energy deficiency or excess are found, pressure is applied to the points to re-establish the free and harmonious flow of energy. The discussion of kyo and jitsu earlier in this chapter describes the difference in treating an area of deficiency and an area of excess.

Any number of massage technique variations may be effective for AMI. Rather than following a precise protocol, it is more important to keep in mind the intent of the techniques, and choose those that will accomplish your goals. It is also essential in AMI to apply techniques specifically to energy pathways and acupoints.

Principles for Applying Pressure to Acupoints

There are four general principles for applying direct pressure to acupoints. These are (1) weight transfer, (2) stacking the joints, (3) perpendicularity, and (4) good back and neck alignment.

Weight Transfer In acupressure applications, weight transfer refers to applying pressure by shifting the body weight into the point of contact rather than pushing from the shoulders and arms. Pressure through weight transfer has a more comfortable feel to the receiver than that created by tensing the arm and hand muscles. Weight transfer performed using the whole body ensures that the connection between the giver and the receiver involves the entire person.

PRACTICAL APPLICATION

Use a washable marker to trace the primary energy channels of Traditional Chinese Medicine on a practice partner. Locate the useful acupoints described in Table 19.2.

1. Where does each channel begin and end?
2. What path does each channel take as it flows through the body?
3. What anatomical landmarks help you locate specific acupoints?

Stacking the Joints Applying pressure through the joints from bone to bone is called stacking the joints. For example, in applying thumb pressure, the thumb's joints are stacked in line with the wrist, elbow, and shoulder joints. This way the bones absorb much of the force of pressure rather than the joints themselves. When pressure is applied across a joint at an angle, or if the joint is bent, the joint structures and surrounding muscles are stressed. This can cause damage if repeated over time. Correct alignment for stacking the joints to apply thumb pressure is illustrated in Figure 19.5■.

Perpendicularity Applying pressure straight into an acupoint at a 90 degree angle, called perpendicularity, achieves maximum effect. If the line of application is less than or more than 90 degrees, the skin usually slips in one direction or another, lessening the pressure applied to the point itself. This has been likened to trying to pour water into a vase with a narrow neck. Unless you pour the water from directly overhead, some of the water will spill out.

Good Back and Neck Alignment Along with the other three principles, good body alignment ensures that back and neck muscles are not stressed when applying techniques. It is particularly important not to bend from the waist or let the head drop forward.

AMI Practice Sequence for the Back

The principles of acupressure massage integration can be practiced on the back. In this instance, focus is on the Inner and Outer Bladder meridian (Bl), the Gall Bladder meridian (GB), and acupoints Bl-10, GB-20, GB-21, and GB-30. Before practicing, take time to review the flow of these channels and the location of these specific acupoints.

It is common for forms of Asian bodywork to be given on a mat on the floor. This is how it would have been done

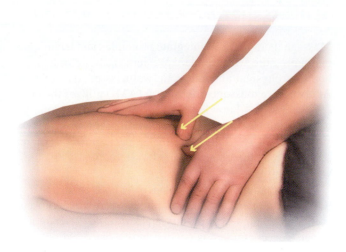

FIGURE 19.5

Correct alignment for stacking the joints to apply thumb pressure to acupoints.

in Asian countries. Acupressure massage integration can be easily adapted for a recipient lying on a massage table. The table is set lower than for Western massage to make it easier to maintain good body mechanics when applying direct pressure into acupoints.

A short practice sequence for acupressure massage of the back is presented here. The sequence offers some ideas for addressing major meridians and acupoints on the back. Western massage techniques can be added for warming, smooth transitions, and finishing as desired. The important point is to be conscious of meridian and acupoint locations and to work with the intention to balance energy, as well as to address areas of kyo and jitsu.

PRACTICE SEQUENCE 19.1

AMI for the Back

20 minutes
Recipient prone

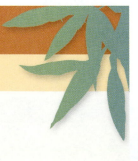

Preliminary Considerations:
• Adjust table height for good body mechanics.
• Screen the recipient for contraindications.
• Position the recipient comfortably in the prone position and undrape the back.

Primary Energy Meridians Affected:
• Bladder—Inner and Outer (Bl)
• Gall Bladder (GB)

Key Acupoints: Bl-10, GB-20, GB-21, GB-30

FIGURE 19.6 Effleurage to the entire back to apply oil. Stand at the side of the table near the recipient's hips to apply oil to the back; feel for areas of kyo and jitsu.

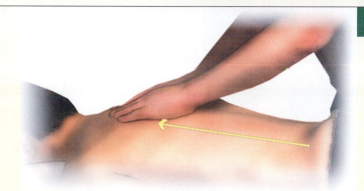

1

Perform Steps 2–10 on one side and then repeat on the other side.

FIGURE 19.7 Pull-ups to side of torso from iliac crest to shoulder. Slide palms up the side of the torso alternating hands while lifting the soft tissues. A. Cover the oblique abdominal muscles, slide fingers between the ribs. B. Pull up over the scapula and tops of the shoulders.

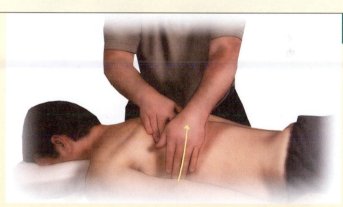

2

A

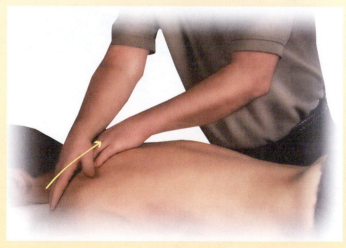

B

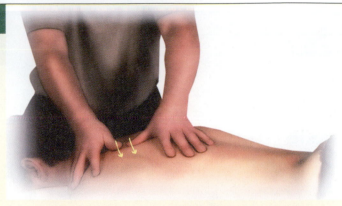

FIGURE 19.8 Thumb petrissage to the paraspinal muscles up the back from hip to shoulders. Use the thumbs to press into the soft tissues while sliding away from the spine; pressure on Inner then Outer Bladder Meridians; focus on upper back between spine and medial border of scapula. Transition to low back.

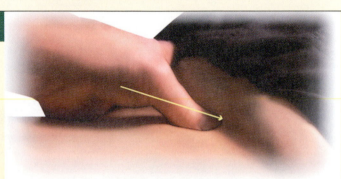

A

FIGURE 19.9 A. Thumb press the sacral notches. B. Press with fingertips into GB-30; press 2–3 times.

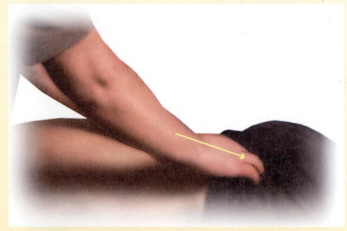

B

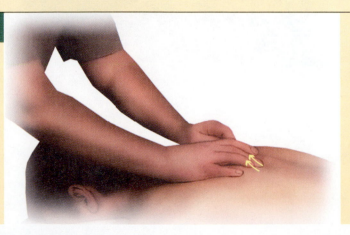

FIGURE 19.10 Fingertips knead along paraspinal muscles from the sacrum to the top of the shoulder; one hand on the Inner Bladder Meridian and the other on the Outer Bladder Meridian. Take note of tightness in different areas of the back.

6

FIGURE 19.11 A. Thumb press across top of shoulder. B. Press GB-21 repeatedly to disperse energy; massage the top of the shoulder.

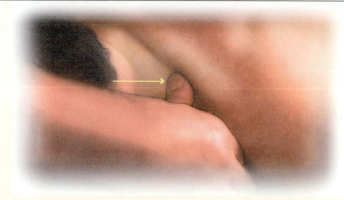

A

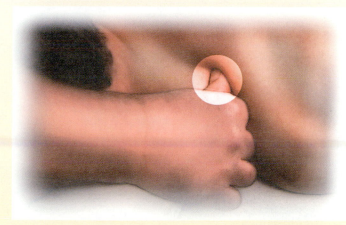

B

7

FIGURE 19.12 Thumb press Inner and Outer Bladder Meridians in upper back between shoulder blades; press into areas of kyo or excess found there.

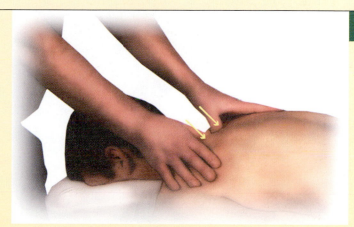

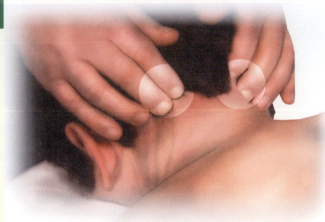

FIGURE 19.13 Press with fingertips into Bl-10 and GB-20 at the base of the skull; press individually and then with fingertips to all points along the occipital ridge at the same time.

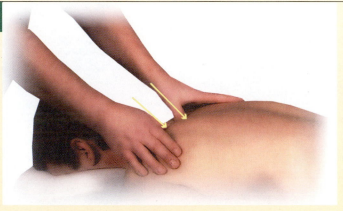

FIGURE 19.14 A. Thumb presses between shoulder blades on Inner and Outer Bladder Meridian acupoints. B. Apply friction to areas of muscle tightness.

A

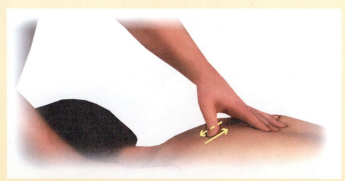

B

10

FIGURE 19.15 Stripping effleurage to shoulder as smoothing and transition technique. Apply with thumbs sliding away from each other.

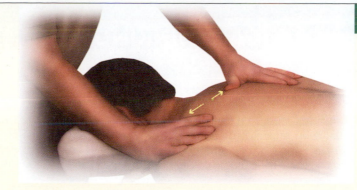

Finish the sequence with Steps 11–12 applied bilaterally to the back.

11

FIGURE 19.16 Rhythmic sliding compression down both sides of the spine, with palmar friction back up to shoulders.

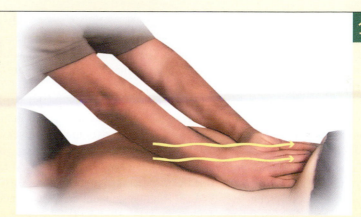

12

FIGURE 19.17 Superficial friction with palms along back. Hands are perpendicular to the spine; apply friction with palms shifting hands back and forth as they move first down the spine to the hips and back up to the shoulders.

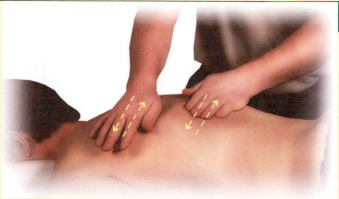

After you perform the Practice Sequence, evaluate how well you did by filling out Performance Evaluation Form 19.1, AMI for the Back. The form can be found in Appendix F, Performance Evaluation Forms on page A-40 and on your DVD.

CRITICAL THINKING

Think about the theoretical foundations for different forms of Eastern bodywork, especially concepts related to energy, energy channels, and special points. Analyze how these theories are applied in traditional bodywork of different parts of Asia: China, India, and Thailand.

1. How does each of these theories explain the intent of body-work sessions?

2. What manual techniques were developed to address health goals?
3. How would you describe what is common in these systems? What is unique in each system?

QI GONG

Qi gong means *energy exercise* in Chinese. The overall objective of these ancient exercises is to stimulate the healthy and balanced flow of Qi in the body. Practiced regularly, qi gong aims to prevent illness, improve health, and promote longevity.

Qi gong is also a body-mind practice that develops coordination, body awareness, and concentration. It focuses the mind and coordinates posture, breathing, and movement. Performed regularly, qi gong improves overall well-being and can be a valuable self-care practice for massage practitioners (see the Qi Gong Twenty Form Routine segment on your DVD). It is a useful supplement to Asian Bodywork Therapy since it has the same goal, that is, to improve the flow of Qi in the body's energy channels.

Two examples of simple qi gong forms from the Dao Yin Shen Gong style illustrate basic qi gong principles. They are Gliding Phoenix and Spring for the Crane and Deer. See Figures 19.18■ and 19.19■.

Qi Gong Forms

Qi gong exercises consist of a variety of choreographed movements that involve bending, stretching, reaching, stepping, and other movements designed to harmonize the flow of Qi. Each movement, sometimes referred to as a form, has its own benefits. Different forms are strung together for a continuous flow of movement. Qi gong is often performed to music to pace the movements and inspire a gentle, flowing quality. The slow and fluid movements of qi gong bring the mind into a meditative state for rejuvenation and relaxation.

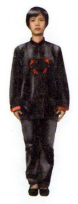
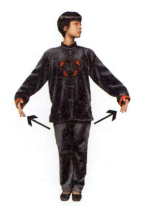
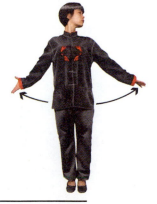
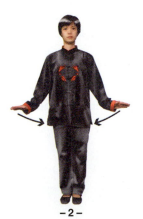
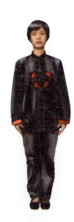

—— 1 ——   – 2 –

FIGURE 19.18

Gliding Phoenix.

Beginning position: Legs straight and together, arms at sides of body.

1. Rise up onto the balls of the feet keeping the legs naturally straight, and rotate your head to the left fully; raise arms to the sides at a 45 degree angle and rotate the arms externally to full extension, bringing scapulae towards the spine (inhale).
2. Lower your heels to the ground and lower arms to the side of the body naturally; return head to center (exhale).

Perform movements 1 and 2 to the right side. (Left and right = 1 cycle). Perform two breathing cycles.

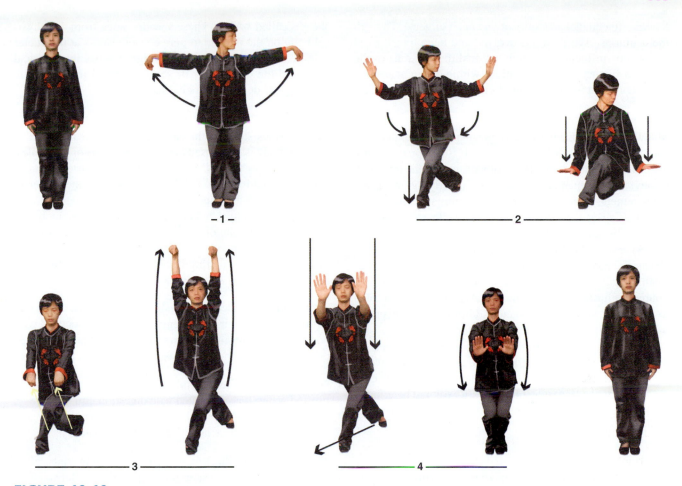

FIGURE 19.19

Spring for the Crane and Deer.

Beginning position: Legs straight and together, arms at sides of body.

1. Gradually raise arms to sides at shoulder height and flex wrists to press Tia Yuan, Da Ling and Shen Men points; hands should be hooked with thumb over index finger; rotate head left (inhale).
2. Step the right foot back crossed behind the left foot and bend the knees; elbows sink down and wrists flex; hands face forward; keep looking left. Lower the body and the hands; end in a squat looking left (exhale).
3. Gradually raise your body, straighten right leg behind left leg, keeping left leg bent softly; raise wrists and arms from front of body to sides of ears with hooked hands, thumb over index finger; extend arms to full extension (inhale).
4. Release tension and relax, softly lower arms and palms from front to sides of body; right foot returns to center. End with hands at sides and legs together (exhale).

Alternate left and right sides (one cycle). Perform two cycles.

Individual qi gong forms are designed to stimulate specific energy channels and acupoints. Some exercises also aim at specific therapeutic effects, for example, to improve range of motion in a certain area, or to improve function of a certain organ. Some have a more general effect on overall health.

BREATHING

Qi gong movements are coordinated with deep, even abdominal breathing. Breathing is through the nose and is gentle and quiet. Most upward and inward movements of the arms and head are done on the inhalation, while most downward and outward movements occur on the exhalation. The breath sets the pace for the rhythmic movement of qi gong, alternating in and out, up and down.

AYURVEDA

Ayurveda refers to the traditional health and healing practices of India. The term Ayurveda combines two Sanskrit words, *ayu* or life and *veda* or knowledge. Thus Ayurveda is knowledge of life, or more to the point, knowledge of the principles of living a long and healthy life. It is one of the oldest systems of health and healing in the world.

Ayurveda is said to have been passed down to mortals from Brahma the creator to the seers on earth, who started an oral tradition passed on from generation to generation. This knowledge has been written down through the ages, first in the ancient text of the *Rig Veda* (c.1700 BCE), and later in two treatises from about 1000 BCE called the *Charaka*

Samhita (medicine) and *Sushrut Samhita* (surgery). Through the centuries, Ayurdeva has evolved and been transformed by various influences, including Muslim invasions of the eleventh century, healing traditions within different areas of India, and most recently by modern science and technology.

Ayurvedic Health Practices

Many Ayurvedic practices focus on enhancing overall health and on prevention of illness and disease. Some practices aim toward increasing longevity. Another aspect is the treatment of physical and mental disorders. An underlying goal is the achievement of our full potential as human beings. Thus Ayurveda spans the entire scope of the wellness perspective and is holistic in nature.

Ayurvedic health practices include a vegetarian diet, cleansing and detoxifying the body, movements and postures (hatha yoga), breathing exercises, meditation, and massage. Sources of further information about Ayurveda can be located in Appendix H, References and Additional Resources, on page A-74.

Ayurveda is a complex philosophy of health and healing unique to India. A complete description of this philosophy is not within the scope of this text. However, a few basic concepts relevant to Ayurvedic massage are explored here. Table 19.3■ is a glossary of some basic terms used in Ayurveda.

The Physical Body—Koshas, Doshas, and Chakras

In Ayurveda, human beings are seen as having a material body, as well as subtle energy bodies that surround and move through the physical aspect. A person has five layers or sheaths called *koshas*. These sheaths range from the physical body on the outside to pure consciousness at the center (Figure 19.20■). Ayurvedic massage touches the physical body and the outer layer of subtle energy directly, while affecting the deeper layers indirectly.

PHYSICAL BODY—KOSHA 1

The outermost kosha is the *annamaya* or physical body. The physical body is composed of the three *doshas* or principles, seven *dhatus* or tissues, and three *malas* or waste products. These evolved from the five basic elements of the universe: earth, air, fire, water, and ether.

Within the physical body are 16 *srotas* or channels that allow for the circulation or movement of substances such as air, food, lymph, blood, urine, feces, sweat, and cellular level nutrients. Also circulating through the srotas are the three doshas called *Vata, Pitta,* and *Kapha.*

Vata   Vata, also called Vayu, is the wind principle, composed of the elements of air and ether or space. It is associated with bodily movement and the nervous system. Vata is located primarily in the pelvic and leg regions, and its seat is the colon.

Pitta   Pitta is the bile principle, composed of the elements of fire and water. It is associated with digestion, thirst, courage, and thinking. Pitta is located primarily in the abdominal region and in blood and skin, and its seat is the stomach.

Kapha   Kapha is the mucus principle, composed of the elements of earth and water. It is responsible for lubrication, and controls patience. Kapha is located primarily in the upper body, and its seat is the lungs.

TABLE 19.3	Glossary of Basic Ayurvedic Terms
Term	**Meaning**
Ayurveda	Knowledge of long and healthy life
Chakras	Seven energy centers: Root, Sacral, Solar Plexus, Heart, Throat, Third Eye, Crown
Dhatus	Types of tissues or fluids in the body: lymph, blood, muscle, bone, fat, marrow, and sexual fluids
Doshas	Three governing principles: Vata, Pitta, Kapha
Elements	Components of all matter: earth, air, fire, water, and ether
Koshas	Five body sheaths: Physical body, subtle energy, mind, intellect, bliss
Malas	Waste products of digestion: urine, feces, sweat
Marma point	Subtle junctions between consciousness and matter
Nadis	Energy channels for Prana flow
Prakriti	Constitution: Vata, Pitta, Kapha, Vata-Pitta, Pitta-Kapha, Vata-Kapha, Sama
Prana	Subtle energy
Shakti	Creative spiritual life force or love
Srotas	Sixteen circulatory channels in the body
	1–3 control flow of water, food and breath
	4–10 support major tissues of the body
	11–13 control waste removal
	14 carries thought from heart to mind
	15–16 carry menstrual fluid and lactate
Vayu	Subtle energy

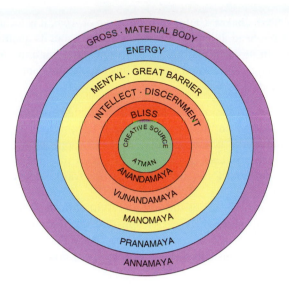

FIGURE 19.20

Five layers or sheaths called koshas in Ayurvedic philosophy.

TABLE 19.4	The Three Major Doshas—Basic Constitutional Types
Dosha	Characteristics
Vata	Thin frame, very tall or short, odd proportions, narrow hips and shoulders, dry skin and hair, cold hands and feet, high metabolism, quick, endurance poor, aversion to cold weather, tendency for irregular bowels, painful joints, acute allergies, and worry.
Pitta	Medium frame, medium height, proportionate, medium hips and shoulders, oily skin and hair, competitive, hot, fiery, endurance medium, aversion to hot weather, tendency for heartburn, skin rashes, inflammatory diseases, irritability.
Kapha	Large frame, solid build, broad hips and shoulders, easy going, low metabolism, endurance strong, hold weight and water, methodical, tendency for allergies and congestion, and resists change.

CONSTITUTIONAL TYPES

The proportion of the three doshas differs from person to person. A person's innate natural healthy dosha mix is his or her *prakriti* or body constitution. There are seven constitution types:

1. Vata
2. Pitta
3. Kapha
4. Vata-Pitta
5. Pitta-Kapha
6. Vata-Kapha
7. Sama

In the rare Sama constitutional type, the three doshas are found in equal proportion. The doshas are in dynamic relationship to each other. When they are in proper balance, the result is health. When they are imbalanced, there is dysfunction and disease. The main goal of Ayurvedic medicine and health practices is to maintain and restore balance according to an individual's unique constitutional makeup. Major characteristics of the three major constitutional types or prakriti are listed in Table 19.4■.

SUBLE ENERGY—KOSHA 2

The next kosha is the *pranamaya,* which regulates the flow of subtle energy in the body. It is in the pranamaya kosha that the *prana* or subtle energy (also known as the *ten vayus*) flows through nonphysical channels called *nadis.* Nadis lead to important energy centers called *chakras.*

There are seven chakras or concentrations of nadis at different levels of the spine and in the head. Chakra means wheel, and refers to the whirling centers of energy at each level. These centers receive, process, and distribute energy to balance the body, mind, and spirit. The chakras are arranged from gross (bottom, lower functions, physical) to subtle (top, higher functions, mind and awareness). See Figure 19.21■.

The First Chakra Called the Root Chakra or *Muladhara,* it is located at the base of the spine in the perineum. It is governed by the earth element, and its qualities are groundedness, patience, stability, and security. Essential oils associated with it are cinnamon, garlic, and sandalwood, and its herb is mugwort.

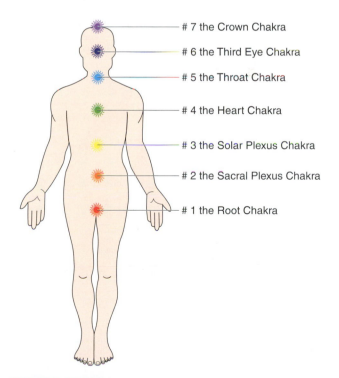

7 the Crown Chakra

6 the Third Eye Chakra

5 the Throat Chakra

4 the Heart Chakra

3 the Solar Plexus Chakra

2 the Sacral Plexus Chakra

1 the Root Chakra

FIGURE 19.21

The seven chakras or energy centers in Ayurvedic philosophy. Courtesy of Rev. Larissa Dahroug, Reiki/MT, Clear & Balanced Energy Work.

The Second Chakra Called the Sacral Chakra or *Svadhisthana*, it is located just below the naval and toward the center of the body. It is governed by the water element, and its qualities are well-being, sexuality, sensuality, pleasure, and abundance. It is the seat of the emotions. Associated essential oils are jasmine and orange blossom, and its herb is cedar.

The Third Chakra Called the Solar Plexus Chakra or *Manipura*, it is directly below the sternum at the solar plexus. It is governed by the fire element, and its qualities are self-worth, self-esteem, and confidence. Associated essential oils are lemon, grapefruit, and juniper, and its herb is rosemary.

The Fourth Chakra Called the Heart Chakra or *Anahata*, it is located in mid-chest. It is governed by the air element, and its qualities are love, peace, unity, purity, and innocence. Associated essential oils are rose, carnation, and lily of the valley, and its herb is lavender.

The Fifth Chakra Called the Throat Chakra or *Vishuddha*, it is located at the throat. It is governed by the ether element, and its qualities are communications, creativity, truthfulness, and integrity. Associated essential oils are chamomile and gardenia, and its herb is wintergreen.

The Sixth Chakra Called the Third Eye or *Ajna*, it is located mid-forehead. It is governed by awareness, and its qualities are intuition, discernment, wisdom, imagination, and knowledge. Associated essential oils are camphor and sweet pea, and its herb is sage.

The Seventh Chakra Called the Crown Chakra or *Sahasrar*, it is located on the top of the head. Its qualities are enlightenment, grace, beauty, serenity, and being one with the universe. Associated essential oils are violet, lavender, and lotus, and its herbs are frankincense and myrrh.

A major goal of the various Ayurvedic health practices is to move the creative spiritual life force or shakti from the Root Chakra to the Crown Chakra or twelve petal lotus. This completes the harmony of body, mind and spirit.

INNERMOST KOSHAS 3–5

Beyond the physical body and the first subtle energy sheath are the mental (*manomaya*), intellect and discernment (*nanamaya*), and the causal (*anandamaya*) sheaths. At the center of the five sheaths is pure consciousness.

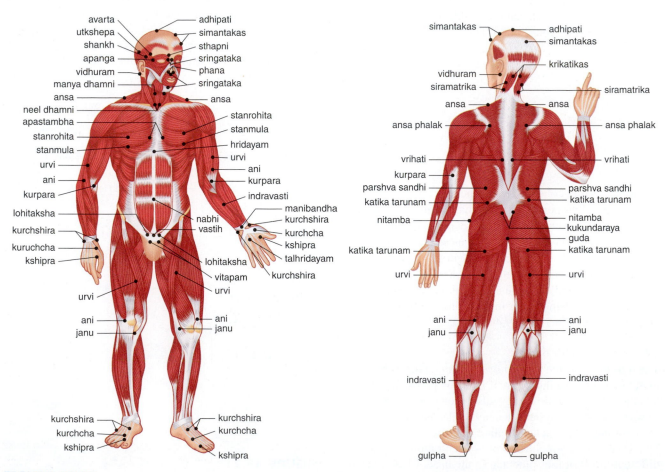

FIGURE 19.22

Major marma point locations.

REALITY CHECK

KELLY

GABRIEL: I have a hard time relating to theories of energy flow in Eastern bodywork. I don't feel energy when I touch people during massage sessions. How do I know anything worthwhile is happening when I practice Eastern bodywork?

KELLY: Those of us from Western cultures aren't as sensitive to the idea of energy as practitioners from Asian cultures. We don't have a concept of Qi, Prana, or life force that compares. Western thinking focuses more on the material aspects. When considering Eastern bodywork, I try to keep an open mind to what others have found over centuries of studying these practices. As far as feeling energy, I have tried to be more aware of energy in my hands as I work. I'm slowly developing a consciousness of its existence. But even if I don't feel energy flowing, I can see physical changes happening like clients relaxing, and muscles letting go of tension. So I can see the effects of these techniques on that level, and if I get the health benefits I'm going for, I don't feel a need to believe all of the theory to value the approach. On the other hand, it is interesting to hear about another culture's perspective. We all experience life so differently.

Marma Points

Marma points are Ayurvedic pressure points. They are considered part of the subtle body, and occur at the junction of the five organic principles of vessels, muscles, ligaments, bones, and joints. The 107 marma points are considered to be junctions between consciousness and matter. They are the locus of *prana* or the vital life force. See Figure 19.22■ for major marma point locations.

Marma points are addressed in different ways in different approaches to Ayurvedic massage. During a massage session, stimulation of marma points can be used to release tension in a congested area. Gentle circular stroking of a marma point with the index or middle finger results in the release of toxins from the area.

Systematic treatment of marma points is called *marma chikitsa*. Marma point therapy is considered a specialization requiring advanced training.

AYURVEDIC MASSAGE

The goal of Ayurvedic massage is to balance the physical and energetic processes that lead to a healthy vibrant life. It begins with attention to physical well-being, which in turn affects subtle energy, and ultimately spiritual consciousness.

The effects of massage in the physical body are familiar to Western massage therapists. These effects include good blood and lymph circulation, muscle relaxation, connective tissue pliability, overall tissue health, and general relaxation. When there is balance in the physical body, effects can occur at deeper levels.

Once balance in the physical body is restored, channels of circulation called *srotas* help to balance the three *doshas*—*Vata, Pitta,* and *Kapha.* At this point Ayurvedic massage begins to move the ten *vayus* or *pranas* that carry life force to both the physical and energetic bodies. Once the vayu function is optimal, the *nadi* system is activated. There are 72,000 nadis in the body that carry subtle energy. Specifically they carry consciousness to the *chakra* system and into the brain centers, where body, mind, and spirit are purified. The goal of this process is full human potential, whereby consciousness is lively in each and every cell. The subtle-body system and the physical body begin to function as one, resulting in perfect physical, mental, and spiritual health. (Douillard 2004, p.1)

Varieties of Ayurvedic Massage

Just as there are variations and specializations within Western massage, several varieties of Ayurvedic massage applications can be identified. These include *Garshana* or dry lymphatic skin brushing, *Abhyanga* or classic herbal oil massage, and *Vishesh* or deep muscular massage. *Udvartana* is an herbal paste and exfoliating lymphatic massage, while the Ayruvedic facial focuses on nourishing the skin and overall energetic balance. Ayurvedic massage is given as part of *panchakarma* or detoxification therapy supervised by an Ayurvedic physician. Two popular adjunct modalities are *Swedana* or herbal steam bath and *Shirodhara* or pouring herbal oil over the forehead.

Several modern spa offerings incorporate knowledge of Ayurvedic practices. These include aromatherapy, stone massage, medicated steam therapy, and various types of herbal showers and baths. Classic Ayurvedic massage is given with oils individualized to a client's prakriti or constitutional type.

Massage Oils

The composition of massage oils in classic Ayurvedic massage is very important. Massage oils are carefully chosen and mixed according to the recipient's constitutional type, the season of the year, and any therapeutic goals. Base oils typically used for Ayruvedic massage are sesame, coconut, almond, olive, mustard, or corn. Some modern blends use a jojoba base.

Essential oils are mixed into the base oil to achieve specific therapeutic goals, for example, relaxation, warming, moisturizing the skin, or relieving congestion. Essential oils are highly concentrated liquids distilled from plant materials such as grasses, leaves, flowers, needles, fruit peels, and roots. They contain volatile aromatic compounds, that is, the distinct scent and essence of the plant. Essential oils are potent. They are used sparingly, and are measured by numbers of drops. They should never be applied to the skin in undiluted form. Be aware of the properties of each essential oil to be put into a mixture.

Some common Ayurvedic oil blends can be purchased premade. For example, a blend especially for relaxation might include a base oil with lavender, rosewood, champa, and tangerine essential oils. A blend for energizing massage might include a base oil with mint, lavender, orange, bergamot, and lime essential oils. Ideally massage oil mixtures are heated and applied warm. This ensures deeper penetration and feels soothing.

Essential oils are the focus of the science and art of aromatherapy. Consult aromatherapy or Ayurvedic references for further information about specific essential oils and their uses. Study essential oils to determine their safe use in different circumstances, and be especially careful during pregnancy. See page 504 in Chapter 17, Spa Applications, for more information about essential oils.

Massage Applications

Ayurvedic techniques for oil massage include sliding or rubbing, kneading, squeezing, and tapping. Rubbing with oil is performed with a flat palm molding to the contour of the body. Fingertips can be used to apply circles in small areas and around joints. Kneading relaxes muscles and resembles kneading bread dough. Squeezing or wringing is performed on the limbs moving proximal to distal. Tapping is applied

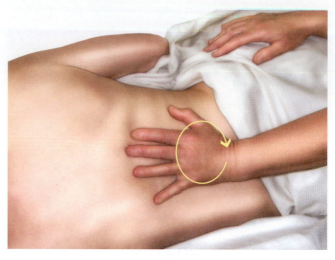

FIGURE 19.24

Ayurvedic massage. Sliding circles at the seat of Vata, recipient in side-lying position.

with cupped hands and is used to activate the nervous system. Fingers and thumbs can be used to stimulate specific points and in small areas.

Ayurvedic massage techniques themselves are familiar to Western massage therapists, but the intent of the application would be quite different. See Figures 19.23■, 19.24■, and 19.25■.

Pressure may vary according to a recipient's constitutional type. Vata types tend to prefer lighter pressure, Pitta types medium pressure, and Kapha types heavier pressure.

Different traditions of Ayurvedic massage apply techniques in different parts of the body in their own unique way.

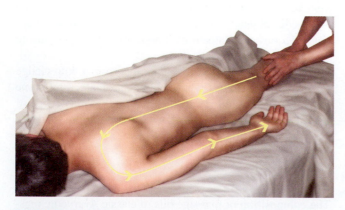

FIGURE 19.23

Ayurvedic massage. Long sweeping stroke from foot around shoulder and down the arm, recipient prone.

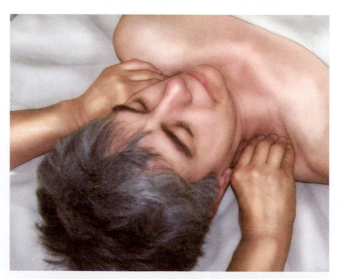

FIGURE 19.25

Ayurvedic massage. Pressing the ansa marma on the front and back of the shoulders with recipient supine.

CASE FOR STUDY

Paul Applies Eastern Bodywork to Enhance a Massage Session

Paul has a client named Don who is experiencing tension in his legs and feet. The Western massage Paul is using has some relaxing effects, but he feels he can get better results by integrating some Eastern bodywork techniques in the sessions. As a martial artist, Don is open to the idea and gives Paul permission to use Eastern bodywork techniques for a few sessions to see the results.

Question:

How might Paul approach integrating Eastern bodywork for the desired effects?

Things to consider:

- What energy channels run through the hips, legs, and feet?

- Where are special points located there?
- What Eastern bodywork techniques can be adapted for an integrated bodywork session?
- Of what importance is intention to the application?

Plan a massage therapy session incorporating Eastern bodywork theory and techniques for addressing Don's therapeutic goals. Describe a possible approach, being specific about concepts and techniques.

_____

_____

_____

One approach to full-body Ayurvedic massage moves from region to region in a systematic sequence. Starting on the back of the body, the lower limbs are massaged from pelvis to toes, then the spine from sacrum to neck, and then the upper limbs from shoulder to fingers. On the front of the body, massage is applied from pelvis to toes, navel to chest, and then collarbone to fingertips.

Some Ayurvedic massage sessions routinely include massage in the side-lying position. The client might start prone, turn to one side, turn to the other side, and end supine. Ayurvedic head and face massage has its own special application.

In another approach called _marma point massage,_ strokes are applied in sequence, with special attention to important marma points. If congestion is felt at a marma point, additional techniques are applied to move energy at that point.

Seasonal massage sessions focus on special needs during each of the four seasons. An example is a Vata balancing massage given in winter. Essential oils would be chosen to balance the dry sluggishness of winter months. For a Pitta constitutional type, these might include bergamot, cypress, geranium, lemongrass, and mogra or Indian jasmine. For other constitutional types the mix might be different.

Ayurvedic massage sessions are typically preceded by a brief interview to determine constitutional type, contraindications including skin allergies, and a recipient's specific goals for the massage. Client preferences are also taken into consideration.

HATHA YOGA

Yoga literally means "joining," and refers to various practices that aim to reunite an individual to pure consciousness. Yoga in its totality is essentially a spiritual practice; however, one aspect called **hatha yoga** has gained popularity in the West as a health and fitness exercise. Hatha yoga is an excellent complement to Ayurvedic massage and a beneficial self-care practice for massage therapists.

Five important aspects of hatha yoga are relaxation, physical exercises or postures called _asanas,_ proper breathing, proper diet, and positive thinking and meditation. The postures are exercises in mind-body coordination and also build strength and flexibility while calming the mind.

A basic relaxation posture is _Savasana_ or the corpse pose. Lie on your back on a mat with your feet apart and arms comfortably away from the body, palms upwards. Close your eyes and take several deep abdominal breaths (Figure 19.26■). Let your mind grow calm and clear.

The Sun Salutation or _Surya Namaskar_ is a good beginning series of postures that can be used later as a warm-up to more difficult postures. It is traditionally performed at dawn, but can be used at any time for limbering and waking up. It begins in a standing position, followed by continuous movement from one posture to the next (Figure 19.27■).

Hatha yoga postures are performed on floor mats from standing, sitting, and lying positions. Traditional postures

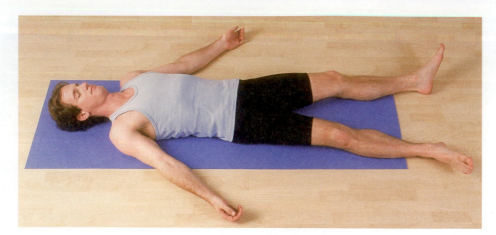

FIGURE 19.26

Hatha yoga corpse pose—savasana.

have varying degrees of difficulty and can be modified for all abilities and ages.

THAI MASSAGE

Traditional bodywork from Thailand is called *nuad boran,* known in the West as **Thai massage.** It has been practiced in Thailand for centuries, passed down through different lineages. It is thought to have come to Thailand originally from India along with Buddhism. Thai massage has become a popular form of bodywork in the West in recent years. The intent is to stimulate the body's self-healing processes and to correct energy imbalances.

Thai massage is based on Ayurvedic medicine. It incorporates knowledge of energy meridians or *sen* lines, pressure points, and hatha yoga postures. It is performed on the floor on a mat. Both giver and receiver are clothed, and no oil is applied. It can be thought of as a combination of pressure techniques, joint mobilizations, and assisted yogalike stretching.

Sen lines are similar to nadis in the Ayurvedic tradition. They also have similar names, for example, *Sen Pingala* is the same as the *Pingala Nadi.* Sen lines are pathways that carry subtle energy. Many pressure points along sen lines are identical with marma points. The exact location of sen lines varies among different lineages of Thai massage. See Figure 19.28■ for an example of a sen line diagram. These diagrams are found on many Buddhist temple walls, such as the famous Wat Po Temple in Bangkok, where the tradition of Thai massage is preserved.

Thai massage sessions typically begin at the feet and move toward the head. The practitioner uses the palms, fingers, thumbs, forearm, and elbow to apply pressure along sen lines and to pressure points. Joint mobilizations and assisted yogalike stretches are interspersed. The session is systematic and flowing from one region to the next. Figures 19.29■ to 19.31■ are examples of Thai massage techniques.

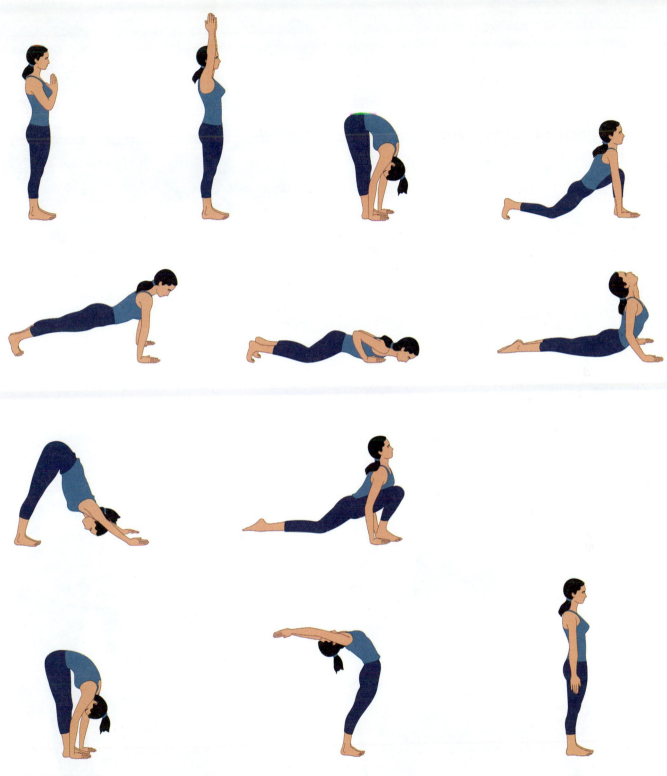

FIGURE 19.27
Hatha yoga Sun Salutation.

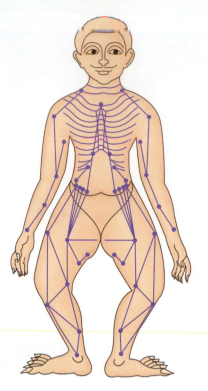

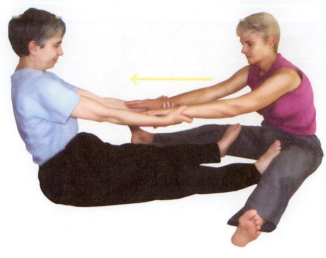

FIGURE 19.30

Wide angle pose (upavistha konasana in hatha yoga), assisted by practitioner on the left during Thai massage session.

FIGURE 19.28

Sen lines in traditional Thai massage.

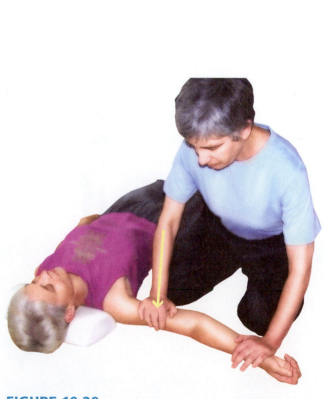

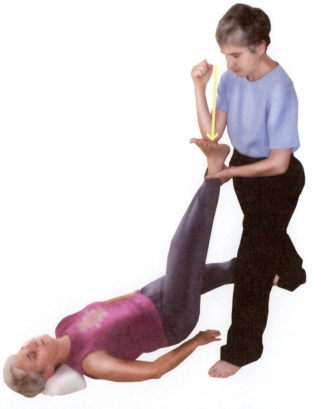

FIGURE 19.31

Reclining hand to foot pose variation (sputa padangushtasana in hatha yoga), and elbow press to marma points on the foot bottom during Thai massage session.

FIGURE 19.29

Press along sen lines and marma points on inner forearm.

CHAPTER HIGHLIGHTS

- Eastern bodywork refers to traditional forms of manual therapy from the continent of Asia.
- Three popular forms of Eastern bodywork are Asian bodywork therapies from China and Japan, Ayurvedic massage from India, and Thai bodywork from Thailand.
  - Their applications and theory are very different from Western massage.
  - They predate modern science and are embedded in whole systems of medicine.
- Similarities in Eastern bodywork forms: holistic view, human beings as part of nature, notion of energy or life force.
- These Eastern manual therapies are used to balance energy and remove obstructions to its free flow in and around the physical body.
- Traditional Chinese medicine originated in China as folk medicine and later evolved into a formalized system of medicine.
  - Earliest known text on TCM is the *Yellow Emperor's Classic of Internal Medicine* written about 500 BCE.
- Yin/Yang symbol has been described as two comets chasing each other.
  - Yin is a dark, deep, dense aspect of the universe; feminine, interior, still, substantial, cool, and contracting in contrast to Yang; the front, interior, medial/interior aspects of the limbs; solid organs that store pure essences extracted from food by the Yang organs.
  - Yang is a light, energetic, and spacious or heavenly aspect of the universe; masculine, exterior, moving, insubstantial, warm and expanding in contrast to Yin; the back, head, exterior, and lateral/posterior aspects of the limbs; hollow organs that transform, digest, and excrete impure products of food and fluids.
  - Five principles of Yin/Yang: interdependence, supporting, opposition, intertransformation, infinitely divisible.
- Qi refers to the life energy of the universe.
  - Chinese character for Qi depicts rice cooking in a pot with steam escaping.
  - TCM harmonizes and balances Qi, and enhances its flow throughout the body.
  - TCM tonifies, disperses, moves, uplifts, and rectifies Qi.
- The Five Elements or *Five Elemental Energies* are Wood, Fire, Earth, Metal, and Water.
  - Wood is Yang, expanding, spring, sunrise, green, wind, and sour taste.
  - Fire is most Yang, fusing, heat, light, summer; laughter, sweat, bitter taste.
  - Earth is Yin, late summer, transformative, rooted, sweet, fragrant.
  - Metal is Yin, autumn, letting go, grief, pungent, dry.
  - Water is most Yin, winter, yielding, conserving, fear, wisdom, salty.
- Sheng and Ko cycles describe relationships among the Five Elements.
  - Sheng is the creation, generating, or promoting cycle.
  - Ko cycle is the controlling or acting cycle.
- Qi travels through the body in a network of energy channels or meridians.
  - There are 12 primary energy channels.
  - Each channel flows in a certain direction, and connects and communicates with other channels.
  - The channels flow through the body according to a natural, daily rhythmic cycle called the Chinese body clock.
- Acupoints are places on energy channels where Qi collects and where it can be accessed and influenced.
  - There are 365 classic acupoints.
  - Acupoints are useful in the diagnosis and treatment of energy imbalances.
- In Japanese shiatsu, the concepts of Kyo and Jitsu indicate acupoints with imbalance of Ki (same as Qi).
  - Kyo means energy deficiency; kyo acupoints feel hollow and soft; kyo acupoints are pressed for 7–10 seconds to tonify them.
  - Jitsu means energy excess; jitsu acupoints feel hard and sensitive; jitsu acupoints are pressed for 3–5 seconds, released, and that press-release repeated about 10 times.
- The traditional pillars assessment in TCM are looking, touching, smelling, listening, and asking.
- Massage can be integrated with the theory and techniques of acupressure to address both the physical and energetic wellness of their clients.
- Acupressure massage integration applies massage techniques region by region along major energy pathways, feeling for signs of deficiency (kyo) or excess (jitsu), and pressing important acupoints; energy balance is restored in areas of kyo and jitsu.
- Qi gong consists of choreographed movements that involve bending, stretching, reaching, stepping, and other movements designed to harmonize the flow of Qi.
- Ayurveda means knowledge of life and is the traditional health and healing practices of India.
- In Ayurvedic theory, human beings are seen as having a material body, as well as subtle energy

bodies that surround and move through the physical aspect.

- The physical body has 16 channels or *srotas* for the circulation of substances such as air, food, lymph, blood, urine, feces, sweat, and cellular level nutrients, and the three principles or *doshas* called Vata, Pitta, and Kapha.
- A person's innate natural healthy dosha mix is his or her body constitution or *prakriti*.
  - ○ Seven constitution types: Vata, Pitta, Kapha, Vata-Pitta, Pitta-Kapha, Vata-Kapha, and Sama.
- Energy centers called *chakras* receive, process, and distribute energy to balance body, mind, and spirit.
  - ○ Chakras from bottom to top (gross to subtle) are Root, Sacral, Solar Plexus, Heart, Throat, Third Eye, and Crown Chakras.
- A major goal of the various Ayurvedic health practices is to move the creative spiritual life force or *shakti*

from the Root Chakra to the Crown Chakra or twelve petal lotus.

- Marma points are Ayurvedic pressure points; the junctions between consciousness and matter.
- In classic Ayurvedic massage, oils are carefully chosen and mixed according to the recipient's constitutional type, the season of the year, and any therapeutic goals.
  - ○ Ayurvedic techniques for oil massage include sliding or rubbing, kneading, squeezing, and tapping.
- Hatha yoga is an Ayurvedic health practice consisting of relaxation, physical exercises or postures called *asanas,* proper breathing, proper diet, and positive thinking and meditation.
- Thai massage is a combination of pressure techniques, joint mobilizations, and assisted yogalike stretching; both giver and receiver are clothed.

EXAM REVIEW

Key Terms

Match the following key terms to their descriptions. For additional study, look up the key terms in the Interactive Glossary on page G-1 and note other terms that compare or contrast with them.

_____ **1.** Acupoints
_____ **2.** Acupressure
_____ **3.** Ayurveda
_____ **4.** Chinese body clock
_____ **5.** Eastern bodywork
_____ **6.** Energy channels
_____ **7.** Five Elements
_____ **8.** Hatha yoga
_____ **9.** Qi
_____ **10.** Thai massage
_____ **11.** Traditional Chinese medicine (TCM)
_____ **12.** Yin and Yang

a. Manual therapies from Asia
b. Life force or energy
c. Way of thinking about relationships among natural phenomena
d. Pressure, joint movements, and assisted yoga
e. Ayurvedic health practice consisting of relaxation, postures called *asanas,* and meditation
f. Points where Qi is easily accessed
g. Healing practices from ancient China
h. Natural, daily, rhythmic cycle of Qi flow
i. Illustrates the relatedness and interconnectedness of all
j. Pressure applied to acupoints to balance energy
k. Pathways for Qi flow
l. Traditional healing from India

Memory Workout

To test your memory of the main concepts in this chapter, complete the following sentences by circling the most correct answer from the two choices provided.

1. An overarching similarity in forms of Eastern bodywork is a (holistic) (mechanistic) perspective, and some notion of (fluid) (energy) that flows throughout the physical body.
2. (Yin) (Yang) is the light, energetic, and spacious or heavenly aspect of the universe.
3. In TCM, if Qi is stagnant, you (move) (uplift) it.
4. In Shiatsu, (kyo) (jitsu) is a point of energy deficiency.
5. Pressure is most effectively applied to an acupoint at a (45) (90) degree angle.
6. In qi gong, most downward and outward movements occur on the (inhalation) (exhalation).
7. In Ayruvedic theory, medium frame and height, aversion to hot weather, and tendency to inflammatory diseases describes the (Pitta) (Kapha) constitutional type.
8. The goal of Ayurvedic health practices is to move the creative spiritual life force or shakti from the (Root) (Sacral) Chakra to the (Crown) (Third Eye) Chakra.
9. In Ayurveda, the (vata) (marma) points are considered to be the locus of the vital life force or prana.
10. Traditional Thai massage is based in principles of (Chinese medicine) (Ayurveda).

Test Prep

The following multiple-choice questions will help to prepare you for future school and professional exams.

1. Which principle of Yin/Yang reminds us that these are relative concepts that cannot exist in isolation?
   a. Infinite divisibility
   b. Mutual supporting
   c. Interdependence
   d. Intertransformation
2. Qi dispersed becomes:
   a. Energy, sunshine, the movement of the wind
   b. Material, rocks, trees, rain drops, human beings
   c. Wood, fire, earth, metal, water
   d. Kyo and jitsu
3. The Yin element felt in late summer and in the change of seasons, and that has a transformative quality, is:
   a. Water
   b. Earth
   c. Wood
   d. Metal
4. Wood feeds Fire, which creates ash residue, which becomes Earth, is an example of the:
   a. Qi cycle
   b. Body clock cycle
   c. Sheng cycle
   d. Ko cycle
5. Tiger's mouth, or LI-4 acupoint, is found on the:
   a. Inside ankle
   b. Dorsal thumb web
   c. Side of the nose
   d. Top of the shoulder
6. The energy channel that runs down the posterior body in double rows on the back is the:
   a. Lung channel
   b. Bladder channel
   c. Large Intestine channel
   d. Gall Bladder channel
7. In Ayurveda, the term *chakra* meaning *wheel* refers to the:
   a. Concentration of acupoints on an energy pathway
   b. Kapha body constitutional type
   c. System of nadis that carry vital energy
   d. Whirling centers of energy at seven levels in the body
8. In Ayurvedic massage, what is mixed into base oils to achieve specific therapeutic goals?
   a. Essential oils
   b. Minerals
   c. Herbs
   d. Vital energy
9. Postures or *asanas* are a major component of:
   a. Qi gong
   b. Acupressure massage integration
   c. Hatha Yoga
   d. Chinese medicine
10. In Thai massage, the pathways that carry energy are called:
    a. Meridians
    b. Sen lines
    c. Nadis
    d. Marma

Video Challenge

Watch the appropriate segment of the video on your DVD and then answer the following questions.

Eastern Bodywork

AMI for the Back

1. What principles of good alignment are demonstrated in the AMI segment of the video?
2. What manual techniques are applied over energy meridians?
3. How does the massage therapist in the video apply pressure to acupoints?

Qi Gong for Self-Care

4. What do you notice in the video about the quality of movement in the qi gong form? How would you describe it?

5. Where is the practitioner looking during the qi gong form demonstrated in the video? How does that affect spinal alignment?
6. What do you notice about the stances in the various qi gong moves demonstrated in the video? How might practicing these stances benefit massage therapists' body mechanics while giving massage?

Comprehension Exercises

The following short answer questions test your knowledge and understanding of chapter topics and provide practice in written communication skills. Explain in two to four complete sentences.

1. Compare and contrast the theories of TCM energy channels, Ayurvedic nadis, and Thai sen lines. What are the similarities and differences? What is their role in their respective forms of Eastern bodywork?
2. Compare qi gong and yoga as body-mind practices. What are the goals of each? How do they differ in practice?
3. How do the applications of the manual techniques in different forms of Eastern bodywork differ?

For Greater Understanding

The following exercises are designed to take you from the realm of theory into the real world. They will help give you a deeper understanding of the subjects covered in this chapter. Action words are underlined to emphasize the variety of activities presented to address different learning styles and to encourage deeper thinking.

1. Receive a bodywork session from a practitioner who specializes in an Eastern bodywork form. Compare and contrast your experience with Western massage.

2. Integrate knowledge of TCM energy channels and acupoints into a Western massage. Apply sliding techniques along energy channel lines, and press important acupoints as you address different regions. Focus on your intent to balance energy as you apply techniques.

3. Practice qi gong exercises or hatha yoga postures. Relate these practices to associated forms of Eastern bodywork.

20 Special Populations and Adaptations

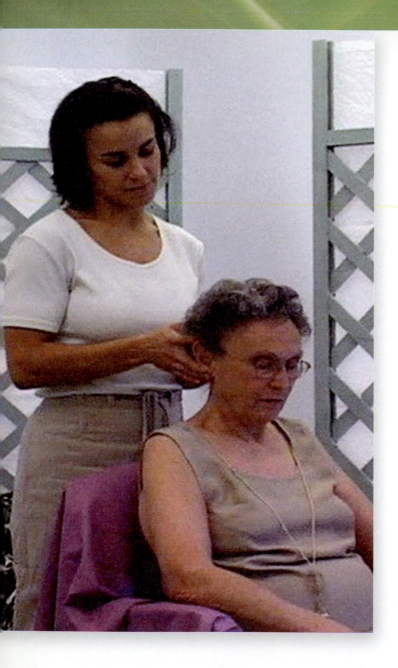

 CHAPTER OUTLINE

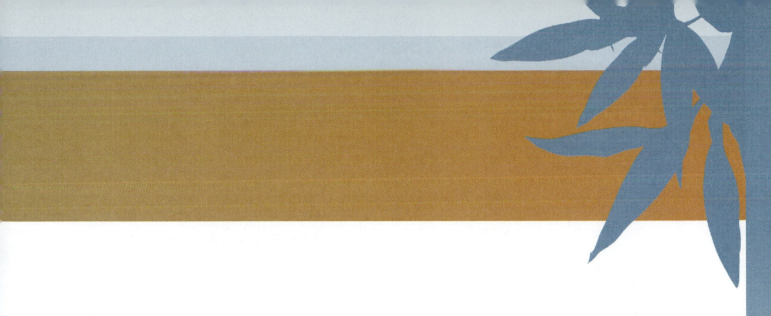

LEARNING OUTCOMES

After studying this chapter, you will have information to:

1. Plan massage sessions to meet the needs of athletes.
2. Provide massage safely to healthy women with low risk pregnancies.
3. Massage infants for optimal growth and development.
4. Provide safe and effective massage to the elderly.
5. Plan massage to address the needs of the terminally ill and dying.
6. Adapt massage sessions for people with visual, hearing, and mobility impairments.

7. Accommodate large and small clients.
8. Accommodate clients with amputations and prosthetic limbs.
9. Provide massage safely to clients with internal and external medical devices.
10. Recognize the rewards and challenges of serving special populations.

KEY TERMS

MASSAGE *in* ACTION

On your DVD, explore:

- Postevent Sports Massage for Run/Walk Event
- Pregnancy Massage
- Infant Massage
- Massage for the Elderly in a Semireclining Position
- Gentle Hand and Arm Massage

INTRODUCTION

A **special population** is a group of people with some distinctive life circumstance that sets them apart from a normal adult population. They include athletes, pregnant women, infants, the elderly, and people with various physical impairments and diseases. Whatever it is that makes a special population "special" can influence their goals for massage and may require adaptations to the session for safety or comfort. Contraindications might be different for members of a special population, and so more information about their individual circumstances is needed in planning massage sessions.

There is a difference between massage for special populations and clinical applications of massage. Clinical applications are distinguished by a focus on helping the client heal from or manage a specific pathology or injury and are provided in clinical settings. On the other hand, special populations are encountered in all settings, and individuals may be interested in massage for reasons having nothing to do with their "special" circumstances.

Do not assume that someone with a medical condition is coming for massage to treat that condition. He or she may just want to relax or may be getting massage to enhance his or her general well-being. Always check with new clients about their goals for the massage. You may end up working around a special circumstance rather than addressing it directly.

Adaptations are adjustments or changes to the way things are normally done to meet the unique needs of an individual. Typical adaptations involve communication, positioning, and assistance with dressing and getting on and off the massage table. In some cases, it means giving massage with the client in a bed or chair rather than on the massage table. For others, it requires eliminating or modifying massage applications for safety.

Attitude is important in working with special populations and clients with special needs. Remember that your job is to provide massage for their benefit. Be nonjudgmental and accepting of all clients as human beings. Be sensitive to their feelings about their situation. Be patient and work at the pace necessary for their comfort. Be flexible and open to making modifications. Above all, exercise good judgment and err on the side of doing no harm.

This chapter focuses on special populations commonly seen in massage practices. Massage therapists working in settings open to the general public must be ready to plan massage sessions for whoever walks in the door. Common

sense, experience, and a little knowledge can aid in making the massage session safe and comfortable for these special clients.

ATHLETES

Athletes approach their sports and fitness activities in different ways—personal challenge, recreation, health practice, way of life, or possibly a career. **Sports massage** is a massage application specifically designed to meet the needs of this special population. It is not a set of unique manual techniques, but the application of a variety of techniques aimed at keeping active people healthy and in top form for participation in their sports or fitness activities.

There are five major applications of sports massage.

1. *Recovery* applications enhance physical and mental recovery from strenuous physical activity.
2. *Remedial* applications improve debilitating conditions such as muscle tension and soreness.
3. *Rehabilitation* applications facilitate healing after a disabling injury.
4. *Maintenance* massage is an all-purpose application for recovery, treating debilitating conditions, and overall health and well-being.
5. *Event* applications help athletes to prepare for competition and to recover afterward.

Techniques and Knowledge

Sports massage as practiced in the United States today primarily uses Western massage techniques to meet session goals. For example, effleurage and petrissage are applied with lubricant to increase circulation and for general and specific muscle relaxation. Compressions are typically used to increase circulation in situations where athletes are clothed (e.g., at events). Percussion techniques are mentally stimulating prior to events or practice sessions. Deep transverse friction treats debilitating conditions such as tendinitis, and is used in rehabilitation after injuries. Contemporary forms of bodywork such as myofascial massage, lymphatic facilitation, and trigger point therapy are integrated into sports massage sessions as needed to accomplish therapeutic goals.

Sports massage specialists have well-developed palpation skills and knowledge of musculoskeletal anatomy and kinesiology. Understanding the biomechanics of a client's sport or fitness activity is useful in planning sessions and locating areas of stress. Familiarity with common sports injuries and their treatment is essential to remedial and rehabilitation applications. Massage therapists working with athletes should be well versed in their special needs and be able to plan massage sessions accordingly.

Recovery

A typical recovery massage addresses the tight, stiff, and sore muscles that accompany strenuous exercise, and facilitates healing minor tissue damage. Recovery is a major component of postevent and maintenance sports massage. Focus is on areas stressed in recent activity. Recovery massage targets improved circulation, muscular relaxation, flexibility, and overall stress reduction. Useful adjunct therapies include a hot shower, whirlpool, sauna, and steam room.

Remedial Massage and Rehabilitation

The most common remedial and rehabilitation sports massage applications involve muscle tension and spasms, poor range of motion, trigger points, edema, tendinosis, tendinitis, tenosynovitis, strains, sprains, and general overwork and stress. Deep friction techniques are used for development of healthy scar tissue, and freeing adhesions in connective tissues. Sports massage therapists may team with athletic trainers or physical therapists for rehabilitation applications.

Maintenance

A maintenance sports massage session is an all-purpose massage received regularly to address an athlete's needs at the time. Maintenance sessions last for 60–90 minutes. The intent is to keep the athlete in optimal condition as he or she trains. The foundation for the massage is recovery with remedial massage for problems as needed. Specific goals include:

- Reduce muscle hypertonicity and spasm
- Stretch, broaden, and free adhesions in connective tissue in high stress areas
- Improve overall flexibility and range of motion
- Decrease the impact of delayed-onset muscle soreness and low-grade strains associated with intense training schedules

Injury prevention and anxiety reduction are added benefits from regular massage, and keeping an upbeat outlook is important for an athlete during a competitive season.

Events

Massage given at athletic events is designated as pre-event, interevent, and postevent.

Pre-event Pre-event massage prepares athletes physically and mentally for an upcoming competition, and may be considered part of their warm-up. Pre-event massage is typically 15–20 minutes in duration, has an upbeat tempo, avoids causing discomfort, and concentrates on muscle groups to be used in the performance. Most athletes benefit from a stimulating session to increase their focus and alertness. Athletes are clothed for pre-event massage. Pre-event applications commonly include:

- Compressions
- Direct pressure on stress points
- Friction techniques
- Lifting and broadening
- Percussion, jostling
- Joint mobilizations
- Stretching.

Interevent Interevent massage is given between events at competitions such as track and swim meets. These sessions are short (10–15 minutes), avoid discomfort, and focus on recovery of muscles stressed in the event. It also readies the

athletes for the next performance. It is a combination pre-event and postevent application.

Postevent The primary goal of postevent sports massage is physical and psychological recovery. These sessions are short (10–15 minutes) if given shortly after the event, and longer (30–90 minutes) if given over an hour after the event. The athlete should be cooled down, have taken adequate fluids, and be breathing normally before receiving massage. Pressure is generally lighter than maintenance massage, and the pace is moderate to slow. Special attention is given to muscles used in the past event. Techniques known to increase circulation and promote muscular and general relaxation are emphasized. These include:

- Compression
- Kneading
- Jostling
- Joint movements
- Stretching

If the postevent massage takes place close to the time of the event, the practitioner may also identify and assess injuries received during the competition. The athlete may need first aid and/or be referred to other members of the health care team at the event. Figures 20.1 to 20.5■ show massage techniques typically included in postevent massage.

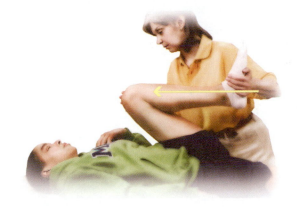

FIGURE 20.1

Knee to chest stretch for posterior hip and leg muscles.

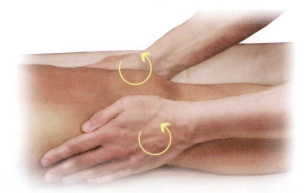

FIGURE 20.2

Circular friction with the heels of the hands to the tendons around the knee.

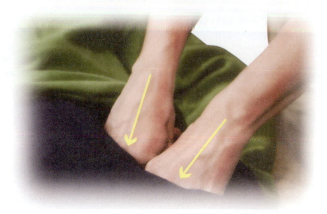

FIGURE 20.3

Compression to the gluteal muscles using the fists.

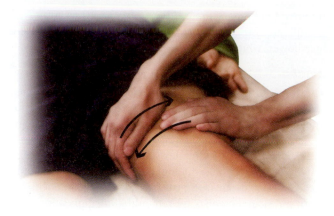

FIGURE 20.5

Horizontal stroking of the thigh muscles.

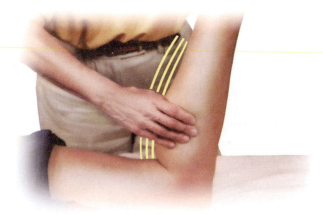

FIGURE 20.4

Shaking the calf muscles.

PREGNANT WOMEN

Providing beneficial and safe massage to pregnant women requires some knowledge of pregnancy itself and of related contraindications and cautions. Massage sessions for healthy women with normal pregnancies involve adaptations for comfort and safety. Particularly important are skills in alternative positioning and draping and massage applications that address common problems of pregnant women.

Massage addresses many of the discomforts experienced by women during the 9-month pregnancy period. Benefits of massage during this time include less fatigue and more energy, less back and leg pain, headache relief, better sleep, and stress reduction. Many women experience improved mood, and less anxiety and depression. Pregnant women experience a dramatic change in size, weight, and shape over a relatively short period of time. In a typical preg-

CRITICAL THINKING

Think about the needs of athletes directly before and after competitive events and in between events. Compare and contrast their needs in each situation, and analyze how massage sessions might be used to address those needs.

1. What are the goals of massage in each situation?
2. Which massage techniques are effective in meeting those goals?
3. Which massage applications are best avoided in each situation?

View the video of Practice Sequence 20–1, Postevent Sports Massage for Run/Walk Event, on your DVD to guide you through a sports massage session. After you perform the Practice Sequence, evaluate how well you did by filling out Performance Evaluation Form 20–1, Postevent Sports Massage for Run/Walk Event. The form can be found in Appendix F, Performance Evaluation Forms, on page A-44 of this book and on your DVD.

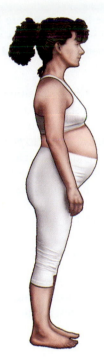

FIGURE 20.6

Typical pregnancy posture.

nancy posture a woman's head is forward, chest back, belly forward, and lower back curved (Figure 20.6■). Massage can ease some of the stresses on the body experienced over the 9-month pregnancy period.

Contraindications

Giving massage to women with high-risk pregnancies should only be done by massage therapists with specialized advanced training, or avoided altogether if contraindicated. Therefore, it is important to identify high-risk situations and screen for warning signs of possible medical problems.

High-risk pregnancies are those in which the mother or fetus is at higher than normal risk for complications or negative developments. The following conditions are considered high-risk pregnancies:

- Mother's age (under 15 or over 35)
- Mother extremely underweight or overweight
- Mother with chronic illness (e.g., diabetes, heart disease)
- Mother with history of pelvic inflammatory disease (PID), endometriosis, or sexually transmitted disease (STD)
- History of miscarriage or preterm delivery
- More than five previous pregnancies—completed or not
- Twins, triplets, or other multiples
- Fetal abnormalities
- Serious complications: gestational diabetes, pregnancy-induced hypertension (PIH), pre-eclampsia, eclampsia, ectopic pregnancy (fertilized egg implants outside of the uterus)

Screen for warning signs for contraindications before every massage session. Do not give massage if a pregnant client has any of the following signs:

- Morning sickness, nausea, vomiting
- Vaginal bleeding or discharge
- Fever
- Decrease in fetal movement in past 24 hours
- Diarrhea
- Abdominal pain
- Excessive swelling in the arms or legs

Some signs that require immediate medical attention are:

- Chest discomfort or pain
- Pain in one or both arms, back, neck, jaw, or stomach
- Labored breathing
- Breaking into a cold sweat
- Nausea, lightheadedness, dizziness
- Seizure, convulsions, loss of consciousness
- Pitting edema (pressure leaves indentation in tissues)
- Swelling in the hands or face

Uterine contractions may indicate that the birth process has begun. If they continue, stop the massage, and advise the client to contact her health provider immediately.

Of course, all of the normal contraindications and cautions apply to pregnant women. Find out what medications a client is taking. Ask if there have been any new or adverse reactions to them recently. Modify massage applications accordingly, especially for medications that affect circulation or sensation.

Pregnancy Massage Application

Once you identify that a pregnancy is normal, you can proceed with the massage with some adaptations. Considerations focus on the safety of the mother and the fetus, and may call for restrictions on massage applications. Some restrictions are for the entire pregnancy, others are in certain trimesters. The position of the fetus in late pregnancy results in stresses on muscles and joints, internal organs, and major blood vessels along the spine (Figure 20.7■).

CREATING A COMFORTABLE ENVIRONMENT

The environment for pregnancy massage should be comfortable and relaxing. Keep the space well ventilated and with fresh air if possible. The temperature can be cooler than usual for massage, between 68–72 degrees Fahrenheit. Avoid strong scents in the air. Play music relaxing to the client.

An accessible bathroom is a must. Suggest that the client urinate just before beginning a massage session. Be prepared to stop the session and help the client off of the table to go to the bathroom and then to get back on again. Having a robe handy is practical for this purpose.

A step stool is useful for getting up onto the table. Be present if needed to assist the recipient and help her get into a comfortable position. A woman may require more assistance with this in the later stages of pregnancy.

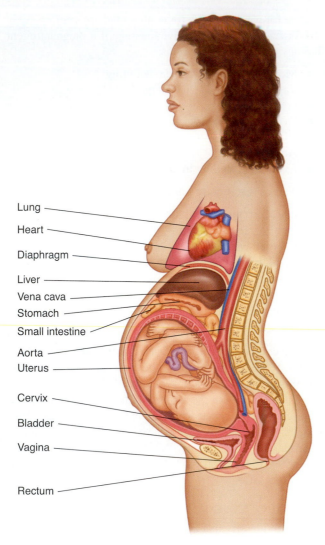

Lung

Heart

Diaphragm

Liver

Vena cava

Stomach

Small intestine

Aorta

Uterus

Cervix

Bladder

Vagina

Rectum

FIGURE 20.7

Position of the fetus in late pregnancy results in stresses on the mother's body.

Provide a glass of water for the client. Keep tissues and extra towels in reach.

POSITIONING OPTIONS

The primary purpose of positioning is to make the pregnant woman comfortable and safe during massage applications. In addition, positioning itself can be effective in reducing stress in the client's back and legs. The preferred positions for pregnancy massage are semireclining, side-lying, and seated. Although the supine and prone positions may be tolerated very early in the pregnancy, some experts recommend avoiding them altogether.

A general rule of thumb for positioning pregnant women is to fill in any spaces you find with bolsters, pillows, or rolled-up towels. The recipient should feel secure and supported all around.

There are massage tables and bolstering systems designed specifically for pregnant women. These have both positive and negative features and are beyond the scope of this text. Focus here is on adaptations that can be made for pregnant women when using standard massage tables and bolstering with pillows.

Semireclining Semireclining position, or half-sitting, is a good alternative to lying supine. Bolsters and pillows may be used to prop the recipient into a half-sitting position. Additional bolsters may be used to prop up the legs. A towel rolled up and placed under the right hip, will shift weight slightly to the left, taking pressure off major blood vessels. Some massage tables have an adjustment to convert a flat tabletop into one with an inclined back support. A disadvantage of semireclining is limited access to the back of the body.

Side-Lying The side-lying position offers better access to more of the body. It does, however, require turning over to reach both left and right sides. If turning over is a problem, especially later in pregnancy, ask the client to lie on the side most comfortable for her.

In the side-lying position, the client's back and buttocks are near the edge of the table. This allows room for the arms, legs, and bolsters on the table top. The top leg is bent. Pillows are placed under the head, the top arm and leg, and around the belly if needed for support. Prop up the leg so that the hip, knee, and ankle are in a horizontal line (Figure 20.8■).

Seated The seated position can also be useful. The client sits on a chair placed at the side of the table and leans forward into pillows for support. The arms are crossed and placed on the pillows with the forehead resting on them. This provides bracing for massage on the back. The client can sit up straight for massage of the arms and hands. A hospital gown or other clothing opened in the back provides draping and access to the back of the body.

Changing position during a massage session might also make sense. If a client becomes uncomfortable after some time in a particular position, change to a different position. If massaging a client in semireclining position, consider ending in the seated position with massage of the back. For safety, assist the client as needed when changing position, especially later in pregnancy.

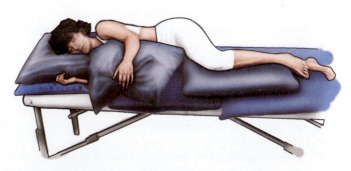

FIGURE 20.8

Side-lying position and bolstering for pregnancy massage.

TABLE HEIGHT

Adjust the table height to allow for your good body mechanics with the client in different positions. When the client is semireclining, a lower table height allows easier access to the head and shoulders. When the client is side-lying, a higher table height is sometimes better since techniques are applied more horizontally, rather than downward vertically. If you expect to specialize in pregnancy massage, or work with other special populations, a mechanically adjustable table would be good to have.

CAUTIONS AND ADAPTATIONS

Unscented oils and lotions are the safest choice for pregnant women. Avoid heavily scented products. Some essential oils that promote relaxation, such as lavender and chamomile, may be used if the client is not adversely sensitive to smells. See page 506 in Chapter 17, Spa Applications, for more information about using essential oils on pregnant women.

Deep abdominal massage is contraindicated throughout pregnancy and in the weeks after delivery. In the second and third trimesters, gentle effleurage, passive touch, and some forms of energy bodywork may be performed safely on the abdomen. Use a broad flat hand to apply light effleurage in a clockwise direction over the enlarged abdomen.

Avoid aggressive or heavy pressure techniques applied to connective tissues. These include ligaments, tendons, and fascial tissues that are all affected by the hormone relaxin, which softens ligaments in the body in preparation for birth and can result in unstable joints. Stretching techniques are generally contraindicated.

Watch for excessive edema and varicose veins in the legs. Pregnant women are at higher risk for blood clots due to changes in blood chemistry during this time. Blood flow to and from the legs is restricted during pregnancy, especially in the third trimester. This creates a prime environment for blood clots.

Massage to the legs may be contraindicated if circulation is excessively poor, if the mother has been inactive or on bed rest by doctor's orders, or if she has varicose veins. Some advise avoiding massage to the legs altogether (except possibly the feet) during the third trimester (Werner 2005).

Advise pregnant clients to refrain from eating a meal for about 2 hours before a massage if possible. This is especially important later in the pregnancy.

Traditional Chinese medicine (TCM) prohibits certain techniques during pregnancy. Among these are pressure to acupoints LI-4 in the web of the thumb, and Sp-6 above the inside ankle (see Figure 19.4 on page 558). If there is worry about miscarriage, also avoid pressure on the Yin Channels on the inside of the lower legs. See Table 19.2 on page 560 for more information about acupoints and pregnancy.

TRIMESTER CONSIDERATIONS

The first and third trimesters are the most tenuous for the fetus. In the first trimester, the attachments to the mother are just becoming established. In the third trimester, the fetus and mother are preparing for eventual detachment and delivery. The fragility of these times calls for special attention and care.

First Trimester In the first trimester use only gentle relaxation massage techniques. Avoid pressure over the abdomen, sacrum, and low back. Stroking and kneading of the buttocks, legs, shoulders, and arms help relieve general tension. Head, face, and neck massage are also relaxing and pleasurable. Omit joint movements and stretching techniques, especially in the lower body. To be most conservative, avoid pressure to LI-14 and Sp-6 acupoints and stimulation of the area on the feet between the ankle and the heel.

Second Trimester In a normal pregnancy, the second trimester is the safest and easiest part. Most women experience less nausea in this period. However, connective tissues continue to loosen and prohibitions on joint movements and stretching still apply. Use positioning to help relax muscles which have begun to tighten and possibly spasm. Gentle stroking of the abdomen is permissible at this point. Attention to lower back muscles and along the muscle attachments on the iliac crest with circular friction and fingertip kneading can help relieve tightness there.

Third Trimester In the third trimester, discomfort increases as the fetus gains weight and the mother's body prepares for delivery. Massage sessions focus on comfort and relaxation. Watch for signs of poor circulation, swelling, and varicose veins in the legs. Omit massage of the legs if the client has been inactive and/or signs of poor circulation are evident. Refer the client to her health care provider if you notice pitting edema. Assist the client on and off the table and as needed for undressing and dressing.

Contraindications in late pregnancy related to blood clots in the legs continue for 8–10 weeks postpartum. In addition, the side-lying position may continue to be the most comfortable position for a new mother even after delivery, especially if she is breast feeding the baby.

Massage techniques can be adapted for the side-lying position. For example, the foot of the upper leg is readily accessible for massage (Figure 20.9■). The upper arm is also accessible and supported (Figure 20.10■). Effleurage and petrissage techniques on the back are relaxing (Figure 20.11■).

View the video of Practice Sequence 20–2, Pregnancy Massage, on your DVD to guide you through a pregnancy massage session. After you perform the Practice Sequence, evaluate how well you did by filling out Performance Evaluation Form 20–2, Pregnancy Massage. The form can be found in Appendix F, Performance Evaluation Forms, on page A-46 of this book and on your DVD.

PRACTICAL APPLICATION

Practice positioning a practice partner in semireclining, side-lying, and seated position as if he or she were pregnant. Try out different approaches to massage applications appropriate for pregnancy massage.

1. How many bolsters do you need and where are they placed for greatest security and comfort?
2. What is the best table height for each positioning alternative, taking into consideration your body mechanics?
3. How are massage applications adapted for different client positions?

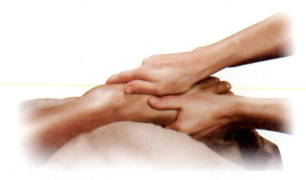

FIGURE 20.9

Foot massage in side-lying position.

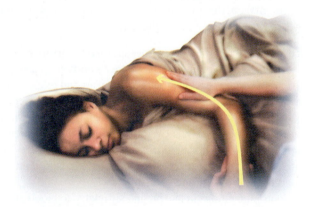

FIGURE 20.10

Massage to the upper arm in side-lying position.

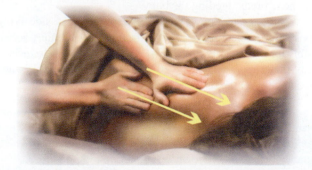

FIGURE 20.11

Long effleurage strokes on the back in side-lying position.

INFANTS

Infant massage given by parents and other caregivers is an excellent way to provide the kinesthetic and tactile stimulation essential for the healthy growth and development of infants. A significant body of evidence confirms that massage not only contributes to the healthy development of normal infants, but also is effective in promoting recovery of preterm, cocaine-exposed, HIV-exposed, and other high-risk infants.

Infant massage has other benefits, including release of tension and learning to relax. It promotes bonding with parents, aids digestion and elimination, improves sleep, and eases growing pains. Massage helps calm colicky babies. In addition, touching and handling her baby promotes the mother's milk production by stimulating the secretion of the hormone prolactin. Massage can also provide fathers with an opportunity to touch and interact with their babies in a way that is satisfying and also builds confidence in handling small children.

Massage practitioners may include training in infant massage in their services to pregnant clients and their families before or after delivery. Dolls may be used to introduce massage techniques before the baby is delivered.

Infant Massage Application

Infant massage is about interacting socially as much as it is about applying massage techniques. Caregivers maintain eye contact and talk or sing to the child throughout the massage (Figure 20.12■). Massage can be a time of playful interaction that enhances the infant's emotional, social, and physical development.

Be sure the space for infant massage is safe, secure, and warm. Minimize distractions such as noise and bright lights. Turn off the television and radio. Have all supplies in reach. Use unscented natural oil or lotion. Place a towel under the infant for the massage.

It is important that the massage giver be relaxed and comfortable throughout the session. Givers may sit on the floor with legs extended and back straight, perhaps supported against a wall or piece of furniture. The infant is placed

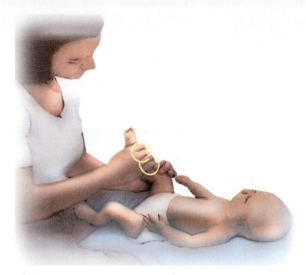

FIGURE 20.12

Make eye contact and talk to the baby during massage.

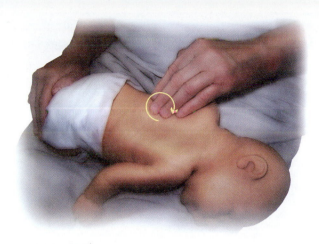

FIGURE 20.13

Infant positioned prone across the caregiver's legs.

supine on or between the giver's legs or prone across the legs (Figure 20.13■). If the infant is on a bed or table, be sure that he or she cannot fall off. Infants can be very active during massage.

Infant massage is a simple, gentle, yet firm application of stroking, pressing, squeezing, and movement of the limbs. Use enough pressure to engage the tissues and avoid a light tickling touch. Infant massage is less specific than massage for adults. The idea is to provide pleasurable stimulation through touch and movement.

Massage techniques are applied systematically from the chest to the back. Some examples are sliding techniques on the forehead (Figure 20.14■), and joint movements of the arms (Figure 20.15■). Abdominal massage along with bringing the knees to the chest in rhythmic repetitions aids bowel movements (Figures 20.16■ and 20.17■).

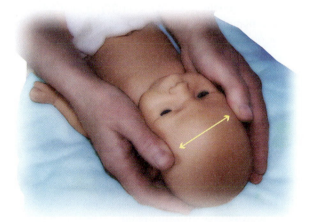

FIGURE 20.14

Thumb slides across the forehead.

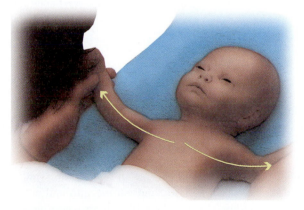

FIGURE 20.15

Joint movement for the shoulders.

View the video of Practice Sequence 20–3, Infant Massage, on your DVD to guide you through an infant massage session. After you perform the Practice Sequence, evaluate how well you did by filling out Performance Evaluation Form 20–3, Infant Massage. The form can be found in Appendix F, Performance Evaluation Forms, on page A-47 of this book and on your DVD.

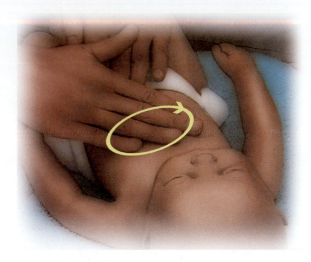

FIGURE 20.16

Abdominal massage in clockwise direction.

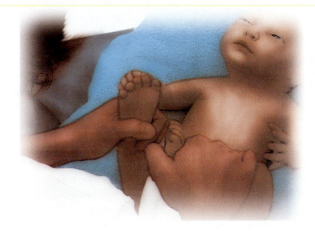

FIGURE 20.17

Bringing infant's knees to the chest in rhythmic repetitions.

THE ELDERLY

The elderly, defined as people 70 years and older, are a rapidly growing special population. Massage has many benefits for elders, including helping them keep the strength and flexibility needed to do activities of daily living (ADL) that contribute to maintaining independence. ADLs include things such as getting in and out of a chair, dressing and undressing, climbing stairs, and getting into and out of a bathtub. Another physical benefit is improved digestions and elimination.

Massage helps ease the pain of loss, frustration, and fear about the future. Loss of work, home, spouse, family, friends, independence, and financial security can result in anxiety and worry. The caring touch and relaxing benefits of massage help ease these emotional pains.

Massage also provides an avenue for social interaction, especially for elders in nursing homes or homebound. The personal interaction with the practitioner helps reduce feelings of social isolation, and the inherent touch of massage provides a special connection to others.

Some of the common problem conditions experienced by the elderly that massage can help alleviate are insomnia, loss of appetite, constipation, immobility, poor circulation, and decreased immune system functioning. Massage can address skin problems such as loss of elasticity and dryness, bedsores, and physical discomfort and pain. Massage reduces chronic stress, chronic depression, and feelings of being alone and useless.

Some of the research about elders and massage in clinical settings is reviewed in Chapter 8, Clinical Applications of Massage, on page 282. Studies have shown massage to be beneficial to those hospitalized for a number of conditions, including heart disease, cancer, and psychiatric problems. The benefits of back massage to institutionalized elderly included relaxation, improved communication, and a reduction in the common dehumanizing effects of institutional care.

There is promising research on massage for the agitated elderly in institutions and for those with Alzheimer's disease and dementia. Several studies have found reduction in certain agitated behaviors with regular 10-minute massage. Massage performed in the studies can be characterized as using light pressure, even rhythm, and slow strokes.

Physiological Age

Elders are perhaps the most distinctive population to work with. Individuals in this age group are more different from each other than those in other age groups. By the time people have reached 70-plus years of age, they exhibit the accumulated effects of a lifetime of good and poor health habits, diseases and injuries, and life experiences. They are more likely to have chronic health problems and to be taking medications. Care should be taken in learning about each individual and in planning his or her massage sessions.

It is useful to think about older adults in terms of physiological age, rather than chronological age. **Physiological age** describes a person's health status relative to the norm in different age groups. For example, a 60-year-old person in good physical condition could be described as having the body of a normal 50-year-old.

People age at different rates depending on their genetic makeup, lifelong health habits, and unique life events. Traumatic events such as car accidents, work accidents, and sports injuries take their toll over time. Diseases experienced earlier in life may have effects later. An example is the incidence of post–polio syndrome affecting people 40–50 years after the acute phase of the disease. Negative factors can often be offset with healthy habits such as good nutrition and regular exercise.

Elders may be thought of as falling into one of three categories: robust, age appropriate, and frail.

Robust Elders These individuals show few outward signs of impaired health, look younger than their chronologic age, and are mentally sharp and physically active. Robust elders can generally be treated like the typical middle-aged recipient of massage. Information obtained on a health questionnaire can help you identify any areas of caution that are not obvious.

Age-Appropriate Elders People who show some of the typical signs of aging are considered age appropriate. Age-appropriate elders will have some problems associated with aging. Information from a health questionnaire is useful to identify contraindications and areas of caution. Use pillows and bolsters to ensure maximum comfort and the least stress on joints. Limit the prone position to 15–20 minutes. After the session, help the recipient sit up or at least stay near the massage table until he or she is sitting up. Leave the room only when you are sure that the recipient is not lightheaded and can get off the table safely.

Frail Elders Frail elders look and feel fragile to the touch and need special care. Check with their physicians before massaging the very frail. Frail elders will probably need assistance getting on and off the table (see Figure 12.15 on page 369). You might find it necessary to massage them in a regular chair or on their beds. Limit the session to 15–20 minutes until you know that they can handle longer sessions. Watch them carefully in the prone position on the table to be sure that they can lie there comfortably. Be extra gentle in lifting frail elders, avoiding pulling on their arms to help them up. Cradle their bodies to help them change position.

Positioning Options for the Elderly

Lying supine and prone as usual for full-body massage is a good option for most robust and many age-appropriate elders, although the prone position would normally be limited to a maximum of 20 minutes. The side-lying position puts stress on the hip and shoulder on the table, and is a less desirable option in most cases.

Better positioning options for many age-appropriate and most frail elderly clients is either the seated (Figure 20.18■) or the semireclining positions (Figure 20.19■). These positions allow more social interaction between the elderly person and the massage therapist, including eye contact. They also diminish the problem many elderly have with dizziness

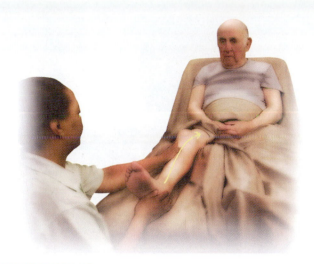

FIGURE 20.19
Semireclining position for massage for the elderly.

when changing from a horizontal to a more vertical position, as in standing up after lying down.

Guidelines for Massage of Older Adults

There are no special massage techniques that slow the aging process. However, there are certain points to keep in mind when working with older adults and especially with the elderly.

Do include the following in a massage session for healthy aging:

- Techniques to improve circulation in the extremities. Effleurage moving distal to proximal enhances venous return, and relaxing the muscles with kneading and jostling improves local circulation (Figure 20.20■).
- Kneading, compression, and other petrissage movements that help keep muscle and connective tissue pliable and elastic (Figure 20.21■).
- Joint movements and stretches of the lower extremities for improved mobility and flexibility. Spend time on the feet to relieve soreness, improve circulation, and mobilize joints. Mobilizing the legs and feet can help increase kinesthetic awareness, and thereby improve movements such as walking and climbing stairs (Figure 20.22■).

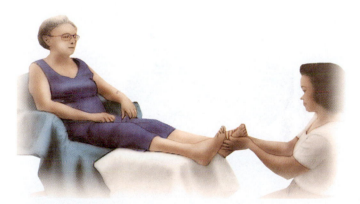

FIGURE 20.18
Seated position for massage for the elderly.

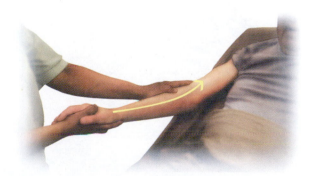

FIGURE 20.20
Effleurage on the extremities improves general circulation.

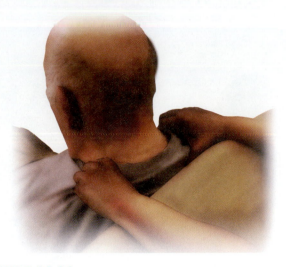

FIGURE 20.21

Kneading relaxes the shoulders.

- Movements and stretches for the shoulders to help maintain some important daily living functions, such as getting dressed and undressed and reaching for things overhead. The hands may benefit from special attention to help them to stay mobile and sensitive.
- Passive motion and stretches for the cervical muscles to help maintain normal range of motion in the head and neck. With declining peripheral vision, the ability to turn the head to see things in the environment is important. This is essential for the safety of elders who drive motor vehicles.
- Techniques that focus on lengthening the front of the body, especially abdominal and pectoral muscles, to help maintain an erect posture. Exercises are also needed to keep postural muscles strong and to avoid a bent-over or collapsed condition later in life.
- Abdominal massage for the viscera, which may be important for sedentary elders to improve digestion and elimination. Use gentle but firm pressure, always going clockwise during circular movements (Figure 20.23■).

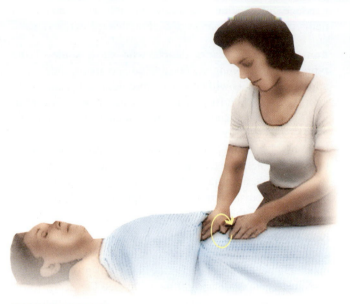

FIGURE 20.23

Abdominal massage improves digestion.

- Back massage is relaxing and comforting. It can be done even from a semireclining position if the client leans forward to allow access (Figure 20.24■).

Cautions and Adaptations

Some problem conditions are more common in older adults and warrant special awareness. Massage is rarely contraindicated totally, but certain cautions apply with the conditions discussed below. It is important to take a thorough health history to identify the conditions that are contraindicated or for which cautions are warranted. Always consult the person's physician when in doubt about a condition or disease mentioned by a recipient of massage.

- Massage may be contraindicated with certain medications. If you work regularly with older adults and elders, it would be wise to have a reference book that explains

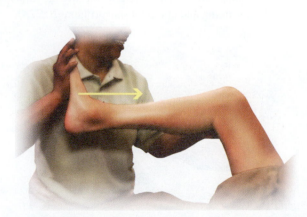

FIGURE 20.22

Joint movements in the legs improve mobility.

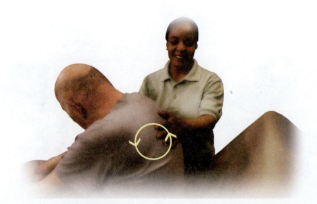

FIGURE 20.24

Superficial stroking of the back is relaxing and comforting.

the effects and possible side effects of common medications. Books written specifically about massage and medications are listed under Chapter 20 in Appendix H, References and Additional Resources, on page A-75. See Table 9.1 on page 304 for at-a-glance information about medications. Check with the recipient's physician if in doubt about the advisability of him or her receiving massage while taking a certain medication.

- Elders typically have thin and delicate skin and bruise more easily than younger people. Pressure used in massage should be gentle to moderate depending on the recipient's general condition. Use enough oil or lotion to prevent skin tearing.

- Watch for varicose veins in the legs, and do not perform deep effleurage or strong kneading over them. Light effleurage and jostling movements are better for circulation in this case. Elevating the legs slightly when the recipient is supine will help venous return during the massage.

- Deep vein thrombosis (DVT) and thrombophlebitis are two serious contraindications that may affect legs of elderly people. With these conditions, the legs will sometimes show typical signs of inflammation, that is, redness, heat, swelling, pain. There may be a cordlike hardness or a deep aching in the calf, or pitting edema in the skin. However, there may not be any signs of the underlying condition. Avoid massage of the legs if DVT is suspected.

- Older adults and elders may have diagnosed or undiagnosed atherosclerosis, or hardening of the arteries. This is especially dangerous in the cerebral arteries, which pass through the neck. Avoid deep work in the lateral neck area. Avoid movements that put the neck in hyperextension or increase the cervical curve, since this position may further occlude blood vessels to the head and cause fainting.

- Use great care in performing mobilizing techniques and stretches around artificial joints. In the elderly, joint replacements are particularly common in the hip and knee. After a hip replacement, avoid movements involving abduction and circumduction in that joint. Consult the recipient's health care provider for instructions. Extreme care should be taken in the case of any joint replacement because of the potential instability of the joint or decreased range of motion due to scar tissue.

- In the case of cancer patients, always check with the physician before performing massage. Observe appropriate cautions with those receiving chemotherapy or radiation cancer treatments.

- Older adults and elders tend to have problems in their joints, including osteo- and rheumatoid arthritis. Massage of the area should be avoided if the joint is inflamed. When there is no inflammation, massage of the surrounding muscles is indicated to help relieve stress on the joint. Holding and warming arthritic and sore joints can be soothing. Heat is contraindicated if there is swelling.

- Because massage is commonly done directly on the skin, practitioners may detect possible skin cancers of which recipients are unaware. Basal and squamous cell carcinoma and malignant melanoma usually appear on sun-exposed areas of the body, including the face, arms, and chest. Malignant melanoma may develop at the site of a mole. Report any lesion or suspicious-looking skin condition to the recipient, or to the caregiver in the case of frail elders. Suggest that it be checked by a general physician or dermatologist. Do not massage directly over the site. See Chapter 6, Anatomy & Physiology, Pathology, and Kinesiology, beginning on page 137, for illustrations of integumentary system pathologies.

THE TERMINALLY ILL

Massage is used to bring caring and comforting touch to the terminally ill and dying. It is a valuable complementary therapy in hospital, hospice, and home care. Simple massage techniques may be used by health practitioners and taught to nonprofessional caregivers to aid those seriously ill or approaching the end of their lives.

From the wellness perspective, even those with terminal illnesses or nearing death continue to strive for optimal well-being in their unique life circumstances. Although massage will not cure or save someone from imminent death, it can help improve physical function and ease some of the pain and anxiety felt. It has been observed that "attentive nurturing touch can be a significant therapeutic factor in treating despondency in the aging and/or the ill because of its multiple psycho-social, mental, emotional, and physical benefits" (Nelson 1994, p. 12). Nurturing touch provides food for the soul, as well as for the body and mind.

General relaxation, improved circulation of blood and lymph, reduced muscular tension, and skin stimulation are effects of massage with benefits for everyone. These effects are relevant to the special needs of those who have been physically inactive or bedridden for a long period of time. Massage helps alleviate problems with insomnia, digestion, constipation, difficulty in breathing, and skin degeneration. It can help prevent bedsores.

View the video of Practice Sequence 20–4, Massage for the Elderly in a Semireclining Position, on your DVD. After you perform the Practice Sequence, evaluate how well you did by filling out Performance Evaluation Form 20–4, Massage for the Elderly in a Semireclining Position. The form can be found in Appendix F, Performance Evaluation Forms, on page A-49 of this book and on your DVD.

People who are terminally ill and dying experience emotional distress for a number of reasons. They may feel isolation, grief from the loss of freedom and friends, fear of abandonment, fear of the disease or aging, or fear of dying. Depression is common among the seriously ill and elderly and may be caused or deepened by touch deprivation. Touch is essential nourishment for optimal well-being at all stages of life.

Gentle relaxation massage is known to reduce anxiety, provide a sense of connection, and generate feelings of general well-being. Massage may also facilitate a release of pent-up feelings, frustrations, sadness, and emotional energy. Pain that is aggravated by stress may be lessened with relaxing massage.

Near the end of life, massage can provide comforting touch and communicate care and love in a nonverbal way. The quality of touch for the dying should be gentle and the techniques simple, such as stroking and holding (Figure 20.25■). When death is near, smooth, soothing touch is used as a form of comfort and a means of nonverbal communication. Some technical skills are needed to avoid causing pain or damaging delicate tissues.

In hospice and home-care situations, family members and other caregivers can be taught simple ways of giving massage to the dying person. This has benefits for both parties, since it offers caregivers something active to do with their loved one and provides a means of connection even for those who may not be able to speak.

Adaptations for the Terminally Ill

A medical profile of the recipient is essential in working with the seriously ill and dying to protect both the recipient and you. As with any other massage, identify contraindications and areas of caution before proceeding with a session. It may also be useful to understand the symptoms expected as a specific disease or condition progresses.

Specific techniques are less important than other essential skills when working with this special population. Intuition and sensitivity to others are important qualities for giving massage to the terminally ill and dying. "If you develop the ability to 'see' an individual rather than just

looking at a body, and if you reach out to that individual with a caring and open heart . . . out of your real and pure contact with the individual, you will intuitively know what to do and how to proceed" (Nelson 1994, p. 43).

Other recommended characteristics and abilities include being touch oriented, able to adapt, open-hearted, able to focus energy, willing to face death, and able to focus on the individual. Important skills include:

- Sensitive massage
- Active holding
- Listening and feedback
- Visualization and guided fantasy
- Guided meditation
- Shared breathing
- Communicating with the dying

While some of these skills seem outside of the normal scope of a massage practitioner, they are useful in working with this special population.

In planning massage sessions for the terminally ill or dying, there are no specific procedures to follow or ironclad rules to memorize. Each individual will be different in how he or she experiences dying and in how massage might be of benefit. However, there are some general guidelines to keep in mind.

In general, massage sessions with the dying should be softer, gentler, and shorter than a regular massage session. A person may only be able to benefit from 10–20 minutes of contact. Techniques may vary from simple hand holding to full-body massage. Massage may be given with the receiver lying on a standard massage table, sitting in a chair or wheel chair, or lying in bed. Patients may be in hospital beds with tubes or IVs in their bodies. Massage practitioners in these situations need to be versatile and able to adapt to the circumstances. Listening and feedback skills are important since communication may be a great need for someone facing death. The key is to be caring, supportive, and accepting.

Hand and arm massage is a useful approach for getting to know a new patient or client. The hands are a familiar place of contact with other people. The hands are easily accessible, relatively safe to massage, and benefit from the application of lotion. Having the hands touched is comforting in itself and affords the opportunity for eye contact while talking. Simple techniques such as sliding (Figure 20.26■), kneading (Figure 20.27■), and joint movements (Figure 20.28■) can be very effective. Hand and arm massage is also easy for volunteers in nursing homes and hospices to learn.

Self-Care

Working with the terminally ill and dying can be physically and emotionally challenging. It is important to practice conscious self-care to help maintain your own well-being.

The actual massage techniques used with the seriously ill or elderly tend to be simple and light and easy on the practitioner's hands. However, maintaining good body mechanics may be difficult when working with people in chairs or

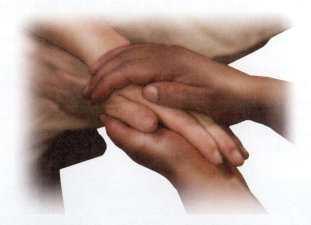

FIGURE 20.25

Holding the hand is a simple and gentle way to touch a dying person.

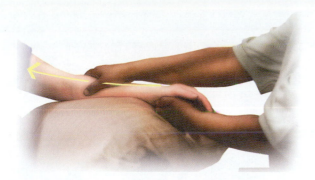

FIGURE 20.26

Applying lotion to the arm with sliding technique.

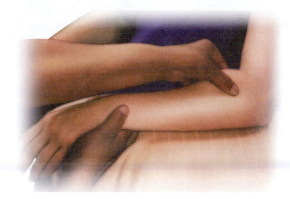

FIGURE 20.27

Kneading the forearm muscles.

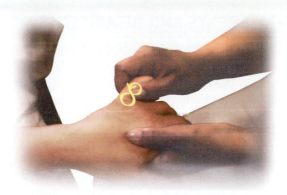

FIGURE 20.28

Joint movement of the fingers.

in beds. The general principles of good mechanics apply here also, and you need to find ways to keep your back straight and spine and neck in good alignment.

If the recipient has a communicable disease, proper precautions and hygiene should be observed. Although seemingly awkward, either latex or another type of glove should be worn if necessary for protection.

Maintaining emotional well-being involves a variety of factors. It helps to have confronted your own issues and fears around illness and death to a point of acceptance. Conscious awareness of how you feel when you are with someone seriously ill or nearing death can help you work through those feelings later with a friend, coworker, or supervisor.

 View the video of Practice Sequence 20–5, Gentle Hand and Arm Massage, on your DVD. After you perform the Practice Sequence, evaluate how well you did by filling out Performance Evaluation Form 20–5, Gentle Hand and Arm Massage. The form can be found in Appendix F, Performance Evaluation Forms, on page A-51 of this book and on your DVD.

CASE FOR STUDY

Keisha Prepares to Give Massage to a Client at the End of Life

Keisha's longtime client is coming close to the end of her life, ending a battle with inoperable cancer. The client has asked Keisha to provide her massage while she is in hospice care. Keisha agrees to do this and has scheduled her first session.

Question:

How does Keisha prepare for this first session, and how can she adapt her massage for this new situation?

Things to consider:

- Who, besides the client, would Keisha contact to integrate her service with other caregivers?
- How might Keisha find out more about possible contraindications and cautions for massage with this client?
- What about the physical setting would it be helpful for Keisha to know?
- What emotional challenges might Keisha face in this situation?

Write a possible scenario for Keisha's preparation for this massage session.

_____

_____

_____

IMPAIRMENTS AND DISABILITIES

Physical impairments commonly encountered in massage practices include visual, hearing, speech, size, and mobility challenges. These range from mild impairments such as needing a cane while walking to more severe circumstances such as being confined to a wheelchair. The difference between an impairment and disability is a matter of degree. Impairment becomes a **disability** when it severely limits a person's ability to perform daily life activities.

The Americans with Disabilities Act (ADA) is a U.S. Federal civil rights law that prohibits the exclusion of people with disabilities from everyday activities. It went into effect in 1992 and applies to businesses of all sizes. It requires reasonable accommodation to make buildings and services accessible to all. How this applies legally to an individual business is a matter of interpretation, but the principle is clear and ethically sound. Massage therapists have a responsibility to accommodate all of their clients, making reasonable adaptations when possible and safe to do so.

Visual Impairment

Many people wear glasses or contact lenses to correct mild vision problems. Clients wearing glasses will usually remember to take them off before getting on the massage table. If not, take the glasses from the client, and put them in a safe place until the session is over. Ask clients wearing contact lenses to remove them for the massage. If that is not convenient, take care that pressure is not applied to the eyes, especially when lying prone and using a face cradle.

Clients with more severe vision loss require more attention. During their first appointment, assess the situation. Ask them to explain their impairment, and discuss with them the level of assistance they need. Individuals vary on how well they can navigate on their own.

Having a magnifying glass on hand for reading would allow some people to fill out the health history without further assistance. Or a health history interview might be best. At the first visit, verbally describe the office and massage room as you walk them through the space, so that they can become familiar with it. Remove clutter from the floor space to prevent tripping. Show clients where to put their clothes, and where the massage table is from that point. Ask if they would like further assistance, and if so, help them as requested.

There are a few general guidelines when working with the visually impaired.

- Let them know verbally when you are in the room.
- Position yourself in front and to their left when taking them through a space. They may or may not choose to touch your right arm for guidance.
- Describe your surroundings, and indicate where things are using clock face numbers. For example, a chair you can use for dressing is at 11 o'clock about 6 feet ahead.

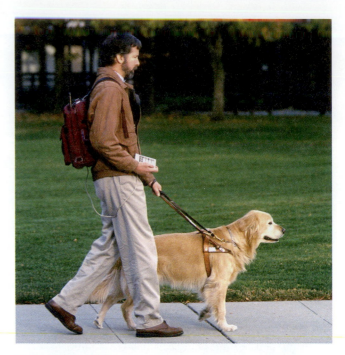

FIGURE 20.29

Do not interact with a service dog unless you have permission from its owner.

- Do not interact with a client's service dog without his or her permission. Discuss with the client where the best place would be for the dog to lie down during the massage (Figure 20.29■).

Hearing Impairment

Hearing loss is common in older adults but can occur at any age. Suspect poor hearing if a client frequently asks you to repeat what you said, asks you to speak louder (if you had been speaking in a normal tone), or seems to be reading your lips. Simply speak more slowly, a little louder, and enunciate clearly. Do not exaggerate your lip movements. Face the client when you speak so that he or she can see your facial expression and read your lips. Maintain good eye contact. Eliminate background noise as much as possible.

Do not shout at someone wearing a hearing aid. If a client wears a hearing aid, ask if he or she would like to remove it during massage. Hearing aids pick up and magnify sounds in the room. If the client does remove the hearing aid, be aware that you will have to speak much louder, or communication will have to be nonverbal. You will need to get his or her attention through touch and move within his or her line of sight so you can make eye contact and your face can be seen. If the hearing aid stays on, keep massage around the head and ears to a minimum since moving the hearing aid can cause annoying feedback.

If you work with a deaf client regularly, consider learning some sign language for common situations. Useful signs would be for hello, ready to start, turn over, finished, and questions about pressure, pain, and other feedback.

Speech Impairment

A person's difficulty communicating verbally can result from a variety of causes. Perhaps he or she has a physical abnormality that affects anatomical structures involved in speech, has had a stroke or head injury, or has a condition such as dementia. Some medications cause slurred speech. People deaf from birth have never heard speech and so may be difficult to understand. And although it is not a physical impairment per se, people speaking English as a second language may have heavy accents, mispronounce words, or use poor grammar, and therefore be hard to understand.

Whatever the cause of poor verbal expression, a little patience and attention will help you communicate adequately with clients. Ask clients to repeat anything you don't understand. Repeat back what you think they mean so that they can confirm it. Listen attentively, and remove background noise that can interfere with your own hearing. Watch their facial expressions and body language.

Distinguish between those who are fully capable mentally (e.g., has a physical impediment to speech) and those whose mental alertness may be clouded by diminished brain function or medication. The former case is a simpler matter of finding a way to communicate, whereas the latter case may require additional considerations.

Size Issues—Large and Small

Massage equipment is designed to accommodate a range of client sizes within normal limits. Tables are typically 6 feet long, 28–32 inches wide, and can safely hold up to about 300 pounds. When clients fall outside of this range, accommodations for their safety and general benefit are in order.

Height Clients over 6 feet tall may extend past the foot of the table when they are supine. Extending the feet over the edge of the table a few inches is usually not uncomfortable. With some table models, you might be able to adjust the face cradle so that the client can use it comfortably as a table extender. The back of the head rests on the cradle with the client face-up, possibly covering or replacing the crescent with a pillow. Consider purchasing a specially made table extender for the foot of the table if you have a tall regular client. This is less of an issue when the client is prone, because several inches are gained when using a face cradle.

People short in stature include those affected by one of the 200 medical conditions know as dwarfism. This special population has a support group called the Little People of America, who provide services and information for adapting to the larger world. "Little people" may need a foot stool to be able to get onto the massage table more easily. They frequently have orthopedic problems in the back and legs that can benefit from massage.

Large Breasts Women with large breasts can be made more comfortable when lying prone with some support. Rolled up towels or small pillows may be positioned to fill in the space above and below the breasts to spread out the weight on the chest area. The face cradle is elevated to maintain a comfortable curvature in the neck. Ready made bolstering systems for women with large breasts are available from different table manufacturers.

Accessing the muscles under breast tissue can be a challenge, especially for women with large breasts. Remember that breast tissue extends from the front of the chest laterally to under the arm pit. If you need to massage the muscles in that area, perhaps the best strategy is to have the client take a side-lying position, so that gravity pulls the breast towards the table. You can hold the upper arm out of the way, while you massage the exposed muscle with the other hand.

Obesity Having a Body Mass Index of 30 or above is the definition of **obesity.** This calculation is based on height, weight, and an estimate of lean body mass. BMI is discussed in more detail on page 80 in Chapter 4, Physical Skills, Fitness, and Self-Care for the Massage Therapist. Obese clients have an unhealthy accumulation of fat tissue in their bodies. It has been estimated that over 25 percent of people in the United States fit this definition, although estimates vary from region to region.

Extremely obese clients typically have mobility problems caused by excess weight and girth. Fitness exercises become more difficult, so inactivity may be a problem. They are likely to have related health issues such as joint pain, diabetes, and heart disease.

Depending on the size of the client, positioning on the massage table may pose challenges. Be sure to know the weight limit for your individual table model. You may need side extenders to accommodate larger girth. Lowering the table in these cases might facilitate better body mechanics for you as you work. Use adequate draping. Giving massage on a floor mat might be a better option for some clients.

It is important to maintain a nonjudgmental and caring attitude. Honor the clients' right to respect and their possible embarrassment about their physical condition. Do not lecture them about the health dangers of being overweight. This is insensitive and outside of the scope of massage therapy. Make the necessary accommodations, and help them reach their wellness goals for the massage session.

Obesity does pose some unique challenges. A factor to consider is the nature of adipose tissue. It has a high proportion of blood capillaries so bruises easily. Palpating anatomical structures deep to the adipose tissue may be difficult. Specific structures that are usually palpable may be inaccessible. Asking a client to flex a particular muscle can help locate it. However, avoid applying deep pressure that can cause pain and bruising.

Carrying excess weight can distort posture and stress the musculature. Relaxation that accompanies massage and the mechanical action of stroking can help relieve some of that stress. In addition, massage reduces anxiety and increases an overall feeling of well-being. It can be a valuable adjunct to any medical weight-loss program.

Avoid abdominal massage with any client who has had weight loss surgery involving the digestive system. People who have significant weight loss may also have skin folds that hang loosely. Do not apply deep pressure to these folds, and avoid pinching the skin when applying techniques to adjacent tissues.

Mobility Challenges

Mobility refers to the ability to go from place to place independently. A person's mobility may be temporarily challenged by injury or illness, or he or she may have a permanent disability that affects mobility.

Accessibility to buildings and offices within buildings is improved with ramps, elevators, wide doors, and automatic doors. Accessible bathrooms are very important for a business like a massage practice. Getting into buildings, moving around in an office space, and getting on and off a massage table are typical mobility issues.

It is relatively easy to accommodate people using canes or crutches. Typically they can negotiate a few stairs and can walk from room to room. Ask if they need assistance, and watch for challenges they may be facing.

Walkers are usually associated with a higher level of impairment (Figure 20.30■). People typically use walkers because of general weakness, problems with balance, or chronic dizziness. Use of the walker may be temporary after surgery, injury, or illness. Or it may be more permanent, such as with the elderly. Those who use walkers in public places may get around fine at home or in small spaces. They will almost certainly need assistance getting on and off a standard massage table.

Wheelchair use indicates a more severe disability. The underlying reason for wheelchair use may be temporary or permanent. There are also different types of wheelchairs, including transfer chairs which require someone else to push, standard models for self-wheeling, and motorized chairs. People who are paralyzed or extremely weak may be strapped into the chair.

In terms of mobility, know about your building's accommodations for outside access and inside maneuverability. Locate the handicapped accessible bathroom. If possible, meet the client at the building entrance to offer assistance, especially at the first appointment.

There are some general guidelines for working with people in wheelchairs. First, respect their autonomy, and do not push a wheelchair without permission. Ask what type of assis-

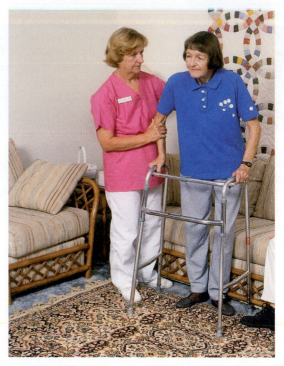

FIGURE 20.30

People using walkers typically have a high level of mobility impairment.

tance they need, since many have the ability to move into and out of the chair on their own. Do not assume the person is helpless, and be sensitive to his or her desire to live as independently as possible. But be ready to help when necessary.

Interview the client to learn the exact cause of his or her disability, which likely involves cautions and possibly contraindications for some massage applications. Sit or kneel so that you are at eye level for the interview in order to make good eye contact.

You and the client may decide that receiving massage in the wheelchair is the best plan. You can wheel the chair to the massage table, and use pillows for support as the client rests his or head and shoulders on the table. Then proceed with seated massage, observing appropriate precautions as needed related to the client's health problems.

PRACTICAL APPLICATION

Role-play massage sessions for clients with different physical impairments and disabilities.

1. Ask appropriate screening questions in the intake interview.

2. Determine what assistance the client may need to prepare for the massage.

3. Position the client appropriately and practice a massage application you might use to meet his or her unique needs.

AMPUTEES AND PROSTHESES

An amputee is a person who has lost one or more arms or legs. People lose limbs for a variety of reasons, such as car and workplace accidents or diseases like diabetes. And an increasing number of returning veterans have lost arms or legs in recent wars. Soldiers, who may have died of their injuries in the past, are returning home and getting rehabilitation services that include technologically advanced prosthetic devices.

Providing massage therapy in the context of treatment for a recent amputee recovering from surgery requires advanced training. However, clients who have lost limbs in the past may come for massage in any setting.

In the intake interview, get information about the limb loss. Ask how long ago it happened. Ask about the cause of the loss, which may uncover contraindications or cautions to be taken, and will help in session planning. If what remains of the limb, commonly called the *stump,* is to receive massage, find out more about the structure. For example, is there anything unusual about the muscles and

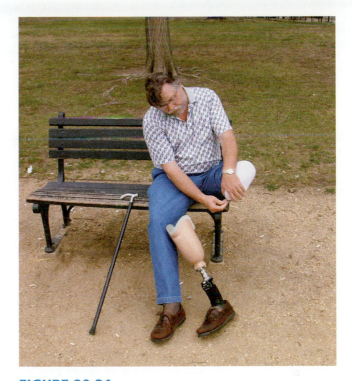

FIGURE 20.31

Amputee and his prosthetic limb.

bones involved? Ask if the stump is numb or sensitive to touch or pressure. The client will probably be able to tell you what will feel uncomfortable and what may feel good to the area. Ask if the client has any goals in mind related to the site of the amputation.

Ask if the client needs assistance in any way, for example, undressing or getting onto the table. Depending on the extent of the loss, the client may be very self-sufficient or may need assistance.

A client with an amputation may experience what is called phantom limb sensation, or phantom limb pain. That is experiencing sensation or pain in a limb that does not physically exist. The missing limb may feel shorter or distorted. The pain is occasional, and the incidence of the sensation usually diminishes over time. This is a neurological condition, and the overall calming effects of massage may help diminish phantom sensations.

Prostheses are artificial appliances that replace missing body parts (Figure 20.31■). The technology of these mechanical and electronic devices, especially those for the upper and lower extremities, can be quite advanced. Clients may or may not want to remove their prosthetic devices for massage. If they wear their devices, ask what precautions to take to avoid damaging them. If the device is removed, look for chafing, irritation, or skin lesions around the area of attachment. Avoid inflamed areas and breaks in the skin.

LUTHER

REALITY CHECK

SONIA: I feel totally inadequate to give massage to someone with special needs. I'm afraid I might say something inappropriate or hurt him or her. Can't I just take appointments from normal people?

LUTHER: I understand how you feel, but we don't always know ahead of time about our clients. And who's to say what normal is? I find that if I am open, honest, and respectful, and err on the side of caution, I do all right. The first time I had a client with a prosthetic leg, I wasn't sure what to do. I just stayed calm and asked her to tell me about her condition. I admitted that I had never massaged someone like her before and would need some direction about what to do and not to do. She had come in for relaxation massage and wasn't looking for anything related to her stump. When she left I did some research about amputees and was more informed the next time she came for an appointment. I've learned a lot through my career and take continuing education on different special populations when I can. You build confidence through experience.

INTERNAL AND EXTERNAL MEDICAL DEVICES

Medical devices may be positioned inside or outside of the body either temporarily or permanently. For example, hospital patients may have temporary urinary catheters or intravenous drips in place during their stays. A more permanent situation might be a heart disease patient with an implanted venous catheter or stent that keeps a blood vessel open.

Pacemakers and Defibrillators

Artificial pacemakers and defibrillators are implanted under the skin in the upper chest with wires attaching to the heart itself. These devices keep the heart beating at a regular rhythm. Avoid massage in the immediate vicinity of an internal or external medical device. Also avoid movements that disturb the device. Use gentle massage techniques in areas that are sensitive around the site of a device.

Colostomy Bag

A colostomy is a surgery in which the colon is attached directly to the anterior abdominal wall, leaving an opening on the abdomen called a *stoma*. Feces leave the colon through the stoma, and are collected in a **colostomy bag** attached to the outside of the body (Figure 20.32■). An ileostomy is similar except that the small intestine is attached to an opening in the abdominal wall. Clients with colostomies lower in the tract can often regulate their bowels. Colostomies and ileostomies may be temporary or permanent depending on the medical situation.

If a client has a colostomy or ileostomy, recommend that he or she not eat for about 2 hours prior to the appointment. Also suggest that he or she empty the bag before the session begins. Do not use lubricant around the stoma or bag opening to avoid weakening the adhesive that keeps the bag in place.

Use the side-lying position instead of prone to avoid pressure on the stoma. A protective pad under the bag area is a prudent step in case of accidental leakage. If a bag leaks or become detached, assist the client as needed to stabilize the situation. Use proper hygienic procedures, and use disposable glove and towels to sanitize any surface that becomes soiled. Keep a calm professional demeanor to minimize embarrassment to the client.

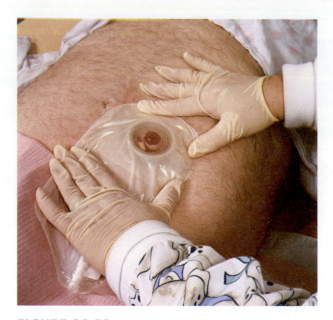

FIGURE 20.32

Colostomy bag attached to the abdomen.

REWARDS AND CHALLENGES

This chapter touched on just some of the many special populations that massage therapists encounter in their careers. Serving special populations can be rewarding and challenging at the same time. It reminds us that each individual is unique and provides the opportunity to practice patience and compassion. It offers an appreciation of the many difficult circumstances life can present. Serving special populations can be mentally stimulating as we learn about different human conditions and plan massage sessions to meet client goals. It challenges us to stretch our minds and learn new skills as we adapt to different situations.

Some massage therapists choose to specialize in a specific population as a special interest or marketing niche. Continuing education offers the opportunity to learn more about individual populations in greater depth.

CHAPTER HIGHLIGHTS

- A special population is a group of people with some distinctive life circumstance that sets them apart from a normal adult population.
  - This special circumstance can influence their goals for massage, may require adaptations to the session for safety or comfort, and may present contraindications.
- Clinical applications focus on treatment for a specific pathology or injury, while special populations may be interested in massage for reasons having nothing to do with their "special" circumstances.
- When working with special populations maintain an open, nonjudgmental, sensitive, and patient attitude.
- Five major applications of sports massage are recovery, remedial, rehabilitation, maintenance, and event.
  - Maintenance massage is an all-purpose massage received regularly that includes recovery and remedial applications.
  - Pre-event massage is upbeat and prepares an athlete for competition; postevent massage focuses on recovery.
- Massage can be given safely to healthy women with low risk pregnancies.
  - Warning signs for contraindications include abdominal pain, discharge, swelling, fever, nausea, and pitting edema.
  - Abdominal massage and joint movements are contraindicated throughout a pregnancy and for several weeks after delivery; other contraindications and cautions apply during different trimesters.
  - Use the side-lying or semireclining positions for pregnancy massage.
- Infant massage provides tactile and kinesthetic stimulation for healthy growth and development.
  - Infant massage is a simple, gentle yet firm application of stroking, pressing, squeezing, and movement of the limbs.

- Massage helps the elderly keep the strength and flexibility needed to do activities of daily living (ADL), and provides pleasurable social interaction.
  - Think of elders in terms of physiological age rather than chronological age.
  - Include massage techniques to improve circulation, promote relaxation, and improve mobility.
- Massage brings caring and comforting touch to the terminally ill and dying, and is a valuable complementary therapy in hospital, hospice, and home care.
  - Near the end of life, massage can provide comforting touch and communicate care and love in a nonverbal way.
  - Massage sessions with the dying should be softer, gentler, and shorter than a regular massage session.
- Physical impairments commonly encountered in massage practices include visual, hearing, speech, and mobility challenges.
- When clients fall outside of a normal size range, accommodations for their safety and general benefit are in order.
  - Excessively obese clients may be better positioned on a floor mat for massage.
- Assist clients with amputated limbs as needed, and watch for irritated or chafed skin at the site of attachment of prosthetic devices.
- Avoid sites around internal and external medical devices.
  - Position clients with colostomy bags in the side-lying position, and be prepared for hygienic cleanup if a bag leaks.
- Working with special populations challenges us to stretch our minds and learn new skills as we adapt to different situations.

EXAM REVIEW

Key Terms

To study the key terms listed at the beginning of this chapter, match the appropriate lettered meaning to each numbered key term listed below. For additional study, look up the key terms in the Interactive Glossary on page G-1 and note other terms that compare or contrast with them.

_____ 1. Adaptations
_____ 2. Colostomy bag
_____ 3. Disability
_____ 4. High-risk pregnancies
_____ 5. Infant massage
_____ 6. Mobility
_____ 7. Obesity
_____ 8. Physical impairment
_____ 9. Physiological age
_____ 10. Special population
_____ 11. Sports massage

a. Distinctive life circumstance that sets them apart from the norm
b. A person's age relative to his or her health status
c. Adjustments to the way things are normally done to meet the unique individual needs
d. Visual, hearing, speech, size, and mobility challenges
e. The mother or fetus is at higher than normal risk for complications or negative developments
f. An application specifically designed to meet the needs of athletes
g. External medical device
h. Provides kinesthetic and tactile stimulation for healthy growth and development
i. Unhealthy accumulation of fat tissue
j. An impairment that severely limits a person's ability to perform daily life activities
k. The ability to go from place to place independently

Memory Workout

To test your memory of the main concepts in this chapter, complete the following sentences by circling the most correct answer from the two choices provided.

1. Pre-event sports massage applications are typically (upbeat and stimulating) (calming and mild).
2. Use (unscented) (fragrant) oils and lotions when giving massage to pregnant women.
3. The pressure used for infant massage is gentle but (deep) (firm).
4. (Age appropriate) (Robust) elders show few outward signs of impaired health.
5. Programs designed to provide high quality palliative care to the dying are called (nursing homes) (hospice).
6. Perhaps the most important skill for people giving massage to the dying is their ability to (listen) (speak with authority).

7. When guiding a visually impaired person through a space, position yourself in front and to their (left) (right).
8. A person who comes for massage using a walker for balance, will (almost certainly) (not necessarily) need assistance getting onto and off of a standard massage table.
9. When giving massage to an extremely obese client, consider (raising) (lowering) your massage table to facilitate better body mechanics for you as you work.
10. If a client has a colostomy or ileostomy, recommend that he or she not eat for about two hours (after) (prior to) the massage appointment.

Test Prep

The following multiple-choice questions will help to prepare you for future school and professional exams.

1. Improving a debilitating condition such as muscle soreness and tension is the goal of what sports massage application?
   a. Pre-event
   b. Postevent
   c. Remedial
   d. Rehabilitation
2. If a pregnant woman has been on bed rest by a doctor's orders, massage of the legs is:
   a. Beneficial
   b. Contraindicated
   c. Indicated
   d. Welcomed by the recipient
3. In a normal pregnancy, which trimester is the safest and easiest part?
   a. First
   b. Second
   c. Third
   d. No significant difference
4. The following technique promotes bowel movement in infants:
   a. Foot massage
   b. Milking the legs
   c. Bringing the knees to the chest repeatedly
   d. Back massage
5. To avoid tearing or bruising skin that has thinned over time, it is advisable to use:
   a. Less pressure
   b. More pressure
   c. Generous amount of lotion or oil
   d. Both a and c

6. Which of the following is most important when giving massage to the terminally ill?
   a. Critical thinking
   b. Technical skill
   c. Using a wide variety of techniques
   d. Intuition and sensitivity
7. When speaking to someone with a hearing impairment do not:
   a. Speak more slowly
   b. Exaggerate your lip movements
   c. Speak a little louder
   d. Face the person directly
8. To better access chest muscles in women with large breasts, have them lie in this position.
   a. Side-lying
   b. Supine
   c. Prone
   d. Seated
9. When someone comes for massage in a wheelchair, the best approach is to:
   a. Give assistance before being asked to
   b. Assume they are helpless
   c. Ask about what assistance they might need
   d. Assume they have developed skills for complete independence
10. Pacemakers are medical devices that are typically:
    a. Hung externally on the chest
    b. Hung externally on the abdomen
    c. Implanted into the abdomen
    d. Implanted in the chest

Video Challenge

Watch the appropriate segment of the video on your DVD and then answer the following questions.

Special Populations and Adaptations

Postevent Sports Massage
1. In the postevent sports massage video, what did you notice about positioning that is different from standard relaxation massage? Why do you think it is done this way?

Pregnancy Massage
2. What massage techniques are shown in the video for addressing tight muscles in the low back of a pregnant woman?

Infant Massage
3. In the video showing infant massage, what techniques are used to massage the arms and legs? How does this differ from massage of the average adult?

Massage for the Elderly
4. In the video showing massage of an elderly person, how was he positioned and draped? What challenges did this present to the massage therapist in terms of the massage application and of maintaining good body mechanics?

Gentle Hand and Arm Massage
5. What qualities of touch can you see in the massage application demonstrated in the video? In what other ways does the massage therapist convey caring?

Comprehension Exercises

The following short answer questions test your knowledge and understanding of chapter topics and provide practice in written communication skills. Explain in two to four complete sentences.

1. Explain some of the restrictions on massage applications for pregnant women. Relate those restrictions to the physiology of pregnancy.

2. Describe how skin changes as we age. What precautions should be taken during massage to avoid damage to the skin of an elderly recipient?

3. What questions would you include in an intake interview with a man who is wearing a prosthetic device on his leg? How might his answers impact session plans?

For Greater Understanding

The following exercises are designed to take you from the realm of theory into the real world. They will help give you a deeper understanding of the subjects covered in this chapter. Action words are underlined to emphasize the variety of activities presented to address different learning styles and to encourage deeper thinking.

1. Observe treatment of athletes at a sports medicine rehabilitation center. Note the roles of physical therapists, athletic trainers, and massage therapists in the setting. How are the roles different? How are they similar? How did different therapists use massage? What adjunct therapies were offered?

2. Observe people of a variety of ages in a public place such as a park or shopping mall. Note differences in the way they move, their posture, and other visible characteristics. Compare and contrast children, young adults, older adults, and the elderly. Describe any physical impairments you observe.

3. Interview a health professional who is working or who has worked with the terminally ill or dying. Ask the individual about the type of setting and his or her personal challenges working in that environment. What were the patients' greatest needs? Inquire about the role of massage, if any, where he or she worked, and the potential benefits of massage for this special population. Discuss your findings with a study partner or group.

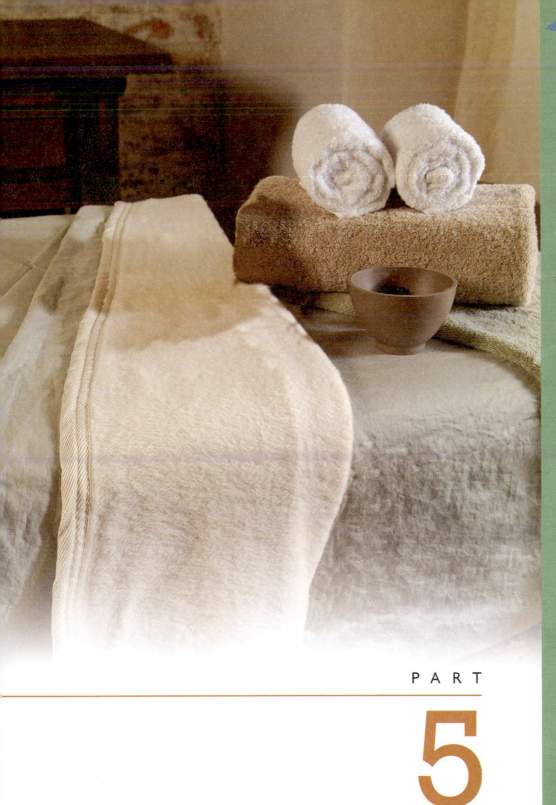

PART

5

Career and Practice Development

21   Career Plans and Employment

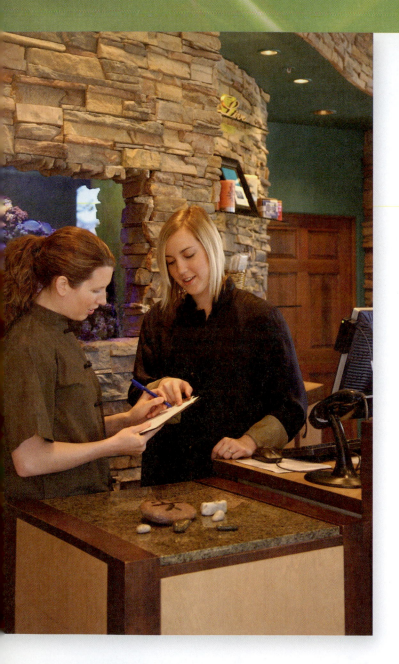

 CHAPTER OUTLINE

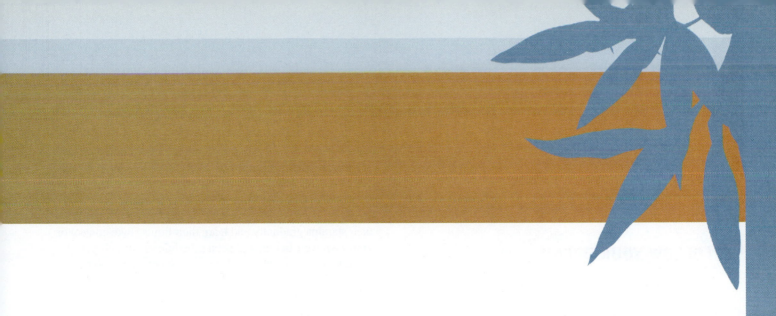

 ## LEARNING OUTCOMES

After studying this chapter, you will have information to:

1. Develop career plans for the first year after graduation.
2. Create a vision and identity for a massage practice.
3. Identify the benefits and drawbacks of employment and self-employment.
4. Design a résumé, business card, and brochure.
5. Locate and secure employment as a massage therapist.

 ## KEY TERMS

Employee *612*

Income goal *615*

Independent contractor *613*

Mission statement *615*

Practice identity *616*

Private practice *613*

Résumé *617*

Self-employed *613*

Sole proprietor *613*

Vision *612*

MASSAGE *in* ACTION

On your DVD, explore:

- Developing a Business Plan
- Employment Interview
- Getting Started in Your Career

FOLLOW YOUR DREAM

Career plans begin with a dream—imagining the possibilities for your future as a massage therapist. Making that dream come true takes planning, effort, and perseverance. Career plans provide direction to achieving success step-by-step.

As described in Chapter 1, there are many career possibilities for massage therapists. Some work full time and some part time. Some look for certain settings such as spas, health clubs, integrative health care clinics, or private practice. Some prefer to focus on specific populations such as athletes, the elderly, people with certain diseases, or those in rehabilitation from musculoskeletal injuries. Others focus on a specific type of massage and bodywork, such as Western massage, Asian bodywork therapy, reflexology, or chair massage. Many choose eclectic practices with a variety of clients and types of massage. There are many options.

A good place to begin career plans is to formulate your practice vision and identity. Focus for now on the first year after graduation. You can always revise the plan later on as you become more experienced and your vision evolves, but it is important to make a decision and choose a place to start.

VISION

All aspects of your practice flow from your vision. Your **vision** is how you see your practice in its broad scope. It includes whether you work full time or part time, your practice format, the setting you are working in, your clients, what kind of massage you offer, and your income goals. The clearer the vision, the more likely you will be to achieve your career dreams one year after graduation and for each year of your practice into the future. A worksheet for outlining your practice vision is provided in Figure 21.1■.

Part-Time or Full-Time Work

Massage therapists can have successful careers working full time or part time. Full-time work can be thought of as earning most or all of your income doing massage therapy. However, it is not as simple as a 40-hour workweek. For a private practice, figure full-time work in terms of client load at about 15–20 clients per week, spending 90 minutes on setup, massage, and cleanup for an hour appointment. That comes to 22–30 hours per week. Add in another 1–2 hours per day for related activities, such as client notes, bookkeeping, and

marketing your practice. Full-time employment may be 4–5 days per week, seeing several clients each day at a place such as a spa, health club, or other facility.

It is important to keep in mind that because massage therapy is physically and emotionally demanding, taking more than 20 clients per week for 1-hour massage can put you at risk for injury, stress, and burnout. While some massage therapists may be able to handle more clients per week safely, massage therapists starting out are wise to build their stamina gradually and learn their limits. Take control of your own well-being, and set a schedule that is full yet reasonable. Figure on at least 1 day of rest per week and a minimum of 2–3 weeks of vacation per year. When you plan your budget for the year, figure in your scheduled holidays and vacation time.

Part-time work as a massage therapist can be a fulfilling way to supplement other income. Some massage therapists choose part-time work because they have another job that they do not want to give up, family responsibilities, or other time commitments. Part-time work ranges anywhere from 1–10 clients per week and accounts for part of your income or part of a total household income. You might work 2 nights at a spa, or take a few private clients per week. There are a variety of options for the part-time massage therapist.

Some massage therapists start out working part time while keeping a steady job doing something else, and then gradually develop a full-time practice. Some work part time in two different careers or jobs, or part time while pursuing advanced education. Formulating a career plan takes into consideration whether working full time or part time as a massage therapist is the goal and how best to go about making that happen. Flexible scheduling is a major benefit of a career in massage therapy.

Employment or Private Practice

Practice formats include regular employment and self-employment in private practice. Many massage therapists have a combined practice, for example, part-time employment combined with a private practice for a full-time career. Each practice format has its upsides and downsides.

Regular employment can be found in spas, resorts, integrative health care clinics, and other settings that offer massage. The Internal Revenue Service (IRS) glossary says that an **employee** "works for an employer. Employers can control when, where, and how the employee performs the work" (www.irs.gov). Employers set prices, assign work schedules, book clients, provide equipment and supplies, advertise services, and generally take care of the business side of the practice. Employers may also dictate the type of massage offered to clients, set a dress code, or impose other restrictions. Massage therapist employees perform massage as scheduled and, in some cases, may be required to do other work such as paperwork, cleaning, or staffing a reception desk.

The upsides of regular employment are a stable hourly wage; low or no expenses for space, equipment, and supplies; potential for health insurance and vacation benefits;

FIGURE 21.1

Vision worksheet.

Vision of Massage Therapy Practice for

_____
Name of massage therapist / Practice

Dates _____ to _____
     Month/Day/Year   Month/Day/Year

Size

    ☐ Full time—hours/clients per week _____

    ☐ Part time—hours/clients per week_____

Format

    ☐ Employee (preferred setting) _____
    ☐ Self-employed (private practice—sole proprietor/independent contractor)
    ☐ Combination

      _____ % employed (# days/clients per week _____)

      _____ % self-employed (#days/clients per week _____)

Mission Statement (Purpose/Focus and Competitve Edge)

_____

_____

_____

_____

    Annual Income Goal

    ☐ <$5,000   amount $ _____

    ☐ $ 5,000–10,000   amount $ _____

    ☐ $10,000–20,000   amount $ _____

    ☐ $20,000–30,000   amount $ _____

    ☐ $30,000–40,000   amount $ _____

    ☐ $40,000–50,000   amount $ _____

    ☐ >$50,000   amount $ _____

and having much of the business of massage taken care of by the employer. In addition, employers pay a portion of social security taxes (FICA). Downsides include no control over massage fees, less time flexibility, and less control over the schedule and work environment. Employees do not take home all of the fees that clients pay, but also do not have the extra expenses, responsibilities, and risks that self-employed massage therapists do.

You are considered **self-employed** if you carry on your practice as a sole proprietor or an independent contractor. Self-employment is sometimes referred to as being in **private practice.**

As a **sole proprietor,** you are the legally recognized business owner—the employer and employee rolled into one. This form of practice offers maximum flexibility for creating your own workspace, choosing clientele, controlling the type of massage offered, setting the schedule, and determining fees. You also have sole responsibility for building an adequate client base, complying with government regulations, completing paperwork and bookkeeping, and paying required taxes. Being a sole proprietor means being a self-starter and self-motivator and taking responsibility for getting things done.

An **independent contractor** performs services for another person or business, but is not an employee. Independent contractors are self-employed. They are contracted to accomplish a certain result, but are not under the direct control of an employer. An example of an independent contract situation for a massage therapist would be if a business hired a massage therapist to come to its office or workplace to give chair massage to employees on Employee Appreciation Day.

CASE FOR STUDY

Roberta and Her Dream Practice

Roberta has participated in sports all her life, from junior soccer to high school volleyball. She loves to work out and enjoys being around athletes. Her dream practice as a massage therapist is to work with athletes either in a health club, professional sports setting, or private practice.

Question:

What can Roberta do to increase her chances of achieving her dream practice after graduation?

Things to consider:

- What expertise will potential employers and clients look for on her résumé?
- Could her grades in any particular subjects be important to a potential employer?
- How important might it be for her to keep up her own fitness level?
- What part-time jobs might she get for general experience in sports settings?
- What kind of volunteer work might she do to demonstrate experience with sports massage to a potential employer?
- What type of specialty training might she seek out?
- How can she create a professional identity to match her dream?
- What might her mission statement look like?

Ideas for realizing Roberta's dream practice:

_____

_____

_____

Some businesses use the independent contractor format rather than taking on the added expense of hiring massage therapists as employees. This applies to massage therapists who hire other massage therapists in order to expand their practices. The United States has labor laws that define when this is legal and when it is not, that is, when persons can be considered independent contractors and when they must be treated as employees.

Just declaring someone an independent contractor does not make him or her one in the eyes of the law. The courts have developed a strategy called the "dominant impression test" to distinguish between employees and independent contractors. No single factor determines status, but several factors taken together are considered for their overall effect. The following are some factors that help define employment:

- Instructions given about when, where, and how to perform the work
- Training provided
- Integration into the business operation
- Services rendered personally by the worker
- Set work hours and schedule
- Oral or written reports required
- Significant tools, material, and equipment furnished
- Right to discharge the worker at will
- Work performed on the business premises
- Ongoing relationship
- Working for or supplying services to only one business

The National Employers' Association offers a discussion of this issue in an article called "Employers beware, you can't have your cake and eat it too!" It looks at the implication of different provisions of the Labor Relations Act (www.neasa-sa.com).

Why is it important for massage therapists to understand the difference between employees and independent contractors? One reason is to know if you are being treated fairly and legally by a potential employer. Massage therapists can be taken advantage of by employers who are just trying to avoid the responsibility and expense of having additional employees. Another reason is that if you want to expand your business by hiring other massage therapists, you will want to know the applicable labor laws. The U.S. government imposes monetary penalties on businesses that misrepresent employee status. Consult a lawyer for advice on whether a dominant impressions test for a certain situation points to employment or an independent contractor arrangement.

How do you determine which format is best for you starting out in your career? Only you can decide, but these are some factors to consider. Look for employment if you want to focus on clients rather than business tasks, or if you are looking for steady work with some benefits. Employment gives you immediate income with minimal or no startup costs. Also, if you have little work or business experience, you can learn the basics by working for someone else first.

Consider self-employment if you are self-motivated and like your independence. It helps to have prior business experience, good contacts or a natural ability to network, and the necessary skills to build a business from the ground up. Startup money is important to get a practice off and running. Private practices are not built in a day, but hard work and perseverance can lead to satisfying results.

Some massage therapists have short-term and longer-term plans, which might entail starting out with part-time employment while building knowledge and skills with an eye

TABLE 21.1	Comparison of Employment and Self-Employment Requirements, Upsides, and Downsides			
Practice Format	Requirements	Upsides		Downsides
Employment	• Successful interview • Meet employer expectations and obey policies • Cooperate with coworkers • Be reliable in attendance • Satisfy customers and employer	• Stable hourly wage • Low overhead • Employer pays portion of FICA • Employer advertises and schedules clients • Employer handles government regulations such as business or massage establishment license • Potential health insurance & vacation benefits • Shared client-base building with employer		• No control over fees, schedule, environment • Less time flexibility • Imposed dress code
Self-Employment 　Sole proprietor 　Independent contractor	• Business skills • Self-motivation • Discipline • Perseverance • Patience • Ability to satisfy clients	• Control over fees, policies and procedures and type of massage offered • Create own environment • Personal choice about clientele • Set own schedule		• Income less predictable • Expenses for space, equipment, and supplies • Keep own records • Build own client base • Provide own health insurance • Pay self-employment tax

toward building a private practice in the future. Table 21.1■ compares different practice formats.

Mission Statement

A useful approach to clarifying your vision is to write a **mission statement.** A mission statement consists of one to three sentences defining the purpose of your practice and your main strategy for achieving competitive advantage. It answers the questions, "What is the focus of this practice?" and "Why would clients come to me (or why would an employer hire me) instead of someone else?"

A good mission statement narrows your focus and keeps you on a straight path toward your goal. A personal mission statement can lead you to employment in a particular setting or working with a certain type of client. A mission statement for a private practice serves as a reference point for the many decisions that must be made, and it defines who you are as a massage therapist. In a combined practice, your mission statement may have two different parts, or you may maintain a coherent mission throughout your practice. Box 21.1● contains some examples of mission statements.

Since your mission statement directs your path, it is worth taking time to create one that truly reflects your current interests and talents. Write several drafts of your statement until it seems right for you at this time in your career.

Income Goal

An **income goal** specifies how much money you need or want from the practice in a certain time period, such as a year. This figure will guide you in many important choices, such as whether to work full time or part time, whether to accept a certain job, or how many clients need to be scheduled per week. Income goals go hand in hand with mission statements in filling out the vision of a viable massage therapy practice.

Since massage therapists work both part time and full time, the range for potential income is wide. Income goals should be as realistic as possible. For example, a person in private practice has to build a client base, so the income for the first year or two will probably be less than it will be once the practice matures.

Projecting your personal expenses for the first year helps you determine how much money you need to bring in. That involves calculating, month by month, such expenses as rent, food, transportation, health care, personal services, recreation, loan payments, and other essentials. Be as realistic and detailed as possible. Since the cost of living differs in different parts of the country, and for cities and smaller towns, these projections will vary for different people.

For the first year, figure in startup costs for the practice. Startup costs are discussed in detail on page 635 in Chapter 22, Private Practice and Finances. Take into consideration the income from another job or business and whether you share personal expenses with someone else. When all things are considered, determine how much you need to make from the massage therapy practice to pay the bills and have some discretionary money.

BOX 21.1   Examples of Mission Statements

Employed

My mission as a massage therapist is to apply my training to help clients achieve optimal wellness within the spa environment. Continuing education and active membership in professional associations keep my knowledge and skills about massage and bodywork in spas up-to-date and responsive to consumer trends.

My mission as a massage therapist is to apply my skills as part of an integrative team of health professionals in a medical practice environment. Advanced training in manual methods of pain management and musculoskeletal conditions provide me with knowledge and skills necessary to treat patients in rehabilitation.

Self-Employed

My mission as a massage therapist is to apply my knowledge and skills to help clients achieve optimal wellness. Affordable massage therapy is offered in a clean, pleasant, and relaxing environment. This is a community-centered and family-based private practice welcoming people of all ages.

My mission is to help clients heal from illness and injury through massage therapy. Advanced approaches to healing through manual therapies are applied in a caring and competent manner. Collaboration with other health professionals ensures safe and effective treatment.

The mission of Office Oasis Massage is to relieve the stress of office workers by providing high-quality chair massage at a convenient time and place. In addition to relaxation, therapeutic applications focus on muscular aches and pains resulting from sitting at a desk for a major part of the workday. We create an oasis for rejuvenation in the midst of the workplace.

The mission of Gold Medal Sports Massage is to improve athletes' performance, and to prevent and treat sports-related injuries through massage therapy. Athletes receive personal attention from highly skilled sports massage professionals who understand their needs and competitive drive. We earn the athletes' confidence by producing observable results.

REALITY CHECK

KELLY

MAURICE: I'm trying to write a vision for my future practice, but can't quite get a clear picture. I just want to get a job as a massage therapist when I graduate. Isn't that enough?

KELLY: I would encourage you to look further than just getting a job somewhere where you may or not be happy in the longer term. Let yourself dream a little about your ideal situation after you graduate. What type of settings are you attracted to? What settings would you not like to work in? Look around at massage therapists who have built practices that you admire. Find a role model about whom you can say, "Yes, that's what I want to be doing in the future." Your vision will become clearer to you as you get a sense of the possibilities.

IDENTITY

Practice identity flows from your vision and is the image you project to the world. It includes such things as business name and logo, credentials, résumé, business cards and stationery, and a website. It includes your dress and office decoration.

Even the color and quality of your sheets and the music you play reflect your practice identity.

Business Name and Logo

Your business name should take into consideration your vision and your potential market. It could be as simple as your name, for example, Robin P. Jones or Alex Lipinsky. A practice name could include your location, for example, Granite City Massage Therapy. Or it might contain some natural characteristic you want associated with your practice, for example, sky, water, clouds, rain, or earth. It might suggest the type of massage and bodywork you offer, such as quiet space, workplace oasis, or relief center. If you are choosing a business name that is not your own name, check with state or local authorities, and the U.S. Patent and Trademark Office to make sure the name is not already taken (www.uspto.gov).

A *logo* is a symbol that identifies you and your practice at a glance. Your logo could be original artwork that you commissioned, paid for, and trademarked, or it could be chosen from clip art in the public domain. Printers usually have books of clip art from which people can choose a design or graphic for their business cards and stationery. Some people use stylized versions of their initials for their logos. Your business name and logo are used on business cards, stationery, brochures, and your website.

Credentials

Information about credentials and the ethics related to their use are found on page 13 in Chapter 1, The Massage Therapy Profession, and page 650 in Chapter 23, Business Ethics.

Remember that credentials are titles awarded for achievements and meeting professional standards. Use them correctly to advertise yourself to potential clients, other health professionals, and the general public. Credentials can be sought and earned to build an identity in concert with your mission.

Résumé

A **résumé** is a written summary of education, experience, achievements, professional memberships, and other information relevant to application for a job, volunteer position, or other occasion where someone wants a snapshot of your identity. A résumé contains selected pieces of information and not your entire personal history. It is formatted so that the reader can easily scan it at a glance for pertinent information.

It is important to have an up-to-date résumé on hand. In addition to accompanying job applications, résumés can be displayed on websites for massage therapy practices, among other uses. Figure 21.2■ shows typical categories and content for massage therapists' résumés.

The basic elements of a résumé include general information such as name, address, phone number, e-mail and/or

FIGURE 21.2

Sample of résumé content.

```
                            Name
                        Mailing Address
                     City, State, Zip Code
                       Telephone Number
                     E-mail Address/Website

                           RÉSUMÉ

[Optional: Mission Statement or Employment Goal]

EDUCATION (reverse chronological order)
    Certificate/Date                  School Name
                                       Massage Program Name
                                       City/State

    Degree/Date                        College Name
                                       City/State
                                       Major/Minor

    Diploma/Date                       High School Name
                                       City/State


EMPLOYMENT (reverse chronological order)
    Dates                              Employer or Self-Employed
                                       City/State
                                       Job title/Responsibilities
    Dates                              Employer or Self-Employed
                                       City/State
                                       Job title/Responsibilities

PROFESSIONAL AFFILIATIONS, LICENSE, CERTIFICATIONS, HONORS
    Date                               Massage License, State, Number
    Date                               Certification Name, Organization, City/State
    Date                               Professional Organization Membership, Level
    Date                               Award, Organization

VOLUNTEER EXPERIENCE
    Date                               Organization
                                       City/State
                                       Responsibilities

    Date                               Organization
                                       City/State
                                       Responsibilities


LEISURE ACTIVITIES
    Activities

        References available upon request.
```

website address. Current practice is *not* to include your age, year of birth, marital status or family information, or social security number.

A detailed résumé contains dates, places, degrees, job titles, and credentials. It shows the depth of your knowledge and skills, past responsibilities and accomplishments, areas of expertise, and other elements for your identity as a massage therapist.

Education and training are listed in reverse chronological order. This section lists dates of attendance or graduation, school name and place, name of the course of study or program, and the degree or certificate earned. Program accreditation can be indicated. Sometimes formal education like college attendance is separated from massage therapy training.

Work experience is also listed in reverse chronological order. This section lists dates, employers' names, job titles and responsibilities, and special achievements. It is often useful to list your military service and record. Massage therapy experience and other types of work may be separated into two different sections.

Credentials, including occupational licenses and specialty certifications, professional memberships, and special awards and achievements, are listed to build your identity further. Potential employers will be looking for required licenses and training in desired specialties. Professional memberships show a level of commitment to the profession, and awards indicate outside recognition of your achievements.

Volunteer experience is important for those with limited work experience and also shows an altruistic commitment to the community. Volunteer work relevant to massage therapy includes activities such as outreach programs and officer or committee work in professional associations. Community volunteer experience might include work with the American Red Cross, a local food pantry, or an animal shelter.

Optional information includes hobbies, leisure activities, and other interests. These further define you as a person and may help your résumé stand out in a pile of otherwise similar résumés.

RÉSUMÉ DESIGN

Good résumés are simple in design and concise—one or two pages. They use a consistent format for margins and headings, and leave plenty of white space to avoid looking crowded. The font chosen for the text is easily readable. Word processing features such as bold, italics, underlining, and capital letters are used conservatively to prevent too much visual distraction.

Remember that résumés are designed to be read at a glance. The main divisions within a well-organized résumé stand out and are easily located. Reverse chronological order is used for items such as education and work experience, so that the most recent items are on top, and work history is traced backward by skimming down the list.

Unfamiliar abbreviations, symbols, or initials after a name are avoided, and entries are spelled out fully for the reader. For example, the initials *LMP*, used in some states, should be spelled out as *Licensed Massage Practitioner*. The same applies to organization names; for example,

AMTA should be spelled out as *American Massage Therapy Association*, and *ABMP* as *Associated Bodywork and Massage Professionals*.

Grammatical style is consistent, especially elements such as verb tense and punctuation. Grammar, spelling, and typographical errors are avoided by looking over the résumé carefully. Remember that your résumé is part of your identity and should reflect your best efforts.

BUILDING AN IMPRESSIVE RÉSUMÉ

The résumé can serve as a vehicle for planning professional growth. A look at your current résumé can bring to mind ideas for what education, work or volunteer experience, certification, or other addition would make it more attractive to a potential employer or client. Seek opportunities that demonstrate professional development and add them as they are completed. Use your mission statement as a guide. Keep the résumé in electronic form so that it can be updated easily and as often as needed.

Be sure that everything that appears on your résumé is true, and there is nothing misleading. Honesty and accuracy are expected in an ethical massage therapist.

Business Cards and Stationery

Business cards may be the single most important marketing device for building a client base. Business cards give clients and prospective clients essential information about you and how to contact you for appointments. They reflect who you are as a massage therapist.

A business card packs a lot of information into 2.5 × 3 inches of space. A typical card has your name and/or business name, address if you have an office, phone number to call for appointments, and other contact information such as e-mail address and website. It may list the type of massage and bodywork you offer and important certification and license information. The design may include a logo or graphic element. A sample business card design is shown in Figure 21.3■.

As with résumés, readable and simple business cards are best. Use fonts large enough for everyone to read. Do not

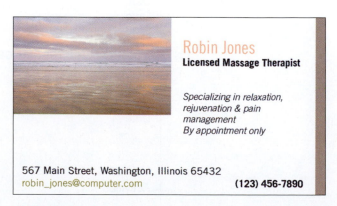

Robin Jones
Licensed Massage Therapist

*Specializing in relaxation, rejuvenation & pain management
By appointment only*

567 Main Street, Washington, Illinois 65432
robin_jones@computer.com   **(123) 456-7890**

FIGURE 21.3

Sample of a business card design.

let design elements and color detract from the essential information. However, a unique and attractive design may make a favorable impression.

Remember that most clients want to think that their massage therapist is professional, trustworthy, and competent. A well-designed business card communicates that impression.

A spa, health club, clinic, or other business that employs massage therapists may provide standard business cards with its name and logo. Since you still have to build a client base at a place of employment, business cards are important to have available there, too.

Although stationery may not be important for massage therapists who are employed full time, anyone in private practice should have stationery on hand for official correspondence. The design, color, and general impression should match business cards, brochures, and website elements to present a coherent identity.

Brochures and Websites

Brochures and websites give potential clients more detailed information about massage therapists and their private practices. With word processing programs and digital photography, a massage therapist can create attractive brochures that reflect a practice identity. A simple trifold brochure can be printed on standard 8.5 × 11 heavyweight paper and copied in color.

A typical brochure for a massage therapy practice might have a cover page with the name and/or business name, address, phone number to call for appointments, and other contact information such as e-mail address and website. Photos of the massage therapist, the reception area and massage room, and other relevant images can be included. Other ideas include descriptions of the type of massage and bodywork offered, more detail on credentials, possible goals for massage sessions, policies, appointment times, and fees. Plan on updating a brochure about once per year.

Websites serve the same general purpose as brochures and may be more accessible to potential clients. Someone thinking about making an appointment with you may want to check your website for a better sense of you and your practice. Poten-tial employers may also check out your website. Websites can hold more information than brochures, such as complete résumés, testimonials, fuller explanations of services, and more photos. They can have special features such as links to other sites that have information about the type of massage therapy you offer.

Developing technology is making website creation more user-friendly and economical. Check out websites for other massage therapists as you plan your website design to see what the options are. Make sure that your website reflects your practice identity and that your image and information is consistent throughout your marketing materials. Website designers can be hired to help you set up your website. Some professional associations offer website hosting as a service to members. More information about marketing a private practice can be found on page 630 in Chapter 22, Private Practice and Finances.

GETTING EMPLOYMENT

Getting employment as a massage therapist is a step-by-step process that begins with finding the job opening and then interviewing successfully. It entails locating openings, filling out job applications, submitting résumés, writing cover letters, presenting references, getting interviews, and interviewing well.

Your school's placement department may have a listing of local employers and openings for massage therapists. Job postings for massage therapists can also be found in places such as local newspapers, professional journals and magazines, and some websites listing employment opportunities. Networking with other massage therapists can lead to hearing about job opportunities.

As you survey the job market, think about the vision for your practice and whether it leads you toward certain types of jobs or settings. If possible, narrow your search to the types of jobs that best fit your career plan. You can also be proactive in identifying where you would like to work, and then inquiring about how to go about getting a job there.

Once a potential job situation is identified, your focus is on getting a job interview. Steps to the interview typically

CRITICAL THINKING

Analyze the identity or image of several different massage practices in your area. Look at résumés, business cards, brochures, and websites.

1. What do they say to potential clients about the massage therapist and his or her practice?

2. Is the image presented consistent with the reality of the practice?

3. Can you think of ways to create a more attractive identity for this practice?

4. What ideas would you consider using to create the identity of your own future practice?

involve filling out a job application and/or submitting a résumé and references.

A job application is a preprinted form used by companies to get essential information for screening job applicants. It gives employers a standard format to more easily compare applicants and narrow down the pool before looking at résumés. Even though much of the information asked for may be on your résumé, do not write in "see résumé." The purpose of the form is for employers to easily see relevant information to determine if they want to look at your résumé. If the application is incomplete, they may not look any further. Fill in all information neatly and accurately. An employer may also want to see if you can read and follow directions, and how good are your written communication skills, such as grammar and spelling.

If the application asks why you want the job, take time to think about your answer. Let the employer know that you understand the job requirements, that you are familiar with the company and want to work there, and that you are a good match for the job. Be honest about your schooling and credentials. Misrepresentation is not only unethical but may have legal consequences. Many states require massage therapists to disclose prior criminal offenses to obtain licenses. Do not lie about past convictions on your job application. That is fraud and would later be grounds for immediate dismissal.

A potential employer may also ask for your résumé. If possible, submit it with a cover letter written in business letter format on good stationery. In the letter, introduce yourself, detail your qualifications, and state your interest in the job. Try to find out who is actually doing the hiring, and address the letter to that person. Show your knowledge about the company and the nature of the job. An employer will be impressed that you did your homework. Be sure to include your contact information and good times to call you.

References are good to have. These are people who know you personally, can recommend your work, and give a prospective employer information about you. References can be former employers, coworkers, people from volunteer and community work, teachers, or anyone who can give relevant information about your work, character, and factors relevant to the job. Never use family members as references. Later in your career, satisfied clients may also be willing to write letters of recommendation.

Keep two to three letters of reference on hand to include with a résumé or take to an interview. Prospective employers may want to contact your references personally for verification and for further information. It is a good idea to call your references to ask their permission to use their names and to let them know what job you've applied for and when they might expect to be contacted by the employer.

Your answering machine or voice mail message should be one that you would want a prospective employer to hear. Remember that employers may call to arrange an interview or to ask questions.

Once prospective employers know that you are a job candidate, they notice how you dress and act. The impression you make stays with you. Even before a job interview, appear neat and well groomed to a potential employer, for example, when dropping off a résumé or inquiring about a place like a spa or clinic (Figure 21.4■).

Realize that employers often use the Internet to check job applicants. Internet search engines can find your name in newspaper articles, official notices, and in other website postings. Social networking sites may also be able to be accessed by others. Be aware of your Internet profile, and do not post anything that might be embarrassing if seen by a potential employer.

A direct call to a manager or person hiring for a job may be useful. You can inquire if your information was received and if you need to send anything else. This gives the person a chance to hear your voice and talk to you personally.

Successful Job Interviews

Job interviews are a two-way street. The massage therapist is evaluating whether the job offers what he or she is looking for, and the employer is determining whether the massage therapist has the knowledge and skills for the position and will fit well into the work environment

Before going for an interview, write down questions you would like answered about the job, benefits, pay, and other important factors. The following are things you might want to consider.

- What types of clients/patients come to the spa/clinic/office? What are they looking for from massage therapy? Does that fit your knowledge and skills, mission and identity?
- What exactly will your duties be? Will anything else in addition to doing massage therapy be required?
- How many massages will you be expected to do in a day? How much time will you have between massages?

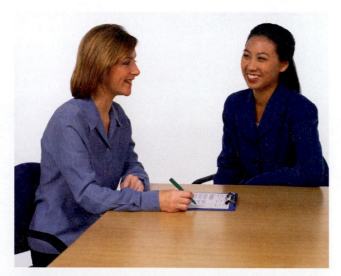

FIGURE 21.4
Appear professional and organized for a job interview.

- What paperwork is involved? Are SOAP notes required?
- Will you interact with other health professionals?
- What is your likely schedule? What days and times?
- What is the dress code? Are uniforms required and provided?
- What are the policies about sick days and vacations?
- Who will your supervisor be?
- What are the terms of your wages? Is this true employment or would you be as an independent contractor? How often are you paid? Is there a policy about tips?
- Are there any benefits (e.g., health insurance, 401k or other retirement plan, vacation pay)?
- Do they have an employee policy manual?
- Are there any additional perks (e.g., use of spa or health club, free parking)?

To further prepare for the interview, plan what you will wear. Choose clothes that fit well into the environment in which you would be working. Find out in advance if you will be expected to give the interviewer a massage. If so, arrive dressed appropriately or be ready to change into proper clothes for giving massage.

Review the materials you sent to the employer. Bring copies to the interview so that you can refer to them if you forget something. Bring letters of recommendation if you did not send them before. Also bring your massage therapy license if one is required in the employer's area. Arrange any papers you bring to the interview neatly in a folder so that you appear organized. To boost confidence and practice your verbal responses, role-play the interview with another massage therapist or friend.

On the day of the interview, arrive a little early to settle in and relax. Greet the interviewer by name if you know it. Be prepared to answer the following common interview questions:

- "Tell me a little about yourself and your background in massage."
- "How did you hear about this job?"
- "What types of massage therapy are you trained in?"
- "What makes you qualified for this job?"
- "Why do you want this job?"
- "How do you think you'll fit in here?"
- "When are you available to work?"
- "What are your salary requirements?"

A massage therapist often is asked to give a massage to the interviewer or someone else connected to the employer. This is reasonable since the employer is hiring the massage therapist for his or her skills. Before the massage session, ask if the employer or hiring person would like you to do a health history interview, or if the person receiving the massage has a file you can review. Even if the employer or interviewer says to go ahead with the massage without a health history, do a brief verbal screening for contraindications and ask the person to clarify what he or she wants from the mas-

sage. It is important to know the employer or interviewer's expectations so you can plan the session accordingly. He or she may be looking for specific things in your massage.

Be very careful in responding to questions and requests. A potential employer may be testing to see how well you keep professional boundaries, or how you handle inappropriate behavior. Be confident and act professionally at all times.

ILLEGAL INTERVIEW QUESTIONS

It is wise to be informed about interview questions that courts have determined to be discriminatory in nature and illegal to ask. Federal and state laws attempt to ensure that job candidates are hired based solely on their qualifications for the job. Discrimination in hiring typically is prohibited based on certain factors such as marital status, family responsibilities, plans for pregnancy, child care arrangements, age, gender, sexual orientation, nationality, ethnic background, and disability. Comments about one's weight, height, and grooming are also not appropriate. See the National Labor Relations Board (www.nlrb.gov) and the U.S. Equal Employment Opportunity Commission (www.eeoc.gov) websites and similar agencies in your state for further information on illegal hiring practices.

Appropriate questions are directly related to job qualifications and are usually general in nature. The following are acceptable questions:

- "Do you have any responsibilities that will limit what days or times you can work?"
- "Are you prepared to perform four or five massages in a day?"
- "If you are hired, could you provide verification of your right to work in the United States?"
- "Do you have training in working with the elderly?"

If you think the interviewer has asked an illegal question, you have various options for responding. It may have been an innocent mistake by an untrained interviewer or a truly discriminatory inquiry.

Depending on the situation, you can steer your answer more toward what you think the interviewer is trying to get at or what you want the person to know about you. For example, a good response to "How old are you?" might be "After I finished high school I completed my massage training and am well prepared for the responsibilities of this job." Or you could respond "Is there an age requirement for the job?" This question steers the interviewer back to job qualifications.

If you feel there is potential for illegal discrimination for some reason, it is wise to practice your responses to illegal questions. Planning ahead and good communication skills will help you complete job interviews with confidence.

AFTER THE INTERVIEW

If the job is offered to you after the interview, your possible responses are yes, no, or I have to think about it. Before you accept a job offer, be sure that the job meets your require-

PRACTICAL APPLICATION

Role-play job interviews with a study partner or friend. Use specific job postings to add some reality to the exercise. Write out expected questions and even some illegal questions for your interviewer to ask. Practice your responses aloud. Rehearse your responses until you have confidence in your ability to answer them well.

Keep in mind that the purpose of a job interview is not only to answer questions posed by the interviewer, but also to ask questions that will allow you to determine if the job you are applying for is right for you. What questions will you ask your interviewer to find out more about the job expectations, the working environment, clients, benefits, and so on?

Now switch roles with your study partner.

1. Critique each other's answers to the interview questions. Constructively brainstorm together about how your answers could be improved.
2. Take careful note of which types of questions were the most difficult to answer and plan to practice these until you are satisfied that you can answer them well.

ments in terms of your vision and income goals. If you have done your homework and are sure the job is everything you have been looking for, do not be afraid to say yes right away. If you have any doubts, take time to talk it over with friends or family and think about your decision.

If the job is not offered to you right away, feel free to call back in a day or two to see how things stand. They may have hired someone else or may have more interviews to do. Calling to inquire shows continued interest and keeps your name visible.

If you do not get the job, call and ask if the employer or hiring person would share with you why you were not hired or what would have made you a more desirable candidate. The company may have found someone more qualified or who was available for more days or hours. Take it as a learning experience to increase your chances of success in the future.

CHAPTER HIGHLIGHTS

- A massage therapist's career plans begin with formulating the vision and identity of a future practice.
  - The practice may be full time or part time and may consist of regular employment, self-employment, or a combination of the two.
  - The mission statement defines the purpose of the practice and the main strategy for achieving a competitive advantage.
  - Income goals specify how much money is needed or wanted from the practice in a certain period of time, such as a year.
- Practice identity flows from the vision and is the image projected to the world.
  - Business cards present a lot of information in a small space and are important for building a client base.
  - Brochures and websites are useful for displaying more detailed information.
- Getting employment as a massage therapist entails locating openings, filling out job applications, submit-

ting résumés, writing cover letters, presenting references, getting interviews, and interviewing well.
  - A résumé summarizes relevant education, experience, and professional achievements and is essential when looking for employment.
  - A cover letter for a résumé should explain why you are qualified for the job and reflect your suitability for the place of employment.
  - References provide outside verification of your past performance and give you credibility.
- Job interviews are for massage therapists to evaluate whether the jobs offer what they are looking for and for employers to determine if the massage therapists have the qualifications for the positions.
- Preparation for an interview involves writing your questions about the job and practicing answers to probable questions from the interviewer.
  - Giving a massage is often part of a job interview for massage therapists.

- Project confidence and be professional at all times. Be aware of illegal questions from interviewers and respond tactfully.
- Accept a job offer right away if you are sure you want it, but do not be afraid to say no or ask for time to think about it if you are not sure.

- Call the employer if you do not hear back from the company within a few days.
- If you do not get the job, try to find out why, and consider it a learning experience for future success.

EXAM REVIEW

Key Terms

To study the key terms listed at the beginning of this chapter, match the appropriate lettered meaning to each numbered key term listed below. For additional study, look up the key terms in the Interactive Glossary on page G-1 and note other terms that compare or contrast with them.

_____ 1. Employee
_____ 2. Income goal
_____ 3. Independent contractor
_____ 4. Mission statement
_____ 5. Practice identity
_____ 6. Private practice
_____ 7. Résumé
_____ 8. Self-employed
_____ 9. Sole proprietor
_____ 10. Vision

a. Defines the purpose of your practice and describes your main strategy for achieving competitive advantage
b. The image you project about your practice
c. You carry on your practice as a sole proprietor or an independent contractor; also called private practice
d. How much money you need or want from your practice in a certain time period
e. The legally recognized owner of a one-person business
f. Someone who works for an employer
g. How you see your practice in its broad scope
h. Written summary of education, experience, achievements, professional memberships, and other information relevant to application for a job
i. You carry on your practice as a sole proprietor or an independent contractor; also called self-employed
j. Performs services for another person or business, but is not an employee

Memory Workout

To test your memory of the main concepts in this chapter, complete the following sentences by circling the most correct answer from the two choices provided.

1. Employees have less (control) (security) than self-employed massage therapists have.
2. You are considered self-employed if you carry on your practice as a sole (proprietor) (employer) or an independent (contractor) (employee).
3. A mission statement consists of one to three sentences defining the (layout) (purpose) of your practice and your main strategy for achieving (competitive) (therapeutic) advantage.
4. As with résumés, (elaborate and trendy) (readable and simple) business cards are best.
5. Massage therapists in private practice should have (stationery) (notepads) on hand for official written correspondence.
6. Websites serve the same general purpose as (business cards) (brochures).
7. A job application is a preprinted form used by companies to get essential information for (screening) (interviewing) job applicants.
8. Misrepresentation on a job application is not only unethical, but may have (legal) (emotional) consequences.
9. References are people who know you personally and who can (recommend) (describe) your work.
10. It is (illegal) (reasonable) for a potential employer to ask for a massage as part of a job interview.
11. Federal and state laws attempt to ensure that job candidates are hired based solely on their (qualifications) (aspirations) for the job.
12. If a job is not offered to you right away after an interview, feel free to call back in a (day) (month) or two to see how things stand.

Test Prep

The following multiple-choice questions will help to prepare you for future school and professional exams.

1. Which of the following offers immediate income with minimum startup costs?
   a. Sole proprietor
   b. Employee
   c. Independent contractor
   d. Private practice
2. Which of the following is *not* part of a mission statement for a massage therapy practice?
   a. Focus of the practice
   b. Purpose of the practice
   c. Income goal
   d. Competitive advantage
3. A logo is:
   a. Part of your practice identity
   b. A symbol that identifies your practice at a glance
   c. Original or clip art
   d. All of the above
4. On a résumé, education and work experience are typically listed in:
   a. Chronological order
   b. Reverse chronological order
   c. Alphabetical order
   d. Order of importance
5. The single most important marketing device for building a client base will most likely be your:
   a. Diploma
   b. Résumé
   c. Business card
   d. Brochure
6. Which of the following would not be appropriate to list as your references as part of a job application?
   a. Family members
   b. Teachers
   c. Former employers
   d. Satisfied clients
7. Which of the following is *not* appropriate for a prospective employer to do during a job interview?
   a. Ask about your qualifications for the job
   b. Ask for a sample massage session
   c. Ask about your marital status and children
   d. Ask about your ability to work a certain schedule
8. If you have limited job experience, which of the following would likely impress a prospective employer the most as evidence of your character and sense of responsibility?
   a. Music or other collection
   b. Professional image you project
   c. Good grades in school
   d. Volunteer work in the community

Video Challenge

Watch the appropriate segment of the video on your DVD and then answer the following questions.

Career Plans and Employment

Developing a Business Plan

1. What were the initial visions of the massage therapists interviewed in the video of their future practices? How did they change with time?

2. What does the massage therapist in the video say about having small goals? How did that lead her in the direction she wanted to go?

Employment Interview

3. According to the video, how should you prepare for a job interview?

Comprehension Exercises

The following short answer questions test your knowledge and understanding of chapter topics and provide practice in written communication skills. Explain in two to four complete sentences.

1. What is the purpose of developing a vision of your future massage therapy practice? What are the essential elements of that vision?

2. Compare employees and independent contractors. What does the government look for in determining which category best fits a particular job? What is the dominant impression test?

3. What are some questions you might have for a potential employer during a job interview? Why would you be asking questions at this time?

For Greater Understanding

The following exercises are designed to take you from the realm of theory into the real world. They will help give you a deeper understanding of the subjects covered in this chapter. Action words are underlined to emphasize the variety of activities presented to address different learning styles and to encourage deeper thinking.

1. Write a mission statement for your future massage therapy practice. Take into account your current interests, talents, and employment goals. Write your mission statement in positive language so that it may inspire you and keep you on track to meet your overall career goals.

2. Develop a personal budget for a year listing projected expenses and total income, including income from various jobs and contributions from spouse or family. Given your circumstances, determine how much money you need to make from your massage therapy practice to cover bills and have some discretionary income. This is your income goal for your massage therapy practice.

3. Develop a list of job opportunities for massage therapists in your area. How many job postings could you find? How many fit your vision for your practice?

22 Private Practice and Finances

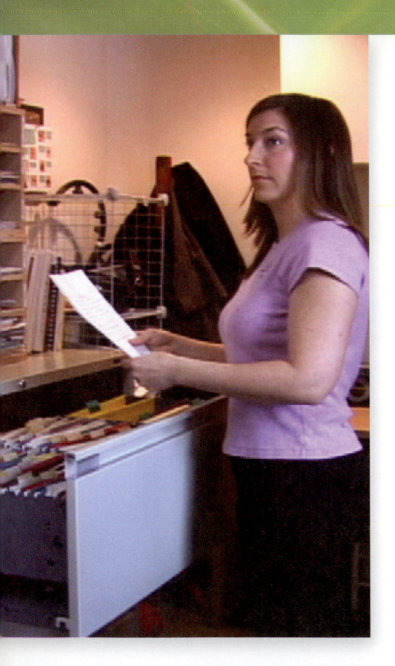

 CHAPTER OUTLINE

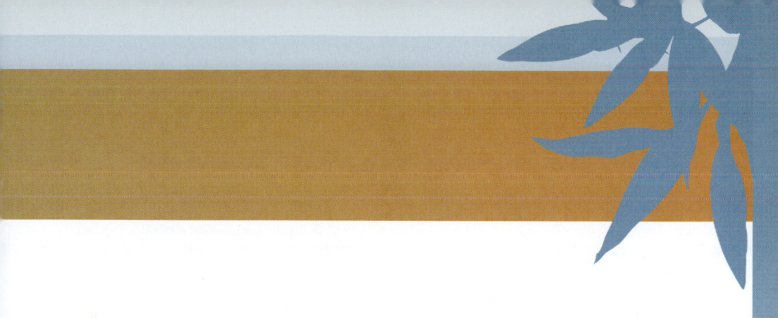

LEARNING OUTCOMES

After studying this chapter, you will have information to:

1. Develop a business plan for a private practice in massage therapy.
2. Create a marketing strategy to build a client base.
3. Organize a massage practice office.
4. Enter into contracts with knowledge and forethought.
5. Establish policies for practice management.

6. Create a filing system for keeping client records.
7. Project startup costs for a massage therapy practice.
8. Project first-year income and expenses.
9. Design a bookkeeping system for tax purposes.
10. Manage practice finances on a daily basis.

KEY TERMS

MASSAGE *in* ACTION

On your DVD, explore:

- Business Plan
- Advertising
- First-Year Budget
- Bookkeeping

PRIVATE PRACTICE

A self-employed massage therapist is said to have a private practice. A private practice can be small and part time, with a few clients per week, or it can be large and full time and serve many clients each week. A private practice in massage therapy has much in common with other small businesses that sell products and services to the public. For example, a massage therapy practice is regulated as a business and has responsibilities for keeping financial records for tax purposes. It also markets services to the public to build a client base. This chapter provides an overview of the business side of having a private practice in massage therapy.

BUSINESS PLAN OVERVIEW

A **business plan** spells out the details of putting the practice vision into operation. A business plan has four major parts: description of the business, marketing, management, and finances. The major elements of a business plan for a massage therapy practice are summarized in Box 22.1●. Further information about developing a business plan is available from the U.S. Small Business Administration (www.sba.gov). The remainder of this chapter discusses these elements in more detail.

DESCRIPTION OF THE BUSINESS

The vision developed in your career plan (see page 612 in Chapter 21, Career Plans and Employment) lays the foundation for the description of your private practice, that is, your business. The mission statement is a good opening for the description. Express the size of the business in terms of whether it is full time or part time, how many clients are planned on average per week, and the total number of clients per year. State your income and profit goals. Looking at the income and profit goals in relation to the number of clients is essential. Remember that income from clients minus business expenses and taxes is the real profit from the practice. It is the profit that you put into your pocket. Do the math to see if your expectations about how much money you will make from your practice are realistic. Finances are discussed in more detail later in the chapter.

BOX 22.1 Private Practice Massage Therapy Business Plan

Section 1: Description of the Business

- Vision
  - Mission
  - Size (full time or part time; number of clients per week or month)
  - Income and profit goals
  - Legal structure (sole proprietor, partnership, corporation)
- Location
  - Home, space rental, or traveling practice
  - Applicable ordinances and zoning laws

Section 2: Marketing

- Market research
- Client sources
- Advertising and promotions
  - Business card
  - Brochure
  - Website
  - Other

Section 3: Management

- License, insurance, contracts
- Policies
- Office space
- Appointments
- Client records

Section 4: Finances

- Startup budget
- First-year budget
- Bookkeeping
- Taxes
- Banking

Legal Structure

The concept of sole proprietor was introduced in Chapter 21, Career Plans and Employment, on page 613 to distinguish employment from self-employment. Sole proprietor is the most common legal structure chosen for massage therapy practices, especially when starting out. Other choices are partnership and corporation. Major differences in the three structures have to do with who owns the business, who takes profits and losses, who is responsible for legal matters, and what taxes apply. Box 22.2● summarizes the characteristics of the three possible legal structures.

It is outside of the scope of this book to delve deeply into the pros and cons of partnerships and corporations for massage therapy practices. If you want to know more, someone experienced in business, such as a lawyer or accountant, can help sort out the issues. Information is also available from the U.S. Small Business Administration (www.sba.gov).

BOX 22.2 Options for Legal Structures*

Sole Proprietor

- Owned by one person who makes all decisions and who takes all profits and losses.
- Owner is personally liable for any lawsuits that arise from the business.
- Registered in the state as a sole proprietor.
- Owner pays income taxes on the business profits as personal income.

Partnership

- Two or more owners who make decisions and share profits.
- All partners are liable for lawsuits that arise from the business.
- Legal contract called a "partnership agreement" defines the responsibilities of each partner.
- Partners pay income taxes on their share of the profits as personal income.

Corporation

- A corporation is a legal entity or "person" under the law and is composed of stockholders operating under one company name. Stockholders own the corporation and elect a board of directors to manage the company.
- The corporation is liable for lawsuits that arise from the business. Stockholders have limited liability and cannot have their personal assets taken to pay a judgment from a lawsuit.
- Corporations are registered by states in the United States and must abide by that state's laws related to corporations. Laws differ in different states.
- Main disadvantage in some types of corporations is that corporate profits are taxed twice—once as a corporation and again as dividends to individual stockholders on their personal income tax.
- Types of corporations
  - *C Corporation* sells ownership as shares of stock; limited liability for stockholders; income taxed twice.
  - *Subchapter S Corporation* limits the number of stockholders to 75; has limited liability; income taxed only once as personal income of the owners.
  - *Professional Corporation* for professionals in practice together; special rules apply.
  - *Nonprofit Corporation* or 501c (3) set up with mission to improve society; tax exempt; no profits shared by stockholders.
  - *Limited Liability Company* (LLC) combines best features of partnerships and corporations; limited personal liability; income taxed once.

*See U.S. Small Business Administration [www.sba.gov] and U.S. Internal Revenue Service [www.irs.gov] for more information about legal structures for businesses.

For the purposes of this text, a sole proprietor legal structure will be assumed. A sole proprietor makes all decisions, takes all profits and losses, is personally liable for lawsuits, and pays income taxes on business profits as personal income.

Location

Location can make or break a business. Marketing research can tell you where your potential clients are and how much competition will be in a certain area. Municipal ordinances regulating massage therapy and local zoning laws may limit where a massage therapy business can be located.

Options for massage therapy practice locations include a home office, space in a commercial building or within another business space, and a storefront. These options may be limited by law in some locations, for example, in some places home businesses are prohibited. Each of these potential places has advantages and disadvantages to consider.

Many massage therapists have satisfying practices in their homes. The main advantages here are low overhead and a short commute. Home-based practices require a separate space dedicated to massage and, ideally, separate entrances and bathrooms. Mixing of personal and business space should be avoided as much as possible. Having strangers in their homes may not appeal to some massage therapists. In addition, zoning laws may prohibit home businesses, or a variance may be required. Despite all the potential difficulties, home-based practices can be quite successful with careful planning.

Renting space is another option. A room in an office building or within another business may be all you need. Rooms within spas, salons, health clubs, and medical offices can offer a nice reception area and give valuable exposure to potential clients. Sometimes massage therapists rent rooms to other massage therapists. If an acceptable schedule can be worked out, sharing space with another massage therapist can be a good startup alternative. Note that this is not a legal partnership, but simply a space-sharing arrangement.

Storefront rental is a larger financial commitment. The advantage is that foot traffic in the area may result in more clients as people walk by and see your business signs. You can design the space as you like it and even rent space to other massage therapists or other compatible businesses. It is also a more complex situation, complete with a landlord, more possible legal restrictions, more initial financial outlay for altering the space to fit your needs, more upkeep expenses, and usually a greater monthly financial liability. A storefront may be a good option for a suburban or small-town practice.

An alternative to having a fixed location is to have an on-the-road practice in which you go to your clients' locations. You can see private clients in their own homes, or in places such as hotels and resorts, nursing homes, or the workplace. An individual client may contract with you for massage, or you may have an arrangement as an independent contractor to provide massage to patrons or employees of another business in its space. A traveling practice eliminates overhead for space, but requires a means of transportation and possibly special equipment for easy transport.

MARKETING

A market is defined as a group of people with the potential interest of buying a given product or service. **Marketing** is the process of identifying these potential customers and meeting their needs and wants. In marketing yourself, you identify potential clients who want what you have to offer.

In a sense, everyone is a potential client, so you must decide to whom to market your services. Options are to try to appeal to a broad, diverse market or to narrow your focus to a group with specific needs. When starting out, it might be wiser to market to a broader audience and narrow your focus later, if you want to, once your client base has grown.

Marketing also takes into consideration your competitive advantage, which is the reason people would come to you for massage instead of someone else. Factors that may give you an advantage are quality, expertise, price, location, variety of services, special skills, convenience, or environment. From the business point of view, it is useful to think of clients as customers or consumers.

Market Research

Market research is the process of collecting relevant information for identifying and reaching potential customers. The following are basic market research questions for massage therapists.

- Who are my potential clients? Who is interested in receiving the massage therapy that I offer?
- What do they hope to gain by receiving massage?
- Who in my area can afford massage?
- How do potential clients find out about massage therapists in the area?
- Who else is providing massage in the area? Who do they seem to be targeting or attracting?
- Is there an untapped or underserved market in the area?
- What are my strengths and/or preferences in massage therapy, and how do they match up with potential markets?
- How can I develop my own niche or loyal client base?
- Who is the target audience for my massage practice?

Answers to these questions are found in a variety of sources. To begin with, the Wellness Massage Pyramid discussed on page 4 in Chapter 1, Introduction to Massage Therapy, offers insight into the broad range of reasons that people might need or want massage therapy. Consumer research conducted by associations and organizations provides insight about massage consumers. An example is the annual *Massage Therapy Consumer Survey Fact Sheet* from the American Massage Therapy Association (www.amtamassage.org).

Magazine and journal articles can show what the general public is looking for from massage therapy and the latest trends. Organizations or support groups for people with certain illnesses or disabilities may promote massage to their members. The local library or phone book has information about who in a geographic area is already providing massage

and whom they are targeting, as well as potential competing practices at spas, salons, health clubs, YMCAs, integrative health care facilities, chiropractic offices, and other places.

Once potential clients are identified, you can make decisions about how best to reach them, and position your practice as the best choice for their needs.

Building a Client Base

A primary source of clients in a personal service like massage is word of mouth, that is, recommendations from other clients, friends, and family. Referrals from health professionals such as personal trainers, chiropractors, physical therapists, and doctors can also be important.

Professional associations and independent groups offer special massage therapist locator services to the general public. Potential clients often check the Internet to locate massage therapists in their areas, and so subscribing to one of these services may be beneficial.

Networking in the community helps potential clients get to know you. Many massage therapists join their local chamber of commerce, or service clubs such as Rotary International and Lions Clubs International. Besides being supporting members, massage therapists can give presentations about massage to these community organizations. Special interest groups such as sports clubs, senior centers, and support groups are also open to having speakers come to talk to them. Good presentation skills, as discussed on page 65 in Chapter 3, Professional and Personal Development, are useful in marketing private practices.

Getting your name and face out to the public is the key. People need to know that you are in the area and how to contact you for an appointment.

Advertising and Promotions

Advertising is a paid public announcement providing information about a product or service to potential customers. Ads may be in print or electronic media and range in size from what can fit on the side of a pen to an outdoor billboard.

The purpose of advertising is to attract potential clients to a specific business or person, and convince them that their needs or wants can be fulfilled by the service advertised. Ads remind potential clients of needs or wants and may even create a desire for the service that did not exist before. Ads convince potential clients that a certain business or person is the right one to fulfill their desires.

The most cost-effective advertising investments for a startup massage practice are business cards, brochures, websites, and phone directory yellow pages ads. In smaller towns, ads in the local newspaper may be worthwhile. Visible signs with basic information also let potential customers know that you are in the area. Perhaps the most expensive and least effective advertising for most small practices are big-city newspapers, and television and radio ads, unless there are local channels or stations that serve the immediate area in which your practice is located.

Advertising opportunities can be found in a variety of public places. For example, a public sports facility may have advertising space around a lobby bulletin board, or a local movie theater may show ads for community businesses on the screen before the feature starts. Some fund-raising groups sell space in ad books or souvenir programs and encourage their supporters to do business with sponsors who bought ads. These types of advertising build awareness of your existence and can make your name familiar in the community over a period of time. Buy such ads in places where you think your potential clients will see them. When someone thinks of massage therapy, your name will come up in association.

Promotions are ways to encourage people to pick up the telephone and make those appointments. Promotions include giving discounts to new clients for their first massage, or a discounted package for a series of sessions, for example, five sessions for the cost of four. Some massage therapists offer seasonal discounts around the holidays or for special groups such as teachers, police, and firefighters. Gift certificates can also bring in new clients.

Advertising and promotion ideas abound in a free market environment. A lot can be learned from becoming more aware of how other businesses market their services. Some may work for a massage therapy practice and some may not. Box 22.3● lists some ideas for building a client base.

BOX 22.3 Building a Client Base

Sources of Clients
- Word of mouth from other clients, friends, and family
- Referrals from other health professionals
- Referrals from massage therapist locator services
- Networking in the community (chambers of commerce, service groups, special interest groups)

Advertising
- Business cards
- Signs on a place of business
- Yellow pages phone book
- Website
- Brochure
- T-shirts, caps, pens, bags, or other objects with name and contact information for a business
- Refrigerator magnets with business name and information
- Signage on cars and vans
- Printed signs for placement on bulletin boards or in windows
- Advertisements in newspapers, magazines, or newsletters
- Direct-mail coupons
- Announcements on local radio or television stations

Promotions
- Discount for new clients
- Packages of sessions at special price
- Seasonal promotions
- Discount for special groups
- Gift certificates

In any case, care must be taken in marketing and advertising to avoid unethical practices. Many of the ethical pitfalls in this area of business are discussed in Chapter 23, Business Ethics, on page 649. To summarize ethical advertising:

- Tell the truth and avoid deception
- Be professional
- Do not make guarantees
- Use testimonials sparsely
- List prices honestly
- Honor copyright and trademark rights

MANAGEMENT

Management involves activities necessary to keep the business running smoothly. Obtaining licenses and insurance, defining policies, and negotiating contracts are examples. Massage office design and upkeep, making appointments, and maintenance of client files are also important management functions. All the behind-the-scenes operations that make it possible for the massage therapist to provide a therapeutic experience for clients falls into the category of management. This section discusses some of the basic management details of a massage therapy practice.

Licenses and Insurance

Certain licenses may be required to start a private massage practice. First, an occupational license to practice massage therapy must be obtained from the state or local government where applicable. This applies to employment, as well as to having a private practice.

Second, a business license may be required by a city or county. Some places have special massage establishment licenses and space requirements. Zoning may limit where a massage business can be located. Before you sign a rental contract, make sure that massage is legally allowed in that location and get the required permits.

Insurance protects you financially. *Professional liability insurance* covers you for liability for incidents arising from the massage therapy itself. Criminal acts or actions outside of the scope of massage therapy as legally defined are usually excluded. Injuries occurring when practicing without a required license may also not be covered. Read your professional liability insurance policy to clearly understand what it includes.

Premise liability insurance, also called "slip and fall" insurance, is for accidents to clients and visitors on the business premises not related to massage. *Renters' insurance* covers the cost of equipment, supplies, and other objects lost or damaged due to fire, theft, or flood.

Contracts

Setting up a private practice usually entails some legal agreements or contracts. Examples are rental agreements, phone and Internet service, credit cards, linen service, cleaning service, and bills of sale. Independent contractor agreements are used when a massage therapist provides massage services to another business. It is important to understand the basic elements of contracts to ensure that agreements entered into support your business plans and expectations.

A **contract** is an official written agreement between two or more people. The terms of a contract may be upheld in court if one party is considered to have breached or violated the agreement. Lawsuits arise when agreements are either not clear or have not been kept.

A contract must have a clear statement of the terms of the agreement, that is, person A agrees to this, and person B agrees to that. The length of the agreement should be specified from beginning date to ending date. What happens if one party breaches the agreement may be clarified, such as arbitration or mediation. Grounds for termination and method of termination should be spelled out. Acknowledgment of understanding of the agreement, the date of the agreement, and parties to the agreement and their signatures appear on the contract. Guidelines for legal agreements include:

- Always put contracts in writing and have them signed and dated by all legally responsible parties.
- Never sign a significant contract, for example, partnership, rental, or lease, without a lawyer looking it over first.
- Always read contracts before you sign them, so that you know what you are agreeing to. You will be held responsible whether you have read it or not.
- If you write the contract, use the simplest language possible so all parties understand what they are agreeing to; avoid legalese when possible.
- Have legal counsel review the contract if it involves a significant amount of money.
- Don't be afraid to suggest changes to a contract presented to you. If all parties agree to a change, simply strike out the words you do not want, write in alternate terms if appropriate, and have each party initial the change.
- For a contract involving a lot of money, add a witness, who is a neutral party, to the signing of the agreement.

Massage therapists who work as independent contractors usually have a stock contract that they fill in for different situations. This contract is an agreement by a massage therapist to provide massage services for a separate legal entity. It states the fee per massage session or time worked, date(s) of service, place, and how and when payment is made. It may stipulate conditions such as how clients are solicited and scheduled, reporting mechanisms, and type of massage provided. There may be a cancellation provision. Both parties sign the contract and keep copies for future reference.

Verbal agreements may be legally binding but are hard to enforce. People may have different understandings of the agreement or may remember details differently. Always get agreements related to your business in writing and signed. Laws related to contracts vary by state.

Practice Policies

Practice policies clarify expectations and specific points of the agreement between the massage therapist and the client. Policies set the ground rules for what happens given a particular situation. They should be given to clients and signed as part of the general client contract.

There are many types of policies. Pricing policies list fees for different services and posting them may be required by law. Payment policies specify when payment is due, for example, before or after a session. Method of acceptable payment is clarified, for example, cash, check, debit card, or credit card. Other financial policies include insufficient funds/returned check policy and a health insurance reimbursement policy. Some massage therapists have a satisfaction or money-back guarantee.

Late arrival policies clarify what happens when a client comes late for an appointment. One approach is that clients pay for the time periods they have scheduled. If clients are late, their massages end at the originally designated times, and the clients owe the originally agreed-upon fees. Another approach may be that a client who is over 30 minutes late for an appointment does not receive a massage and is charged as if he or she were a no-show.

A cancellation policy may be that 24-hour notice is required or $25 will be charged for the missed appointment. It may also be that no penalty is incurred if the time slot is subsequently filled. A missed appointment policy may be that clients pay in full for missed appointments or, alternatively, that clients pay 50 percent of the original fee for missed appointments.

Conduct policies clarify to clients that the massage provided is nonsexual massage and that any attempt to sexualize a session will be grounds for termination of the massage without a refund of fees. Hygiene policies might specify that clients are expected to come for massage clean and free of strong scents from products like perfumes and cologne or that clients are expected to shower immediately prior to a massage.

A health history disclosure and update policy might be that clients agree to disclose medical conditions and medications as requested to screen for contraindications. They might also be expected to keep the massage therapist updated on any changes in conditions and medications.

A termination policy might state that the massage therapist reserves the right to terminate a session if he or she believes that the safety or health of the client or massage therapist would be threatened if the session were continued. A confidentiality and privacy policy reiterates that the massage therapist will not talk to anyone, including health care providers and insurance companies, without the client's permission. It also states that client health and session records will be kept secure and only seen by those needing to see them.

A scope of practice statement defines what type of massage therapy is offered and for what purposes. It is good to make clear that the massage therapist applies massage within his or her scope of practice and will refer clients as needed to an appropriate massage therapist or health care professional. Explanation of scope of practice is often followed by a consent form.

Waiver of liability can be attached to a policies document. In waivers, clients agree to hold the massage therapist harmless for unpredictable negative reactions or results. This may benefit the massage therapist in the event of a lawsuit, but waivers do not usually hold in cases of proven negligence.

Clearly stating policies in writing promotes greater understanding of expectations and defines important aspects of the therapeutic relationship. Signed copies should be kept in clients' files and additional copies be given to them to take home. A summary of types of policies important to a massage therapy practice appears in Box 22.4●.

Massage Practice Office Space

Massage practice spaces have some common requirements whether in the home or in a commercial building. There should be space set aside for a reception area, massage therapy room, business office, and bathrooms.

The reception area is where clients are greeted and can wait if they are early for an appointment. A reception area typically has one or two chairs, a small table, lamp, and decorations. Framed certificates may hang on the wall. The area should be inviting, comfortable, and partitioned off from the massage therapy room.

The massage therapy room must be large enough for all of the equipment and supplies needed for massage sessions. At a minimum, it should hold a massage table and sitting stool on wheels, with adequate space for movement around the table. Storage cabinets hold linens, lotions, and other supplies, and a covered container keeps dirty linens separate. An accessible tabletop is necessary for lubricants, small hand tools, hot packs, and other objects used during massage. A stepping stool may be useful for short or less mobile clients to get onto the table.

The room should also have a chair and clothes rack for clients' belongings. A small wall mirror is useful for clients to check their hair or makeup after massage. Anatomy charts, certificates, or artwork may be hung on the walls. The floor covering should be easily washable.

Office space is set aside for working on and keeping financial records, client files, and other aspects of the business side of the practice. Office furniture includes a desk and chair and a locking file cabinet. Basic office equipment includes a telephone and answering machine, with optional computer, printer, and copier. Storage space is needed for office and cleaning supplies. Figure 22.1■ shows a basic layout for a massage therapy office.

BOX 22.4	Types of Policies Important for a Massage Therapy Practice

Financial Policies

- Pricing/fees
- Payment due
- Methods of payment
- Insurance reimbursement
- Insufficient funds or returned checks
- Satisfaction or money back guarantee

Client Behavior Policies

- Late arrival
- No-show or missed appointment
- Cancellation
- Conduct or unacceptable behavior
- Hygiene
- Health history disclosure and update

General Practice Policies

- Schedule of days and times for appointments
- Services and types of massage therapy offered
- Scope of practice
- Referral
- Termination
- Confidentiality
- Consent for massage applications
- Waiver of liability

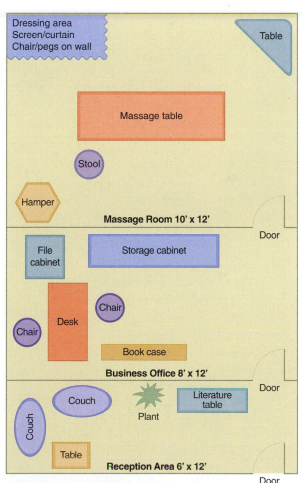

FIGURE 22.1

Basic massage practice office area.

PRACTICAL APPLICATION

Visit several massage therapy practices and carefully observe the offices. Sketch their office spaces using approximate dimensions. Answering the following questions will help you focus on the elements that constitute a well-designed massage therapy office space.

1. What colors, smells, lighting, or other factors do you remember from your visits to massage therapy offices? Which ones made a favorable or unfavorable impression on you?

2. What was it about the offices' atmosphere, comfort, and safety practices that impressed you?
3. Which elements did the offices have in common?
4. What were the elements that left you with a positive impression?

Now design your own massage office space. Include reception area, massage room, business office, and location of bathrooms. Incorporate elements that will positively influence clients coming to you for massage.

A bathroom should be accessible for client use. Some massage ordinances also require showers. Check local massage ordinances for requirements related to massage establishments.

Appointments

Making and keeping appointments is an important time-management function. A massage therapist should have a separate appointment book for his or her private practice. This can also serve as a supporting document for tax purposes.

An appointment book can be the pencil-and-paper variety or can be in electronic form. A drawback of electronic record keeping is the potential for a glitch that wipes out appointment information. On the other hand, a traditional appointment book can be lost. Keeping a backup of all electronic information is vital for responsible record keeping.

Generally, the days of the week and times appointments are scheduled should be consistent and a matter of policy. Resist the temptation when starting out to take appointments whenever clients want them. If clients are informed of your days and times of operation, they generally find a time that works for them. Switching appointment times to fit clients' schedules should be kept to a minimum.

Leave at least 30 minutes between appointments if you have one massage room in a location. If traveling to an appointment, plan enough time for travel plus setup and takedown.

Client Records

Create a folder with essential information for each regular client. File folders with fasteners at the top keep papers in order. On one side of the folder, attach a cover sheet with contact information such as name, address, telephone number, and e-mail address. A signed policy agreement and waiver, and HIPAA (Health Insurance Portability and Accountability Act) confidentiality statement, if applicable,

are underneath. On the other side, fasten the initial health history form and SOAP notes for massage sessions. Financial records are usually kept in separate files from session records (Figure 22.2■).

Client records must be kept secure and locked to ensure client confidentiality, and in some cases may require compliance with HIPAA regulations (www.hhs.gov/ocr/hipaa). See page 112 in Chapter 5, Ethics and the Therapeutic Relationship, for more on HIPAA requirements. Electronic systems are available for client records. Computer programs for keeping client files have been developed and can be found on the Internet and in advertisements in professional journals. Back up electronic files daily for preservation in case of file corruption, and use passwords for client record security.

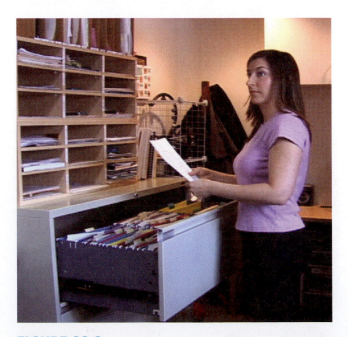

FIGURE 22.2

Client files are kept in alphabetical order in locked file cabinets.

Keep accurate, honest, adequate client records. Keep client records secure and confidential. Abide by laws related to record keeping, for example, those set forth by HIPAA. Schedule record keeping into your practice time. Doing paperwork is an important part of a massage therapy practice.

FINANCES

The financial viability of a massage therapy practice is fundamental to its success. That means setting income goals and profit projections, budgeting for income and expenses, tracking money coming in and going out, and paying taxes. Once you understand the basics of business finances and put them into practice, it can be rewarding to watch your massage therapy business grow and prosper.

Income and profit goals are part of the vision for your private practice. *Gross* income means how much money is collected from clients, while *net* income is what is left over after expenses and taxes. After subtracting expenses from income, a negative number means the business had a *loss* for the year, and a positive number shows your *profit*. The concept is simple, but keeping expenses low enough in relation to income in order to generate a profit is the challenge of having a private practice. More about planning for profit is discussed later in the chapter in the section on figuring the first-year budget.

Startup Costs

Startup costs are the initial expenses involved in setting up a massage therapy practice. Many of these costs are incurred before the first client walks in the door. Startup costs include buying basic equipment such as a massage table and related equipment, linens, and lotions; getting a license to practice; securing professional liability insurance; printing business cards; purchasing basic office supplies; establishing telephone service and an answering machine; and paying a security deposit and the first month's rent. Other costs fall into the "nice to have" category rather than the essential things. Nonessential expenses can be put off until money is available.

Startup costs are related to the type of private practice being developed. Some types of practices have lower startup costs than others. Typical startup costs for a massage practice are listed in Box 22.5•.

Startup cash may come from a variety of sources. Some massage therapists use their personal savings or borrow from family members. Some work at other jobs with steady income, and start out as part-time massage therapists, gradually building their practices. A smaller number of massage therapists take out loans from banks or credit unions. Some startup costs can be covered by credit cards, but these often incur high interest payments that eat into profits. Starting out with the least amount of debt at the lowest interest rate is a good financial goal.

BOX 22.5 | **Typical Startup Cost Categories**

Licensing Costs
- Occupational license (application, exam, fingerprinting, other)
- Massage establishment license
- Business permit or license

Professional Association Membership

Insurance
- Professional liability
- Premise liability ("slip and fall")
- Health insurance
- Auto insurance
- Other insurance

Business Checking Account

Communication Services
- Phone installation or connection
- Computer connection to Internet

Massage Equipment
- Massage table and accessories
- Massage chair and accessories
- Heater for hot packs
- Freezer for cold packs
- Other equipment

Office Furniture and Equipment
- Light fixtures
- Computer and printer
- Sound system for music
- Answering machine

Supplies
- Linens (sheets and towels)
- Oils
- Hot and cold packs
- Appointment book/system
- Forms and folders for client records
- Miscellaneous office supplies
- Decorations for office

Marketing and Advertising
- Business cards
- Brochures
- Website
- Stationary

Legal and Professional Fees
- Attorney
- Bookkeeper
- Accountant
- Other

Office Setup
- Security deposit
- First month's rent
- Communications installation
- Utilities deposit

CRITICAL THINKING

Write a business plan for your future massage therapy practice. Refer back to your notes about your practice identity and mission statement in writing your business plan. Present your plan to the class and solicit feedback and suggestions. Review and revise your plan as you think of better approaches.

Now list the startup costs for a private practice you currently have in mind. Ask yourself these questions:

1. How do you plan to get the money needed for the startup?
2. Are there any ways to reduce startup costs to increase your profits in the beginning?

First-Year Budget

The first-year budget forecasts income and expenses for the initial 12 months of operation. Month-by-month budgeting is usually the most useful. Develop a month-by-month chart or spreadsheet that shows monthly expenses and projected income from the practice.

Projecting income for the first year can be tricky. Income will be a factor of the number of clients seen per week multiplied by the fees collected per session. Research the going rate for massage in your area. When starting out, you might want to consider staying on the lower side of the cost range to attract clients, especially if there is a lot of massage available in your area. On the other hand, if you are one of a few massage therapists, or if you have a unique service, you may want to charge the average rate or more.

Expect a gradual growth in clients and massage sessions over the initial 12-month period. Figure no more than six clients per week in the first 6 months, gradually working up to 10–15 per week by the end of the year. Be conservative. Allow for cancellations. It is better to have more income than predicted. Remember to plan for vacation time, holidays, and sick days during the first year. Projecting 4 weeks of down time is recommended.

Projecting monthly expenses allows you to determine how much income you need to break even, or make a profit, in any given month. **Fixed costs,** sometimes called *overhead,* are expenses you have whether you see clients or not, for example, rent and utilities. Fluctuating operating expenses, or **variable costs,** such as laundry and massage supplies, depend on the number of clients seen.

Some experts recommend putting enough money in the bank to cover at least 3 months' fixed costs before you start your practice. This is called a **cash reserve** and should be figured in startup costs. Ideally, a cash reserve should be built up and maintained throughout a practice to cover unforeseen events such as illnesses or family emergencies. Deficits in 1 month can be made up in subsequent months, or profits in 1 month can help offset expected expenses in coming months. By the end of the year, income hopefully will outpace expenses to yield a profit.

A **salary draw** is the money taken out of the practice monthly for your personal use. Some experts recommend not expecting a salary draw for the first six months of a new practice. This allows for income to be put back into the business to cover operating expenses and build the cash reserve. To make this possible, some massage therapists build up savings, borrow money, depend on a spouse or family for support, or keep part-time jobs to cover personal expenses until their practices starts turning a good profit.

Keeping expenses low is paramount. Income minus expenses predicts your cash flow, or how much cash you have on hand at any one time. If your expenses outpace your income, and you have no savings to back you up, your practice will eventually fail. Careful monitoring of income and expenses can help you make adjustments as your practice evolves. Consider the first-year budget as a working plan for developing the business side of your practice. A sample spreadsheet for developing a first-year budget appears in Figure 22.3■.

Income Taxes

Massage therapists pay income tax on the profits from their private practices, in addition to taxes related to employment. This means that they must keep accurate records of income from their private clients, as well as receipts from business expenses.

The following information is an overview of the subject of income taxes; however, a professional tax preparer is recommended for specific questions about any individual situation. The Internal Revenue Service (IRS) has information booklets on matters related to taxes that are updated every year (www.irs.gov). Some IRS publications and forms that massage therapists may find useful are listed in Box 22.6●.

The *tax year* for sole proprietor businesses like massage therapy practices is the calendar year beginning January 1 and ending December 31. *Taxable income* is the total income from a massage therapy practice minus qualified business expenses. All fees collected, as well as tips, are considered taxable income. Tips are taxable income for employed massage therapists as well.

Massage therapists who do not sell products usually use the *cash method* of accounting. Under the cash method, income is reported in the tax year it is received, and expenses are deducted in the tax year they are paid for. A different system called the *accrual method* is sometimes used by businesses. In the accrual method, income is reported in the tax

PROJECTED INCOME

Source	Jan	Feb	Mar	April	May	June	July	Aug	Sept	Oct	Nov	Dec
Massage fees												
Tips												
Miscellaneous												
Monthly Totals												

PROJECTED EXPENSES

Expense	Jan	Feb	Mar	April	May	June	July	Aug	Sept	Oct	Nov	Dec
Loan payment												
Rent												
Phone												
Utilities												
Bank fees												
Linen service												
Cleaning												
Bookkeeper												
Insurance												
Memberships												
Continuing Education												
Business travel												
Estimated taxes												
Salary draw												
Miscellaneous												
Monthly Totals												

FIGURE 22.3

Sample budget spreadsheet form for first year of business.

year it is earned, even though payment may be received in a later year, and expenses are deducted in the tax year they are incurred, whether or not they are paid in that year. (See IRS Publication 583, *Starting a Business and Keeping Records.*)

Qualified business expenses reduce the amount of taxable income. Most expenses related to maintaining a practice/business are deductible, for example, equipment and supplies, office rent, continuing education, and license

CASE FOR STUDY

Jim and his Startup Plans

Jim wants to build a private massage practice after graduation, but realizes that will take money he does not have right now. He is willing to get part-time employment as a massage therapist as he builds his own business. His mission is "to apply my knowledge and skills to help clients achieve optimal wellness. Affordable massage therapy is offered in a clean, pleasant, and relaxing environment. This is a community-centered and family-based private practice welcoming people of all ages."

Question:

What strategies can Jim use to minimize startup costs and build his own private practice over time?

Things to consider:

- How can Jim decide how many days to devote to employment and how many to building his private practice during the first year?

- Employment in what type of setting(s) would contribute most to his long-range plans for his private practice?
- What are the options for his initial private practice location to minimize overhead?
- How can he build a solid client base for his private practice successfully and ethically?
- In what ways can he best and most inexpensively get his name out into the community?
- What could his contingency plans be if (a) his private practice grows more rapidly than expected or (b) his private practice grows more slowly than expected?

Ideas for accomplishing his first-year goals:

_____

_____

_____

REALITY CHECK

MARIA

BARRY: I have some great ideas for a private practice but the financial aspects and record keeping seem too complicated. Do you have any suggestions for how to approach this side of having a private practice?

MARIA: Going into private practice is essentially starting a small business. Keep things simple, and get some help with record keeping and taxes. Set aside time every week to put income and expenses in a bookkeeping ledger, and keep all expense receipts. Consider it part of your practice, like seeing a client. Look ahead to tax time, and track all deductible expenses and taxable income. Consider using a computer program for record keeping. In learning how to use the program, you will get a better picture of the financial side of having a private practice.

BOX 22.6	**Useful IRS Publications and Forms***

IRS Publications
- Your Federal Income Tax—For Individuals (Publication 17)
- Starting a Business and Keeping Records (Publication 583)
- Tax Guide for Small Businesses (Publication 334)
- Instructions for Schedule C or C-EZ
- Business Expenses (Publication 535)
- Tax Withholding and Estimated Tax (Publication 505)
- Reporting Tip Income (Publication 531)
- Employee's Daily Record of Tips & Report to Employers (Publication 1244)
- Travel, Entertainment, Gift & Car Expenses (Publication 463)
- Business Use of Your Home (Publication 587)

Forms for Filing Income Taxes
- Form 1040 Individual Income Tax Return
- Schedule C Profit or Loss from Business (sole proprietorship)
- Schedule SE (Form 1040) Self-Employment Tax
- Form 1065 (partnership)
- Form 2553 Election by a Small Business Corporation
- Form 1120S U.S. Income Tax Return for an S Corporation

*IRS forms and publications can be obtained online from www.irs.gov, or by calling the IRS toll free number, or from the U.S. Post Office during tax season. Tax laws are changed yearly so obtain the latest publication available.

---

fees. Mileage to and from clients' homes or other travel may be deductible; however, travel to and from a place of employment is not deductible. Keeping good records and receipts related to business expenses is essential for an accurate calculation of deductions. Check with a tax preparer for further information on allowed deductions. (See IRS Publication 535, *Business Expenses*.)

Form 1040 is used to file U.S. income taxes for individuals and covers both employment and self-employment. Form 1040 is a summary form to which other forms and schedules are attached, for example, W-2 forms to report wages and tips from employment. Schedule C reports small business income and expenses. Form 1099 is similar to a W-2 form from an employer but is used to report income as an independent contractor.

Various other forms are attached to the 1040 as needed to complete the filing. A tax preparer can help you figure out which forms are required for a specific case. (See IRS Publication 17, *Your Federal Income Tax for Individuals*.)

Self-employment tax (SE tax) is a social security and Medicare tax for individuals who work for themselves. It applies to social security coverage for retirement, disability, survivor, and Medicare benefits. SE tax applies if your net earnings from self-employment are $400 or more. SE tax is in addition to your regular income tax, and was slightly over 15 percent in 2009. Some SE tax may be claimed as a business expense, but rules change yearly. (See Schedule SE [Form 1040], *Self-Employment Tax*.)

Estimated tax payments may be due to the IRS four times a year in April, June, September, and January. This is another financial matter to discuss with your tax preparer, preferably at the beginning of the tax year and every quarter thereafter. Estimated tax payments, similar to withholding for employment income, estimate the tax that will be owed at the end of the year. Since you are your own employer, you have the responsibility for paying estimated tax. Estimated tax payments should appear on the budget as an expense. (See IRS Publication 505, *Tax Withholding and Estimated Tax*.)

Using a tax preparation professional is recommended unless you have all income from regular employment or an otherwise simple tax situation. Costs for tax preparation are qualified business expenses.

Tax preparation is made easier with a good bookkeeping system. The tax preparer takes the numbers provided by you and fills in tax forms. An accountant who is a tax preparer can also give you advice on deductions and other ways to reduce income tax owed at the end of the year. Setting up a bookkeeping system is addressed later in this chapter.

Income taxes are an integral part of the financial planning of a private practice in massage therapy—not an afterthought. Good planning can reduce any confusion and stress surrounding bookkeeping and taxes. It is all part of the business side of having a massage therapy practice.

Bookkeeping

Bookkeeping involves keeping accurate records of income and expenditures for tax purposes and tracking payments made by clients, as well as calculating how the business side of the practice is doing financially. The bookkeeping system chosen for a specific practice depends on how large the practice is and how skilled the massage therapist is with numbers.

BOOKKEEPING SYSTEMS

One choice for bookkeeping is a simple handwritten ledger. The advantage of pencil-on-paper systems is that they are inexpensive and easy to learn. The process of making entries by hand can lead to a better understanding of how ledgers work. It is estimated that "half of all new businesses use hand-posted ledgers the first year, and some never see a need for anything else" (Kamoroff 2003, p. 42). For most sole proprietor massage therapists, a handwritten bookkeeping system is adequate.

Published bookkeeping ledgers typically have a page for listing details of daily expenditures and daily receipts or income. There is sometimes a section for expenditures broken out by category of deduction such as rent, postage, and telephone. Keeping running totals for expenditures and income provides a check of profits at a glance and is handy at tax time (Figure 22.4■).

FIGURE 22.4

Sample of a weekly bookkeeping ledger.

Week of ______________ **2**__ __ __
Month/Day to Month/Day

Total Receipts for the Week*			
Day	**Notes — Fees & Tips**	**$ Amount**	
Sun			
Mon			
Tues			
Wed			
Thurs			
Fri			
Sat			
	Total This Week		
	Previous Total		
	Total for Year to Date		

*A receipt book or notations in an appointment book serve as supporting documents for the daily receipt totals in the ledger.

Expenditures for the Week*				
Date	**Paid To**	**Check#/Credit**	**$ Amount**	

*Receipts for goods and services purchased, reflected in cancelled checks and credit card bills, are support documents for expenditures listed.

Expenditures by Deduction Category*								
#	**Category**	**Total This Week**		**Previous Total**		**Total for Year to Date**		
1	Rent							
2	Phone							
3	Utilities							
4	Linen service/laundry							
5	Equipment							
6	Massage supplies							
7	Office supplies							
8	Advertising							
9	Travel							
10	Professional dues							
11	Continuing education							
12	Miscellaneous							

*Expense categories are set up by an accountant or bookkeeper and reflect the usual expenses of the business.

Often these record books include additional useful information such as a tax calendar, allowable deductions, instructions for making entries, calculation of net worth, and tax information sheets. The *Dome Simplified Weekly/Monthly Bookkeeping Record* is an example of a handwritten system available from office supply stores.

Computer programs for bookkeeping are also available, for example, QuickBooks® (www.quickbooks.intuit.com). Some programs are designed specifically for massage therapists' needs. Computer programs do essentially the same things as hand-posted ledgers. Their advantages are that they are faster, provide clean-looking reports, and do the math for you. Some software programs integrate banking and bookkeeping and can generate totals and reports easily. Mastering the software may take some time, but for larger practices, bookkeeping by computer may make sense.

Accountants and bookkeepers can also be hired to help track finances. A*ccountants* are trained in the principles of setting up and auditing financial accounts and are responsible for reporting financial results in accordance with government and regulatory authority rules. Accountants can set up bookkeeping systems and prepare taxes. *Bookkeepers* record day-to-day transactions in systems chosen by the business owner. They take care of the paperwork involved in recording expenditures and receipts, and may also balance the checkbook. Bookkeepers still have to be provided with necessary checks, bills, receipts, and other records from the business.

TRACKING CLIENT PAYMENTS

Massage fees collected plus tips received equal income from a private practice. A simple way to track client payments is to keep a handwritten receipt book. A typical receipt lists the amount of money received, method of payment (cash, check, or charge), date, service rendered, client's name, and the person who took the payment and filled out the receipt. The client gets one copy, while a carbon copy stays in the receipt book. The receipt book can serve as a supporting document for bookkeeping and tax reporting purposes.

As a backup record, a daily accounting of income can be made right in an appointment book. For each appointment kept, write the amount the client paid plus tip. Also note when appointments are canceled or missed. This provides a valuable cross-check and record of the daily activity of the practice.

One-write systems are useful for offices with more than one massage therapist, or for tracking payment histories of individual clients. These systems include a running daily income ledger for the office, individual client ledger cards that can be filed alphabetically, and individual receipts for each transaction. These are sometimes called pegboard systems.

There are also computer systems for tracking client payments. Whatever system is used, receipts should be entered into the bookkeeping system daily.

Banking

It is important to keep a separate business checking account for a private practice. This keeps personal and business finances clearly separate and makes bookkeeping simpler. There is also less chance of confusion if audited for income taxes.

Compare fees and features for business accounts before choosing a bank. Choose a bank convenient for making frequent deposits. Establishing a banking relationship may be useful if seeking a business loan or for credit card processing in the future.

A few important rules apply to banking. First, pay all business bills by check, from a petty cash account, or a credit card designated for the business. Second, deposit all income, checks and cash, into the business account. Third, when taking money out of the business account for personal use, write a check to yourself payable to "cash" or write "personal draw" on the memo line. This way personal draws or withdrawals can be tracked more easily (Kamoroff 2003).

Set aside time every month to balance the business bank account and review financial records. It is recommended that bank statements and canceled checks be kept for at least 7 years.

HEALTH INSURANCE BILLING AND REIMBURSEMENT

Few insurance companies cover massage therapy in their policies. As a result of public demand and changes in health care regulations, some of the more progressive managed care plans (Health Maintenance Organizations [HMOs], Preferred-Provider Organizations [PPOs]) cover massage therapy if the client has a referral and a prescription from a medical doctor or if the treatment is part of a prescribed physical therapy regimen. In a small number of states in the United States (Maryland, New Hampshire, Utah, Washington) coverage of massage therapy is mandated in health care plans offered by employers. Many automobile insurance policies include Personal Injury Protection (PIP) clauses, which cover massage therapy services. Workers' Compensation claims frequently will be covered if prescribed by a medical doctor. Medicare and Medicaid generally do not cover massage therapy.

A massage therapist who is an employee of a healthcare business, such as a physical therapy or chiropractic practice, a spa, or a licensed massage therapy business, most likely will not have to assume the task of dealing with insurance companies. That will be handled by an administrative staff member or possibly the owner of the business. In order to maintain the records required for insurance company reimbursement to the business, however, the massage therapist needs to be capable of certain tasks, such as conducting and recording client assessments, keeping charts current, writing treatment plans, and, in general, keeping accurate and up-to-date records.

For the massage therapist in his or her own practice, the decision to accept clients with insurance coverage requires careful thought. The additional paperwork, record keeping, billing, and waiting for reimbursement (which may never arrive or be severely discounted when it does) can become a financial quagmire for a small business. The massage therapist must gain entry to the list of approved providers of the HMO or PPO in order to have services covered, which often are paid at a reduced rate. It is important to have the client sign a medical release form so that there can be communication between the insurance company, the massage practitioner, and the client's other health care providers. Equally vital is keeping the physician's prescription for the client in a secure file.

Massage therapists who accept clients using insurance to pay their bills should be educated about relevant insurance company policies and procedures. It is dishonest and illegal to misrepresent the nature of treatment or the number of sessions given to a client. Adequate records should be kept to substantiate charges billed. It is unethical, and may be illegal in some places, to charge insurance companies more than clients who are paying out of pocket.

Since massage therapists are not considered primary heath care providers (PHCP), a diagnosis from a PHCP is usually necessary for insurance billing. These referrals are for a specific pathology, and massage billed to an insurance company should be related to treatment for the stated condition. "According to standard insurance definitions, treatment is warranted until the condition is corrected or maximum improvement is made" and also includes instruction for self-care and prevention of future occurrences of the same problem (Benjamin and Sohnen-Moe 2003, p. 207). Massage sessions for maintenance and prevention are not usually included in insurance plans and should not be billed as treatment.

Standardized Forms and Billing Codes

A standardized form, the CMS-1500 (replacing the HCFA-1500 form), is used for billing all insurance companies, as well as Medicare and Medicaid. Using one form instead of many different types is efficient and a time saver for health care professionals. To ensure legibility (and readability by the optical character recognition software that scans each form), the form should be filled out in black ink using a typewriter or computer. It is important to be sure that each client's intake form and other documentation contain all the information required on the CMS-1500 form.

Filling out a CMS-1500 form requires knowledge of ICD-9-CM (International Classification of Disease, 9th Revision, Clinical Modification) codes, CPT (current procedural terminology) codes, and place of service codes. Because they change frequently, actual code numbers are not listed or discussed in this text.

- *ICD-9-CM Codes* Every health condition (diseases, symptoms, complaints, etc.) can be assigned a category and given a code using this system first instituted by the World Health Organization (WHO) and published in the United States by the National Center for Health Statistics, a component of the Centers for Disease Control and Prevention (CDC). A diagnosis, and thus an ICD-9-CM code, can be provided only by a physician. Be sure when accepting a client's prescription that the ICD-9-CM code is included. You will need to enter it on the CMS-1500 form.
- *CPT Codes* All services health care practitioners provide to patients, such as medical, surgical, and diagnostic procedures, are assigned a five-digit alphanumeric code. Developed, maintained, and copyrighted by the American Medical Association (AMA), these codes provide a uniform way of communicating information to insurance companies, who then determine the amount of reimbursement to be paid to practitioners based on the coding. CPT codes change frequently, and there are a specific few that apply to massage therapy. When submitting bills to insurance companies, it is important to use only those codes that are within your scope of practice. Code books can be purchased from the AMA (www.ama-assn.org), but it may be more cost-effective and efficient simply to verify the proper codes to use with each insurance company you are billing.
- *Place of Service Codes* These are generally two-digit codes that indicate where the provided services took place, such as office, hospital, rehabilitation facility, and so on.

Billing insurance companies (and getting paid) can be difficult and stressful. The following are a few keys to success.

- Verify that the client's insurance company reimburses for massage therapy.
- Provide accurate documentation.
- Use correct code numbers.
- Follow the doctor's prescription.
- Stay within your scope of practice.
- Fill out the CMS-1500 form correctly and fully.

In addition, inform your clients in writing that they will be responsible for any charges not paid by their insurance companies.

CHAPTER HIGHLIGHTS

- A self-employed massage therapist is said to have a private practice with a business side, much like other businesses.
- A business plan spells out the details of a practice and includes sections on business description, marketing, management, and finances.
- A business description explains the practice vision and identity, as well as legal structure and plans for location.
  - Most massage therapists start out as sole proprietors, with office locations in the home, in a commercial space, or traveling to the clients' homes or workplaces to give massage.
- Marketing is the process of identifying potential clients and their needs or wants using market research.
- In building a client base, it is important to find ways to make yourself visible to the public and provide contact information.
  - Business cards are a key tool for obtaining new clients.
  - Paid advertising may help, as well as promotions to encourage people to make appointments.
- Management includes activities necessary to run the business.
  - Acquiring necessary licenses, insurance, and contracts lays the foundation.
  - Written policies clarify expectations related to fees, hours of operation, payment, conduct, scope of practice, client health information and confidentiality, and other aspects of the client relationship.
- Massage practice spaces typically have a reception area, massage therapy room, office, and bathrooms.
  - Spaces should be attractive, comfortable, safe, and comply with local ordinances.
- Appointments may be listed by hand in an appointment book or in electronic form.
- Client records with basic information, health histories, and session notes should be kept well organized and secure.
- A good financial goal is to start out in practice with the least amount of debt as possible at the lowest interest rate.
- Planning a first-year budget helps forecast income and expenses and is essential for making good financial decisions.

- Tracking monthly income and expenses closely is essential for financial viability.
- Keeping fixed and variable costs to a minimum maximizes profits in the end.
- A salary draw is the money taken out of the business for your personal use.
- Income taxes must be paid annually on profits from the business.
  - Taxable income for a sole proprietor is the total income (fees and tips) from the practice minus qualified business expenses.
  - Estimated taxes are paid to the IRS four times per year.
  - The IRS publishes many useful instruction booklets.
  - Hiring a professional tax preparer is recommended for massage therapists with private practices.
- Bookkeeping systems record financial transactions related to the practice.
- Financial records should be kept up-to-date and accurate.
  - Set aside time every month to balance the business bank account and review financial records.
- Some insurance plans cover massage therapy, including automobile insurance policies with PIP clauses and Workers' Compensation. Medicare and Medicaid generally do not cover massage therapy at this time.
- A physician's prescription for massage therapy is necessary for insurance claims to be paid.
- When billing insurance companies for massage services, company polices and procedures should be followed and treatment reported honestly.
  - It is unethical, and may be illegal in some places, to charge insurance companies more than clients who are paying out of pocket.
  - Accurate and up-to-date records need to be kept to support insurance claims and substantiate charges billed.
  - The CMS-1500 form is a standardized form used to bill all insurance companies. Massage providers need to be familiar with ICD-9-CM codes, CPT codes, and place of service codes in order to fill out forms correctly.
- Clients should be informed in writing that they will be responsible for charges not paid by their insurance companies.

EXAM REVIEW

Key Terms

Match the following key terms to their descriptions. For additional study, look up the key terms in the Interactive Glossary on page G-1 and note other terms that compare or contrast with them.

_____ 1. Business plan
_____ 2. Cash reserve
_____ 3. Contract
_____ 4. Estimated tax
_____ 5. Fixed costs
_____ 6. Marketing
_____ 7. Promotions
_____ 8. Salary draw
_____ 9. Self-employment tax
_____ 10. Startup costs
_____ 11. Variable costs

a. Expenses such as rent and utilities
b. Process of identifying potential customers and meeting their needs and wants
c. Money taken out of the practice on a regular basis for your personal use
d. Spells out the details of putting your practice vision into operation
e. Fluctuating operating expenses
f. A social security and Medicare tax for individuals who work for themselves
g. The initial expenses involved in setting up a massage therapy practice
h. An official written agreement between two or more people
i. Include giving discounts to new clients for their first massage
j. Putting enough money in the bank to cover at least 3 months' fixed costs
k. Payments sent to the IRS four times a year

Memory Workout

To test your memory of the main concepts in this chapter, complete the following sentences by circling the most correct answer from the two choices provided.

1. Income from clients minus (personal) (business) expenses equals the real profit from the practice.
2. The main advantages of a (home) (storefront) practice are low rent and a short commute.
3. (Promoting) (Marketing) is the process of identifying potential clients and meeting their needs and desires.
4. Advertising is a (free) (paid) public announcement providing information about goods and services to potential clients.
5. (Gift certificates) (Fee schedules) are an example of a promotion to attract clients.
6. To help avoid lawsuits, contracts should be (written down) (made verbally in good faith).
7. Practice (policies) (brochures) clarify expectations and points of agreement between the massage therapist and the client.
8. Reception areas should be (open to) (partitioned from) the massage therapy room.
9. Starting out with the least amount of (income) (debt) at the lowest interest rate is a good financial goal.
10. Money put away to cover fixed costs when starting out, or later in case of emergency, is called (a cash reserve) (petty cash).
11. Money taken out of the practice for personal use is called a (salary draw) (business expense).
12. (Taxable) (Spendable) income includes all fees collected plus tips received.
13. Charging more for a massage when an insurance company is paying the bill is considered (unethical) (good business).

Test Prep

The following multiple-choice questions will help to prepare you for future school and professional exams.

1. The most common legal structure for massage practices starting out is:
   a. Sole proprietor
   b. Partnership
   c. Limited Partnership
   d. Corporation

2. A primary source of clients in a personal service like massage is:
   a. Newspaper advertising
   b. Radio advertising
   c. Word of mouth from satisfied clients
   d. Direct mailing advertising

3. Insurance that covers you for liability for incidents arising from massage therapy itself is called
   a. Premise liability insurance
   b. Catastrophic insurance
   c. "Slip and fall" insurance
   d. Professional liability insurance

4. How often should electronic files and records be backed-up?
   a. At least once a week
   b. At least monthly
   c. Daily
   d. Biweekly

5. Money left over after expenses are paid is called
   a. Gross income
   b. Net income
   c. Profit
   d. Both b and c

6. Expenses incurred whether you see clients or not are called
   a. Fixed costs
   b. Variable costs
   c. Startup costs
   d. Reserve

7. When you are self-employed, estimated tax payments are typically sent to the IRS
   a. Two times a year
   b. Four times a year
   c. When taxes are filed
   d. When requested in writing

8. In addition to regular income tax, massage therapists in private practice pay an additional tax to cover social security and Medicare. This tax is referred to as:
   a. Reserve tax
   b. Variable tax
   c. Net income tax
   d. Self-employment tax

Video Challenge

Watch the appropriate segment of the video on your DVD and then answer the following questions.

Private Practice and Finances
1. What do the massage therapists interviewed in the video say about who helped them get started in their practices? What kind of help did they get?

Advertising
2. What ideas for marketing and advertising a massage therapy practice are presented in the video?

First-Year Budget
3. What does the video say about the importance of figuring startup costs and developing a first-year budget?

Comprehension Exercises

The following short answer questions test your knowledge and understanding of chapter topics and provide practice in written communication skills. Explain in two to four complete sentences.

1. List the four sections of a business plan, and explain what information goes into each section. Why is a business plan important for starting and maintaining a successful massage therapy practice?

2. Define *market research*. List at least five useful market research questions.
3. Explain why a good bookkeeping system is essential for a massage therapy practice. What are the elements of a good bookkeeping system?

For Greater Understanding

The following exercises are designed to take you from the realm of theory into the real world. They will help give you a deeper understanding of the subjects covered in this chapter. Action words are underlined to emphasize the variety of activities presented to address different learning styles and to encourage deeper thinking.

1. Conduct market research for the area in which you plan to open a private practice. Who is already practicing in the area? What kind of massage therapy are they offering? How do they advertise their services? What type of competitive advantage might you develop?

2. List the startup costs for a private practice you currently have in mind. How do you plan to get the money needed for the startup? Are there any ways to reduce startup costs to increase your profits in the beginning?

3. Develop a first-year budget for a private practice you currently have in mind. Use a month-by-month format. List all fixed and variable expenses you can think of. Determine your cash flow for each month.

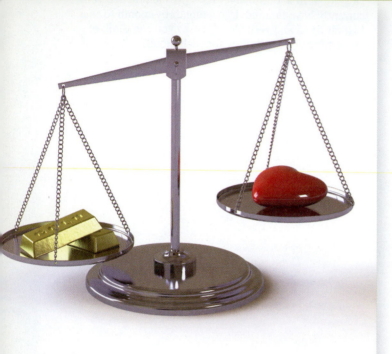

 CHAPTER OUTLINE

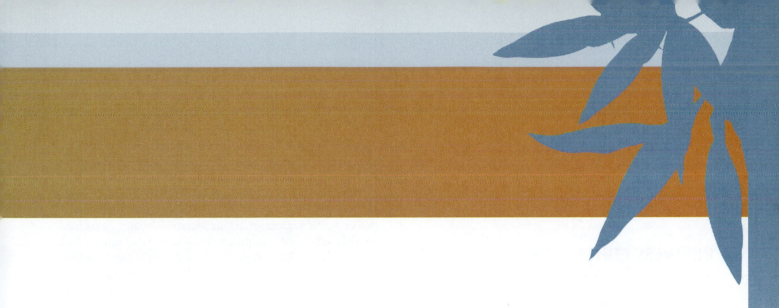

LEARNING OUTCOMES

After studying this chapter, you will have information to:

1. Follow consumer protection laws.
2. Present your credentials honestly.
3. Make truthful claims for massage therapy.
4. Abide by copyright and trademark laws.
5. Set fair policies related to money.

6. Sell products with integrity.
7. Make and take referrals properly.
8. Increase client base ethically.
9. Report unethical behavior appropriately.

KEY TERMS

Business ethics *648*

Copyright *652*

Deceptive advertising *649*

Defamation *656*

Endorsements *651*

Guarantee *651*

Massage establishment
  ordinances *648*

Occupational license *648*

Qualifying statements *652*

Trademarks *652*

MASSAGE *in* ACTION

On your DVD, explore:

- Claims for Massage Therapy
- Tips and Gifts
- Selling Products

BUSINESS ETHICS

Business ethics are moral and legal considerations related to commercial transactions (i.e., buying and selling of goods and services) and fair treatment of consumers. Because public safety and financial interests are involved, state and local governments enact business practices and consumer protection laws that give many ethical principles legal force.

Massage therapists, and the spas and clinics that employ them, are selling massage as a health service to customers. So in addition to treating people ethically as *clients* in the therapeutic relationship, they should also be treated fairly as *consumers* who pay money for advertised services.

Because massage therapy consumers are also clients, business ethics related to massage practices are stricter in some ways than in other commercial venues. The ethics of the therapeutic relationship give the massage therapist a fiduciary responsibility not necessarily present in other business transactions. For example, salespeople in clothing stores, or servers in restaurants, do not have the same responsibilities to their customers as massage therapists do to their clients. It is a responsibility of all massage therapists to put their clients' well-being above their own personal gain. This is a departure from usual business thinking.

Health professionals usually speak of having a *practice* rather than a *business*. The concept of a practice blends the professional aspects related to relationships with clients and the business aspects of the operation. The professional and business sides together make up a massage therapy practice.

A massage therapist's practice is the totality of his or her work. A practice may range from 5–20 regular private clients a week. It may include work in several locations, for example, a few clients at a home office, a few days as an employee of a spa, and a shift at a chiropractor's office. Or a person may be a practicing massage therapist for 20 hours per week and a spa manager for 20 hours. A small, part-time practice may include 2 days' work at a spa. Depending on where they work and the hats they are wearing, massage therapists can have more or less involvement in the business side of massage.

LOCAL AND STATE REGULATIONS

It is a basic ethical principle that massage therapists comply with local and state laws. Therefore, knowledge of applicable laws is fundamental to developing ethical massage practices.

There are four general types of laws to be aware of: those related to occupational licenses, zoning ordinances, business licenses, and special massage establishment licenses.

An **occupational license** is a credential issued by a government that gives a person permission to practice a profession in its jurisdiction. In the United States, state governments issue occupational licenses, although in the absence of a state license, some cities and counties issue their own occupational licenses. Forty-two states plus the District of Columbia currently regulate massage therapy. Usually states have specific educational requirements and possibly others, such as passing a written examination and not having a criminal record. Licensing laws also specify scope of practice and advertising policies. Having a license for one location does not automatically mean that you can practice in a different place. Having a current occupational license, if it is required, in the location where you are working is a basic ethical principle. More on occupational licensing can be found on page 14 in Chapter 1, The Massage Therapy Profession.

A zoning ordinance is a law that specifies what type of housing or what kind of business can be in a particular location. For example, some areas are zoned for residential housing (e.g., single- or multifamily), and some for certain types of businesses such as retail or manufacturing. Massage businesses are sometimes zoned in light industrial or adult entertainment areas, especially if a locality has had problems with massage parlors. Zoning for massage should be checked before signing a lease or other contract for practice space. Some places prohibit small businesses, such as massage therapy practices, from operating out of private homes. Zoning variances that allow exceptions to the law may be available if applied for and approved. Zoning ordinances are passed by local governments like towns, cities, or counties.

A business license may be required by a town or city government to operate a commercial enterprise in that jurisdiction. This way, government agencies know who is doing business in their area and can ensure that the businesses are complying with all related laws.

Some local governments have enacted special **massage establishment ordinances,** primarily to try to stop massage parlors being used as a cover for prostitution. In localities where a massage establishment license is required, even health clubs and spas must have a license to offer massage therapy. Since an establishment is a place with an address, massage therapists who work for someone else or who have home visit practices are usually exempt from getting massage establishment licenses.

Establishment ordinances cover a variety of topics such as where the business can be located, hours of operation, shower and toilet facilities, sanitation, posted prices, and other factors related to the business operation. Some have requirements for STD (sexually transmitted disease) tests for persons performing massage, for clothes that may not be worn (e.g., see-through garments), unlocked massage room doors, unannounced inspection, prohibitions on serving liquor, and other regulations obviously aimed toward curbing prostitution, and not for legitimate massage therapists.

As offensive as some of these laws are, massage therapists must work for their revision rather than avoid getting a license to operate their practices. It has become easier to change restrictive establishment and zoning laws as more states adopt occupational licensing that limits the practice of massage to trained and ethical practitioners.

ADVERTISING

Advertising involves disseminating information about your massage therapy practice to potential clients. Advertising takes many forms and includes handing out business cards, putting flyers on community bulletin boards, displaying brochures, putting ads in newspapers and magazines, having a telephone directory yellow pages listing, or posting a website on the Internet. Possibilities for advertising are discussed in more detail on page 630 in Chapter 22, Private Practice and Finances.

The ethical principles of advertising are based on values of honesty and integrity. **Deceptive advertising** involves misleading the public about credentials, the nature of the service, its benefits, or how much it costs. The Federal Trade Commission (FTC) defines deceptive advertising as a "representation, omission or practice that is likely to mislead the [reasonable] consumer" (FTC Policy 1983) (www.ftc.gov/bcp/policystmt/ad-decept.htm). Consumer protection laws are designed to protect the public from unsafe products and services, and from deceptive advertising. Local regulations and licensing laws may also affect how massage therapy may be advertised.

Professional Image

The words and images used in advertising should convey a sense of professionalism, such as the ad shown in Figure 23.1■. Some of the ethical principles of therapeutic relationships also apply to advertising, for example, those related to professional boundaries and confidentiality.

Using sexual suggestion in advertising text or images is highly unethical and may also be illegal. Unfortunately, many allusions to relaxation and pleasurable touch, which are perfectly ethical benefits of massage, also have sexual overtones. In the United States, the word "masseuse" has become associated with prostitution, so "massage therapist" is the preferred term for a professional massage practitioner.

Ads in big city phonebooks are instructive of what to avoid in advertising. For example, "taste of paradise, female masseuse, 24 hours, outcalls available" with a photo of a seductive-looking woman in a flirtatious pose does not say "professional massage" to the reader. Another example of the type of advertising to avoid is "Angela's magic hands, full body sensual massage, beautiful female masseuses, 'it doesn't get any better than this,'" with a photo of a woman's hands with long nails. "Jeannie Pampers, 'get pampered at your own place'" is less obvious but still suggestive.

Photos should show professional massage with good draping. If using photos of actual clients, get written permission to use their photos or names. Professional associations and photo dealers may have stock photos that can be used in ads.

Giving the wrong impression in advertising can result in unwanted calls from people looking for prostitution. Have colleagues, family, or friends review your ads to evaluate

CASE FOR STUDY

Harry the Natural Salesman

Harry is a natural salesman and promoter, and he is putting those skills to use in building his massage practice. In his advertising, he claims that his massage can cure a variety of modern-day ills and always includes six endorsements from satisfied clients. He figures that getting potential clients to make appointments is most important and that all of his customers can only benefit from getting massage.

Question:

Is Harry's style of advertising ethical?

Things to consider:

- Are there any legal implications with Harry's style of advertising related to claims for massage and the use of endorsements?
- Would this style of advertising be permitted under massage therapy licensing laws?

- If Harry's ads are successful in attracting clients, aren't they acceptable from a business point of view?
- How does his style of advertising live up to values of honesty, integrity, and professionalism?
- Is this situation covered in a code of ethics or standards of practice for massage therapists?
- Who might be affected by this style of advertising, either positively or negatively?
- What is Harry's major motivation with this style of advertising?
- What are the most important considerations in this situation?
- What decision would maintain the highest standards?

Your reasoning and conclusions:

_____

_____

_____

_____

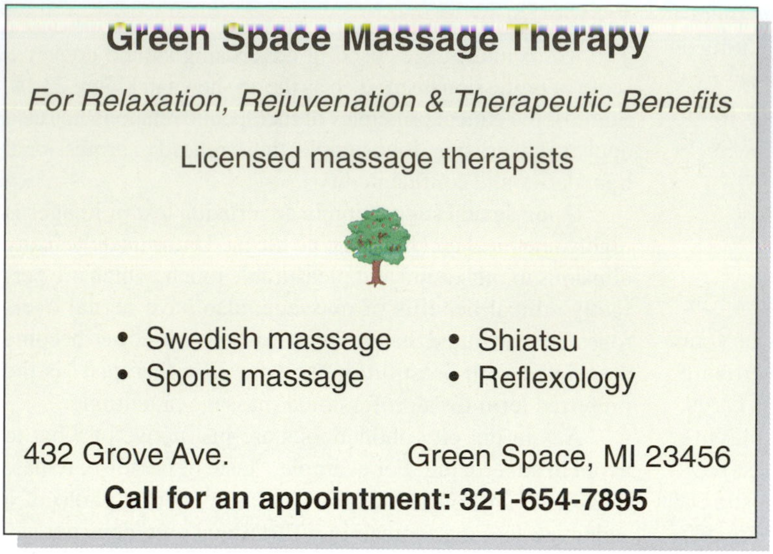

Green Space Massage Therapy

For Relaxation, Rejuvenation & Therapeutic Benefits

Licensed massage therapists

- Swedish massage
- Sports massage
- Shiatsu
- Reflexology

432 Grove Ave.   Green Space, MI 23456

Call for an appointment: 321-654-7895

FIGURE 23.1
Massage therapy advertising should convey a professional image.

their professional image. What seems cute or clever to you may give the wrong impression about your massage therapy practice.

CREDENTIALS

Credentials are professional designations or titles given to massage therapists by organizations such as schools, certification commissions, licensing agencies, and other legitimate institutions. Credentials should be represented honestly in advertising. The general public, clients, employers, and other health professionals rely on credentials to assess a person's training and qualifications.

Obviously, it is unethical to lie about your credentials. It is more likely that a massage therapist would mislead the public by being vague about qualifications or by wording his or her qualifications incorrectly in an advertisement. The ethical question to ask is, "Will the public be misled about my qualifications

if I use this wording?" Since massage therapists are recognized health professionals, they should display their credentials using the same conventions as other similar professions.

The credential received upon graduation from an entry-level massage program is usually a *certificate of completion* or a *diploma*. The correct way to word that credential in advertising would be "Graduate of ABC Massage School" or "Diploma from ABC Professional Massage Program."

Certification and *certified* are perhaps the most ambiguous terms used as credentials by massage therapists. Being "certified" is currently used to mean anything from completing a weekend workshop in some massage technique, to finishing a 500-hour program, to completing extensive training in a specialty, passing an examination, and keeping up with continuing education. This can be confusing to the general public.

A person from the general public who hears that someone is "certified" in some massage system expects it to be backed

PRACTICAL APPLICATION

Knowing the correct ways to maintain a professional image and advertise your massage therapy practice is often a matter of knowing what *not* to do. In your community, observe what other massage therapists do to promote their massage practices. Keep your eyes and ears open for examples of good and bad advertising, professional and unprofessional images, appropriate and inappropriate use of credentials, and the use of guarantees, endorsements, and claims made in advertising.

Ask yourself whether the examples you find in your community reflect well or ill upon the massage practitioner. Take note of good examples that you might emulate, without violating another practitioner's copyright, trademark, or patent.

1. Find examples of deceptive advertising in a newspaper or magazine. What makes the advertisements misleading?
2. Find examples of professional and unprofessional advertising for massage in newspapers, magazines, and the telephone book. What makes some examples unprofessional?
3. Find examples of credentials displayed both correctly and questionably in advertising by massage therapists. What makes the use of credentials questionable?
4. Find examples of guarantees, endorsements, and claims made in advertising. Analyze their legitimacy. Should the massage therapist have such elements in his or her advertising? Would you?

by considerable training and acquired expertise. In addition, other health professions generally reserve the term *certification* for lengthy programs aimed at competence in a specialty.

National certification and *board certification* are understood as being conferred after one completes a program of study and passes a written and/or performance examination. Adherence to a code of ethics and continuing education are often required. This level of certification is given by an independent, nonprofit organization or commission whose mission is to provide these credentials for the benefit of the public. Passing a profession's "boards" is often a prerequisite for getting an occupational license.

So when is it ethical for a massage therapist to say that he or she is *certified*? Certification boards usually designate titles for those certified by their organization, for example, "Nationally Certified in Therapeutic Massage and Bodywork" or "Certified Rolfer" (Rolf Institute). Some use the word *registered* to mean much the same thing, as in "Registered Polarity Practitioner" (American Polarity Therapy Association). In any case, the title designates the practitioner as having acquired competence and continuing education in the subject and using the title exactly as it is given is correct.

On the other hand, it is misleading to say that you are certified after having completed a weekend workshop in a certain technique, whether or not the presenter or organization giving the workshop says that you are certified. It is more accurate to say that you have completed so many hours of training in a particular subject. The certificate you receive at the end of the workshop is just that, a certificate of completion for the course of study.

The use of initials after a name is also a matter of judgment. Initials after a name are generally understood to signify an earned academic degree, board certification, or licensing. Academic degrees are AA, BS, MS, PhD, or some variation. NCTMB means Nationally Certified in Therapeutic Massage and Bodywork. In some states, LMT is used to designate Licensed Massage Therapist. In some Canadian provinces, RMT is used to mean Registered Massage Therapist. There are other variations for initials used by massage therapists, and it is wise to check on which designations are correct in your situation.

Initials are not meant to signify an occupation. The initials "MsT" (used to mean "massage therapist") and "CMT" (used to mean having a diploma from a massage program) are misleading. Information should be spelled out if using only initials would be misleading, for example, use the terms "massage therapist," and "graduate massage therapist." It may be more informative to spell out "licensed massage therapist" followed by the license number in states or local areas where licensing is required. Some states require a person's license number to appear on all advertising.

Guarantees and Endorsements

Honesty in advertising means describing the service or product truthfully and avoiding unfounded guarantees and claims. A **guarantee** is a promise that something will work as stated,

usually with the implication that the money will be refunded if it does not.

The problem with making guarantees is that no one can predict the outcome of a particular massage session or series of sessions. There are too many variables involved. Statements like "guaranteed to reduce stress" or "guaranteed relief after one session" border on fraudulent. Using a ploy like "guaranteed to work or your money back" is not appropriate for a professional health service.

Some have suggested that massage therapists might use "satisfaction guaranteed or your money back" to show confidence in their service. The therapeutic result is not guaranteed, but the client's satisfaction, which is easier to substantiate, is ensured (Benjamin and Sohnen-Moe 2003).

Endorsements or testimonials are anecdotes from someone besides the massage therapist, usually clients, about how well the massage worked for them. The Federal Trade Commission (FTC 1980) defines an endorsement as "any advertising message . . . which consumers are likely to believe reflects the opinions, beliefs, findings, or experience of a party other than the sponsoring advertiser."

Some examples of massage therapy endorsements are: "My tension headaches went away after one massage." "I shaved 10 minutes off my marathon time with sports massage." "My insomnia dissolved, and I sleep like a baby after receiving massage from ABC Massage." Endorsements may be made by individuals, organizations, or experts.

While these statements by particular clients may be true, they may also be misleading. The FTC (1980) states that endorsements "may not contain any representations which would be deceptive, or could not be substantiated if made directly by the advertiser." Making claims for massage therapy is discussed in a following section.

Endorsements are best used sparingly, if at all. They are not a substitute for the results of research on the effects of massage. Acceptable strategies for advertising are discussed on page 630 in Chapter 22, Private Practice and Finances.

Prices and Bait Advertising

If a price is stated in an advertisement, the massage therapist must honor it in most cases. Exceptions would be if it is an obvious typographical mistake by the printer of a one-time ad (e.g., $6 instead of $65 for an hour-long massage) and would present an undue financial hardship. A mistake on a brochure should be fixed by hand and/or by having the brochure reprinted. It is wise to add in print that prices are subject to change to allow for raising prices in the future, especially in a brochure that someone may keep for a period of time.

If offering a special price or discount, the conditions should be clearly stated. For example, include the time period for the offer (e.g., November 20 through December 24, 2010), the specific service covered, and special conditions such as "daytime appointments only."

Bait advertising is unethical and illegal. Bait advertising is "an alluring but insincere offer to sell a product or service which the advertiser in truth does not intend or want to sell" (FTC 2000). The purpose of bait advertising is to generate leads to potential customers, or to sell something else at a higher price, which is called bait and switch. For example, it would be unethical to advertise $10 for a 30-minute massage, and then pressure the client to switch to a $60 hour massage instead. Other ethical considerations related to pricing are discussed later in the chapter.

CLAIMS FOR MASSAGE THERAPY

Claims that massage therapists make for their work must be honest and truthful. This includes claims made in advertising or directly spoken to a client, and those stated explicitly or implied. Exaggerated claims, like promising a client that massage can cure pain in five sessions, are almost always unfounded and dishonest.

Furthermore, the FTC requires that claims made in advertising are substantiated claims, that is, "that advertisers and ad agencies have a reasonable basis for advertising claims before they are disseminated" (FTC 1984). Businesses are required to possess information substantiating such claims as "research shows" or "doctors recommend."

Scientific research is perhaps the most reliable evidence for claims about the various benefits of massage. Legitimate claims may also be backed by knowledge in textbooks and articles, logical deduction from facts, and personal experience. However, claims are legitimately made for massage therapy itself and not for how it will affect any particular client.

Massage therapists are admonished to "accurately inform clients, other health practitioners, and the public of the scope and limitations of their discipline," and to "acknowledge the limitations of and contraindications for massage and bodywork and refer clients to appropriate health professionals" (NCBTMB 2008). For example, a client who comes for massage to lose weight or "melt fat" would be better referred to a nutritionist or personal trainer.

It is the responsibility of massage therapists to become knowledgeable about the potential effects and benefits of massage and to stay up-to-date on the latest research and knowledge in the field. This can be accomplished through reading and studying journals, pursuing continuing education, and looking up research on various topics of interest. Massage therapists who practice critical thinking examine evidence for the benefits of massage and do not accept everything they read or hear without question.

Qualify claims about massage therapy by citing sources of information. **Qualifying statements** that can be made when speaking to clients include "in a pathology and massage text it says . . . ," "a recent research study found that . . . ," "from my experience I've noticed that . . . ," "according to the manufacturer, this product . . . ," and "other clients have reported that. . . ." Having to qualify statements forces massage therapists to become more aware of how they know

what they know. It is wise to check out claims made by vendors selling something or claims for new or unique techniques. Do not make claims you cannot reasonably substantiate or that you know or suspect are false.

COPYRIGHTS, TRADEMARKS, AND PATENTS

Copyright, trademarks, and patents offer legal protection for intellectual property rights. It is a matter of ethics that these protections be respected by individuals and businesses.

Copyright laws protect written, musical, and artistic works from unauthorized use and are designated by the symbol ©. Copyrights are administered in the United States by the U.S. Copyright Office at the Library of Congress in Washington, DC (www.copyright.gov).

According to copyright laws, a person cannot copy brochures, flyers, pamphlets, business logos, artwork, books or significant parts of books, and other materials written or prepared by someone else without the author's or copyright holder's express permission. A work receives copyright protection immediately from the time it exists in fixed form. Protected use includes reproduction, derivative works, and distribution of copies. Authors and artists may sign over copyright for their work to someone else, such as a publisher.

When developing advertising materials and other documents, copyrighted works may be used for ideas and for reference, but should not be copied exactly and used as one's own. For example, it would be unethical to take someone else's unique brochure and just replace that person's name with yours without permission.

Some brochures are available for purchase and have a space for printing a business name and contact information. It is all right to buy these brochures for distribution, but unethical to copy them rather than ordering more from the publisher.

Fair use of a copyrighted work is allowed. "Fair use" allows limited use of copyrighted materials for education and research purposes. This does not apply to whole works or significant parts of works such as whole chapters in a book. Any use that takes away from the copyright holder's potential market for selling the work is not fair use. For example, if an author creates drawings of self-massage techniques to give to clients for home care and makes them available for purchase in notepad format, it would be unethical and illegal for you to photocopy them for your clients. If however, they are published in a book, and the author clearly states that they may be copied for clients, then this use does not violate copyright law.

Trademarks offer exclusive use of a name or symbol to identify unique goods and services and use the symbol™ or ® for registered trademarks. Trademarks distinguish a particular brand or company from others. Trademarks are handled by the U.S. Patent and Trademark Office in Washington, DC. States in the United States (www.uspto.gov) and Canadian provinces may also have laws that protect trademarks such as names and logos for businesses that operate within their jurisdictions.

Trademarks include unique business names like "Wellspring Massage Therapy" or "Morristown Spa and Massage," along with the logo or identifying design used on documents and in advertising. Trademarks for services are also called *service marks* (sm). The business that uses the name or logo first and consistently on materials associated with the business has the right to the trademark. Most states have offices where the names of businesses can be researched to see if they are already in use. It is wise to register the name of your practice or business to protect it from use by someone else.

Artwork for logos and text for advertising may be in the "public domain" meaning that they are commonly available or have been created for pubic distribution. Books of stock logos are available at printing companies, and professional associations may have text and designs for advertising available for general use. Using words and artwork in the public domain is an ethically safe and economical alternative to developing your own unique materials.

Massage and bodywork systems such as Rolfing®, Jin Shin Do®, and Feldenkrais Method® are registered trademarks. Massage therapists may not use trademarked names in their advertising or descriptions of their work unless they hold credentials from the trademark organizations that allow them to use the designation.

Patents are protections for inventions and include utility and design patents. The inventor of a massage tool, machine, or other product related to massage may apply for a patent from the U.S. Patent and Trademark Office. Patented inventions may not be copied by others for sale.

FEES AND PRICING

The exchange of money is an integral part of massage therapy practices and must be done with honesty and integrity. Key principles are fair compensation, clarity, and consistency.

Fair compensation is determined partially by the usual rate for massage in a particular location. What are others charging? Generally speaking, massage costs more in big cities than in rural areas or areas with lower costs of living. A house call usually costs more than in-office massage. A massage therapist with more training and/or experience may command a rate at the higher end of the scale than one just out of school. In many ways "fair" is determined by what the market will bear, that is, what people are willing to pay.

Once established, a pricing policy should be clearly stated in promotional materials, and posted prominently in the place of business. Simplicity is best, but different rates for different session lengths (usually 30, 60, or 90 minutes), or sessions for which special training is required (e.g., lymphatic drainage massage or sports massage), are appropriate.

Be sure that policies regarding when payment is expected and what form it can take (cash, check, credit/debit card) are clear. Tell clients before a session begins what rate will be charged. If a session goes longer than expected, it is the massage therapist's responsibility, and the client would not ordinarily be charged extra.

Consistent pricing is a matter of fairness. Charging one person less than another can be complicated, even when offering discounts for friends and family. Treating discounted sessions with less professionalism is unethical.

Special pricing such as sliding scales and prepaid plans require careful thought. Sliding scales are problematic and

CASE FOR STUDY

Lilly's Pricing System

Lilly is just beginning to build her massage therapy practice. She worries about being competitive with other massage therapists in the area and has difficulty asking for money from clients. The going rate for massage seems so high to her. She never publishes her rates and changes her rates according to what she thinks the client can afford or will be willing to pay.

Question:

Is Lilly's pricing system ethical?

Things to consider:

- Are there any legal implications for Lilly's pricing system? Do local licensing laws require posting rates?
- Does Lilly have the right to charge what she wants for her massage?

- How does her system of pricing live up to values of fairness and integrity?
- Is this situation covered in a code of ethics or standards of practice for massage therapists?
- Who might be affected by her system of pricing?
- What is Lilly's major motivation for this pricing system?
- What are alternative pricing strategies?
- What are the most important considerations in this situation?
- What decision would maintain the highest standards?

Your reasoning and conclusions:

_____

_____

_____

_____

are avoided by most practitioners. If a sliding scale is adopted, establish objective guidelines, for example, based on a person's or family's income. Prepaid plans can be good for marketing, but be sure to state the terms clearly. An example of a prepaid plan is a package of six prepaid sessions for the price of five sessions. Make time limits clear, like "must be used within 1 year" or by a certain expiration date.

Charging more for a massage when an insurance company is paying is considered unethical and may also be illegal. While it is true that practices using third-party payments have more paperwork to complete, those costs are typically absorbed in general operation costs.

TIPS AND GIFTS

Tips are gratuities (i.e., given in gratitude) over and above the cost of a massage session given directly to the massage therapist. Whether a tip is given and the amount is determined at the discretion of the client. Accepting tips in an ethical way calls for some careful thought.

Soliciting or accepting tips for massage therapy poses ethical questions not relevant to other service occupations. Complicating factors are that massage therapy is given in a variety of settings with different customs related to tipping (e.g., spas, salons, medical settings, and private offices), that massage therapists may have independent practices or may be employees, and that massage involves a therapeutic relationship with clients which presents special responsibilities.

Accepting tips can be ethical if they do not negatively influence the therapeutic relationship, if they are truly optional, and if tippers and nontippers receive the same level of care. Tips are most appropriate in settings where it is customary to give gratuities for services, such as at salons, spas, hotels, and resorts.

In places where tipping is customary, owners of the businesses are usually not tipped. Employees or independent contractors who receive less than the cost of the massage are commonly tipped. In private massage practices, where the practitioner sets the price of the massage, tips should not be expected.

Tips for massage are problematic in settings such as medical clinics, chiropractic offices, and private practices. Tipping health professionals is not customary. Tipping may be confusing and awkward for clients in settings considered to be health care related, rather than personal service or recreation related.

It is appropriate to let clients know if tipping is customary in a certain setting. A sign that states "Tips appreciated" lets clients know that it is a place where tips are accepted. However, clients must never feel that they need to give a tip to receive high-quality service. Tips should never be solicited personally by massage therapists.

Turn down tips that have expectations attached and tips that are too large. Tips that seem too large (e.g., $25 for a $60 massage) may involve transference on the part of the client or may be an attempt to gain favor. Such tips cross

professional boundaries and should not be accepted. On the other hand, a client who offers a larger than usual tip in appreciation for pain relief or doing well in a big race after receiving sports massage may simply be expressing his or her gratitude, and accepting the tip causes no harm. These are judgment calls for the massage therapist to make. It is acceptable to adopt a "no tipping" policy in a private practice.

Gifts are a similar situation. Nonmonetary gifts that are tokens given in appreciation or at special times like the holidays may be appropriate to accept. Gifts given to gain favor compromise the therapeutic relationship and cross boundaries, and should be politely refused. Never accept a gift from a client whom you suspect has a romantic interest in you. Gifts with high monetary value are also inappropriate to accept. Trust your intuition to tell you that something does not seem right, or ask advice about it from a colleague or friend who understands the professional implications involved.

According to the IRS, tips are taxable income and should be reported when filing income tax returns. Monetary gifts would be considered tips. Keep a record of all tips received.

REALITY CHECK

ROB

SASHA: I really look forward to getting tips from my clients at the health club. I count on that added income. I have some stingy clients who never tip, and I don't feel like giving them my best. Should I drop some hints to them about leaving a tip? Maybe they don't know I expect one.

ROB: Given your expectations, I can understand why you feel the way you do. But let's look at this from an ethical point of view. First, your clients probably view you as a health professional, and may not think of tipping you anymore than they would a physical therapist. Calling them "stingy" sounds really judgmental. Does the health club have a tipping policy displayed at the appointment desk? Soliciting tips directly, even by hinting, is unacceptable. Tipping is always at the discretion of the client. It is unethical to tie the level of service you provide to the tip you may or may not receive afterward. This is all about expectations and attitude. I suggest figuring your projected income without any tips. At the health club, I'd prefer to get paid at a good rate, like the other professionals working there, and not worry about tips.

SELLING PRODUCTS

Some massage therapists sell products in conjunction with their massage practices. Massage-related products include massage oils and lotions, tools for self-massage such as foot rollers, support pillows, hot and cold packs, and books and videos. Having products for sale can be a valuable service to clients and is not unethical as long as clients do not feel pressured to buy them from you. Your role as a massage therapist would be to inform clients about the benefits of the products with the opportunity to buy them, if desired. There are clearer boundaries if products for sale are not displayed in the massage room, but are in a reception or sales area (Figure 23.2■).

Selling products is often part of a spa or salon business, and employees may be expected to "push" the products for sale. This is problematic for massage therapists who are cautioned not to use the power differential in the therapeutic relationship for their personal gain. As stated earlier, educating clients and making products available is acceptable; however, talking clients into products they may not want or need is not.

Be particularly aware of your conflict of interest if you are part of a multilevel marketing program. It is not ethical to use your massage clients to meet sales goals. Clients who feel pressured into buying products outside of their interest in receiving massage may also feel taken advantage of and seek massage elsewhere.

Be especially mindful if you are selling nutritional supplements, herbal preparations, or vitamins. Do not confuse being trained in selling a product by its manufacturer or distributor with having professional education in nutrition. To keep clear boundaries between your massage practice and nutritional sales, make separate appointments to talk to clients about these other products, preferably in a space different from the massage office.

Know that your massage clients may see you as a health expert and may therefore give unwarranted trust in your judgment about nutrition. Make it clear that you are not an expert in nutrition unless you have additional academic training and credentials in that field. If clients feel that you are prescribing supplements for a specific medical condition, you may be perceived as practicing medicine without a license. You may also be liable if the client has a negative reaction to a product you sold to him or her.

REFERRALS

It is expected that massage therapists make referrals to other health professionals when clients have needs outside of the therapists' scope of practice, or when massage may not be the best treatment for a specific condition. A client's needs may also be beyond a particular massage therapist's training or expertise, and referral to a massage therapist with advanced or specialized training might be best for the client.

Keeping a list of other health professionals (including doctors, chiropractors, naturopathic physicians, physical therapists, athletic trainers, and massage therapists) that you believe are competent and ethical is a good practice. When making referrals give the client two or three names from which to choose. Become familiar with websites that list certified practitioners of specific massage and bodywork systems or that list massage therapists and their specialties. Refer clients to those sites if appropriate.

It is unethical for health practitioners to reward each other for referrals in a quid pro quo manner with either money or gifts. For example, it would be unethical for a chiropractor to give a massage therapist $10 for every referral he or she makes to the chiropractor. This violates the principle of avoiding conflict of interest. Massage therapists are advised to "refuse any gifts or benefits which are intended to influence a referral, decision or treatment that are purely for personal gain and not for the good of the client" (NCBTMB 2008).

The same principles apply when accepting referrals. Do not accept clients on referral that have conditions outside of your scope, and do not reward referrals made to you. Clients should be able to trust that referrals are made in their best interests and not for monetary gain. A thank you note for referrals is an appropriate acknowledgment. However, because of confidentiality issues, you might consider omitting the name of the client and just give a simple "thank you for a recent referral."

CLIENT BASE

Building a base of regular clients is the foundation of success for massage therapists, whether they are in private practice or employed somewhere like a spa. Clients will come back to massage therapists whom they respect and trust, and who give them good service.

There are a few ethical pitfalls in attracting and keeping clients. Previous sections have discussed making false claims

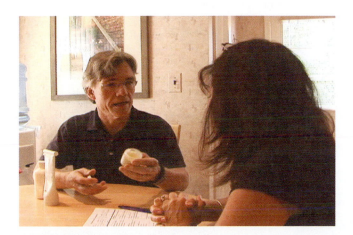

FIGURE 23.2

Educate clients about products related to massage therapy and the clients' health goals without pressuring them to buy.

and exceeding scope of practice. Another pitfall is trying to build yourself up by speaking poorly of another massage therapist. A wise person once said, "You don't make yourself taller by cutting down your neighbor." It is better to concentrate on the quality of what you offer than criticize a colleague to a client.

If you are employed somewhere like a spa or clinic, the clients you see there are shared by you and the larger business. It is considered unethical, and may be a violation of an employment agreement, to solicit clients seen at an employer's place for your private practice. For example, it would be unethical to say to a client, "Why don't you come for massage at my home office instead of here?" The temptation is there, since you might make more money by seeing a client in your own space.

The issue of "stealing" clients can be a murky one, since clients have free choice regarding from whom they receive massage. They also can get attached to their massage therapists, much the same as they do to the people who cut their hair. What if a regular client requests to see you at your place for the sake of convenience? If your employment agreement explicitly prohibits seeing the company's clients at another place, then this would be unethical.

What if you are leaving an employer and your clients want to keep seeing you for massage? It would be unethical to actually make an appointment for your private practice while on your employer's premises. However, providing information about your practice, if directly asked by a client, would in most circumstances be all right. Then the client can take the initiative to call you if he or she prefers to continue as your client. The key principles here are "no solicitation," the "client's initiative," and any prior employment agreement. In complex cases like these, it is best to apply the ethical decision-making model described on page 98 in Chapter 5, Ethics and the Therapeutic Relationship, to determine the most ethical path.

DEFAMATION

Defamation is a legal term for injury to a person or an organization's reputation. Defamation is known as *libel* if written and as *slander* if spoken. It is highly unethical to defame the character or reputation of a client or another massage therapist or health professional.

Defamation can also result in a civil lawsuit if the person defamed experiences a loss of some kind. A court may award a plaintiff monetary damages if the statements were untrue and/or made with malice or intent to harm. To avoid such issues, do not repeat malicious gossip.

Defamation laws differ slightly in different jurisdictions but usually include accusations of criminal conduct and allegations that negatively affect a person's business or profession. Stating that a person has a disease or has engaged in

CASE FOR STUDY

Rochelle and Client Choice

Rochelle started out giving massage at a local beauty salon as an independent contractor. There was a verbal agreement that she could use a spare room for appointments and split the receipts 60/40 with the salon owners. After a while, Rochelle decided that she would leave the salon and take a job at a local spa that offered better working conditions and employee benefits. She would receive a bit less income from each massage, but she figured that it was to her advantage overall. Another massage therapist is taking Rochelle's place at the salon. Massage rates are a little higher at the spa than at the salon.

Question:

Is it ethical for Rochelle to solicit her salon clients to come to the spa for massage instead of to the salon?

Things to consider:

- Are there any legal implications in this situation?
- Was there an explicit or implicit agreement with the salon about whose customers the massage clients were?

- What values are involved in a decision to solicit those clients?
- Is this situation covered in a code of ethics or standards of practice for massage therapists?
- Who might be affected by Rochelle's solicitation, either positively or negatively?
- What is Rochelle's major motivation for soliciting these clients?
- What are alternative courses of action?
- What are the most important considerations in this situation?
- What decision would maintain the highest standards?

Your reasoning and conclusions:

_____

_____

_____

_____

certain sexual activity, thus damaging his or her reputation, may also be defamation.

Descriptive statements and opinions about situations are two different things. For example, it would be better to say to a coworker that a client came for massage smelling like beer and talking with a slur than to call him a "drunk" or "lush." If the descriptive statement was made in confidence as a matter of information to protect other massage therapists, or to describe to a supervisor why you refused to work with a client at a specific appointment, it might not qualify as defamation with damages. A court of law would make its own judgment.

Remember that a client may ask to see his or her records, so what is written in them should be thought out carefully to avoid accusations of libel. It is an especially sensitive situation to report perceived misbehavior by a client, or to record something not related to the massage itself that was told in confidence in a session. It is wise to stick with accurate objective descriptions and tell a coworker or colleague immediately after something unusual happens.

It is also defamation to criticize or malign another massage therapist or health professional. If you do not trust the competence of a colleague, and for some reason wish to reveal your view to someone else, state the facts and then your opinion separately. For example, "Two of my clients have complained about massage therapist 'G' using too much pressure and bruising them. I believe that she is being insensitive."

SAFETY AND WELFARE OF CLIENTS

Massage therapists are responsible for the safety and well-being of their clients during massage sessions and while clients are on the premises. It is unethical to put clients in danger through carelessness.

Provide regular maintenance for massage tables, chairs, and other equipment. Make sure surfaces are sanitary and massage procedures hygienic. Massage offices should be well lighted and free from obstacles that could cause accidents.

Massage therapists are guilty of negligence if an accident or injury is caused by their carelessness. If the cause is something a trained practitioner is expected to know, the massage therapist may be guilty of malpractice.

To protect themselves and their clients financially, massage therapists should carry accident (slip and fall) insurance, as well as professional liability insurance. Carrying certain types of insurance may be a condition for maintaining a license to practice.

REPORTING UNETHICAL BEHAVIOR

What should massage therapists do when they suspect another massage therapist of unethical behavior? What kinds of actions are important to report? How much evidence is enough to accuse someone of wrongdoing? To whom do they report their suspicions? These are some important questions to ask before accusing someone of something that may affect that person's future as a massage therapist.

Before reporting suspected unethical behavior, a person should be clear about the facts of the case and reasonably sure that something unethical happened. If the unethical behavior is relatively minor, and the person unaware that he or she is behaving unethically, talking to the offender about the situation may be the best response. For example, if someone starts talking inappropriately about a client, make a statement such as, "This seems like gossip to me; I'd rather not continue this conversation."

Reminding a coworker or colleague of an ethical principle may be enough to stop the unethical behavior. For example, if coworkers are leaving client files open on a desk, remind them that files are confidential and should be kept secure. Friendly reminders are usually accepted well.

If, however, the situation involves physical or emotional harm to a client, or to another health professional, then more official action may be required. Professional associations, certification commissions, and licensing agencies have procedures for reporting misconduct by professionals. Unethical conduct can result in disciplinary action

CRITICAL THINKING

If your state has occupational licensing, explain in writing the process for reporting misconduct by a massage therapist. Then answer the following questions:

1. In your state, what constitutes professional misconduct?
2. What disciplinary actions might happen to a massage therapist who is proven to have engaged in misconduct?

3. How do the standards of practice and code of ethics for massage practitioners protect both the practitioner and the consumer?

against the offender, which ranges from letters of reprimand, to probation, to losing a membership or license. These actions would follow due process, investigation, and a hearing.

Passing along secondhand information is less desirable than convincing the person harmed, or a firsthand witness, to file a complaint. However, if the allegations are serious enough, and there is strong evidence for them, then they could be reported with or without firsthand information. The organization or agency receiving the report can determine if it wants to follow through with a hearing.

Where does someone report suspected unethical behavior? If there is legal jurisdiction, then the licensing agency should be contacted. If it involves a business practice such as deceptive advertising or a payment dispute, then a complaint can also be filed with the Better Business Bureau. The Federal Trade Commission has a complaint procedure in place for consumer protection (www.ftc.gov). Local and state governments may also have procedures for consumer complaints.

BEYOND GRADUATION— AN INVITATION

The journey to becoming a successful massage therapist in some ways never ends. Beyond graduation loom the challenges of getting employment or setting up a private practice. But the reward of having meaningful and satisfying work that sustains you through the years is worth the effort.

The following "invitation" is based on similar oaths from other health professions. It summarizes important ideas to keep in mind as you start out in your new chosen profession.

Invitation to Massage Therapists

Welcome into the ranks of therapeutic massage and bodywork professionals.

May you remember your days at school with fondness and appreciation.

May you honor your teachers and all who helped you through your training.

May you serve your fellow creatures with compassion and humility.

May you always hold the best interests of your clients above your own personal gain.

May you behave honestly and honorably in your practice.

May you continue to seek knowledge and skill in your profession—there is always more to learn.

May you join your colleagues in protecting the practice of massage therapy.

May you value always the healing benefits of touch.

And over all, may you find fulfillment and meaning in the work of your hands.

PJB

CHAPTER HIGHLIGHTS

- Business ethics are moral and legal considerations related to commercial transactions.
- Business practices and consumer protection laws give ethical principles legal force.
- A massage therapy practice blends professional aspects related to client relationships with business aspects of the operation; in this sense, a client is also a customer.
- Massage therapists must comply with local and state laws, including occupational licensing laws, zoning ordinances, and business license and establishment license requirements.
- Design advertising to be professional and avoid deception.
  - Display credentials honestly and correctly.
  - Limit guarantees or promises about massage therapy, and use endorsements and testimonials sparingly.
  - Advertised prices must be honored, discounts defined clearly, and bait advertising avoided.
- Claims for massage therapy must be honest and truthful, and backed up by research if possible.
  - Qualify claims by citing sources of information such as textbooks or experience.
- Copyright, trademark, and patent laws protect intellectual property rights. Never claim another person's work as your own, and do follow principles of fair use.
  - Massage therapists may not use trademarked names for massage and bodywork unless they hold proper authorization.
- Charging more for a massage when an insurance company is paying is considered unethical and may also be illegal.
- Accepting tips or gifts is acceptable under certain circumstances.
  - Tips are taxable income to be reported when filing income tax returns.
  - Refuse tips and gifts if there are unethical expectations attached, and never accept gifts from clients who may have romantic intentions.

- Selling products as part of a massage practice may be ethical if done properly.
  - Educating clients about useful products is acceptable, but pressuring them to buy is not.
  - Massage clients should not be used to meet sales quotas.
  - Special care about scope of practice is warranted when selling nutritional products.
- Refer clients to other qualified health professionals for treatment beyond the scope of a massage therapist's own knowledge and skills.
  - Receiving money or gifts from another health professional for referrals is considered a conflict of interest and is unethical.
- When building a client base, emphasize the quality of your service, rather than criticizing other massage therapists.
- Do not solicit clients of an employer's business for your own private practice.
- Defamation—injury to another's reputation—is called libel if written and slander if spoken. Defamation can result in a civil lawsuit if the person defamed experiences a loss.
  - It is safer to keep to descriptive statements of something that happened rather than give interpretations or opinions.
  - Clients are entitled to see their records, so massage therapists should be especially careful about what is written in them.
- It is unethical to put clients in danger through carelessness or negligence.
  - Keep premises and equipment clean and well maintained.
- Massage therapists should talk to each other about minor or unintentional unethical behaviors.
- Report suspected serious unethical behavior by other massage therapists to proper authorities, such as a state licensing agency or the local police.

EXAM REVIEW

Key Terms

Match the following key terms to their descriptions. For additional study, look up the key terms in the Interactive Glossary on page G-1 and note other terms that compare or contrast with them.

_____ 1. Business ethics
_____ 2. Copyright
_____ 3. Deceptive advertising
_____ 4. Defamation
_____ 5. Endorsements
_____ 6. Guarantee
_____ 7. Massage establishment ordinance
_____ 8. Occupational license
_____ 9. Qualifying statements
_____ 10. Trademarks

a. Anecdotes from someone besides the massage therapist about how well the massage worked for them
b. Credential issued by a government that gives a person permission to practice a profession in its jurisdiction
c. Local government regulations that cover hours of operation, sanitation, and other aspects of a massage therapy business
d. A promise that something will work as stated, usually with the implication that the money will be refunded if it does not
e. Moral and legal considerations related to commercial transactions and fair treatment of consumers
f. Citing sources of information to substantiate claims about the benefits of massage therapy
g. Offer exclusive use of a name or symbol to identify unique goods and services
h. Protects written, musical, and artistic works from unauthorized use
i. Misleading the public about credentials, the nature of the service, its benefits, or how much it costs
j. Legal term for injury to a person or an organization's reputation

Memory Workout

To test your memory of the main concepts in this chapter, complete the following sentences by circling the most correct answer from the two choices provided.

1. Business ethics are moral and legal considerations related to (commercial) (banking) transactions.
2. Massage therapists can mislead the public by being (truthful) (vague) about their qualifications or by wording their qualifications (incorrectly) (in Latin).
3. Information should be (left) (spelled) out completely if using initials after a name would be misleading.
4. The FTC states that endorsements "may not contain any representation which would be deceptive, or could not be (broadcast) (substantiated)."
5. Advertising something for a certain price, and then pressuring the client/customer to buy something more expensive is called (bait) (smart) advertising.
6. Claims about massage should be qualified by citing (sound bites) (sources) of information.
7. Massage therapists may not use (trademarked) (copyrighted) names for forms of bodywork, unless they have earned the appropriate credentials.
8. Tips that should be turned down are ones with (gratitude) (expectations) attached, or that are too (large) (small).
9. Do not confuse being trained in selling a nutritional product by its manufacturer or distributor with having (sales experience) (professional education) in nutrition.
10. It is unethical for health professionals to (reward) (thank) each other for referrals.
11. It is unethical to (solicit) (talk to) clients seen first at an employer's business.

Test Prep

The following multiple-choice questions will help to prepare you for future school and professional exams.

1. Consumer protection laws are designed to:
   a. Ensure a minimum level of training for professionals
   b. Regulate where certain types of businesses can be located
   c. Protect the public from unsafe products and deceptive advertising
   d. Protect employees from unfair employment situations

2. When a seller makes a promise that something will work as stated, with the implication that the money will be refunded if it does not, it is called:
   a. Endorsement
   b. Guarantee
   c. Testimonial
   d. Bait advertising

3. Which of the following is the most ethical method of advertising to clients that you have graduated from a massage therapy program?
   a. Spelling out "Graduate of ABC Massage Therapy School"
   b. Using the initials "GMT" after your name to designate "graduate massage therapist"
   c. Using the initials "CMT" after your name to designate "certified massage therapist"
   d. Any of the above

4. Which of the following offers legal protection for the exclusive use of a name or symbol to identify unique goods and services?
   a. Copyright
   b. Trademark
   c. Patent
   d. Licensing

5. When is it ethical to pressure massage clients to buy goods you have for sale?
   a. When you must meet a sales goal
   b. When you are sure that they will benefit from the product
   c. When you need to reduce inventory
   d. Never

6. Slander is:
   a. Gossiping about someone
   b. Publicly criticizing someone's behavior
   c. Causing injury to someone's reputation by something written
   d. Causing injury to someone's reputation by something spoken

7. If an accident or injury results from carelessness, it is called:
   a. Libel
   b. Negligence
   c. Unfortunate
   d. An act of God

8. When is it ethical to give reduced service to a client who never leaves a tip?
   a. At spas where tipping is customary
   b. When a "tips accepted" sign is clearly visible
   c. When saving energy for clients who do tip
   d. Never

Video Challenge

Watch the appropriate segment of the video on your DVD and then answer the following questions.

Business Ethics

Claims for Massage Therapy

1. What are the ethical principles related to advertising discussed in the video?

Tips and Gifts

2. What do the massage therapists in the video say regarding when accepting tips is ethical and when to turn them down?

Selling Products

3. What types of products might massage therapists sell to clients? What are some ethical principles related to selling products mentioned in the video?

Comprehension Exercises

The following short answer questions test your knowledge and understanding of chapter topics and provide practice in written communication skills. Explain in two to four complete sentences.

1. What types of laws must massage therapists be aware of for building ethical practices? What is the over-reaching ethical principle related to laws?

2. What does the law say about making claims for a product or service? How do you qualify claims made for massage? Give an example.

3. When is it *not* ethical to accept tips from clients? What is the ethical principle related to soliciting tips?

For Greater Understanding

The following exercises are designed to take you from the realm of theory into the real world. They will help you give a deeper understanding of the subjects covered in this chapter. Action words are underlined to emphasize the variety of activities presented to address different learning styles and to encourage deeper thinking.

1. Tell the class or a study partner about a time you were treated unfairly or dishonestly in a business transaction. Analyze what happened in ethical and legal terms. Were consumer protection laws or any other laws broken?

2. Speak to the class or a study partner about a time you were given a gift that didn't feel right to you (i.e., with expectations attached or too costly given your relationship with the person). Analyze the person's motivation and your response. Was the outcome positive or negative? Would you act differently today?

3. Tell the class or study partner about a time you felt pressured to buy something. Analyze the motivation of the seller and how you felt being pressured.

4. Obtain a copy of an employment agreement for a massage therapist at a spa or clinic. Analyze provisions for soliciting clients, and discuss it in terms of fairness or unfairness.

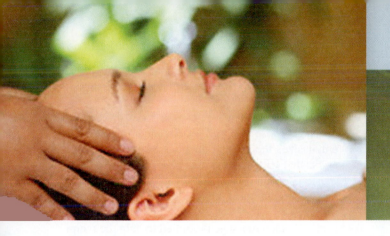

25 Forms of Therapeutic Massage and Bodywork

The therapeutic massage and bodywork forms described in this Appendix are some of the major systems practiced today. Descriptions include a summary of their origins and history, techniques and applications, the theory on which they are based, and some resources for further information. Noncommercial websites are listed when available, and books for forms that do not have relevant websites are also cited. Readers are encouraged to check the Internet for websites appearing after publication of this text.

Many of the forms of massage and bodywork listed are root systems from which other forms or spin-offs have been derived. Because the field of massage therapy is an emerging profession with a large entrepreneurial component, there are several trademarked forms (e.g., Rolfing®). Spin-offs of originals may also be trademarked, or there may be generic spin-offs without trademarks. For further explanations of these and other forms of massage and bodywork, see *Discovering the Body's Wisdom* by Mirka Knaster (New York: Bantam Books, 1996).

1. *Alexander Technique*
   Origin: Alexander Technique was developed by an Australian named Frederick Matthias Alexander (1869–1955), who practiced in London in the early 1900s. Alexander, a Shakespearean actor, cured himself of loss of voice through correction of faulty posture in the head and neck. He later worked with other actors and public speakers using the same method to improve their vocal abilities.
   Technique: Alexander Technique is a form of contemporary bodywork in which a teacher guides the student through various movements such as sitting, walking, and bending. The emphasis is on achieving balance in the head-neck relationship, called Primary Control. Poor habitual patterns are replaced by light, easy, simple, and integrated movement.
   Theory: Proper body alignment and movement patterns are achieved by heightened kinesthetic awareness and conscious movement.
   Websites: Alexander Technique (www.alexandertechnique.com)
   Alexander Technique International (www.ati-net.com)

American Society for the Alexander Technique (www.alexandertech.org)

2. *Aromatherapy Massage*
   Origin: The use of natural plant essences for health and therapeutic effects is ancient. The modern term "aromatherapie" was coined by a French chemist named Rene Maurice Gattefosse (1881–1950) as he studied the use of fragrant oils for their healing properties in the 1920s–1930s. Later, Madame Marguerite Maury (1895–1968) started prescribing essential oils for her patients and is credited with the modern use of essential oils for massage. She wrote an important aromatherapy guide in French in 1961 that was translated into English in 1964.
   Technique: Aromatherapy massage involves the use of essential oils in massage oil blends for their therapeutic effects. Techniques of Western massage, Ayurvedic massage, and other systems of soft tissue manipulation may be used in the application of aromatherapy massage oils.
   Theory: Essential oils are highly concentrated aromatic extracts that are cold-pressed or steam distilled from plants such as grasses, leaves, flowers, fruit peels, wood, and roots. Each essential oil has a specific therapeutic effect such as relaxing, boosting immune system, relieving congestion, or soothing muscular aches and pains. Common massage blends contain essential oils such as peppermint, lavender, citrus, tea tree, and rosemary.
   Website: National Association for Holistic Aromatherapy (www.naha.org)

3. *Ayurvedic Massage*
   Origin: Ayurvedic massage is one of the healing practices of ancient India. Vedic scriptures of India dating back to 3000 BCE describe healing practices, including massage with oil.
   Technique: Ayurvedic massage techniques include rubbing, kneading, squeezing, tapping, and pulling or shaking the body. Emphasis is given to massage of the head and feet. Sessions are invigorating and the recipient changes position several times during a

session. Pressure is applied to *marmas*, or pressure points on the body.

Theory: Ayurvedic massage is based in traditional Ayurvedic medicine of India. Massage is thought to remove obstructions to the flow of *vayu* (wind) through *siras*, or wind-carrying vessels, to reduce pain, relieve tension, and encourage more natural breathing patterns. Massage oils are chosen according to body type, the atmosphere, and the season.

Reference: *Ayurvedic Massage: Traditional Indian Techniques for Balancing Body and Mind* by Harish Johari (Rochester, VT: Healing Arts Press, 1996).

Website: National Ayurvedic Medical Association (www.ayurveda-nama.org)

4. *Clinical Massage Therapy*
See Medical Massage

5. *Craniosacral Therapy (CST)*
Origin: Craniosacral therapy stems from the work of an osteopath named Dr. William Garner Sutherland (1873–1954) in the early 1900s. Dr. Sutherland developed the basic theory of CST, including cranial suture movement, rhythmic motion of cerebrospinal fluid (i.e., Breath of Life), and the relationship between craniosacral rhythm and health. John E. Upledger, DO, has continued development of this work and added the concept of somatoemotional release (SER) of negative emotions stored in traumatized tissues. The Upledger Foundation was established in 1987 to study CST.

Technique: Craniosacral therapy is a form of contemporary bodywork that uses gentle compression to realign the skull bones and stretch related membranes to balance the craniosacral rhythm (CSR) and improve function of the nervous system.

Theory: CST is based in Western anatomy and physiology and osteopathic science. The craniosacral system (i.e., cranium, spine, and sacrum) is connected by a fascial membrane called the dura mater that houses the brain and central nervous system. Cerebral spinal fluid is pumped throughout the system, creating a pulse or CSR. CST techniques aim to balance the CSR so that cerebral spinal fluid flows freely through the system. Once this is achieved, the body's own healing mechanism can function properly.

Websites: The Upledger Institute
(www.upledger.com)
Craniosacral Therapy Association of North America (www.craniosacraltherapy.org)

6. *Esalen Massage*
Origin: Esalen massage was developed at the Esalen Institute in Big Sur, California, in the 1970s. Its development grew out of the Human Potential Movement and counterculture of the 1960s. Esalen massage was popularized in the classic *The Massage Book* by George Downing, published in 1972.

Technique: Esalen massage is a form of Western massage loosely based in Swedish massage. It emphasizes the sensual qualities of massage and is associated with scented oils, incense, and New Age music. It initially was performed without draping, but accepted draping standards are now observed in most settings.

Theory: Esalen massage is applied to help the recipient get in touch with his or her senses and inner self, and is considered a meditative and personal growth experience. General health benefits of Swedish massage apply to Esalen massage.

Reference: *The Massage Book* by George Downing (New York: Random House, 1998; 1st edition, 1972).

Website: Esalen Institute (www.esalen.org)

7. *Feldenkrais Method®*
Origin: The Feldenkrais Method was developed by Moshe Feldenkrais (1904–1984), who was an engineer, physicist, judo master, and mathematician. In efforts to heal himself of a knee injury, Feldenkrais developed a system of movement reeducation. The Feldenkrais Method came to light during the human potential movement of the 1970s–1980s.

Technique: The Feldenkrais Method is a form of contemporary bodywork consisting of functional integration (i.e., hands-on table work in which the practitioner uses his or her hands to communicate new sensory movement patterns to the recipient through passive movements). In Awareness Through Movement, a teacher leads a group through structured movement experiences performed on the floor.

Theory: The Feldenkrais Method is based in Western anatomy and physiology. Integrated movement patterns are established by reeducating the sensorymotor nervous system through repeated movements.

Websites: Feldenkrais Guild® of North America
(www.feldenkrais.com)
International Feldenkrais Federation
(www.feldenkrais-method.org)

8. *Infant Massage*
Origin: Massage has been given to infants from time immemorial by their mothers, grandmothers, and other caregivers. Instances of infant massage are found among native tribes in Africa, South Pacific Islands, and North America, in ancient and modern India, and folk cultures of Europe. Recent interest in infant massage was revived by Vimala Schneider in the 1980s and by the research of Dr. Tiffany Fields at the University of Miami in the 1990s.

Technique: Infant massage is a specialty within Western massage and consists of simple techniques such as stroking, kneading, twisting, and pressing performed with gentle pressure. Some passive joint movements are incorporated. Eye contact and communication with the infant are emphasized.

Theory: Infant massage is based in Western anatomy, physiology, and theories of child development. It aims to help the infant relax, improve circulation and other body functions, improve immune function, and promote neurological development. Research confirms the necessity of touch and movement for healthy human development and the benefits of massage for premature infants.

Reference: *Infant Massage: A Handbook for Loving Parents* by Vimala Schneider McClure, revised edition (New York: Bantam Doubleday Dell, 2000).

Websites: International Institute of Infant Massage (www.infantmassageinstitute.com)
Loving Touch Foundation (www.lovingtouch.com)
Touch Research Institute (www.miami.edu/touch-research)

9. *Lomi-Lomi*

Origin: Lomi-lomi is a traditional massage of the natives of the Hawaiian Islands practiced for centuries. Different styles of lomi-lomi were developed within families. Typically a tutu (i.e., grandmother) or other respected family member was the keeper of the tradition. Its modern form was popularized by Aunty Margaret Machado of Kona, Hawaii, in the 1970s–1980s.

Technique: Lomi-lomi is a form of traditional native massage consisting of pressing and squeezing techniques performed with the fingers, palm, and elbow. Kukui nut, macadamia, or coconut oil may be used. The recipient lies on a mat, or in modern times a massage table, to receive lomi-lomi. Associated methods include baths, bone adjusting techniques, and prayer.

Theory: Lomi-lomi is based in traditional Hawaiian culture, and emphasizes letting go of stress, offering unconditional love, and opening the heart to harmony, acceptance, and healing.

Reference: *Hawaiian Lomi-Lomi: Big Island Massage* by Nancy S. Kahalewai (Hilo, HI: Island Massage Publishing, 2000).

Website: Aunty Margaret Homepage (http://homepages.hawaiian.net/kea/aunty.html)

10. *Manual Lymph Drainage*

Origin: Manual techniques applied to enhance lymphatic system function and treat lymphedema were developed as early as the 1880s. Emil and Astrid Vodder developed their manual lymph drainage (MLD), or Vodder Method, in the 1930s in France. In the 1970s, Hungarians Michael and Ethel Foldi combined Vodder's MLD with other modalities to create a treatment for lymphedema called complete decongestive therapy (CDT).

Technique: Lymphatic massage is a specialized form of Western massage consisting of gentle techniques applied to the superficial skin layers to stretch the tissue and open the superficial lymphatic vessels so that lymph fluid can enter the vessels more easily. Classic Vodder techniques include stationary circles, scoop, pump, rotary, and light effleurage applied rhythmically and in specific directions.

Theory: Lymphatic massage is based on Western anatomy and physiology and knowledge of the lymphatic system. Techniques are applied in a way to enhance the movement of lymph fluid into superficial vessels and through the system. Lymphatic massage improves immune function, reduces areas of edema, and aids injury healing.

Websites: Academy of Lymphatic Studies (www.acols.com)
Dr. Vodder School North America (www.vodderschool.com)

11. *Medical Massage*

Origin: Massage has been used to treat ailments from time immemorial all over the globe. Historically in Western medicine, it has been called medical rubbing, frictions, massage, massotherapeutics, and physiotherapy. Medical massage is emerging in the twenty-first century as a specialty within the broader field of therapeutic massage and bodywork. It is sometimes called *clinical massage.*

Technique: Medical massage is a specialty of Western massage in which soft tissue manipulation and related techniques are applied in the treatment of pathological conditions. A subspecialty is the treatment of musculoskeletal dysfunction.

Theory: Medical massage is based in Western anatomy, physiology, kinesiology, and pathology. Traditional and contemporary massage techniques are used as appropriate in treatment plans.

References: *Basic Clinical Massage Therapy: Integrating Anatomy and Treatment* by James H. Clay and David M. Pounds (Philadelphia: Lippincott Williams & Wilkins, 2003).
Clinical Massage Therapy: Understanding, Assessing and Treating over 70 Conditions by Fiona Rattray and Linda Ludwig (Toronto: Talus Incorporated, 2000).
Massage for Orthopedic Conditions by Thomas Hendrickson (Philadelphia: Lippincott, Williams & Wilkins, 2003).
Medical Massage by Ross Turchaninov and Connie Cox (Scottsdale, AZ: Stress Less Publishing, 1998).

12. *Myofascial Massage*

Origin: Manual techniques that target the myofascial tissues were developed in the 1950s by Ida Rolf (1896–1979) in her system of Rolfing®, and by osteopath Robert Ward as myofascial release technique in the 1960s. Since then several systems of bodywork that treat myofascial tissues have been developed.

Technique: Myofascial massage techniques apply traction to the skin and underlying tissues to slowly and gently push, pull, and stretch fascial tissues and break fascial adhesions. They are applied without oil so that restrictions can be palpated and techniques applied without slipping.

Theory: Myofascial massage is based in Western anatomy and physiology. It focuses on connective or myofascial tissues that surround muscles, nerves, blood vessels, and all organs of the body. Restrictions in fascial tissues can cause a variety of dysfunctions, including limited mobility, postural distortion, poor cellular nutrition, and pain. Myofascial massage produces a softening of tissues and freeing of fascial restrictions.

Reference: *The Myofascial Release Manual* (3rd ed.) by Carol J. Manheim (Thorofare, NJ: Slack, Inc., 2001).

13. *Polarity Therapy*

Origin: Polarity Therapy was developed by Randolph Stone (1890–1981) in the 1930s–1950s. Stone combined Western knowledge with theories from Chinese and Ayurvedic medicine, particularly regarding energy balancing. Upon his retirement in 1973, Stone's successors taught polarity therapy throughout the United States. The American Polarity Therapy Association was founded in 1984.

Technique: Polarity therapy is an eclectic form of energy bodywork. Most polarity therapy techniques consist of placing the hands in different positions on the body to affect the free flow of energy. Other techniques include pressing, gentle rocking, and brushing.

Theory: Polarity therapy techniques aim to remove obstructions to the free flow of energy in the body. Stone developed his own esoteric theories of energy flow after studying Chinese and Ayurvedic medicine.

Website: American Polarity Therapy Association (www.polaritytherapy.org)

14. *Reflexology*

Origin: Modern reflexology was developed by Eunice Ingham Stopfel (1889–1974), who combined the theory of zone therapy with compression massage of the feet and hands. She mapped the feet for their corresponding zones of reference and developed pressure techniques for stimulating points on the feet to affect specific organs and structures of the body. She started her work in the 1930s and taught throughout the United States in the 1950s–1960s.

Technique: Reflexology is performed primarily on the feet. Pressure is applied to areas of the feet to stimulate other parts of the body. Reflexology techniques include thumb walking, finger walking, hook and backup, along with Western massage and joint movements applied to the feet.

Theory: Reflexology is based in zone therapy, which postulates that 10 longitudinal zones of the body end in the feet and the hands. Pressure to a zone in the feet causes stimulation of the entire zone. Reflexology charts map out which specific organs or body structures will be affected by pressure on specific areas of the feet. Reflexology is thought to normalize function, improve circulation, and promote relaxation. Knowledge of Western anatomy, physiology, and pathology are important in reflexology.

Websites: Reflexology Association of America (www.reflexology-usa.org)
International Council of Reflexologists (www.icr-reflexology.org)

15. *Rolfing® Structural Integration*

Origin: Rolfing was developed by Ida P. Rolf (1896–1979), and brought to public recognition during the 1970s within the human potential movement. The Rolf Institute® of Structural Integration was founded in 1971 and provides training and certification for Rolfing practitioners.

Technique: Rolfing is a form of contemporary Western bodywork, also called structural integration. It includes soft tissue manipulation and movement education. In Rolfing, myofascial tissues are manipulated so that they lengthen and glide, to balance the body around its vertical axis, achieving proper alignment or posture. In the process of working with deep myofascial tissues, past emotional trauma is also released.

Theory: Rolfing is based in Western anatomy and physiology, especially of fascial tissues, and psychology.

Website: The Rolf Institute for Structural Integration (www.rolf.org)

16. *Shiatsu (Namikoshi)*

Origin: Shiatsu evolved from traditional Japanese massage called Amma. Tokujiro Namikoshi (1905–2000) developed a system of finger pressure to treat various ailments. He founded the first Shiatsu Institute of Therapy on Hokkaido in 1925, and the Japan Shiatsu Institute in Tokyo in 1940. His son, Toru Namikoshi (1931–), popularized Shiatsu in Japan and throughout the world in the 1950s–1970s.

Technique: Shiatsu is a form of Asian bodywork therapy. Shiatsu literally means finger pressure (shiatsu) in Japanese. Pressure is applied along energy (ki) meridians and to acupoints with the thumbs, fingers, or elbows. The recipient is either lying on a mat on the floor or on a bodywork table.

Theory: Shiatsu, as developed by Namikoshi, combines traditional Chinese medicine and Western anatomy and physiology. Important acupoints are pressed to elicit desired results and to enhance the balance and flow of ki, or energy.

Website: American Organization of Bodywork Therapies of Asia (www.aobta.org)

17. *Sports Massage*

Origin: Sports massage can be traced to ancient Greece and Rome where massage was given in the gymnasia and public baths. Massage prepared athletes for exercise and helped in recovery from competition. In the late nineteenth century, rubbers and athletic masseurs used massage in the training of athletes. Sports massage was revived in the 1970s within the context of Western massage.

Technique: Sports massage is a specialty within Western massage. Western massage techniques are applied to enhance athletic performance, prevent injuries, prepare for and recover from competition, and in rehabilitation of injuries. Modern sports massage given at events emphasizes the technique of compression and other forms of petrissage. Individual practitioners may add other bodywork approaches to achieve the goals of the athlete.

Theory: Sports massage is based in Western anatomy, physiology, kinesiology, pathology, and sports science.

Reference: *Understanding Sports Massage* (2nd ed.) by Patricia J. Benjamin and Scott Lamp (Champaign, IL: Human Kinetics, 2005).

18. *Stone Massage*

Origin: Stones have been used in healing practices all over the world, including Asia. Healing or hot stone massage is a treatment that gained popularity in North American spas in the 1990s–2000s.

Technique: Stone massage is a form of contemporary bodywork and spa treatment. Stones of various sizes, shapes, and textures are used as massage tools and as a form of thermal therapy. As massage tools, stones are used instead of the hands to apply pressure during techniques such as effleurage. As thermal therapy, stones may be heated and placed on the body over certain anatomical structures or in patterns over energy centers and meridians or cooled and used as cryotherapy to reduce swelling and cool tissues.

Theory: Stone massage is practiced as an eclectic form of bodywork incorporating Western anatomy and physiology with traditional Asian medicine. Geological properties of various kinds of stones are considered. Hot stones applied to the body impart weight and heat that promotes relaxation, normal body function, and energy balancing.

References: *Healing Stone Massage.* Video with Carollanne Crichton (Real Bodywork, 2001). *Japanese Hot Stone Massage* by Mark Hess and Shogo Mochizuki (Kotobuki Publications, 2002).

19. *Swedish Massage*

Origin: Swedish massage and related techniques were developed in Europe in the early 1800s and brought to North America in the 1860s. It can be traced historically to the work of two men: Pehr Henrick Ling (1776–1839) of Sweden and Johann Mezger (1838–1909) of Amsterdam. The heyday of Swedish massage in the United States was the 1930s–1950s, when it was offered in health clubs, salons, and as part of physiotherapy.

Technique: Swedish massage is a form of traditional Western massage. The five classic technique categories of Swedish massage soft tissue manipulation are effleurage (stroking, sliding), petrissage (kneading, compression), tapotement (percussion), friction, and vibration. Joint movements and hydrotherapy are also within the scope of Swedish massage.

Theory: Swedish massage is based in Western anatomy, physiology, and pathology. It is applied to support the normal function of the human body and its systems, as well as enhance its innate healing capacity. *See* Western Massage.

20. *Thai Massage*

Origin: Nuad bo-Rarn means *ancient massage* in the language of Thailand. It has been practiced for over 2,500 years. At the Temple of the Reclining Buddha in Bangkok, 200-year-old stone engravings illustrate the energy lines and points and techniques of this ancient practice. Thai massage is passed down in families and also taught at schools of traditional Thai medicine.

Technique: In Thai massage, the practitioner uses passive movement, assisted yoga stretches, and pressure techniques to stimulate energy channels called *sen lines* and release tension in the body. Application is gentle and rhythmic. Recipients lie on floor mats to receive Thai massage.

Theory: Thai massage is based on Ayurvedic (India) medicine and was influenced by yoga, as it evolved in ancient Thailand. Techniques stimulate the free flow of energy through channels.

Website: Institute of Thai Massage (www.thai-massage.org)

21. *Therapeutic Touch (TT)*

Origin: Therapeutic Touch was developed by Delores Krieger, a professor of nursing, and her teacher, Dora Kunz, in the 1960s–1970s. It is a modification of the ancient practice of laying on of the hands.

Technique: Therapeutic Touch is a system of energy bodywork performed in five steps: (1) centering of the practitioner, (2) assessment of the energy field of the recipient with the palms of the hands, (3) clearing blockages, imbalances, or congestion of energy with sweeping hand movements, (4) establishing harmony in the energy field using the mind, and (5) smoothing out the energy field by sweeping the hands outward toward the periphery of the field.

Theory: Therapeutic Touch is based in theories of bioelectricity and electromagnetic energy fields. The sweeping hand movements of TT move energy to create balance and harmony in a person's energy field. Imbalances, blockages, and congestion in the energy field are thought to result in disease and dysfunction. TT is used in the treatment of many different ailments.

Website: Nurse Healers–Professional Associates International (www.therapeutic-touch.org)

22. *Trager® Approach*

Origin: Trager Approach, also known as psychophysical integration, was developed by Milton Trager, MD (1908–1997). After earning a medical degree after World War II, Trager opened a practice in Hawaii in 1959 and gave a public demonstration of his work in 1973.

Technique: The Trager Approach is a system of contemporary Western bodywork that combines tissue and joint mobilization, relaxation, and movement reeducation. The practitioner applies continuous rhythmic movement to different joints in the body with the recipient lying on a table. Recipients recreate the easy, light, free movements of the table work in a system of active exercise called Mentastics.

Theory: Trager focuses on creating the sensations of lighter, easier, and freer movement through affecting neurological mechanisms of the body. It imparts an experience of deep relaxation and greater joint mobility.

Website: Trager International (www.trager.com)

23. *Trigger Point Therapy*

Origin: A precursor to trigger point therapy (also called neuromuscular therapy) was developed by a natural healer named Stanley Lief in the 1920s. Trigger point therapy was brought to public attention through the work of Janet Travell, MD (1901–1997), an expert in myofascial pain, and her treatment of Presidents Kennedy and Johnson in the 1960s. Fitness expert Bonnie Prudden developed a popular system of trigger point therapy called Myotherapy® in the 1970s.

Technique: Neuromuscular therapy is a form of contemporary Western massage in which trigger points (i.e., hyper-irritable taut bands in the myofascial tissues) are located and deactivated using ischematic compression. Pressure is applied to trigger points for about 30 seconds using the thumb, fingers, or small hand tool. A stretch of the affected muscle follows application of pressure on trigger points.

Theory: A trigger point is a taut band or irritable spot in myofascial tissue that causes muscle pain at the trigger point and in its referral zones. It also causes muscle shortening and decreased strength. Under a microscope, trigger points appear to be bands of contracted muscle tissue.

References: *Myofascial Pain and Dysfunction: The Trigger Point Manual,* Volume 1—*Upper Half of the Body* (2nd ed.) by J. G. Travell and D. G. Simons (Baltimore, MD: Williams & Wilkins, 1999).

Myofascial Pain and Dysfunction: The Trigger Point Manual, Volume 2—*The Lower Extremities* by J. G. Travell and D. G. Simons (Baltimore, MD: Williams & Wilkins, 1992).

Website: Bonnie Prudden Myotherapy (www.bonnieprudden.com)

24. *Tuina*

Origin: The origin of Tuina, or Chinese medical massage, is clouded in the mists of time. It developed from the same roots as acupuncture in Chinese medicine. Tuina is written about in several ancient medical texts, and a Tuina department was set up in the Imperial Health Administration in the Tang Dynasty (618–907 CE). Tuina for infants and children became popular in the Qing Dynasty (1644–1911 CE).

Technique: Tuina is a form of Chinese medical massage (i.e., Asian bodywork therapy). Techniques of Tuina include stroking, pushing, grasping, pressing, palm-rubbing, twisting, pinching, rubbing, rolling, tapping, stretching, kneading, lifting, and holding. Techniques are applied to stimulate acupoints and affect blood circulation. Tuina also includes joint manipulation, herbal remedies, and therapeutic exercise.

Theory: Tuina is based in theory of Chinese medicine including *qi* or energy, energy channels, and yin-yang. Modern Tuina incorporates knowledge of Western anatomy, physiology, and pathology. Tuina is used to treat ailments recognized by Chinese medicine, as well as Western pathology.

Reference: *Chinese Tuina Therapy* by Wang Fu (Bejing, China: Foreign Languages Press, 1994).

Website: Traditional Chinese Medicine and Acupuncture Health Information Organization (www.tcm.health-info.org/tuina/tcm-tuinamassage.tm)

25. *Western Massage*

Origin: Western massage can be traced to health and healing practices of ancient Greece and Rome. Techniques of soft tissue manipulation were further developed through the centuries in Europe and

North America. Western massage today is an outgrowth of Swedish massage, massage used in Western medicine, and various contemporary systems of massage and bodywork.

Description: Western massage techniques include classic Swedish massage techniques, plus various forms of contemporary massage (e.g., trigger point therapy, myofascial massage, lymphatic drainage massage, and other forms of massage therapy based in Western anatomy, physiology, and pathology). Western massage practitioners tend to be eclectic, incorporating various techniques, including energy approaches, with classic Swedish massage.

Theory: Western massage is based in Western anatomy, physiology, and pathology. It aims to enhance the normal functioning of the body and its systems, including the innate healing power in each person.

Websites: American Massage Therapy Association (www.amtamassage.org)

Associated Bodywork and Massage Professionals (www.abmp.com)

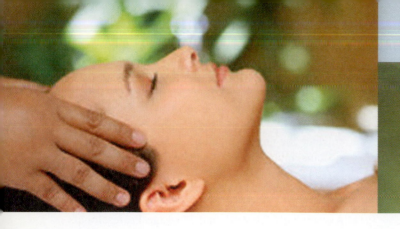

Personal Care and Health Professionals

This is a guide to personal care and health professionals who interact with massage therapists in typical work settings. Licensing of these occupations varies from state to state in the United States and from country to country throughout the world.

PERSONAL CARE PROVIDERS

Barbers specialize in men's grooming (e.g., cutting hair and beards, shaving facial hair).

Cosmetologists specialize in women's grooming (e.g., styling hair; giving facials, manicures, and pedicures; and applying cosmetics); sometimes called beauticians, hairstylists.

Estheticians specialize in nonmedical skin care.

SPORTS, FITNESS, AND RECREATION PROFESSIONALS

Athletic trainers (ATs) focus on prevention and treatment of injuries common in sports; typically they have college degrees, have completed an internship, and have professional certification. *See* National Athletic Trainers' Association (www.nata.org).

Coaches organize sports teams and train individual athletes; responsibilities include teaching sports skills, organizing practices, developing strategies, and directing play during competitions.

Personal trainers are health and fitness specialists hired by individuals to develop exercise programs, and supervise and motivate them to achieve their fitness goals; different levels of training for personal trainers range from workshops to college degrees, usually in exercise physiology; professional certification from different organizations. *See* National Strength and Conditioning Association (www.nsca-cc.org) and National Council on Strength and Fitness (www.ncsf.org/certexam).

HEALTH CARE PROFESSIONALS

Conventional

Medical doctors (MDs) are trained in conventional medicine; diagnose and treat diseases of the human body/mind primarily with drugs, surgery, and referral to therapists.

Nurses (RNs, LPNs) specialize in direct patient care, including treatment, education, record keeping, and providing emotional support for patients and their families; *RN* means registered nurse and *LPN* means licensed practical nurse; RN and LPN represent different levels of training and licensure. *See* American Nurses Association (www.nursingworld.org).

Osteopaths (DOs) historically traced disease to imbalances in the musculoskeletal structure of the human body and rejected use of drugs and surgery; in many places today, including the United States, they have expanded their scope of practice to conventional medicine; different philosophies prevail in different countries. *See* American Osteopathic Association (www.osteopathic.org).

Physiatrists are physicians who specialize in physical medicine and rehabilitation and focus on restoring musculoskeletal function; typically have 8 years of graduate and postdoctorate medical training. *See* American Academy of Physical Medicine and Rehabilitation (www.aapmr.org).

Psychologists study the human mind, including behavior and thinking; clinical psychologists provide mental health care to clients. *See* American Psychological Association (www.apa.org).

THERAPISTS[1]

Occupational therapists (OTs) help clients who have disabilities to better perform activities of daily living and work tasks; teach people with permanent disabilities to use adaptive equipment; typically have college degrees. *See* American Occupational Therapy Association (www.aota.org).

[1]These practitioners focus on the application of specific modalities for rehabilitation and in the treatment of diseases and injuries. A doctor's prescription must be obtained for treatment by these professionals in most cases. Licenses are required to practice in most states.

Physical therapists (PTs) use exercise, hydrotherapy, and other modalities to restore function and reduce pain from injury and illness; typically have college degrees; in some places called *physiotherapists. See* American Physical Therapy Association (www.apta.org).

Physical therapist aides or assistants (PTAs) help administer physical therapy treatments to patients under the direction of a physical therapist and perform some clerical tasks; trained on the job or in associate/vocational degree programs. *See* American Physical Therapy Association (www.apta.org).

Respiratory therapists (RTs) evaluate, treat, and care for patients with respiratory disorders; use oxygen, respiratory physiotherapy, and other modalities. *See* American Association for Respiratory Care (www.aarc.org).

Complementary and Alternative (CAM)

Acupuncturists provide treatment based in Chinese medicine (Oriental medicine); use needles, pressure, and other methods to stimulate traditional energy points. *See* American Association of Oriental Medicine (www.aaom.org).

Chiropractors (DCs) or chiropractic physicians address misalignment of the musculoskeletal structure to affect the nervous system and treat diseases. *See* Chiropractic Association (www.amerchiro.org).

Homeopaths or homeopathic physicians treat medical conditions using homeopathic preparations; based on the Law of Similars; not regulated in the United States. *See* National Center for Homeopathy (www.homeopathic.org).

Naturopaths or naturopathic physicians (NDs) use natural remedies such as herbs, nutritional supplements, and other natural modalities to treat human diseases; licensed in 14 states. *See* American Association of Naturopathic Physicians (www.naturopathic.org).

Osteopaths (DOs) *See* Conventional health care professionals.

THERAPISTS[2]

Aromatherapists use essential oils from plants to evoke good health and healing.

Art therapists are mental health professionals that use the creative processes of art to improve physical, mental, and emotional well-being.

Bodywork practitioners or bodyworkers apply manual techniques and movement therapy for holistic well-being; includes massage therapists.

Equine therapists or equitherapists use horses and the movement of horses in treatment of a variety of physical and mental conditions.

Hypnotherapists use the mental therapy of hypnosis in treating a variety of conditions.

Massage therapists apply soft tissue manipulation and related therapies to improve health and promote healing.

Music therapists use music in the treatment of a variety of human ills.

Recreation therapists or therapeutic recreation specialists plan, organize, and conduct recreation programs for special populations, and teach people with various disabilities to participate in leisure activities for social, physical, and mental health.

Further information may be found in the U.S. Department of Labor, *Occupational Outlook Handbook,* which lists the nature of the work, typical work conditions, training necessary, earnings, and additional sources of information. The website for the Bureau of Labor Statistics is www.bls.gov. Another resource is the National Center for Complementary and Alternative Medicine (NCCAM) at the National Institutes of Health at www.nccam.nih.gov.

---

[2]These practitioners focus on the application of specific modalities in the treatment of diseases and injuries and to improve health. Several of these occupations are off-shoots of more established professions, and some require board certification and licenses to practice in certain jurisdictions. All are holistic and are considered complementary or alternative therapies.

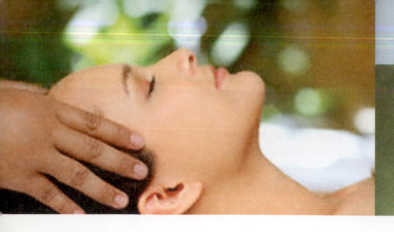

Organizations and Publications

ORGANIZATIONS

American Massage Therapy Association (AMTA)
500 Davis Street, Suite 900
Evanston, IL 60201-4695
(877) 905-2700 or (847) 864-0123
www.amtamassage.org

American Organization for Bodywork Therapies of Asia
  (AOBTA)
1010 Haddonfield-Berlin Road, Suite 408
Voorhees, NJ 08043
(856) 782-1616
www.aobta.org

American Polarity Therapy Association (APTA)
122 North Elm Street, Suite 512
Greensboro, NC 27401
(336) 574-1121
www.polaritytherapy.org

Associated Bodywork & Massage Professionals (ABMP)
25188 Genesee Trail Road
Golden, CO 80401
(800) 458-2267
www.abmp.com

Canadian Touch Research Center
760 Saint-Zotique Street East
Montreal, Quebec, Canada H2S 1M5
(514) 272-2254
www.ccrt-ctrc.ca

Center for Compassionate Touch
610 East University Street
Springfield, MO 65807
(417) 844-8514
www.compassionate-touch.org

Commission on Massage Therapy Accreditation (COMTA)
5335 Wisconsin Avenue, NW, Suite 440
Washington, D.C. 20015
(202) 895-1518
www.comta.org

Federation of State Massage Therapy Boards
7111 West 151st Street, Suite 356
Overland Park, KS 66223
(913) 681-0380 or (888)-70-FSMTB
www.fsmtb.org

International Association of Infant Massage Instructors (US)
P.O. Box 6370
Ventura, CA 93006
www.iaim-us.com

International Institute of Reflexology, Inc.
5650 First Avenue North
P.O. Box 12642
St. Petersburg, FL 33733-2642
(727) 343-4811
www.reflexology-usa.net

International Loving Touch Foundation (infant massage)
4133 S.E. Division Street
Portland, OR 97292
(800) 929-7492 or (503) 253-8482
www.lovingtouch.com

International Spa Association (ISPA)
2365 Harrodsburg Road, Suite A325
Lexington, KY 40504
(888) 651-4772 or (859) 226-4326
www.experienceispa.com

Massage Therapy Alliance of Canada (MTAC)
1200 West 73rd #180
Vancouver, BC, Canada V4N 2V7
(604) 873-4467
www.cmta.ca

Massage Therapy Foundation
500 Davis Street, Suite 900
Evanston, IL 60201-4695
(847) 869-5019
www.massagetherapyfoundation.org

National Center of Complementary and Alternative
   Medicine
National Institutes of Health
9000 Rockville Pike
Bethesda, Maryland 20892
www.nccam.nih.gov

National Certification Board for Therapeutic Massage and
   Bodywork (NCBTMB)
1901 South Meyers Road, Suite 240
Oakbrook Terrace, IL 60181
(800) 296-0664 or (630) 627-8000
www.ncbtmb.com

National Certification Commission for Acupuncture and
   Oriental Medicine (NCCAOM)
76 South Laura Street, Suite 1290
Jacksonville, FL 32202
(904) 598-1005
www.nccaom.org

National Association of Nurse Massage Therapists
   (NANMT)
28 Lowry Drive
P.O. Box 232
West Milton, OH 45383
(800) 262-4017
www.nanmt.org

Nurse Healers–Professional Associates International
   (Therapeutic Touch) (NH-PAI)
Box 419
Craryville, NY 12521
(877) 32NHPAI or (518) 325-1185
www.therapeutic-touch.org

Rolf Institute of Structural Integration®
5055 Chaparral Court, Suite 103
Boulder, CO 80301
(800) 530-8875 or (303) 449-5903
www.rolf.org

The Stone Institute LLC—Reflexology
2025 Zumbehl Road #20
St. Charles, MO 63303
636-724-8686
www.thestoneinstitute.org

TouchPro Institute (Professional Chair Massage)
584 Castro Street, #555
San Francisco, CA 94114
(800) 999-5026
www.TouchPro.com

Touch Research Institutes (TRI)
University of Miami School of Medicine
P.O. Box 016820
Miami, FL 33101
(305) 243-6781
www.miami.edu/touch-research

PERIODICAL PUBLICATIONS

Peer-Reviewed Journals

International Journal of Therapeutic Massage &
Bodywork: Research, Education & Practice (Open
access publication of the Massage Therapy Foundation):
   www.massagetherapyfoundation.org
Journal of Bodywork and Movement Therapies
   www.elsevier.com

Trade Publications

Massage Therapy Journal
   www.amtamassage.org/journal/home.html
Massage & Bodywork
   www.massageandbodywork.com
Massage Magazine
   www.massagemag.com
Massage Today
   www.massagetoday.com

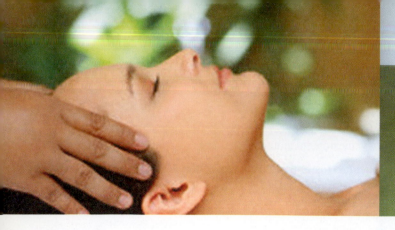

Code of Ethics and Standards of Practice for Massage Therapists

NATIONAL CERTIFICATION BOARD FOR THERAPEUTIC MASSAGE AND BODYWORK CODE OF ETHICS

Revised August 3, 2008

NCBTMB certificants and applicants for certification shall act in a manner that justifies public trust and confidence, enhances the reputation of the profession, and safeguards the interest of individual clients. Certificants and applicants for certification will:

I. Have a sincere commitment to provide the highest quality of care to those who seek their professional services.

II. Represent their qualifications honestly, including education and professional affiliations, and provide only those services that they are qualified to perform.

III. Accurately inform clients, other health care practitioners, and the public of the scope and limitations of their discipline.

IV. Acknowledge the limitations of and contraindications for massage and bodywork and refer clients to appropriate health professionals.

V. Provide treatment only where there is reasonable expectation that it will be advantageous to the client.

VI. Consistently maintain and improve professional knowledge and competence, striving for professional excellence through regular assessment of personal and professional strengths and weaknesses and through continued education training.

VII. Conduct their business and professional activities with honesty and integrity, and respect the inherent worth of all persons.

VIII. Refuse to unjustly discriminate against clients and/or health professionals.

IX. Safeguard the confidentiality of all client information, unless disclosure is requested by the client in writing, is medically necessary, is required by law, or necessary for the protection of the public.

X. Respect the client's right to treatment with informed and voluntary consent. The certified practitioner will obtain and record the informed consent of the client, or client's advocate, before providing treatment. This consent may be written or verbal.

XI. Respect the client's right to refuse, modify, or terminate treatment regardless of prior consent given.

XII. Provide draping and treatment in a way that ensures the safety, comfort, and privacy of the client.

XIII. Exercise the right to refuse to treat any person or part of the body for just and reasonable cause.

XIV. Refrain, under all circumstances, from initiating or engaging in any sexual conduct, sexual activities, or sexualizing behavior involving a client, even if the client attempts to sexualize the relationship unless a preexisting relationship exists between an applicant or a practitioner and the client prior to the applicant or practitioner applying to be certified by NCBTMB.

XV. Avoid any interest, activity, or influence which might be in conflict with the practitioner's obligation to act in the best interests of the client or the profession.

XVI. Respect the client's boundaries with regard to privacy, disclosure, exposure, emotional expression, beliefs, and the client's reasonable expectations of professional behavior. Practitioners will respect the client's autonomy.

XVII. Refuse any gifts or benefits that are intended to influence a referral, decision, or treatment, or that are purely for personal gain and not for the good of the client.

XVIII. Follow the NCBTMB Standards of Practice, this Code of Ethics, and all policies, procedures, guidelines, regulations, codes, and requirements promulgated by the National Certification Board for Therapeutic Massage and Bodywork.

NATIONAL CERTIFICATION BOARD FOR THERAPEUTIC MASSAGE AND BODYWORK STANDARDS OF PRACTICE

Adopted February 6, 2000; Implemented September 15, 2000; Revised August 3, 2008

Background

The purpose of the National Certification Board for Therapeutic Massage and Bodywork (NCBTMB) is to foster high standards of ethical and professional practice in the delivery of services through a recognized credible certification program that assures the competency of practitioners of therapeutic massage and bodywork.

These Standards of Practice ensure that certificants and applicants for certification are aware of, and committed to, upholding high standards of practice for the profession. Also, the Standards of Practice are meant to assist members of the general public, including consumers, other health care professionals, and State and Municipal Regulatory Agencies or Boards with understanding the duties and responsibilities of NCBTMB certificants and applicants for certification.

The NCBTMB developed and adopted the Standards of Practice to provide certificants and applicants for certification with a clear statement of the expectations of professional conduct and level of practice afforded the public in, among other things, the following areas: Professionalism, Legal and Ethical Requirements, Confidentiality, Business Practices, Roles and Boundaries, and Prevention of Sexual Misconduct. These Standards of Practice were approved and ratified by the NCBTMB Board of Directors, representatives of the certificant population, and key stakeholders of the NCBTMB.

Preamble

These Standards of Practice for the profession of therapeutic massage and bodywork are the guiding principles by which certificants and applicants for certification conduct their day-to-day responsibilities within their scope of practice. These principles help to assure that all professional behaviors are conducted in the most ethical, compassionate, and responsible manner. Through these Standards of Practice, NCBTMB seeks to establish and uphold the highest standards, traditions, and principles of the practices that constitute the profession of therapeutic massage and bodywork. The Standards are enforceable guidelines for professional conduct, and therefore, are stated in observable and measurable terms intended as minimum levels of practice to which certificants and applicants for certification are held accountable. Upon submission of the application for the National Certification Examinations, each applicant for certification must agree to uphold and abide by the NCBTMB Code of Ethics, Standards of Practice, and applicable policies. Certificants or applicants for certification's failure to comply with the Code of Ethics and the Standards of Practice as provided herein constitutes professional misconduct and may result in sanctions, or other appropriate disciplinary actions, including the suspension or revocation of certification.

NCBTMB certificants and applicants for certification are obligated to report unethical behavior and violations of the Code of Ethics and/or the Standards of Practice they reasonably and in good faith believe have been performed by other NCBTMB certificants and applicants for certification to NCBTMB.

These Standards of Practice reflect NCBTMB's clear commitment that certificants and applicants for certification provide an optimal level of service and strive for excellence in their practice. This includes remaining in good standing with NCBTMB, committing to continued personal and professional growth through continuing education, and understanding and accepting that personal and professional actions reflect on the integrity of the therapeutic massage and bodywork profession and NCBTMB. Certificants and applicants for certification are responsible for showing and maintaining professional compliance with the Standards of Practice. NCBTMB requires certificants and applicants for certification to conduct themselves in a highly professional and dignified manner. NCBTMB will not consider and/or adjudicate complaints against certificants and applicants for certification that are based solely on consumer related issues or are based on competitive marketplace issues.

As the therapeutic massage and bodywork profession evolves, so, too, will the Standards of Practice. The Standards of Practice are, therefore, a live and dynamic document and subject to revision in keeping with the changing demands and expectations of the therapeutic massage and bodywork profession.

Standards of Practice

STANDARD I: PROFESSIONALISM

The certificant or applicant for certification must provide optimal levels of professional therapeutic massage and bodywork services and demonstrate excellence in practice by promoting healing and well-being through responsible, compassionate, and respectful touch. In his/her professional role the certificant or applicant for certification shall:

a. Adhere to the NCBTMB Code of Ethics, Standards of Practice, policies, and procedures

b. Comply with the peer review process conducted by the NCBTMB Ethics and Standards Committee regarding any alleged violations of the NCBTMB Code of Ethics and Standards of Practice

c. Conduct him/herself in a manner in all settings meriting the respect of the public and other professionals

d. Treat each client with respect, dignity, and worth

e. Use professional verbal, nonverbal, and written communications

f. Provide an environment that is safe and comfortable for the client and which, at a minimum, meets all legal requirements for health and safety

g. Use standard precautions to ensure professional hygienic practices and maintain a level of personal hygiene appropriate for practitioners in the therapeutic setting

h. Wear clothing that is clean, modest, and professional

i. Obtain voluntary and informed consent from the client prior to initiating the session

j. If applicable, conduct an accurate needs assessment, develop a plan of care with the client, and update the plan as needed

k. Use appropriate draping to protect the client's physical and emotional privacy

l. Be knowledgeable of his/her scope of practice and practice only within these limitations

m. Refer to other professionals when in the best interest of the client and practitioner

n. Seek other professional advice when needed

o. Respect the traditions and practices of other professionals and foster collegial relationships

p. Not falsely impugn the reputation of any colleague

q. Use the initials NCBTMB only to designate his/her professional ability and competency to practice therapeutic massage and bodywork, or the initials NCTM only to designate his/her professional ability and competency to practice therapeutic massage

r. Remain in good standing with NCBTMB

s. Understand that the NCBTMB certificate may be displayed prominently in the certificant's principal place of practice

t. Use the NCBTMB logo and certification number on business cards, brochures, advertisements, and stationery only in a manner that is within established NCBTMB guidelines

u. Not duplicate the NCBTMB certificate for purposes other than verification of the practitioner's credentials

v. Immediately return the certificate to NCBTMB if certification is revoked

w. Inform NCBTMB of any changes or additions to information included in his/her application for NCBTMB certification or recertification.

STANDARD II: LEGAL AND ETHICAL REQUIREMENTS

The certificant or applicant must comply with all the legal requirements in applicable jurisdictions regulating the profession of therapeutic massage and bodywork. In his/her professional role the certificant or applicant shall:

a. Obey all applicable local, state, and federal laws

b. Refrain from any behavior that results in illegal, discriminatory, or unethical actions

c. Accept responsibility for his/her own actions

d. Report to the proper authorities any alleged violations of the law by other certificants or applicants for certification

e. Maintain accurate and truthful records

f. Report to NCBTMB any criminal conviction of, or plea of guilty, nolo contendere, or no contest to, a crime in any jurisdiction (other than a minor traffic offense) by him/herself and by other certificants or applicants for certification

g. Report to NCBTMB any pending litigation and resulting resolution related to the certificant or applicant for certification's professional practice and the professional practice of other certificants or applicants for certification

h. Report to NCBTMB any pending complaints in any state or local government or quasi-government board or agency against his/her professional conduct or competence, or that of another certificant, and the resulting resolution of such complaint

i. Respect existing publishing rights and copyright laws, including, but not limited to, those that apply to NCBTMB's copyright-protected examinations.

STANDARD III: CONFIDENTIALITY

The certificant or applicant for certification shall respect the confidentiality of client information and safeguard all records. In his/her professional role the certificant or applicant for certification shall:

a. Protect the confidentiality of the client's identity in conversations, all advertisements, and any and all other matters unless disclosure of identifiable information is requested by the client in writing, is medically necessary, is required by law or for purposes of public protection

b. Protect the interests of clients who are minors or who are unable to give voluntary and informed consent by securing permission from an appropriate third party or guardian

c. Solicit only information that is relevant to the professional client/therapist relationship

d. Share pertinent information about the client with third parties when required by law or for purposes of public protection

e. Maintain the client files for a minimum period of four years

f. Store and dispose of client files in a secure manner.

STANDARD IV: BUSINESS PRACTICES

The certificant or applicant shall practice with honesty, integrity, and lawfulness in the business of therapeutic massage and bodywork. In his/her professional role the certificant or applicant shall:

a. Provide a physical setting that is safe and meets all applicable legal requirements for health and safety

b. Maintain adequate and customary liability insurance

c. Maintain adequate progress notes for each client session, if applicable

d. Accurately and truthfully inform the public of services provided

e. Honestly represent all professional qualifications and affiliations

f. Promote his/her business with integrity and avoid potential and actual conflicts of interest

g. Advertise in a manner that is honest, dignified, accurate and representative of services that can be delivered and remains consistent with the NCBTMB Code of Ethics and Standards of Practice

h. Advertise in a manner that is not misleading to the public and shall not use sensational, sexual, or provocative language and/or pictures to promote business

i. Comply with all laws regarding sexual harassment

j. Not exploit the trust and dependency of others, including clients and employees/coworkers

k. Display/discuss a schedule of fees in advance of the session that is clearly understood by the client or potential client

l. Make financial arrangements in advance that are clearly understood by and safeguard the best interests of the client or consumer

m. Follow acceptable accounting practices

n. File all applicable municipal, state, and federal taxes

o. Maintain accurate financial records, contracts and legal obligations, appointment records, tax reports, and receipts for at least four years.

STANDARD V: ROLES AND BOUNDARIES

The certificant or applicant for certification shall adhere to ethical boundaries and perform the professional roles designed to protect both the client and the practitioner, and safeguard the therapeutic value of the relationship. In his/her professional role the certificant or applicant for certification shall:

a. Recognize his/her personal limitations and practice only within these limitations

b. Recognize his/her influential position with the client and not exploit the relationship for personal or other gain

c. Recognize and limit the impact of transference and countertransference between the client and the certificant

d. Avoid dual or multidimensional relationships that could impair professional judgment or result in exploitation of the client or employees and/or coworkers

e. Not engage in any sexual activity with a client

f. Acknowledge and respect the client's freedom of choice in the therapeutic session

g. Respect the client's right to refuse the therapeutic session or any part of the therapeutic session

h. Refrain from practicing under the influence of alcohol, drugs, or any illegal substances (with the exception of a prescribed dosage of prescription medication which does not significantly impair the certificant)

i. Have the right to refuse and/or terminate the service to a client who is abusive or under the influence of alcohol, drugs, or any illegal substance.

STANDARD VI: PREVENTION OF SEXUAL MISCONDUCT

The certificant or applicant for certification shall refrain from any behavior that sexualizes, or appears to sexualize, the client/therapist relationship. The certificant or applicant for certification recognizes the intimacy of the therapeutic relationship may activate practitioner and/or client needs and/or desires that weaken objectivity and may lead to sexualizing the therapeutic relationship. In his/her professional role the certificant or applicant shall:

a. Refrain from participating in a sexual relationship or sexual conduct with the client, whether consensual or otherwise, from the beginning of the client/therapist relationship and for a minimum of six months after the termination of the client/therapist relationship unless a preexisting relationship exists between a certificant or applicant for certification and client prior to the certificant or applicant for certification applying to be certified by NCBTMB

b. In the event that the client initiates sexual behavior, clarify the purpose of the therapeutic session, and, if such conduct does not cease, terminate or refuse the session

c. Recognize that sexual activity with clients, students, employees, supervisors, or trainees is prohibited even if consensual

d. Not touch the genitalia

e. Only perform therapeutic treatments beyond the normal narrowing of the ear canal and normal narrowing of the nasal passages as indicated in the plan of care and only after receiving informed voluntary written consent

f. Only perform therapeutic treatments in the oropharynx as indicated in the plan of care and only after receiving informed voluntary consent

g. Only perform therapeutic treatments into the anal canal as indicated in the plan of care and only after receiving informed voluntary written consent

h. Only provide therapeutic breast massage as indicated in the plan of care and only after receiving informed voluntary consent from the client.

Glossary of Terms Used in This Document

Acceptable Accounting Procedures: Rules, conventions, standards, and procedures that are widely accepted among financial accountants.

Boundary: A boundary is a limit that separates one person from another. Its function is to protect the integrity of each person.

Competency: Study and development of a particular professional knowledge base and skills associated with and applied in practice within that knowledge base.

Countertransference: A practitioner's unresolved feelings and issues which are unconsciously transferred to the client.

Dignity: The quality or state of being worthy, honored or esteemed.

Dual Relationships: An alliance in addition to the client/therapist relationship, such as social, familial, business, or any other relationship that is outside the therapeutic relationship.

Genitalia, Female: Labia majora, labia minora, clitoris, and vaginal orifice.

Genitalia, Male: Testes, penis, and scrotum.

Impugn: To assail by words or arguments, oppose or attack as false.

Integrity: Honesty. Firm adherence to a code of values.

Multidimensional Relationships: Overlapping relationships in which therapist and client share an alliance, in addition to the therapeutic relationship.

Progress Notes: Notes written, by a practitioner certified by NCBTMB, and kept in a separate client file that indicates the date of the session, areas of complaint as stated by client, and observations made and actions taken by the practitioner.

Scope of Practice: The minimum standards necessary for safe and effective practice and the parameters of practice determined by the certificant's professional training and education, and, when applicable, regulatory bodies.

Sexual Activity: Any verbal and/or nonverbal behavior for the purpose of soliciting, receiving, or giving sexual gratification.

Sexual Harassment: Sexual harassment consists of unwelcome sexual advances, requests for sexual favors, and other verbal or physical conduct of a sexual nature when: 1. Submission to such conduct is made either explicitly or implicitly a term or condition of an individual's employment; 2. Submission to, or rejection of, such conduct by an individual is used as the basis for employment decisions affecting such individuals; or 3. Such conduct has the purpose or effect of unreasonably interfering with an individual's work performance or creating an intimidating, hostile, or offensive working environment.

Therapeutic Breast Massage: Manipulation of the non-muscular soft tissue structure of the breast up to and including the areola and nipple.

Transference: The displacement or transfer of feelings, thoughts, and behaviors originally related to a significant person, such as a parent, onto someone else, such as a massage therapist (or doctor, psychotherapist, teacher, spiritual advisor).

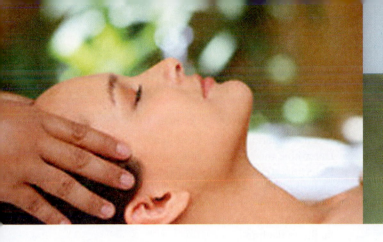

Goal-Oriented Planning

LONG-TERM PLANNING—INITIAL SESSION AND ONGOING EVALUATION

1. Gather information from the client.
   - Review intake form
   - Review health history form
   - Conduct interview
2. Collect information through observation and measurement.
   - Observe client (e.g., general posture, motion, expression, stress level)
   - Conduct tests and measurements related to stated goals or complaint
3. Assess the overall situation and establish long-term goals.
   - Identify wellness goals that can be addressed with massage
   - Identify problems for which massage is indicated
   - Identify contraindications and cautions
   - Prioritize goals together with the client
4. Develop an action plan to achieve long-term goals.
   - Suggest frequency and length of massage sessions
   - Determine general massage approaches to use
   - Set a date for evaluating progress on specific goals
   - Suggest home care to help achieve goals (e.g., self-massage, hot and cold applications, stretching, exercises, relaxation techniques)
5. Implement the long-term plan.
   - Make appointments
   - Provide client with information or tools for home care
6. Evaluate progress toward long-term goals.
   - Write SOAP notes to document the long-term plan
   - Adjust the long-term plan as needed to achieve original client goals and/or set new or modified goals
   - Set date for evaluating progress toward long-term goals

INDIVIDUAL SESSION PLANNING

1. Gather information from the client, and review previous documentation.
   - Review intake and health history forms
   - Review notes from previous sessions
   - Presession interview
   - Ask about changes in health status or medications
   - Ask about progress or regression since last session
2. Collect information through observation and measurement.
   - Observe the client (e.g., general posture, motion, expression)
   - Palpation and simple measurements during the session
3. Assess the situation and set session goals.
   - Identify current client state and next step to reach long-term goals
   - Prioritize goals for the session
   - Determine cautions and contraindications for this session
4. Develop a general plan for the session.
   - Plan session organization including body areas to be addressed, and in what order to apply massage
   - Choose general approach to use in the session (e.g., relaxation massage, trigger points, myofascial massage, lymph drainage massage, polarity therapy, etc.)
   - Determine use of adjunct methods (e.g., hot or cold applications, aromatherapy, electronic vibration device)
5. Implement the session plan.
   - Apply massage and related techniques
6. Evaluate progress toward the session goals.
   - Ongoing evaluation during session
   - Postsession evaluation (e.g., postsession observations, postsession client interview)
   - Ongoing adjustments during the massage session
   - Write SOAP notes to document the session

TREATMENT PLANNING— FOR TREATMENT AND RECOVERY FROM ILLNESS OR INJURY

1. Gather information from client related to the illness, injury, or complaint.
   - Review intake form
   - Review medical history
   - Review medical diagnosis if available
   - Conduct initial interview
     Onset of condition
     Symptoms
     Degree of pain
     Functional limitations
     Activities of daily living (ADL) affected
     First aid or home remedies applied
     What seems to make it better or worse

2. Collect information related to the illness or injury through observation and measurement.
   - Observe general state of client (e.g., facial expression, voice quality, energy level)
   - Take measurements relative to the complaint or diagnosed condition (e.g., standing posture, sitting posture, walking gait, body mechanics, range of motion at specific joints)
   - Visual observation of skin (e.g., color, bruises, swelling, pitting, scars, moles, wounds, rashes)
   - Palpation of soft tissues in specific areas (e.g., texture [degree of oiliness or dryness], temperature, pliability, firmness, adhesion, fibrosis, puffiness, springiness)
   - Palpation of muscle and tendon structures (e.g., firmness, shape, tension, atrophy or wasting, taut bands in muscle tissue, trigger points, taut tendons)

   - Palpation of movement (e.g., ease of movement, crepitations)
   - Orthopedic tests for specific pathologies

3. Assess the situation and set treatment goals.
   - Determine the condition of tissues
   - Determine function or loss of function
   - Identify contraindications and cautions for massage therapy
   - Determine how massage can alleviate symptoms or facilitate healing
   - Set anatomical, physiological, and/or functional treatment goals

4. Develop a treatment action plan.
   - Suggest the frequency and length of massage sessions
   - Choose a general approach to reach goals (e.g., Western massage, myofascial massage, neuromuscular therapy, lymphatic massage, foot reflexology, polarity therapy)
   - Set a date for evaluating progress on specific goals
   - Suggest home care (e.g., self-massage, hot and cold applications, stretching, exercises, relaxation techniques)

5. Implement the treatment plan.
   - Make appointments
   - Provide client with information or tools for home care

6. Evaluate progress toward healing and recovery.
   - Adjust the treatment plan as needed to achieve goals for healing and recovery
   - Write SOAP notes to document the treatment plan

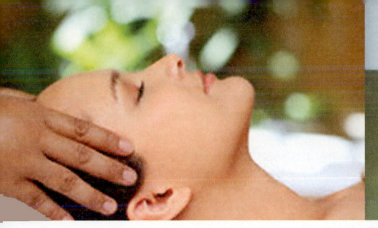

Performance Evaluation Forms

INSTRUCTIONS

Use these Performance Evaluation Forms to track your progress in learning massage techniques and to prepare for upcoming practical exams. Rate yourself, or have a practice partner rate you, on how well you did performing the Practice Sequences and techniques presented throughout this textbook. The instructor can also use these forms to measure your accomplishments.

There is a Performance Evaluation Form in this appendix for individual Western massage techniques, joint movements, Qi Gong Twenty Form Routine, and every Practice Sequence in this textbook and/or on the companion DVD. If you prefer, the Performance Evaluation Forms can be downloaded from your DVD.

HOW TO EVALUATE YOUR PERFORMANCE

Before the performance evaluation, look over the form to see what elements are listed. This helps identify what the evaluator will be looking for. Review the chapters for descriptions of techniques listed and other important information related to their application. Make notes about points you want to remember.

Review the DVD video for the Practice Sequence or techniques you are going to evaluate. Look closely for items mentioned on the evaluation form.

When practicing for a practical exam, add items emphasized by your instructor in class if you do not see them listed on the form. Note that some elements are common to almost all forms, for example, client communication, positioning, draping, and body mechanics. Others are unique to a particular form of massage and bodywork.

Evaluation is done by using a rating scale from 0 to 5. While this is somewhat subjective, it provides a measurement for seeing progress over time. Be honest about how you are doing. Work on skills that need improvement. Aim for achieving ratings of good (4) or excellent (5) for all items listed.

PERFORMANCE EVALUATION FORM 11–1

Hygienic Hand Washing

Student: _____ Date: _____

Scoring Key: 0 = incorrect; 1 = very poor; 2 = poor; 3 = adequate; 4 = good; 5 = excellent

1. Wet hands and forearms up to elbows. Water flows from elbows to hands and off of fingertips.

   0   1   2   3   4   5

2. Scrub nails to loosen dirt. Clean the surface and under the nails.

   0   1   2   3   4   5

3. Apply soap and create soapy lather up to the elbows. Include finger and thumb webs.

   0   1   2   3   4   5

4. Rub hands and arms for at least 15 seconds.

   0   1   2   3   4   5

5. Rinse off soap from fingertips to elbows. Water flows off of elbows.

   0   1   2   3   4   5

6. Dry hands thoroughly with paper towels.

   0   1   2   3   4   5

7. Use the same paper towel to turn off the faucet, and if applicable, open the door handle to the massage room.

   0   1   2   3   4   5

8. Discard the paper towel in a proper receptacle.

   0   1   2   3   4   5

Total points _____ / 8 = _____ Average Rating

Evaluated by: _____

PERFORMANCE EVALUATION FORM 13–1

Individual Western Massage Techniques

Student: _____   Date: _____

Scoring Key: 0 = incorrect; 1 = very poor; 2 = poor; 3 = adequate; 4 = good; 5 = excellent

Effleurage

1. Basic sliding effleurage

   0   1   2   3   4   5

2. Stripping

   0   1   2   3   4   5

3. Shingles effleurage

   0   1   2   3   4   5

4. Bilateral tree stroking

   0   1   2   3   4   5

5. Three-count stroking of the trapezius

   0   1   2   3   4   5

6. Mennell's superficial stroking

   0   1   2   3   4   5

7. Nerve strokes

   0   1   2   3   4   5

8. Knuckling

   0   1   2   3   4   5

Petrissage

9. Basic two-handed kneading

   0   1   2   3   4   5

10. One-handed kneading

   0   1   2   3   4   5

11. Alternating one-handed kneading

   0   1   2   3   4   5

12. Circular two-handed petrissage

   0   1   2   3   4   5

13. Fingers-to-thumb petrissage

   0   1   2   3   4   5

14. Skin lifting and rolling

   0   1   2   3   4   5

15. Compression

   0   1   2   3   4   5

16. Rolling

   0   1   2   3   4   5

Friction

17. Superficial warming friction with the palms

    0   1   2   3   4   5

18. Superficial warming friction—sawing (ulnar friction)

    0   1   2   3   4   5

19. Superficial warming friction with the knuckles

    0   1   2   3   4   5

20. Cross-fiber deep friction

    0   1   2   3   4   5

21. Circular deep friction

    0   1   2   3   4   5

22. Deep transverse (Cyriax) friction

    0   1   2   3   4   5

Tapotement

23. Hacking

    0   1   2   3   4   5

24. Cupping

    0   1   2   3   4   5

25. Clapping

    0   1   2   3   4   5

26. Slapping

    0   1   2   3   4   5

27. Tapping

    0   1   2   3   4   5

28. Pincement

    0   1   2   3   4   5

29. Quacking

    0   1   2   3   4   5

30. Squishes

    0   1   2   3   4   5

Vibration

31. Deep vibration with the fingertips

   0   1   2   3   4   5

32. Light effleurage with vibration

   0   1   2   3   4   5

33. Shaking—coarse vibration

   0   1   2   3   4   5

34. Jostling—coarse vibration

   0   1   2   3   4   5

Touch without movement

35. Passive touch

   0   1   2   3   4   5

36. Direct pressure with thumb or fingers

   0   1   2   3   4   5

Total points _____ / 36 = _____ Average Rating

Evaluated by: _____

PERFORMANCE EVALUATION FORM 13–2
Joint Movements

Student: _____   Date: _____

Scoring Key: 0 = incorrect; 1 = very poor; 2 = poor; 3 = adequate; 4 = good; 5 = excellent

Neck

1. Simple mobilizing movements of the neck

    0   1   2   3   4   5

2. Finger push-ups

    0   1   2   3   4   5

3. Suboccipital release

    0   1   2   3   4   5

4. Wave movement

    0   1   2   3   4   5

5. Stretch in lateral flexion

    0   1   2   3   4   5

6. Stretch in rotation

    0   1   2   3   4   5

7. Stretch in forward flexion

    0   1   2   3   4   5

8. Cross-arm stretch

    0   1   2   3   4   5

Shoulder girdle

9. Wagging the arm

    0   1   2   3   4   5

10. Shaking the arm

    0   1   2   3   4   5

11. Passive shoulder roll

    0   1   2   3   4   5

12. Scapula mobilizing

    0   1   2   3   4   5

13. Horizontal flexion

    0   1   2   3   4   5

14. Overhead stretch

    0   1   2   3   4   5

Elbow

15. Wagging the arm

    0   1   2   3   4   5

16. Pronate and supinate the hand

    0   1   2   3   4   5

17. Circling the forearm

    0   1   2   3   4   5

18. Overhead stretch

    0   1   2   3   4   5

Wrist

19. Passive movement through range of motion

    0   1   2   3   4   5

20. Wagging

    0   1   2   3   4   5

21. Flexion

    0   1   2   3   4   5

22. Extension

    0   1   2   3   4   5

Hand

23. Mobilizing knuckles with figure-8s

    0   1   2   3   4   5

24. Scissoring metacarpals

    0   1   2   3   4   5

25. Hyperextend the fingers

    0   1   2   3   4   5

Chest

26. Gentle rocking of rib cage

    0   1   2   3   4   5

27. Overhead stretch

    0   1   2   3   4   5

Hip

28. Rocking the leg

    0   1   2   3   4   5

29. Passive movement through range of motion

    0   1   2   3   4   5

30. Knee to chest flexion

    0   1   2   3   4   5

31. Straight leg flexion

    0   1   2   3   4   5

32. Diagonal adduction

    0   1   2   3   4   5

33. Hyperextension

    0   1   2   3   4   5

Knee

34. Wag the leg

    0   1   2   3   4   5

35. Leg toss

    0   1   2   3   4   5

36. Circling the lower leg

    0   1   2   3   4   5

37. Heel to buttocks stretch

    0   1   2   3   4   5

Ankle

38. Dorsiflexion of foot

    0   1   2   3   4   5

39. Passive movement of ankle through its full range of motion

    0   1   2   3   4   5

40. Side-to-side mobilizing

    0   1   2   3   4   5

41. Stretch in dorsiflexion

    0   1   2   3   4   5

42. Stretch in plantarflexion

    0   1   2   3   4   5

Foot

43. Figure-8s with toes

    0   1   2   3   4   5

44. Scissoring metatarsals

    0   1   2   3   4   5

45. Uncurling toes with effleurage

    0   1   2   3   4   5

46. Stretch toes in hyperextension

    0   1   2   3   4   5

47. Widening stretch at metatarsals

    0   1   2   3   4   5

48. Fingers between toes

    0   1   2   3   4   5

Methods of Stretching

49. Simple static stretch

    0   1   2   3   4   5

50. Contract-relax-stretch (CRS)

    0   1   2   3   4   5

51. CRS using reciprocal inhibition

    0   1   2   3   4   5

52. Active assisted stretch

    0   1   2   3   4   5

Total points _____ / 52 = _____ Average Rating

Evaluated by: _____

PERFORMANCE EVALUATION FORM 14–1
Full-Body Western Massage

Student: _____ Date: _____

Scoring Key: 0 = incorrect; 1 = very poor; 2 = poor; 3 = adequate; 4 = good; 5 = excellent

1. Professional demeanor.

   0   1   2   3   4   5

2. Client communication: health history interview, explanations, feedback.

   0   1   2   3   4   5

3. Positioning and draping.

   0   1   2   3   4   5

Recipient Prone

4. Back—apply oil, application of massage techniques.

   0   1   2   3   4   5

5. Lower limbs and buttocks—apply oil, application of massage techniques.

   0   1   2   3   4   5

6. Finish and transition—rock and light effleurage over drape; turn over.

   0   1   2   3   4   5

Recipient Supine

7. Lower limbs—apply oil, application of massage techniques.

   0   1   2   3   4   5

8. Upper limbs and chest—apply oil, application of massage techniques.

   0   1   2   3   4   5

9. Abdomen—apply oil, application of massage techniques.

   0   1   2   3   4   5

10. Neck and shoulders—apply oil, application of massage techniques.

    0   1   2   3   4   5

11. Face and Head—application of massage techniques.

    0   1   2   3   4   5

12. Finish—brush off front, hold feet, announce end of session.

    0   1   2   3   4   5

13. Safety, use of pressure, avoidance of endangerment sites.

    0   1   2   3   4   5

14. Body/hand mechanics and ease of movement around the table.

    0   1   2   3   4   5

15. Overall application (timing, pacing, rhythm, flow, quality of touch).

    0   1   2   3   4   5

Total points _____ / 15 = _____ Average Rating

Evaluated by: _____

PERFORMANCE EVALUATION FORM 15–1

Seated Massage

Student: _____ Date: _____

Scoring Key: 0 = incorrect; 1 = very poor; 2 = poor; 3 = adequate; 4 = good; 5 = excellent

1. Positioning the recipient on the massage chair.

    0   1   2   3   4   5

2. Client communication—health history interview; explanations, feedback.

    0   1   2   3   4   5

3. Establish contact and squeeze shoulders.

    0   1   2   3   4   5

4. Upper back—compressions and thumb pressure to paraspinal muscles.

    0   1   2   3   4   5

5. Shoulders—broad forearm compression and elbow pressure to points.

    0   1   2   3   4   5

6. Finish shoulders and transition to arms—squeeze along shoulders and down arms bilaterally.

    0   1   2   3   4   5

7. Arm—position arm hanging down, knead, reposition.

    0   1   2   3   4   5

8. Forearm—thumb pressure, circular friction, squeezes.

    0   1   2   3   4   5

9. Wrist, hand, fingers—circular friction, squeezes.

    0   1   2   3   4   5

10. Joint mobilizing wrist, hand, and fingers.

    0   1   2   3   4   5

11. Stretch arm overhead.

    0   1   2   3   4   5

12. Neck muscles—kneading, thumb pressure, and circular friction to points.

    0   1   2   3   4   5

13. Scalp mobilization and light tapotement to head.

    0   1   2   3   4   5

14. Finish session with brush off from head to hips.

    0   1   2   3   4   5

15. Body/hand mechanics and ease of movement around the massage chair.

    0   1   2   3   4   5

16. Overall application (safety, timing, pacing, rhythm, flow, quality of touch).

    0   1   2   3   4   5

Total points _____ / 16 = _____ Average Rating

Evaluated by: _____

PERFORMANCE EVALUATION FORM 16–1
Hot Application on Upper Back

Student: _____   Date: _____

Scoring Key: 0 = incorrect; 1 = very poor; 2 = poor; 3 = adequate; 4 = good; 5 = excellent

1. Positioning and draping.

   0   1   2   3   4   5

2. Client communication: health history interview, explanations, feedback.

   0   1   2   3   4   5

3. Check heat source for temperature.

   0   1   2   3   4   5

4. Place heat barrier on upper back—sheet or towel of appropriate thickness.

   0   1   2   3   4   5

5. Instructions about effects of heat and how to give feedback if the application becomes too hot.

   0   1   2   3   4   5

6. Apply heat source, cover, and ask for feedback—apply more heat barriers if necessary.

   0   1   2   3   4   5

7. Get feedback every 3–4 minutes about heat intensity—add or take away barriers to maintain therapeutic heat level.

   0   1   2   3   4   5

8. Remove heat and check skin for redness.

   0   1   2   3   4   5

9. Body/hand mechanics and ease of movement around the table.

   0   1   2   3   4   5

10. Overall application (safety, timing, pacing, rhythm, flow, quality of touch).

   0   1   2   3   4   5

Total points _____ / 10 = _____ Average Rating

Evaluated by: _____

PERFORMANCE EVALUATION FORM 16–2

Cold Application for Knee

Student: _____   Date: _____

Scoring Key: 0 = incorrect; 1 = very poor; 2 = poor; 3 = adequate; 4 = good; 5 = excellent

1. Positioning and draping.

   0   1   2   3   4   5

2. Client communication: health history interview, explanations, feedback.

   0   1   2   3   4   5

3. Place cold barrier on knee—sheet or towel of appropriate thickness.

   0   1   2   3   4   5

4. Instructions about effects of cold, and how to give feedback if the cold becomes too intense.

   0   1   2   3   4   5

5. Apply cold source, cover, and ask for feedback—apply more cold barriers if necessary.

   0   1   2   3   4   5

6. Get feedback every 3–4 minutes about cold intensity—add or take away barriers to maintain therapeutic cold level.

   0   1   2   3   4   5

7. Remove cold source, and check for redness and swelling.

   0   1   2   3   4   5

8. Body/hand mechanics and ease of movement around the table.

   0   1   2   3   4   5

9. Safety, use of pressure, avoidance of endangerment sites.

   0   1   2   3   4   5

10. Overall application (safety, timing, pacing, rhythm, flow, quality of touch).

   0   1   2   3   4   5

Total points _____ / 10 = _____ Average Rating

Evaluated by: _____

PERFORMANCE EVALUATION FORM 16–3

Ice Massage for Elbow

Student: _____   Date: _____

Scoring Key: 0 = incorrect; 1 = very poor; 2 = poor; 3 = adequate; 4 = good; 5 = excellent

1. Positioning and draping.

    0   1   2   3   4   5

2. Client communication: health history interview, explanations, feedback.

    0   1   2   3   4   5

3. Massage forearm muscles—kneading, muscle stripping, transverse friction over tendons, direct pressure to tender points.

    0   1   2   3   4   5

4. Instructions about effects of ice, stages of feeling cold, and how to give feedback if the cold becomes too intense.

    0   1   2   3   4   5

5. Ice massage to tendons around elbow—continuous circular movement of ice, medium pressure, 10 minutes.

    0   1   2   3   4   5

6. Get feedback periodically about cold intensity and stages of feeling.

    0   1   2   3   4   5

7. Remove cold source and apply superficial friction with towel.

    0   1   2   3   4   5

8. Body/hand mechanics and ease of movement around the table.

    0   1   2   3   4   5

9. Safety, use of pressure, avoidance of endangerment sites.

    0   1   2   3   4   5

10. Overall application (safety, timing, pacing, rhythm, flow, quality of touch).

    0   1   2   3   4   5

Total points _____ / 10 = _____ Average Rating

Evaluated by: _____

PERFORMANCE EVALUATION FORM 18–1

Lymphatic Facilitation for the Lower Extremity

Student: _____   Date: _____

Scoring Key: 0 = incorrect; 1 = very poor; 2 = poor; 3 = adequate; 4 = good; 5 = excellent

1. Positioning and draping.

    0   1   2   3   4   5

2. Client communication: health history interview, explanations, feedback.

    0   1   2   3   4   5

3. L stroke on both sides of neck—finger placement, L direction, snap back, repetitions.

    0   1   2   3   4   5

4. L stroke on terminus—finger placement, L direction, snap back, repetitions.

    0   1   2   3   4   5

5. Clearing the cisterna chyle—instruction for forceful breaths, 5–6 breaths

    0   1   2   3   4   5

6. Clearing the inguinal catchment area—hand placement, direction of movement, repetition.

    0   1   2   3   4   5

7. Clearing the thigh with long strokes—full hand placement, skin stretch, slide, snap back, repetitions.

    0   1   2   3   4   5

8. Clearing the popliteal catchment area—hand placement under knee, lift and stretch, release and return to start, repetitions.

    0   1   2   3   4   5

9. Clearing the lower leg with long strokes—full hand placement, skin stretch, slide, snap back, repetitions.

    0   1   2   3   4   5

10. Clearing the tarsals, metatarsals, and toes—hand placement, skin stretch, snap back, repetitions.

    0   1   2   3   4   5

11. Principles of lymphatic facilitation—light touch, slow gentle repetitions, appropriate direction, skin snaps back

    0   1   2   3   4   5

12. Body/hand mechanics and ease of movement around the table.

    0   1   2   3   4   5

13. Safety, use of pressure, avoidance of endangerment sites.

    0   1   2   3   4   5

14. Overall application (safety, timing, pacing, rhythm, flow, quality of touch).

    0   1   2   3   4   5

Total points _____ / 14 = _____ Average Rating

Evaluated by: _____

PERFORMANCE EVALUATION FORM 18–2

General Reflexology Session

Student: _____   Date: _____

Scoring Key: 0 = incorrect; 1 = very poor; 2 = poor; 3 = adequate; 4 = good; 5 = excellent

1. Positioning the recipient.

    0   1   2   3   4   5

2. Client communication—health history interview, foot examination for structural and skin problems, explanations, feedback.

    0   1   2   3   4   5

3. Warm-up—variety of massage and joint movement techniques.

    0   1   2   3   4   5

4. Spinal twist—three quick twists at pelvis, waist, and diaphragmatic guidelines.

    0   1   2   3   4   5

5. Spinal reflex—thumb rolling sacrum to C-1, foot position on lateral edge.

    0   1   2   3   4   5

6. Toe rotations—rotate each toe, compress tip with snap, work from medial to lateral.

    0   1   2   3   4   5

7. Bidirectional thumb walking on plantar surface—thumb walking technique, elbows flap, apply in horizontal lines from base of toes to heel.

    0   1   2   3   4   5

8. Pressure along diaphragm guidelines—apply medial to lateral.

    0   1   2   3   4   5

9. Lymphatic drainage on dorsum ending with ankle rotation—stretch dorsum skin row by row, end at ankle joint, use fingers to rotate ankle.

    0   1   2   3   4   5

10. Press-and-flex medial and lateral ankle—finger position, roll ankle into pressure points.

    0   1   2   3   4   5

11. Press-and-flex on shoulder reflex—roll foot into pressure points.

    0   1   2   3   4   5

12. Hook and backup on the hypothalamus/pituitary gland reflex—thumb position, pressure application

    0   1   2   3   4   5

13. Finish with general foot massage.

    0   1   2   3   4   5

14. Knowledge of reflex and guideline locations.

    0   1   2   3   4   5

15. Overall application (safety, timing, pacing, rhythm, flow, quality of touch).

    0   1   2   3   4   5

Total points _____ / 15 = _____ Average Rating

Evaluated by: _____

PERFORMANCE EVALUATION FORM 18–3

Myofascial Massage of the Back

Student: _____   Date: _____

Scoring Key: 0 = incorrect; 1 = very poor; 2 = poor; 3 = adequate; 4 = good; 5 = excellent

1. Positioning and draping.

    0   1   2   3   4   5

2. Client communication: health history interview, explanations, feedback.

    0   1   2   3   4   5

3. Initial contact—place hands over sheet on upper and lower back, and rock gently.

    0   1   2   3   4   5

4. Skin lifting—simple lift and lift adding movement, slow steady lift 1 to 2 minutes per spot.

    0   1   2   3   4   5

5. Skin rolling—skin lift and roll, slow steady movement in multiple directions over same spot.

    0   1   2   3   4   5

6. Cross-handed stretch for subcutaneous fascia—hold for 2 to 3 minutes or until tissues release.

    0   1   2   3   4   5

7. Fascial mobilization in 1 direction using palm—engage tissues, shift horizontally, hold tension steadily for 2 to 5 minutes until a shift is felt, move from spot to spot.

    0   1   2   3   4   5

8. Facial mobilization shifting direction—engage tissues, shift horizontally in direction of resistance or least resistance, shift direction as tissues dictate.

    0   1   2   3   4   5

9. Pin and stretch—pin tissues with one hand while the other pulls away, slow steady tension, hold for 2 to 3 minutes or until tissues release.

    0   1   2   3   4   5

10. Deep fascial mobilization—use reinforced fingertips or forearm; engage deep fascia, shift tissues horizontally, hold steady for 2 to 5 minutes or until tissues release.

    0   1   2   3   4   5

11. Finish with redraping and passive touch—letting tissues rest.

    0   1   2   3   4   5

12. Body/hand mechanics and ease of movement around table.

    0   1   2   3   4   5

13. Safety, use of pressure, avoidance of endangerment sites.

    0   1   2   3   4   5

14. Overall application (timing, pacing, rhythm, flow, quality of touch).

    0   1   2   3   4   5

Total points _____ / 14 = _____ Average Rating

Evaluated by: _____

PERFORMANCE EVALUATION FORM 18–4

Trigger Point Therapy for Tension Headaches

Student: _____   Date: _____

Scoring Key: 0 = incorrect; 1 = very poor; 2 = poor; 3 = adequate; 4 = good; 5 = excellent

1. Positioning and draping.

   0   1   2   3   4   5

2. Client communication: health history interview, explanations, feedback.

   0   1   2   3   4   5

3. Initial contact and warming neck—gently squeeze posterior cervical muscles, effleurage along cervical and shoulder muscles, traction with head in neutral position.

   0   1   2   3   4   5

4. Locating TrPs—checking common trigger point locations in cervical and shoulder muscles, using feedback from recipient

   0   1   2   3   4   5

5. General treatment of TrPs—pressing, monitoring pain, slow application, hold for 30 to 90 seconds and repeat, follow-up with massage and stretching.

   0   1   2   3   4   5

6. Direct pressure to TrPs in upper trapezius—locating, applying direct pressure.

   0   1   2   3   4   5

7. Pincer technique to SCM muscle—turn head, avoid endangerment site.

   0   1   2   3   4   5

8. Direct pressure to TrPs in posterior and suboccipital muscles—using fingertips or thumbs, position head for access.

   0   1   2   3   4   5

9. Stretches for neck muscles—forward flexion, lateral flexion, rotation, traction.

   0   1   2   3   4   5

10. Finishing—wave-like movement in posterior cervical muscles, cat paw.

    0   1   2   3   4   5

11. Body/hand mechanics

    0   1   2   3   4   5

12. Overall application (safety, timing, pacing, rhythm, flow, quality of touch).

    0   1   2   3   4   5

Total points _____ / 12 = _____ Average Rating

Evaluated by: _____

PERFORMANCE EVALUATION FORM 18–5

Lymphatic Facilitation for the Head and Neck

Student: _____ Date: _____

Scoring Key: 0 = incorrect; 1 = very poor; 2 = poor; 3 = adequate; 4 = good; 5 = excellent

1. Positioning and draping.

   0   1   2   3   4   5

2. Client communication: health history interview, explanations, feedback.

   0   1   2   3   4   5

3. L stroke on both sides of neck—finger placement, L direction, snap back, repetitions.

   0   1   2   3   4   5

4. L stroke on terminus—finger placement, L direction, snap back, repetitions.

   0   1   2   3   4   5

5. L stroke under mandible—finger placement, L direction, snap back, repetitions.

   0   1   2   3   4   5

6. L stroke on face—hand placement, L direction, snap back, repetitions.

   0   1   2   3   4   5

7. L stroke near eyes—finger placement, L direction, snap back, repetitions.

   0   1   2   3   4   5

8. L stroke on forehead—finger placement, L direction, snap back, repetitions.

   0   1   2   3   4   5

9. L stroke on temples and side of head—finger placement, L direction, snap back, repetitions.

   0   1   2   3   4   5

10. L stroke on lateral neck toward terminus—finger placement, L direction, snap back, repetitions.

   0   1   2   3   4   5

11. Finishing—effleurage to arms, kneading shoulders, passive touch.

   0   1   2   3   4   5

12. Principles of lymphatic facilitation—light touch; slow, gentle repetitions; appropriate direction; skin snaps back.

   0   1   2   3   4   5

13. Body/hand mechanics.

   0   1   2   3   4   5

14. Overall application (safety, timing, pacing, rhythm, flow, quality of touch).

   0   1   2   3   4   5

Total points _____ / 14 = _____ Average Rating

Evaluated by: _____

PERFORMANCE EVALUATION FORM 18–6

General Session of Polarity Therapy

Student: _____   Date: _____

Scoring Key: 0 = incorrect; 1 = very poor; 2 = poor; 3 = adequate; 4 = good; 5 = excellent

Polarity Therapy Techniques

1. The cradle.

    0   1   2   3   4   5

2. Neck stretch.

    0   1   2   3   4   5

3. Tummy rock.

    0   1   2   3   4   5

4. Leg pull.

    0   1   2   3   4   5

5. Inside ankle press (right foot).

    0   1   2   3   4   5

6. Outside ankle press (right foot).

    0   1   2   3   4   5

7. Inside ankle press (left foot).

    0   1   2   3   4   5

8. Outside ankle press (left foot).

    0   1   2   3   4   5

9. Pelvis and knee rock (right side.)

    0   1   2   3   4   5

10. Arm shoulder rotation (right side).

    0   1   2   3   4   5

11. Thumb web—forearm stimulation (right side).

    0   1   2   3   4   5

12. Elbow milk—abdominal rock (right side).

    0   1   2   3   4   5

13. Pelvic rock (right side).

    0   1   2   3   4   5

14. Pelvis and knee rock (left side).

    0   1   2   3   4   5

15. Arm shoulder rotation (left side).

    0   1   2   3   4   5

16. Thumb web—forearm stimulation (left side).

    0   1   2   3   4   5

17. Elbow milk—abdominal rock (left side).

    0   1   2   3   4   5

18. Pelvic rock (left side).

    0   1   2   3   4   5

19. Occipital press.

    0   1   2   3   4   5

20. Cranial polarization.

    0   1   2   3   4   5

21. Navel-third eye.

    0   1   2   3   4   5

22. Brushing off to finish—back and front.

    0   1   2   3   4   5

Polarity Therapy Session

23. Client positioning and instructions.

    0   1   2   3   4   5

24. Client communication: health history interview, explanations, feedback.

    0   1   2   3   4   5

25. Practitioner body mechanics.

    0   1   2   3   4   5

26. Transitions from technique to technique.

    0   1   2   3   4   5

27. Quality of touch and energy sensitivity.

    0   1   2   3   4   5

28. Overall effect.

    0   1   2   3   4   5

Total points _____ / 28 = _____ Average Rating

Evaluated by: _____

PERFORMANCE EVALUATION FORM 19–1

A M I for the Back

Student: _____   Date: _____

Scoring Key: 0 = incorrect; 1 = very poor; 2 = poor; 3 = adequate; 4 = good; 5 = excellent

1. Positioning and draping.

   0   1   2   3   4   5

2. Client communication—health history interview, explanations, feedback.

   0   1   2   3   4   5

3. Oil application and warm-up—effleurage to entire back.

   0   1   2   3   4   5

4. Hand-over-hand effleurage to entire back—reach to opposite side, stroke up and down the back alternately, parallel to spine.

   0   1   2   3   4   5

5. Pull-ups around side of torso from iliac crest to the shoulder—flat palms.

   0   1   2   3   4   5

6. Circular fingertip kneading along paraspinal muscles—hip to shoulders.

   0   1   2   3   4   5

7. Alternate thumb petrissage along paraspinal muscles—shoulder to sacrum.

   0   1   2   3   4   5

8. Thumb press sacral notches.

   0   1   2   3   4   5

9. Press GB-30—with fingertips, 2–3 times.

   0   1   2   3   4   5

10. Fingertip kneading along paraspinals on Inner and Outer Bladder Meridians—sacrum to top of shoulder.

    0   1   2   3   4   5

11. Thumb press across top of shoulder—press GB-21 repeatedly, finish with kneading.

    0   1   2   3   4   5

12. Thumb press between shoulder blades Inner and Outer Bladder Meridians—press into areas of kyo or excess.

    0   1   2   3   4   5

13. Effleurage over upper shoulder area.

    0   1   2   3   4   5

14. Rhythmic sliding compression down the paraspinal muscles, sliding back to start—palms on either side of spine, compression movement from shoulders to sacrum.

    0   1   2   3   4   5

15. Press points at base of skull—Bl-10, BG-20 and all points with spread fingertips.

    0   1   2   3   4   5

16. Pull-ups from shoulder to buttocks—reach across, pull up around torso, fingertips between ribs.

    0   1   2   3   4   5

17. Thumb petrissage to paraspinal muscles from sacrum to shoulder—search for tightness in mid-back area, thumb presses or deep friction to tight spots.

    0   1   2   3   4   5

18. Thumb presses between shoulder blades to acupoints on Inner and Outer Bladder Meridians.

    0   1   2   3   4   5

19. Rhythmic sliding compression from shoulders to hips, palmar friction back to start—palms on either side of spine, compression movement from shoulders to sacrum.

    0   1   2   3   4   5

20. Effleurage to entire back.

    0   1   2   3   4   5

21. Fingertip kneading along paraspinal muscles from shoulders to buttocks.

    0   1   2   3   4   5

22. Circular palmar petrissage over entire back—tissues lift.

    0   1   2   3   4   5

23. Hourglass effleurage around tops of shoulders.

    0   1   2   3   4   5

24. Superficial friction with palms over paraspinal muscles.

    0   1   2   3   4   5

25. Overall application (safety, timing, pacing, rhythm, flow, quality of touch).

    0   1   2   3   4   5

Total points _____ / 25 = _____ Average Rating

Evaluated by: _____

PERFORMANCE EVALUATION FORM 19–2

Qi Gong Twenty Form Routine

Student: _____   Date: _____

Scoring Key: 0 = incorrect; 1 = very poor; 2 = poor; 3 = adequate; 4 = good; 5 = excellent

1. Mind on Dan Tian

   0   1   2   3   4   5

2. Mind and Heart at Ming Men

   0   1   2   3   4   5

3. Lao Gong Gather Qi

   0   1   2   3   4   5

4. Mind on Yun Quan Point

   0   1   2   3   4   5

5. Guide Qi Flow on Ren and Du Channels

   0   1   2   3   4   5

6. Gliding Phoenix

   0   1   2   3   4   5

7. Light Boat Sails Smoothly

   0   1   2   3   4   5

8. Pick the Stars

   0   1   2   3   4   5

9. Open the Magic Door

   0   1   2   3   4   5

10. Crane and Deer Appear in the Spring

   0   1   2   3   4   5

11. Wash Your Clothes

   0   1   2   3   4   5

12. Dragon Coils at the Sea

   0   1   2   3   4   5

13. Dust Your Boots

   0   1   2   3   4   5

14. Clear the Blockage

   0   1   2   3   4   5

15. Push the Stone Tablets

   0   1   2   3   4   5

16. Phoenix Pays Tribute

    0   1   2   3   4   5

17. Monk Nodding

    0   1   2   3   4   5

18. Adjust Breathing Left

    0   1   2   3   4   5

19. Adjust Breathing Right

    0   1   2   3   4   5

20. Adjust Breathing in the Center and Ending Position

    0   1   2   3   4   5

Total points _____ / 20 = _____ Average Rating

Evaluated by: _____

PERFORMANCE EVALUATION FORM 20–1

Postevent Sports Massage for Run/Walk Event

Student: _____ Date: _____

Scoring Key: 0 = incorrect; 1 = very poor; 2 = poor; 3 = adequate; 4 = good; 5 = excellent

1. Positioning the recipient.

    0   1   2   3   4   5

2. Client communication—health history interview, explanations, feedback.

    0   1   2   3   4   5

Athlete Supine

3. Initial contact and leg mobilizing.

    0   1   2   3   4   5

4. Thigh muscles—broaden/lift, knead, shake, jostle.

    0   1   2   3   4   5

5. Stretch hamstrings—knee to chest.

    0   1   2   3   4   5

6. Knee—circular friction to tendons.

    0   1   2   3   4   5

7. Lower leg muscles—position leg, squeeze.

    0   1   2   3   4   5

8. Ankle and foot mobilizing—joint movements at ankle, foot, and toes.

    0   1   2   3   4   5

9. Foot muscles—squeeze/press.

    0   1   2   3   4   5

10. Finish—light strokes from hip to foot.

    0   1   2   3   4   5

Athlete Prone

11. Stretch quadriceps—heel to buttocks.

    0   1   2   3   4   5

12. Buttocks muscles—compressions with fist.

    0   1   2   3   4   5

13. Thigh muscles—compressions, lift and wring, shaking, jostling.

    0   1   2   3   4   5

14. Lower leg muscles—shake, squeeze.

    0   1   2   3   4   5

15. Ankle—dorsiflex and press into foot bottom.

    0   1   2   3   4   5

16. Finish leg—light strokes from ankle to hip.

    0   1   2   3   4   5

17. Upper body—compressions over back and shoulders.

    0   1   2   3   4   5

18. Finish session—brush off from shoulders to feet.

    0   1   2   3   4   5

19. Body/hand mechanics and ease of movement around the table.

    0   1   2   3   4   5

20. Overall application (safety, timing, pacing, rhythm, flow, quality of touch).

    0   1   2   3   4   5

Total points _____ / 20 = _____ Average Rating

Evaluated by: _____

PERFORMANCE EVALUATION FORM 20–2
Pregnancy Massage

Student: _____   Date: _____

Scoring Key: 0 = incorrect; 1 = very poor; 2 = poor; 3 = adequate; 4 = good; 5 = excellent

1. Positioning and draping.

   0   1   2   3   4   5

2. Client communication: health history interview, explanations, feedback.

   0   1   2   3   4   5

3. Apply oil and effleurage to top leg.

   0   1   2   3   4   5

4. Hip and leg muscles—effleurage, petrissage.

   0   1   2   3   4   5

5. Feet—squeeze, press, joint movement.

   0   1   2   3   4   5

6. Back and shoulders—warming effleurage.

   0   1   2   3   4   5

7. Paraspinal muscles—circular friction.

   0   1   2   3   4   5

8. Shoulder and neck muscles—effleurage, petrissage.

   0   1   2   3   4   5

9. Finish back—superficial friction.

   0   1   2   3   4   5

10. Arm—effleurage, petrissage.

   0   1   2   3   4   5

11. Finish side—passive touch.

   0   1   2   3   4   5

12. Assist recipient in turning over or in getting off of the table.

   0   1   2   3   4   5

13. Body/hand mechanics and ease of movement around the table.

   0   1   2   3   4   5

14. Safety, use of pressure, avoidance of endangerment sites.

   0   1   2   3   4   5

15. Overall effectiveness (timing, pacing, rhythm, flow, quality of touch).

   0   1   2   3   4   5

Total points _____ / 15 = _____ Average Rating

Evaluated by: _____

PERFORMANCE EVALUATION FORM 20–3
Infant Massage

Student: _____ Date: _____

Scoring Key: 0 = incorrect; 1 = very poor; 2 = poor; 3 = adequate; 4 = good; 5 = excellent

1. Positioning the infant supine and prone.

   0   1   2   3   4   5

2. Communication—eye contact, talking, smiling.

   0   1   2   3   4   5

3. Quality of touch—gentle, firm.

   0   1   2   3   4   5

Infant Supine

4. Fingertip circle over head.

   0   1   2   3   4   5

5. Thumb slides over forehead and along nose.

   0   1   2   3   4   5

6. Apply oil with butterfly strokes across the chest.

   0   1   2   3   4   5

7. Squeeze and milk the arms.

   0   1   2   3   4   5

8. Thumb strokes to palm and fingers.

   0   1   2   3   4   5

9. Squeeze and milk the legs.

   0   1   2   3   4   5

10. Thumb strokes to foot bottoms.

   0   1   2   3   4   5

11. Stroking to abdomen clockwise.

   0   1   2   3   4   5

12. Shoulder movement—cross arms and open out.

   0   1   2   3   4   5

13. Hip and leg movement—bend and straighten legs.

   0   1   2   3   4   5

Infant Prone

14. Circular fingertip friction along paraspinal muscles.

    0   1   2   3   4   5

15. Scoop from shoulders to heels.

    0   1   2   3   4   5

16. Turn baby over and finish supine with passive touch to head—eye contact and smile.

    0   1   2   3   4   5

17. Body/hand mechanics and ease of movement.

    0   1   2   3   4   5

18. Overall application (safety, timing, pacing, flow, quality of touch).

    0   1   2   3   4   5

Total points _____ / 18 = _____ Average Rating

Evaluated by: _____

PERFORMANCE EVALUATION FORM 20–4

Massage for the Elderly in Semireclining Position

Student: _____   Date: _____

Scoring Key: 0 = incorrect; 1 = very poor; 2 = poor; 3 = adequate; 4 = good; 5 = excellent

1. Positioning and draping.

   0   1   2   3   4   5

2. Client communication: health history interview, explanations, feedback.

   0   1   2   3   4   5

3. Establish contact and mobilize the feet.

   0   1   2   3   4   5

4. Apply lotion to foot and leg.

   0   1   2   3   4   5

5. Thigh muscles—compressions, effleurage, petrissage.

   0   1   2   3   4   5

6. Lower leg muscles—knead, press.

   0   1   2   3   4   5

7. Passive movements to leg—rocking, knee flexion.

   0   1   2   3   4   5

8. Apply lotion to arm.

   0   1   2   3   4   5

9. Arm muscles—squeezes.

   0   1   2   3   4   5

10. Hands—thumb strokes to back of hand and palm.

   0   1   2   3   4   5

11. Mobilizing hand and wrist joints.

   0   1   2   3   4   5

12. Finish arm—long effleurage and brush off.

   0   1   2   3   4   5

13. Shoulders—knead.

   0   1   2   3   4   5

14. Neck muscles—knead.

   0   1   2   3   4   5

15. Upper and lower back—superficial friction.

   0   1   2   3   4   5

16. Scalp mobilizing and circular friction over temples.

   0   1   2   3   4   5

17. Connecting with light tapotement over head, arms, legs.

    0   1   2   3   4   5

18. Finish session with brush off from head to feet.

    0   1   2   3   4   5

19. Body/hand mechanics and ease of movement around the table/chair.

    0   1   2   3   4   5

20. Overall application (safety, timing, pacing, flow, quality of touch).

    0   1   2   3   4   5

Total points _____ / 20 = _____ Average Rating

Evaluated by: _____

PERFORMANCE EVALUATION FORM 20–5
Gentle Hand and Arm Massage

Student: _____   Date: _____

Scoring Key: 0 = incorrect; 1 = very poor; 2 = poor; 3 = adequate; 4 = good; 5 = excellent

1. Positioning the recipient.

    0   1   2   3   4   5

2. Client communication: health history interview, explanations, feedback.

    0   1   2   3   4   5

3. Quality of touch—gentle, firm, adapted to recipient's condition.

    0   1   2   3   4   5

4. Apply lotion to entire arm.

    0   1   2   3   4   5

5. Upper arm—stroke and knead.

    0   1   2   3   4   5

6. Lower arm—stroke and knead.

    0   1   2   3   4   5

7. Joint mobilizing with pressing and rolling.

    0   1   2   3   4   5

8. Hand and fingers—thumb circles over wrist, squeeze hand and fingers, thumb slides.

    0   1   2   3   4   5

9. Joint mobilizing wrist, hand, and fingers.

    0   1   2   3   4   5

10. Connecting arm with gentle squeezes from shoulder to hand.

    0   1   2   3   4   5

11. Finish session holding hands.

    0   1   2   3   4   5

12. Overall application (safety, timing, pacing, flow, quality of touch).

    0   1   2   3   4   5

Total points _____ / 12 = _____ Average Rating

Evaluated by: _____

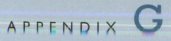
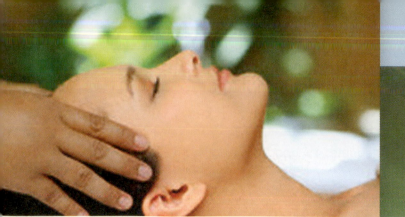

Intake, Health History, and Note Forms

New Client Information Form

Date _____

Name _____ Gender: ☐ Male ☐ Female

Address _____

City _____ State _____ Zip _____

Home Phone _____ Cell Phone _____

Work Phone _____ E-Mail Address _____

Age _____ Date of Birth _____ Occupation _____

Primary Health Care Provider _____

Address _____ City _____ State _____ Zip _____

Phone _____

Insurance Company _____ Policy # _____

ID # _____ Group # _____ Claim # _____

Phone Number _____

Emergency Contacts:

1st Name _____ Relationship _____

Phone Number(s) _____

2nd Name _____ Relationship _____

Phone Number(s) _____

(1 of 3)

Policies, Privacy, and Consent Form (Sample)

General Policies

1. Massage sessions are available by appointment only from 9:00 AM–6:00 PM, Tuesday–Saturday.

2. Payment is due at the time of the massage appointment.

3. Fees are $65 for a 60-minute appointment, $90 for a 90-minute appointment.

4. Payments must be in cash or check. Credit cards are not accepted.

5. Appointments are reserved for the time slot chosen. Clients arriving late for their appointments will receive massage as possible during the remainder of their reserved time.

6. There is a 24-hour cancellation policy. Clients will be charged for missed appointments.

7. Client records are kept secure and confidential (see Privacy Policy, below).

8. Clients are expected to exhibit good hygiene and are asked to minimize the use of perfume, cologne, and heavily scented personal products.

9. The use of cell phones or beepers is not allowed during the massage session, except in special circumstances agreed upon beforehand by the massage therapist.

10. Massage sessions may be terminated at any time the massage therapist has reason to believe that a client is sexualizing the massage, or uses inappropriate or threatening language or behavior.

11. This office follows the Code of Ethics and Standards of Practice of the American Massage Therapy Association (www.amtamassage.org).

Privacy Policy

Your massage therapy records are kept in the strictest confidence by this office. All client records are kept in a secure place, and only those who need to see a client's file for legitimate business or professional purposes have access to them. Your records will not be released to third parties, including health care providers and insurance companies, without your written consent. Records may be surrendered if required by law.

(2 of 3)

General Agreement and Consent

I, _____, understand that the massage therapy given to me by _____ is for the purpose of general health and wellness, relaxation, improved circulation, pain management, and other effects supported by experience and research. Massage therapy is performed here within the scope of practice of massage therapists in this state.

I understand that massage therapists do not diagnosis medical conditions, nor do they prescribe medical treatments or medications, nor do they perform spinal manipulation or chiropractic adjustments.

I understand that massage therapy is not a substitute for examination by a medical provider, and that it is recommended that I seek medical attention first for any illness, injury, or disorder that I might have.

I understand that massage therapy can be a valuable complement to health care provided by medical doctors, chiropractic physicians, naturopathic physicians, practitioners of traditional Chinese medicine, and psychiatrists and psychologists. I agree to keep my massage therapist informed of any medical treatment I am receiving with the understanding that it may impact the massage therapy I receive.

I have stated all my known medical conditions, treatments, and medications, and I agree to keep the massage therapist updated on any changes.

My signature below confirms my agreement to the general policies, privacy policy, and consent statements above.

Name _____ Date _____

Witness _____ Date _____

(3 of 3)

Health History for Massage Therapy—Wellness

Name _____ Date of initial visit _____

Address _____ Phone _____

Occupation _____ Date of birth _____

Sports/physical activities/hobbies _____

The following information will be used to help plan safe and effective massage sessions. Please answer the questions to the best of your knowledge.

1. Have you had professional massage before?   Yes   No

2. Do you have any difficulty lying on your front, back, or side?   Yes   No
   If yes, please explain _____

3. Do you have allergic reactions to oils, lotions, ointments, liniments, or other
   substances put on your skin?   Yes   No
   If yes, please explain _____

4. Do you wear contact lenses ☐ dentures ☐ a hearing aid ☐?

5. Do you sit for long hours at a workstation, computer, or driving?   Yes   No
   If yes, please describe _____

6. Do you perform any repetitive movement in your work, sports, or hobby?   Yes   No
   If yes, please describe _____

7. Do you experience stress in your work, family, or other aspect of your life? Yes   No
   If yes, how do you think it has affected your health?

   muscle tension ☐ anxiety ☐ insomnia ☐ irritability ☐ other _____

8. Is there a particular area of the body where you are experiencing tension,
   stiffness, or other discomfort?   Yes   No
   If yes, please identify _____

9. Do you have any particular goals in mind for this massage session?   Yes   No
   If yes, please explain _____

In order to plan a massage session that is safe and effective, we need some general information about your medical history.

10. Are you currently under medical supervision?   Yes   No
    If yes, please explain _____

11. Are you currently taking any medication?   Yes   No
    If yes, please list _____

(1 of 2)

12. Please check any condition listed below that applies to you:

_____	contagious skin condition	_____	phlebitis
_____	open sores or wounds	_____	joint disorder
_____	easy bruising	_____	rheumatoid arthritis
_____	recent accident or injury	_____	osteoporosis
_____	current fever	_____	epilepsy
_____	swollen glands	_____	headaches
_____	allergies	_____	cancer
_____	heart condition	_____	diabetes
_____	high or low blood pressure	_____	decreased sensation
_____	circulatory disorder	_____	recent surgery
_____	noncontagious skin condition	_____	joint disorder
_____	varicose veins	_____	artificial joint
_____	atherosclerosis	_____	elective surgeries

Comments:

_____

_____

_____

13. For women: Are you pregnant?   Yes   No
    If yes, how many months? _____

14. Is there anything else about your health history that you think would be useful for your massage practitioner to know to plan a safe and effective massage session for you?

_____

_____

_____

_____

I understand that these massage sessions are for general wellness purposes and that I should see a doctor or other appropriate health care provider for diagnosis and treatment of any suspected medical problem. Also, that it is my responsibility to keep my massage practitioner informed of any changes in my health, and any medications that I may begin to take in the future.

Signature _____ Date _____

(2 of 2)

Health History for Massage Therapy Treatment

Name _____ Date of initial visit _____

Address _____ Phone _____

Occupation _____ Date of birth _____

Name of physician _____ Phone _____

Other health care provider _____

Referred by _____

1. Have you had massage therapy before?	Yes	No

2. For women: Are you pregnant?   Yes   No
   If yes, how many months? _____

3. Do you have any difficulty lying on your front, back, or side?   Yes   No
   If yes, please explain _____

4. Do you have allergic reactions to oils, lotions, ointments, liniments, or other
   substances put on your skin?   Yes   No
   If yes, please explain _____

5. Do you wear contact lenses ☐ dentures ☐ a hearing aid ☐?

6. Do you sit for long hours at a workstation, computer, or driving?   Yes   No
   If yes, please describe _____

7. Do you perform any repetitive movement in your work, sports, or hobby?   Yes   No
   If yes, please describe _____

8. Do you experience stress in your work, family, or other aspect of your life?   Yes   No

   How would you describe your stress level?

   Low Medium High Very high

   If high, how do you think stress has effected your health?

   muscle tension ☐ anxiety ☐ insomnia ☐ irritability ☐ other _____

9. Is there a particular area of the body where you are experiencing tension,
   stiffness, or other discomfort?   Yes   No
   If yes, please identify _____

In order to plan a massage session that is safe and effective, we need some general information about your medical history.

10. Are you currently under medical supervision?   Yes   No
    If yes, please explain _____

11. Are you currently taking any medication?   Yes   No
    If yes, please list _____

(1 of 2)

12. Please check any condition listed below that applies to you:

_____ Skin condition (e.g., acne, rash, skin cancer, allergy, easy bruising, contagious condition)
_____ Allergies
_____ Recent accident, injury, or surgery (e.g., whiplash, sprain, broken bone, deep bruise)
_____ Muscular problems (e.g., tension, cramping, chronic soreness)
_____ Joint problems (e.g., osteoarthritis, rheumatoid arthritis, gout, hypermobile joints, recent dislocation)
_____ Lymphatic condition (e.g., swollen glands, nodes removed, lymphoma, lymphedema)
_____ Circulatory or blood conditions (e.g., atherosclerosis, varicose veins, phlebitis, arrhythmias, high or low blood pressure, heart disease, recent heart attack or stroke, anemia)
_____ Neurologic condition (e.g., numbness or tingling in any area of the body, sciatica, damage from stroke, epilepsy, multiple sclerosis, cerebral palsy)
_____ Digestive conditions (e.g., ulcers)
_____ Immune system conditions (e.g., chronic fatigue, HIV/AIDS)
_____ Skeletal conditions (e.g., osteoporosis, bone cancer, spinal injury)
_____ Headaches (e.g., tension, PMS, migraines)
_____ Cancer
_____ Emotional difficulties (e.g., depression, anxiety, panic attacks, eating disorder, psychotic episodes). Are you currently seeing a psychotherapist for this condition? Yes No
_____ Previous surgery, disease, or other medical condition that may be affecting you now (e.g., polio, previous heart attack or stroke, previously broken bones)
_____ Elective surgery or procedures

Comments:

_____

_____

_____

13. Is there anything else about your health history that you think would be useful for your massage practitioner to know to plan a safe and effective massage session for you?

_____

_____

_____

14. Has your physician or other health care provider recommended massage for any of the conditions listed above?   Yes   No
If yes, please explain _____

15. Do you have any particular goals in mind for this massage session related to any of the conditions mentioned above?   Yes   No
If yes, please explain _____

I understand that I should see a doctor or other appropriate health care provider for diagnosis and treatment of any suspected medical problem. It may be beneficial for my massage practitioner to speak to my doctor about my medical condition to determine how massage may help the healing process, and to avoid worsening the condition. I will be asked for permission to contact my doctor, if the massage practitioner thinks that it might be useful. I also understand that it is my responsibility to keep my massage practitioner informed of any changes in my health, and any medications that I may begin to take in the future.

Signature _____ Date _____

Intake Form for Outreach Events

Massage Therapist _____ Date _____

WELCOME! To ensure a safe and healthy experience of massage therapy, please tell your massage therapist the following:

- If you have a medical condition that may be adversely affected by massage
- If you are taking medication that affects circulation or ability to sense pain
- If you have high or low blood pressure
- If you have had a serious illness or injury recently
- If you are pregnant
- Any areas the massage therapist should avoid

Your signature below indicates that you have given the massage therapist the information requested and give your consent to receive massage. The massage therapist and the sponsoring organization are not responsible for unforeseeable adverse reactions to the massage received.

Name   Time

1. _____ _____

    print   signature

2. _____ _____

    print   signature

3. _____ _____

    print   signature

4. _____ _____

    print   signature

5. _____ _____

    print   signature

6. _____ _____

    print   signature

7. _____ _____

    print   signature

8. _____ _____

    print   signature

9. _____ _____

    print   signature

10. _____ _____

    print   signature

Form # _____ MT Initials _____

SOAP NOTE CHART
CONTINUING MASSAGE SESSION

Practitioner's Name _____ Date _____

Client's Name _____

S: Reason for massage, complaints, reports

O: Observations, qualitative/quantitative measurements

A: Primary and secondary goals for the session;
contraindications

P: Duration of massage; areas addressed; techniques
used; results; suggested home care

Practitioner Signature _____ Date _____

_____

Symbols:

Primary 1°   Secondary 2°   Change Δ   Increase ↑   Decrease ↓   Tension ≡
Adhesion **X**   Pain **P**   Numbness ∿∿   Inflammation ✳   TrP ⊗

Short Intake and Note Form

Client _____ Date _____

Address _____ Phone _____

Massage Therapist _____

Please answer the following questions to ensure a comfortable and safe massage session:

1. What is your primary goal for this massage?

   ☐ Relaxation, stress reduction

   ☐ Relieve muscle tension, specify area: _____

   ☐ General health and well-being

   ☐ Other, please specify _____

2. Have you had any illness, accidents, or injury recently?   Yes   No

   If so, please explain briefly _____

   _____

3. Are you experiencing any of the following today? Check all that apply.

   ☐ pain or soreness   ☐ numbness or tingling   ☐ dizziness

   ☐ stiffness   ☐ swelling   ☐ nausea

4. Do you have any allergies, especially to oils or lotions?   Yes   No

   If so, please explain briefly _____

   _____

5. For women—Are you pregnant?   Yes   No   Maybe

6. Have you taken any medications today?   Yes   No

   If so, please list _____

I have answered the above questions to the best of my ability. I acknowledge that massage therapy does not include medical diagnosis and that I should see an appropriate health care provider to diagnose and treat medical problems. I give my consent for the massage session.

Signature _____ Date _____

Plan: _____

_____

Comments: _____

_____

_____

Short Note Chart

Client's Name _____

Date _____ Practitioner's Name _____

S: Comments, complaints, reports, recent illness or injury, medications

O: Visual observations, palpation

P: Length of session, routine given, significant modifications

C: General comments

MT Initials_____

Date _____ Practitioner's Name _____

S: Comments, complaints, reports, recent illness or injury, medications

O: Visual observations, palpation

P: Length of session, routine given, significant modifications

C: General comments

MT Initials _____

Date _____ Practitioner's Name/Initials_____

S: Comments, complaints, reports, recent illness or injury, medications

O: Visual observations, palpation

P: Length of session, routine given, significant modifications

C: General comments

MT Initials _____

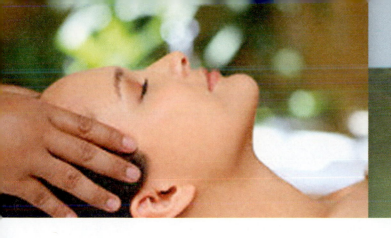

References are the sources of quotes and specific content in the chapters.

Additional Resources are valuable sources for further information.

CHAPTER 1

References

American Massage Therapy Association. (2004). *Consumer survey fact sheet.* Evanston, IL.

American Massage Therapy Association. (2004, May/June). Study shows massage ranks first among spa treatments. *Hands-On,* p. 1.

Huitt, W. G. (2004). Maslow's hierarchy of needs. Retrieved: July 2008 from http://chiron.valdosta.edu/whuitt/col/regsys/maslow.html.

Massage Therapy Foundation, 1999, *Massage Therapy Research Agenda*

National Center for Complementary and Alternative Medicine. (2004). *NCCAM Newsletter, 11*(3).

White House Commission on Complementary and Alternative Medicine Policy. (2002). *Final report.* Washington, DC: Department of Health and Human Services. Retrieved from www.whccamp.hhs.gov

Additional Resources

American Massage Therapy Association (www.amtamassage.org)

Associated Bodywork and Massage Professionals (www.abmp.com)

American Organization of Bodywork Therapies of Asia (www.aobta.org)

American Polarity Therapy Association (www.polaritytherapy.org)

Barnes, P.M., Powell-Griner, E., McFann, K., and Nahin, R. (2004, May 27). *Complementary and alternative medicine use among adults: United States, 2002.* (Advance Data *Report No. 343*). Hyattsvill, MD: U.S. Department of Health and Human Services, Centers for Disease Control and Prevention.

Knaster, M. (1996). *Discovering the body's wisdom: A comprehensive guide to more than fifty mind-body practices.* New York: Bantam Books.

Hospital-Based Massage Network (www.hbmn.com)

International Association of Infant Massage (www.iaim.net)

International Spa Association (www.experienceispa.com)

Massage Therapy Foundation (www.massagetherapyfoundation.org)

National Association of Nurse Massage Therapists (www.nanmt.org)

National Center of Complementary and Alternative Medicine at the National Institutes of Health, Washington, DC. (www.nccam.nih.gov)

Rolf Institute® of Structural Integration (www.rolf.org)

Touch Research Institute at the University of Miami (www.miami.edu/touch-research)

Wellness Associates (www.thewellspring.com)

White House Commission on CAM Policy Report (www.whccamp.hhs.gov)

CHAPTER 2

References

AMTA National Historian's Report. (1987, Fall). AMTA membership 1943–1987. *Massage Therapy Journal,* pp. 12–15.

Armstrong, D., and Armstong, E. M. (1991). *The great American medicine show: Being an illustrated history of hucksters, healers, health evangelists, and heroes from Plymouth Rock to the present.* New York: Prentice Hall.

Benjamin, P. J. (2002). Breast massage: Old becomes new again. *Massage Therapy Journal, 41* (1), 154–158.

Benjamin, P. J. (2001). Genuine Swedish massage applied to slim down. *Massage Therapy Journal, 40* (2), 152–154.

Benjamin, P. J. (1986, Fall). National historian's report: Annual convention programs. *Massage Therapy Journal*, pp. 8–9.

Ellison, M. A. (1909). *A manual for students of massage* (3rd ed.). London: Baillere, Tindall and Cox.

Frierwood, H. T. (1953, September–October). The place of health service in the total YMCA program. *Journal of Physical Education.*

Graham, D. (1902). *A treatise on massage: Its history, mode of application and effects* (3rd ed.). Philadelphia: Lippincott.

Haggard, H. W. (1932). *The lame, the halt, and the blind: The vital role of medicine in the history of civilization.* New York: Blue Ribbon Books.

Johnson, W. (1866). *The anatriptic art.* London: Simpkin, Marshall & Co.

Joya, M. (1958). *Mock Joya's things Japanese.* Tokyo: Tokyo News Service.

Kellogg, J. H. (1895). *The art of massage: Its physiological effects and therapeutic applications.* Battle Creek, MI: Modern Medicine Publishing.

Ling, P. H. (1840a). The general principles of gymnastics. In The collected works of P. H. Ling. (1866). Stockholm, Sweden. Translated by Lars Agren and Patricia J. Benjamin. Unpublished.

Ling, P. H. (1840b). Notations to the general principles. In The collected works of P. H. Ling. (1866). Stockholm, Sweden. Translated by Lars Agren and Patricia J. Benjamin and published in *Massage Therapy Journal,* Winter 1987.

Ling, P. H. (1840c). The means or vehicle of gymnastics. Translated by R. J. Cyriax. In *American Physical Education Review, 19*(4), April 1914.

Livingston, H., and Maroni, A. (1945). *Everyday beauty culture.* Bloomington, IL: McKnight & McKnight.

McKenzie, R.T. (1915). *Exercise in education and medicine* (2nd ed.). Philadelphia: Saunders.

Mitchell, S.W. (1877). *Fat and blood and how to make them.* Philadelphia: J. B. Lippincott & Co.

M'Lean, T. (1914.) *Picturesque representations of the dress and manners of the Chinese.* London: Howlett & Brimmer.

Murphy, M. C. (1914). *Athletic training.* New York: Scribner's.

Nissen, H. (1889). *A manual of instruction for giving Swedish movement and massage treatment.* Philadelphia: F. A. Davis.

Perrone, B., Stockel, H. H., and Krueger, V. (1989. *Medicine women, curanderas, and women doctors.* Norman: University of Oklahoma Press.

Pollard, D. W. (1902). *Massage in training.* Unpublished thesis, International Young Men's Christian Association Training School, Springfield, MA.

Puderbach, P. (1925). *The massage operator.* Butler, NJ: Dr. Benedict Lust.

Taylor, G. (1900. *Health by exercise . . . showing what exercises to take . . . including the process of massage.* New York: The Improved Movement Cure Institute. (Original work published 1860)

Thomas, N. (2003). *Cook: The extraordinary voyages of Captain James Cook.* New York: Walker & Company.

Williams, R. J. (1943). Second annual national YMCA health service clinic. *Journal of Physical Education, 41.*

Zhang, Y. (Director). (2000). *Shower* [Film]. Sony Pictures Entertainment, Inc.

Additional Resources

Baumgartner, A.J. (1947). *Massage in athletics.* Minneapolis, MN: Burgess.

Calvert, R. N. (2002). *The history of massage: An illustrated survey from around the world.* Rochester, VT: Healing Arts Press.

Esalen Institute (www.esalen.org)

Esalen massage (Video). (1999). Big Sur, CA: Esalen Institute. (www.esalen.org)

Erz, A. A. (c. 1924). Ad for book *The medical question: The truth about official medicine and why we must have medical freedom.* Butler, NJ: Nature Cure Publishing.

Hawaiian lomi-lomi: Level 1 (Video). Venture, CA: Hawaiian Healing Arts. (www.lomi-lomi.com)

Massage Magazine (www.massagemag.com)

Massage Therapy Foundation (www.massagetherapyfoundation.org)

Massage Therapy Foundation Research Database (www.massagetherapyfoundation.org/researchdb.html)

Murphy, W. (Ed.) (1995). *Healing the generations: A history of physical therapy and the American Physical Therapy Association.* Lyme, CT: Greenwich Publishing Group.

Roth, M. (1851). *The prevention and cure of many chronic diseases by movements.* London: John Churchhill.

CHAPTER 3

References

American heritage dictionary of the English language (2000). (4th ed.). New York: Houghton Mifflin.

Benjamin, B. E., and Sohnen-Moe, C. (2003) *The ethics of touch.* Tucson, AZ: SMA.

Bixler, S., and Dugan L. S. (2001). *5 steps to professional presence: How to project confidence, competence, and credibility at work.* Avon, MA: Adams Media Corporation.

Booher, D. (1994). *Communicate with confidence: How to say it right the first time and every time.* New York: McGraw-Hill

Cole, K. (2002). *The complete idiot's guide to clear communication.* Indianapolis, IN: Alpha.

Goleman, D. (1995). *Emotional intelligence: Why it can matter more than IQ.* New York: Bantam Books.

Hahn, P. R. (2003). *The everything writing well book: Master the written word and communicate clearly.* Avon, MA: Adams Media Corporation.

Levine, M. (2002). *A mind at a time.* New York: Simon & Schuster.

McCormick, A. R., and McCormick, M. D. (1997). *Horse sense and the human heart: What horses can teach us about trust, bonding, creativity and spirituality.* Deerfield Beach, FL: Health Communications.

Makely, S. (2005). *Professionalism in health care: A primer for career success* (2nd ed.). Upper Saddle River, NJ: Prentice Hall.

McIntosh, N. (1999). *The educated heart: Professional guidelines for massage therapists, bodyworkers and movement teachers.* Memphis, TN: Decatur Bainbridge Press.

CHAPTER 4

References

Chuen, L. K. (1991). *The way of energy: Mastering the Chinese art of internal strength with chi kung exercise.* New York: Simon & Schuster.

Heckler, R.S. (1997). *Holding the center: Sanctuary in a time of confusion.* Berkeley, CA: Frog. Kagan, J., Snidman, N., Arcus, D., and Reznick, J. S. (1998). *Galen's prophecy: Temperament in human nature.* Boulder, CO: Westview Press.

Marieb, E. N. (2009). *Essentials of human anatomy and physiology* (9th ed.). Upper Saddle River, NJ: Pearson Prentice Hall

Schlosberg, S. (2005). *The ultimate workout log.* Boston: Houghton Mifflin Company.

Additional Resources

Bloom, B. (Ed.). (1956). *Taxonomy of educational objectives: Handbook I. Cognitive domain.* New York: Longman.

Chuckrow, R. (1998). *The tai chi book: Refining and enjoying a lifetime of practice.* Boston: YMAA Publication Center.

Csikszentmihalyi, M. (1997). *Finding flow: The psychology of engagement with everyday life.* New York: Basic Books.

Greene, E., and Goodrich-Dunn, B. (2004). *The psychology of the body.* Philadelphia: Lippincott Williams & Wilkins.

Hall, S. (1991). *Basic biomechanics.* St. Louis, MO: Mosby.

Mipham. (2003). *Turning the mind into an ally.* New York: Penguin Putnam.

National Heart, Lung, and Blood Institute website (www.nhlbisupport.com/bmi/bmicalc.htm)

Seiger, L., Kanipe, D., Vanderpool, K., and Barnes, D. (1998). *Fitness and wellness strategies* (2nd ed.). New York: McGraw-Hill.

Simpkins, C. A., and Simpkins, A. (2000). *Simple Confucianism: A guide to living virtuously.* Boston: Tuttle.

Travis, J. W., and Ryan, R. S. (2004). *Wellness Workbook* (3rd ed.). Berkeley, CA: Celestial Arts.

CHAPTER 5

References

Benjamin, B. E., and Sohnen-Moe C. (2003). *The ethics of touch.* Tucson, AZ: SMA.

Greene, E., and Goodrich-Dunn B. (2004). *The psychology of the body.* Philadelphia: Lippincott Williams & Wilkins.

Kisch, R. M. (1998). *Beyond technique: The hidden dimensions of bodywork.* Dayton, OH: BLHY Growth Publications.

McIntosh, N. (2005). *The educated heart: Professional guidelines for massage therapists, bodyworkers, and movement teachers* (2nd ed.). Philadelphia: Lippincott, Williams & Wilkins.

Taylor, K. (1995). *The ethics of caring.* Santa Cruz, CA: Hanford Mead.

Additional Resources

American Massage Therapy Association (www.amtamassage.org)

Associated Bodywork and Massage Professionals (www.abmp.com)

HIPAA Guidelines (www.hhs.gov/ocr/hipaa)

National Certification Board for Therapeutic Massage and Bodywork (www.ncbtmb.org)

National Certification Commission for Acupuncture and Oriental Medicine (www.nccaom.org)

Purtilo, R. (1993). *Ethical dimensions in the health professions* (2nd ed.). Philadelphia: W. B. Saunders.

CHAPTER 6

Additional Resources

Beaman, N., and Fleming-McPhilips, L. (2007). *Pearson's anatomy and physiology for medical assisting* (Vol. II). Upper Saddle River, NJ: Pearson Prentice Hall.

Biel, A. (2001). *Trail guide to the body: How to locate muscles, bones, and more* (2nd ed.). Boulder, CO: Books of Discovery.

Colbert, B., Ankney, J., and Lee, K. T. (2007). *Anatomy and physiology for health professions.* Upper Saddle River, NJ: Pearson Prentice Hall.

Fremgen, B. F., and Frucht, S. S. (2009). *Medical terminology: a living language* (4th ed.). Upper Saddle River, NJ: Pearson Prentice Hall.

Marieb, E. N. (2009). *Essentials of human anatomy and physiology* (9th ed.). Upper Saddle River, NJ: Pearson Prentice Hall

Mulvihill, M. L., Zelman, M., Holdaway, P., Tompary, E., and Raymond, J. (2006). *Human diseases, a systemic approach* (6th ed.). Upper Saddle River, NJ: Pearson Prentice Hall.

Rice, J. (2008). *Medical terminology: A word-building approach* (6th ed.). Upper Saddle River, NJ: Pearson Prentice Hall.

Werner, R. (2008) *A massage therapist's guide to pathology* (4th ed.). Philadelphia: Lippincott Williams & Wilkins.

CHAPTER 7

References

Andrade, C., and P. Clifford. (2001). *Outcomes-based massage.* Philadelphia: Lippincott Williams & Wilkins.

Barr, J. S., and N. Taslitz. (1970). Influence of back massage on autonomic functions. *Physical Therapy,* 50.

Bauer, W. C., and Dracup, K. A. (1987). Physiological effects of back massage in patients with acute myocardial infarction. *Focus on Critical Care, 14*(6), 42–46.

Brown, C. C., ed. (1984). *The many facets of touch.* Johnson & Johnson Baby Products Company.

Cady, S. H., and Jones, G. E. (1997). Massage therapy as a workplace intervention for reduction of stress. *Perceptual and Motor Skills, 84*(1), 157–158.

Crosman, L. J., Chateauvert, S. R., and Weisburg, J. (1985). The effects of massage to the hamstring muscle group on range of motion. *Massage Journal,* 59–62.

Curties, D. (1999). *Breast massage.* Toronto: Curties-Overzet Publications.

Cyriax, J. H., and Cyriax, P. J. (1993). *Illustrated manual of orthopedic medicine* (2nd ed.). Boston: Butterworth & Heinemann.

de Bruijn, R. (1984). Deep transverse friction: Its analgesic effect. *International Journal of Sports Medicine,* 5(suppl.), 35–36.

DeDomenico, G., and Wood, E. C. (1997). *Beard's Massage* (4th ed.). Philadelphia: W. B. Saunders.

Diego, M .A., Field, T., Hernandez-Reif, M., Shaw, J. A., Rothe, E. M., Castellanos, D., and Mesner, L.

(2002). Aggressive adolescents benefit from massage therapy. *Adolescence, 37,* 597–607.

Drinker, C. K., and Yoffey, J. M. (1941). Lymphatics, lymph and lymphoid tissue: Their physiological and clinical significance. Cambridge: Harvard University Press.

Elkins, E. C., Herrick, J. F., Grindlay, J. H., et al. (1953). Effects of various procedures on the flow of lymph. *Archives of Physical Medicine, 34,* 31.

Ernst, E. (1998). Does post exercise massage reduce delayed onset muscle soreness? A systematic review. *British Journal of Sports Medicine, 32,* 212–214.

Fakouri, C., and Jones, P. (1987). Relaxation: Slow stroke back rub. *Journal of Gerontological Nursing, 13*(2), 32–35.

Field, T. (2000). *Touch therapy.* London: Churchill Livingstone.

Field, T. M., Fox, N., Pickens, J., Ironsong, G., and Scafidi, F. (1993). Job stress survey. Unpublished manuscript. Touch Research Institute, University of Miami School of Medicine. Reported in *Touchpoints: Touch Research Abstracts, 1*(1).

Fraser, J., and Kerr, J. R. (1993). Psychophysiological effects of back massage on elderly institutionalized patients. *Journal of Advanced Nursing, 18,* 238–245.

Greene, E. (1996). Study links stress reduction with faster healing. *Massage Therapy Journal, 35*(1), 16.

Greene, E. and Goodrich-Dunn, B. (2004). *The psychology of the body.* Philadelphia: Lippincott, Williams & Wilkins.

Hasson, D., Arnetz, B., Jelvis, L., and Edelstam, B. (2004). A randomized clinical trial of the treatment effects of massage compared to relaxation tape recordings on diffuse long-term pain. *Psychotherapy and Psychosomatics, 73,* 17–24.

Ironson, G., Field, T. et al. (1996). Massage therapy is associated with enhancement of the immune system's cytotoxic capacity. *International Journal of Neuroscience,* 84: 205–217.

Juhan, D. (1987). *Job's body: A handbook for bodywork.* Barrytown, NY: Station Hill Press.

Kaard, B., and Tostinbo, O. (1989). Increase of plasma beta endorphins in a connective tissue massage. *General Pharmacology, 20*(4), 487–489.

Kelly, D. G. (2002). *A primer on lymphedema.* Upper Saddle River, NJ: Prentice Hall.

Knaster, M. (1996). *Discovering the body's wisdom.* New York: Bantam.

Kresge, C. A. (1983). Massage and sports. In O. Appenzeller and R. Atkinson (eds.), *Sports medicine: Fitness, training, injuries* (pp. 367–380). Baltimore: Urban & Schwarzenberg.

Labyak, S. E., and Metzger, B. L. (1997). The effects of effleurage backrub on the physiological components of relaxation: A meta-analysis. *Nursing Research, 46,* 59–62.

Martini, F. H., and Bartholomew, M. S. (1999). *Structure & function of the human body*. Upper Saddle River, NJ: Prentice-Hall.

Menard, M. B. (2009). *Making sense of research: A guide to research literacy for complementary practitioners* (2nd ed.). Toronto: Curties-Overzet Publications.

Mitchell, J. K. (1894). The effect of massage on the number and haemoglobin value of the red blood cells. *American Journal of Medical Science, 107*, pp. 502–515.

Montageu, A. (1978). *Touching: The human significance of the skin* (2nd ed.). New York: Harper & Row.

Mortimer, P. S., Simmonds, R., Rezvani, M. et al. (1990). The measurement of skin lymph flow by isotope clearance: Reliability, reproducibility, injection dynamics, and the effects of massage. *Journal of Investigative Dermatology, 95,* 666–682.

Moyer, C. A., Rounds, J., and Hannum, J. W. (2004). A meta-anaylsis of massage therapy research. *Psychological Bulletin, 130,* 3–18.

Ottenbacher, K. J., Muller, L., Brandt, D., Heintzelman, A., Hojem, P., and Sharpe, P. (1987). The effectiveness of tactile stimulation as a form of early intervention: A quantitative evaluation. *Developmental and Behavioral Pediatrics, 8,* 68-76.

Pemberton, R. (1939). Physiology of massage. In *American Medical Association Handbook of Physical Therapy* (3rd ed.). Chicago: Council of Physical Therapy.

Rattray, F. S. (1994). *Massage therapy: An approach to treatments*. Toronto, Ontario: Massage Therapy Texts and MA Verick Consultants.

Rattray, F., and L. Ludwig (2000). *Clinical massage therapy: Understanding, assessing and treating over 700 conditions*. Toronto, Canada: Talus Incorporated.

Rich, G. J. (2002). *Massage therapy: The evidence for practice*. New York: Mosby.

Robbins, G., Powers, D., and Burgess, S. (1994). *A wellness way of life* (2nd ed.). Madison, WI: Brown & Benchmark.

Travell, J. G., and Simons, D. G. (1983). *Myofascial pain and dysfunction: The trigger point manual*. Baltimore: Williams & Wilkins.

Travell, J. G., and Simons, D. G. (1992). *Myofascial pain and dysfunction: The lower extremities*. Vol. 2. Baltimore: Williams & Wilkins.

Walach, H., Guthlin, C., and Konig, M. (2203). Efficacy of massage therapy in chronic pain: a pragmatic randomized trial. *Journal of Alternative and Complementary Medicine, 9,* 837–46.

Walton, T. (2006, Summer). Cancer & massage therapy: Essential contraindications. *Massage Therapy Journal, 45*(2), pp. 119–133.

Wood, E. C., and Becker, P. D. (1981). *Beard's massage* (3rd ed.). Philadelphia: W. B. Saunders.

Yates, J. (2004). *A physician's guide to therapeutic massage* (3rd ed.). Toronto, Canada: Curties-Overzet Publications

Zeitlin, D. et al. (2000). Immunological effects of massage therapy during academic stress. *Psychosomatic Medicine, 62,* 83–87.

Additional Resources

Anatomy and pathology for bodyworkers (Video). Santa Barbara, CA: Real Bodywork. (www.deeptissue.com)

Anderson, K. N., and Anderson, L. E. (1990). *Mosby's pocket dictionary of medicine, nursing and allied health*. St. Louis: C. V. Mosby Company.

Bell, A. J. (1964). Massage and the physiotherapist. *Physiotherapy, 50,* 406–408.

Benjamin, P. J., and Lamp, S. P. (2005). *Understanding sports massage* (2nd ed.). Champaign, IL: Human Kinetics.

Claire, T. (1995). *Bodywork: What type of massage to get, and how to make the most of it*. New York: William Morrow.

Dychtwald, K. (1977). *Body-mind*. New York: Jove Publications.

Greene, E. (1996). Study links stress reduction with faster healing. *Massage Therapy Journal, 35*(1), 16.

MacKenzie, J. (1923). *Angina pectoris*. London: Henry Frowde and Hodder and Stoughton.

Massage Therapy Foundation (www.massagetherapyfoundation.org)

Massage Therapy Practice Magazine (www.massagetherapypractice.com)

Massage Therapy Research Consortium (www.massagetherapyresearchconsortium.com)

National Center for Complementary and Alternative Medicine (www.nccam.nih.gov)

National Library of Medicine (ncbi.nlm.nih.gov/PubMed)

Nurse-Healers–Professional Associates International (www.therapeutic-touch.org)

Schultz, R. L., and R. Feitis (1996). *The endless web: Fascial anatomy and physical reality*. Berkeley, CA: North Atlantic Books.

Stillerman. E. (1992). *Mother-massage*. New York: Delta/Delcorte.

Thomas, C. L. (ed.). (1985). *Taber's cyclopedic medical dictionary*. Philadelphia: F. A. Davis.

Touch Research Institute (www.miami.edu/touch-research)

CHAPTER 8

References

Archer, P. (2007). *Therapeutic massage in athletics*. Philadelphia: Lippincott Williams Wilkins.

Badger, C. (1986). The swollen limb. *Nursing Times* (England), *82*(31), 40–41.

Bauer, W. C., and Dracup, K. A. (1987). Physiological effects of back massage in patients with acute myocardial infarction. *Focus on Critical Care, 14*(6), 42–46.

Beeken, J. et al. (1998). Effectiveness of neuromuscular release massage therapy on chronic obstructive lung disease. *Clinical Nursing Research, 7*(3), 309–325.

Benjamin, B. E. (1995). Massage and body work with survivors of abuse: Part I. *Massage Therapy Journal, 34*(3), 23–32.

Bunce, I. H., Mirolo, B. R., Hennessy, J. M. et al. (1994). Post-mastectomy lymphedema treatment and measurement. *Medical Journal Australia, 161,* 125–128.

Chamness, A. (1996). Breast cancer and massage therapy. *Massage Therapy Journal,* 35(1, Winter).

Cherkin, D. C., Eisenberg, D. et al. (2001). Randomized trial comparing traditional Chinese medical acupuncture, therapeutic massage, and self-care education for chronic low back pain. *Archives of Internal Medicine 161*(8), 1081–1088.

Corwin, E. J. (1996). *Handbook of pathophysiology.* Philadelphia: Lippincot.

Culpepper-Richards, K. (1998, July). Effect of a back massage and relaxation intervention on sleep in critically ill patients. *American Journal of Critical Care, 7*(4), pp. 288–299.

Curties, D. (1999). *Breast massage.* Toronto, Canada: Curties-Overzet Publications.

Curties, D. (1999). *Massage therapy and cancer.* Toronto, Canada: Curties-Overzet Publications.

Curtis, M. (1994). The use of massage in restoring cardiac rhythm. *Nursing Times* (England), *90*(38), 36–37.

de Bruijn, R. (1984). Deep transverse friction; its analgesic effect. *International Journal of Sports Medicine, 5,* 35–36.

Fakouri, C., and Jones, P. (1987). Relaxation: Slow stroke back rub. *Journal of Gerontological Nursing, 13*(2), 32–35.

Ferrell-Torry, A. T., and Glick, O. J. (1993). The use of therapeutic massage as a nursing intervention to modify anxiety and the perception of cancer pain. *Cancer Nursing, 16*(2), 93–101.

Field, T. (2000). *Touch therapy.* London: Churchill Livingston.

Field, T. M., Morrow, C., Valdeon, C. et al. (1992). Massage reduces anxiety in child and adolescent psychiatric patients. *Journal of the American Academy of Child and Adolescent Psychiatry, 31*(1), 125–131.

Field, T. M., Schanberg, S. M., Scafidi, F., et al. (1986). Tactile/kinesthetic stimulation effects on preterm neonates. *Pediatrics, 77*(5), 654–658.

Frazer, J., and Kerr, J. R. (1993). Psychophysiological effects of back massage on elderly institutionalized patients. *Journal of Advanced Nursing, 18,* 238–245.

Hammer, W. I. (1993). The use of transverse friction massage in the management of chronic bursitis of the hip and shoulder. *Journal of Manipulation and Physical Therapy, 16*(2), 107–111.

Heidt, P. (1981). Effect of therapeutic touch on anxiety level of hospitalized patients. *Nursing Research, 30*(1), 32–37.

Hernandez-Reif, M., Ironson, G., Field, T. et al. (2004, July). Breast cancer patients have improved immune and neuroendocrine functions following massage therapy. *Journal of Psychosomatic Research,* 57(1):45–52.

Joachim, G. (1983). The effects of two stress management techniques on feelings of well-being in patients with inflammatory bowel disease. *Nursing Papers, 15*(5), 18.

Karpen, M. (1995). Dolores Kreiger, PhD, RN: Tireless teacher of Therapeutic Touch. *Alternative & Complementary Therapies,* April/May, 142–146.

Keller, E., and Bzdek, V. M. (1986). Effects of therapeutic touch on tension headache pain. *Nursing Research, 35*(2), 101–106.

Kelly, D. G. (2002). *A primer on lymphedema.* Upper Saddle River, NJ: Prentice Hall.

Kramer, N. A. (1990). Comparison of therapeutic touch and casual touch in stress reduction of hospitalized children. *Pediatric Nursing, 16*(5), 483–485.

Kurz, W., Wittlinger, G., Litmanovitch, Y. I. et al. (1978). Effect of manual lymph drainage massage on urinary excretion of neurohormones and minerals in chronic lyphedema. *Angiology, 29,* 64–72.

Longworth, J. D. (1982). Psychophysiological effects of slow stroke back massage in normotensive females. *Advances in Nursing Science, 4,* 44–61.

MacDonald, G. (1995, Summer). Massage for cancer patients: A review of nursing research. *Massage Therapy Journal,* 53–56.

Mitchinson, A. R., Kim, H. M., Rosenburg, J. M., Geisser, M., Kirsh, M., Cikrit, D., and Hinshaw, D. B. (2007). Acute postoperative pain management using massage as an adjuvant therapy. *Archives of Surgery, 142*(12), pp. 1158–1167.

Moyer, C. A., Rounds, J., and J. W. Hannum (2004). A meta-anaylsis of massage therapy research. *Psychological Bulletin, 130,* 3-18.

Premkumar, K. (1999). *Pathology A to Z: A handbook for massage therapists* (2nd ed.). Calgary, Canada: Van Pub Books.

Preyde, M. (2000). Effectiveness of massage therapy for subacute low-back pain: A randomized controlled trail. *CMAJ, 162*(13), 1815–1820.

Puustjarvi, K., Airaksinen, O., and Pontinen, P. J. (1990). The effects of massage in patients with chronic tension headache. *Acupuncture Electrotherapy Research, 15*(2), 159–162.

Quinn, C., Chandler, C., and Moraska, A. (2002). Massage therapy and frequency of chronic tension headaches. *American Journal of Public Health, 92*(10), 1657–1660.

Rhiner, M., Ferrell, B. R., Ferrell, B. A., and Grant, M. M. (1993). A structured non-drug intervention program for cancer pain. *Cancer Practice, 1,* 137–143.

Sims, S. (1986). Slow stroke back massage for cancer patients. *Nursing Times, 82,* 47–50.

Sunshine, W., Field, T. et al. (1996). Fibromyalgia benefits from massage therapy and transcutaneous electrical stimulation. *Journal of Clinical Rheumatology, 2*(1), 18–22.

Walton, T. (2006, Summer). Cancer & massage therapy: Essential contraindications. *Massage Therapy Journal, 45*(2), pp. 119–133.

Weinrich, S. P., and Weinrich, M. C. (1990). The effect of massage on pain in cancer patients. *Applied Nursing Research, 3,* 140–145.

Werner, R. (2005). *A massage therapist's guide to pathology* (3rd ed.). Philadelphia: Lippincott Williams Wilkins.

Wheeden, A., Scafidi, F., Field, T. et al. (1993). Massage effects on cocaine-exposed preterm neonates. *Developmental and Behavioral Pediatrics, 14*(5), 318–322.

Witt, P. L., MacKinnon, J. (1986). Trager psychosocial integration: A method to improve chest mobility of patients with chronic lung disease. *Physical Therapy, 66*(2), 214–217.

Yates, J. (1999). *A physician's guide to therapeutic massage: Its physiological effects and treatment applications* (2nd ed.). Vancouver, BC: Massage Therapists' Association of British Columbia.

Zanolla, R., Monzeglio, C., Balzarini, A., and Martino, G. (1984). Evaluation of the results of three different methods of postmastectomy lymphedema treatment. *Journal of Surgical Oncology, 26,* 210–213.

Additional Resources

Canada Institute of Palliative Massage. *AIDS massage* (Video). Nelson, British Columbia, Canada: Sutherland Massage Productions. (www.sutherlandmassageproductions.com)

Benjamin, P. J. (2006, Summer). Loosening the grip: How massage can sooth chronic tension headaches. *Massage Therapy Journal, 45*(2), pp. 51–58.

Born, B.A. (2005) *The essential massage companion: Everything you need to know to navigate safely through today's drugs and diseases.* Berkley, MI: Concepts Born.

Canada Institute of Palliative Massage. *Cancer massage* (Video). Nelson, British Columbia, Canada: Sutherland Massage Productions. (www.sutherlandmassageproductions.com)

Canada Institute of Palliative Massage. *Massage for children with Down syndrome* (Video). Nelson, British Columbia, Canada: Sutherland Massage Productions. (www.sutherlandmassageproductions.com)

Canadian Massage Therapy Research Network (www.cmtrn.ca)

Canadian Touch Research Center (www.ccrt-ctrc.ca)

Macdonald, G. (1999). *Medicine hands: Massage therapy for people with cancer.* Tallahassee, FL: Findhorn Press.

Massage Therapy Foundation (www.massagetherapyfoundation.org)

Massage Therapy Practice Magazine (www.massagetherapypractice.com)

Massage Therapy Research Consortium (www.massagetherapyresearchconsortium.com)

Menard, M. B. (2003). *Making sense of research: A guide to research literacy for complementary practitioners.* Toronto: Curties-Overzet Publications.

National Center for Complementary and Alternative Medicine (www.nccam.nih.gov)

National Library of Medicine (ncbi.nlm.nih.gov/PubMed)

Nurse-Healers–Professional Associates International (www.therapeutic-touch.org)

Rattray, F., and L. Ludwig (2000). *Clinical massage therapy: Understanding, assessing and treating over 700 conditions.* Toronto, Canada: Talus Incorporated.

Touch Research Institute (www.miami.edu/touch-research)

CHAPTER 9

References

Rattray, F., and Ludwig, L. (2000). *Clinical massage therapy: Understanding, assessing and treating over 70 conditions.* Toronto, Canada: Talus Incorporated.

Additional Resources

Persad, R. (2001). *Massage therapy & medications.* Ontario, Canada: Curties-Overzet Publications.

Thomas, C. L. (ed.). (1985). *Taber's cyclopedic medical dictionary.* Philadelphia: F. A. Davis.

Werner, R. (2005). *Massage therapist's guide to pathology* (3rd ed.). Philadelphia: Lippincott Williams & Wilkins.

Wible, J. (2004). *Pharmacology for massage therapy.* Philadelphia: Lippincott Williams & Wilkins.

Yates, J. (2004). *A physician's guide to therapeutic massage* (3rd ed.). Toronto: Curties-Overzet Publications.

CHAPTER 10

References

Biel, A. (2001). *Trail guide to the body: How to locate muscles, bones, and more* (2nd ed.). Boulder, CO: Books of Discovery.

Chaitow, L. (1997). *Palpation skills: Assessment and diagnosis through touch.* New York: Churchill Livingston.

Hoppenfeld, S. (1976). *Physical examination of the spine and extremities.* Upper Saddle River, NJ: Prentice Hall.

Lowe, W. (2001). *Functional assessment in massage therapy* (3rd ed.). Sisters, OR: Orthopedic Massage Education & Research Institute (www.omeri.com).

Rattray, L., and Ludwig, L. (2000). *Clinical massage therapy: Understanding, assessing, and treating over 70 conditions.* Toronto: Talus Incorporated.

Thompson, D. L. (2005). *Hands heal: Communication, documentation, and insurance billing for manual therapists* (3rd ed.). Philadelphia: Lippincott Williams & Wilkins.

Yates, J. (2004). *A physician's guide to therapeutic massage* (3rd ed.). Toronto: Curties-Overzet.

Additional Resources

Associated Bodywork and Massage Professionals. (2001). *Successful business handbook.* Evergreen, CO: Author.

American Massage Therapy Association. (2002). *The business of massage.* Evanston, IL: Author.

Benjamin, P. J., and Tappan, F. M. (2005). *Tappan's handbook of healing massage techniques.* Upper Saddle River, NJ: Prentice Hall.

Greenman, P. (1989). *Principles of manual medicine.* Baltimore: Williams & Wilkins.

Holey, E., and Cook, E. (2003). *Evidence-based therapeutic massage: A practical guide for therapists.* London: Churchill Livingston.

Lowe, W. (2004). *Orthopedic massage: Theory and technique.* St. Louis, MO, Mosby.

Sohnen-Moe, C. M. (1997). *Business mastery* (3rd ed.). Tucson, AZ: Sohnen-Moe Associates.

U.S. Department of Health and Human Services, HIPAA Privacy Rules (www.hhs.gov/ocr/hipaa)

CHAPTER 11

Additional Resources

Dixon, M. W. (2001). *Body mechanics and self-care manual.* Upper Saddle River, NJ: Prentice Hall.

Field, T. (2001). *Touch.* Cambridge, MA: The MIT Press.

Frye, B. (2000). *Body mechanics for manual therapists: A functional approach to self-care and injury prevention.* Stanwood, WA: Freytag Publishing.

McIntosh, N. (1999). *The educated heart: Professional guidelines for massage therapists, bodyworkers and movement teachers.* Memphis, TN: Decatur Bainbridge Press.

National Certification Board for Therapeutic Massage and Bodywork (2000) Standards of Practice. Retrieved March 2008 (www.ncbtmb.org).

U.S. Department of Health and Human Services, Centers for Disease Control and Prevention (www.cdc.gov.).

CHAPTER 12

Additional Resources

Benjamin, B. E., and Sohnen-Moe, C. (2003). *The ethics of touch.* Tucson, AZ: SMA Inc.

Dixon, M. W. (2001). *Body mechanics and self-care manual.* Upper Saddle River, NJ: Prentice Hall.

Field, T. (2001). *Touch.* Cambridge, MA: The MIT Press.

Frye, B. (2000). *Body mechanics for manual therapists: A functional approach to self-care and injury prevention.* Stanwood, WA: Freytag Publishing.

McIntosh, N. (1999). *The educated heart: Professional guidelines for massage therapists, bodyworkers and movement teachers.* Memphis, TN: Decatur Bainbridge Press.

Montagu, A. (1978). *Touching: The human significance of the skin* (2nd ed.). New York: Harper & Row.

National Certification Board for Therapeutic Massage and Bodywork (2000) Standards of Practice. Retrieved March 2008 (www.ncbtmb.org).

National Certification Board for Therapeutic Massage and Bodywork (www.ncbtmb.org)

CHAPTER 13

References

Cyriax, J. H., and Cyriax, P. J. (1993). *Illustrated manual of orthopedic medicine* (2nd ed.). Boston: Butterworth & Heinemann.

McMillan, M. (1925). *Massage and therapeutic exercise.* Philadelphia: W. B. Saunders.

Rattray, L., and Ludwig, L. (2000). *Clinical massage therapy: Understanding, assessing, and treating over 70 conditions.* Toronto: Talus Incorporated.

Additional Resources

Benjamin, P. J. (2007). "Hidden hardware: What's under your client's skin?" *Massage Therapy Journal, 46*(1), pp. 106–115.

Cailliet, R. (1981). *Shoulder pain* (2nd ed.). Philadelphia: F. A. Davis.

Graham, D. (1884). *Practical treatise on massage.* New York: Wm. Wood and Co.

Hoffa, A. J. (1900). *Technik der massage* (3rd ed.). Verlagsbuchhandlung, Stuttgart: Ferdinand Enke. As translated by F. M. Tappan and Ruth Friedlander.

Kellogg, J. H. (1895). *The art of massage: Its physiological effects and therapeutic applications.* Battle Creek, MI: Modern Medicine Publishing Co.

Roth, M. (1851). *The prevention and cure of many chronic diseases by movements.* London: John Churchill.

Werner, R. (2005). *A massage therapist's guide to pathology* (3rd ed.). Philadelphia: Lippincott, Williams & Wilkins.

CHAPTER 14

Additional Resources

Body massage for the day spa (Video). (1997) Erica Miller Professional Education Series. Mile Ranch, British Columbia: Spa Expertise Canada LTD.

Born, B. A. (2005). *The essential massage companion.* Berkley, MI: Concepts Born.

Classical and innovative European facial massage (Video). (1988). Erica Miller Professional Education Series. Mile Ranch, British Columbia, Canada: Spa Expertise Canada LTD.

Curties, D. (1999). *Breast massage.* Moncton, New Brunswick, Canada: Curties-Overzet Publications.

Head, neck & shoulder massage (Video). (2003). Massage Master Class™ Series. Riverside, CT: At Peace Media. (www.atpeacemedia.com).

Japanese hand massage (Video). (2001). With Shogo Mochizuki. Boulder, CO: Kotobuki Publications.

Therapeutic massage (Video). Santa Barbara, CA: Real Bodywork. (www.deeptissue.com)

Werner, R. (2005). *A massage therapist's guide to pathology.* Philadelphia: Lippincott Williams & Wilkins.

CHAPTER 15

References

Field, T. M., Fox, N., Pickens, J., Ironsong, G., and Scafidi, F. (1993). Job stress survey. Unpublished manuscript, Touch Research Institute, University of Miami School of Medicine. Reported in Touchpoints: Touch Research Abstracts, 1(1).

Hodge, M., Robinson, C., Boehmer, J., and Klein, S. (2002). "Employee outcomes following work-site acupressure and massage." Chapter 9 in *Massage therapy: The evidence for practice.* New York: Mosby.

No author (1996). Massage helps lower stress of working, taking final exams. *Massage, 62* (July/August), p. 148.

Palmer, D. (1995). The death of on-site massage? *Massage Therapy Journal, 34*(3), pp. 119–120.

Additional Resources

Benjamin, P. J. (1994). *On-site therapeutic massage: Investment for a healthy business.* Information brochure. Rockford, IL: Hemingway Publications.

Chair massage with Connie Scholl (Video). Riverside, CT: At Peace Media. (www.atpeacemedia.com)

Japanese chair massage (Video). (2002) By Shogo Mochizuki. Boulder, CO: Kotobuki Publications.

TouchPro Institute (www.touchpro.org)

CHAPTER 16

References

Barclay, J. (1994). *In good hands: The history of the chartered society of physiotherapy 1894–1994.* London: Butterworth-Heinemann.

Belanger, A.Y. (2002). *Evidenced-based guide to therapeutic physical agents.* Philadelphia: Lippincott Williams & Wilkins.

Croutier, A. L. (1992). *Taking the waters: Spirit, art, sensuality.* New York: Abbeyville Press.

Graham, R. L. (1923). *Hydro-hygiene: The science of curing by water.* New York: Thompson-Barlow Company.

Miller, E. T. (1996). *Day spa techniques.* Albany, NY: Milady Publications.

Additional Resources

Benjamin, P. J. (2004). "Massage and sweatbaths among the ancient Maya." *Massage Therapy Journal,* Spring, pp. 148–154.

Day Spa 1: Hydrotherapy Treatments (Video). (1997) Erica Miller Professional Education Series. Mile Ranch, British Columbia, Canada: Spa Expertise Canada Ltd.

Fowlie, L. (2006) *An introduction to heat and cold as therapy.* Toronto: Curties-Overzet Publications.

Hecox, B., Mehreteab, T. A., and Weisberg, J. (1994). *Physical agents: A comprehensive text for physical therapists.* Norwalk, CT: Appleton & Lange.

Knight, K. L. (1995). *Cryotherapy in sport injury management.* Champaign, IL: Human Kinetics.

Monastersky, R. (2002). "Plumbing ancient rituals: Sweatbaths in Maya cities provide a window into lives long ago." *Chronicle of Higher Education.* 17 May 2002, pp. A22–23.

Persad, R. S. (2001). *Massage therapy & medications: General treatment principles.* Toronto: Curties-Overzet.

CHAPTER 17

References

Buckle, J. (2007). *Clinical aromatherapy, essential oils in practice.* New York: Churchill Livingstone.

Calistoga Spas (2008). "The Mud Baths." Retrieved 10 May 2008 from www.calistogaspas/mud-baths/.

Glen Ivy Hot Springs Spa (2008). "Hot Springs Spa, History." Retrieved 10 May 2008 from www.glenivy .com/index.php/resort/C8/ .

Minton, M. (2008b). "Mud: Dig it!" Retrieved 10 May 2008 from www.massagemag.com/spa/treatment/mud/php.

NAHA (2005a). "About aromatherapy." Retrieved 15 May 2008 from www.naha.org/about_aromatherapy.htm.

NAHA (2005b). "Aromatherapy regulation." Retrieved 15 May 2008 from www.naha.org/faq_regulation.htm#11.

Ody, P. (2002). *Essential guide to natural home remedies.* London, England: Kyle Cathie Limited.

Ody, P. (1993). *The medicinal herbal.* New York: Dorling Kindersley.

Price, S., and Price. L. (2007). *Aromatherapy for health professionals* (3rd ed.). Philadelphia: Churchill Livingstone Elsevier

Pure Essential, Inc. (2007). "Esssential oils and perfume notes." Retrieved 15 May 2008 from www.essential-oil .org/essential_oils_notes.asp

Rose, J. (1999). *375 Essential oils and hydrosols.* Berkeley, CA: Frog Ltd.

Shutes, J., and Weaver, C. (2008). *Aromatherapy for body-workers.* Upper Saddle River, NJ: Pearson Prentice Hall

Tisserand, R. B. (1985). *The art of aromatherapy.* Essex, England: Saffron Walden: C. W. Daniel Company Ltd.

Williams, A. (2007). *Spa bodywork, a guide for massage therapists.* Philadelphia: Lippincott, Williams & Wilkins.

Worwood, V. A. (1999). *The fragrant heavens.* Novato, CA: New World Library.

Additional Resources

Ahava—Dead Sea mud (www.ahava.com)

Innovative Spa (www.innovativespa.com)

Massage Warehouse and Spa Essentials (www.massagewarehouse.com)

QE Health (formerly the Queen Elizabeth Hospital) in Rotorua www.rotoruanz.com/attractions/spa_wellness .php) (www.qehealth.co.nz)

Spa Elegance (www.spaelegance.com)

SpaEquip (www.spaequip.com)

Torf Spa—organic moor mud from Europe (www.torfspa.com)

Universal Companies (www.universalcompanies.com)

Water Werks (www.vichyshower.com)

CHAPTER 18

References

Carter, M., and Weber, T. (1997). *Healing yourself with foot reflexology.* Englewood Cliffs, NJ: Prentice-Hall.

Stone, P. (2004). A snapshot of the history of reflexology. *Massage Therapy Journal* online edition. www.amtamassage.org

Stone, P. (2006, Summer). Keeping step: Your guide to adding reflexology to your business. *Massage Therapy Journal* online edition. www.amtamassage.org

Stone, P. (2004). *History of reflexology.* St Charles, MO, author.

Stone, Randolph. (1987). *Dr. Randolph Stone's Polarity Therapy: The complete collected works.* Harlan Tarbell, Illustrator. Sebastopol, CA: CRCS Publications.

Stone, Randolph. (1991). *Health building: The conscious art of living well.* Sebastopol, CA: CRCS Publications.

Travell, J. G., and Simons, D. G. (1999). *Myofascial pain and dysfunction: The trigger point manual,* Volume 1—*Upper half of the body* (2nd ed.). Baltimore: Williams & Wilkins.

Travell, J. G., and Simons, D. G. (1992). *Myofascial pain and dysfunction: The trigger point manual,* Volume 2—*The lower extremities.* Baltimore: Williams & Wilkins.

Additional Resources

Advanced myofascial release (Video). (2000) Santa Barbara, CA: Real Bodywork (www.deeptissue.com)

American Commission for Accreditation of Reflexology Education and Training (www.acaret.org)

American Polarity Therapy Association (www.polaritytherapy.org)

American Reflexology Certification Board (www.arcb.net)

Anderson, K. N., and Anderson, L. E. (1990). *Mosby's pocket dictionary of medicine, nursing, & allied health.* St. Louis: C. V. Mosby.

Archer, P. (2007). *Therapeutic massage in athletics.* Philadelphia: Lippincott Williams & Wilkins.

Badger, C. (1990). Treating lymphoedma. *Nursing Times,* 92(11), pp. 84–88.

Barnes, J. F. (1987). Myofascial release. *Physical Therapy Forum,* September 16.

Benjamin, P. J. (2006 Summer). Loosen the grip: How massage can soothe chronic tension headaches. *Massage Therapy Journal, 45*(2), pp. 50–59.

Benjamin, P. J. (1989a). Eunice Ingham and the development of foot reflexology in the United States. Part one: The early years—to 1946. *Massage Therapy Journal*, Spring, pp. 38–44.

Benjamin, P. J. (1989b). Eunice Ingham and the development of foot reflexology in the United States. Part two: On the road 1946–1974. *Massage Therapy Journal*, Winter, pp. 49–55.

Byers, D. C. (2001). *Better health with foot reflexology. Revised.* St. Petersburg, FL: Ingham Publishing.

Cantu, R. I., and Grodin, A. J. (1992). *Myofascial manipulation: Theory and clinical application.* Gaithersburg, MD: Aspen Publishers.

Casley-Smith, J. R., and Casley-Smith, J. R. (1994). *Modern treatment of lymphedema.* Adelaide, Australia: Henry Thomas Laboratory, Lymphoedma Association of Australia.

Chaitow, L. (1996). *Modern neuromuscular techniques.* London: Churchill Livingston.

Chikley B. (1999). *Lymph drainage therapy: Study guide for Level I.* France: UI and self-published, 1996.

Claire, T. (1995). *Bodywork: What type of massage to get and how to make the most of it.* New York: William Morrow.

Deep tissue and neuromuscular therapy: The torso (Video). Santa Barbara, CA: Real Bodywork. (www.deeptissue.com)

Deep tissue and neuromuscular therapy: The extremities (Video). Santa Barbara, CA: Real Bodywork. (www.deeptissue.com)

Findley, T. W., and Schleip, R. (2007). *Fascial research: Basic science and implications for conventional and complementary health care.* New York: Elsevier.

First International Fascia Research Congress (www.fascia2007.com)

Fitzgerald, W. H., and Bowers, E. F. (1917). *Zone therapy.* Columbus, OH: I. W. Long.

Foldi, E., and Foldi, M. (1999). *Textbook of Foldi School, Austria.* Self-published, English translation by Heida Brenneke.

Gordon, R. (1979). *Your healing hands: The polarity experience.* Santa Cruz, CA: Unity Press.

Guyton, A. C. (1991). *Textbook of medical physiology.* Philadelphia: Saunders.

International Council of Reflexologists (www.icr-reflexology.org)

Issel, C. (1993). *Reflexology: Art, science, and history.* Sacramento, CA: New Frontier Publishing

Juhan, D. (1987). *Job's body.* Barrytown, NY: Station Hill Press.

Kasseroller, R. (1998). *Compendium of Dr. Vodder's manual lymph drainage.* Heidelberg, Germany: Karl F. Haug Publishers.

King, R. K. (1996). *Myofascial massage therapy: Towards postural balance.* Self-published training manual by Bobkat Productions, Chicago.

Knaster, M. (1996). *Discovering the body's wisdom.* New York: Bantam Books.

Kunz, K., and Kunz, B. (2007). *Complete reflexology for life.* New York, NY: Dorling Kindersley Limited.

Kurz, I. (1986). *Textbook of Dr. Vodder's Manual Lymphatic Drainage,* Vol. III, *Treatment* (3rd ed.). Heidelberg, Germany: Karl F. Haug Publishers.

Kurz, I. (1986). *Textbook of Dr. Vodder's Manual Lymphatic Drainage,* Vol. II: *Therapy* (3rd ed.). Heidelberg, Germany: Karl F. Haug Publishers.

Manheim, C. (2001). *The myofascial release manual* (3rd ed.). Thorofare, NJ: Slack Inc.

Martini, F. H., and Bartholomew, E. F. (2000). *Essentials of anatomy & physiology* (2nd ed.). Upper Saddle River, NJ: Prentice Hall.

Massage Therapy Foundation (www.massagetherapyfoundation.org)

Mense, S., and Simons, D. G. (2001). Myofascial pain caused by trigger points. Chapter 9 in *Muscle pain: Understanding its nature, diagnosis, and treatment.* Philadelphia: Lippincott, Williams & Wilkins.

Myofascial Release (www.myofascial-release.com)

Natural Therapies Certification Board (www.ntcb.org)

Paoletti, S. (2006). *The fasciae.* Seattle, WA: Eastland Press. English edition.

Pishinger, E. A. (1991). *Matrix and matrix regulation: Basis for a holistic theory in medicine.* Portland, OR: Medicina Biologica.

Prudden, B. (1980). *Pain erasure: The Bonnie Prudden way.* New York: M. Evans.

Prudden, B. (1984). *Myotherapy: Bonnie Prudden's complete guide to pain-free living.* New York: Ballantine Books.

Quinn, C., Chandler, C., and Moraska, A. (2002, October). Masage therapy and frequency of chronic tension headaches. *American Journal of Public Health, 92*(10), pp. 1657–1661)

Reflexology Association of America (www.reflexology-usa.org)

Reflexology for the feet and hands with Geri Riehl (Video). (2001). Santa Barbara, CA: Real Bodywork. (www.deeptissue.com)

Reflexology with Rhonda Funes, Volume 1: *The feet* (Video). (2001). Massage Master Class™ Series. Riverside, CT: At Peace Media. (www.atpeacemedia.com)

Reihl, S. (2001). *Beginning myofascial release.* Instructional video produced by Real Bodywork.

Rolf Institute of Structural Integration (www.rolf.org)

Scheumann, D. W. (2002). *The balanced body: A guide to deep tissue and neuromuscular therapy* (2nd ed.). Philadelphia: Lippincott, Williams & Wilkins.

Schultz, R. L., and Feitis, R. (1996). *The endless web: Fascial anatomy and physical reality.* Berkeley, CA: North Atlantic Press.

Siedman, M. (1982). *Like a hollow flute: A guide to polarity therapy.* Santa Cruz, CA: Elan Press.

Siegel, A. (1986). *Live energy: The power that heals.* Bridgeport, Dorset, England: Prism Press/Colin Spooner.

Sills, Franklin. (2002). *The polarity process: Energy as a healing art.* Berkeley, CA: North Atlantic Books.

Stephenson, N. L. N., Swanson, M., Dalton. J., Keefe, F. J., and Engelke, M. (2007, January). Partner-delivered reflexology: effects on cancer pain and anxiety. *Oncology Nursing Forum, 34*(1).

Swartz, M. A., and Fleury, M.E. (2007). Intersitital flow and its effects in soft tissues. *Annual Review of Biomedical Engineering, 9,* pp. 229–256.

Tibshraeney-Morten, L. (2008). *Moving the energy: Reflexology and meridian therapy.* Seminole, FL: JLM Publishing.

Travell, J. G., and Rinzler, S. H. (1952). The myofascial genesis of pain. *Postgraduate Medicine, 11,* 425–434.

Wittlinger, H., and Wittlinger, G. (1998). *Textbook of Dr. Vodder's manual lymphatic drainage,* Vol. I: *Basic course.* 6th English Translation revised and edited by Robert Harris, Heidelberg. Germany: Karl F. Haug Publishers.

CHAPTER 19

References

Douillard, J. (2004). *The Encyclopedia of aurvedic massage.* Berkeley, CA: North Atlantic Books.

Johari, H. (1996). *Ayurvedic massage: Traditional Indian techniques for balancing body and mind.* Rochester, VT: Healing Arts Press.

National Certification Commission for Acupuncture and Oriental Medicine (www.nccaom.org)

Parks, W. (2007). *Integrating acupressure with Will Parks* (Video).

Additional Resources

American Organization for Bodywork Therapies of Asia (www.aobta.org)

Beresford-Cooke, C. (1999). *Shiatsu theory and practice.* Edinburgh: Churchill Livingstone.

Capra, F. (1999). *The tao of physics: An exploration of the parallels between modern physics and eastern mysteries.* Boston: Shambhala Publications.

Cheng, X. (1993). *Chinese acupuncture and moxibustion.* Beijing, China: Foreign Languages Press.

Connelly, D. (1979). *Traditional acupuncture: The law of the five elements,* Columbia, MD: Center for Traditional Acupuncture.

Deadman, P. (1998). *A manual of acupuncture.* East Sussex, England: Journal of Chinese Medicine Publications.

Henshall, K. (1992). *A guide to remembering Japanese characters.* Rutland, VT: Charles E. Tuttle Company.

Jarmey, C., and Mojay, G. (1991). *Shiatsu: The complete guide.* Hammersmith, London: Thorsons.

Jarrett. L. (2000). *Nourishing destiny: The inner tradition of Chinese medicine.* Stockbridge, MA: Spirit Path Press.

Jwing-Ming, Y. (2005). *Qigong massage: Fundamental techniques for health and relaxation.* Boston: YMAA Publication Center.

Kuhn, A. (2004). *Natural healing with qigong: Therapeutic qigong.* Boston: YMAA Publication Center.

Maciocia, G. (1998). *The foundations of Chinese medicine: A comprehensive text for acupuncturists and herbalists.* Edinburgh: Churchill Livingstone.

Maciocia, G. (1994). *The practice of Chinese medicine: The treatment of diseases with acupuncture and Chinese herbs.* Edinburgh: Churchill Livingstone.

Masunaga, S., and Ohashi, W. (1977). *Zen Shiatsu: How to harmonize yin and yang for better health.* Tokyo: Japan Publications.

Moyers, B. The mystery of chi, Volume 1: Healing and the mind (Video). Video series. Ambrose Video.

Namikoshi, T. (1969). *Shiatsu: Japanese finger-pressure therapy.* Tokyo: Japan Publications.

Namikoshi, T. (1981). *The complete book of shiatsu therapy.* Tokyo: Japan Publications.

Ni, M. (1995). *The yellow emperor's classic of medicine: A new translation of the Nei Jing Suwen with commentary.* Boston: Shambhala.

Tedeschi, M. (2000). *Essential anatomy for healing and the martial arts.* Tokyo: Weatherwill.

Wang, J. (1994). The history of massage in mainland China (Video). American Organization for Bodywork Therapies of Asia (AOBTA), Video 13, Boston, MA convention.

Wang, J. (1999). To treat before sick. From *Pulse,* Voorhees, NJ: AOBTA.

Yuen, J. (2001). *Light on the essence of Chinese medicine: The Nei Jing Su Wen.* New England School of Acupuncture, Boston, MA.

Yang, J. M. (2005). *Qigong massage: Fundamental techniques for health and relaxation.* Boston: YMAA Publication Center.

Zukav, G. (1980). *The dancing WuLi masters: An overview of the new physics.* New York: Bantam Books.

CHAPTER 20

References

Nelson, D. (1994). *Compassionate touch: Hands-on caregiving for the elderly, the ill, and the dying.* Barrytown, NY: Station Hill Press.

Rattray, F., and Ludwig, L. (2000). *Clinical massage therapy.* Toronto: Talus Incorporated.

Werner, R. (2005). A massage therapist's guide to pathology (3rd ed.). Philadelphia: Lippincott Williams & Wilkins.

Additional Resources

ABC's of geriatric massage (Video). Day-Break Massage Institute (www.daybreak-massage.com).

Aging Research Centre (ARC) (www.arclab.org)

AIDS massage (Video). Canada Institute of Palliative Massage. Nelson, British Columbia, Canada: Sutherland Massage Productions. (www.sutherlandmassageproductions.com)

American Society on Aging (www.asaging.org)

Archer, P. (2007). *Therapeutic massage in athletics.* Philadelphia: Lippincott Williams & Wilkins.

Benjamin, P. J., and Lamp, S. P. (2005). *Understanding sports massage* (2nd ed.). Champaign, IL: Human Kinetics.

Born, B. A. (2005.) *The essential massage companion.* Berkley, MI: Concepts Born.

Cancer massage (Video). Canada Institute of Palliative Massage. Nelson, British Columbia, Canada: Sutherland Massage Productions. (www.sutherlandmassageproductions.com)

Center to Advance Palliative Care (www.capc.org)

Curties, D. (1999). *Breast massage.* Moncton, New Brunswick, Canada: Curties-Overzet Publications.

Day-Break Geriatric Massage Institute (www.daybreak-massage.com)

Dieter, J. N. I., and Emory, E. K. (2002). "Supplemental tactile and kinesthetic stimulation for preterm infants." Chapter 7 in *Massage therapy: The evidence for practice.* Rich, G. J. (ed.). New York: Mosby.

Ellis, V., Hill, and Campbell, H. (1995). Strengthening the family unity through the healing power of massage. *Journal of Hospice & Palliative Care, 12,* pp. 19–20.

Evans, W., and Rosenberg, E. H. (1991). *Biomarkers.* New York: Simon & Schuster.

Fakouri, C., and Jones, P. (1987). Relaxation: Slow stroke back rub. *Journal of Gerontological Nursing, 13*(2), pp. 32–35.

Fanslow, C. (1984). Touch and the elderly. In *The many facets of touch,* edited by C. C. Brown. Skillman, NJ: Johnson & Johnson Baby Products Company.

Field, T. (2000). "Enhancing growth." Chapter 1 in *Touch Therapy.* New York: Churchhill Livingston.

Field, T. (2001). *Touch.* Cambridge, MA: MIT Press.

Field, T., Hernandez-Reif, M., Hart, S., Teakston, H., Schanberg, S., Kuhn, C., and Burman, I. (1999). Pregnant women benefit from massage therapy. *Journal of Psychosomatic Obstetrics and Gynecology, 1920,* pp. 31–38.

Field, T., Hernandez-Reif, M., Taylor, S., Quintino, O., and Burman, I. (1997). Labor pain is reduced by massage therapy. *Journal of Psychosomatic Obstetrics and Gynecology, 18,* pp. 286–291.

Frazer, J., and Kerr, J. R. (1993). Psychophysiological effects of back massage on elderly institutionalized patients. *Journal of Advanced Nursing, 18,* pp. 238–245.

Gach, M. R. (1990). *Acupressure's potent points: A guide to self-care for common ailments.* New York: Bantam Books.

Gentle touch infant massage (Video). (2003) Goldhil Home Media.

Howdyshell, C. (1998). Complementary therapy: Aromatherapy with massage for geriatric and hospice care for a holistic approach. *Hospice Journal, 13,* pp. 69–75.

Infant massage: A gift of love (Video). (1999) With Cheryl Brenman. Sedona, AZ: Brenman Productions.

Infant massage lessons for dads: The power of a father's touch (Video). (2003) with John G. Louis. Acuforce International, Inc.

Infant massage: The power of touch (Video). (1995). View Video.

International Loving Touch Foundation (www.lovingtouch.com)

International Association of Infant Massage Instructors (www.iaimi.com)

Kunz, K., and Kunz, B. (1991). *The complete guide to foot reflexology.* Englewood Cliffs, NJ: Prentice-Hall.

Living Arts massage practice for infants (Video). Gaiam/Living Arts. (www.gaiam.com)

Living Arts massage practice for pregnancy (Video). (2000) With Michelle Kluck. Gaiam/Living Arts. (www.gaiam.com)

Lundberg, P. (1992). *The book of shiatsu.* New York: Simon & Schuster.

Martini, F. H. and Bartholomew, E. F. (2000). *Essentials of Anatomy & Physiology* (2nd ed.). Upper Saddle River, NJ: Prentice Hall.

Massage for sports health care: For enhanced athletic performance and recovery (Video). (1998) Champaign, IL: Human Kinetics. (www.humankinetics.com)

Miesler, D. W. (1990). *Geriatric massage techniques: Topics for bodyworkers no. 2.* Guerneville, CA: Day-Break Productions.

National Council on Aging (NCOA) (www.ncoa.org)

National Hospice and Palliative Care Organization (www.nhpco.org)

National Hospice Foundation (www.hospiceinfo.org)

National Institute on Aging at the National Institutes of Health (www.nia.nih.gov)

Nelson, D. (1994). *Compassionate touch: Hands-on caregiving for the elderly, the ill and the dying.* New York: Station Hill Press.

Nelson, D. (2001). *From the heart through the hands: The power of touch in caregiving.* Forres, Scotland: Findhorn Press.

Older, J. (1982). *Touching is healing.* New York: Stein & Day.

Osborne-Sheets, C. (1998) *Pre- and perinatal massage therapy: A comprehensive practitioner's guide to pregnancy, labor, postpartum.* San Diego, CA: Body Therapy Associates.

Persad, R. (2001). *Massage therapy & medications: General treatment principles.* Toronto: Curties-Overzet Publications.

Pre- and Perinatal Massage Therapy (www.bodytherapyassociates.com)

Remington, R. (2002). "Hand massage in the agitated elderly." Chapter 8 in *Massage therapy: The evidence for practice* by G. J. Rich (ed.). New York: Mosby.

Ruebottom, A., Lee, C., and Dryden, P. J. (1989). Massage for terminally ill AIDS patients. International Conference on AIDS, June.

Schneider, Vimala (1982). *Infant massage: A handbook for loving parents.* New York: Bantam Books.

Sports massage (Video). Nelson, British Columbia, Canada: Sutherland Massage Productions. (www.sutherlandmassageproductions.com)

Stillerman, E. (1992). *Mother-massage: A handbook for relieving the discomforts of pregnancy.* New York: Delta/Delcorte.

U.S. Administration on Aging (AoA) (www.aoa.gov)

Wible, J. (2004). *Pharmacology for massage therapy.* Philadelphia: Lippincott Williams & Wilkins.

CHAPTER 21

Additional Resources

Internal Revenue Service (www.irs.gov)

Makely, S. (2005). *Professionalism in health care: A primer for career success* (2nd ed.). Upper Saddle River, NJ: Prentice Hall.

Mariotti, S. (2007). *Entrepreneurship: Starting and operating a small business.* Upper Saddle River, NJ: Prentice Hall.

National Employers Association (neasa-sa.com)

National Labor Relations Board (www.nlrb.gov)

U.S. Equal Employment Opportunity Commission (www.eeoc.gov)

CHAPTER 22

References

American Massage Therapy Association. (2005). *Massage therapy consumer survey fact sheet.* Evanston, IL: Author.

Benjamin, B.E., and Sohnen-Moe, C. (2003). *The ethics of touch.* Tucson, AZ: SMA.

Internal Revenue Service. (2005). *Business expenses,* IRS Publication 535.

Internal Revenue Service. (2006). *Self-employment tax,* Schedule SE (Form 1040).

Internal Revenue Service. (2006). *Starting a business and keeping records,* IRS Publication 583.

Internal Revenue Service. (2006). *Tax withholding and estimated tax,* IRS Publication 505.

Internal Revenue Service. (2005). *Your federal income tax—For individuals,* IRS Publication 17.

Kamoroff, B. B. (2003). *Small time operator: How to start your own business, keep your books, pay your taxes, and stay out of trouble.* Laytonville, CA: Bell Springs Publishing.

Picchoine, N. (1990). *Dome simplified weekly bookkeeping record: A simple, complete, and practical business record as required by federal and state laws.* Warwick, RI: Dome Publishing.

Additional Resources

Internal Revenue Service (www.irs.gov)

Madison-Mahoney, V. (updated 2008) *Manipulate your future: Comprehensive guide to massage therapy insurance billing.* (www.thebodyworker.com/massage-insurance-billing.htm)

Mariotti, S. (2007). *Entrepreneurship: Starting and operating a small business.* Upper Saddle River, NJ: Prentice Hall.

QuickBooks® (www.quickbooks.intuit.com)

U.S. Small Business Administration (www.sba.gov)

CHAPTER 23

References

Federal Trade Commission. (1980). *FTC guides concerning use of endorsements and testimonials in advertising.*" Retrieved September 2, 2009 from ww.ftc.gov/bcp/guides/ensorse.htm.

Federal Trade Commission. (1984). *FTC policy statement regarding advertising substantiation.* Retrieved September 3, 2009 from www.ftc.gov/bcp/guides/ad3subst.htm

Federal Trade Commission (1983). *FTC statement on deception.* Retrieved September 2, 2009 from www.ftc.gov/bcp/policystmt/ad-decept.htm

Federal Trade Commission. (2000). *Guides against bait advertising.* Retrieved September 2, 2009 from www.ftc.gov/bcp/guides/baitads-gd.htm

National Certification Board for Therapeutic Massage and Bodywork. (2001). Code of ethics. Retrieved September 5, 2009 from www.ncbtmb.com/handbooks/2002/code_of_ethics.htm

U. S. Copyright Office. (2000). *Circular 1: Copyright basics.* Retrieved September 9, 2009 from www.copyright.gov/circs/circ1.html

Additional Resources

Benjamin, B. E., and Sohnen-Moe, C. (2003). *The ethics of touch.* Tucson, AZ: SMA.

Better Business Bureau (www.bbb.org)

Federal Trade Commission (www.ftc.gov)

Internal Revenue Service (www.irs.gov)

National Certification Board for Therapeutic Massage and Bodywork (www.ncbtmb.com)

U.S. Copyright Office (www.copyright.gov)

U.S. Patent and Trademark Office (www.uspto.gov)

Interactive Glossary

This interactive glossary defines terms used in the text and also suggests relationships between terms. Look for the words **See**, **Compare to**, and **Contrast with**, which designate relationships among different terms.

Abdominal breathing is a method of breathing focusing on movements of the diaphragm; also called diaphragmatic breathing. During inhalation the diaphragm pushes downward, allowing the lungs to fill with air; the abdominal wall expands, while the chest and shoulders remain relatively still. During exhalation the diaphragm relaxes and the abdominal wall contracts slightly, pushing the air out. Used for relaxation and in body–mind practices such as qi gong. See *Qi gong*.

Accountability is a trait in which individuals accept responsibility for their actions, do not make excuses for repeated mistakes, and apologize sincerely for and correct mistakes that they have made. See *Work ethic*.

Accreditation is recognition awarded to institutions or education programs by a nongovernmental organization that sets standards of excellence; accredited schools have undergone a peer evaluation to confirm that the accreditation standards are met. Contrast with *Certification*.

Active assisted stretch is a method of stretching in which a practitioner provides additional force in the direction of an active stretch being performed by a recipient. See *Stretching*. Contrast with *Simple static stretch* and *Contract–relax–stretch*.

Active listening is a communication skill that involves reflecting back to the speaker what the listener thinks was said; accomplished by paraphrasing or restating the words to clarify their meaning. Contrast with *Affirmative listening*.

Active movements are initiated and powered voluntarily by a person with no or some assistance from a practitioner. Types of active movements are free, assistive, and resistive. Contrast with *Passive movements*.

Active range of motion (AROM) refers to the evaluation of motion at a joint while a person actively moves that joint through its range; observations include degree of motion possible, restrictions or shortening, and any discomfort experienced; used to collect objective information for *Goal-oriented planning*.

Active trigger points are always tender, prevent full lengthening, weaken the muscle, and refer pain on direct compression. See *Trigger point therapy* and *Trigger points*.

Activities of daily living (ADLs) are common physical activities performed in everyday life that contribute to living independently; examples are getting up out of a chair, dressing and undressing, climbing stairs, eating, and getting in and out of a bathtub. See *Special population*.

Acupoints are part of the theory of Asian bodywork therapy that refers to places along energy channels where Qi can collect and be accessed and influenced by applying pressure; also called acupuncture points and acupressure points. There are 365 classic acupoints located along the major energy channels. See *Acupressure*, *Energy channels*, *Qi*.

Acupressure is a Western term for a form of Asian bodywork therapy based on Chinese medicine in which energy channels and acupuncture points (acupoints) are stimulated to balance the flow of energy or Qi. See *Asian bodywork therapies*.

Acupressure massage integration (AMI) is a bodywork adaptation in which principles and techniques of acupressure are integrated with standard Western massage to address both the physical and energetic wellness of clients. See *Acupressure* and *Western massage*.

Adaptations are adjustments or changes to the way things are normally done in a massage therapy session to meet the unique needs of an individual client. See *Special population*.

Affirmative listening is a communication skill that involves letting the speaker know that you are paying attention; accomplished by occasional verbal cues and body language. Contrast with *Active listening*.

Age-appropriate elders are people over age 70 who show some of the typical signs of aging. Contrast with *Robust elders* and *Frail elders*.

Aleiptes is a historical term used in ancient Greece to describe the people in the gymnasium who rubbed athletes with oil.

Alternative therapy refers to methods or systems of healing outside of mainstream medicine. Contrast with *Complementary therapy* and *Integrative health care*.

American Organization for Bodywork Therapies of Asia (AOBTA®) is a professional membership association that certifies ABT practitioners and instructors and promotes excellence in ABT education. See *Asian bodywork therapies*.

Ammashi is a historical term for a practitioner of traditional Japanese massage; occupation for the blind in nineteenth- and twentieth-century Japan. See *Asian bodywork therapies*.

Anatomical position is the body posture used when describing the positions and relationships of structures in the human body; in the anatomical position, a person is standing erect with arms at the sides, legs together, toes pointing forward, palms of the hands facing forward, and the head is centered with eyes looking straight ahead.

Anmo is a term from Chinese medicine meaning to press or rub, and refers to Chinese massage; three categories of anmo are Pu Tong Anmo or general massage, Tuina Anmo or push grab massage, and Dian Xue Anmo or cavity press massage. Compare to *Acupressure* and *Acupressure massage integration*.

Aromatherapy is the therapeutic use of the preparation of fragrant essential oils extracted from plants. See *Ayurvedic massage*.

Asian bodywork therapies (ABTs) are forms of massage and bodywork whose theoretical basis is traditional Asian (Chinese) medicine. See *Acupoints* and *Energy channels*.

Assertive behavior is a confident authoritative manner that demands obedience or attention. See *Intervention model*.

Assessment refers to the practitioner's conclusions from the subjective and objective information gathered during goal-oriented planning; for primary health care providers it includes a diagnosis of the problem; from a wellness perspective it may identify long- and short-term goals for the client; written in the A section of *SOAP notes*.

Assisted movement is a type of active movement in which a person initiates the movement, while another person helps him or her complete it. See *Active movements*.

Associated trigger point is a term referring to secondary or satellite trigger points. See *Trigger point therapy*, *Trigger points*, *Secondary trigger points*, and *Satellite trigger points*.

Attendance is an aspect of work ethic reflected in showing up when expected or when scheduled for work. See *Reliability* and *Work ethic*.

Ayurvedic massage is a system of soft tissue manipulation based in traditional theories of health and disease from India (i.e., Ayurvedic medicine). See *Massage and bodywork traditions*.

Bait advertising is an attractive but insincere offer to sell a product or service which the advertiser does not intend or want to actually sell; purpose is to generate leads to potential customers, or to sell something else at a higher price, an illegal practice called bait and switch. See *Business ethics*.

Bath attendant is a historical term describing persons who assisted patrons of public baths and natural healing resorts; included giving a superficial rubdown after a bath; late nineteenth- and early twentieth-century Europe and North America.

Benefits are positive outcomes. The benefits of massage are experienced by recipients when the effects of massage support their general health and well-being. Contrast with *Effects of massage*.

Biomechanical analysis is the examination of the body in motion; takes into account principles of motion and the structure and function of the human body, especially the muscle and skeletal systems; a branch of kinesiology and an important aspect of sports medicine; used to collect objective information for goal-oriented planning. See *Gait analysis*.

Biomechanics is the study of movement in living organisms. See *Biomechanical analysis*.

Bipedal locomotion is the act of moving from one place to another on two feet. See *Gait analysis*.

Body awareness is the ability to sense where your body is in space while at rest and in motion and to coordinate movement with mind; entails an integration of body and mind so that a person exists as an embodied being.

Body-centered therapy refers to methods of healing that work primarily through the physical body, but which affect the whole person—body, mind, emotions, and spirit.

Body charts are diagrams of the human figure that are marked by clients to locate problem areas and to indicate the nature of a complaint; offer a visual and kinesthetic way to give subjective information. See *Interview skills*.

Body mechanics refers to the posture and biomechanics of the practitioner when performing massage. Good body mechanics protect the practitioner from injury and maximize the efficiency of technique applications. Compare to *Self-care*.

Body-mind effects of massage result from the interplay of body, mind, and emotions in health and disease. Compare to *Effects of massage* and *Holistic*.

Body language is communication through physical presence; includes posture, hand gestures, eye contact, and facial expression. See *Communication skills*.

Body-mind practices are physical exercises useful for improving various aspects of physical fitness with the added benefit of developing coordination, body awareness, concentration, and relaxation; examples are yoga, tai chi, qi gong, and pilates. See *Self-care*.

Body polish is a gentle form of exfoliation using soft granules such as those found in crushed almonds or grape seed meal. See *Exfoliants* and *Exfoliation*.

Body systems are a level of body organization characterized by several organs and tissues working together to perform specific body functions; for example, the cardiovascular system.

Bodywork is a general term for practices involving touch and movement in which the practitioner uses manual techniques to promote health and healing of the recipient. The healing massage techniques described in this text are considered forms of bodywork. Compare to *Manual therapy* and *Massage*.

Body wraps are spa services that involve applying a substance to the body, after which the person is wrapped in sheets, blankets, and/or a plastic covering; the primary purpose is to detoxify the body by stimulating blood and lymph circulation. Contrast with *Exfoliation*.

Bolsters are long narrow pillows or cushions used to support or prop clients into position for massage.

Boundaries refer to practices that clearly delineate and maintain practitioner and client roles within the therapeutic relationship. See *Therapeutic relationship*.

Boundary crossing is a transgression of personal or professional boundaries that may or may not be experienced as harmful. See *Personal boundaries* and *Professional boundaries*.

Boundary violation is a transgression of personal or professional boundaries that causes harm; leaves a sense of being violated, which is stronger than feeling annoyed or uncomfortable; personal or professional integrity is compromised in some way. See *Personal boundaries* and *Professional boundaries*.

Bow and arrow stance is a leg position used when facing the head or foot of the table; both feet face the direction of movement, the front leg is bent more than the rear leg, and the torso is upright; power is generated by shifting the weight from the back leg to the front leg while keeping the back in alignment. See *Body mechanics*. Contrast with *Horse riding stance*.

Bracing refers to offering a counterresistance to prevent movement in the opposite direction when applying force to the body; for example, having a seated client lean into pillows to bace against pressure during massage of the back.

Business ethics is the study of moral behavior relative to commerce and consumers. Contrast with *Professional ethics*.

Business license is a document that grants permission to operate a commercial enterprise in a certain legal jurisdiction; allows government agencies to know who is doing business in their area, and can ensure that they are complying with all related laws. Compare to *Massage establishment license*.

Business plan is a document that spells out the details of putting a business or practice vision into operation; four major parts: a description of the business, marketing, management, and finances. See *Private practice*.

CAM is an acronym for complementary and alternative medicine. See *Alternative therapy* and *Complementary therapy*.

Carrier oils are base oils in which essential oils must be diluted before applying to the body. See *Aromatherapy* and *Ayurvedic massage*.

Cash reserve is money set aside to cover emergencies and deficits in income at certain time periods; recommended to have at least three months' fixed costs in reserve when starting a massage practice; should be figured in start-up costs. See *Startup costs* and *First year budget*.

Catchments are concentrations of lymph nodes; major catchment areas include the inguinal and axillary lymph nodes. Lymphatic facilitation techniques direct lymph fluids toward catchment areas. See *Lymphatic facilitation* and *Watersheds*.

Cautions are areas of potential danger that require thoughtful consideration and possible modifications of technique application. Compare to *Contraindications* and *Endangerment sites*.

Cells are the basic unit of all living organisms and make up all tissues and organs in the body. Contrast with *Body systems*.

Centered refers to finding your focal point or point of organization from which being and movement occur and to staying there; has a physical and psychological dimension; opposite is being scattered, off balance, and moving from the periphery. Compare to being *Grounded*.

Certificate program is a course of study in a particular subject for which a certificate of completion is awarded. Contrast with *Certification*.

Certification is a type of credential given after extensive education in a specific subject and may also include examinations, continuing education, and renewal. Contrast with *Certificate program*.

Chinese body clock is a concept in Chinese medicine that refers to the natural, rhythmic cycle of the flow of Qi in the body's energy channels; at a specific time of day, each channel has a peak flow when its Qi is at its maximum and a valley when its Qi is at its minimum. See *Energy channels* and *Qi*.

Chronological age refers to the number of years a person has been alive. Contrast with *Physiological age*.

Client-centered massage focuses on the recipient's unique situation, needs, and goals as the basis for treatment planning, as opposed to recipe-based or formula massage. Compare to *Evidence-based practice* and *Principle-based therapy*.

Clinical massage therapy describes applications of massage for the treatment of pathologies; also called *Medical massage*.

Clinical reasoning is the cognitive process used to plan treatment for a health problem or medical condition; involves problem definition, information collection, data analysis, therapeutic application planning and implementation, and outcomes evaluation. See *Goal-oriented planning*.

Clinical supervision is formal consultation with a specially trained supervisor about problems and ethical issues that come up in the therapeutic relationship; an opportunity for massage therapists to process what is happening in their practices and their experiences with clients. See *Professional ethics* and *Therapeutic relationship*.

Codes of ethics list the acceptable and encouraged moral behavior of members of a profession. Compare to *Standards of practice*.

Cold packs are temperature therapy devices for applying cold to the body; can be ice or some other material that maintains a cold temperature. See *Cryotherapy* and *Temperature therapy*. Contrast with *Hot packs*.

Collagen is a fibrous structural protein found in bones, cartilage, and connective tissue; binds structures together and gives them strength; the most abundant protein in the body. See *Fascia* and *Fascial anatomy*. Contrast with *Elastin*.

Collector vessels collect lymph from the I/T vessels and connect to the transport vessels or lymphangia; are generally only one or two cells thick and do not contain valves. See *Lymphatic facilitation*. Contrast with *Initial/terminal lymph vessels* and *Transport vessels*.

Colostomy bag is a medical device attached to the outside of the body to collect feces directly from the colon after a person has undergone a colostomy.

Comforting touch is a term used in reference to massage for the terminally ill and dying; refers to touching another person with the intention of providing physical and emotional comfort. Compare to *Nurturing touch* and *Palliative care*.

Communication skills are the means of information exchange among people, and include verbal (i.e., speech and writing) and nonverbal (i.e., body language, facial expression, touch) methods.

Communication through touch is achieved by the contact and different qualities of touch applied during massage, or before or after the session when greeting or saying good-bye to a client.

Compassion is the awareness of the suffering of others coupled with the wish to relieve it; combines empathy with a dedication to service to others. See *Empathy* and *Emotional intelligence*.

Complementary therapy refers to healing methods that are used as secondary treatments to enhance the effectiveness of primary treatments and that contribute to a patient's recovery. See *CAM*. Compare to *Alternative therapy* and *Integrative health care*.

Competencies is an educational term referring to applications of knowledge and skills essential to the practice of a profession; define education in terms of what a practitioner can actually do, rather than just having completed a number of hours in certain subjects. See *Accreditation*.

Competitive advantage is a marketing concept that identifies the reasons customers would come to someone for a service or product instead of going elsewhere; competitive advantage factors for massage therapists include quality, expertise, price, location, selection or variety, level of service, convenience, and environment. See *Marketing* and *Mission statement*.

Concentration is the ability to sustain attention on something for a period of time; length of time for concentration before being distracted is called attention span; can be improved with practice. See *Meditation*.

Confidentiality is an ethical principle that upholds a client's right to privacy and prohibits giving information about a client to others without the client's permission. See *HIPAA privacy rules* and *Therapeutic relationship*.

Conflict resolution is a social skill used in solving problems or differences between two people or groups; options for resolution include collaboration, accommodation, compromise, avoidance, and force.

Conscious self-care refers to taking personal responsibility for seeking physical and emotional aid when needed from colleagues, a supervisor, or friends and family; supports health and well-being related to the practice of a profession such as massage therapy. See *Self-care*.

Contact refers to the sense presence of the massage therapist's hands on the client's body. When contact is good, the client feels a full, confident, deliberate, and warm connection to the massage therapist. Compare to *Touch*.

Contemporary massage and bodywork is a general category for systems of manual therapy that were developed in the twentieth century (e.g., myofascial massage, trigger point therapy, polarity therapy). See *Bodywork* and *Massage therapy*.

Continuing education is education beyond entry-level training in an occupation or profession; often needed for license or certification renewal.

Continuing session notes are a form of documentation that record the session-by-session history of a client's visits. See *SOAP notes*.

Continuity offers a sense of continuous touch throughout a massage session; avoids abrupt removal of touch. See *Organization*. Compare to *Flow*.

Contract is a legal agreement between two or more people; may be verbal or written; the terms of a contract may be upheld in court if one party breaches or violates the agreement; lawsuits arise when agreements are either not clear or have not been kept.

Contract–relax–stretch (CRS) is a facilitated stretching technique in which the practitioner gets into position to apply the stretch, but first asks the client to contract the muscle to be stretched against a resistance. Immediately following the targeted muscle's relaxation, the stretch is applied. See *Resisted movements* and *Stretching*.

Contraindications   are conditions or situations that make receiving massage inadvisable because of the harm that it might do. See *Do no harm*. Compare to *Cautions*.

Copyright   laws protect written, musical, and artistic works from unauthorized use; designated by the symbol ©; copyrights are administered in the United States by the U.S. Copyright Office at the Library of Congress in Washington D.C. Compare to *Patents* and *Trademarks*.

CPT codes   are medical codes used to process insurance claims; acronym for Current Procedural Terminology.

Countertransference   is a psychological phenomenon that occurs when a practitioner responds to a client as if the practitioner were relating to someone important in his or her past (e.g., mother) and transferring those positive or negative feelings onto the therapeutic relationship. Contrast with *Transference*.

Courtesy   is polite behavior that is expected in social situations; shows respect for others and exhibits thoughtfulness about their feelings, comfort, and safety; good manners. See *Social skills*.

Credentials   refers to titles, certificates, or other forms of recognition that testify to the accomplishments of the person holding them; allow others to evaluate a person's background in a given field; are awarded by schools, organizations, or government agencies to individuals meeting their criteria for the credential.

Critical thinking   is a higher level thinking process that aims to discover the truth about something; weighs reasons to believe against reasons to doubt; looks for objective evidence, confirmation of claims, errors, distortions, false information, and exaggerations; looks beneath the surface for authenticity and honesty; takes into consideration the thinker's own prejudices and beliefs. See *Intellectual skills*.

Cryotherapy   refers to temperature therapy modalities below body temperature (e.g., cold packs and ice). See *Temperature therapy*. Contrast with *Thermotherapy*.

Cyriax friction   is a form of deep transverse friction popularized by James Cyriax and used in rehabilitation of injuries. See *Deep friction* and *Deep transverse friction*.

Dan Tian   is a concept in Chinese medicine that refers to a place just below the navel and about one-third of the way from front to back; the physical and energetic center of the body that provides a point of organization and balance. See *Qi gong*.

Dao Yin   is an ancient Chinese term used to describe Qi gong; means "to guide." See *Dao Yin Yang Shen Gong* and *Qi gong*.

Dao Yin Yang Sheng Gong   is a specific system of Qi gong; combines historical Qi gong movements, martial arts movements, and movements from other styles of Qi gong and tai chi; roughly translated as exercises to preserve, nourish, and restore life. See *Dao yin*, *Qi gong*, and *Sheng*.

Deceptive advertising   is advertising that misleads the public about the nature of goods or services offered for sale, their benefits, prices, or credentials; violates values of honesty and integrity; violates consumer protection laws. See *Business ethics*.

Deep fascia   is an intricate series of dense connective sheets and bands that hold the muscles and other structures in place throughout the body. See *Fascia* and *Fascial anatomy*. Contrast with *Subcutaneous fascia*.

Deep friction   is a type of friction in which the practitioner's fingers do not move over the skin, but instead move the skin over the tissues underneath. Cross-fiber and circular friction are types of deep friction. Contrast with *Superficial friction*. Compare to *Deep transverse friction*.

Deep transverse friction   is a specific type of deep friction used in rehabilitation to break adhesions, facilitate healthy scar formation, and treat muscle and tendon lesions. It is performed across the tissues, causing broadening and separation of fibers. Deep transverse friction was popularized by James Cyriax. See *Cyriax friction*.

Defamation   is a legal term for injury to a person or an organization's reputation; known as libel if written and as slander if spoken.

Defense mechanisms   are behaviors or thoughts that help people cope with unwanted feelings such as fear, anxiety, guilt, and anger; common types are projection, denial, repression, displacement, and resistance; often unconscious.

Demonstrations   are a method of presentation that show an audience how something is done or how something works by actually performing the action while giving a verbal description or explanation. Contrast with *Explanation* and *Persuasion*.

Diaphragm relaxation   is a reflexology technique in which thumb pressure on the diaphragm reflex is deepened by flexing the recipient's toe over the point of pressure. See *Foot reflexology*. Compare to *Press-and-flex*.

Diploma   is a document that states that a specific person has successfully completed a course of study; typically designates the school name, location, course of study, number of hours completed, and date of graduation, and is signed by school officials.

Direct pressure,   or direct static pressure, is the application of force to compress tissues in a specific spot; it is applied with a thumb, finger, elbow, or knuckle. It can be considered a form of compression without movement and has also been called static friction. See *Touch without movement* and *Western massage*.

Direct therapeutic effects   of clinical massage focus on the healing of a diagnosed medical condition or easing of its symptoms. Contrast with *Indirect therapeutic effects*.

Disability is a physical or mental condition that severely limits a person's ability to perform daily life activities. See *Special population*.

Discharge notes are a form of documentation containing a final summary of a client's progress, and any comments about the course of treatment. See *Documentation*.

Do no harm is one of the most basic ethical principles of giving therapeutic massage; it means avoiding actions that may harm clients and protecting their health and safety. See *Cautions*, *Contraindications*, and *Endangerment sites*.

Documentation is the process of writing session records for future reference; also called note-taking or charting; may refer to the documents themselves; kept on paper or in electronic form. See *SOAP notes*.

Draping refers to the use of sheets, towels, or other materials to cover recipients of massage to preserve their privacy and modesty, to maintain professional boundaries, and for warmth. Compare to *Boundaries*.

Dry brushing is an exfoliation technique using brushes or fiber tools. See *Exfoliation*. Contrast with *body polish*.

Dual relationship is any relationship other than the primary one of practitioner and client. See *Professional ethics*. Compare to *Boundaries* and *Therapeutic relationship*.

Duties are obligations to act in a particular way; responsibilities that arise out of being in a certain position in relationship to others, or as the result of some action. See *Professional ethics*.

Eastern bodywork refers to traditional forms of manual therapy from the continent of Asia. See *Bodywork* and *Massage Therapy*.

Eclectic practitioners combine two or more systems of massage and bodywork into their own unique approach to manual therapy.

Effectiveness of a massage performance refers to the degree to which intended goals are achieved and to which the recipient is satisfied. Compare to *Effects of massage*.

Effects of massage refer to changes that occur in the body, mind, and emotions of the recipient as a result of soft tissue manipulation. See *Long-term effects*, *Multiple-dose effects*, *Short-term effects*, and *Single-dose effects*.

Effleurage is a Western massage technique category that includes movements that slide or glide over the body with a smooth, continuous motion. See *Swedish massage* and *Western massage*.

Elastin is a protein found in elastic fibers that make up flexible body tissues such as the skin and fascia; more elastin fibers in a tissue results in greater ability for that tissue to stretch and then return to its original length when the stretch is released. See *Fascia*. Contrast with *Collagen*.

Elders are adults age 70 years and older. See *Chronological age*. Contrast with *Physiological age*.

Emollient is a substance that makes the skin soft and supple. See *Body polish*.

Emotional distress refers to feelings or emotions typically considered to be negative (e.g., isolation and loneliness, grief, depression, fear, and anger).

Emotional intelligence is defined by a set of skills related to five domains: knowing one's emotions, managing emotions, motivating oneself, recognizing emotions in others, and handling relationships; works with intellectual and physical skills for full maturity and success as a professional.

Empathy is recognizing emotions in others; is the basis for creating rapport, and is the root of caring. Compare to *Compassion*.

Employee is a person who works for an employer who controls when, where, and how the employee performs the work; defined by IRS and U.S. Labor Laws. Contrast with *Self-employed* and *Independent contractor*.

Endangerment sites are areas of the body where delicate body structures are less protected and, therefore, may be more easily damaged when receiving massage. See *Do no harm*. Contrast with *Contraindications*.

Endorsements are anecdotes from someone besides the advertiser about how well a product or service worked for them; reflects the opinions, beliefs, findings, or experience of a party other than the sponsoring advertiser; also called *Testimonials*. See *Business ethics*.

Energetic effects of massage refer to balancing and improving the flow of energy in the body through soft tissue manipulation. Compare to *Acupressure* and *Polarity therapy*. Contrast with *Mechanical effects*.

Energy channels are part of the theory of Asian bodywork therapy that refers to the pathways for the flow of Qi in the body; there are 12 major energy channels; called meridians in some forms of Asian bodywork therapy. See *Chinese body clock* and *Qi*.

Energy flow is part of the theory of polarity therapy that states that all natural healing techniques are effective because they support the individual's innate capacity for health by stimulating the free and balanced flow of life energy; polarity therapy techniques are designed to have a positive effect on the subtle life energy of the body. See *Polarity therapy*. Compare to *Removing obstructions*.

Environment for massage includes the room, air quality, lighting, sound, dressing arrangements, equipment, and overall cleanliness and neatness of the space in which a session is given.

Equipment refers to items used in a massage practice that are relatively costly and that last for several years, such as massage tables and massage chairs.

Ergonomics is the applied science of equipment and furniture design intended to maximize productivity by reducing fatigue, discomfort, and overwork injuries. See *Repetitive strain injuries*, *Worker productivity*, and *Workplace wellness programs*.

Esalen massage is a genre of bodywork based on a simplified form of Swedish massage, whose main purpose is to enhance nonverbal connection with the inner self and with others. It emphasizes the sensual aspects of massage. It was developed at the Esalen Institute in Big Sur, California, in the 1970s as part of the human potential movement. See *Human potential movement*.

Essential oils are volatile plant oils extracted from certain aromatic plants that have both physiological and psychological effects on the human body and mind. See *Aromatherapy*.

Estimated tax payments are paid to the IRS quarterly (four times a year) based on the amount of income tax expected to be owed at the end of the year; similar to withholding for employment income; estimated tax payments should appear on the annual budget as an expense.

Ethical decision-making model is a step-by-step process of thinking through an ethical question or ethical dilemma; involves critical thinking and problem solving; takes into consideration both external and internal standards in making an ethical choice of action.

Ethical dilemmas are a type of ethical question in which two or more principles are in conflict and where something of value will be compromised regardless of the choice of action; involves selecting the lesser harm or greater good. Contrast with *Ethical questions*.

Ethical judgment is consistency in making good ethical decisions; strengthened by awareness, learning, and experience; improves with critical thinking and evaluating results. Compare to *Ethical decision-making model*.

Ethical questions are problems related to the morality of certain actions; require judgment to determine the most ethical choice. See *Ethical decision-making model*.

Ethical standards are statements designating the generally accepted and encouraged moral behavior of members of a profession; appear as codes of ethics and standards of practice documents developed by professional associations. See *Codes of ethics*.

Ethics is the study of the nature of moral behavior, of right and wrong; examines choices for behavior, and uses a decision-making process to determine the degree of morality of certain actions. See *Business ethics* and *Professional ethics*.

Event is a term used in sports massage to describe massage applications that help the athlete prepare for and recover from a specific competitive event. See *Interevent, Preevent, Postevent*, and *Sports massage*.

Evidence-based practice is founded on verifiable objective evidence for the effectiveness of certain therapies; considers scientific research, the practitioner's experience and judgment, and the recipient's values and preferences. Compare to *Client-centered massage* and *Principle-based therapy*.

Exfoliants are substances or processes that remove dead skin cells. See *Body polish*.

Exfoliation is the process of peeling and sloughing off dead skin cells from the surface of the body.

Explicit agreements are understandings between people that are spoken or written; agreements that are in the open and can be verified. Compare to *Contract*. Contrast with *Implicit agreements*.

Fascia is loose, irregular connective tissue found throughout the body; composed of three primary elements: ground substance, collagen, and elastin. Fascia holds structures together giving them their characteristic shapes, offers support, and connects the body as a whole. See *Collagen, Elastin*, and *Fascial anatomy*.

Fascial anatomy includes fascial structures that shape the body such as the body straps or retinaculae that give the body contour, and fascial sheaths that surround muscles and link muscle groups. See *Fascia*.

Fascial restrictions are places where fascial tissues are less pliable, shortened, or adhering. Fascial restrictions limit mobility and cause postural distortion, poor cellular nutrition, pain, and a variety of other dysfunctions. See *Myofascial massage*.

Fiduciary is a legal term used to describe a relationship in which person A has placed a special trust in person B, who is then obligated to watch out for person A's best interests. See *Duty* and *Therapeutic relationship*.

Fingerwalking is a variation of the reflexology technique of *thumbwalking* in which the fingertips are used to apply pressure while they "walk" along an area of the body. See *Foot reflexology*. Compare to *Thumbwalking*.

Finishing techniques are used at the end of a massage session to reconnect parts of the body that have been worked on more specifically, or to further sedate or stimulate the recipient; effleurage, tapotement, and passive touch are common finishing techniques. See *Organization*. Contrast with *Opening techniques*.

First impressions are the thoughts, beliefs, and feelings about others formed immediately upon meeting them for the first time. See *Professional demeanor* and *Professional image*.

First-year budget is a document that forecasts income and expenses for the initial twelve months of operation of a business or practice. See *Startup costs*.

Five Elements within the context of traditional Chinese medicine are Wood, Fire, Earth, Metal, and Water; Five Element Theory describes relationships among the elements as a way of using natural phenomena to explore and treat our psyche, spiritual state, anatomy, physiology, and the dynamics of the disease process as a whole; the Five Elements are used to describe flow of Qi and the cycle of life. See *Ko Cycle* and *Sheng Cycle*.

Fixed costs are expenses incurred whether a massage therapist see clients or not, for example, rent and utilities; sometimes called overhead. See *First-year budget*. Contrast with *Variable costs*.

Flow is the continuous, gentle sense of movement or quality of a massage session achieved through an orderly sequence and smooth transitions from one part of the body to the next. See *Transition techniques*. Contrast with *Pacing* and *Rhythm*.

Folk and native massage traditions are found all over the world among families, tribes, and villages. They are based on tradition and experience and often involve herbal remedies, rituals, and religious beliefs. See *Massage and bodywork traditions*.

Foot reflexology is based on the theory that pressure applied to specific areas on the feet, called reflexes, produces a change in a corresponding part of the body. See *Reflexology*.

Form 1040 is an IRS form used to file U.S. income taxes for individuals; covers both employment and self-employment; a summary form to which other forms and schedules are attached; must be filed annually by April 15.

Frail elders are people over age 70 who look and feel fragile to the touch. Contrast with *Robust elders* and *Age appropriate* elders.

Free active movements or free exercises are performed entirely by a person with no assistance from a practitioner. See *Active movements*.

Friction is a massage technique category that includes movements that rub one surface over another repeatedly and includes superficial and deep friction. See *Deep friction*, *Superficial friction*, and *Western massage*.

Full-body Western massage refers to a massage session lasting from 30 to 90 minutes, in which traditional Western massage techniques are combined into a routine to address the whole body. These sessions are generally wellness oriented and aim to improve circulation, relax the muscles, improve joint mobility, induce general relaxation, promote healthy skin, and create a general sense of well-being. Compare to *Swedish massage*. Contrast with *Acupressure* and *Acupressure massage integration*.

Full-time work is earning most or all of your income in one job or occupation; for massage therapists full-time is 15–20 clients per week or working 4–5 days in employment, or some comparable combination. Contrast with *Part-time*.

Gait analysis is the examination of biomechanics while walking or running; looks at normal gait and deviations from normal; used to collect information for goal-oriented planning. See *Biomechanics* and *Bipedal locomotion*.

General contraindications are conditions or situations that make receiving *any* massage inadvisable because of the harm that it might do. See *Contraindications*. Contrast with *Local contraindications*.

General membership organization is an organization that welcomes practitioners of different forms of massage and bodywork; can be further categorized into *professional associations* and *member services organizations*. Contrast with *Specialty associations*.

Gentle art describes the quality of polarity therapy in which nothing is ever forced; the giver invites the receiver to enter a deeply relaxed state and invites the muscles to relax. See *Polarity therapy*. Compare to *Love* and *Understanding*.

Goal-oriented planning is a type of session planning that focuses on meeting specific client needs, rather than giving a standardized massage routine; client goals provide the focal point for organizing massage sessions and choosing appropriate techniques. See *Session planning*.

Gong is a Chinese word that can be translated to mean exercise. See *Qi gong*.

Greek gymnasia were centers in ancient Athens and Sparta run by the state for free men and youths that contained facilities for exercises, frictions, and baths. Compare to *Roman baths* and *Turkish baths*.

Ground substance is a gel-like mucopolysaccharide, the same liquid that forms interstitial or intercellular fluid. See *Fascia*.

Guarantee is a promise that something will work as stated, usually with the implication that the money charged will be refunded if it does not. See *Business ethics*. Contrast with *Endorsement*.

Guidelines are landmarks used in foot reflexology to help in locating specific reflexes on the feet; five important guidelines are neck/shoulder, diaphragm, waist, pelvic, and the longitudinal tendon. See *Foot reflexology*. Compare to *Reflexology chart*.

Hand mechanics are body mechanics that minimize strain on the fingers, thumb, and wrist. See *Self-care*.

Hatha yoga is an Ayurvedic practice that includes relaxation, physical exercises or postures called *asanas*, proper breathing, proper diet, and positive thinking and meditation. See *Body-mind practices*. Compare to *Thai massage*.

Healing means enhancing health and well-being. It is the process of regaining health or optimal functioning after an injury, disease, or other debilitating condition. "To heal" means to make healthy, whole, or sound; restore to health; or free from ailment.

Health care settings are places where patients are treated for illnesses and injuries.

Health history is an interview of a client taken during the initial visit that provides information about medical conditions and health issues to be aware of before giving massage; may be verbal or written on a form. See *Contraindications* and *Do no harm*.

Health-service operator is a historical term used in the YMCA for practitioners trained in physical therapeutics or physiotherapy; included massage, hydrotherapy, electrotherapy, light, relaxation techniques, and exercise; goals focused on health, fitness, and general well-being; early to mid-twentieth-century North America.

High-risk pregnancies include those in which the mother or fetus is at higher than normal risk for complications or negative developments. See *Pregnancy* and *Trimesters*.

HIPAA privacy rules specify how medical records must be secured, who may have access to medical records, and under what conditions records may be shared with others; an acronym for the Health Insurance Portability and Accountability Act of 1996. See *Confidentiality*.

Holistic   refers to those approaches to health and healing that take into account the wholeness of human beings, including body, mind, emotions, and spirit. See *Holistic massage*.

Holistic massage   refers to forms of massage that take into account the wholeness of human beings (i.e., body, mind, emotions, and spirit). See *Holistic*.

Holistic self-care plan   includes those activities that support development as a massage therapist and minimize factors that lead to illness and injury, for example, having a plan for physical, mental, and emotional health and fitness, and avoiding undue stress and burnout. See *Conscious self-care*.

Home-visit practice   refers to a massage therapy business in which the massage therapist travels to clients' homes to provide massage; convenient for clients. See *Business plan* and *Private practice*.

Hook-and-backup   is a reflexology technique used to apply deep pressure to a specific area or reflex; the thumb is placed directly on the targeted spot, bending at the first joint to apply pressure, and then pulled to the side across the spot to deepen the pressure. See *Foot reflexology*. Compare to *Direct pressure*. Contrast with *Thumbwalking*.

Horse riding stance   is a leg position used when facing the table directly; both feet face the table with head and back in alignment; knees are bent equally to lower the body into position; weight is shifted from side to side as techniques are applied. Contrast with *Bow and arrow stance*.

Hospice   programs provide compassionate care at the end of life; typically involve a team-oriented approach to medical care, pain management, and emotional and spiritual support tailored to the needs of the dying; are provided in freestanding facilities, hospitals, nursing homes, and other long-term care facilities. Compare to *Palliative care*.

Hospital-based massage   is a specialty in which massage is integrated into the regular hospital setting such as in the pediatric ward, cancer unit, or cardiac care.

Hot packs   are temperature therapy devices for applying heat to the body; may be wet or dry applications. See *Temperature therapy* and *Thermotherapy*. Contrast with *Cold packs*.

Human meaning   of different body regions refers to the special significance individuals give to certain parts of the body. This may be related to what each region allows him or her to do and to be in this world, or there may be significant social and emotional associations. See *Holistic*.

Human potential movement   was a historical social movement in the 1960s–1970s in the United States that advocated exploring the limits of human potential and spawned many forms of massage and bodywork. See *Esalen massage*.

Hydrotherapy   is the use of water in different forms for its therapeutic effects. See other hydrotherapy facilities, *Sauna*, *Steam room*, and *Whirlpool bath*. See also *Temperature therapy*.

Hygienic hand washing   is a thorough hand-washing procedure that can prevent the transfer of pathogens during massage. Compare to *Sanitation*.

Hypothalamus   is the part of the brain that controls many physiological functions; plays a major role in the regulation of homeostasis. See *Aromatherapy*.

Hypothesis   is an unproven theory about how something works or what will happen in a certain situation; forms the basis of a scientific study. See *Research literacy* and *Scientific method*.

Ice massage   involves rubbing ice directly on the skin using an ice cube or ice cup; applied in a circular motion until the area is numb. See *Cryotherapy*. Contrast with *Cold pack*.

Implicit agreements   are understandings between people that may be unspoken and unwritten; agreements assumed or taken for granted. Contrast with *Explicit agreements*.

Income goal   is part of a business plan that specifies the desired net income for a projected annual budget. See *First-year budget*.

Income tax   is a tax paid to a government based on income from employment and/or profits from a business; taxable income from a private practice equals gross income minus qualified business expenses; tips are considered taxable income; U.S. income tax is filed annually with the Internal Revenue Service on form 1040. See *Estimated tax* and *Self-employment tax*.

Independent contractor   is a form of self-employment in which a person performs services for another person or business, but is not an employee; is contracted to accomplish a certain result, but is not under the direct control of an employer. See *Self-employed*. Contrast with *Employee*.

Indication   is a term used in the treatment model to mean that when a specific medical condition is present, a particular modality is indicated or advised to alleviate the condition. Massage is indicated as a treatment for a number of medical conditions. Contrast with *Contraindications*.

Indirect therapeutic effects   of clinical massage focus on enhancing the effectiveness of a primary treatment, or creating a more favorable environment for healing. Contrast with *Direct therapeutic effects*.

Infant massage   involves soft tissue manipulation and joint movements designed to enhance the growth and development of newborns and children. See *Tactile stimulation*.

Informed voluntary consent   is a procedure used to ask for explicit permission from a client to touch a certain body area or perform a specific technique. See *Boundaries* and *Professional ethics*.

Infusions are liquids produced by steeping herbs or botanicals in boiling water; oil may be used for an infusion in place of water. See *Body wraps*.

Initial note is a type of documentation that includes the client's stated reason for massage or their complaint, related subjective and objective information, agreed upon long-term goals, and a general plan. See *Long-term planning* and *Documentation*.

Initial/terminal (I/T) lymph vessels are the smallest lymph vessels with walls that are only one cell thick; the entry point for metabolic and cellular waste, proteins, and excess fluids. See *Lymphatic facilitation*. Contrast with *Collector vessels* and *Transport vessels*.

Intake is the process of gathering relevant information from a new client. See *Interview skills*.

Intake notes are comprehensive records that include the client's stated reason for massage or specific complaint, related subjective and objective information, agreed upon long-term goals, and a general plan is the process of gathering relevant information from a new client. See *Interview skills*.

Integrative health care is an approach to healing in which mainstream medicine and alternative healing methods are offered as equal options for treating patients. Contrast with *CAM*.

Integrative medicine center is a health care facility that offers a team approach to the treatment of illness and injury; includes a variety of Western medical health care providers, traditional and indigenous healers, and CAM practitioners in a collaborative effort.

Intellectual skills are thinking or cognitive abilities; six levels identified by educators include knowledge, comprehension, application, analysis, synthesis, and evaluation. Contrast with *Emotional intelligence*.

Intention is the aim that guides the action, that is, what the practitioner hopes to accomplish; refers to effects the practitioner is aiming for when applying techniques.

Interconnections refer to the anatomical and physiological wholeness and integrity of the human body; important to keep in mind during regional and full-body massage. See *Holistic*.

Interevent is a sports massage application given between events at competitions; gives attention to psychological recovery and also readiness for the upcoming performance; combines preevent, postevent, and recovery sports massage to meet an athlete's needs. See *Sports massage*. Compare to *Postevent*, *Preevent*, *Recovery*.

Interstitial space refers to the area between cells that is structured by collagen fibers and that contains fluid and various molecules to be returned to circulation; sometimes called the matrix. See *Lymphatic facilitation* and *Matrix*.

Intervention model is a procedure used to clarify a possible misunderstanding of intention by a client (e.g., sexual intent), and to make a decision whether to stop or continue with a massage session. See *Boundaries* and *Professional ethics* and *Sexual misconduct*.

Interview skills are communication skills used to elicit useful information from clients; used in initial client interviews and taking health histories. See *Intake*.

Introduction is a social process in which one person presents another person to a third person giving some basic information such as name and other relevant facts; also self-introduction to another person. See *Social skills*.

Intuition is a direct perception of the truth, independent of any rational process; lets us respond to our environment without calling rational problem solving into play; related to instinct. Contrast with *Intellectual skills*.

Jitsu is a concept from Asian bodywork therapy that describes an area of energy excess; felt in the tissues as hardness, resistance; manual techniques are applied to disperse the excess energy and sedate areas of jitsu. See *Acupressure massage integration*. Contrast with *Kyo*.

Joint manipulations sometimes called adjustments or chiropractic adjustments, refer to techniques that take a joint beyond its normal range of motion and that are specific attempts to realign a misaligned joint, usually using a thrusting movement. Joint manipulations are not part of Western massage and are not within the scope of this text. Contrast with *Joint movements*.

Joint movements are techniques that involve motion in the joints of the body and include mobilizing techniques and stretching. See *Mobilizing techniques* and *Stretching*.

Kinesiology is the study of human movement; it looks at the combined action of the muscular, skeletal, and nervous systems that result in movement. Compare to *Biomechanics*.

Ko Cycle is a concept within the Five Element Theory that looks at relationships among the Five Elements; also called the controlling or acting cycle; each Element controls another and is also controlled by another Element. The Ko Cycle balances the Sheng Cycle to avoid unrestrained growth. See *Five Elements*. Contrast with *Sheng Cycle*.

Kyo is a concept from Asian bodywork therapy that describes an area of energy deficiency; felt in the tissues as a soft, hollow spot with no tone; manual techniques are applied to strengthen or tonify kyo areas. See *Acupressure massage integration*. Contrast with *Jitsu*.

Latent trigger points are painful only when pressed. See *Trigger point*. Contrast with *Active trigger points*.

Limbic system is located within the cerebrum and plays a major role in a variety of emotions, such as pleasure, fear, sorrow, sexual attraction, and anger; also involved in memory and olfaction. See *Hypothalamus*.

Listening means making a conscious effort to hear what someone is trying to communicate; allows you to gather information, understand others better, and take in new ideas; helps build good relationships. See *Active listening* and *Affirmative listening*.

Local contraindications   are conditions or situations that make receiving massage on a particular part of the body inadvisable because of the harm that it might do. See *Contraindications*. Contrast with *General contraindications*.

Logo   is a symbol or graphic that identifies a person or business at a glance; can be original artwork or clip art in the public domain; if original, can be registered as a trademark for protection of use. See *Trademarks*.

Long stroke   is a lymphatic facilitation technique similar to effleurage but applied with light pressure and stretching of the skin in the desired direction of lymph flow; applied with repetition and "snap back"; generally used on the extremities. See *Lymphatic facilitation*. Contrast with *L-stroke*.

Long-term effects   of massage refer to changes that start during a massage session and that last for a longer period of time, such as a few days or weeks. Or they may be more lasting changes that occur from massage received regularly over a period of time. See *Effects of massage*. Contrast with *Short-term effects*.

Long-term planning   is a form of goal-oriented planning in which the goal is to accomplish a client's specific health objectives over a series of massage sessions; long-term refers to more than one massage session, or the interval between an initial session and a progress session to check the extent to which goals have been reached. See *Goal-oriented planning*. Contrast with *Session planning*.

Love   is a basic principle in polarity therapy that recognizes a caring so powerful that it carries with it no agenda, no end result that must be obtained. The practitioner does his or her work simply, always responding to the felt need, and yet without attachment to healing. See *Polarity therapy*. Compare to *Understanding*.

Lower body regions   for the purposes of massage, are commonly identified as hips and buttocks, upper and lower legs, and feet. See *Regional massage*. Contrast with *Upper body regions*.

L-stroke   is a lymphatic facilitation technique in which the skin is stretched tracing the L pattern; applied with repetition and "snap back"; moves lymph toward desired direction and catchment area. See *Lymphatic facilitation*. Contrast with *Long stroke*.

Lubricants   are topical substances used in some massage sessions to enhance the effects of techniques and to minimize skin friction. Common lubricants include vegetable and mineral oils, jojoba, lotions, and combinations of these substances.

Lymph   is a clear fluid that contains water, protein molecules, cellular components, and fatty acids that need to be transported back into blood circulation; the fluid in lymphatic vessels. See *Lymphatic facilitation*.

Lymphatic facilitation (LF)   is a light and gentle massage technique used to facilitate the removal of excess fluid that collects in tissues after trauma and inflammation; assists the function of the lymphatic system by the appli-cation of slow, light, and repetitive strokes that help move lymph fluid through the system of vessels and nodes. See *Long stroke* and *L-stroke*.

Maintenance   is a sports massage application with the goals of enhancing recovery from strenuous exertion, treating debilitating conditions, and helping the athlete maintain optimal health. See *Sports massage*. Compare to *Recovery*, *Rehabilitation*, and *Remedial massage*.

Manual therapy   refers to healing methods applied with the practitioner's hands touching or moving the recipient's body. See *Massage*.

Marketing   is the process of identifying potential customers or clients and meeting their needs and wants. See *Business plan*.

Massage   is the intentional and systematic manipulation of the soft tissues of the body to enhance health and healing; joint movements and stretching are commonly performed as part of massage; primary characteristics of massage are touch and movement. See *Swedish massage* and *Western massage*.

Massage and bodywork traditions   are systems of manual therapy that have been passed down from generation to generation within groups of people; these traditions are typically defined as originating from a specific ethnic group, geographic location, or civilization. Compare to *Asian bodywork therapies*, *Ayurvedic massage*, and *Western massage*.

Massage chair   is a specially designed piece of equipment that provides comfortable support for receiving massage in a seated upright position; includes support for the legs, arms, and face. See *On-site massage* and *Seated massage*.

Massage chair adjustments   include the height of the chest pad; the angle of the face cradle; and the height and/or angle of the seat, the kneeling pads, and the armrest. See *Positioning*.

Massage establishment license   is a business license to operate a commercial space where customers come for massage; typically requires revealing the owner(s), detailing hygiene and safety standards, posting services and prices, and affirming that all practitioners in the establishment have the required occupational licenses. See *Business license*. Compare to *Zoning ordinance*.

Massage operator   is a historical term for massage practitioner in early twentieth-century United States. Contrast with *Masseuse and Masseur*.

Massage therapist   refers to a person who has graduated from a massage therapy program and has met accepted standards for competency in the field; has obtained occupational licensing where required and/or national certification; and upholds the ethical standards of the profession. Contrast with *Practitioner*.

Massage therapy   is a general term for health and healing practices involving touch and movement, which are based in massage and related manual techniques. It is sometimes used synonymously with the term *bodywork*. The term *massage therapy* has been adopted by some massage practitioners to define their profession, which is a licensed profession in many states. See *Manual therapy*.

Masseur is the historical French term for a male massage therapist; twentieth-century Europe and North America. Contrast with *Masseuse*.

Masseuse is the historical French term for a woman massage therapist; twentieth-century Europe and North America; corrupted in mid-twentieth-century United States by association with prostitution. Contrast with *Masseur*.

Matrix is a descriptive term for *interstitial space*; referred to as a prelymphatic channel in many manual lymph drainage texts; structured by collagen fibers that form "scaffolding" within which fluids carrying nutrients, gases, wastes, and inorganic and organic material flow. See *Interstitial space* and *Lymphatic facilitation*.

Mechanical effects of massage refer to changes that occur on the gross level of the physical structure and that result from the physical forces of massage, such as compression, stretching, shearing, broadening, and vibration of body tissues. Contrast with *Energetic effects*, *Mind–body effects*, *Physiological effects*, and *Reflex effects*.

Mechanotherapy is a historical term for a tradition of bodywork also known as medical gymnastics and physical therapeutics; cure of diseases through movement including active and passive exercises; sometimes used machines to perform movements; early twentieth-century Europe and North America. Compare to *Bodywork* and *Massage therapy*.

Medical gymnast is a historical term for a practitioner trained in medical gymnastics or Swedish movement cure; used active and passive movements to treat disease; late nineteenth- and early twentieth-century Europe and North America. See *Swedish movement cure*.

Medical massage See *Clinical massage therapy*.

Medical rubbing is a term from the eighteenth and nineteenth centuries for frictions and rubbing used in conventional medical treatments. Compare to *Massage*.

Medical spa is a type of spa that integrates spa services with conventional and complementary therapies for healing mind and body. See *Spa*.

Meditation is a practice designed to improve the ability to concentrate or pay focused attention; basic meditation technique involves choosing something like a word or object to place attention on, and when the mind wanders, bringing it back to the object of attention. See *Concentration*.

Melting refers to the feeling of softening or "giving" in myofascial tissues as adhesions are broken, and tissues become softer and more pliable with the application of myofascial techniques. See *Fascial restrictions* and *Myofascial massage*.

Member services organization is a general membership organizations whose major mission is to provide benefits such as professional liability insurance, group health insurance, publications, and information of interest to their members, may also promote the interests of members related to licensing and legislation. Contrast with *Professional associations*.

Mind–body effects of massage refer to the interplay of mind, body, and emotions during massage applications, for example, in the relaxation response. Contrast with *Energetic effects*, *Mechanical effects*, *Physiological effects*, and *Reflex effects*.

Mineral spring spa is a type of spa located at a natural mineral or hot springs site, which uses the spring water in treatments offered. See *Spa*.

Mission statement is a part of the vision outlined in a business plan that defines the purpose of the business and the main strategy for achieving competitive advantage; states the focus of the business. See *Vision* and *Competitive advantage*.

Mobility refers to the ability to go from place to place independently. See *Disability* and *Special population*.

Mobility restrictions are limits to the ability to go from place to place by walking, running, or other forms of locomotion; may be due to overuse and shortening of muscles, lack of use, aging, recuperation from an extended illness or injury, or a sedentary lifestyle. See *Bipedal locomotion* and *Disability* and *Special population*.

Mobilizing techniques are free and loose nonspecific joint movements within the normal range of joint motion. Compare to *Stretching*. Contrast with *Joint manipulations*.

Modality is a method of treating a medical condition; massage is considered a modality in the tradition of physiotherapy, along with other modalities such as ice packs, hot packs, ultrasound, or whirlpool baths.

MRSA stands for methicillin-resistant Staphylococcus aureus, which is a drug-resistant bacterial infection typically found on the skin but which can occur elsewhere in the body. See *Sanitation*.

Muds are derived from soils and marine sediments and applied to the body for deep skin cleansing and the removal of waste products; their drawing action also can stimulate local blood and lymphatic flow. See *Body wraps*. Contrast with *Peat*.

Multiple-choice questions are inquiries that give clients a choice of descriptors in answer to a question; gives clients choices that they might not have thought of themselves and have meaning for the interviewer. See *Interview skills*. Contrast with *Open-ended questions* and *Rating scale*.

Multiple-dose effects of massage refer to changes that occur over time from repeated massage applications. See *Effects of massage*. Contrast with *Single-dose effects*.

Myofascial massage is a general term for manual techniques aimed at releasing restrictions in superficial fascia, in deep fascia surrounding muscles, and in fascia related to overall body alignment; restores mobility in the body's fascia and softens connective tissue that has become rigid; also called myofascial release and myofascial unwinding. See *Fascia* and *Fascial restrictions*.

National certification refers to a credential given by a nongovernmental, nonprofit organization that attests to a person's competency in a given profession; usually involves qualifying by education and/or experience, passing a written examination and/or performance evaluation, and abiding by a code of ethics; is renewed periodically and usually requires a certain amount of continuing education; sometimes referred to as *Board certification*.

Natural healing refers to a philosophy that shows preference for methods of healing derived from nature, the belief in an innate healing force, and a holistic view of human life. See *Natural healing arts* and *Massage and bodywork traditions*.

Natural healing arts are methods of healing derived from nature, for example, nutritious food, herbs, water therapy, exercise, relaxation, fresh air, sunshine, and massage. See *Natural healing*.

Naturopathic physician's office is a health care facility offering naturopathic medicine. See *CAM*.

Net income refers to all of the money earned in a private practice, including fees and tips, minus business expenses and taxes; results in a *profit* if income is more than expenses. See *First-year budget* and *Income tax*. Contrast with *Salary draw*.

Neuromuscular therapy (NMT) is a form of contemporary massage focused on deactivating myofascial trigger points. See *Trigger point therapy*.

Neutral position refers to a hand position in which the wrist is neither flexed nor extended. See *Hand mechanics* and *Self-care*.

Nonverbal communication is connecting with another person without using words; touch is a form of nonverbal communication that can convey comfort, nurturing, and caring. See *Comforting touch*, *Nurturing touch*, and *Palliative care*.

Nurturing touch is a term used in reference to massage for the terminally ill or dying; refers to touching another person with the intention of satisfying the innate human need for touch by another person. Compare to *Comforting touch*, *Palliative care*, and *Touch deprivation*.

Nutrition refers to the intake of food and drink to nourish the body and mind. See *Self-care*.

Obesity is defined as having a Body Mass Index (BMI) of 30 or above. Compare to *Physical fitness*.

Objective information refers to what the practitioner observes about the client during goal-oriented planning; includes observations, qualitative and quantitative measurements, and results of orthopedic tests; written in O section of *SOAP notes*.

Observation is the act of noticing a client's condition using the eyes, ears, nose, and hands; used to collect information for goal-oriented planning. See *Objective information*.

Occupational licensing is permission granted to qualified practitioners to accept compensation for massage in a specific governmental jurisdiction; is awarded by the government agency that regulates professions in the jurisdiction; is required to practice. Compare to *Certification*.

On-site massage refers to a massage practice format in which the practitioner goes to where the potential clients are (e.g., at work, in stores, at airports, on the street), making massage more accessible; typically given with the client on a specially designed massage chair. See *Massage chair* and *Seated massage*.

Open-ended questions are inquiries that steer clients to specific topics, but leave space for them to answer in their own words; rather than dictating the form of response, the interviewer listens to what the client has to say in answer to a simple question. See *Interview skills*. Contrast with *Multiple-choice questions* and *Rating scales*.

Opening techniques refer to the initial touching of the recipient during a massage session; used to establish contact and sometimes also to apply oil and warm tissues. See *Organization* and *Warming techniques*.

Optimism is an aspect of emotional intelligence that means expecting that things will turn out all right in the end, despite setbacks and difficulties; an optimistic attitude helps a person persevere when the going gets rough; contrast with being pessimistic, or expecting failure. See *Emotional intelligence*.

Organization of a session refers to the overall structure of a massage session into beginning, middle, and end; the progression from one section of the body to another and the ordering of techniques into sequences; organization includes the use of opening techniques, transitions, and finishing techniques. See *Session* and *Session Planning*.

Organs are anatomical structures composed of different types of tissue that work as a unit to perform specific functions in the body, for example, the heart. Compare to *Body systems*.

Orthopedic tests are methods of assessing pathology in musculoskeletal structures, movement and locomotor disorders, and sources of soft-tissue pain and dysfunction; used to gather objective information in treatment planning. See *Objective information*.

Pacing refers to the speed of performing techniques, which may vary from very slow to very fast for different effects. Contrast with *Continuity*, *Flow*, and *Rhythm*.

Palliative care refers to methods of reducing symptoms and discomfort associated with certain diseases or their treatment; also care given to the terminally ill or dying for physical comfort and emotional support. Compare to *Hospice*. Contrast with *Treatment*.

Palpation is the act of sensing information about the client through touch; is about the "feel" of tissues and of movement at joints; used to collect objective information for goal-oriented planning. See *Objective information* and *Palpatory sensitivity*.

Palpatory sensitivity is the ability to use the sense of touch to locate anatomical structures, feel the condition of the tissues, and feel changes in tissues. See *Objective information*.

Part-time work is earning a portion of your income from a particular job or occupation; for a massage therapist, part-time ranges anywhere from one to ten clients per week, or one or two days or nights at place of employment, or some comparable combination. Contrast with *Full-time*.

Passive movements are body movements initiated and controlled by the practitioner, while the recipient remains relaxed and receptive. Contrast with *Active movements*.

Passive range of motion (PROM) refers to the evaluation of motion at a joint while it is passively moved through its range by a therapist; observations include degree of motion possible, restrictions or shortening, and any discomfort experienced; used to collect objective information for *Goal-oriented planning*.

Passive touch is simply laying the fingers or one or both hands on the body. Passive touch may impart heat to an area, have a calming influence, or help balance energy. See *Finishing techniques* and *Touch without Movement*.

Patents are legal protections for inventions and include utility and design patents; administered by the U.S. Patent and Trademark Office; patented inventions may not be copied by others for sale. Compare to *Copyright* and *Trademarks*.

Peat is organic soil that contains minerals, organic matter, water, and trapped air; has therapeutic properties when applied to the skin. Contrast with *Muds*.

Peer-reviewed journals are journals that only publish research reports that meet certain standards and that have been evaluated by experts in the field; different from trade magazines. See *Research literacy*.

Perpendicularity is one of the general principles for applying pressure to acupoints; means applying pressure directly into an acupoint at a 90-degree angle. Compare to *Stacking the joints* and *Weight transfer*.

Personal boundary is a limit established by a person to maintain his or her own integrity, comfort, or well-being. See *Boundaries* and *Boundary crossing*.

Personal care settings are places where personal grooming, relaxation, and rejuvenation services to patrons are provided. Compare to *Spa*.

Personal hygiene involves looking neat and smelling clean to inspire the confidence and trust of clients. See *Professional demeanor* and *Professional image*.

Personal temptation is an attraction to unethical actions. Contrast with *Ethical dilemmas*.

Person-centered massage refers to maintaining awareness of the whole person during a session, as opposed to focusing strictly on the pathology (i.e., pathology centered). Compare to *Client-centered massage*.

Petrissage is a massage technique category that includes movements that lift, wring, or squeeze soft tissues in a kneading motion; or press or roll the soft tissues under or between the hands. See *Swedish massage* and *Western massage*.

Phasic muscles are movers that cause movement against gravity; tend to weaken when postural muscles are shortened. Contrast with *Postural muscles*.

Physical effects of aging are the changes that occur in the mind–body as people get older; examples include decreased strength, slower nerve conduction, less efficient circulation, loss of tissue elasticity, thinner and dryer skin, loss of bone mass, diminished senses, and less efficient immune system. See *Chronological age* and *Physiological age*.

Physical fitness refers to optimal function of the physical body; elements include cardiovascular fitness, muscular strength and endurance, flexibility, and body composition. See *Conscious self-care* and *Self-care*.

Physical impairments commonly encountered in massage practices include visual, hearing, speech, size, and mobility challenges. Contrast with *Disability*.

Physiological age describes the age of an individual according to his or her overall state of health and disease compared to typical age characteristics; influenced by genetic makeup, lifelong health habits, and unique life events such as car accidents and diseases; example is a 60-year-old person having the body of a typical 50-year-old. Contrast with *Chronological age*.

Physiological effects of massage refer to biochemical processes at the cellular, tissue, organ, and organ system levels that result from massage applications. Contrast with *Energetic effects, Mechanical effects, Mind–body effects*, and *Reflex effects*.

Plan refers to the activities and applications chosen to achieve results for meeting client goals; a final step in goal-oriented planning; written in P section of *SOAP notes*. See *Goal-oriented planning*.

Polarity therapy is a form of bodywork that uses simple touch and gentle rocking movements with the intention to balance life energy, to remove obstructions to the free flow of energy, and to encourage relaxation. It was developed by Randolph Stone in the mid-twentieth century. See *Removing obstructions*.

Policies are rules set down to guide the operation of a business or practice; practice policies for massage therapists include pricing, late arrivals, missed appointments, conduct, and confidentiality. See *Private practice* and *Therapeutic relationship*.

Portable massage table is one that can be carried from place to place or set up and taken down easily. See *Equipment*.

Positioning the receiver refers to placing the recipient of massage in a position (e.g., supine, prone, side-lying, seated) to maximize his or her comfort and safety. Bolsters and other props may be used to support specific body areas.

Postevent is a sports massage application given after an athlete competes; the primary goal is physical and psychological recovery of the athlete and may include first aid for minor injuries. See *Sports massage*. Contrast with *Interevent* and *Preevent*.

Postural muscles are muscles that stabilize and support the body against gravity; tend to shorten and tighten under strain and are overworked if upright posture is unbalanced. Contrast with *Phasic muscles*.

Posture analysis   is the evaluation of body alignment; evaluation of standing, sitting, and sleeping postures; used to collect information for goal-oriented planning. See *Objective information*. Contrast with *Gait analysis*.

Power differential   refers to the difference in authority between a massage therapist and a client in the therapeutic relationship; massage therapists have more power in the relationship by virtue of training, experience, and perception of greater authority. See *Professional ethics* and *Therapeutic relationship*.

Practice clients   are family and friends of students who agree to allow students of massage to practice techniques on them; a type of dual relationship; special type of client for whom professional boundaries and ethical considerations apply. See *Professional ethics*.

Practice identity   is that part of a business plan which creates the image you project to the world; includes business name and logo, credentials, résumé, business cards and stationery, website, dress, and office decoration. See *Business plan*.

Practitioner   refers to someone trained in massage techniques and who uses massage in the practice of his or her profession. See *Massage therapist*.

Preevent   is a sports massage application given before an athlete competes; the purpose of preevent massage is to help the athlete prepare physically and mentally for the upcoming event; may be part of the athlete's warmup routine. See *Sports massage*. Contrast with *Interevent* and *Postevent*.

Pregnancy   refers to the time a woman carries a fetus before birth, which is normally for 9 months after fertilization. See *Pregnancy massage*, *Pregnancy posture*, and *Trimesters*.

Pregnancy massage   refers to massage and bodywork adapted to meet the needs of pregnant women and relieve some of the discomforts related to the pregnant state. See *Adaptations* and *Special population*.

Pregnancy posture   refers to the typical posture of a pregnant woman; may be described as head forward, chest back, belly out, hips tilted forward, locked knees, and feet turned out; causes stress on the body. See *Pregnancy*, *Pregnancy massage*, and *Trimesters*.

Press-and-flex   is a reflexology technique in which direct pressure is applied to reflexes by moving the foot into the finger or thumb. See *Foot reflexology*. Compare to *Direct pressure*.

Pressure   is related to the force used in applying techniques and to the degree of compaction of tissues as techniques are applied. The amount of pressure used in massage will depend on the intended effect and the tolerance or desires of the recipient. See *Cautions*.

Primary trigger points   are trigger points activated by acute or chronic overload of a muscle. See *Trigger points*

and *Trigger point therapy*. Contrast with *Secondary trigger points*.

Principle-based therapy   refers to treatment plans that take into consideration the pathology being treated, the condition of the individual, and the therapeutic potential of different treatment methods; allows for variation; different from protocol or formula approaches. Compare to *Client-centered massage* and *Evidence-based practice*.

Private practice   refers to self-employment as a heath care practitioner; combines both the business and professional sides of being a practitioner. Contrast with *Employee*.

Private-practice settings   are places where massage is given; settings include one-room massage office, massage clinic with two or more rooms, in an office building or a storefront; a dedicated massage room can be set aside in a residence for a home-based practice where not prohibited by zoning laws. See *Private practice*.

Problem solving   is a systematic approach to finding a solution to a problem using critical thinking skills; starting point is some issue, question, or dilemma for which there are choices for responding; time and effort are taken to gather information needed to make an informed choice or formulate a solution; information gathered is analyzed and evaluated, and finally a solution is determined. See *Intellectual skills*.

Professional associations   are nonprofit organizations run by elected leadership, whose mission is to promote their profession, to represent their members and the profession in the larger world, to offer services to members, and to set standards; typically have an IRS designation as 501(c)(6) corporations (United States), that is, nonprofit professional association. Contrast with *member services organization*.

Professional boundaries   are limits that clarify the nature of the therapeutic relationship and the roles of massage therapist and client; five types of professional boundaries are physical, emotional, intellectual, sexual, and energetic. See *Boundaries*.

Professional demeanor   refers to the appearance, language, and behavior of practitioners, all of which meet professional standards and inspires trust and respect. Compare to *Professional image*.

Professional ethics   is the study of moral behavior related to a certain occupation. See *Therapeutic relationship*, *Confidentiality*, and *Dual relationship*.

Professional image   means projecting a professional presence in dress, grooming, posture, and language; identifies a person as someone clients can have confidence in and trust; should be clean, neat, modest, and appropriate for the work setting. See *Personal hygiene*.

Professionalism   is a state of mind, a way of being, knowing, and doing that reflects a sense of being individuals who value their work and hold themselves to the highest standards of their occupations; projecting a professional image. Compare to *Professional demeanor* and *Professional image*.

Professional library includes the resources practitioners have accessible within their own offices, including some basic sources of information about conditions, pathologies, and special populations commonly encountered in their massage practices. See *Professionalism*.

Progress notes are for special sessions that reevaluate a client's progress related to his or her long-term goals; contain more assessment information than regular session notes and may identify new goals and plans. See *Documentation*.

Promotions are methods to encourage people to act to buy goods or services; includes discounts, specials, and gift certificates. Contrast with *Advertising*.

Prone refers to the positioning of a client lying facedown on a massage table. Contrast with *Semireclining* and *Supine*.

Proprioceptors are sensory organs embedded in tendons and muscles that detect the amount of stretch or tension that is occurring. See *Body awareness* and *Kinesiology*.

PSOAP is a variation of a SOAP note that separates the problem, complaint, or referral diagnosis into the first P section; recommended if one routinely accepts referrals from health care providers. See *SOAP notes*.

Psychotherapy is a health profession that treats problems and disorders related to the mind and emotions; sometimes referred to as "talk therapy"; outside of the scope of practice of massage therapists. See *Defense mechanisms* and *Transference*.

Punctuality is an aspect of work ethic that means showing up for work on time or early. See *Work ethic*. Compare to *Attendance*.

Qi is a term from traditional Chinese medicine that means life force or energy; everything in the universe is produced and sustained by the movements and the changes of Qi; Qi is a continuous form of energy that takes material form when it condenses and nonmaterial form when it disperses; also spelled "chi" and referred to as "ki" in Japanese. See *Acupressure*, *Energy channels*, and *Qi gong*.

Qi gong is a Chinese term that means energy exercise, or exercise based on the theory of the natural energy of Qi; exercises consist of a variety of choreographed movements that involve bending, stretching, reaching, stepping, and other movements designed to harmonize the flow of Qi in the body. See *Energy channels*, *Gong*, and *Qi*.

Qualifying statements are explanations that accompany claims for a product or service and identify the source of information for the claim; sources may include reading, logic, experience, hearsay, or scientific research. See *Advertising* and *Business ethics*.

Qualities of touch are related to contact and vary from soft and gentle to hard and rough. See *Contact* and *Touch*.

Randolph Stone (1890–1981) was the man who originally developed polarity therapy in the mid-1900s; he was trained in the natural healing methods of chiropractic, naturopathy, and osteopathy, and studied healing methods from India. See *Polarity therapy*.

Range of motion refers to the direction and distance a joint can move to its full potential. See *Joint movements* and *Kinesiology*.

Rating scales are rough measurements of things from the client's subjective view; use numbers to measure the degree or level of the client's experience of some factor related to their goals; example: a scale from 1 to 10. See *Interview skills*. Contrast with *Multiple choice questions* and *Open-ended questions*.

Recipe-based massage is a formulaic massage in which every client receives exactly the same treatment (i.e., the same techniques applied in the same way) for a particular medical condition. Contrast with *Principle-based massage*.

Reciprocal inhibition is a facilitated stretching technique in which the practitioner gets into position to apply the stretch, but first asks the client to contract the target muscle's antagonist against a resistance; target muscle relaxes as its antagonist contracts; immediately following the antagonist's relaxation, the stretch is applied. See *Stretching*. Compare to *Resisted movements*.

Reconstruction aide is a historical term for a practitioner trained to help rehabilitate wounded soldiers using corrective exercise and massage; antecedent of physical therapists; active in early twentieth century during and after World War I.

Recovery is a sports massage application that focuses on enhancing the physical and mental recovery from strenuous physical activity. See *Sports massage*. Contrast with *Maintenance* and *Rehabilitation*.

Reference zone is a trigger point therapy concept meaning the area of the body that feels pain or has another reaction when its related trigger point is activated. See *Active trigger points*, *Satellite trigger points*, and *Trigger points*.

Reflex effects of massage refer to functional changes in the mind and body mediated by the nervous system, and also the largely unexplained phenomenon in which pressing or massaging one part of the body is believed to have a normalizing effect on an entirely different part of the body. See *Reflexology*. Contrast with *Energetic effects*, *Mechanical effects*, *Mind–body effects*, and *Physiological effects*.

Reflexology is a form of bodywork based on the theory of zone therapy, in which specific spots on the feet or hands are pressed to stimulate corresponding areas in other parts of the body. See *Foot reflexology*.

Reflexology chart is a diagrammed map of the feet showing the location of reflexes on the feet according to the theory of reflexology; identifies which part of the body is affected by pressing a specific spot on a foot. See *Foot reflexology* and *Reflexology*.

Regional massage is focused on a particular area of the body, which provides an opportunity for greater specificity. See *Specificity*. Contrast with *Full-body Western massage*.

Rehabilitation refers to massage applications to treat injuries; a sports massage application to facilitate healing after a disabling injury. Contrast with *Event, Maintenance, Recovery,* and *Remedial massage.*

Relaxin is a hormone excreted in the first trimester of pregnancy that softens ligaments in the body, causing joints to become more mobile; helps prepare the woman's body for delivery later on; results in unstable joints for the duration of the pregnancy. See *Pregnancy massage* and *Trimesters.*

Reliability is an aspect of a work ethic that means people can depend on you to do what you say you are going to do, when you are supposed to do it; if you are reliable, people will have trust and confidence in you. See *Work ethic.* Compare to *Accountability.*

Remedial massage is a sports massage application that focuses on improving debilitating conditions and minor injuries. See *Sports massage.* Contrast with *Event, Maintenance,* and *Rehabilitation.*

Removing obstructions is a basic principle in polarity therapy referring to eliminating barriers to the free flow of energy; an obstruction is an area of the body where there seems to be a stagnation or a holding pattern that interferes with a free flow of energy. See *Energy flow* and *Polarity therapy.*

Repetitive strain injuries (RSIs) are musculoskeletal injuries caused by repeated stress on specific muscles and joints; result in aching, tenderness, swelling, tingling, numbness, weakness, loss of flexibility, and spasms in the muscles affected; can result in chronic pain, loss of mobility, and eventually, disability. See *Ergonomics, Seated massage,* and *Workplace wellness programs.*

Research literacy refers to knowledge and skills needed to understand and use scientific research; includes an understanding of the scientific method, locating research articles, and reading, analyzing, and evaluating research studies. Compare to *Evidence-based practice* and *Principle-based therapy.*

Resisted movements are a type of active movement in which a person initiates the movement, while a second person offers resistance, thereby challenging the muscles used; sometimes used in rehabilitation to restore strength to a muscle. Contrast with *Assisted movements.*

Résumé is a document that provides a summary of training, experience, and credentials in an occupation or profession; used to present qualifications for a job, volunteer position, or whenever a summary of past accomplishments is required; also known as CV (curriculum vitae). Contrast with *Transcript.*

Rhythm refers to a recurring pattern of movement with a specific cadence, beat, or accent and may be described as smooth, flowing, or uneven. Contrast with *Flow* and *Pacing.*

Rights are claims to certain treatment or to protection from certain treatment; expected to be honored by others, and enforced by standards or laws if necessary. See *Professional ethics.* Compare to *Duties.*

Robust elders are people age 70 and older who show few outward signs of impaired health, look younger than their chronological ages, are mentally sharp, and physically active. Contrast with *Age-appropriate* and *Frail elders.*

Rocking motions are basic polarity therapy techniques involving small, gentle oscillations of a small area of the body, or large, vigorous oscillations that move the entire body; rocking motions induce relaxation, lower muscle tone, reduce pain, and encourage an increase in the active range of motion afterward. See *Polarity therapy.* Compare to *Energy flow.*

Rolling is a reflexology technique in which a thumb or finger is rolled into a reflex point to apply pressure. See *Foot reflexology.* Contrast with *Fingerwalking* and *Thumbwalking.*

Roman baths were public institutions in the ancient Roman Empire that consisted of a space for undressing, an exercise court, a warm room, a type of steam room, and a cold pool; might also have a swimming pool. Compare to *Greek gymnasia* and *Turkish baths.*

Rubber is a historical term for an unschooled massage practitioner who gave rubdowns to athletes; learned their skills on the job, or from other rubbers; early twentieth-century Europe and North America. Compare to *Masseuse* and *Masseur.*

Rubdown is a term used in athletic venues for superficial skin friction with the hand, a brush, a coarse towel, or a horsehair glove; popular in the nineteenth and early twentieth centuries. Contrast with *Western massage.*

Salary draw is the money taken out of a business or practice monthly for the owner's personal use. Contrast with *Net income.*

Sanitation refers to taking precautions that prevent the spread of disease and to following good hygiene practices. See *Do no harm.*

Satellite trigger points are trigger points that become active because they are in a muscle in a zone of reference of another trigger point. See *Associated trigger point* and *Reference zone.*

Sauna is a thermohydrotherapy facility; typically a wood-lined room heated without steam, and with very dry air; patrons sit on wooden benches. See *Thermotherapy.* Contrast with *Steam room.*

Schedule C is an IRS income tax form that reports small business income and expenses; attaches to *Form 1040.*

Scientific method is a systematic way of testing theories through gathering and analyzing relevant information to see if it supports the theory in question. It is based on observations rather than on authority or anecdotes. See *Hypothesis* and *Research literacy.*

Scope of practice describes the legally allowed, or professionally defined, methods used by a certain profession, as well as its intention in performing them. Different professions have different scopes of practice as defined by law or by the profession. Massage techniques fall within the scope of practice of several professions. See *Professional ethics.*

Screening interview is conducted to check for contraindications and cautions before giving massage to a new client. See *Intake notes*.

Scrubs are manual exfoliation methods using salts or coarser organic substances. See *Exfoliants*. Contrast with *Body polish*.

Seated massage refers to massage given with the recipient seated in an ordinary or a special massage chair; called on-site massage when the chair is taken to a public place such as an office or commercial establishment; also called chair massage. See *Massage chair* and *On-site massage*.

Secondary trigger points are trigger points that become active because of their reaction to a muscle containing a primary trigger point. See *Trigger point therapy* and *Trigger points*. Contrast with *Primary trigger points*.

Self-awareness is an aspect of emotional intelligence that involves recognizing a feeling as it happens and its accompanying emotion or impulse to act. See *Emotional intelligence*.

Self-care refers to actions massage practitioners take for their own well-being and to promote their longevity in the profession; includes physical self-care such as physical fitness and good body mechanics and emotional self-care such as in dealing with grief, anger, and confusion. See *Conscious self-care* and *Holistic self-care plan*.

Self-disclosure is revealing personal information about the self; self-disclosure by a therapist can be a boundary crossing in the therapeutic relationship. See *Professional boundaries*.

Self-employed describes operating a business as a sole proprietor or independent contractor; a person is his or her own employer; called being in private practice for a massage therapist. See *Private practice* and *Independent contractor*. Contrast with *Employee*.

Self-employment tax (SE tax) is a social security and Medicare tax for self-employed individuals; applies to social security coverage for retirement, disability, survivor, and Medicare benefits; SE tax must be paid if net earnings from self-employment are $400 or more; SE tax is in addition to the regular income tax. See *Income tax*.

Self-reflection is an aspect of critical thinking that takes into consideration the thinker's own prejudices and beliefs in determining the truth about something. See *Critical thinking*.

Semireclining refers to the positioning of a client who is supine on a massage table into a half-sitting position by placing pillows under the upper body; the upper body is at about a 45-degree angle to the lower body. Contrast with *Side-lying*, *Prone*, and *Supine*.

Service is a value in which we hold our clients' well-being above our own desire for money, power, and worldly recognition; means that the primary motivation for being a massage therapist is to help people achieve their personal wellness goals. See *Professional ethics* and *Values*.

Session refers to a period of time in which massage is given to a recipient by a practitioner. Sessions have logical organization, have a wellness or a treatment purpose, and generally vary from 10 minutes to 2 hours. See *Goal-oriented planning* and *Session planning*.

Session planning is the logical process of thinking through a specific massage session; includes collecting relevant information, assessing the situation and setting goals, choosing massage applications, performing the massage, and evaluating results. See *Goal-oriented planning*.

Sexual misconduct refers to any sexualizing of the relationship between a massage therapist and a current client; can occur before, after, or during a massage session, and can be perpetrated by the massage therapist or by the client; forms of sexual misconduct range from those involving speech and body language to inappropriate touch to sexual contact to sexual assault. See *Intervention model*.

Sheng is a Chinese term meaning "life." See *Dao Yin Yang Shen Gong*. Compare to *Sheng Cycle*.

Sheng Cycle is a concept within the Five Element Theory that looks at relationships among the elements; also called the creation, generating, or promoting cycle; in the Sheng Cycle, each Element supports the next, for example, the Ko Cycle balances the Sheng Cycle to avoid unrestrained growth. See *Five Elements*. Contrast with *Ko Cycle*.

Shiatsu is a general term for Japanese bodywork based on Chinese meridian theory and Western science, in which *tsubo* (i.e., acupoints) are pressed to balance the flow of energy or *ki*. Compare to *Acupressure*.

Short-term effects of massage are physiological and psychological changes that occur during a massage session. See *Effects of massage*. Contrast with *Long-term effects*.

Side-lying refers to the positioning of a client on his or her left or right side for massage; pillows under the upper arm and leg support the body for client comfort. Contrast with *Prone*, *Semireclining*, and *Supine*.

Simple static stretch is a passive stretch characterized by slow, sustained, and even application. See *Passive movements* and *Stretching*.

Simplified notes are forms of documentation that contain minimum information; used at venues such as health fairs, trade shows, sports events, and outreach events where people receive a short standard massage routine and will not be seen again by the practitioner. Contrast with *SOAP notes*.

Single-dose effects of massage refer to changes that occur from one massage application. See *Effects of massage*. Contrast with *Multiple-dose effects*.

Skilled touch refers to abilities related to physical contact; four dimensions important to massage therapists include contact, qualities, communication, and palpation. See *Contact* and *Palpation*.

SOAP notes are a standard form for documenting therapeutic sessions; SOAP is an acronym for Subjective,

Objective, Assessment, and Plan. See *Documentation*. Contrast with *Simplified notes*.

Sobardoras are traditional Hispanic healers trained by apprenticeship to use massage in treating ailments; also use ritual, herbal remedies, and bone-setting manipulation techniques; part of the healing tradition of curanderas.

Social skills are methods of interacting with other people that promote harmony, understanding, and connection, while peacefully solving problems such as disagreements, misunderstandings, and reconciliation after harm done; primary goal is building good relationships. See *Conflict resolution* and *Emotional intelligence*.

Sole proprietor is a form of self-employment in which a person is the legally recognized business owner, the employer and employee combined. See *Self-employment*.

SOTAP is a form of documentation for therapeutic sessions; variation of SOAP notes; acronym for Subjective, Objective, Treatment, Assessment, and Plan; provides a separate T section for recording the massage and related techniques used in the session. See *Documentation*. Contrast with *SOAP notes*.

Spa refers to a business that offers personal care services in an environment that focuses on overall well-being and renewal of mind, body, and spirit; emphasis on natural therapies and spa treatments using natural substances. See *Personal care*.

Special population is a group of people with some distinctive life circumstance that sets them apart from a normal adult population; include athletes, pregnant women, infants, the elderly, and people with various physical impairments and diseases. See *Adaptations* and *Disability*.

Specialty associations are organizations composed of practitioners of a particular style of massage or bodywork or those who work in a particular setting. Contrast with *General membership organization*.

Specialty certification refers to certification in a specific massage and bodywork system; involves some combination of education, skill development, internship, written and performance tests, ethical code, continuing education, and/or periodic renewal. See *Certification*.

Specificity refers to targeting a specific muscle or small area and applying massage techniques to structures there; different from broad or general massage applications. See *Palpatory sensitivity*.

Sports, fitness, and recreation centers are facilities whose main purpose is to provide opportunities for physical exercise and sports, but which also provide support services like massage.

Sports massage is the science and art of applying massage and related techniques to ensure the health and well-being of the athlete and to enhance athletic performance; major applications of sports massage are recovery, remedial, rehabilitation, maintenance, and event (i.e., pre-, inter-, and postevent).

Sports medicine center refers to a rehabilitation facility specializing in athletic injuries and improvement of sports performance.

Stabilizing hand refers to the hand providing a brace or backstop during the application of reflexology techniques. See *Foot reflexology* and *Bracing*. Contrast with *Working hand*.

Stacking the joints is one of the general principles for applying pressure to acupoints; means lining the joints up so that pressure travels from bone to bone and not across joints. Compare to *Perpendicularity* and *Weight transfer*.

Standards of practice are documents developed by professional associations that outline acceptable ethical professional conduct. Contrast with *Codes of ethics*.

Startup costs are the initial expenses involved in setting up a business like a massage therapy practice. See *First-year budget*.

Steam room is a hydrotherapy facility; typically a room tiled from floor to ceiling and with benches for sitting; steam comes out from jets in the walls and fills the space with wet heat. See *Hydrotherapy* and *Thermotherapy*. Contrast with *Sauna*.

Stone massage involves the use of hot or cold stones applied to the body for therapeutic purposes.

Stress-control strategies include good time management, adequate rest and relaxation, and anxiety reduction techniques, including massage. See *Holistic self-care plan*.

Stretching is a type of joint movement performed to the limit of a joint's normal range in a specific direction. Stretching elongates the muscles and connective tissues that cross the joint and helps relax the muscles involved. Contrast with *Mobilizing techniques*.

Subcutaneous fascia is a continuous layer of connective tissue over the entire body between the skin and the deep fascia. See *Fascia* and *Myofascial massage*. Contrast with *Deep fascia*.

Subjective information refers to what clients report to the therapist during goal-oriented planning; includes complaints and comments about their conditions and how they feel; written in S section of *SOAP notes*. Contrast with *Objective information*.

Substantiated claims for a product or service have a credible basis or evidence in their support; unsubstantiated claims for products or services are illegal according to consumer protection laws. See *Advertising* and *Business ethics*.

Superficial friction is a type of friction in which the hand rubs briskly back and forth over the skin to improve circulation in superficial tissues and to create heat. Contrast with *Deep friction*.

Supine refers to the positioning of a client lying face-up on a massage table. Contrast with *Prone* and *Semireclining*.

Swedish massage is a genre of bodywork that includes traditional Western massage, Swedish movements, hydrotherapy, heat lamps, and other modalities; a popular form of massage in health clubs, spas, and resorts.

Contrast with *Western massage* and *Swedish movement cure*.

Swedish Movement Cure   refers to Pehr Ling's system of medical gymnastics that was developed in the early 1800s and that, along with Mezger's massage, is the forerunner of today's Western massage. Contrast with *Swedish massage*.

Table skills   include a variety of actions required to position and drape a client properly on a massage table. See *Draping* and *Positioning*.

Tactile stimulation   refers to the stimulation of the tactile nerves in the skin through touch and movement; essential for the healthy growth and development of infants; provided by infant massage. See *Infant massage*.

Tapotement   is a massage technique category consisting of brisk percussive movements that are performed in rapid, rhythmic fashion; forms include hacking, rapping, cupping, clapping, slapping, tapping, and pincement. See *Swedish massage* and *Western massage*.

Technique   refers to the technical aspects of the application of massage or how the body moves while performing massage; a broader concept of the term *technique* also includes the intent. See *Intention*.

Telltack   is a historical term for a practitioner of a vigorous type of bodywork given at the Turkish baths or hammam; nineteenth- and twentieth-century Middle East, Near East, Europe, and North America. See *Turkish baths*.

Temperature therapy   involves the application of hot and cold modalities for their therapeutic effects (e.g., hot packs, ice). See *Hydrotherapy*.

Tenting   is a technique that prevents clients from getting rolled up in the drape. See *Table skills*.

Terminus   refers to the hollow space just lateral to the left and right attachments of the sternocleidomastoid (SCM) muscles on the clavicle; at the terminus lymphatic facilitation techniques are applied to increase the flow of lymph into the thoracic ducts, thus clearing the area. See *Lymphatic facilitation*.

Tissues   of the body form when like cells group together to perform one activity, for example, muscle cells combine to form muscle tissue; come together to form body organs. See *Organs* and *Body systems*.

Thai massage   is traditional bodywork from Thailand; its intent is to stimulate the body's self-healing processes and to correct energy imbalances. Compare to *Ayurvedic massage*. Contrast with *Swedish massage*.

Therapeutic relationship   is a model for understanding the separate and unique roles of the practitioner and the client in the therapeutic setting. See *Boundaries* and *Standards of Practice*.

Therapeutic Touch   is a form of manual therapy in which the energy field of the recipient is rebalanced, thus promoting health and healing. See *Energetic effects*.

Thermotherapy   refers to temperature therapy modalities above normal body temperature (e.g., hot packs). See *Temperature therapy*. Contrast with *Cryotherapy*.

Thixotropy   is a characteristic of fascia in which fascial tissues can change from a more solid to a more liquid gel consistency. Fascia becomes more pliable with movement, stretching, and increase in temperature. See *Fascia* and *Myofascial massage*.

Thumbwalking   is a reflexology technique performed by bending the thumb at the first joint, pressing into the tissues, and then straightening the thumb, moving from spot to spot on the foot; action is repeated as the thumb "walks" in line along the foot. See *Foot reflexology*. Compare to *Fingerwalking*. Contrast with *Hook-and-backup*.

Time management   is a personal skill of scheduling daily and weekly activities to reflect personal priorities; involves identifying goals and priorities for a certain period of time and plotting a schedule accordingly; includes keeping to the schedule developed. See *Holistic self-care plan*.

Tips   are gratuities (i.e., given in gratitude) over and above the cost of a service; given directly to the person providing the service; given at the discretion of the person receiving the service; are taxable income reported to the IRS on income tax forms. See *Income tax*.

Topical substance   is a liniment, oil, lotion, cream, or combinations of these used in massage. See *Lubricants*.

Touch   means "to come into contact with"; massage practitioners touch their clients or patients in many ways, but primarily with their hands; touch may happen on a physical or an energetic level. See *Palpation*, *Tactile stimulation*, and *Touch deprivation*.

Touch deprivation   is a physical and psychological condition resulting from a lack of healthy, pleasurable touch; can lead to emotional distress; can be relieved by the caring touch of massage. See *Nurturing touch* and *Palliative care*.

Touch without movement   is a massage technique in which the practitioner comes in contact with the recipient either physically or energetically, but no perceptible movement occurs that fits into the five traditional classic massage categories. Two common types of touch without movement are passive touch and direct static pressure. See *Swedish massage* and *Western massage*.

Trademarks   offer exclusive use of a name or symbol to identify unique goods and services; use the symbol ™ or ® for registered trademarks; distinguish a particular brand or company from others; handled by the U.S. Patent and Trademark Office in Washington, D.C.; may also be regulated on the state (United States) or provincial (Canada) level. Compare to *Copyright*.

Traditional Chinese medicine (TCM)   is a system of healing based on ancient Chinese medicine, and includes concepts such as yin/yang, the Five Elements, energy (Qi), and energy channels. Compare to *Acupressure* and *Qi gong*.

Trained masseuses   is a historical term for massage practitioners who took courses of study in private schools and hospital programs in the early 1900s, differentiating themselves from the many untrained massage practitioners of the time. Compare to *Masseuses* and *Masseurs*.

Transcript is a detailed record of a student's performance while in school, including specific subjects studied, grades, attendance, date of graduation, honors, school information, and other facts; an original transcript carrying the school seal is usually required for official purposes such as obtaining a license to practice. Contrast with *Diploma*.

Transference is a psychological phenomenon that occurs when a client responds to a practitioner as if the client were relating to someone important in his or her past (e.g., father), and transferring those positive or negative feelings onto the therapeutic relationship. Contrast with *Countertransference*.

Transition techniques serve to provide continuity and flow from one section of the body to another during a massage session. See *Organization*. Contrast with *Finishing techniques*.

Transport vessels, or lymphangia, are lymph system vessels that carry lymph fluid from the collector vessels to the thoracic ducts; are segmented with each segment referred to as a lymphangion, which is bounded by a valve on each end and which contracts to move fluid through the vessel. See *Lymphatic facilitation*. Contrast with *Collector vessels* and *Initial/terminal lymph vessels*.

Treatment refers to interventions aimed at alleviating a specific medical condition. Contrast with *Palliative care*.

Treatment model is a concept that explains the intention of using specific interventions or modalities to alleviate medical conditions. Contrast with *Wellness model*.

Treatment planning is a form of goal-oriented planning in which the goal is alleviation of symptoms, or facilitation of healing of a pathological condition; used for medical, clinical, and orthopedic massage applications; sometimes called a *Plan of care*. See *Goal-oriented planning*.

Trigger point therapy involves the identification and deactivation of painful fibrous nodules in muscle and connective tissue called trigger points; manual TrP techniques include ischemic compression, deep friction, deep stripping, and stretching. See *Trigger points*.

Trigger points are small, hyperirritable spots in muscle or related connective tissue that are felt as taut bands of tissue that elicit pain if pressed and that refer pain to other areas in predictable patterns. See *Reference zone* and *Trigger point therapy*.

Trimesters refers to the three stages of pregnancy, each trimester lasting about 3 months; the first, second, and third trimesters each have specific implications for the mother and the fetus related to massage applications. See *Pregnancy* and *Pregnancy massage*.

Triptai is a historical term used in ancient Greece for someone who specialized in rubbing; massage has been called the *anatriptic art*; *anatriptic* means to "rub up" or toward the body's center.

Turkish baths are public institutions modeled after Roman baths, which were brought to the West from the Middle East during the Renaissance Period; became popular in large cities in Europe and America. Compare to *Roman baths*.

Understanding is a basic principle of polarity therapy referring to the practitioner being open to the recipient's experience and to the effects of polarity therapy; it calls for knowledge of the broader picture in terms of the physiological and psychological reactions happening in a session. See *Polarity therapy*. Compare to *Love*.

Universal precautions are procedures that aim to prevent the transmission of serious communicable disease; also called standard or sanitary precautions. See *Sanitation*.

Upper body regions, for the purposes of massage, are commonly identified as face, head, neck, upper and lower back, shoulders, arms and hands, and chest and abdomen. See *Regional massage*. Contrast with *Lower body regions*.

Values are principles, traits, or qualities considered worthwhile or desirable; protected by ethical standards and codes of ethics. See *Ethics* and *Ethical standards*.

Variable costs are fluctuating operating expenses and depend on the number of clients seen; examples: laundry and massage supplies. Contrast with *Fixed costs*.

Verbal skills describe the ability to communicate by means of the spoken word; includes good articulation and voice quality; delivery of spoken word more important than content in some cases. See *Communication skills* and *Voice quality*.

Vertical position is the common position during seated massage; clients are supported on their buttocks, lower legs, and chest instead of lying facedown on a horizontal surface. See *Massage chair* and *Seated massage*.

Vibration is a Western massage technique category that includes oscillating, quivering, or trembling movements; or movement of soft tissues back and forth, or up and down, performed quickly and repeatedly. Vibration may be described as fine or coarse (e.g., shaking, jostling). See *Swedish massage* and *Western massage*.

Vision is an element of a business plan that describes the broad scope of the proposed business; for a massage practice, it would include mission, size, format, location, and income goals. See *Business plan*.

Voice quality is an aspect of verbal communication that includes the pitch, tone, volume, clarity, and richness of the sound of someone's speech; can affect a person's image or how they are perceived by others.

Warming techniques are used to raise the temperature of tissues, increase superficial circulation, and prepare an area for more specific massage applications. See *Opening techniques*, and *Organization*. Contrast with *Finishing techniques*.

Watersheds describe superficial lymphatic drainage patterns in different areas of the body. Lymph traveling in the lymphangia moves within its watershed or drainage area toward the catchments or concentrations of lymph nodes nearby. See *Catchments* and *Lymphatic facilitation*.

Weight transfer is one of the general principles for applying pressure to acupoints; means applying pressure by shifting the body weight into the point of contact rather than pushing from the shoulders and arms. Compare to *Perpendicularity* and *Stacking the joints*.

Wellness refers to a condition of optimal physical, emotional, intellectual, spiritual, social, and vocational well-being. See *Wellness profession*.

Wellness center refers to a facility that offers fitness activities, rehabilitation programs, massage therapy, and classroom instruction in preventing disease and developing a healthy lifestyle; often connected to a hospital.

Wellness massage is massage performed with the intention of promoting the receiver's general well-being; it goes beyond the treatment of specific conditions to help the receiver achieve high-level wellness. See *Wellness Massage Pyramid*.

Wellness Massage Pyramid is a model for understanding the possible contributions of massage therapy to high-level wellness. Pyramid levels from the base to the top are treatment, recovery, prevention, neutral zone, health maintenance, personal growth, and life enjoyment. See *Wellness massage*.

Wellness model is a concept that explains good health and well-being as aimed at living a healthy, vibrant, and meaningful life; it goes beyond the idea of health as the absence of disease and emphasizes personal responsibility; also called the wellness perspective. See *Wellness*. Contrast with *Treatment model*.

Wellness movement is a twentieth-century phenomenon within health care and fitness that emphasizes taking responsibility for health and well-being and that addresses holistic health of body, mind, emotions, and spirit. See *Holistic* and *Wellness Massage Pyramid*.

Wellness profession is a profession or occupation with a scope of practice that spans the breadth of the wellness model from treatment and recovery to personal growth and life enjoyment; focus is on attaining high-level wellness. See *Wellness*.

Western massage is a form of soft tissue manipulation developed in Europe and the United States over the past 200 years; technique categories commonly used to describe Western massage are effleurage, petrissage, tapotement, friction, vibration, touch without movement, and joint movements. Compare to *Swedish massage*.

Whirlpool bath is a hydrotherapy device consisting of a water-filled tub that has air or water jets causing movement or churning of the water; typically contains hot water; may be private or communal; may be large enough to sit or lie down in or small enough for a part of the body. See *Hydrotherapy* and *Thermotherapy*.

Worker productivity refers to the amount and quality of work employees can accomplish in a certain period of time; is affected negatively by work time lost due to illness or injury. See *On-site massage* and *Workplace wellness programs*.

Work ethic is an attitude that positions one's job as a high priority in life and that promotes applying oneself to high-quality performance; taking pride in one's work. See *Accountability*, *Attendance*, *Punctuality*, and *Reliability*.

Working hand refers to the hand applying a reflexology technique. See *Foot reflexology*. Contrast with *Stabilizing hand*.

Workplace wellness programs are employer-sponsored programs that make services and activities available to employees to improve their overall health and well-being. See *On-site massage* and *Worker productivity*.

Written correspondence is a form of communication that utilizes basic writing skills such as correct spelling, punctuation, grammar, sentence construction, and organization of thought; forms include memos, e-mails, and business letters. See *Communication skills*.

Yang is the masculine principle in Chinese medicine; the light, energetic, and ethereal aspect of the universe; characterized as exterior, moving, nonsubstantial, warm, expanding, and opposing but also supporting Yin; the Chinese character for Yang is a hillside in full sun. Contrast with *Yin*.

Yin is the feminine principle in Chinese medicine; the dark, deep, dense aspect of the universe; characterized as interior, still, substantial, cool, and contracting in contrast to Yang; the Chinese character for Yin depicts the shady side of a hill or mountain. Contrast with *Yang*.

Zone therapy is a foundation theory of reflexology stating that pressure on certain places in the body provides therapeutic reactions in other parts of the body in predictable patterns; there are 10 longitudinal zones running from the head to the hands and feet. See *Foot reflexology*, *Reflexology*, and *Reflexology chart*.

Zoning ordinance is a local law that specifies what type of housing or what kind of business can be in a certain location. Compare to *Massage establishment license*.

Index

I - 1

Pearson Education, Inc.

YOU SHOULD CAREFULLY READ THE TERMS AND CONDITIONS BEFORE USING THE CD-ROM PACKAGE. USING THIS CD-ROM PACKAGE INDICATES YOUR ACCEPTANCE OF THESE TERMS AND CONDITIONS.

Pearson Education, Inc. provides this program and licenses its use. You assume responsibility for the selection of the program to achieve your intended results, and for the installation, use, and results obtained from the program. This license extends only to use of the program in the United States or countries in which the program is marketed by authorized distributors.

LICENSE GRANT

You hereby accept a nonexclusive, nontransferable, permanent license to install and use the program ON A SINGLE COMPUTER at any given time. You may copy the program solely for backup or archival purposes in support of your use of the program on the single computer. You may not modify, translate, disassemble, decompile, or reverse engineer the program, in whole or in part.

TERM

The License is effective until terminated. Pearson Education, Inc. reserves the right to terminate this License automatically if any provision of the License is violated. You may terminate the License at any time. To terminate this License, you must return the program, including documentation, along with a written warranty stating that all copies in your possession have been returned or destroyed.

LIMITED WARRANTY

THE PROGRAM IS PROVIDED "AS IS" WITHOUT WARRANTY OF ANY KIND, EITHER EXPRESSED OR IMPLIED, INCLUDING, BUT NOT LIMITED TO, THE IMPLIED WARRANTIES OR MERCHANTABILITY AND FITNESS FOR A PARTICULAR PURPOSE. THE ENTIRE RISK AS TO THE QUALITY AND PERFORMANCE OF THE PROGRAM IS WITH YOU. SHOULD THE PROGRAM PROVE DEFECTIVE, YOU (AND NOT PEARSON EDUCATION, INC. OR ANY AUTHORIZED DEALER) ASSUME THE ENTIRE COST OF ALL NECESSARY SERVICING, REPAIR, OR CORRECTION. NO ORAL OR WRITTEN INFORMATION OR ADVICE GIVEN BY PEARSON EDUCATION, INC., ITS DEALERS, DISTRIBUTORS, OR AGENTS SHALL CREATE A WARRANTY OR INCREASE THE SCOPE OF THIS WARRANTY.

SOME STATES DO NOT ALLOW THE EXCLUSION OF IMPLIED WARRANTIES, SO THE ABOVE EXCLUSION MAY NOT APPLY TO YOU. THIS WARRANTY GIVES YOU SPECIFIC LEGAL RIGHTS AND YOU MAY ALSO HAVE OTHER LEGAL RIGHTS THAT VARY FROM STATE TO STATE.

Pearson Education, Inc. does not warrant that the functions contained in the program will meet your requirements or that the operation of the program will be uninterrupted or error-free.

However, Pearson Education, Inc. warrants the diskette(s) or CD-ROM(s) on which the program is furnished to be free from defects in material and workmanship under normal use for a period of ninety (90) days from the date of delivery to you as evidenced by a copy of your receipt.

The program should not be relied on as the sole basis to solve a problem whose incorrect solution could result in injury to person or property. If the program is employed in such a manner, it is at the user's own risk and Pearson Education, Inc. explicitly disclaims all liability for such misuse.

LIMITATION OF REMEDIES

Pearson Education, Inc.'s entire liability and your exclusive remedy shall be:

1. the replacement of any diskette(s) or CD-ROM(s) not meeting Pearson Education, Inc.'s "LIMITED WARRANTY" and that is returned to Pearson Education, or

2. if Pearson Education is unable to deliver a replacement diskette(s) or CD-ROM(s) that is free of defects in materials or workmanship, you may terminate this agreement by returning the program.

IN NO EVENT WILL PEARSON EDUCATION, INC. BE LIABLE TO YOU FOR ANY DAMAGES, INCLUDING ANY LOST PROFITS, LOST SAVINGS, OR OTHER INCIDENTAL OR CONSEQUENTIAL DAMAGES ARISING OUT OF THE USE OR INABILITY TO USE SUCH PROGRAM EVEN IF PEARSON EDUCATION, INC. OR AN AUTHORIZED DISTRIBUTOR HAS BEEN ADVISED OF THE POSSIBILITY OF SUCH DAMAGES, OR FOR ANY CLAIM BY ANY OTHER PARTY.

SOME STATES DO NOT ALLOW FOR THE LIMITATION OR EXCLUSION OF LIABILITY FOR INCIDENTAL OR CONSEQUENTIAL DAMAGES, SO THE ABOVE LIMITATION OR EXCLUSION MAY NOT APPLY TO YOU.

GENERAL

You may not sublicense, assign, or transfer the license of the program. Any attempt to sublicense, assign or transfer any of the rights, duties, or obligations hereunder is void.

This Agreement will be governed by the laws of the State of New York.

Should you have any questions concerning this Agreement, you may contact Pearson Education, Inc. by writing to:

Director of New Media
Higher Education Division
Pearson Education, Inc.
One Lake Street
Upper Saddle River, NJ 07458

Should you have any questions concerning technical support, you may contact:

Product Support Department: Monday–Friday 8:00 A.M. –8:00 P.M. and Sunday 5:00 P.M.-12:00 A.M. (All times listed are Eastern). 1-800-677-6337

You can also get support by filling out the web form located at http://247.prenhall.com

YOU ACKNOWLEDGE THAT YOU HAVE READ THIS AGREEMENT, UNDERSTAND IT, AND AGREE TO BE BOUND BY ITS TERMS AND CONDITIONS. YOU FURTHER AGREE THAT IT IS THE COMPLETE AND EXCLUSIVE STATEMENT OF THE AGREEMENT BETWEEN US THAT SUPERSEDES ANY PROPOSAL OR PRIOR AGREEMENT, ORAL OR WRITTEN, AND ANY OTHER COMMUNICATIONS BETWEEN US RELATING TO THE SUBJECT MATTER OF THIS AGREEMENT.